ASTHMA IN THE WORKPLACE

ASTHMA IN THE WORKPLACE

Second Edition, Revised and Expanded

edited by

I. LEONARD BERNSTEIN
University of Cincinnati College of Medicine
Cincinnati, Ohio

MOIRA CHAN-YEUNG
University of British Columbia and Vancouver General Hospital
Vancouver, British Columbia, Canada

JEAN-LUC MALO
Université de Montréal and Sacré-Coeur Hospital
Montréal, Quebec, Canada

DAVID I. BERNSTEIN
University of Cincinnati College of Medicine
Cincinnati, Ohio

MARCEL DEKKER, INC.

NEW YORK · BASEL

ISBN: 0-8247-1963-8

This book is printed on acid-free paper.

Headquarters
Marcel Dekker, Inc.
270 Madison Avenue, New York, NY 10016
tel: 212-696-9000; fax: 212-685-4540

Eastern Hemisphere Distribution
Marcel Dekker AG
Hutgasse 4, Postfach 812, CH-4001 Basel, Switzerland
tel: 41-61-261-8482; fax: 41-61-261-8896

World Wide Web
http://www.dekker.com

The publisher offers discounts on this book when ordered in bulk quantities. For more information, write to Special Sales/Professional Marketing at the headquarters address above.

Current printing (last digit):
10 9 8 7 6 5 4 3 2 1

PRINTED IN THE UNITED STATES OF AMERICA

To Professor Jack Pepys, the Father of Occupational Asthma.

Preface

Medical interest in occupationally induced lung diseases has been focused chiefly on dust-induced disorders since the earliest description of miners' lung disease by both Agricola and Paracelsus in the middle of the sixteenth century. It is therefore not surprising that contemporary textbooks of occupational lung disease have emphasized ailments that, until recently, were very common in industrialized countries and could be detected by progressive x-ray changes, permanent loss of pulmonary function, and unique structural histological characteristics. Although occupational asthma was recognized as early as the eighteenth century, its importance as an industrial hazard was not widely appreciated until the technological era that emerged after the end of World War II. The post–World War II literature concerning occupational asthma throughout the world continues to increase steadily each year, and industrial specialists have recognized that it may now be one of the most common work-related diseases. Recent journal reviews, book chapters, and monographs also document the proliferation in the number of specific causes of occupational asthma and the overall increase in prevalence. Indeed, occupational asthma is now more prevalent than pneumoconiotic lung disease in most developing countries (see Chapter 15.)

The diagnosis of occupational asthma is often difficult because of multiple causality in many industrial environments, the variability of symptoms and patterns of late-phase asthmatic reactions, the requirements for special diagnostic procedures, and the unpredictability of onset and persistence of symptoms. On the other hand, outbreaks of occupational asthma in specific work settings may provide ideal, mini-epidemiological paradigms of naturally occurring asthma. Such outbreaks provide excellent opportunities for investigating the source, the characteristics of the emission–dispersion cycle, and the health impact of inciting agents. Environmental sampling for monitoring the concentration of both chemicals and proteins is available in many industrial situations where occupational asthma has occurred (Chapters 13 and 17). The ready access to such integrated data in a defined setting provides an ideal milieu and investigational model for further advancement of knowledge about the pathophysiological pathways and natural history of asthma.

These expanded opportunities have attracted the collaborative interests of allergists, immunologists, pulmonologists, immunotoxicologists, occupational health specialists, aerosol scientists, industrial hygienists, and epidemiologists. In addition, the economic and social hardships imposed on workers who have refractory symptoms associated with occupational asthma require consultation with medicolegal experts. These interactions have clearly established that the features of occupational asthma are unique and often at odds with medical dogma derived from the surveillance, diagnosis, and prevention of dust-induced lung disorders. Combined with the recent upsurge of scientific interest and literature in the pathophysiology of asthma in the general population, these considerations convinced us that a textbook dealing exclusively with occupational asthma was overdue. The enthusiastic response to publication of the first edition of *Asthma in the Workplace* and the number of literature citations attributed to it have more than justified preparation of a second edition.

As is the case with most new fields of medical expertise, discovery and research in occupational asthma have continued at a rapid pace and have served as the impetus for this updated and revised edition. In addition, coverage of several specific areas of interest that had not yet clearly evolved prior to publication of the first edition has been either added or expanded.

Because new advances in occupational asthma are international in scope, the coalition of editors and individual contributors in this book is a reflection of this orientation. The common goal of this cooperative effort was to prepare an authoritative, educational resource for primary care physicians, occupational health specialists, allergists, and pulmonologists. A reference book of this type was considered particularly germane for primary care providers because current mandates for early detection and reporting of occupational asthma require that these physicians develop skills that lead to early recognition of this disease. To this end, special emphasis has been given to an algorithm of clinical diagnosis, immunological evaluation, and physiological methods of evaluation (Chapters 8, 9, 10, and 11) as a practical guide for primary care physicians. Special chapters on medicolegal aspects, compensation, assessment of disability, prevention, and surveillance (Chapters 15, 16, and 17) address the social outcomes of workers disabled by asthma and should serve as useful reference sources for occupational health physicians, workers' compensation administrators, private insurers, attorneys, adjudicators, and legislators. The chapters concerning epidemiology and disease entities have been prepared to provide sufficient in-depth information for occupational health and other medical subspecialists primarily concerned with asthma in the workplace. This second edition also describes new entities that either are relevant in differential diagnosis or are often associated with OA. The former include Chapter 33 ("Hypersensitivity Pneumonitis and Organic Dust Toxic Syndromes") and Chapter 34 ("Building-Related Illnesses"). The relationship of conditions frequently associated with occupational asthma is reviewed in Chapters 18 and 19 ("Upper Airways Involvement" and "Occupational Urticaria").

The book is organized into three main sections. Part I, "General Considerations," contains chapters on historical background, epidemiology, pathophysiology, and natural history. Notable additions are chapters on genetics and animal models. Recent research advances concerning the role of genetic polymorphisms in asthma have also been reported in several established occupational asthma syndromes. The role of animal models as predictors of risk assessment has expanded significantly since the first edition.

Part II, "Assessment and Management," includes chapters that delineate the basic guidelines for clinical and objective evaluation, environmental monitoring, and prevention of occupational asthma. Medicolegal aspects, assessment of disability, and surveillance strategies are also discussed in this section.

Detailed information about specific agents (including a variety of high-molecular-weight and chemical agents) that induce asthma or asthma-like diseases is found in Part III, "Specific Disease Entities." New chapters on occupational asthma caused by enzymes, latex, and flour appear in the second edition because of recently heightened recognition of their importance. The increasing prevalence of irritant-induced asthma (RADS) warranted a revised and expanded chapter (Chapter 30). Separate chapters (Chapters 31 and 32) concerning asthma-like disorders (cotton, other textiles, and grain dusts) are also presented in this part of the book.

Part IV contains several compendiums. Chapter 35 contains two comprehensive tables that list the major protein and chemical inducers of occupational asthma, the chief workplaces in which these occur, key literature references, the approximate number of documented cases in each category, and other pertinent immunological and physiological data.

The second compendium (Chapter 36) is a description of the U.S. National Occupational Exposure Survey (NOES) Data Base obtained as a result of a survey conducted in 4490 manufacturing facilities in the United States. Detailed information in this data base includes: specific causative agents and the respective job processes and occupations in which workers are likely to be exposed, total numbers of exposed workers classified by gender, and the actual number of workers reporting significant symptoms. This data base has been transferred to several high-density hard disks that may be used in either IBM- or MacIntosh-compatible personal computers. To illustrate how such data may be used, representative examples of hardcopy printouts are included in this compendium. Information about the availability and cost of the NOES Data Base may be obtained by writing to: David H. Pedersen, Ph.D., Environmental Health Specialist, Division of Surveillance, Hazard Evaluation and Field Studies, 4676 Columbia Parkway, R-19, Cincinnati, Ohio 45229-1998, fax (513) 641-4489.

The third compendium (Chapter 37) contains a description of a French telematic information system (Minitel) on occupational asthma. Minitel was designed to generate a data base for detection of occupational asthma by primary care practitioners and health professionals interested in this field. It was prepared by the team in Montpellier under the principal supervision of Henriette Dhivert-Donnadieu and Philippe Godard, and it is now operating in France. As a result of a cooperative agreement between Minitel and the Occupational Lung Committee of the American Academy of Allergy, Asthma and Immunology, the complete Minitel data base is now available on floppy disk compatible with either IBM-compatible or MacIntosh computers. A copy of the disk may be obtained by writing to: Learning Resource Center, American Academy of Allergy, Asthma and Immunology, 611 E. Wells Street, Milwaukee, Wisconsin 53202.

In a sense, the preparation of individual chapters by multiple authors is similar to meta-analyses that compare different published medical data pertaining to a given research question. As often occurs with meta-analyses, agreement at times is incomplete. Above all, the authors and editors have attempted to balance opposing views as objectively as possible. In most cases, this balancing process was successful in arriving at editorial consensus. Where this was not possible, the data appear with the caveat that a controversy exists and resolution is not possible, because definitive data are either not yet available or under investigation. These critical assessments have been rewarding educational experiences for the editors and authors. We hope that this joint effort will not only provide pragmatic information for current clinical applications but also serve as a foundation for significant new research information that will most assuredly advance the discipline during the forthcoming millennium.

I. Leonard Bernstein
Moira Chan-Yeung
Jean-Luc Malo
David I. Bernstein

Introduction

In his classic treatise *On Asthma: Its Pathology and Treatment* (William Wood and Co, New York, 1882), Henry Hyde Slater discusses the etiology of asthma in a most interesting way. He notes: "There are many irritants of asthma, whose modus operandi is not very clear . . . . How do they act? To what class do they belong? Let me endeavor to answer these questions with regard to some of these doubtful irritants . . . ." This is followed by commentaries about cold, heat and thunder, overexertion, laughing, and, lastly, coughing and sneezing. Eventually, Dr. Slater remarks that among the "agents of circumstances tending to provoke asthma . . . chemical and mechanical irritants . . . dust, smoke, pungent fumes, sulfite vapors, cold air are irritants of this kind."

It is noteworthy that nowhere in this classic text on asthma is the word "occupation" mentioned. But, of course, this was before occupational medicine had become the necessary partner of the industrial revolution. Nowadays things are different, and occupational health is part of the public health focus. Nonetheless, it appears that occupational asthma may not be on the "radar screen" of practitioners.

This volume is a landmark in the history of asthma. Its editors achieved much with their first edition. This second, expanded edition is a major landmark and a tool for those who see and treat patients suffering from occupational asthma.

The contributors, who come from many disciplines and many countries, present us with what are among the most authoritative discussions of all the issues relevant to occupational asthma.

Asthma is a complex, multi-faceted disease that results from many causes. Readers of this book will undoubtedly be equipped to contribute to the further reduction of asthma-related morbidity.

Claude Lenfant, M.D.
Director
National Heart, Lung, and Blood Institute
National Institutes of Health
Bethesda, Maryland

Contents

Contents

Contributors

Margaret R. Becklake, M.B., B.Ch., M.D., F.R.C.P. Department of Medicine, Department of Epidemiology and Biostatistics, and Department of Occupational Health, Respiratory Epidemiology Unit, McGill University, Montréal, Quebec, Canada

David I. Bernstein, M.D. Division of Immunology, Department of Medicine, University of Cincinnati College of Medicine, Cincinnati, Ohio

I. Leonard Bernstein, M.D. Division of Immunology, Department of Internal Medicine, University of Cincinnati College of Medicine, Cincinnati, Ohio

Jonathan A. Bernstein, M.D. Department of Internal Medicine, University of Cincinnati College of Medicine, Cincinnati, Ohio

Paul Blanc, M.D., M.S.P.H. Division of Occupational and Environmental Medicine, Department of Medicine, University of California–San Francisco, San Francisco, California

Piera Boschetto, Ph.D., M.D. Section of Hygiene and Occupational Medicine, Department of Clinical and Experimental Medicine, University of Ferrara, Ferrara, Italy

Jean Bousquet, M.D. Respiratory Disease Clinic, Hôpital Arnaud de l'Aiguelongue, Montpellier, France

Stuart Brooks, M.D. Department of Environmental and Occupational Health, College of Public Health, University of South Florida, Tampa, Florida

Sherwood Burge, M.Sc., M.D., F.R.C.P., F.F.O.M., D.I.H. Occupational Lung Disease Unit, Birmingham Heartlands Hospital, Birmingham, England

Brian T. Butcher, Ph.D. Department of Research and Professional Education, Arthritis Foundation, Atlanta, Georgia

Gaetano Caramori, M.D. Research Center on Asthma & COPD, Section of Respiratory Diseases, Department of Clinical and Experimental Medicine, University of Ferrara, Ferrara, Italy

André Cartier, M.D. Faculty of Medicine, Université de Montréal and Respiratory Division, Sacré-Coeur Hospital, Montréal, Quebec, Canada

Moira Chan-Yeung, M.B., F.R.C.P.(C), F.R.C.P.   Respiratory Division, Vancouver General Hospital, and Department of Medicine, University of British Columbia, Vancouver, British Columbia, Canada

B. Lauren Charous, M.D.   Allergy and Respiratory Care Center, Milwaukee Medical Clinic and Medical College of Wisconsin, Milwaukee, Wisconsin

David C. Christiani, M.D., M.P.H.   Departments of Environmental Health and Epidemiology, Harvard School of Public Health, and Department of Medicine and Pulmonary & Critical Care Unit, Massachusetts General Hospital, Harvard Medical School, Boston, Massachusetts

Yvon Cormier, M.D.   Department of Medicine, Laval University and Hôpital Laval, Ste-Foy, Quebec, Canada

Henriette Dhivert-Donnadieu, M.D.   Clinique des Maladies Respiratoires, Hôpital Arnaud de Villeneuve, Montpellier, France

Leonardo M. Fabbri, M.D.   Research Center on Asthma & COPD, Section of Respiratory Diseases, Department of Clinical and Experimental Medicine, University of Ferrara, Ferrara, Italy

William Gerald Gaines, Jr., M.D., M.P.H.   Department of Occupational and Environmental Medicine, Scott and White Clinic, Texas A&M Health Sciences Center and School of Rural Public Health, and Texas A&M/National Science Foundation Industry–University Cooperative Ergonomics Research Center, College Station, Texas

Denyse Gautrin, Ph.D.   Department of Social and Preventive Medicine and Department of Medicine, Université de Montréal, Montréal, Quebec, Canada

Philippe Godard, M.D.   Clinique des Maladies Respiratoires, Hôpital Arnaud de Villeneuve, Montpellier, France

Susan Gordon, Ph.D.   Department of Occupational and Environmental Medicine, Imperial College School of Medicine at the National Heart and Lung Institute, London, England

Leslie C. Grammer, M.D.   Department of Medicine, Northwestern University Medical School, Chicago, Illinois

Dick Heederik, Ph.D.   Department of Environmental Sciences, Environmental and Occupational Health Group, Wageningen University and Research Center, Wageningen, The Netherlands

Anthony Johnson, M.B.B.S., F.R.A.C.P., M.O.H.S.   Institute of Respiratory Medicine, Royal Prince Alfred Hospital, Sydney, Australia

Meryl Karol, Ph.D.   Department of Environmental and Occupational Health, University of Pittsburgh, Pittsburgh, Pennsylvania

Susan M. Kennedy, Ph.D.   Department of Occupational Hygiene, University of British Columbia, Vancouver, British Columbia, Canada

Helena Keskinen, M.D.   Finnish Institute of Occupational Health, Helsinki, Finland

Jacques Lesage, M.Sc.   Research Institute in Occupational Health and Safety, Montréal, Quebec, Canada

James T. Li, Ph.D., M.D.   Department of Allergy and Internal Medicine, Mayo Clinic, Rochester, Minnesota

Gary M. Liss, M.D., M.S., F.R.C.P.(C)   Ontario Ministry of Labour and Department of Public Health Sciences, University of Toronto, Toronto, Ontario, Canada

Boris D. Lushniak, M.D., M.Ph.   National Institute of Occupational Safety and Health, Cincinnati, Ohio

Jean-Luc Malo, M.D.   Department of Medicine, Université de Montréal and Sacré-Coeur Hospital, Montréal, Quebec, Canada

Cristina Elisabetta Mapp, M.D.   Laboratory of Respiratory Pathophysiology, Section of Occupational Medicine, Department of Environmental Medicine and Public Health, University of Padova, Padova, Italy

C. G. Toby Mathias, M.D.   Group Health Associates and Departments of Environmental Health and Dermatology, University of Cincinnati Medical Center, Cincinnati, Ohio

Dick Menzies, M.D., M.Sc., F.R.C.P.(C)   Department of Medicine, Epidemiology, and Biostatistics, McGill University, Montréal, Quebec, Canada

James A. Merchant, M.D., Dr.P.H.   Departments of Preventive Medicine and Environmental Health, University of Iowa, Iowa City, Iowa

François-Bernard Michel, M.D.   Department of Respiratory Diseases, University Medical School and Hôpital Arnaud de Villeneuve, Montpellier, France

Gianna Moscato, M.D.   Division of Allergy/Immunology, Salvatore Maugeri Foundation, Institute for Rehabilitation and Care, Medical Center of Pavia, Pavia, Italy

Benoit Nemery, Ph.D., M.D.   Laboratory of Pneumology, Katholieke Universiteit Leuven, Leuven, Belgium

Anthony J. Newman Taylor, M.B.B.S., M.Sc., M.R.C.P., M.F.O.M., F.R.C.P., F.F.O.M.
Department of Occupational and Environmental Medicine, Imperial College School of Medicine at the National Heart and Lung Institute, London, England

Roy Patterson, M.D.   Division of Allergy/Immunology, Department of Medicine, Northwestern University Medical School, Chicago, Illinois

David H. Pedersen, Ph.D.   Division of Surveillance, Hazard Evaluation and Field Studies, National Institute for Occupational Safety and Health, Cincinnati, Ohio

Jack Pepys, M.D.[†]   Royal Postgraduate Medical School, London, England

Guy Perrault, Ph.D.   Research Institute in Occupational Health and Safety, Montréal, Quebec, Canada

Brigitte Perrin, M.D.   Respiratory Disease Clinic, Hôpital Arnaud de l'Aiguelongue, Montpellier, France

Anthony Pickering, F.R.C.P., F.F.O.M., D.I.H.   Department of Occupational and Environmental Medicine, Northwest Lung Centre, Wythenshawe Hospital, Manchester, England

Charles E. Reed, M.D.   Department of Internal Medicine, Mayo Clinic, Rochester, Minnesota

Hal B. Richerson, M.D.   Department of Internal Medicine, College of Medicine, University of Iowa, Iowa City, Iowa

Cecile S. Rose, M.D., M.P.H.   Department of Occupational and Pulmonary Medicine, National Jewish Medical and Research Center, and University of Colorado, Denver, Colorado

Katherine Sarlo, Ph.D.   Department of Human and Environmental Safety, The Procter & Gamble Company, Cincinnati, Ohio

David A. Schwartz, M.D., M.P.H.   Department of Internal Medicine, University of Iowa, Iowa City, Iowa

Joseph A. Seta[†]   Division of Surveillance, Hazard Evaluation, and Field Studies, National Institute for Occupational Safety and Health, Cincinnati, Ohio

Mark C. Swanson   Allergic Disease Research Laboratory, Mayo Clinic, Rochester, Minnesota

Susan M. Tarlo, B.S., M.B., F.R.C.P.(C)   Occupational Lung Disease Clinic, University of Toronto, Toronto, Ontario, Canada

Olivier Vandenplas, M.D.   Department of Chest Medicine, University Hospital of Mont-Godinne, Yvoir, Belgium

---

[†]Deceased.

Katherine M. Venables, M.Sc., M.D., F.R.C.P., F.F.O.M., M.F.P.H.M.   Department of Occupational and Environmental Medicine, Imperial College School of Medicine at the National Heart and Lung Institute, University of London, London, England

Randy O. Young   Division of Surveillance, Hazard Evaluation, and Field Studies, National Institute for Occupational Safety and Health, Cincinnati, Ohio

C. Raymond Zeiss, M.D.   Division of Allergy/Immunology, Department of Medicine, Northwestern University Medical School and VA Chicago Health Care System/Lakeside Division, Chicago, Illinois

1
Definition and Classification of Asthma

I. Leonard Bernstein and David I. Bernstein
University of Cincinnati College of Medicine, Cincinnati, Ohio

Moira Chan-Yeung
Vancouver General Hospital and University of British Columbia, Vancouver, British Columbia, Canada

Jean-Luc Malo
Université de Montréal and Sacré-Coeur Hospital, Montréal, Quebec, Canada

PRIOR DEFINITIONS

To avoid ambiguity about defining occupational asthma in this book, an editorial basis for consensus was sought by analyzing two principal prior definitions of occupational asthma:

Any Agent Specific to the Workplace.   Several definitions in this category have been proposed, respectively, by Brooks, Sheppard, Parkes, and Newman Taylor. All of these definitions specify that the causal agent is specific to the workplace.

1. "Occupational asthma is a disorder in which there is generalized obstruction of the airways, usually reversible, caused by inhalation of a substance or material that a worker manufactures or uses directly or is incidentally present at the worksite" (1).
2. "Although the term 'occupational asthma' usually refers to new onset asthma caused by workplace exposure, exacerbations of preexisting asthma are an equally important cause of workplace morbidity ... extreme sensitivity of airways to chemical, physical and pharmacologic stimuli is a characteristic feature of asthma. Thus, many agents encountered in the workplace that have little or no effect on nonasthmatic workers can cause pronounced symptomatic bronchoconstriction in workers with asthma" (2).
3. "Occupational asthma, therefore, is caused by some specific agent or agents in the form of dust, fumes or vapors in an industrial environment" (3).
4. "Occupational asthma is variable airways narrowing causally related to exposure in the working environment to airborne dust, gases, vapors or fumes" (4).

Sensitizing Agents Specific to the Workplace.   These definitions specify not only that the agent has to be present in the workplace but that it also exerts its effects through "sensitization." Such definitions have been proposed by Cotes and Steal, Burge, and Chan-Yeung and Malo.

1

1. "Occupational asthma is caused by exposure at a place of work to a sensitizing bronchoconstrictor substance" (5).
2. "Occupational asthma is asthma which is due in whole or in part to agents met at work. Once occupational sensitization has occurred . . . " (6).
3. "Occupational asthma will be defined as asthma caused by specific agents in the workplace. This will exclude bronchoconstrictions induced by irritants at work, exercise and cold air" (7).

EDITORIAL CONSENSUS DEFINITION

After deliberating about the diversity of opinion represented in the above opinions, the editors adopted the following definition, which allows sufficient latitude to include both immunological and nonimmunological causes of asthma in the workplace: *Occupational asthma is a disease characterized by variable airflow limitation and/or airway hyperresponsiveness due to causes and conditions attributable to a particular occupational environment and not to stimuli encountered outside the workplace. Two types of occupational asthma are distinguished by whether they appear after a latency period:*

1. *Immunological. This category is characterized by work-related asthma appearing after a latency period and encompasses: (1) work-related asthma caused by most high- and certain low-molecular-weight agents for which an immunological (IgE mediated) mechanism has been proven; and (b) occupational asthma induced by specific occupational agents (e.g., western red cedar) and appearing after a latency period but for which neither an IgE- nor a non-IgE-mediated immunological mechanism has been identified.*
2. *Nonimmunological. This classification describes irritant-induced asthma or reactive airways dysfunction syndrome (RADS), which may occur after single or multiple exposures to nonspecific irritants at high concentrations.* Activation of preexistent asthma or airway hyperresponsiveness by nontoxic irritants or physical stimuli in the workplace ordinarily is excluded by this definition. This type of occurrence is explained in Part II.

A history of preexistent asthma does not preclude the possibility that either type of occupational asthma may develop after an appropriate workplace exposure. Special modifications of the above definition of occupational asthma may be required for practical applications in epidemiological surveillance studies (e.g., an epidemiological case definition) or for medical/legal purposes. These special definitions are discussed in more detail in Chapters 15 and 17.

CLASSIFICATION

Occupational exposure can result in two major categories of variable airways limitation: occupational asthma and occupational asthma-like disorders. Occupational asthma, defined above, constitutes the main topic of this book. The recently described RADS, which follows a single or multiple exposure(s) to high concentrations or spill(s) of an irritant product (e.g., chlorine gas, anhydrous ammonia, fire smoke), is considered occupational asthma according to our definition. However, it might more properly be designated as irritant-induced asthma. Affected workers develop variable reversible airways limitation and hyperresponsiveness for varying periods of time after the initial exposure. This syndrome is discussed in Chapter 25.

The second variety of occupational variable airways limitation is an occupational asthma-like disorder. An asthma-like disorder typically presents with symptoms of chest tightness associated with a cross-shift change in FEV_1 but without persistent bronchial hyperresponsiveness and eosinophilia. However, cross-shift decreases of FEV_1 may predict later development of chronic airflow limitation. The chief prototype of this is byssinosis, a textile dust disease, which affects the airways of workers exposed to cotton, flax, hemp, jute, or sisal (see Chapter 26). Symptoms of obstructive airflow limitation occurring after exposure to grain dusts are also included in this category (see Chapter 27).

REFERENCES

1. Brooks SM. Occupational asthma. In: Weiss EB, Segal MS, Stein M, eds. Bronchial Asthma. Boston: Little, Brown, 1985:461–469.
2. Sheppard D. Occupational asthma and byssinosis. In: Murray JF, Nadel JA, eds. Textbook of Respiratory Medicine. Philadelphia: WB Saunders, 1988:1593–1605.
3. Parkes WR. Occupational Lung Disorders. London: Butterworths, 1982:415–453.
4. Newman Taylor AJ. Occupational asthma. Thorax 1980; 35:241–245.
5. Cotes JE, Steal J. Oxford: Blackwell Scientific Publ., 1987:345–372.
6. Burge PS. Occupational asthma. In: Barnes P, Rodger IW, Thomson NC, eds. Asthma: Basic Mechanisms and Clinical Management. London: Academic Press, 1988:465–482.
7. Chan-Yeung M, Malo J-L. Occupational asthma. Chest 1987; 81:130S–136S.

2
Historical Aspects of Occupational Asthma

Jack Pepys[†]
Royal Postgraduate Medical School, London, England

I. Leonard Bernstein
University of Cincinnati College of Medicine, Cincinnati, Ohio

INTRODUCTION

The recognition and acceptance of occupational asthma as an important and distinct entity has depended upon clarification of the term "asthma" and upon means of establishing its occupational relationship. Asthma translated literally means "panting," that is, a symptom rather than a clinical disorder. Hippocrates (460–370 B.C.) cites its presence in metal workers, fullers, tailors, horsemen, farmhands, and fishermen. The use of the term asthma to describe a clinical disorder is attributed to Aretaeus in the first century A.D. Maimonides, known as Rambam, discussed the disorder in a "Treatise on Asthma" in 1190. The paroxysmal nature of the disorder interspersed with periods of freedom was described by van Helmont in 1662 and by Floyer in 1698.

Observation of relationships of diseases to occupations has been influenced by socioeconomic factors, according to Sigerist (1). In antiquity industry was small scale, employed ancient technology, and was frequently conducted outdoors. Early examples of occupational respiratory problems can be seen in a citation from an ancient Egyptian papyrus (Papyrus Sallier) describing "the weaver engaged in home work [who] is worse off in the house than the women: doubled up with his knees drawn up to his stomach, he cannot breathe," and in Roman times in a report by Pliny stating that "persons employed in the manufactories in preparing minimum [native cinnabar, red lead] protect the face with masks of loose bladder skin, in order to avoid inhaling the dust, which is highly pernicious: the covering being at the same time sufficiently transparent to admit of being seen through." There was little development in reports on occupational diseases in the Middle Ages.

With the development of trade and the need for precious and other metals in the fifteenth century, occupational diseases became of medical interest and were mainly concerned with mining and traumatic injuries and termed morbi metallici. Ellenbog in 1473 wrote a short pamphlet entitled "On the Poisonous and Wicked Fumes and Smokes" encountered by goldsmiths and others. Paracelsus (1493–1541) wrote the first monograph

---

[†]Deceased.

on occupational diseases arising from his interest in chemistry and this was devoted mainly to mining.

Occupational disease in general came of age when Bernardino Ramazzini published in 1713 his great classic landmark in occupational diseases, *De morbis artificum diatriba* (2). This contained important contributions to occupational respiratory disease affecting bakers, handlers of old clothes, and workers with flax, hemp, and silk, and in a section on "Diseases of sifters and measurers of grain" the description corresponds with the features of farmer's lung, the classical example of extrinsic allergic alveolitis (bronchioloalveolitis). Such subjects may also have an asthmatic component of their illness and some may be mainly or solely asthmatic. Whereas Ramazzini was referred to as the historical source of information on farmer's lung when the main cause, *Micromonospora faeni*, was being identified (3), it was of interest to learn of a much earlier comparable description by Olaus Magnus in 1555 of respiratory disease due to threshing of grain (Fig. 1).

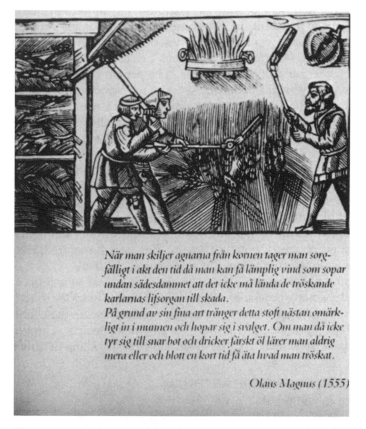

Närr man skiljer agnarna från kornen tager man sorg-
fälligt i akt den tid då man kan få lämplig vind som sopar
undan sädesdammet att det icke må lända de tröskande
karlarnas lifsorgan till skada.
På grund av sin fina art tränger detta stoft nästan omärk-
ligt in i munnen och hopar sig i svalget. Om man då icke
tyr sig till snar bot och dricker färskt öl lärer man aldrig
mera eller och blott en kort tid få äta hvad man tröskat.

Olaus Magnus (1555)

Figure 1 "When sifting the chaff from the wheat, one must carefully consider the time when a suitable wind is available that sweeps away the harmful dust. This fine-grained material readily makes its way into the mouth, congests in the throat, and threatens the life organs of the threshing men. If one does not seek instant remedy by drinking one's beer, one may never more, or only for a short time, be able to enjoy what one has threshed."—Olaus Magnus, 1555.

Ramazzini, in addition to his incisive and always topical description of diseases due to various occupations, made another great contribution. He wrote, "The Divine Hippocrates informs us, that when a Physician visits a Patient, he ought to inquire into many things, by putting questions to the Patient and Bystanders" and adds, "To which I would presume to add one Interrogation more: namely, what Trade is he of?", thus providing an indispensable dictum for occupational disease. This should, of course, include "What other occupations have you had?"

The next step in occupational diseases and priority in their description arose with the Industrial Revolution in the United Kingdom in the 1800s. Charles Turner Thackrah published in 1832 a fine book on the effects of arts, trades, and professional and civic status and habits of living on health and longevity (4). A review of this book at the time in the *Edinburgh Medical and Surgical Journal* concluded that "English literature has until now been destitute of a single general treatise on the diseases of trades and professions." Thackrah used the term asthma only twice, with reference to maltsters and coffee roasters and to hatters and hairdressers. These were thought to have chronic bronchitis, "the chronic pulmonary catarrh of Laennec." He also mentions the production of respiratory symptoms in pharmacists grinding to powder ipecacuanha, the Brazilian shrub used as an expectorant from early in 1648. The affected persons had to stay out of buildings where this was being done. Thomas Dover used ipecacuanha together with opium to form Dover's powder, widely used, even recently, for coughs and colds.

Thackrah was concerned with respiratory problems in flax mills and, like Patissier in France, described mill fever on the initial exposure followed by troublesome cough and observed "that the respiratory symptoms evinced a great and easily excited irritability." The noises of flax mills made auscultation of the workers difficult, and Thackrah describes the usefulness of the "pulmometer" in diseases of the lungs. This consisted of "a large graduated glass jar, inverted over, and filled with water. The person blows through a tube, the lower end of which is under the jar, making however but one expiration at each trial. The air bubbling up displaces of course the water at the upper part of the vessel, and as this is marked from above downward, the subsidence of the water indicates the quantity of air expired." The spirometer was developed in 1836.

Just as Ramazzini instructed that questions about occupation should be put, so Thackrah stated dogmatically, "If any object, that the cure not the causes or prevention of disease, is the business of the medical practitioner, I would reply that the scientific treatment of a malady requires a knowledge of its nature, and the nature is imperfectly understood without knowledge of the cause." In other words, precise etiologic diagnosis is required, most pertinent to occupational asthma, and to be discussed further.

Major contributions to the recognition of extrinsic causes of asthma in general were made, among others, by Bostock in 1819 (5), Blackley in 1873 (6), and Salter in 1860 (7). Literature on occupational diseases in the United States began in 1837, instigated by the New York Medical Society. The first chairs in industrial hygiene were created in 1910 in New York and in Milan.

OCCUPATIONAL CAUSES OF ASTHMA—EARLY 1900s TO 1960s

Among the limited examples of asthma related to specific occupational causes are those due to both high- (mainly protein) and low-molecular-weight (mainly chemical) allergens.

In chronological order, the first comprise castor bean dust (8), western red cedar (9), endemic asthma due to castor bean dust (10), atopy to acacia (gum arabic) (11), mayfly (Ephemerida) (12), asthma due to gum acacia (13), tragacanth (14), wood dust (15), and locust (16). Among low-molecular-weight chemical allergens are platinum halide salts (17), platinum salts (18), chromium (19), chromates (20), phthalic anhydride (21), sulfonechloramides (22), platinum salts (23,24), toluene diisocyanate (25), chrome, nickel, and aniline (26), and rubber, lacquer, and shellac (27).

The reason for the above arbitrary and limited selection of references is to show the great increase in reports on occupational asthma and its causes, in particular low-molecular-weight chemicals, from about 1960 onward. For example, in 1980, more than 200 causes had been identified and more than 2000 new substances were being synthesized each year (28). The comprehensive discussion on occupational asthma by Brooks (9) has 347 references, and the other chapters in this volume will increase these numbers.

DEVELOPMENTS IN DIAGNOSIS

Ramazzini initiated the clinical diagnosis of the occupational nature of asthma by asking "What is your occupation?" Support for this may be obtained by pulmonary function tests in relation to work, as suggested by Thackrah using the pulmometer, and in etiological terms by skin and other immunological tests. The gold standard for identifying a particular occupational agent as the probable cause of asthma is the response to exposure under controlled and appropriate conditions, and most attention will be paid to its development. The use of bronchial provocation tests with common protein allergens was pioneered by Colldahl (29). A new era in which such tests are made with low-molecular-weight chemical compounds was opened by Gelfand (27). He investigated respiratory allergy due to chemical compounds encountered in the rubber, lacquer, shellac, and beauty culture industries. Almost all of his subjects were atopic with evidence of sensitivity to common allergens. He elicited immediate skin and bronchial reactions to solutions of ethylenediamine, monoethanolamine, ammonium thioglycolate, and hexamethylenetetramine. These were administered as a fine mist, and Gelfand states that "in many instances, spraying the material into the air near the patient would result in immediate symptoms," The duration of the inhalation tests was not stated. In the case of a granular product, hexamethylenetetramine, unsuitable for an aerosol test, the lacquer and hair spray product as used by the public was tested. The reactions elicited, lasting one-half to 2 hr, were an "uncontrollable paroxysmal cough, blocking or running of the nose, as well as precipitation of asthmatic breathing." The latter required injection of adrenaline. The sera of two patients who gave positive reactions to ethylenediamine gave positive reactions to passive transfer test. Gelfand's description of the severity of reactions is not encouraging for similar tests, though the results had useful etiological diagnostic value. As for isocyanates, he states, "This chemical is too toxic for either skin or provocative inhalation testing."

In 1964, Gandevia reported on "respiratory symptoms and ventilatory capacity in men exposed to isocyanate vapour" (30). He found, as did Gelfand, that work exposure to toluene diisocyanate (TDI) elicited more cough than wheeze, suggestive of bronchitis, and that subjects regularly had nocturnal symptoms, now recognized to be a feature of occupational asthma. None had a past history of allergy. In 1967, Gandevia and Milne investigated asthma in workers handling western red cedar (31). Aqueous solutions of an extract elicited bronchial provocation test asthmatic reactions occurring after 4–6 hr, again at night, and recurring on successive nights thereafter, with normal findings during the daytime. Such subjects would not notice improvement when off work over weekends, which can otherwise be so useful in diagnosing occupational asthma. This sequence of reactions corresponded with the clinical histories of affected workers of rhinitis and cough at the end of the day's work or early at night followed by later nocturnal asthma.

The next study of this sort was made by Popa and colleagues in 1969, who investigated "bronchial asthma and asthmatic bronchitis determined by simple chemicals" using skin, serological, and bronchial provocation tests (32). The low-molecular-weight substances were tested as aerosols inhaled for 5 min except for a test with the fume from a heated urea formaldehyde resin. A decrease in the FEV_1 of 10% was taken as positive, a lower value than the 20% decrease required at present. Two patterns of asthmatic reaction were elicited. In one group of subjects an immediate reaction was associated with immediate intradermal and passive transfer reactions to ethylenediamine, sulfathiazole, and chloramine. These corresponded with the clinical history. In another group, the inhalation test reactions came on after 2–12 hr. Skin tests, intradermal and patch, gave delayed 24- to 48-hr reactions, but no immediate reactions, leading to the hypothesis of a delayed hypersensitivity mechanism, as yet still subject to confirmation and a topic of much interest. The provocation test reactions corresponded to the clinical histories of dyspnea at the end of the shift and persisting for 1–2 hr, only to recur during the night as a "classic nocturnal asthma." An explanation is needed for their finding of negative bronchial reactions to common environmental allergens to which most of the subjects had given positive intradermal tests.

OCCUPATIONAL-TYPE BRONCHIAL PROVOCATION TESTS

The above findings raised challenging questions about low-molecular-weight chemicals as causes of occupational asthma but left open the urgent need for safe, acceptable, and reproducible procedures for definitive and analytical bronchial tests. Faced with the problems of the unsuitability of many agents for use as aerosols and the possibilities of irritant, toxic, highly potent allergenicity, and other adverse effects, Pepys et al. developed a pragmatic, simulated occupational type of test. This was suggested by a patient with severe occupational asthma who was occupied in varnishing boats for the Oxford-Cambridge boat race using a two-part varnish consisting of polyurethane resin to which toluene diisocyanate (TDI) was added prior to use. He was tested as shown in Figure 2 by painting on a surface with the polyurethane resin, which gave no reaction. This was followed the next day by painting with the mixture of polyurethane and TDI, which elicited an unequivocal and reproducible nonimmediate reaction (33).

This form of test avoids artificiality in the nature of the exposure, the duration of which may be as little as a few breaths with certain substances and in all cases far less than the ordinary work exposure, usually of many hours each day. It is, in essence, a small piece of real life and is fully acceptable, when made with care under controlled conditions, on ethical grounds and for clinical, etiological diagnosis. Indeed, failure to establish a precise cause and leave the subject to continued exposure is undesirable. The testing is time consuming but potentially precise in identifying causes in complex exposures. The simulated occupational type of test was a landmark in future studies. Examples will be given of the various patterns of reaction, immunochemical, and other findings in response to dusts, powders, fumes, gaseous emanations, and aerosols (34).

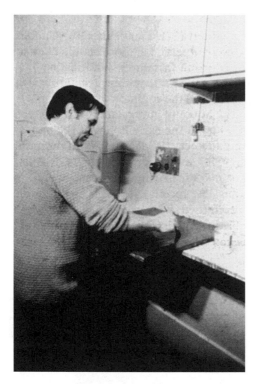

Figure 2   Occupational-type test for toluene diisocyanate (TDI) (gaseous emanations) sensitivity. Repeated application of polyurethane varnish with and without TDI activator in proportions as used. Atmospheric concentration in test cubicle was 0.00173–0.0018 ppm. (From Ref. 33.)

PATTERNS OF ASTHMATIC REACTION

The various patterns reported by Gelfand (27), Gandevia (30), Gandevia and Milne (31), and Popa et al. (32) were observed in more detail. They consisted of (1) an immediate reaction starting in minutes and lasting $1\frac{1}{2}$–2 hr, and of nonimmediate reactions, (2) an uncommon reaction starting after about 1 hr and lasting 4–5 hr, (3) the common late reaction starting after several hours and lasting 12 hr or more, and (4) a nocturnal reaction coming on after about 16 hr in the early hours of the morning and capable of recurring without any further challenge and with decreasing intensity at the same time each night for several or many nights. Isolated single reactions or late reactions or combined reactions were found. Care was needed regarding late reactions, which could develop after negative immediate reactions even to very limited challenges. Furthermore, as Gandevia (30) noted, recurrent reactions can result in persistence of asthma when off work over weekends or longer, thus giving an impression of nonoccupational asthma. Such findings showed that it is also necessary to ensure than any recurrent reactions due to previous work exposure shall have ceased before starting the tests, as otherwise a false-positive result may be elicited. In the course of these tests it was shown that sodium cromoglycate could inhibit both immediate and dual reactions, whereas corticosteroid inhalation had no effect on the immediate reaction but was very effective in inhibiting the late reaction (34).

These patterns are identical to those elicited by common protein environmental allergens, and they corresponded to the common clinical histories of occupational asthma often starting with respiratory symptoms at the end of the day or elicited by exercise, followed later by asthmatic attacks at the end of the day and at night and in some cases later by immediate attacks on work exposure.

SIMULATED OCCUPATIONAL PROVOCATION TESTS

A number of reports have been published on the results of occupational-type tests with a variety of different exposures to gaseous emanations, fumes, and dusts of natural organic origin and of inorganic and organic chemical origin, mainly of low molecular weight. Other methods of testing aimed at quantitative aspects and many other identified causes appear in subsequent chapters. It is noteworthy that the pragmatic occupational-type exposures are capable of giving very reproducible reactions and can suffice for clinical etiological purposes (see Figs. 6,7). Points of special interest will be cited. The test for sensitivity to TDI as made by Pepys et al. (33) is an example of its versatility. Of the subjects concerned, two were employed soldering television wires. They were tested as if at work by soldering the relevant wire coated or uncoated with a polyurethane film and the resin flux for 10 min. The coated wire liberated toluene diisocyanate fumes, and a late asthmatic reaction was elicited. The specific sensitivity was confirmed by a painting test for 30 min with polyurethane varnish mixed with the TDI activator (see Fig. 2).

The environmental effect of reactive chemicals was shown by the production of asthma in workers in a storeroom in East London (36). In the absence of possible causes, questions were asked about neighboring enterprises. It transpired that an adjacent factory making polyurethane foam was exhausting its products near the ventilation system of the storeroom. TDI was found in the ventilation filters, the portal of entry into the storeroom. Provocation tests by painting with polyurethane resin plus TDI established TDI as the cause. These workers were subsequently compensated by the neighboring factory. The initial presenting patient was so sensitive that he had only to approach the area to develop severe asthma that day.

In the case of amino-ethyl ethanolamine (37), a flux component for aluminum wire soldering was identified as the cause in a test consisting of three to four inhalations of the fumes, confirming the findings of Sterling (38).

In testing with dusty or powdered agents, the material was mixed with well-dried lactose, starting with a low concentration and increasing for daily tests until a reacting concentration was found. This was tipped from one receiver to another, simulating the inhalation exposure at work (Fig. 3). In two subjects working with piperazine, late reactions were elicited by this method (39). These reactions were inhibited by sodium cromoglycate when it was inhaled before and 4 hr after the challenge and before the late reaction had begun to present.

Tests for sensitivity to wood dusts were made by the tipping method using the wood dusts themselves and gave specific late reactions (40). Chan-Yeung et al. (41), studying sensitivity to western red cedar, have shown that a low-molecular-weight organic acid in western red cedar, plicatic acid, is an allergen.

The acceptability of this form of occupational-type test is shown by its use in tests for sensitivity to platinum halide salts, which are of extremely high allergenicity. Starting with microgram amounts in 250 g of lactose (Fig. 3), the concentration was increased gradually, one test per day, up to 40 mg/kg, which elicited reactions to the dust after

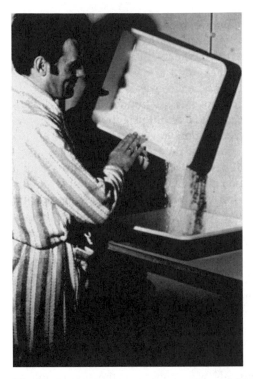

Figure 3 Occupational-type test for sensitivity to dust/powder agents mixed with lactose or un-mixed, e.g., for wood dusts. Repeated tipping under controlled conditions and with increasing concentrations. Stippled areas in Figures 4–7 show duration of challenges.

carefully monitored exposures of 4–30 min. This elicited immediate, dual and isolated late asthmatic reactions. Skin testing was approached with caution in view of severe reactions to scratch and intradermal tests (18,42,43). Skin prick tests starting with a 10^{-6} concentration up to 10^{-3} are effective for demonstrating sensitivity (44), and subsequently specific IgE antibodies were shown in the majority by RAST (45). A number of points of basic serological and immunochemical interest (47) were present in the findings on platinum salt allergy. Passive transfer tests in humans and monkeys showed the presence in unheated serum of long-term specific IgE antibodies and also in heated serum of short-term heat-stable antibodies, presumably IgG-STS, capable of giving immediate reactions to the platinum halide salt itself and without any need for conjugation with a carrier protein for the making of the test (46). A possible role for heat-stable, short-term sensitizing antibody to low-molecular-weight chemicals merits examination.

The capacity of low-molecular-weight chemicals in themselves to elicit immediate reactions and react with specific IgE antibodies or in PK tests has been shown for a number of other occupational allergens, such as chlorhexidine (48), the anhydrides (49,50), azo and anthraquinone dyes (51), sulfonechloramides (22), and ethylenediamine and para-phenylenediamine (32).

An important area of future research on the allergenic effects of reactive low-molecular-weight chemicals is shown by the capacity of the platinum halide salts to create in affected subjects neoantigens in human serum albumin, against which specific IgE antibody is formed. This antibody can react with neoantigens in serum albumin resulting from combination with other unrelated chemical haptens. Thus, in platinum salt–sensitive workers, 4 out of 38 gave positive RASTs to human serum albumin compared with 3 out of 116 nonsensitive subjects. Tests with dinitrophenyl-HSA gave positive RASTs with 8 out of 38 sera and with 4 of the 116 nonsensitive subjects (52).

Similar findings have been made in a patient allergic to nickel sulfate (53,54) and in patients allergic to the phthalic anhydrides (55), trimellitic acid anhydride (56), and diisocyanates (57). This phenomenon has been described as autoantibodies induced by extrinsic, low-molecular-weight chemical allergens, i.e., extrinsically determined auto-allergy (EDAA) (58). Evidence for a possible active role of such IgE antibodies to neoantigens in human serum albumin in biological reactions is the elicitation of an immediate reaction to a skin prick test with human serum albumin in a subject sensitive to trimellitic acid who had IgE antibodies to HSA (A. Newman Taylor, personal communication). Similar findings have been shown in guinea pigs sensitized to TDI in which reaginic antibodies were induced against both the TDI and guinea pig serum albumin neoantigens. Skin tests with guinea pig serum albumin elicited immediate reactions (59).

A great advantage of low-molecular-weight chemicals is their known chemical structure. This can provide basic immunochemical information. For example, skin prick tests with a wide range of platinum salts (47) showed that allergenicity in eliciting reactions was related to the number of chlorine molecules in the test material. Chlorine is a leaving ligand and is loosely bound to the platinum. By contrast, palladium encountered in the refining of platinum is poorly, if at all, allergenic, and in this case the chlorine molecules are firmly bound. Investigations of this sort would be very useful with other agents containing chlorine, such as amprolium chloride, capable of eliciting immediate skin test reactions and for the identification of other possibly relevant ligands. In the context of chlorine itself it is remarkable that chlorhexidine becomes potently allergenic for inducing sensitivity and eliciting reactions by simple dilution in chlorinated water (48).

An investigation of asthma in four workers from the same firm manufacturing ampicillin and exposed also to benzyl-penicillin and 6-amino-penicillanic acid showed differences in their sensitivities (60). Tests by dust inhalation (see Fig. 3) of mixtures with lactose elicited characteristic and reproducible late asthmatic reactions. In one case the reactions were elicited by commercial preparations of 6-amino-penicillanic acid and ampicillin but not by purified preparations, showing sensitivity to an unidentified impurity present in both products (Figs. 4, 5). In another subject typical late reactions coming on after 3–4 hr and lasting more than 16 hr were elicited by both commercial and purified ampicillin (Fig. 6). Both commercial and purified preparations of 6-amino-penicillanic acid elicited quite different reactions to the ampicillin, coming on after 10 hr and maximal at 16 hr (Fig. 7). The difference between the two materials is the addition of phenylglycine acid chloride as a side chain to the 6-amino-penicillanic acid to make ampicillin. Identical asthmatic reactions were given after oral administration of a dose of the relevant antibiotic (Fig. 8). Immediate-type reactions to phenyl-glycine being made in large amounts have also been reported (61). Figures 6 and 7 show the reproducibility of the reactions in the occupational-type test.

Two female asthmatic hairdressers were tested as if at work by mixing in a mortar a hair-bleaching agent with hydrogen peroxide (62). One gave an acute immediate and the other a late reaction. The cause in a mixture of 11 unnamed ingredients provided by the maker was identified as potassium persulfate. The immediate reactor also gave a immediate skin reaction to application of a drop of solution to unbroken skin, an example of contact urticaria. The late reactor to the bleach was also sensitive to henna, which on

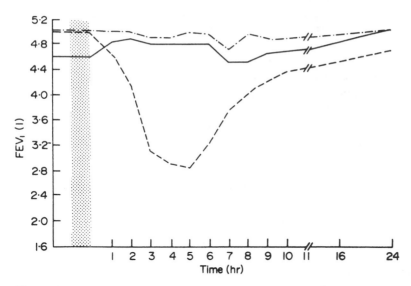

Figure 4 Occupation-type test as in Figure 3 with mixture of 1 g of 6-amino-pennicillanic (6APA) acid in 250 g lactose. (—), Lactose control test; (— —), lactose plus commercial 6APA; (—·—), lactose plus purified 6APA. *Note*: Late asthmatic reaction to commercial and not purified 6APA, i.e., die to a contaminant. (From Ref. 60.)

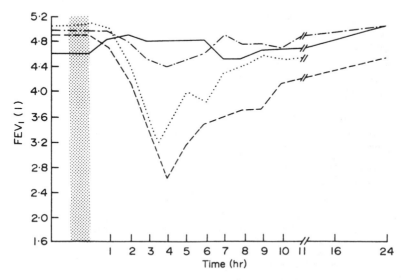

Figure 5 Occupational-type test as in Figure 3 with mixture of 1 g ampicillins in 250 g lactose in patient in Figure 4. (—), Lactose control; (— —), lactose plus commercial unpurified ampicillin; (·······), lactose plus another unpurified ampicillin; (—·—), lactose plus purified ampicillin. *Note*: Late asthmatic reaction to contaminant in unpurified ampicillin as with 6APA in Figure 4. (From Ref. 60.)

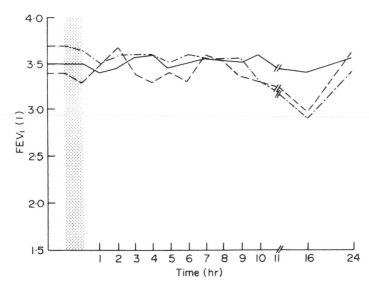

Figure 6 Occupational-type test as in Figure 3 with mixture of 10 g of 6APA, commercial and purified in 250 g lactose. (—), Lactose control; (—·—), lactose plus purified 6APA; (— —), lactose plus commercial 6APA. *Note*: Late, reproducible, 16-hr reactions to both purified and unpurified 6APA, i.e., reacting agent in 6APA molecule. (From Ref. 60.)

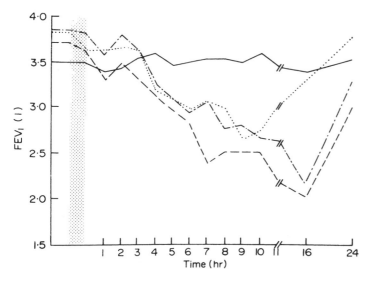

Figure 7 Occupational-type test as in Figure 3 with mixture of 10 g of purified commercial ampicillins in 250 g lactose in same patient as Figure 6. (—), Lactose control; (— —), lactose plus commercial unpurified ampicillin; (—·—), lactose plus purified ampicillin; (······), lactose plus another unpurified ampicillin. *Note*: Late, reproducible 3–4-hour onset asthmatic reactions to purified and unpurified ampicillins, more severe than 6APA reactions (Fig. 6) and attributable to addition of phenyl-glycine to 6APA nucleus to form ampicillin. (From Ref. 60.)

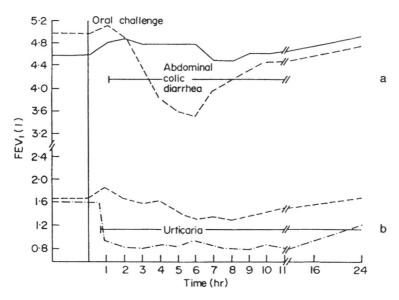

Figure 8 Oral challenge with capsules of (a) commercial ampicillin (2 × 500 mg) in patient (Figs. 6, 7) and (b) benzyl penicillin (2 × 500 g) in another subject. *Note*: Reproducible late asthmatic reactions to ampicillin, plus gastrointestinal reactions to ingested allergen in (a) and to benzyl penicillin in (b) plus urticaria. Similar reactions were observed to oral challenges in subjects giving late reactions to tests with other inhaled and possibly ingested dusts. (From Ref. 60.)

testing in the same way gave an immediate nasal and conjunctival reaction and a positive immediate skin prick test reaction.

A worker who developed asthma while making salbutamol noticed an association with an intermediate product termed "glycol compound" [(2-*N*-benzyl-*N*-*tert*-butyl-amino)-4′-hydroxy-3′-hydroxymethyl acetophenone diacetate]. Provocation tests with the powder and lactose mixture (see Fig. 3) elicited a late asthmatic reaction to the glycl compound and less so to a benzyl compound. Salbutamol itself, the final product, caused no reaction on challenge and was effective when used for relief of symptoms (63).

A major role in the chemical cause of occupational asthma is played by the development of synthetic resins to take the place of colophony and its derivatives, mainly acrylics, epoxy resins, and polyurethanes. The first polyurethane foams were made during World War II by I.G. Farben in Germany, using toluene diisocyanate as an activator. It has been calculated that 2.2 million tons are likely to be used in the United States in the next 10 years involving many thousands of workers. Occupational-type tests were made with epoxy resin systems containing phthalic acid anhydride, trimellitic acid anhydride, and triethylene tetramine (64). Their sensitivity could be shown by the test consisting of as little as a single breath of fume from heated materials. Their diagnostic value was shown in a patient thought to have asthma due to TDI to which he, however, gave a negative reaction; an acute immediate reaction was given to a heated cured resin containing phthalic acid anhydride. In another subject, painting with a liquid bisphenol A resin to which triethylene tetramine was added gave a late asthmatic reaction to the mixture but not to the resin alone. Sensitivity to trimellitic acid anhydride (TMA) was demonstrable in yet another by one breath of the invisible fume from heated epoxy paint, which elicited a dual asthmatic reaction. TMA is remarkable in that it causes three different syndromes with different immunological findings (65). Immediate reactions are present with positive skin tests and IgE and other antibodies to TM-human serum albumin. Late respiratory reactions coming on 4–12 hr after exposure occurred in patients with negative skin tests and high total antibody levels but not IgE antibody to TM-human serum albumin. In the third pulmonary disease/anemia syndrome, very high levels of antibody to TM-human serum albumin are present but no IgE antibody.

Asthma due to the fumes from the soldering of Multicore—a tin-lead alloy containing cores of wood resin flux—has been shown to result from colophony, a pine resin widely used for soft soldering in the electronics industry and for other purposes (66). The active material in the resin is mainly abietic acid. Immediate asthmatic reactions, late and dual, were elicited by one breath to 3-min exposure in tests made on separate days of the fumes from heating of the Multicore or the colophony resin. Up to 20% of the workers were sensitized (67), and many showed the value of frequent monitoring of the peak flow rate to show occupational effects. Affected subjects may develop symptoms in the neighborhood of pine trees that emanate resins into the air, and they can react to unheated colophony (68).

There is as yet no explanation in general for isolated late reactions or the recurrent nocturnal reaction, in contrast to immediate and many dual reactions where specific IgE antibody is present as shown by skin and serological tests. The above list of agents and reactions to occupational-type tests will be expanded considerably in the chapters to follow, as will discussions and results of tests with other methods of exposure, because of their importance in establishing etiological diagnosis in occupational asthma.

FUTURE OF OCCUPATIONAL ASTHMA

Greater recognition of occupational asthma is leading to improved environmental control and avoidance of the use of potent causal agents. Points of importance include greater understanding of the immunochemical properties of such agents, on the one hand, and of factors predisposing to sensitization of exposed subjects, on the other. Examples of the former are the role of halide molecules, notably chlorine, behaving as leaving ligands, in bestowing sensitizing and eliciting capacity. This is shown by platinum halide salts in humans (47) and in experimental animals (69) and by the striking effect of chlorine on allergenicity of chlorhexidine (48). The well-defined structure of low-molecular-weight chemical allergens offers many opportunities for establishing more basic information like this.

Of the factors predisposing to sensitization, with the induction of specific IgE antibody, atopy has been taken to be or prime importance, supported by clinical observations with common environmental protein allergens and by investigations showing that atopies are more readily sensitized than nonatopics to allergen aerosol (70). Atopy in immunological terms can be defined as the predisposition to sensitization to common allergens as shown by immediate skin prick test reactions (71). From 30 to 40% of apparently asymptomatic subjects belong in the atopic group so defined and present a problem in deciding whether occupational exposure to potential allergens should be permitted. Recent findings, however, emphasize the importance of cigarette smoking in its own right and as an additive factor to atopy in favoring IgE sensitization to a variety of occupational agents (72). Zetterstrom et al. (73) found that cigarette smokers had raised serum levels of IgE and a higher rate of sensitization to isphaghula. Similar sensitizations are reported to tetrachlorophthalic anhydride (74), platinum halide salt (75), and *Bacillus subtilis* enzymes (76).

This effect of smoking may be attributable to increased permeability of the bronchial epithelium (77) and to immunological effects. A striking contrast is the finding in extrinsic allergic alveolitis occurring mainly in nonatopic subjects, farmer's lung, bird fancier's lung, and seasonal disease in Japan, that nonsmokers are more likely to develop precipitating antibodies and clinical disease (78–81). Uncertainty about the relationships between atopy and work are discussed by Nordman (82).

ACTIONS OF REGULATORY BODIES

In 1956 the U.S. Department of Labor noted 100 occupations apparently associated with the development of asthma. The problem was to recognize this by law with rights of compensation. France in 1960 was the first country to do so and related it to the manufacturing and handling of penicillin. Additions were made in 1967 of tropical woods, followed in 1972 by low-molecular-weight chemicals, paraphenylenediamine and ethanolamine, and in 1973 by isocyanates and biological enzymes, and further agents have been added since then. In Germany a law was passed in 1961 accepting "bronchial asthma enforcing the cessation of the professional occupation or any other paid employment," with special emphasis on flour and TDI.

The United Kingdom bowed much later to the pressures of the clinical and etiological diagnoses being made from the findings with isocyanates and platinum salts. The contents of the report on occupational asthma under the Social Security Act of 1975 illustrate the approach to the problems of recognition for medicolegal purposes. The question examined was "whether there is any condition resulting from exposure to industrial asthma-inducing agents which should be prescribed under the Act." The main problem, it was stated, was that of separating asthmatics whose asthma is unrelated to their occupation from those whose asthma has been initiated by a sensitizing agent encountered at work. The first and most important step was the detailed clinical and occupational history, and the four key diagnostic points consisted of (1) a sensitizing agent is present at work, (2) the patient has been exposed for some time before the asthma develops, (3) the symptoms improve when away from work, and (4) exposure to a much smaller dose than the work exposure causes the symptoms to recur.

The last two points are relevant to the foregoing discussion. Symptoms can persist for some time after cessation of exposure in the form of recurrent nocturnal asthma (30,83–85) and also in response to ordinary environmental exposure to the causal agents. For example, a patient sensitive to ampicillin developed asthma at night after visiting the town where the factory was; a TDI-sensitive patient had the same problem in the neighborhood of the factory, and colophony-sensitive patients can react to pine trees and even to unheated colophony and turpentine (68). The acceptance of responses to minimal reexposure emphasizes the importance of provocation studies to provide definitive evidence, especially in relation to new substances or where the cause is in doubt so that established knowledge cannot, for practical purposes, be assumed to suffice for the diagnosis.

The report concluded with a list of seven causal agents regarded as the most clearly established causes of occupational asthma (86). These were platinum salts, isocyanates, acid anhydride and amine hardening agents, fumes from the use of resin as a soldering flux, proteolytic enzymes, animals and insects in laboratories, and dusts arising from milling and handling flour and from harvesting, drying, transporting, and storing grains. A further seven additions made in 1986 were antibiotics, cimetidine, wood dusts, isphaghula, castor bean dust, ipecacuanha (a hark back to Thackrah and Dover's powder), and azo-dicarbonamide. The last nine additions in 1990 were glutaraldehyde, persulfate salts or henna arising from their use in the hairdressing trade, crustaceans or fish or products arising from these in the food-processing industry, reactive dyes, soybeans, tea dust, green coffee bean dust, fumes from stainless steel welding, and, finally, a catchall addition to the list consisting of "any other sensitizing agent inhaled at work."

OCCUPATIONAL ASTHMA—RECENT DEVELOPMENTS, 1993–1998

The second edition of *Asthma in the Workplace* appears 5 years after the first edition and in the last year of this millennium. Unfortunately, Dr. Jack Pepys can no longer personally witness the rapid evolution of the discipline he helped to pioneer, but it would have been a great source of satisfaction to him that some of his predictions about the future of occupational asthma either have already transpired or are beginning to emerge in the relatively short period of time since the original publication of this book.

In the past 5 years the recognition curve of occupational asthma has assumed a much steeper slope, as evidenced by at least a 100% increase in literature citations reviewed in this text. Prospective surveillance programs continue to demonstrate that occupational asthma is by far the most common disorder among all occupationally induced lung diseases (87). Commensurate with this upward trend, there also appears to be an increased awareness among adjudication officials that disability and compensation must be evaluated apart from classical fibrogenic and restrictive lung diseases (88). Longitudinal surveillance of several worksites confirms that early detection and removal from exposure are the optimal means of preventing long-term disability. When specific causal relationships can be established, employers may be able to alter the manufacturing process itself, which, in some cases, may attenuate or abolish the risks of high exposure (89). However, exhaustive environmental control measures to eliminate human exposure may not suffice to completely prevent occupational asthma due to agents such as diisocyanates even in an optimally engineered plant (89).

As morbidity and mortality statistics of asthma continue to rise in the world's developed nations, the perception that occupational allergens, nonspecific triggers, and irritants are important contributory factors has been noted in several evidentiary-based guideline documents on the diagnosis and management of asthma (90,91). Technological progress in the identification of both high- and low-molecular-weight agents in the workplace environment has expanded: these developments are discussed in detail in Chapters 13 and 14. The role of nonspecific irritants in the induction of nonimmunological occupational asthma has been explored more extensively since the first edition of this book was published. First described by Brooks et al. in 1985, many case reports, case series, and several epidemiological studies of reactive airways dysfunction syndrome (RADS) have appeared in the recent literature and are reviewed in the current edition (92–95). A number of new cases have been described after multiple exposures to both high and low levels of the same workplace irritants (see Chapter 25). Of particular interest is additional information derived from bronchoalveolar lavage and biopsy investigations about the histopathological features of RADS. Although the overall microscopic anatomical changes of RADS are identical to asthma, unique differences between RADS, immunologically induced occupational asthma, and naturally occurring asthma have been identified (93,96). Epithelial desquamation is a common feature but it is more intense in the acute phase of RADS and is often accompanied by a higher percentage of bronchoalveolar neutrophils.

Some investigators have not observed as many bronchoalveolar eosinophils in chronic stages of RADS. Subepithelial fibrosis is more prominent in RADS than in other forms of occupational or nonoccupational asthma. These findings, coupled with the chronic persistence of airway hyperresponsiveness, have firmly established RADS as a prototype of nonimmunological asthma. Future research in the various clinical stages of RADS and their corresponding pathophysiological mechanisms will undoubtedly expand because RADS or RADS-like illnesses may ultimately provide clues that help to explain the continued increase in incidence of asthma in industrial urban centers.

Better understanding of risk factors has evolved over the past 5 years. In the case of protein allergens, the extent and distribution of exposure are foremost among risk assessment (97). The significance of these risk factors is illustrated by the rapid appearance of respiratory sensitization among 5–10% of health workers soon after universal barrier control management of AIDS patients mandated the usage of latex gloves (98,99). In his historical review, Dr. Jack Pepys emphasized the role of halides in conferring allergenicity to certain chemicals such as platinum salts and chlorohexidine. This concept has been extended to other reactive organic chemicals and their analogs. As a result there has been renewed interest in predictive animal models based on structure-activity relationships of haptenic allergenicity. For example, systematic immunological investigations of acid anhydride chemicals have demonstrated that ring structure, position of double bonds, and methyl group substitution may be critical determinants of IgE-mediated sensitization (100). A computer-assisted analysis of respiratory sensitization based on chemical structure has also been developed as a means of predicting human allergenicity (101). Preexistent atopy also continues to be an important determinant of IgE-mediated asthma induced by workplace high-molecular-weight allergens (102,103). In some instances, new workers who are atopic may already be presensitized to occupational protein allergens (e.g., laboratory animals) prior to entering the workplace. Interestingly, Brooks et al. recently proposed that atopy is also a risk factor in the ''not so sudden'' form of RADS (104). Except for platinum salts, atopy does not appear to be a prerequisite for sensitization to many low-molecular-weight chemicals. Nevertheless, genetic susceptibility has been explored further and may predispose individuals to sensitization by specific low-molecular-weight chemicals such as TDI and trimellitic anhydride, both of which demonstrate associations between specific HLA class II genes (105,106). Smoking is a well-established risk factor for IgE-mediated occupational asthma induced by high-molecular-weight substances and a few chemicals such as platinum salts and tetrachlorophthalic anhydride (107,108). Occupational exposure to environmental tobacco smoke also presents a substantial risk to workers (109). However, a susceptibility role of smoking has not been proven in workers who develop asthma after exposure to low-molecular-weight agents (e.g., TDI, western red cedar), for which immunological mechanisms do not entirely account for all the pathophysiological consequences induced by these chemicals (108).

The pathogenesis of the inflammatory milieu of immunological occupational asthma is in many respects similar to that of nonoccupational asthma, especially in those instances where TH2 cytokines, IgE antibodies, and immediate hypersensitivity mediator pathways are involved (110). However, T cells and their proinflammatory secretions are also prominent in non-IgE-mediated polyisocyanate asthma in which specific T-cell proliferation, activated T cells, and increased ratios of CD8+ T cells and T-cell-derived proinflammatory cytokines and chemokines have all been recently demonstrated (111–113). The unique aerobiological components (source, release, dispersion, impact) components of occupational asthma have stimulated design of many new rodent models that more accurately simulate the human paradigm (100,114–117). These have been designed to investigate many important components of occupational asthma: (1) deposition of antigens (115); (2) structure-function relationships (100); (3) prediction of human sensitization (114); (4) contrasting effects of sensitizing and IgG antibodies (117); and (5) the role of cytokines, chemokines, and mediators in the inflammatory response (118,119). Advances in respiratory physiological technology also enable the assessment of airway obstruction and nonspecific bronchial responsiveness in nonanesthetized animals (119).

The diagnosis of occupational asthma requires a combination of: (1) recognition of the source and dispersion of the causative agent; (2) characteristic symptoms; and (3) specific and nonspecific functional abnormalities related to the worksite. In the case of high-molecular-weight allergens, skin prick tests are the preferred diagnostic correlates of IgE sensitization (120). The role of IgG antibodies is more problematic but some investigators suggest that they could be used as biomarkers of exposure (121). What would have been especially gratifying to Dr. Pepys is that controlled, specific bronchial provocation remains the "gold standard" of diagnosis, although in many instances this can only be accomplished as a workplace challenge. Of particular interest to him would have been recent reports about the role of cytokine and chemokine networks in the pathogenesis of late or dual-phase bronchial challenge responses (110,111). He also would have been impressed that occupational asthma has evolved into an excellent model of human asthma because it affords a unique opportunity of examining pathophysiological processes during the initial phases of exposure, subsequent elicitation of symptoms after reexposure, and sequential changes on a prospective basis (122).

REFERENCES

1. Sigerist HE. (1936). Historical background of industrial and occupational diseases. Bull NY Acad Med 1936; 12:597–609.
2. Ramazzini B. De morbis artificum diatriba. Chicago: University of Chicago Press, 1940 (translated by WC Wright).
3. Pepys J, Jenkins PA, Festenstein GH, Gregory PJ, Lacey ME, Skinner FA. Thermophilic actinomycetes as a source of "farmer's lung hay" antigens. Lancet 1963; 2:607–611.
4. Thackrah CT. (1832). The Effects of the Principal Arts, Trades and Professions, and of Civic States and Habits of Living on Health and Longevity, with Suggestions for the Removal of Many of the Agents Which Produce Disease and Shorten the Duration of Life. Reprint. Edinburgh: Livingstone, 1957.
5. Bostock J. Case of a periodical affection of the eyes and chest. Med Chir Trans 1819; 10: 161.
6. Blackley CH. Experimental Researchers on the Causes and Nature of Catarrhus Aestivas (Hay Fever or Hay Asthma). London: Bailliere, Tindall & Cox, 1873.
7. Salter HH. On Asthma, Its Pathology and Treatment. London: Churchill, 1860.
8. Bernton HS. On occupational sensitisation to the castor bean. Am J Med Sci 1923; 165:196–202.
9. Brooks SM. Occupational asthma. In: Weiss EB, Segal MS, Stein M, eds. Bronchial Asthma, Mechanisms and Therapeutics, 2nd ed. Boston: Little, Brown, 1985: 461–493.
10. Figley, KD, Elrod RM. Endemic asthma due to castor bean dust. JAMA 1928; 90:79–82.
11. Spielman AD, Baldwin HS. Atopy to acacia (gum arabic). JAMA 1933; 101:444–445.
12. Figley KD. Mayfly (Ephemerida) hypersensitivity. J Allergy 1940; 11:376–387.
13. Sprague PH. Bronchial asthma due to sensitivity to gum acacia. Can Med Assoc J 1942;47: 253.

14. Gelfand HH. The allergenic properties of vegetable gums. A case of asthma due to tragacanth. J Allergy 1943; 14:203–219.
15. Ordman D. Bronchial asthma caused by inhalation of wood dust. Ann Allergy 1949; 7: 492–496.
16. Frankland AW. Locust sensitivity. Ann Allergy 1953; 11:445–453.
17. Karasek ST, Karasek M. The use of platinum paper. Report of Illinois State Commission of Occupational Disease, 1911:97.
18. Vallery-Radot P, Blamoutier R. Sensibilisation au chloroplatinite de potassium: accidents graves de choc survenus a la suite d'une cutireaction avec ce cel. Bull Soc Med Hop Paris 1929; 222–230.
19. Joules H. Asthma from sensitisation to chromium. Lancet 1932; 2:182–183.
20. Card WI. A case of asthma sensitivity to chromates. Lancet 1935; 2:1348.
21. Kern RA. Asthma and allergic rhinitis due to sensitisation to phthalic anhydride. Report of a case. J Allergy 1939; 10:164–165.
22. Feinberg SM, Watrous BM. Atopy to simple chemical compounds, sulphonechloramides. J Allergy 1945; 16:209–220.
23. Hunter D, Milton R, Perry KMA. Asthma caused by the complex salts of platinum. Br J Ind Med 1945; 2:92–98.
24. Roberts AE. Platinosis: 5 year study of effects of soluble platinum salts on employees in platinum laboratory and refinery. Arch Ind Hyg 1951; 4:549–559.
25. Woodbury JW. Asthmatic syndrome following exposure to tolylene di-isocyanate. Ind Med Surg 1956; 25:540–543.
26. Tolot F, Broudeur P, Meulat G. Troubles pulmonaires asthmatiformes chez des ouvriers ex-poses a l'inhalation de chrome, nickel, aniline. Arch Mol Prof. 1957; 18:291–293.
27. Gelfand HH. Respiratory allergy due to chemical compounds encountered in the rubber, lacquer, shellac and beauty culture industries. J Allergy 1963; 34:374–381.
28. Newman Taylor AJ. Occupational asthma. Thorax 1980; 35:241–245.
29. Colldahl H. Study of provocation tests on patients with bronchial asthma. Acta Allergol 1952; 5:133–142, 154–162.
30. Gandevia B. Respiratory symptoms and ventilatory capacity in men exposed to isocyanate vapour. Aust Ann Med 1964; 13:157–166.
31. Gandevia B, Milne J. Occupational asthma and rhinitis due to western red cedar (*Thuja plicata*), with special reference to bronchial reactivity. Br J Ind Med 1970; 27:235–244.
32. Popa V, Teculescu D, Stanescu D, Gavrilescu N. Bronchial asthma and asthmatic bronchitis determined by simple chemicals. Dis Chest 1969; 56:395–404.
33. Pepys J, Pickering CAC, Bresin ABX, Terry DJ. Asthma due to inhaled chemical agents— tolylene di-isocyanate. Clin Allergy 1972; 2:225–236.
34. Pepys J, Hutchcroft BJ. Bronchial provocation tests in etiologic diagnosis and analysis of asthma. Am Rev Respir Dis 1975; 112:829–859.
35. Pepys J, Davies RJ, Breslin ABX, Hendrick DJ, Hutchcroft B. The effects of inhaled beclo-methasone dipropionate (Becotide) and sodium cromoglycate on asthmatic reactions to prov-ocation tests. Clin Allergy 1974; 4:13–24.
36. Carroll KB, Secombe CJP, Pepys J. Asthma due to nonoccupational exposure to toluene (tolylene) di-isocyanate. Clin Allergy 1976; 6:99–104.
37. Pepys J, Pickering CAC. Asthma due to inhaled chemical fumes—amino-ethyl-ethanolamine in aluminum soldering flux. Clin Allergy 1972; 2:197–204.
38. Sterling GM. Asthma due to aluminum soldering flux. Thorax 1967; 22:533–537.
39. Pepys J, Pickering CAC, Loudon HWG. Asthma due to inhaled chemical agents—piperazine hydrochloride. Clin Allergy 1972; 2:189–196.
40. Pickering CAC, Batten JC, Pepys J. Asthma due to inhaled wood dusts—western red cedar and Iroko. Clin Allergy 1972; 2:213–218.
41. Chan-Yeung M, Giclas PC, Henson PM. Activation of complement responsible for asthma due to western red cedar (*Thuja plicata*). J Allergy Clin Immunol 1980; 65:331–337.

42. Freedman SO, Krupey J. Respiratory allergy caused by platinum salts. J Allergy 1968; 42: 233–237.
43. Levene GM, Calnan GD. Platinum sensitivity and treatment by specific hyposensitisation. Clin Allergy 1971; 1:75–82.
44. Pepys J, Pickering CAC, Hughes EG. Asthma due to inhaled chemical agents—complex salts of platinum. Clin Allergy 1972; 2:391–396.
45. Cromwell O, Pepys J, Parish WE, Hughes EG. Specific IgE antibodies to platinum salts in sensitised workers. Clin Allergy 1979; 9:109–118.
46. Pepys J, Parish WE, Cromwell O, Hughes EG. Passive transfer in man and the monkey of type I allergy due to heat labile and heat stable antibody to complex salts of platinum. Clin Allergy 1979; 9:99–108.
47. Cleare MJ, Hughes EJ, Jacoby B, Pepys J. Immediate (type I) allergic responses to platinum compounds. Clin Allergy 1976; 6:183–195.
48. Layton GT, Stanworth DR, Amos HE. Factor influencing the immunogenicity of the hapten drug chlorhexidine in mice. II. the role of the carrier and adjuvants in the induction of IgE and IgG anti-hapten responses. Immunology 1986; 59:459–465.
49. Maccia CA, Bernstein IL, Emmett EA, Brooks SM. In vitro demonstration of specific IgE in phthalic anhydride hypersensitivity. Am Rev Respir Dis 1976; 113:701–704.
50. Howe W, Venables K, Topping MD, Dally M, Hawkins R, Law JS, Newman Taylor AJ. Tetrachlorophthalic acid anhydride asthma: evidence for specific IgE antibody. J Allergy Clin Immunol 1983; 71:5–11.
51. Alanko K, Keskinen H, Bjorksten F, Ojanin S. Immediate type hypersensitivity to reactive dyes. Clin Allergy 1978; 8:25–31.
52. Murdoch RD, Pepys J, Hughes EG. IgE antibody responses to platinum group metals: a large scale refinery survey. Br J Ind Med 1986; 43:37–43.
53. Malo J-L, Cartier A, Doepner M, Nieboer E, Evans S, Dolovich J. Occupational asthma caused by nickel sulphate. J Allergy Clin Immunol 1982; 69:55–59.
54. Dolovich J, Evans SL, Nieboer E. Occupational asthma from nickel sensitivity. I. Human serum albumin in the antigenic determinant. Br J Ind Med 1984; 41:51–55.
55. Bernstein DI, Gallagher JS, D'Souza L, Bernstein IL. Heterogeneity of specific IgE responses in workers sensitised to acid anhydride compounds. J Allergy Clin Immunol 1984; 74:794–801.
56. Zeiss CR, Levitz D, Pruzansky JJ, Patterson R. Antibody to haptenized human serum albumin and human secretory IgA in workers exposed to trimellitic anhydride (TMA). J Allergy Clin Immunol 1982; 69:123 (abstract).
57. Butcher BT, Mapp C, Reed MA, O'Neill CE, Salvaggio JL. Evidence for carrier specificity of IgE antibodies detected in sera of isocyanate exposed workers. J Allergy Clin Immunol 1982; 69:123 (abstract).
58. Pepys J. Autoantibodies induced by extrinsic, low molecular weight chemical allergens. Proc XII Int Cong Allerg Clin Immunol, St Louis: CV Mosby, 1986:204–208.
59. Sarlo K. Inhalation sensitisation of guinea pigs to toluene di-isocyanate: generation of antibodies that recognise toluene di-isocyanate and guinea pig serum albumin. Toxicology 1989; 9:72 (abstract).
60. Davies RJ, Hendrick DJ, Pepys J. Asthma due to inhaled chemical agents: ampicillin, benzyl penicillin, 6-amino-penicillanic acid and related substances. Clin Allergy 1974; 4:227–247.
61. Kammermeyer JK, Matthews, KP. Hypersensitivity to phenyl-glycine acid chloride. J Allergy Clin Immunol 1973; 52:73–84.
62. Pepys J, Hutchcroft BJ, Breslin ABX. Asthma due to inhaled chemical agents—persulphate salts and henna in hairdressers. Clin Allergy 1976; 6:399–404.
63. Fawcett IW, Pepys J, Erooga MA. Asthma due to "glycyl compound" powder—an intermediate in production of salbutamol. Clin Allergy 1976; 6:405–409.
64. Fawcett IW, Newman Taylor AJ, Pepys J. Asthma due to inhaled chemical agents—epoxy resin systems containing phthalic acid anhydride, trimellitic acid anhydride and triethylenetetramine. Clin Allergy 1977; 7:1–14.

65. Zeiss CR, Wolkonsky P, Chacon R, Tuntland PA, Levitz D, Pruzansky JJ, Patterson R. Syndromes in workers exposed in trimellitic anhydride: a longitudinal clinical and immunologic study. Ann Intern Med 1983; 98:8–12.

66. Fawcett IW, Newman Taylor AJ, Pepys J. Asthma due to inhaled chemical agents—fumes from "Multicore" soldering flux and colophony resin. Clin Allergy 1976; 6:577–585.

67. Burge PS. Occupational asthma, rhinitis and alveolitis due to colophony. In: Pepys J, ed. Clinics in Immunology, Vol. 4. Occupational Respiratory Allergy, London: WB Saunders, 1984:55–81.

68. Burge PS, Wieland A, Robertson AS, Weir D. Occupational asthma due to unheated colophony. Br J Ind Med 1986; 43:559–560.

69. Murdoch RD, Pepys J. Immunological responses to complex salts of platinum. II. Enhanced IgE antibody responses to ovalbumin with concurrent administration of platinum salts in the rat. Clin Exp Immunol 1985; 58:478–485.

70. Salvaggio JE, Kayman H, Leskowitz S. Immunologic responses of atopic and normal individuals to aerosolised dextran. J Allergy 1966; 38:31–40.

71. Pepys J. Atopy. In: Gell PGH, Coombs RRA, Lachmann PJ, eds. Clinical Aspects of Immunology, 3rd ed. Oxford: Blackwell Scientific Publications, 1975:877–902.

72. Editorial. Smoking, occupation, and allergic lung disease. Lancet 1:965.

73. Zetterstrom O, Osterman K, Machads L, Johanson SGO. Another smoking hazard: raised serum IgE concentration and increased risk of occupational allergy. Br Med J 1981; 283:1215–1217.

74. Venables KM, Topping MD, Howe W, Luczynska CM, Hawkins R, Newman Taylor AJ. Interaction of smoking and atopy in producing specific IgE antibody. Br Med J 1985; 290:201–204.

75. Venables KM, Dally MB, Nunn AJ, Stevens JF, Stephens R, Farrer N, Hunter JV, Stewart M, Glyn-Hughes E, Newman Taylor AJ. Smoking and occupational allergy in workers in a platinum refinery. Br Med J 1989; 299:939–941.

76. Greenberg M, Milne JE, Watt A. A survey of workers exposed to dusts containing derivatives of *Bacillus subtilis*. Br Med J 1970; 11:629–633.

77. Hulbert WC, Walker DC, Jackson A, Hogg JC. Airway permeability to horseradish peroxidase in guinea pigs: the repair phase after injury by cigarette smoke. Am Rev Respir Dis 1981; 123:320–326.

78. Morgan DC, Smyth JT, Lister RW, Pethybridge RJ. Chest symptoms and farmers' lung: a community survey. Br J Ind Med 1973; 30:259–265.

79. Morgan DC, Smyth JT, Lister RW, Pethybridge RJ, Gilson JC, Callaghan P, Thomas GO. Chest symptoms in farming communities with special reference to farmers' lung. Br J Ind Med 1975; 32:228–234.

80. Warren CPW. Extrinsic allergic alveolitis: a disease commoner in non-smokers. Thorax 1977; 32:567–569.

81. Arima K, Ando M, Yoshida K, Sakata T, Sugimoto M, Araki S, Fusatsuka M. Suppressive effects of cigarette smoking on the prevalence of summer-type hypersensitivity pneumonitis caused by *Trichosporon cutaneum* and specific antibody response to the antigen. Am Rev Respir Dis 1990; 141:A316 (abstract).

82. Nordman H. Atopy and work. Scand J Work Environ Health 1984; 10:481–485.

83. Davies RJ, Green M, Schofield NM. Recurrent nocturnal asthma after exposure to grain dust. Am Rev Respir Dis 1976; 114:1011–1019.

84. Newman Taylor AJ, Davies RJ, Hendrick DJ, Pepys J. Recurrent nocturnal asthmatic reactions to bronchial provocation tests. Clin Allergy 1979; 9:213–219.

85. Henrick DJ, Lane DJ. Occupational formalin asthma. Br J Ind Med 1977; 34:11–18.

86. Occupational asthma. Department of Health and Social Security (Social Security Act, 1975). Her Majesty's Stationery Office, 1981, Cmnd 8121.

87. Sallie B, Ross D, Meredith S, et al. SWORD '93: Surveillance of work-related and occupational respiratory disease in the UK. Occup Med 1994; 44:177–182.

88. Dewitte JD, Chan-Yeung M, Malo J-L. Medicolegal and compensation aspects of occupational asthma. Eur Respir J 1994; 7:969–980.
89. Bernstein DI, Korbee L, Stauder T, Bernstein JA, Scinto J, Herd ZL, Bernstein IL. The low prevalence of occupational asthma and antibody-dependent sensitization to diphenylmethane diisocyanate in a plant engineered for minimal exposure to diisocyanates. J Allergy Clin Immunol 1993; 92:387–396.
90. Spector SL, Nicklas RA, eds. Practice parameters for the diagnosis and treatment of asthma. J Allergy Clin Immunol 1995; 96(Suppl):707–870.
91. National Heart, Lung, and Blood Institute, National Asthma Education and Prevention Program. Expert Panel Report 2: Guidelines for the Diagnosis and Management of Asthma. Bethesda, MD: National Institutes of Health, pub. No. 97-4051, 1997.
92. Brooks SM, Weiss MA, Bernstein IL. Reactive airways dysfunction syndrome (RADS): persistent asthma syndrome after high level irritant exposure. Chest 1985; 88:376–384.
93. Gautrin D, Boulet L, Boutet M, et al. Is reactive airways dysfunction syndrome (RADS) a variant of occupational asthma? J Allergy Clin Immunol 1994; 93:12–22.
94. Gautrin D, Leroyer C, Malo J-L. Longitudinal assessment of workers at risk of chlorine exposure. Am J Respir Crit Care Med 1996; 153:A-185.
95. Sallie B, McDonald C. Inhalation accidents reported to the SWORD surveillance project 1990–1993. Ann Occup Hyg 1996; 40:211–221.
96. Lemière C, Malo J-L, Boutet M. Reactive airways dysfunction syndrome due to chlorine: sequential bronchial biopsies and functional assessment. Eur Respir J 1997; 10:241–244.
97. Houba R, Heederik D, Doekes G, van Run P. Exposure-sensitization relationship for α-amylase allergens in the baking industry. Am J Respir Crit Care Med 1996; 154:130–136.
98. Sussman G, Tarlo S, Dolovich. The spectrum of IgE-mediated responses to latex. JAMA 1991; 265:2844.
99. Heilman DL, Jones RT, Swanson MC, Yunginger JW. A prospective, controlled study showing that rubber gloves are the major contributor to latex aeroallergen levels in the operating room. J Allergy Clin Immunol 1996; 98:325–330.
100. Zhang XD, Lötvall JL, Skerfving S, Welinder H. Antibody specificity to the chemical structures of organic acid anhydrides studied by in vitro and in vivo methods. Toxicology 1997; 118:223–232.
101. Karol MH, Graham C, Gealy R, Macina OT, Sussman N, Rosenkranz HS. Structure activity relationships and computer-assisted analysis of respiratory sensitization potential. Toxicol Lett. 1996; 86:187–191.
102. Botham PA, Lamb CT, Teasdale EL, Bonner SM, Tomenson JA. Allergy to laboratory animals: a follow-up study of its incidence and of the influence of atopy and pre-existing sensitisation on its development. Occup Environ Med 1995; 52:129–133.
103. Bernstein JA, Kraut A, Bernstein DI, Warrington R, Bolin T, Warren CPW, Bernstein IL. Occupational asthma induced by inhaled egg lysozyme. Chest 1993; 103:532–535.
104. Brooks SM, Hammad Y, Richards I, Giovinco-Barbas J, Jenkins K. The spectrum of irritant-induced asthma: sudden and not-so-sudden onset and the role of allergy. Chest 1998; 113: 42–49.
105. Balboni A, Baricordi OR, Fabbri LM, Gandini E, Ciaccia A, Mapp CE. Association between toluene diisocyanate-induced asthma and DQB1 markers: a positive role for aspartic acid at position 57. Eur Respir J 1996; 9:207–210.
106. Young RP, Barker RD, Pile KD, Cookson WOCM, Newman Taylor AJ. The association of HLA-DR3 with specific IgE to inhaled acid anhydrides. Am J Respir Crit Care Med 1995; 151:219–221.
107. Baker DB, Gann PH, Brooks SM, Gallagher J, Bernstein IL. Cross-sectional study of platinum salts sensitization among precious metals refinery workers. Am J Ind Med 1990; 18: 653–664.
108. Venables KM, Chan-Yeung. Occupational asthma. Lancet 1997; 349:1465–1469.
109. Hammond SK, Sorensen G, Youngstrom R, Ockene JK. Occupational exposure to environmental tobacco smoke. JAMA 1995; 274:956–960.

110. Beasley R, Roche WR, Roberts JA, et al. Cellular events in the bronchi in asthma and after bronchial provocation. Am Rev Respir Dis 1989; 139:806–817.

111. Bentley AM, Maestrelli P, Saetta M, Fabbri LM, Robinson DS, Bradley BL, Jeffery PK, Durham SR, Kay AB. Activated T-lymphocytes and eosinophils in the bronchial mucosa in isocyanate-induced asthma. J Allergy Clin Immunol 1992; 89:821–829.

112. Maestrelli P, Del Prete GF, De Carli M, D'Elios MM, Saetta M, Di Stefano AD, Mapp CE, Romagnini S, Fabbri LM. CD8 T-cell clones producing interleukin-5 and interferon-gamma in bronchial mucosa of patients with asthma induced by toluene diisocyanate. Scand J Work Environ Health 1994; 20:376–381.

113. Lummus ZL, Alam R, Bernstein JA, Bernstein, DI. Characterization of histamine releasing factors in diisocyanate-induced occupational asthma. Toxicology 1996; 111:191–206.

114. Sarlo K, Fletcher ER, Gaines WG, Ritz HL. Respiratory allergenicity of detergent enzymes in the guinea pig intratracheal test: association with sensitization of occupationally exposed individuals. Fund Appl Toxicol 1997; 38:44–52.

115. Karol MH, Jin RZ, Lantz RC. Immunochemical detection of TDI adducts in pulmonary tissue of guinea pigs following inhalation exposure. Inhal Toxicol 1997; 9:63–83.

116. Mapp CE, Lapa e Silva JR, Lucchini RE, Chitano P, Rado V, Saetta M, Pretolani M, Karol MH, Maestrelli P, Fabbri LM. Inflammatory events in the blood and airways of guinea pigs immunized to TDI. Am J Respir Crit Care Med 1996; 154:201–208.

117. Dearman RJ, Moussavi A, Kemeny DM, Kimber I. Contribution of CD4+ and CD8+ T lymphocyte subsets to the cytokine secretion patterns induced in mice during sensitization to contact and respiratory chemical allergens. Immunology 1996; 89:502–510.

118. Faccione S, deSiqueira ALP, Jancar S, Russo M, Barbuto JAM, Mariano M. A novel murine model of late-phase reaction of immediate hypersensitivity. Media Inflamm 1997; 6:127–133.

119. Hamelmann E, Vella AT, Oshiba A, Kappler JW, Marrack P, Gelfand EW. Allergic airway sensitization induces T cell activation but not airway hyperresponsiveness in B cell-deficient mice. Proc Natl Acad Sci USA 1997; 94:1350–1355.

120. Bernstein DI, Bernstein IL, Gaines WG Jr, Stauder T, Wilson ER. Characterization of skin prick testing responses for detecting sensitization to detergent enzymes at extreme dilutions: inability of the RAST to detect lightly sensitized individuals. J Allergy Clin Immunol 1994; 49:498–507.

121. Chan-Yeung M. Assessment of asthma in the workplace. Chest 1995; 108:1084–1117.

122. Gautrin D, Infante-Rivard C, Malo J-L. Specific IgE-dependent sensitization and change in bronchial responsiveness in a cohort of apprentices exposed to high-molecular-weight agents. Am J Respir Dis 1998;155:A855.

3
Epidemiological Approaches in Occupational Asthma

Margaret R. Becklake
McGill University, Montréal, Quebec, Canada

Jean-Luc Malo
Université de Montréal and Sacré-Coeur Hospital, Montréal, Quebec, Canada

Moira Chan-Yeung
Vancouver General Hospital and University of British Columbia, Vancouver, British Columbia, Canada

THE ROLE OF EPIDEMIOLOGY

The Discipline of Epidemiology

Epidemiology has been described as a discipline, not a science (1). As a discipline, epidemiology comprises a set of principles and approaches, which in their application to specific domains of knowledge concerning natural events contribute to the body of scientific information that forms the basis for action in that domain. In its application to human ill health, modern epidemiology focuses on the distribution and determinants of health-related states and of disease in populations (2). A determinant has been defined as "an individual characteristic (constitutional, environmental or behavioral) on which the study outcome (in the present context, occupational asthma) depends" (2). It may be causal or not, and can increase or decrease risk. A determinant may also be a primary risk factor, (i.e., it increases incidence) or a secondary risk factor (i.e., it increases severity and/or triggers symptoms) (3).

The determinants of disease are usually considered under two broad headings, environmental factors and host factors. In the context of occupational asthma, the environmental factors of interest are those that are encountered in the workplace. Included are all exposures encountered in the workplace, whether to gaseous or airborne particulate contaminants, or to physical stress, for instance, heat and/or cold, or to any other circumstance unfavorable to health, including factors related to workplace organization.

Historical Perspective

The principles of epidemiology have been applied to the understanding of the nature and causes of work-related illness at least since the days of Ramazzini, who was physician to the trade and crafts workers of Padua, Italy, in the early 1700s (4). By recognizing similarities in patterns of illness in those engaged in similar occupations, he was able to identify certain conditions as work-related, for example, the "asthmatic troubles" that developed in the people who sifted and measured grain, and the work-related shortness of breath of those who worked with cotton. With the social and political upheaval of the nineteenth century that accompanied the Industrial Revolution, and the concentration of labor into factories, the focus shifted from those with common occupations to those in the same or similar workplaces. This period also saw the recognition of diseases such as *byssinosis* (a term introduced in 1887 to describe an asthma-like condition that had become widespread in the cotton mills of North England) and *pneumoconiosis* (introduced to describe the harmful effects of mineral dusts on the lungs), the effects of which were not clearly distinguished from those of tuberculosis infection even as recently as the early decades of the twentieth century.

As the twentieth century moves to a close, the focus has again shifted in terms of both the disease outcomes and the exposures of concern. Thus, pneumoconiosis has yielded to stricter environmental controls (at least in the larger industries in countries with enforcement capability) and tuberculosis to improving socioeconomic conditions as well as to drug therapy, and the work-related diseases now of concern are the airway diseases, including chronic obstructive pulmonary disease and asthma (5,6), and lung cancer (7), all conditions that occur in the general population but may also be caused by work-related exposures. By the 1980s and 1990s, national surveys had documented the fact that occupational asthma accounted for a substantial proportion of work-related lung disease recognized by workmen's compensation boards, ranging from 28% in the United Kingdom (8), to as high as 52% and 63%, respectively, in the Canadian provinces of British Columbia (9) and Quebec (10), while in the database of the Association of Environmental and Occupational Clinics of the United States and Canada, asthma and reactive airway disease acounted for 37.7% of diagnoses related to exposure other than asbestos (11). Likewise, the exposures now of concern are the organic dusts and the many and varied chemicals encountered in modern workplaces as well as the role of the total pollutant burden of dusts. This includes all dusts, even those previously considered "nuisance dusts," as well as their interaction with fumes, gases, and vapors, which may occur even at quite low levels (11). There is also evidence of their interactions with extremes of temperature. In addition, exposure to heat has been shown to be an independent determinant of airway function (12).

When the links between illness and work are obvious, the epidemiological approach is similar to that used in infectious disease epidemiology. Thus, the study of the sentinel case of occupational asthma (13) has much in common with the study of the index case in an outbreak of, for example, typhoid or cholera. When the link to work is less obvious, for instance, for late asthmatic reactions occurring away from work, including at night (14), then the epidemiological approach may be closer to that used in chronic disease epidemiology (6). Community epidemics of asthma due to environmental exposures, whether these are known and recognized or occult, can also be investigated using the approaches of infectious disease epidemiology (15).

The proportional increase in occupational asthma among work-related lung diseases recognized by workmen's compensation boards in Europe and North America has occurred over a period (1970s–1990s) when the prevalence, and probably the incidence, of asthma in the general population, particularly in children, has also been increasing. For instance, in the United States, between 1982 and 1994, overall population rates for asthma increased from under 40/1000 to almost 60/1000 persons of all ages, the increase being greatest in the under-18-year-olds (16) to the extent that the condition has become as much of concern to the public (17) as it is to health care professionals. While environmental factors, particularly those associated with a westernized life-style, have been implicated (18), there is growing support for the view that westernized societies are also becoming more susceptible (19). If so, this may also have contributed to the increasing rates of occupational asthma among work-related lung disease in these societies.

Work-Relatedness of Airway Disease Including Asthma

In a move to acknowledge that the work-relatedness of disease differs for different disease conditions, the International Labor Office (6) suggested the use of several categories to describe these relationships, including (a) conditions caused only by agent-specific exposures; (b) conditions of multifactorial etiology in which work exposures may be the main or one of several etiological factors; (c) conditions to which an individual is susceptible and in which the expression of disease is precipitated by a work-related exposure; and (d) preexisting conditions aggravated by a work-related exposure. Conditions falling into category a are also referred to as occupational diseases by the WHO report, those in categories b, c, and d as work-related diseases, though this terminology is not universal. Currently, the term is used to cover the full spectrum of work-related diseases (8). Asthma occurring at work could be considered in any one of these categories, depending on (a) how it is defined (20), (b) the particular agent under consideration, and (c) the features of the asthma and/or asthma-like reaction it evokes. As a consequence, definitions of occupational asthma vary, not only between clinicians in terms of the clinical diagnosis of occupational asthma (20–24), but also between jurisdictions in terms of attributability for medicolegal purposes (11,25). In the same way, in epidemiological studies, the definition of the term may, and indeed should, vary according to the circumstances and purpose of the study (26,27), as well as the use to be made of the information provided by the study. From the point of view of the individual suffering from work-related asthma, however, the disability experienced is the same, whatever the category of work-relatedness of his or her condition.

Determinants of Occupational Asthma

The classic approach to the study of occupational lung disease focuses on the environmental determinants with careful documentation of exposure levels by objective measurement (28). Objectives usually include the characterization of the exposure-response relationships for the purposes of (a) establishing a causal relation between a given contaminant and the respiratory effect under study, and/or (b) providing the scientific basis for establishing workplace control levels (28). The epidemiological approach to the study of occupational asthma is, however, hampered by the nature of the condition itself for several reasons. First, asthma is usually a nonpermanent condition, all of the markers of which may be absent at any one point in time (see below), including the time when the epidemiological survey is carried out. Second, once an individual is sensitized to an asthmagenic agent or agents in the workplace, he or she reacts to a lower level of exposure than was the case prior to sensitization, often because of the development and persistence of nonspecific bronchial hyperresponsiveness.

As a result, certainly prevalence studies, and possibly even incidence studies, may fail to identify levels responsible for provoking the onset of the condition (even if the affected individual has not quit the workplace location). Furthermore, this level is likely to differ according to whether the mechanism triggering the hyperresponsiveness is allergic and IgE mediated, or irritative through stimulation of irritant receptors, or pharmacological, as was originally postulated for conditions like byssinosis. Theoretically, therefore, the slope and intercept of the exposure-response relationship might differ between individuals in the same workplace according to the mechanism of disease provocation (and therefore host factors). While it seems unlikely that exposure measurements including personal monitoring would ever be sufficiently detailed and accurate to permit between-individual differences in exposure-response relationships to be modeled or measured in epidemiological studies, they nevertheless need to be borne in mind in any discussion of the distribution and determinants of asthma and asthma-like conditions in workplaces.

A 1988 editorial with the provocative title "Why Study the Epidemiology of Asthma?" concluded that research into the causes of asthma should focus on its environmental determinants on the grounds that, despite extensive research on mechanisms, only one known host factor is implicated in the development of asthma, namely atopy (both asthma and atopy may be genetically determined), in contrast to the considerable body of evidence indicating that asthma is in large measure an environmental condition (29). Recognized environmental determinants of asthma include urban/rural differences, community air pollution, exposure to allergens in the home environment, in addition to exposure to some of the many and varied airborne contaminants encountered by men and women in modern workplaces, into which new materials are continually being introduced and in which the combinations of exposures are continually changing.

METHODOLOGICAL ISSUES

Definitions of Occupational Asthma

Primary Definition Versus Diagnostic Criteria

As discussed above, the definition of a disease or condition varies according to the purpose for which information based on the definition is to be used. A 1990 workshop on occupational and environmental asthma adopted the following as a working definition of occupational asthma: "variable airways narrowing causally related to exposure in the environment to airborne dusts, gases, vapors or fumes," but recognized that other and different definitions may be desirable, depending on the circumstances (26). The key word in this definition is *causally*, which was not defined and therefore open to interpretation.

The consensus definition adopted by the editors of this book allows sufficient flexibility to include both immunological and nonimmunological mechanisms, and recognizes that both may coexist (see Chapter 1). A distinction has also usually been made between the primary definition of a medical term and its use as a diagnostic term to describe a particular case when the term implies the presence of certain clinical and/or laboratory features. Thus, for the clinical diagnosis of occupational asthma, these usually include the clinical and/or laboratory information necessary to establish the presence of (a) variable airflow limitation and its relationship to work, (b) immunological status including atopy, (c) nonspecific bronchial hyperresponsiveness, and (d) evidence of exposure or sensitization to an agent specific to the workplace (20). Clearly, also the features considered necessary to establish a clinical diagnosis of occupational asthma are more demanding and restrictive if the diagnosis is to be used for medicolegal purposes, including workmen's compensation, than, for example, for the purpose of a screening examination in workers in a particular workplace that is under suspicion as responsible for causing occupational asthma. In the latter case, the findings might trigger an industrial hygiene survey (20,27), but not necessarily a clinical diagnosis or mandatory withdrawal from the workplace.

Definitions in Epidemiological Studies

Epidemiological studies of occupational asthma, like clinical examinations, are conducted with different objectives in mind; thus, the definition of asthma used will vary according to study question, study design, and study population. Thus, while epidemiologists accept the need for flexibility in the definition of outcome variables, they are nevertheless insistent that once (a) precise definition(s) is (are) formulated for a particular study, these must be meticulously respected. However, clinicians tend to be reluctant to accept information generated by studies using definitions that do not conform to those necessary to describe clinical situations, even though clinical treatises and textbooks on asthma often start with a statement to the effect that there is no generally agreed-upon definition of asthma (30), let alone occupational asthma (20,22–26). To minimize clinical skepticism, the term "asthma-like" has been used in some epidemiological studies (31).

Study Approaches and Design

In this section, study approaches and design are addressed both in general terms (see Fig. 1) (32) and insofar as they relate specifically to the investigation of the epidemiology of occupational asthma; included in the section is a consideration of their strengths and weaknesses as they apply to the investigation of different aspects of occupational asthma (see Table 1). Potential sources of bias are considered later.

Key to the scientific method is the *experiment*, a study design in which the researcher has control over all aspects of the study (28), as illustrated in Figure 1. This includes identification of the entire population eligible for study, characterization of the study pop-

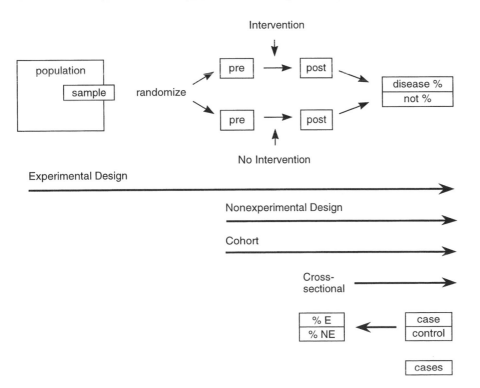

Figure 1   Design of epidemiological studies. (Adapted from Ref. 32 with permission.)

Table 1 Design Used in Epidemiological Studies: Features, Strengths, and Weaknesses

Design	Information provided	Strengths	Limitations	Comment on use
Randomized control trial (RCT)	Evaluation (in terms of efficacy or effectiveness) of treatments, usually drugs, or other interventions; treatment trials may also test hypotheses about mechanisms underlying occupational asthma	All aspects of the study are under the researcher's control	Cases suitable for randomization often not representative of all cases	The design is strengthened if both observer and subject are blinded as to the nature of the intervention. Cases of occupational asthma may be included in drug trials, or be the target of a treatment trial to test a hypothesis
Cohort (prospective)	Incidence (number of new cases), determinants (host and exposure) of new cases over time; natural history of occupational asthma (studies usually workforce based and should include retirees)	Only source of direct evidence on host and exposure factors as determinants of occupational asthma; may be possible to determine the exposure dose that induces asthma, if exposure is measured in sufficient detail, e.g., in a cohort of recruits	Subject to both selection and survivor bias, collectively the healthy worker effect; if follow-up is complete; survivor bias is minimized; loss from cohort likely due to the condition under study, i.e., asthma	Cohort studies in workforces at risk for occupational asthma are resource demanding and are less frequently undertaken than prevalence surveys; attention has more often been focused on host factors than on exposure; follow-up can be facilitated by linkage to workplace medical records or services; cohort studies should include retirees.

Case-control	Additional information on host and/or environmental determinants; if nested in a cohort or prevalence study may provide information on risk and dose-response	Inexpensive of resources; allows detailed study of selected subjects to facilitate contrasts, which will test hypotheses, e.g., matching for exposure to focus on host factors, or vice versa	Representativeness of controls not always easy to achieve except in nested case-control studies	To date, infrequently used in the study of occupational asthma despite their strength in exploring causal factors, host or environmental
Prevalence (cross-sectional)	Prevalence (number of current cases) and potential determinants (host and exposure) at the time of study; usually workforce based	Practical; the "workhorse" of occupational epidemiology; can provide the definition of a cohort to be followed; source of evidence on exposure-response	Unable to distinguish cause and effect; particularly subject to selection and survivor bias because of workplace turnover due to occupational asthma	The most commonly used design in occupational epidemiology; unable to establish whether atopy and/or bronchial hyperresponsiveness measured cross-sectionally preceded or followed the first clinical manifestations of asthma
Case series	Captures clinical experience	Provides material for laboratory study of mechanisms, e.g., inhalation challenge	Unable to provide information on rates or on workplace exposures implicated	Case reports form much of the published scientific literature on occupational asthma

ulation or of an appropriately selected sample prior to randomization for the planned intervention, as well as complete follow-up. Study inferences depend on comparing the exposed with the nonexposed, or those subjected to an intervention compared to those not. Such an approach is possible in studies of animals, plants, or cells, though even in these studies, identification of the target population may be incomplete. In studies of human populations, however, the experimental design is for practical purposes only feasible as the *randomized control trial* (RCT), usually of a treatment, though even in this study design, random sampling of the entire eligible population is not usually achieved. An example of the use of this study design in the investigation of occupational asthma is a recently published paper describing a randomized control trial of the effect of inhaled steroids on recovery from occupational asthma (33). Subjects with occupational asthma are often also included in randomized control trials of asthma management and treatments, but the study population in such studies is seldom confined to cases of occupational asthma.

In most other circumstances, a less than complete experimental design must be accepted as the only practical option, and all such studies are thus classified as *observational.* This is because the key issue of allocation to exposure or not (and the issue that provides the comparisons on the basis of which study inferences are drawn) depends on a variety of circumstances beyond the control of the researcher. For instance, there is good evidence that entry into many workplaces in which airborne contaminants are present is not a random event, but is subject to selection factors, either imposed by others (for instance, by the preemployment examination), or a matter of self-selection by the individual, based on economic, social, or, more usually, health constraints, also called the "healthy" hire effect (34). The "healthy hire" and survivor effects are two aspects of the healthy worker effect (34).

Cohort studies, in which the study population is defined at a given point and is then followed to observe the development of the conditions of interest, are used to estimate incidence, i.e., the development of new cases in a particular time frame. If the population is also stratified according to exposure level, the relationship of incidence to exposure (exposure response) can also be studied. Observational studies, cohort or prevalence, can be strengthened by parallel observations in a nonexposed group. However, even cohort studies, unless they are able to account for those who leave a workplace (i.e., avoid survivor bias), are liable to underestimate rates for occupational asthma. This is because the quit time for the affected subject may be extremely short (for instance, within weeks of starting a particular job), so that the individual is never even recorded as a member of the workforce. This effect, another aspect of the healthy worker effect, can be minimized if the follow-up observations include all who leave the workplace during the study period. A study cohort can also be constituted retrospectively from data obtained in a cross-sectional study. For instance, based on date of onset of asthma symptoms, subjects in a community-based study can be stratified into those whose asthma started prior to or after age 16 years (or prior to or after starting a given job). This would allow exposures that aggravate or induce asthma, respectively, to be studied.

Case-control (or *case-referent*) *studies* are usually used to identify and amplify information about risk factors or risk markers within a population. In this approach, which is closer to the clinical approach than the prevalence or cohort study, cases are identified and compared with noncases to provide additional information about environmental and/ or host factors. For rare conditions, community-based controls are often selected (1). In the investigation of occupational asthma, the case-control design is greatly strengthened if nested in a cohort or prevalence study (1). This permits cases to be matched with controls of similar exposure if the objective of the study is to identify pertinent host factors, or matched with controls with comparable host factors, such as age, if the objective of the study is to identify pertinent exposure characteristics.

Prevalence (cross-sectional) studies, in which the study population is defined and described at the time of the study, give information on case rates at a given point in time (point prevalence) or on case rates up to the time of study (cumulative prevalence). In the case of occupational asthma, prevalence studies are particularly liable to underestimate rates because of the survivor bias referred to under cohort studies.

The term "survey" is also often used. A survey is defined as an investigation in which information is systematically collected but in which the experimental method is not used (2). Many surveys are also epidemiological (i.e., population based) in concept, and the term is most frequently used in association with prevalence studies. In the context of occupational asthma, the term "survey" invariably describes a field study in which data is gathered in a defined workplace or community. Tables 2 and 3 illustrate the type of information on the distribution and determinants of occupational asthma provided by epidemiological surveys of defined workforces or workplaces. The examples were selected from studies of workers exposed to both high (Table 2) and low (Table 3) molecular weight asthmagens, and are discussed in greater detail later.

Clinical case studies, which summarize clinical experience, will always remain a useful source of information, and often provide the starting point for a planned investigation. They do not, obviously, provide information suitable for testing hypotheses concerning risk factors, in particular exposure, or establishing rates.

In a book entitled *The Epidemiology of Work-Related Diseases*, which he edited, McDonald contributes an excellent section on study design to which the reader is referred (34). In this section, he emphasizes the concept of design for a purpose, the purpose being to answer the study question (having regard for the present state of knowledge) and this, in turn, drives the selection of the most appropriate and efficient design (i.e., a design that works) given the appropriate resources. In other words, the choice of design is a matter of compromise between the feasible and the ideal, tempered by the availability of a suitable population and appropriate methods to measure the study outcome and the exposure. To capsulize his advice, McDonald cites Voltaire's admonition "*le mieux est l'ennemi du bien*," with a caution that while "perfectionism can hinder progress, the wrong answer can certainly do so."

Indeed, the importance of the study question cannot be exaggerated, since this drives all aspects of an epidemiological study, from choice of design, population, methods of measurement, and approaches to analysis. Study questions should be clear, unambiguous, and, given the current state of knowledge, relevant to all parties, including the subjects, their medical advisors, and the jurisdictions under which their cases are handled. Study questions must obviously also be ethical, and useful in fields beyond their own. Answers may be yes/no, i.e., a hypothesis was tested [e.g., does the status of inhaled steroids improve the asthmatic state of subjects with occupational asthma once they have left the workplace? (33)], or a number [e.g., what proportion of asthma among adult Canadians is attributable to work-related exposures? (36)], or both [e.g., what are the recent trends in physician diagnosed asthma in Manitoba, Canada? and can they be explained by diagnostic exchange? (37)].

Target Populations

The term "target population" usually refers to the population a particular study seeks to describe and/or to which the results are to be generalized. The term has also been used to

Table 2 Prevalence and Determinants of Asthma Symptoms in Workers Exposed to High-Molecular-Weight Agents: Results of Selected Studies Listed in Decreasing Order of Prevalence

Exposure/industry/occupation	No. studied	Exposure prior to diagnosis (months)	Prevalence of			Determinants of the distribution of asthma symptoms in exposed workforces[c]	Author, year	Ref.
			Work-related asthma[a] (%)	Smoking (%)	Atopy[b] (%)			
Enzymes; detergent industry	98	Intermittent	50	52	64	Exposure level[d]; not smoking or atopy	Mitchell, 1971 Australia	119
Clam/shrimp processors	59	36	26 (8)	49	21	Exposure, atopy	Desjardins, 1995 Quebec	158
Guar gum; carpet manufacture	162	Up to 108	23 (2)	42	24	Exposure, not atopy	Maio 1995 Quebec	61
Snow-crab processors	303	Months	21 (16)	67	11	Smoking, exposure, not atopy	Cartier, 1984 Quebec	57
Locust researcher workers	109	Under 40	11	39	43	Exposure, atopy, not smoking	Burge, 1980 U.K.	159
Laboratory animal workers	141	36	10	n/a	24	Exposure, atopy	Slovak, 1981 U.K.	103
	399	42	8	n/a	22	Exposure, atopy	Gross, 1980 U.S.A.	161
	238	26	7	30	40	Exposure, atopy	Cullinan, 1994 U.K.	95
Bakery workers	344	26	6	57	34	Exposure	Cullinan, 1994 U.K.	94
Latex in hospital workers	289	120[c]	2 (3)	22	25	Skin reactivity to latex	Vandenplas, 1995 Belgium	162

[a]Based on work-related chest symptoms, e.g., wheeze, difficulty with breathing; figures in parentheses are based on the algorithm for case identification (see Fig. 2).
[b]Defined on the basis of a personal history of allergy or skin test reactivity to one or more allergens including the occupational agent(s) under investigation.
[c]Exposure usually defined by job and/or by industrial hygiene measurement of airborne allergen levels (Cartier, 1984; Desjardins 1995; Cullinan 1994, 1994).

describe the collection of individuals about whom the study will make inferences (2). As already mentioned, studies aimed at describing rates of any work-related condition in any occupational groups are liable to be compromised to the extent that they describe survivor populations: the affected individuals who drop out of the workplace affect the numerator, not the denominator, in the calculation. For a population at risk for occupational asthma where employment turnover, and/or job change or rearrangement, is likely to be high, particularly in the short term, this effect is likely to be strong, and this has led to questions being raised as to what is the appropriate denominator for prevalence and/or incidence studies (should it be those ever exposed, those currently exposed, or the average workforce over a given period of time?) and what is the appropriate time frame for data collection (should it be months, years, or decades?) (20,38). Obviously, results will vary with each definition of the denominator and/or time frame, and the choice will depend on the precise objective of the study. For instance, if the objective is to describe incidence, the ideal target population would be a cohort of young apprentices (39) or workers hired at the startup of a new plant (40). If the objective is to describe the prevalence of occupational asthma in a workforce exposed to high-molecular-weight allergens, a shorter time frame, but at least 2 years, might be used, given that about 40% of the subjects develop asthma within 2 years of exposure, and only 20% after 10 years of exposure (10). On the one hand, if the data are being collected in a given workforce to compare with published data on similar workforces, the choice will be made to maximize comparability of these data sets. On the other hand, if the study objective is broader, for instance, to assess the burden of occupational asthma in the general population, then a suitable choice for the rate denominator would be those ever exposed, followed in the longer term, at least for years, and even decades, and the study should also be community, rather than workforce, based (28).

Principles of Measurement in Epidemiological Studies

Inference in science depends on comparisons of measurements made in appropriately selected material. In the case of epidemiological studies of occupational asthma, *inference depends on comparison of population groups* selected because they exhibit differences in health characteristics or have been subject to differences in exposure. The measurements, and obviously the tools used to make the measurements, whether of health outcome or of exposure, should be equally sensitive and/or specific for individuals in the two groups to permit valid inferences to be drawn from their comparison. In other words, every precaution must be taken to minimize measurement differential across the comparison groups since *imprecision in outcome or exposure measurements* can only lead to *attenuation of exposure-response* relationships, and so diminish the chances of showing a relationship between outcome (in the present context, occupational asthma) and exposure (in the present context, workplace contaminants). In addition, whatever outcome measurements are used in a particular study must be repeatable within the same subject, and they must also be valid; i.e., they must measure what they purport to measure. Estimates of within-subject variation (repeatability) are also necessary for calculations of sample size and/or study power. Thus, in any epidemiological study, but particularly in epidemiological studies of occupational asthma, no effort should be spared to assure the quality of the data in terms of reproducibility and validity of the measurements of outcome and response. These are some of the reasons why as eminent a biostatistician as Rothman (41) expresses the view that "an epidemiologic study is properly viewed as an exercise in measurement with accuracy as the goal." He goes on to say that "design strategies are intended to reduce

Table 3 Prevalence and Determinants of Asthma Symptoms in Workers Exposed to Low-Molecular-Weight Agents: Results of Selected Studies Listed in Decreasing Order of Prevalence

Exposure/industry/ occupation	No. studied	Exposure prior to diagnosis (months)	Prevalence of			Determinants of the distribution of asthma symptoms in exposed workforces[c]	Author, year	Ref.
			Work-related asthma[a] (%)	Smoking (%)	Atopy[b] (%)			
Platinum refinery	91	12–24	54	63	33	Smoking, not atopy	Venables, 1989 U.K.	107
Colophony electronics plant	924	24	22	47	n/a	Exposure, atopy, minimal to smoking	Burge, 1979 U.K.	109
Various isocyanates in secondary industry	51	54	20 (12)[d]	52	n/a	Exposure	Séguin, 1987 Quebec	58
Spiramycin	51	n/a	19 (8)[d]	48	39	Exposure	Malo, 1988 Quebec	60
Azodicarbamide	151	n/a	19	43	48	Exposure, not smoking, not atopy	Slovak, 1981 U.K.	123
Phtahllic anhydride	118	1 to 192	18	75	29	Exposure + atopy	Wernfors, 1986 Sweden	125
Toluene diisocyanate secondary industry	241	Within 36 months in most	9.5	51	35	Exposure, probably not atopy	Venables, 1985 U.K.	122
	45	n/a	11	73	18	Exposure	Burge, 1981 U.K.	163

Production of TDI	112	Not given	8.3	Not given	23	Exposure, not atopy	Butcher, 1970 Weill, 1975 USA	121 164
Anhydrides, TCPA	329	Up to 24 months	3.2	50	22	Exposure, not atopy except in first year	Venables, 1985 U.K.	105
Plicatic acid	1320	12–24	3.4	n/a	n/a	Exposure, atopy	Ishizaki, 1973 Japan	124
	652	n/a	4	38	19	Exposure, not atopy	Yeung, 1984 British Columbia	120
							Vedal, 1986 British Columbia	91
	42[d]	13	7[c]	71	n/a	Exposure	Malo, 1994 Quebec	165

[a] Based on various reported work-related chest symptoms e.g. wheeze, difficulty with breathing; figures in brackets based on the algorithm for case identification (see Fig. 2).

[b] Variously defined on the basis of a history of previous allergies or positive skin tests to one or more antigens including the occupational agent(s) under investigation.

[c] Exposure was most often defined by job, in some studies by duration, and in a few by measurement of airborne allergen levels (Malo 1988, 1997; Slovak, 1981).

[d] Refers to subjects considered to have occupational asthma.

to sources of error, both systematic and random. Reduction in random error improves the precision of the measurement, whereas reduction of systematic error improves the validity of the measurement.''

For human epidemiological studies, *the tools used to measure health outcomes* are derived from the tools used in clinical medicine, but adapted and standardized so that the information they furnish is equally repeatable and equally valid in the comparison groups on which the study inferences will be based. Thus, the respiratory symptom questionnaire, a surrogate for the clinical history, is a means to assure that the 'interview' with each study subject is conducted in a standardized fashion, rather than the process being open ended and personalized as is usual in the clinical setting. Likewise, if lung function tests are to be used, the procedure for their administration must be standardized so that each study subject is given the same instructions and the opportunity to perform the same number of trials, rather than this being left to the technician's judgment as would be the case for a clinical test (42). In the case of allergy skin tests, the wheal is often traced onto transparent tape for review and possible remeasurement of the wheal size after the test has been completed.

The *tools used to measure exposure* in the epidemiological studies of occupational asthma vary considerably, depending on the nature of the study, its objectives, the study site(s) and resources available. All of the following have been used with success: (a) self-reported exposure by the subject (5,20,43), (b) industrial hygiene information available for the workplace, either current and collected for the purpose of the study, or gathered from past company or other records (44), and (c) industrial hygiene evaluation of the subject's workplace exposures based on a job/industry history, often using what is called a job exposure matrix or occupational-title-based system (45). Note that in some studies, (a) has been shown to be complementary to (b) and (c), in that it provides information not contained in (b) and (c) (43).

Outcome Measurements

Questionnaires

Many studies have used only questionnaires to assess the frequency of occupational asthma. Indeed, the first study of occupational asthma in grain workers was carried out by Ramazzini in the early 1700s in Italy using a questionnaire (4). The first report of diisocyanate-induced asthma, the most common cause of occupational asthma in developed countries, also exclusively utilized a questionnaire (46). Questionnaires have an obvious advantage of being noninvasive and easy to administer. However, they also have their limitations. First, although questionnaires for epidemiological studies of chronic obstructive lung diseases were developed in the 1960s by the Medical Research Council of Great Britain and by the American Thoracic Society (47), a standardized questionnaire specifically designed for the investigation of asthma has only been developed relatively recently (48). Second, several (49,50), though not all (51), studies show poor correlation between responses to questions on asthma symptoms and the presence or absence of nonspecific bronchial hyperresponsiveness (often considered the hallmark of asthma). Third, bronchial hyperresponsiveness can exist without symptoms (52). Fourth, some asymptomatic subjects with bronchial hyperresponsiveness develop symptoms in subsequent years (52,53). Fifth, questionnaires administered by trained physicians have variable sensitivity and specificity in predicting asthma or occupational asthma (54–56). Finally, subjects may overreport or underreport their symptoms depending on the circumstances where the questionnaire is being administered. From Table 2 it can be seen that the proportion of workers proven to be suffering from occupational asthma by specific challenge tests or by peak flow rate recording varies in different studies, ranging from 8% to 53% of workers who were considered to have occupational asthma by questionnaire. Thus, the questionnaire is a sensitive tool but not a specific one and, while invaluable in analytical (etiological) epidemiological studies in populations at risk for occupational asthma, it is inadequate on its own for clinical case identification.

Immunological Assessment

Assessment of the atopic status of subjects is often included in epidemiological studies of asthma and occupational asthma as atopy is the most important risk factor in asthma. Allergy skin tests using the prick method with common inhalant allergens such as house dust, grain dust mite, cat epidermal antigen, and some local pollens have been found to be invaluable in field studies to assess the atopic status of subjects (57–62). They are easy to perform and do not cause systemic or serious local reactions. Personal and family history of allergy do not correlate well with the tendency of individuals to produce IgE antibodies (63).

Many occupational agents cause asthma by sensitization with the production of specific IgE antibodies. These include mostly high-molecular-weight proteins, which are complete antigens, and some low-molecular-weight agents, such as phthalic anhydride, which act as haptens (64). When appropriate antigens are available, skin tests can be done and blood samples can be taken for the determination of specific IgE antibodies at the time of the survey. These tests provide objective evidence of sensitization. They are useful in screening subjects at risk for developing occupational asthma since immunological sensitization normally occurs first before the development of symptoms.

For many low-molecular-weight compounds including toluene diisocyanate and plicatic acid, the agent responsible for Western red cedar asthma, evidence of immunological sensitization is not a consistent finding. Specific IgE or specific IgG antibodies are found in only a small proportion of patients. Appropriate standardized materials are not available for skin testing or for measurement of specific antibodies. Immunological assessment plays little role in clinical diagnosis or case identification in epidemiological studies of workplaces with these exposures.

Functional Assessment

Measurement of Lung Function.   Measurement of lung function is important in assessing respiratory hazards due to various airborne pollutants. It is usually necessary to perform lung function tests at the plant site and this presents special problems not usually encountered in hospitals or clinic laboratories (42). For example, temperature is an important factor to consider. Low or high temperature in a workplace can greatly affect the results. Rapid testing of many subjects can also increase the temperature of the spirometer. A thermometer should be installed in the spirometer particularly for volume-measuring devices. Inadequate space and lack of electrical power source are also common problems encountered in the field. It is important to have trained technicians to calibrate the equipment and be able to deal with problems with instrumentation. The technicians should also be trained to recognize poor subject performance (65). Poor performance, however, in particular poor reproducibility, may also be an independent marker of airway dysfunction since the forced expiratory maneuver may induce airway narrowing in reactive airways (42,66).

There is an array of available pulmonary function tests. Several factors need to be considered in choosing the lung function tests for each survey undertaken: the cost of equipment, the testing time, the simplicity of the test, and analysis of results, reproducibility, acceptability, and the degree of standardization of the instrument and test procedures. Measurements of peak expiratory flows (PEF), forced expiratory volume in one second (FEV_1), forced vital capacity (FVC), and maximum midexpiratory flow rate (FEF 25–75%) by spirometry fulfill all the criteria mentioned above. However, for most epidemiological studies, measurements of PEF, FEV_1, FVC, and FEV_1/FVC are probably adequate. Measurement of FEF 25–75% has not been useful in our experience. Although it is considered more sensitive, it is more variable compared to FEV_1 and FVC, a disadvantage in much survey work. Nevertheless, it has been shown to be a sensitive measure of small airway abnormality, particularly following exposure to inorganic dusts (67,68), and may prove useful in etiological studies involving complex exposures, for instance to asthmagenic agents with inorganic dusts. Instrument requirement, calibration techniques, test procedures, measurement of test results, and data interpretation should conform to ATS (69) or ERS guidelines.

Pre- and Postshift Spirometric Measurement.   Assessment of FEV_1 pre- and postshift (cross-shift) has been used to confirm work-relatedness of asthma. Initial reports indicated that this test was neither a specific nor a sensitive method for clinical case identification, probably due to a combination of factors such as diurnal variation (levels are lowest in the early hours of the morning, highest in the early hours of the afternoon), measurement or technical errors, and intermittent rather than daily exposure to the sensitizing agent (42,70).

On the other hand, measurement of cross-shift change in lung function has proved a very useful way of detecting acute nonallergic airway response to exposure to occupational agents such as cotton dust and grain dust (71). The cross-shift change in lung function is directly proportional to the level of exposure. Several factors affect cross-shift change in spirometry, such as tobacco smoking, immediate skin test reactivity to common allergens, and initial level of FEV_1 (87). They should be taken into consideration when analyzing and interpreting the results. The most important factor, however, is the time of the day when the spirometric measurements are carried out.

Serial Measurements of Peak Expiratory Flows (PEF).   Serial measurements of peak expiratory flow rate has been shown to be a valuable tool in the assessment of patients with occupational asthma in a clinical setting (72), and they also show a reasonable correlation with the results of specific challenge test (73,74). Nevertheless, their role in the assessment of occupational asthma in prevalence surveys requires further evaluation. Serial PEFR monitoring has been used successfully in several epidemiological surveys (56,59,75,76). However, as yet no study has explored the validity of PEFR monitoring in comparison with specific inhalation challenges for screening subjects with occupational asthma in a large number of subjects in the workplace. There is also the practical problem of subject compliance since the subjects are usually asked to monitor their PEFR at least four times a day at work and at home for 3–4 weeks, a commitment that many find hard to keep. More time is also needed in a field study to explain and instruct the subjects how to measure and register their own peak flow rate properly. Moreover, there might be falsifications in the way subjects record and register the readings. This phenomenon has been demonstrated in some of the snow crab workers (75). The between-observer reproducibility of the interpretation of peak flow rate recordings obtained from surveys is, however, good (77) and comparable to the interpretation carried out in a clinical setting (78).

Nonspecific Challenge Tests.   Increased responsiveness to methacholine or histamine in the absence of airflow limitation can be highly suggestive of asthma. However, its presence does not constitute a clinical diagnosis of occupational asthma. If a subject shows a significant degree of nonspecific bronchial hyperresponsiveness (NSBH) and has evidence of immunological sensitization to a high-molecular-weight agent, it is very likely that he/she will eventually develop an immediate bronchospastic reaction on exposure to the agent. A relationship between NBSH and immunological sensitization was originally suggested by Tiffeneau in 1950 (79). More recently, Cockcroft and co-workers documented this relationship once again (80). They proposed a formula to predict the concentration of a common inhaled allergen that can cause a 20% fall in FEV_1 based on two factors: the diameter of the skin wheal elicited by the prick tests (reflecting the degree of immunological sensitivity) and the PC_{20} of methacholine or histamine (reflecting the degree of NSBH). They confirmed this relationship later in a prospective study (81). Malo and co-workers found that 80% of subjects with immediate skin reactivity to psyllium and increased NSBH showed immediate or dual (immediate combined with late reaction) asthmatic reactions after exposure to psyllium (62).

Measurement of NSBH has been used by a number of investigators in epidemiological surveys of general populations (83,84) and workplace populations (85–87). These studies have shown that methacholine, histamine, and hyperventilation of unconditioned air challenge tests can be carried out in epidemiological settings safely without the presence of physicians. As discussed in another chapter, measurement of NSBH is not specific enough to be used alone in identifying subjects who would attract a clinical diagnosis of asthma. However, when combined with questionnaire information and immunological tests (when feasible), it is very useful for identifying subjects with possible occupational asthma from workplace exposures (60,61,82).

Specific Challenge Tests.   The methodology of specific challenge tests is discussed separately in another chapter. Specific challenge tests with the suspected offending agent have been used successfully in the clinical setting to confirm the diagnosis of occupational asthma. In some jurisdictions, its presence is a requirement for recognizing occupational asthma. These tests are time consuming to conduct (sometimes requiring several days) and are not devoid of danger. They also require supervision by physicians with experience. Very few centers regularly perform these tests. It is not practical to include specific challenge testing in field studies. However, these tests can be used to confirm the diagnosis in subjects suspected to have occupational asthma identified through screening measures and they should be carried out in a laboratory setting with necessary expertise to deal with asthmatic reactions.

Algorithm for Clinical Case Identification (Decision Tree) in Epidemiological Studies of Occupational Asthma.   The Occupational Committee of the American Academy of Allergy and Clinical Immunology has recommended that epidemiological surveys for occupational asthma should include not only whatever screening tests are used, but also should aim at clinical case identification. A stepwise procedure similar to the procedure used in a census sample should be used (88). This scheme is illustrated in Figure 2. This stepwise approach has been used successfully in several workforce-based studies (10). The first two steps have usually been carried out during field studies. Subjects who require further investigation for confirmation of the diagnosis of occupational asthma include those who have questionnaire responses compatible with work-related asthma, evidence of immunological sensitization, and/or NSBH. Serial monitoring of PEF and specific challenge tests should also be conducted on these subjects. It is highly unlikely that subjects without

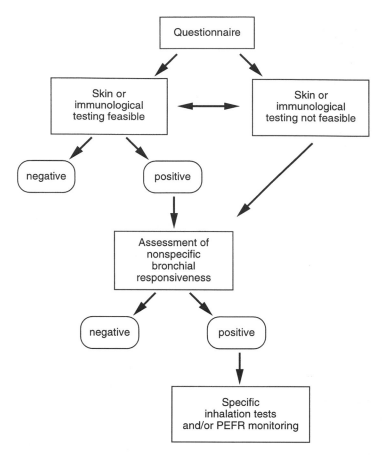

Figure 2 Epidemiological investigation of occupational asthma.

evidence of NSBH and immunological sensitization will react on specific challenge testing to the offending agent.

Assessment of Risk Factors

Exposure Assessment

In occupational epidemiology studies, the strongest evidence of causality is provided by exposure-response relationships. For the pneumoconioses, the key environmental determinant of chronic respiratory effects has been shown to be the cumulative exposure to inorganic dust, measured as the product of the level and the duration of exposure, exposure-response relationships being stronger for this measurement than for either of its components. In occupational asthma, little work has been carried out on quantifying exposure until recently. This is due to the perceived importance of host determinants in asthma, including atopy and genetic markers. The agents responsible are often proteinaceous and exist as dry or wet aerosols. They require different methods of collection, measurement, and analysis, most of which have only been developed recently.

Traditional industrial hygiene techniques are available for measuring several low-molecular-weight chemicals capable of causing asthma, such as isocyanates. Direct-reading monitors are also now available for measurement of chemicals such as formaldehyde, amines, and diisocyanates. However, these methods may not be sensitive enough to detect low, but nevertheless sensitizing, levels. Immunochemical techniques have been developed for quantitating aeroallergens and these have been used in a number of workforce-based studies (89). In general, personal sampling gives a more precise assessment of individual exposure than area sampling. Exposure zoning is a useful sampling strategy for epidemiological studies (21). Personal samplers are now also available to quantitate individual exposure to biological substances in the workplace using immunochemical methods. These new sampling devices have greatly improved the methodology for collecting high-molecular-weight aeroallergens (89).

Several studies have shown that there is a dose-response relationship between the level of exposure to occupational agents and the prevalence of sensitization, and/or NSBH and/or asthma (see Tables 2 and 3). Implicated are exposure to high molecular weight antigens such as flour (93,94) and laboratory animals (95), and low molecular weight antigens such as colophony (96), acid anhydride (97), western red cedar (91,92), and fumes from welding mild steel (98). Once an individual is sensitized to an agent, a minute dose below the permissible exposure limits can bring on an attack of asthma. Concomitant environmental exposures such as to low levels of irritants and cigarette smoke may enhance sensitization to some occupational agents.

In acute challenges with occupational agents in the laboratory, the total dose of the agent (i.e., concentration $\times$ duration of exposure) is the most important determinant of the severity of reaction (99). It is therefore tempting to extrapolate these findings to the actual work situation, i.e., total dose of exposure, rather than to the concentration, which is probably more relevant in causing sensitization.

Exposure to high concentrations of isocyanates (spills) has been shown to induce asthma (100). However, it is less clear whether such spills can lead to the development of isocyanate-induced asthma with a latency period, although an example of this phenomenon has been described (101).

Intermittent exposure to levels higher than the permissible concentration (but not levels encountered in a spill) of an agent may be more important in causing occupational asthma than continuous exposure to low levels of the same agent (100). In this context, a continuous monitoring device with direct readout would be much more useful in assessing exposure than the measurement of 8-hr average, which is often the practice. A great deal more research is required in this area.

Finally, the potential interaction between airborne pollutants must always be borne in mind. Thus, chamber studies have shown that preexposure to low concentrations of ozone can greatly increase bronchial responsiveness to allergen exposure in atopic asthmatic subjects (102).

Host Determinants of Occupational Asthma

While exposure is the single most important determinant of occupational asthma, not all subjects develop occupational asthma given the same degree of exposure. Various host factors (genetically determined) and environmental factors (acquired) have been incriminated. Atopy has been shown to be strongly associated with sensitization to high-molecular-weight agents. However, the positive predictive value of atopy in various studies of occupational asthma is low: 34% in laboratory animal workers (103), 8% in workers exposed to guar gum (61), and 7% to psyllium (62). These findings do not justify routine screening for atopy in high-risk workplaces. Atopic individuals who wish to enter some high-risk workplaces should be advised of this potential risk ahead of time. If they do enter the workplace, regular follow-up examinations for early detection of sensitization and development of nonspecific bronchial hyperresponsiveness (i.e., surveillance for case identification) should be carried out.

The effect of smoking on occupational asthma appears to be dependent on the type of occupational agent. When the agent induces asthma by producing specific IgE antibodies, cigarette smoking enhances sensitization. Venables and co-workers found an interaction between smoking and atopy in workers exposed to laboratory animals (104) and tetrachlorophthalic anhydride (105); atopic smokers had the highest and nonatopic nonsmokers the lowest prevalence of sensitization. Among platinum refinery workers, smoking, not atopy, is the most important risk factor for sensitization (106,107). Cigarette smoking, however, was not associated with increased work-related asthmatic symptoms in workers exposed to detergent enzymes (119). When the agent induces asthma independent of IgE antibodies, nonsmokers may be more frequently affected than smokers as in isocyanate-induced asthma (108), colophony (109), and red cedar asthma (110).

The role of nonspecific bronchial hyperresponsiveness as a host marker in occupational asthma requires more study. In most studies, nonspecific bronchial hyperresponsiveness appears to be an acquired phenomenon rather than a predisposition. This conclusion is based on the demonstration of improvement in nonspecific bronchial hyperresponsiveness in some subjects who leave exposure and worsening of bronchial hyperresponsiveness on reexposure to the offending agent. In a prospective study of western red cedar sawmill workers, none of the four workers who developed red cedar asthma had nonspecific bronchial hyperresponsiveness before development of symptoms (111).

Other genetic markers may be important in occupational asthma. Recently, HLA class II genetic markers were studied in patients with isocyanate-induced asthma (112). The presence of HLA-DQB1*0503 was found to be associated with susceptibility to the development of the disease while the presence of HLA-DQB1*0501 conferred protection. The difference between the two alleles was the occurrence of aspartic acid in DQB1*0503 and valine in DQB1*0501 at residue 57 (113). In patients with asthma due to western red cedar dust exposure, the frequencies of DQB1*0302 and DQB1*604 were found to be significantly elevated compared with exposed controls while DQB1*0501 was significantly reduced in patients compared to controls (114). However, these HLA markers only occurred in up to 30–40% of the affected subjects. Studies of genetic markers should be extended to subjects exposed to other occupational agents and may help us to understand the pathogenic mechanism of occupational asthma.

Upper airway symptoms such as rhinitis and conjunctivitis often precede the occurrence of lower airway symptoms. They can be used as an early marker of occupational asthma. Malo and co-workers have shown that rhinitis and conjunctivitis occurred before the development of asthma in exposure to both high- and low-molecular weight agents (115).

Sources of Bias in Epidemiological Studies of Occupational Asthma

All observational epidemiological studies, and to a much lesser extent experimental studies, including randomized control trials, are potentially subject to bias, and the validity of a study and of its inferences depends on the extent that the sources of bias are minimized. Bias is defined as "deviation of results or inferences from the truth, or processes leading to that deviation" and the definition is further elaborated to include "any trend in the collection, analysis, interpretation, publication or review of data that can lead to conclusions that are systematically different from the truth" (2).

The most important sources of bias are: (a) *selection bias* (refers to study sample being nonrepresentative of the target population in terms of health or exposure characteristics); (b) *information bias* (refers to bias in the health and/or exposure information gathered in the contrasting study groups; for instance, in terms of health information, this usually refers to recall bias with those who attribute their symptoms to exposure at work being more likely to recall any workplace exposures compared to those who report no symptoms; and (c) *confounding bias*. A confounder is defined as "a variable that can cause or prevent the outcome of interest, is not an intermediate variable" (i.e., a step in the process of disease development), "and is associated with [the] factor under investigation" (2). This usually refers to the fact that the variable is unevenly distributed across the comparison groups so that, unless it is possible to take it into account in analysis, its effects cannot be distinguished for the factor under study. For instance, in a study of occupational asthma in which lung function is to be compared in groups exposed to high and low levels of a workplace asthmagen, smoking (known to be associated with lung function level) would be a confounder if smoking rates were higher (or lower) in one group compared to the other. As a result, it would not be possible to separate out the independent effect of the asthmagen of interest unless the information on smoking was available, in which case it could be taken into account in the analysis.

In the investigation of occupational asthma, selection bias is probably the most important, due to the "healthy" worker effect, either because susceptible individuals rarely enter jobs at risk, or because they quit after such short periods that they were never recorded as workers (the "healthy" hire effect), or because at the time of study, those most affected have either already left the workplace, or have rearranged their jobs so as to minimize exposure, or changed jobs and do not therefore appear on the company lists as holding an at-risk job (the "survivor" effect) (34). Examples of the "healthy" hire effect are to be found in studies of laboratory animal workers (21), those exposed to isocyanates at work (58), those who handle spiramycin (76), in grain workers (116), and in foundry workers (117). Examples of the "survivor" effect are also to be found in studies of grain workers (118) and in laboratory animal workers (21). Community-based studies, on the other hand, because they minimize selection bias, have been consistent in showing associations between asthma outcomes and occupational exposures (see below). They have, however, the disadvantage that exposure is of necessity self-reported and therefore a potential source of information bias.

Practical Issues Associated with Occupational Surveys

The key to a successful occupational survey is to obtain cooperation from both management and labor. It should ideally be preceded by discussions with the local occupational health and safety committees (joint management and labor) about local concerns and issues to be addressed by the study. From the onset, the investigator should emphasize the necessity for confidentiality of individual medical results and that no medical information regarding an individual will be released without signed consent. Once the protocol has been agreed upon, it is usually a good idea for the investigator to meet with the workers and explain to them the purpose of the study, test procedures, possible side effects, and the rationale for each test.

Ideally, environmental monitoring should be carried out at the time of the survey to study the effects of current exposure. However, it is also important to obtain results of previous measurements from the management. If measurements of personal sampling are available from past records and are found to be accurate, one can construct cumulative exposure for effects of chronic exposure. To study the effects of acute exposure, personal sampling can also be carried out together with cross-shift measurements of lung function.

Tests carried out in the field may not be conducted under optimal conditions. It is, therefore, very important to have test procedures standardized as much as possible. Calibration of lung function equipment should be done at the worksite daily before testing.

Confidentiality of information should be emphasized to workers to allay their fears. It should be noted that methods used in surveys can only screen for individuals with possible asthma. Further tests are necessary for confirming the diagnosis of occupational asthma. Individuals identified as having possible occupational asthma should be given the opportunity of having confirmatory tests (if those are offered) without losing their jobs. Furthermore, when the diagnosis is confirmed, every effort should be made to help the individual obtain a transfer or find other employment. Without such guarantee ahead of time, it will not be possible to have accurate case identification.

It is also important to have the survey conducted at the worksite and the tests performed in an organized and efficient manner to minimize the time lost from productivity. A well-organized schedule should be made to avoid individuals waiting between tests. At the end of the study, it is a good practice to send individual results directly to the worker and offer to give further explanation if necessary. Advice to the worker and an offer of further testing can be given at the same time. It is also advisable to present the group results to the local occupational health committee for further input before preparation of the final report.

DISTRIBUTION AND DETERMINANTS OF OCCUPATIONAL ASTHMA

Workforce-Based Studies

There is a very rich literature of workforce-based surveys, some initiated by the identification of cluster of cases, either through physician referral or through sentinel programs, others seeking a priori to examine risk factors associated with particular asthmagenic exposures. Tables 2 and 3 summarize the findings from selected studies of workplaces contaminated by high- and low-molecular-weight asthmagens, respectively. All the studies listed were epidemiological in concept, i.e., population (workforce) based; all aimed to record the prevalence by identifying the number of cases as well as the number of subjects at risk, and in all, an analysis was made of the distribution and determinants of occupational asthma, including environmental and host factors. Among the environmental factors examined were exposure level and duration and/or job (as a measure of exposure), and in some the effect of stopping exposure was also studied. Host factors examined included a history of atopy and skin test positivity. Smoking was also examined in most studies and analyzed as a host factor and/or as a cofactor. Note also that the tables are not comprehensive but rather illustrative of the information available to guide both clinical and public health practice. In both tables, the studies are listed in decreasing order of prevalence of questionnaire markers of occupational asthma. Also, in several studies the algorithm for clinical case identification (see above) was followed, and the prevalence rate of cases so identified is included in the tables (in parentheses in column 4), illustrating the differences in the rates between the two definitions, the first essentially for epidemiological (public health) purposes and the second for clinical use (59,61,158,162).

From Table 2, describing workforces exposed to asthmagens of high molecular weight, it is evident that the estimates of prevalences vary considerably, from rates as high as 50% described in an Australian plant manufacturing enzyme detergents when the process was first introduced (119), prior to the introduction of process reformulation to control exposure, to as low as 2% in latex exposed hospital workers (162). While these between-workforce differences are no doubt due in part to technical (methodological) reasons such as differences in the questions used to define occupational asthma, differences in the intensity of the exposure of the different workforces and in the asthmagenic potential of the different agents involved are also likely to have played a role. By contrast, since the definition of asthma within studies was constant, the role of the determinants in the distribution of asthma within a workforce is unlikely to have been affected by this source of bias. It is therefore of interest that in all the studies listed in Table 2, the within-workforce distribution of the questionnaire markers of asthma was related to exposure, and usually, though not in all studies, to atopy or other markers of an allergic diathesis, and to smoking in some studies (57) but not in others (159). The consistency with which exposure relationships are demonstrable is surprising, given the imprecision of the exposure measurements used in most studies. Reasons for the less consistent relationships with atopy and smoking may be in part methodological (due to differences in the definitions of atopy and smoking used), but may also be due in part to different mechanisms operating to produce asthma and asthma-like symptoms in different workers, and/or differences in other features of the workplaces, such as coexposures to environmental tobacco smoke, dust, heat, and other workplace contaminants.

From Table 3, describing workforces exposed to asthmagens of low molecular weight, it is evident that estimates of prevalence also vary considerably and over much the same range as those shown in Table 2. As in Table 2, in all the studies cited in Table 3 in which exposure was examined, level and/or duration (usually defined by job and/or work area) was a determinant of the distribution within a workplace, whereas atopy was either not related to (107,121,123) or only weakly related (105) to the within-workforce distribution, although there were exceptions (109,124,126). Nor was the within-workforce distribution of asthma related to smoking (123), other than trivially (109,126), in the few studies in which it was examined, though a smoking exposure interaction was found for exposure to anhydrides (105). Despite the fact that, in all studies, exposure level was a determinant of the distribution of asthma within a workforce, and though some studies reported specific bronchial challenge tests using the agent concerned in selected subjects, objective measurements of levels of airborne contaminants were infrequently reported (91,96).

Community-Based Studies: Evidence of an Association of Asthma Symptoms with Occupational Exposures

Community-based studies have proved surprisingly powerful in bringing to attention association between occupational exposures and wheezing complaints despite the fact that, in such studies, the potential for misclassification, in terms both of exposure and of outcomes (which are of necessity self-reported) is considerable (127–134). The strength of community-based studies no doubt derives from the fact that they are likely to reach all individuals ever exposed in workplaces at risk, as distinct from only those currently exposed or only those exposed long enough to be registered in any workforce census. The consistency with which relationships between occupational exposures and wheezing complaints can be demonstrated in community-based studies (Table 4) is thus eloquent testimony to health-selection effects that discourage individuals with wheezing complaints from entering workplaces at risk and/or cause them to leave the workplace responsible for inducing their symptoms.

Table 4 Asthma Symptoms in Community-Based Studies: Their Relationship to Work Exposures and Pollution Attributable Proportion (etiological fraction)

City, country, author, year	Subjects: number, age	Exposure (%) Cig.	Exposure (%) Work	Wheezing %	Wheezing OR[a]	PAP[b] (%)	Exposures implicated	Symptoms	Ref.
6 cities, USA Kom, 1987	8515 M and W 25–74 yrs	58	31	6	1.5 1.2 1.6	14	Dust vs. none Fumes vs. none Both vs. none	Persistent wheeze	128
7 cities, France Kryzanowski, 1988	8692 M 7772 W 25–59 yrs	73 28	34 23	17 12	1.6 1.7	17 13	Any vs. none Any vs. none	Wheezing any time	129
Bergen, Norway Bakke, 1991	4469 M and W 15–70 yrs	43	29	29	1.9	16	Dust or gas vs. none	Occasional wheeze	131
Po Valley, Italy Viegi, 1991	1027 M 602 W 18–64 yrs	60 38	31 16	3 4	2.4 2.9	29 27	Any vs. none	Breathless with wheeze or reported asthma	130
Singapore Ng, 1994	2375 M and W 20–54 yrs	42	~59	—	1.7	33	Exposed vs. not	Asthma (recorded in case notes)	134
4 cities, Canada Becklake, 1996	12380 M and W 20–44 yrs	31	49	10	1.9	23	Dust or gas vs. none	Doctor-diagnosed asthma in last year	82
5 regions, Spain Kogevinas, 1996	2646 M and W 20–44 yrs	51	24	24	1.9	3	High vs. low risk at time of diagnosis	Asthma symptoms or treatment	132
New Zealand Fishwick, 1997	1609 M and W 20–44 yrs	21	~5	41	1.6	3	High vs. low risk	Wheezing	133

[a]OR were all adjusted for age and smoking and for gender when data on men and women were combined; additional adjustments were made in some studies for education, socioeconomic status, and air pollution (Kryzanowski, 1988), atopy and race (Fishwick, 1997), and city or area of residence (Kogevinas, 1996; Bakke, 1991).
[b]PAP% = population attributable proportion or etiological fraction.

Table 4 shows the results of selected community-based studies. For all studies listed, both the exposure measurements and the presence of asthma were determined from answers to questionnaires completed by study subjects. In none of the studies was the study objective (and the research question that governed the study design) to investigate these relationships, and yet in all but two studies (131,132), statistically significant relationships were demonstrated for wheezing complaints in relation to occupational exposures to dusts alone or dusts with fumes and/or gases. Three of the recent studies (82,132,133) were carried out following the protocol of the European Community Respiratory Health Survey (135), and in spite of the fact that technical differences are likely to have been minimized for this reason, there are striking differences between them. Thus, the prevalence of wheezing was low, under 5%, in Italy (130) and in the USA (128) compared to New Zealand where the rate was 41% (133), in keeping with high rates of asthma found in that country. By contrast, the population attributable risk was low, approximately 3%, in the studies from Spain and New Zealand compared to 23% in the Canadian study, and estimates of population attributable risk (or etiological fractions) were even higher, 33%, in a case-control study carried out in Singapore though this study design does not allow calculation of the prevalence of wheezing complaints in the general population (134). The wide range of population risks for wheezing complaints attributable to occupational exposures shown in Table 4 is not surprising as these must depend on the local industries, on options for employment, as well, no doubt, as on the population susceptibility. The fact that relationships between exposures and wheezing complaints were demonstrable in different populations in different countries by different researchers, using similar, but not identical study methods, lends strength to the causal hypothesis, i.e., that the wheezing complaints analyzed were the consequence of the occupational exposure (5,28). While wheezing complaints do not constitute a clinical diagnosis of occupational asthma, nevertheless it is among these individuals that one expects to find cases that currently have, or will in the future have, sufficient clinical features to receive a diagnosis of occupational asthma.

Estimates of Incidence of Occupational Asthma from National and Regional Statistics

Estimates of incidence of occupational asthma, important for both public health practice and policy, have been made using various sources of information. These include registers based on mandated or voluntary physician reporting, self-reporting by individuals, medicolegal statistics, and various other national disease or disability registers. Table 5 summarizes the features of, and findings in some of these systems.

The Sentinel Event Notification System for Occupational Risks (SENSOR) was introduced in several states in the United States in the 1980s (13) . The system was based on mandatory and/or voluntary reporting of suspected work-related disease, and linked physicians who identify occupational disease with public health officials with the responsibility for investigating workplaces thought to be at risk. Though confirmation of occupational asthma cases was labor intensive, the system was felt to be successful in increasing health provider awareness. As with infectious disease notification, underreporting was a persistent problem. In the United Kingdom, a sentinel system, modeled on the informal reports of communicable diseases submitted by its Public Health Laboratory Service, was introduced in 1989 (136) and was based on voluntary reporting by selected physicians across the country. Systems based on this model have since been introduced on a trial basis elsewhere, for instance in Canada, in the provinces of Quebec (137) and British

Table 5 Estimates of Annual Incidence of Occupational Asthma from National and Regional Statistics

Country, year	Sources of information	No. of cases	Reference population (million)	Annual incidence per million (range)	Comments	First author, year, ref.
U.K., 1989	Voluntary by physicians	554	Labor force	22 (10–114)	282/554 due to agents receiving WCB benefits	Meredith, 1989 136
Canada, BC, 1991	Voluntary by physicians	124	Labor force 1.05 M	92	82% workers covered; not all cases proven	Contreras, 1994 138
Canada, Québec	Workmen's compensation	~70/yr	n/a	~20	97/213 claims accepted in 1987	Lagier, 1990 10
Canada, Québec, 1992–1993	Voluntary by physicians	287	n/a	121	48% workers covered WCB recognized; one-third of cases reported	Provencher, 1994 137
Sweden, 1990–1992	Registers (self-report)	1010	Census 4.2 M	80 (22–844)[a]	Useful in surveillance and identifying at risk work	Toren, 1996 139
Finland, 1993	Registers of persistent and occupational asthma	8056 386	Labor force 2.02 M	~187	Since 1986 prevalences of asthma and occupational asthma have increased by 21% and 70% respectively	Reijula, 1996 166
Finland, 1981–1989	Occupational disease register	352	Labor force 2.25 M	~156	2-fold increase in registered cases	Reijula, 1994 140

[a]For swedish men across occupational groups.

Columbia (138). Other estimates of incidence of occupational asthma have been derived from national registers of self-reported asthma in Sweden (139), and of registers of persistent and occupational asthma in Finland (140).

As Table 5 shows, there are considerable between-country differences in the estimated incidence of occupational asthma, ranging from 22 per million per year (range 10–114) in the United Kingdom (136) to 187 per million per year in Finland (140,166). No doubt these are due at least in part to differences in the methods used to arrive at these estimates, but they must also be due in part to differences in the profile of the local industries and employment opportunities. The large differences in risk associated with different exposures and/or jobs and/or industries that these show serve to assist public health authorities in where to direct their preventive interventions. Though there may be reservations concerning the validity of between-country differences in the estimates of prevalence and/or incidence for reasons of different methodology, within-country differences are less threatened and can be reasonably accepted as a valid reflection of time trends, perhaps providing one of the few sources of such information. It is therefore of interest that an increase in prevalence and/or incidence over time, in particular the 1980s, was suggested by several studies (140,141,166) and is in keeping with data from general populations also suggesting an increase in the prevalence and/or incidence of asthma (3). The weaknesses of this type of estimate are the potential for both underestimation (not all cases are reported or seen by targeted physicians) and overestimation (not all cases will conform to the clinical and other criteria required for a diagnosis of occupational asthma). Moreover, for the systems that depend on voluntary physician reporting, it is difficult to maintain their collaboration over time.

Of interest is that most of the agents prescribed for disability benefits in the United Kingdom (flour/grain, wood, and other plant dusts, laboratory animals and insects, isocyanates, azodicarbonamide, antibiotics, proteolytic agents, platinum salts, solder flux, and hardening agents) are also among the most frequently implicated agents in other jurisdictions represented in Table 5. Also important is the fact that, in the SWORD reporting system in the United Kingdom, approximately half the cases reported by physicians as occupational asthma had been exposed to agents not prescribed for benefits. In Quebec, a similar percentage of cases was not confirmed for benefits, and the British Columbia report also indicated that a number of cases were not confirmed for benefits.

Cases evaluated for medicolegal benefits are another source used to estimate the incidence of occupational asthma (see also Table 5). Again the variability from country to country depends on several factors, including (a) the means used to confirm the diagnosis; (b) the interest presented by readaptation programs; and (c) real differences in the incidence (142).

Epidemic and Endemic Asthma

The term "environmental asthma" has been used to describe epidemics of asthma affecting communities and attributable to episodes of unusually high environmental pollution by various airborne contaminants (26). Epidemics of this sort are not new. For instance, a 1928 report implicated castor bean dust residue from a Toledo, Ohio, plant expressing plant oils (143). Post–World War II epidemics include: (a) Tokyo-Yokohama asthma, described in the 1950s in American military personnel in Japan, but not in the Japanese, and attributed to high levels of common urban air pollutants (144); (b) New Orleans asthma, described in the 1960s and attributed to simultaneously high levels of several organic pollutants in the city including coffee, grain, and bagasse emitted from local sources (145); (c) Yokkaidu asthma, described in the 1980s and attributed to sulfuric acid mists emitted from a local titanium-manufacturing plant (146); and (d) Barcelona asthma, attributable to soybean dust released during unloading of ships in the Barcelona harbor (147).

In the case of Barcelona asthma, the first outbreak was identified in the emergency room of a city hospital clinic in 1981, though the agent and its source were only identified after several years of study. The first step in this detective story, a retrospective investigation comparing six prior outbreaks with 12 random hospital days, was carried out in 1993. Features in all outbreaks were that most of those affected sought hospital care within a period of hours after the development of symptoms, and in many cases the attacks were severe, requiring assisted ventilation. No etiological hypothesis could be developed on the basis of review of existing data on community pollution levels of smoke and sulfur dioxide. In 1984, after a seventh outbreak, which occurred during a period of high NO_2 pollution, a Collaborative Asthma Group of epidemiologists and clinicians was established. On their advice, a population-based monitoring system was set in place, encompassing the city, and standardized methods of collecting case data were established. As a result, in the eighth outbreak, which occurred in November 1984, a complete description of the episode was possible, covering 43 adults and 22 children who sought emergency room treatment. For the adults, the chance that this episode was a random event was very low. In this episode, the most affected neighborhoods were those close to the harbor and near an industrial area. In the period 1985–1986, six more outbreaks were confirmed by epidemiological investigation, and five of seven outbreaks that had occurred between 1981 and 1984 were also confirmed by retrospective analysis, comparable data now being available. The time clustering of cases was thus confirmed for 12 of the 14 outbreaks, and 23 additional unusual asthma days for the period 1985–1986 were identified that had not been detected by the clinicians. In addition, geographic clustering became evident. This led to the Collaborative Asthma Group to postulate a point source in the harbor or a nearby industrial area and to focus on a specific etiological hypothesis implicating soybean in several well-designed studies. Among these were (a) time-ecological studies to link the asthma episodes with unloading soybean in the harbor and (b) a case-control study that showed measurable specific IgE levels to soybean in 74% of asthma cases seen during the epidemic episodes compared to 4% of asthma cases seen on nonepidemic days. At this point, the evidence for a causal relationship was considered conclusive and community air pollution by soybean dust was recognized as the agent responsible for the Barcelona asthma. Outbreaks of a similar nature were subsequently described in another Spanish port, and after investigation using a similar epidemiological approach, soybean dust was again incriminated as the responsible agent (148).

Asthma episodes less dramatic than the Barcelona epidemic, but nevertheless consistent and so far not fully explained, are the peak incidences of asthma and asthma-like episodes presenting at emergency rooms that have been noted in urban centers in the fall, i.e., September–November, in the Northern hemisphere and April and May in the Southern hemisphere (149). They have been attributed to the rising levels of indoor pollution that accompany the cooler weather as home dwellers close and seal their windows for the winter. Implicated could be any or several or all of the following in varying combinations: mites and fungi, volatile organic compounds, chemical agents, smoke, and cooking fuels (150). The relationship of these episodes to increased levels of the common urban pollutants (151,152) and/or to acid aerosols (151) is also attracting increasing attention.

SCREENING AND SURVEILLANCE

The terms "screening" and "surveillance" are often used interchangeably (153), but in fact they describe different activities with different objectives, which should be clearly distinguished. Thus, screening is directed toward the individual, i.e., it has a clinical focus, whereas surveillance is directed toward the population from which the individual derives, i.e., it has a public health focus.

Screening has been defined as "the presumptive identification of unrecognized disease or defect by the application of tests which can be applied rapidly." In addition, the definition points out that "a screening test is not intended to be diagnostic" (2). Thus screening aims to detect disease before an individual seeks medical advice, that is, at a preclinical stage. Screening is often carried out in the context of a survey of a workforce or occupation group thought to be at risk (see above), in which those identified by the screening procedure are referred for further investigation (see above). The goal of screening is thus secondary prevention, i.e., to detect organ dysfunction and/or disease at a stage when intervention would be beneficial. In the case of occupational asthma, affected individuals have often themselves rearranged or adjusted their jobs to minimize exposure. In addition, for most exposures, the chances of improvement after exposure ceases become less the longer exposure continues after the onset of asthma symptom (see Chapter 7). For not a few individuals detected by screening, this may mean the directive or recommendation to quit their current job and/or workplace, as daunting for the young person in a shrinking job market as to the older individual in a metier that he has pursued for all his working life, and who lacks the skills to adapt to new technologies in the changing workplace. The detection of an index case or cases in a workplace may also trigger public health action in the form of an industrial hygiene investigation of the workplace.implicated. A feature of the SENSOR program in the United States was to link clinicians who identify work-related disease such as asthma with public health officials who can investigate and intervene at specific workplaces and alert other physicians to local settings and/or workplaces at risk (13).

By contrast, *surveillance* is defined as "continued watchfulness over the distribution and trends of disease through the systematic collection, consolidation, and evaluation of morbidity and mortality reports and other relevant data," and perhaps even more important, the timely distribution of data "to all who need to know" (153). Identifying who "needs to know" is clearly important since, by definition, surveillance should trigger public health action. While those who generate the surveillance data are often also those who are responsible for public health action (139), this is not always so (136). National surveys are useful in identifying risk work and in providing estimates of incidence beyond what is provided by the usually smaller workforce- or occupation-based survey where particular work conditions operate, in providing surveillance of time trends, again in workforces or from analysis of national databases, and perhaps even more important, in determining the time trends in national data (Table 6). Examples of this approach to the use of national databases in the form of disease registers are to be found in the reports from Sweden (139) and Finland (140,166), both of which showed increases in the rates of occupational asthma over the 1980s. Despite the potential for bias toward both under- and overestimation, depending on the source of the data, the Swedish self-reported system for registering occupational asthma was considered to be useful and to have provided some important information (139). Ideally, the public health action that findings of this sort might trigger include hygiene surveys in workplaces or occupations identified or suspected

Table 6 Percentage of Adult Asthma Attributable to Work Exposure Based on National Statistics and Panel Studies of Prevalence

Country, year of study	Population number, source	Number of cases (age, yr)	Work-related asthma		Exposure	Information source(s) and comment	Ref.
			%	CI			
USA, 1978	6063 HIS and SSDS[a]	478	15.4	n/a	Job, employer	Questionnaire	Blanc, 1987 167
USA, MI, 1990	Hospital discharge patients	94 (20–65)	3.0[b] 20.2 25.5	n/a	Recognized agents Work symptoms self-attributed	Interviewer for exposure Chart review for asthma	Timmer, 1993 168
USA, CA, 1996	Patient panel study	601 (18–54)	8.8 13.1 14.1	6.5–11.1 10.4–15.8 11.3–16.9	Sensitizers and irritants; high-risk job sensitizer and high-risk job	Telephone interview of job and work exposure 3% (8/255) have WCB benefits	Blanc, 1996 169
Finland, 1993	2.02 M National Register[c]	386 (15–64)	4.8	n/a	Medicolegal criteria	Increase in persistent (21%) and occupational (71%) asthma since 1986	Reijula, 1996 166

[a]1976 Health Interview Survey and 1978 Social Security Administration Disability Survey.
[b]Based on NIOSH criteria for probable (3.0%), possible or probable (20.2%) occupational asthma and self-report opinion on work-relatedness.
[c]National register information on persistent and occupational asthma.

as at risk (but not yet surveyed), and, perhaps even more important, follow-up on previous surveys to determine the effect of any previously implemented preventive interventions.

USES, USEFULNESS, AND APPLICATIONS

Information on the epidemiology (distribution and determinants) of asthma associated with occupational exposures is useful for several purposes (27,28). These include:

1. Establishing prevalence and/or incidence data for public health purposes and as a guide to the need for preventive services and/or surveillance in any industry at risk
2. Addressing etiological questions relating to exposures and personal risk factors
3. Establishing exposure-response relationships to provide the scientific basis for setting environmental control levels
4. Evaluating preventive services or control measures

Although none of this information can be furnished by clinical case studies, all of it bears on each step in the clinical evaluation of a case of occupational asthma. These include establishing the diagnosis, setting prognosis, planning and evaluating management, and taking the appropriate steps in notification.

In terms of study design, the importance of selecting the design most appropriate for answering the particular study question cannot be overemphasized (see Table 1 and Fig. 1). Though all the usual study designs can and have been used in investigating occupational asthma, the emphasis has been on observational studies, all of which are subject to bias due to the "healthy worker" effect. Most information has come from surveys of particular workforces or occupational groups, probably because cohort studies, though stronger, are more difficult to implement, due in large part to the characteristics of work-related asthma with both early and high turnover rates. Emphasis is also placed on the need for the appropriate definition of the study outcome, usually asthma or some marker or surrogate of asthma, and of careful selection of the study population to minimize underestimation of the exposure response effect due to selection bias from the "healthy worker" effect, whether due to "healthy" hire or survivor effects.

Tables 2, 3, and 4 review some of the epidemiological information relating asthma to particular occupational exposures, as well as the role of smoking and atopy as determinants of the distribution of these cases within their respective workforces. These tables also provide estimates of prevalence. This information serves as a guide to public health as well as clinical management of occupational asthma. The data in Tables 2–4 also support the conclusion of the expert committee charged with setting guidelines for epidemiological studies in occupational asthma to the effect that the potential of environmental measurements for evaluating workplace exposures and practices as well as environmental controls has not yet been realized (27). The reader is also referred to this excellent document for further discussion on guidelines and approaches to the epidemiological investigation of occupational asthma.

Table 5 estimates of incidence of occupational asthma in the several industrialized countries for which such data are available; rates vary from as low as 22 per million for the year 1989 in the United Kingdom, based on voluntary physician reporting (136) to ~181 per million for the year 1991 for Sweden, based on self-reporting. Table 6 shows estimates of the percentage of adult asthma due to occupation range from 3% to 29%, while a lower estimate of 6% was made on the basis of patients attending an asthma clinic in a developing country, Zambia (154). While methodological differences are likely to account for a substantial proportion of the between-country differences in estimated rates, the increases in rates over time within countries, e.g., Sweden and Finland, are likely to be valid reflections of what is happening at a time when by and large workplaces are being better maintained and environmental standards better respected. This lends credence to the view that the increase in adult asthma over the past decades may also reflect an increase in the susceptibility of today's populations (19).

SUMMARY

All the information in this chapter has been presented with a view to underlining the role of epidemiology in the public health and clinical evaluation of occupational asthma. Studies with a public health focus include those in which sentinel cases can be identified, as well as those based on national and regional statistics. Studies of this type are currently being carried out in several industrialized countries and can monitor trends as well as triggering prompt industrial hygiene investigations of the workplaces implicated. Many of the agents involved have already been identified as causes of occupational asthma and are common to several countries; others are sufficiently under suspicion to warrant further study; yet others remain to be identified. In addition, several cohort studies, including at least one in which the target population is young apprentices, may reveal relevant early risk factors that could be translated into early secondary prevention. Clinical studies are still (and are likely to remain so for a long time) the commonest source of identification of agents not previously identified as associated with occupational asthma, as well as of workplaces and/or occupations not previously thought to be at risk.

REFERENCES

1. Miettinen OS. Theoretical Epidemiology: Principles of Occurrence Research in Medicine. New York: Wiley, 1985:317–344.
2. Last JM. A Dictionary of Epidemiology, 3rd ed. New York: Oxford University Press, 1995: 1–180.
3. Becklake MR, Ernst P. Environmental factors. Lancet 1997; 350(Suppl II):10–13.
4. Ramazzini B. De morbis artificium diatribas. 1713. WC Wright, trans. Chicago: University of Chicago Press, 1940.
5. Becklake MR. Occupational exposures: evidence of a causal association with chronic obstructive pulmonary disease. Am Rev Respir Dis 1989; 140:S85–S91.
6. World Health Organization. Tenth report of the Joint ILO/WHO Committee on Occupational Health. Epidemiology of Work-Related Diseases and Accidents 1989. Geneva, 1989, Technical report series, 777:1–23.
7. International Agency for Research on Cancer. IARC Monographs on the Evaluation of the Carcinogenic Risk of Chemicals to Humans: Chemicals, Industrial Processes and Industries Associated with Cancer in Humans. IARC, Lyon 1982; 1–29. (suppl 4):1–18.
8. Meredith SK, McDonald JC. Work related respiratory disease in the United Kingdom, 1989–1992: report on the SWORD project. Occup Med 1994; 44:183–189.
9. Chan-Yeung M, Malo JL. Occupational asthma. N Engl J Med 1995; 333:107–112.
10. Lagier F, Cartier A, Malo JL. Statistiques médico-légales sur l'asthme professionnel au Québec de 1986 à 1988. Medico-legal statistics on occupational asthma in Quebec between 1986 and 1988. Rev Mal Respir 1990; 7:337–341.

11. US Department of Health and Human Services. Work-related Lung Disease Surveillance Report 1994. Cincinnati: National Institute for Occupational Safety and Health, 1994. DHHS (NIOSH) Number 94-120.

12. Kauffmann F, Drouet D, Lellouch J, Brille D. Occupasional exposures and 12-year changes among Paris area workers. Br J Ind Med 1982; 39:221–232.

13. Matte TD, Hoffman RE, Rosenman KD, Stanbury M. Surveillance of occupational asthma under the SENSOR model. Chest 1990; 98:173S–178S.

14. Chan-Yeung M. Occupational asthma. Chest 1990; 98:148S–161S.

15. Anto JM, Sunyer J. Epidemiologic studies of asthma epidemics in Barcelona. Chest 1990; 98(Suppl 5):185S–190S.

16. Sears MR. Descriptive epidemiology of asthma. Lancet 1997; 350(Suppl II):1–4.

17. Cowley G, Underwood A. Asthma to be beaten? Newsweek May 16, 1997.

18. Platts-Mills TAE, Carter MC. Asthma and indoor exposure to allergens. N Engl J Med 1997; 336:1382–1384.

19. Seaton A, Godden DJ, Brown K. Increase in asthma: a more toxic environment or a more susceptible population? Thorax 1994; 49:171–174.

20. Becklake MR. Occupational asthma: epidemiology and surveillance. Chest 1990; 98(Suppl 5):165S–172S.

21. Taylor AN. Asthma. In: McDonald JC, ed. The Epidemiology of Work Related Disease. London: BMJ Publishing Group, 1995:117–142.

22. Fish JE. Occupational asthma: a spectrum of acute respiratory disorders. J Occup Med 1982; 24:379–386.

23. Brooks SM. Bronchial asthma of occupational origin: a review. Scand J Work Environ Health 1982; 3:53–72.

24. Venables KM. Epidemiology and the prevention of occupational asthma. Br J Ind Med 1987; 44:73–75 (editorial).

25. Cotes JE, Steel J. Work-Related Lung Disorders. Oxford: Balckwell Scientific Publications. 1987:345–372.

26. Merchant JA. Workshop on environmental and occupational asthma: opening remarks. Chest 1990; 98(Suppl 5):145S–146S.

27. Smith AB, Castellan RM, Lewis D, Matte T. Guidelines for the epidemiologic assessment of occupational asthma. Report of the subcommittee on the epidemiologic assessment of occupational asthma, occupational lung disease committee. J Allergy Clin Immunol 1989; 84: 794–805.

28. Becklake MR. Population studies in risk assessment: strengths and weaknessess. In: Mohr U, ed. Inhalational Toxicology. The Design and Interpretation of Inhalational Studies and Their Use in Risk Assessment. New York: Springer-Verlag, 1988:263–272.

29. Burney P. Why study the epidemiology of asthma? Thorax 1988; 43:425–428.

30. Gross NS. What is this thing called love?—or defining asthma. Am Rev Respir Dis 1980; 121:203–204.

31. Manfreda J, Chan-Yeung M, Dimich-Ward H, Sears MR, Siersted H, Becklake MR, Ernst P, Sweet L, Van Til L, Bowie D, Anthonisen N, Tate RB. Prevalence of asthma in Canada. Am J Respir Crit Care Med 1996, 153:4 (pt 2), A432 (abstract).

32. McDonald JC. Epidemiology. In: Weill H, Turner-Warwick M, eds. Occupational Lung Diseases. New York: Marcel Dekker, 1981:373–403.

33. Malo JL, Cartier A, Côté J, Milot J, Leblanc C, Paquette L, Ghezzo H, Boulet LP. Influence of inhaled steroids on recovery from occupational asthma after cessation of exposure: an 18-month double-blind crossover study. Am J Respir Crit Care Med 1996; 153:953–960.

34. Eisen EA. Healthy worker effect in morbidity studies. Med Lav 1995; 86:125–138.

35. McDonald JC. Methodology. Study design. In: McDonald JC, ed. The Epidemiology of Work-Related Diseases. London: BMJ Publishing Group, 1995:325–351.

36. Becklake M, Ernst P, Chan-Yeung M, Manfreda J, Dimich-Ward H, Sears M, Siersted H. The burden of asthma attributable to work exposures in Canada. Am J Respir Crit Care Med 1996; 153:A433.

37. Manfreda J, Becker AB, Wang PZ, Roos LL, Anthonisen NR. Trends in physician-diagnosed asthma prevalence in Manitoba between 1980 and 1990. Chest 1993; 103:151–157.

38. Diller WF. Facts and fallacies involved in the epidemiology of isocyanate asthma. Bull Eur Physiopathol Respir 1988; 23:551–553.

39. Gautrin D, Infante-Rivard C, Dao TV, Magnan-Larose M, Desjardins D, Malo JL. Specific IgE-dependent sensitization, atopy and bronchial hyperresponsiveness in apprentices starting exposure to protein-derived agents. Am J Respir Crit Care Med 1997; 155:1841–1847.

40. Diem JE, Jones RN, Hendrick DJ, Glindmeyer HW, Dharmarajan V, Butcher BT, Salvaggio JE, Weill H. Five-year longitudinal study of workers employed in a new toluene diisocyanate manufacturing plant. Am Rev Respir Dis 1982; 126:420–428.

41. Rothman KJ. Modern Epidemiology. Boston: Little Brown, 1985.

42. Becklake MR, White N. Sources of variation in spirometric measurements: identifying the signal and dealing with noise. Occup Med: State of the Art Series 1993; 8:241–264.

43. Fonn S, Groeneveld HT, de Beer M, Becklake MR. An environmental and respiratory health survey of workers in a grain mill in the Johannesburg area, South Africa. Am J Ind Med 1993; 24:387–400.

44. Fonn S, Groeneveld HT, deBeer M, Becklake MR. Relationship of respiratory health status to grain dust in a Witwatersrand grain mill: comparison of workers' exposure assessments with industrial hygiene survey findings. Am J Ind Med 1993; 24:401–411.

45. deGrosbois S. Occupational exposures and airway disease: a study to develop a questionnaire for community based studies. PhD thesis, McGill University, Montréal, 1998.

46. Fuchs S, Valade P. Etude clinique et experimentale sur quelques cas d'intoxication par le Desmodur T (diisocyanate de tolulene 1-2-4 et 1-2-6). Arch Mal Profess 1951; 12:191–196.

47. Samet JM. A historical and epidemiological perspective on respiratory symptoms questionnaires. Am J Epidemiol 1978; 198:435–446.

48. Burney PGJ, Laitinen LA, Perdrizet S, Huckauf H, Tattersfield AE, Chinn S, Poisson N, Heeren A, Britton JR, Jones T. Validity and repeatability of the IUATLD (1984) bronchial symptoms questionnaire: an international comparison. Eur Respir J 1989; 2:940–945.

49. Enarson DA, Vedal S, Schulzer M, Dybuncio A, Chan-Yeung M. Asthma, asthmalike symptoms, chronic bronchitis, and the degree of bronchial hyperresponsiveness in epidemiologic surveys. Am Rev Respir Dis 1987; 136:613–617.

50. Dales RE, Nunes F, Partyka D, Ernst P. Clinical prediction of airways hyperresponsiveness. Chest 1988; 93:984–986.

51. Rijcken B, Schouten JP, Weiss ST, Speizer FE, Lende R van der. The relationship between airway responsiveness to histamine and pulmonary function level in a random population sample. Am Rev Respir Dis 1988; 137:826–832.

52. Jansen DF, Timens W, Kraan J, Rijcken B, Postma DS. (A)symptomatic bronchial hyperresponsiveness and asthma. Respir Med 1997; 91:121–134.

53. Laprise C, Boulet LP. Asymptomatic airway hyperresponsiveness: a three-year follow-up. Am J Respir Crit Care Med 1997; 156:403–409.

54. Adelroth E, Hargreave FE, Ramsdale EH. Do physicians need objective measurements to diagnose asthma? Am Rev Respir Dis 1986; 134:704–707.

55. Malo JL, Ghezzo H, L'Archevêque J, Lagier F, Perrin B, Cartier A. Is the clinical history a satisfactory means of diagnosing occupational asthma? Am Rev Respir Dis 1991; 143:528–532.

56. Smith A Blair, Bernstein DI, London MA, Gallagher J, Ornella GA, Gelletly SK, Wallingford D, Newman MA. Evaluation of occupational asthma from airborne egg protein exposure in multiple settings. Chest 1990; 98:398–404.

57. Cartier A, Malo J-L, Forest F, Lafrance M, Pineau L, St-Aubin J-J, Dubois J-Y. Occupational asthma in snow crab-processing workers. J Allergy Clin Immunol 1984; 74:261–269.

58. Séguin P, Allard A, Cartier A, Malo JL. Prevalence of occupational asthma in spray painters exposed to several types of isocyanates, including polymethylene polyphenylisocyanates. J Occup Med 1987; 29:340–344.

59. Bardy JD, Malo JL, Séguin P, Ghezzo H, Desjardins J, Dolovich J, Cartier A. Occupational asthma and IgE sensitization in a pharmaceutical company processing psyllium. Am Rev Respir Dis 1987; 135:1033–1038.

60. Malo JL, Cartier A. Occupational asthma in workers of a pharmaceutical company processing spiramycin. Thorax 1988; 43:371–377.

61. Malo JL, Cartier A, L'Archevêque J, Ghezzo H, Soucy F, Somers J, Dolovich J. Prevalence of occupational asthma and immunological sensitization to guar gum among employees at a carpet-manufacturing plant. J Allergy Clin Immunol 1990; 86:562–569.

62. Malo JL, Cartier A, L'Archevêque J, Ghezzo H, Lagier F, Trudeau C, Dolovich J. Prevalence of occupational asthma and immunologic sensitization to psyllium among health personnel in chronic care hospitals. Am Rev Respir Dis 1990; 142:1359–1366.

63. Vedal S, Chan-Yeung M, Ashley MJ, Enarson D, Lam S. Does a family history or personal history of allergy predict immediate skin test reactivity? Can Med Assoc J 1985; 132:34–37.

64. Maccia CA, Bernstein IL, Emmett EA, Brooks SM. In vitro demonstration of specific IgE in phthalic anhydride hypersensitiviy. Am Rev Respir Dis 1976; 113:701–704.

65. Chan-Yeung M, Lam S, Enarson D. Pulmonary function measurement in the industrial setting. Chest 1985; 88:270–275.

66. Becklake MR. Epidemiology of spirometric test failure. Br J Ind Med 1990; 47:73–74.

67. Wright JL, Churg A. Severe diffuse small airway disease in long term chrysotile asbestos miners. Br J Ind Med 1985; 42:556–559.

68. Kessel R, Redl M, Mauermayer R, Pram GJ. Changes in lung function after working with the shotcrete lining method under compressed air. Br J Ind Med 1989; 46:128–132.

69. American Thoracic Society. Standardization of spirometry. Am J Respir Crit Care Med 1995; 152:1107–1136.

70. Burge PS. Single and serial measurements of lung function in the diagnosis of occupational asthma. Eur J Respir Dis 1982; 63(Suppl 123):47–59.

71. Becklake MR. Relationship of acute obstructive airway change to chronic (fixed) obstruction. Thorax 1994; 149:584–590.

72. Moscato G, Godnic-Cvar J, Maestrelli P, Malo JL, Burge PS, Coifman R. Statement on self-monitoring of peak expiratory flows in the investigation of occupational asthma. J Allergy Clin Immunol 1995; 96:295–301.

73. Côté J, Kennedy S, Chan-Yeung M. Sensitivity and specificity of PC_{20} and peak expiratory flow rate in cedar asthma. J Allergy Clin Immunol 1990; 85:592–598.

74. Perrin B, Lagier F, L'Archevêque J, Cartier A, Boulet LP, Côté J, Malo JL. Occupational asthma: validity of monitoring of peak expiratory flow rates and non-allergic bronchial responsiveness as compared to specific inhalation challenge. Eur Respir J 1992; 5:40–48.

75. Cartier A, Malo J-L, Forest F, Lafrance M, Pineau L, St-Aubin J-J, Dubois J-Y. Occupational asthma in snow crab-processing workers. J Allergy Clin Immunol 1984; 74:261–269.

76. Malo J-L, Cartier A. Occupational asthma in workers of a pharmaceutical company processing spiramycin. Thorax 1988; 43:371–377.

77. Venables KM, Burge P Sherwood, Davison AG, Taylor AJ Newman. Peak flow rate records in surveys: reproducibility of observers' reports. Thorax 1984; 39:828–832.

78. Malo JL, Cartier A, Ghezzo H, Chan-Yeung M. Compliance with peak expiratory flow readings affects the within- and between-reader reproducibility of interpretation of graphs in subjects investigated for occupational asthma. J Allergy Clin Immunol 1996; 98:1132–1134.

79. Tiffeneau R. Hypersensibilité cholinergo-histaminique pulmonaire de l'asthmatique. Relation avec l'hypersensibilité allergénique pulmonaire. Acta Allergol 1958; (Suppl V):187–221.

80. Cockcroft DW, Ruffin RE, Frith PA, Cartier A, Juniper EF, Dolovich J, Hargreave FE. Determinants of allergen-induced asthma: dose of allergen, circulating IgE antibody concentration, and bronchial responsiveness to inhaled histamine. Am Rev Respir Dis 1979; 120:1053–1058.

81. Cockcroft DW, Murdock KY, Kirby J, Hargreave F. Prediction of airway responsiveness to allergen from skin sensitivity to allergen and airway responsiveness to histamine. Am Rev Respir Dis 1987; 135:264–267.

82. Becklake MR, Ernst P, Chan-Yeung M, Dimich-Ward H, Sears MA, Siersted H. The burden of airways disease attributable to work exposures in Canada (abstract). Am J Respir Crit Care Med 1996; 153:4(pt 2):A433.

83. Burney PGJ, Britton JR, Chinn S, Tattersfield AE, Papacosta AO, Kelson MC, Anderson F, Corfield DR. Descriptive epidemiology of bronchial reactivity in an adult population: results from a community study. Thorax 1987; 42:38–44.

84. Woolcock AJ, Peat JK, Salome CM, Yan K, Anderson SD, Schoeffel RE, McCowage G, Killalea T. Prevalence of bronchial hyperresponsiveness and asthma in a rural adult population. Thorax 1987; 42:361–368.

85. Hendrick DJ. Epidemiological measurement of bronchial responsiveness in polyurethane workers. Bull Eur Physiopathol Respir 1988; 23:555–559.

86. Pham QT, Mur JM, Chau N, Gabiano M, Henquel JC, Teculescu D. Prognostic value of acetylcholine challenge test: a prospective study. Br J Ind Med 1984; 41:267–271.

87. Vedal S, Enarson DA, Chan H, Ochnio J, Tse KS, Chan-Yeung M. A longitudinal study of the occurrence of bronchial hyperresponsiveness in western red cedar workers. Am Rev Respir Dis 1988; 137:651–655.

88. Newman Taylor AJ, Venables KM. Clinical and epidemiological methods in investigating occupational asthma. Clin Immunol Allergy 1984; 4:3–17.

89. Reed CE, Swanson MC, Agarwal MK, Yunginger JW. Allergens that cause asthma. Identification and quantification. Chest 1985; 87:40S–44S.

90. Venables KM. Low molecular weight chemicals, hypersensitivity and direct toxicity: the acid anhydrides. Br J Ind Med 1989; 46:222–232.

91. Vedal S, Chan-Yeung M, Enarson D, Fera T, Maclean L, Tse KS, Langille R. Symptoms and pulmonary function in western red cedar workers related to duration of employment and dust exposure. Arch Environ Health 1986; 41:179–183.

92. Brooks SM, Edwards JJ, Apol A, Edwards FH. An epidemiologic study of workers exposed to western red cedar and other wood dust. Chest 1981; 80(Suppl):30–32.

93. Musk AW, Venables KM, Crook B, Nunn AJ, Hawkins R, Crook GDW, Graneek BJ, Tee RD, Farrer N, Johnson DA, Gordon DJ, Darbyshire JH, Newman Taylor AJ. Respiratory symptoms, lung function, and sensitisation to flour in a British bakery. Br J Ind Med 1989; 46:636–642.

94. Cullinan P, Lowson D, Nieuwenshuijsen MJ, Sandiford C, Tee RD, Venables KM, McDonald JC, Taylor AJ Newman. Work related symptoms, sensitisation, and estimated exposure in workers not previously exposed to flour. Occup Environ Med 1994; 51:579–583.

95. Cullinan P, Lowson D, Nieuwenhuijsen MJ, Gordon S, Tee RD, Venables KM, McDonald JC, Taylor AJ Newman. Work related symptoms, sensitisation, and estimated exposure in workers not previously exposed to laboratory rats. Occup Environ Med 1994; 51: 589–592.

96. Burge PS, Edge G, Hawkins R, White V, Taylor AN. Occupational asthma in a factory making flux-cored solder containing colophony. Thorax 1981; 36:828–834.

97. Venables KM. Low molecular weight chemicals, hypersensitivity, and direct toxicity: the acid anhydrides. Br J Ind Med 1989; 46:222–232.

98. Beach JR, Dennis JH, Avery AJ, Bromly CL, Ward RJ, Walters EH, Stenton SC, Hendrick DJ. An epidemiologic investigation of asthma in welders. Am J Respir Crit Care Med 1996; 154:1394–1400.

99. Vandenplas O, Cartier A, Ghezzo H, Cloutier Y, Malo JL. Response to isocyanates: Effect of concentration, duration of exposure, and dose. Am Rev Respir Dis 1993; 147:1287–1290.

100. Butcher BT, Jones RN, O'Neil CE, Glindmeyer HW, Diem JE, Dharmarajan V, Weill H, Salvaggio JE. Longitudinal study of workers employed in the manufacture of toluene-diisocyanate. Am Rev Respir Dis 1977; 116:411–421.

101. Leroyer C, Perfetti L, Cartier A, Malo JL. Can reactive airways dysfunction syndrome (RADS) transform into occupational asthma due to "sensitisation" to isocyanates? Thorax 1998; 53:152–153.

102. Molfino NA, Wright SC, Katz I, Tarlo S, Silverman F, McClean PA, Szalai JP, Raizenne M, Slutsky AS, Zamel N. Effect of low concentrations of ozone on inhaled allergen response in asthmatic subjects. Lancet 1991; 336:199–203.

103. Slovak AJ, Hill RN. Laboratory animal allergy: a clinical survey of an exposed population. Br J Ind Med 1981; 38:38–41.

104. Venables KM, Upton JL, Hawkins ER, Tee RD, Longbottom JL, Newman Taylor AJ. Smoking, atopy and laboratory animal allergy. Br J Ind Med 1988; 45:667–671.

105. Venables KM, Topping MD, Howe W, Luczynska CM, Hawkins R, Taylor AJ Newman. Interaction of smoking and atopy in producing specific IgE antibody against a hapten protein conjugate. Br Med J 1985; 290:201–204.

106. Calverley AE, Rees D, Dowdeswell RJ, Linnett PJ, Kielkowski D. Platinum salt sensitivity in refinery workers: incidence and effects of smoking and exposure. Occup Environ Med 1995; 52:661–666.

107. Venables KM, Dally MB, Nunn AJ, Stevens JF, Stephens R, Farrer N, Hunter JV, Stewart M, Hughes EG, Taylor AJ Newman. Smoking and occupational allergy in workers in a platinum refinery. Br Med J 1989; 299:939–942.

108. Paggiaro PL, Loi AM, Rossi O, Ferrante B, Pardi F, Roselli MG, Baschieri L. Follow-up study of patients with respiratory disease due to toluene diisocyanate (TDI). Clin Allergy 1984; 14:463–469.

109. Burge PS, Perks WH, O'Brien IM, Burge A, Hawkins R, Brown D, Green M. Occupational asthma in an electronics factory: a case control study to evaluate aetiological factors. Thorax 1979; 34:300–307.

110. Chan-Yeung M, Lam S, Koerner S. Clinical features and natural history of occupational asthma due to western red cedar (*Thuja plicata*). Am J Med 1982; 72:411–415.

111. Chan-Yeung M, Kennedy S, Vedal S. A longitudinal study of red cedar sawmill workers. Am Rev Respir Dis 1990; 139:A81.

112. Bignon JS, Aron Y, LYJu, Kopferschmitt MC, Garnier R, Mapp C, Fabbri LM, Pauli G, Lockhart A, Charron D, Swierczewski E. HLA class II alleles in isocyanate-induced asthma. Am J Respir Crit Care Med 1994; 149:71–75.

113. Balboni A, Baricordi OR, Fabbri LM, Gandini E, Ciaccia A, Mapp CE. Association between toluene diisocyanate-induced asthma and DQB1 markers: a possible role for aspartic acid at position 57. Eur Respir J 1996; 9:207–210.

114. Horne C, Quintana PJE, Keown PA, Dimich-Ward H, Chan-Yeung M. Distribution of HLA class II DQB1 alleles in patients with occupational asthma due to western red cedar. Am J Respir Crit Care Med (in press).

115. Malo JL, Lemière C, Desjardins A, Cartier A. Prevalence and intensity of rhinoconjunctivitis in subjects with occupational asthma. Eur Respir J 1997; 10:1513–1515.

116. Zejda JE, Pahwa P, Dosman JA. Decline in spirometric variables in grain workers from start of employment: differential effect of duration of follow up. Br J Ind Med 1992; 49:576–580.

117. Zammit-Tabona M, Sherkin M, Kijek K, Chan H, Chan-Yeung M. Asthma caused by diphenylmethane diisocyanate in foundry workers. Clinical, bronchial provocation, and immunologic studies. Am Rev Respir Dis 1983; 128:226–230.

118. Chan-Yeung M, Ward H Dimich, Enarson DA, Kennedy SM. Five cross-sectional studies of grain elevator workers. Am J Epidemiol 1992; 136:1269–1279.

119. Mitchell CA, Gandevia B. Respiratory symptoms and skin reactivity in workers exposed to proteolytic enzymes in the detergent industry. Am Rev Respir Dis 1971; 104:1–12.

120. Chan-Yeung M, Vedal S, Kus J, Maclean L, Enarson D, Tse KS. Symptoms, pulmonary function, and bronchial hyperreactivity in western red cedar workers compared with those in office workers. Am Rev Respir Dis 1984; 130:1038–1041.

121. Butcher BT, Salvaggio JE, Weill H, Ziskind MM. Toluene diisocyanate (TDI) pulmonary disease: Immunologic and inhalation challenge studies. J Allergy Clin Immunol 1970; 58: 89–100.

122. Venables KM, Dally MB, Burge PS, Pickering CAC, Newman Taylor AJ. Occupational asthma in a steel coating plant. Br J Ind Med 1985; 42:517–524.

123. Slovak AJM. Occupational asthma caused by a plastics blowing agent, azodicarbonamide. Thorax 1981; 36:906–909.

124. Ishizaki T, Sluda T, Miyamoto T, Matsumara Y, Mizuno K, Tomaru M. Occupational asthma from western red cedar dust (*Thuja plicata*) in furniture factory workers. JOM 1973; 15:580–585.

125. Wernfors M, Nielsen J, Schütz A, Skerfving S. Phthalic anhydride-induced occupational asthma. Int Arch Allergy Appl Immunol 1986; 79:77–82.

126. Burge PS, Perks W, O'Brien IM, Hawkins R, Green M. Occupational asthma in an electronics factory. Thorax 1979; 34:13–18.

127. Lebowitz MD. Occupational exposures in relation to symptomatology and lung function in a community population. Environ Res 1977; 14:59–67.

128. Korn RJ, Dockery DW, Speizer FE, Ware JH, Ferris BG. Occupational exposures and chronic respiratory symptoms: a population based study. Am Rev Respir Dis 1987; 130:298–304.

129. Krzyzanowski M, Kauffman F. The relation of respiratory symptoms and ventilatory function to moderate occupational exposure in a general population: results from the French PAARC study of 16000 adults. Int J Epidemiol 1988; 17:397–406.

130. Viegi G, Prediletto R, Paoletti P, Carozzi L, Pede F Di, Vellutini M, Pede C, Giuntini C, Lebowitz M. Respiratory effects of occupational exposures in a general population sample in north Italy. Am Rev Respir Dis 1991; 143:510–515.

131. Bakke P, Eide GE, Hanoa R, Gulsvik A. Occupational dust or gas exposure and prevalences of respiratory symptoms and asthma in a general population. Eur Respir J 1991; 4:273–278.

132. Kogevinas M, Anto JM, Soriano JB, Tobias A, Burney P. The risk of asthma attributable to occupational exposures. Am J Respir Crit Care Med 1996; 154:137–143.

133. Fishwick D, Pearce N, D'Souza W, Lewis S, Town I, Armstrong R, Kogevinas M, Crane J. Occupational asthma in New Zealanders: a population based study. Occup Environ Med 1997; 54:301–306.

134. Ng TP, Hong CY, Goh LG, Wong ML, Koh KTC, Ling SL. Risks of asthma associated with occupations in a community-based case-control study. Am J Ind Med 1994; 25:709–718.

135. Burney PGJ, Luczynska C, Chinn S, Jarvis D. The European Community Respiratory Health Survey. Eur Respir J 1994; 7:954–960.

136. Meredith SK, Taylor VM, McDonald JC. Occupational respiratory disease in the United Kingdom 1989: a report to the British Thoracic Society and the Society of Occupational Medicine by the SWORD project group. Br J Ind Med 1991; 48:292–298.

137. Provencher S, Labrèche FP, Guire L De. Physician based surveillance system for occupational respiratory diseases: the experience of PROPULSE, Québec, Canada. Occup Environ Med 1997; 54:272–276.

138. Contreras GR, Rousseau R, Chan-Yeung M. Occupational respiratory diseases in British Columbia, Canada in 1991. Occup Environ Med 1994; 51:710–712.

139. Toren L. Self reported rate of occupational asthma in Sweden 1990–2. Occup Environ Med 1996; 53:757–761.

140. Reijula K, Patterson R. Occupational allergies in Finland in 1981–91. Allergy Proc 1994; 15:163–168.

141. Blanc P. Occupation and asthma: through a glass darkly. Chest 1997; 110:3–4.

142. Dewitte JD, Chan-Yeung M, Malo JL. Medicolegal and compensation aspects of occupational asthma. Eur Respir J 1994; 7:969–980.

143. Figley KD, Elrod RH. Endemic asthma due to castor bean dust. JAMA 1928; 90:79–82.

144. Phelps HW, Koike S. Tokyo-Yokohama asthma: The rapid development of respiratory distress presumably due to air pollution. Am Rev Respir Dis 1962; 88:55–63.

145. Carroll RR. Epidemiology of New Orleans asthma. Am J Public Health 1968; 58:1677–1683.

146. Kitagawa T. Cause analysis for the Yokkaidu asthma episode. J Air Pollut Control Assoc 1984; 34:743–746.

147. Anto JM, Sunyer J, Rodriguez-Roisin R, Suarez-Cervera M, Vazquez L. Community outbreaks of asthma associated with inhalation of soybean dust. N Engl J Med 1989; 320:1097–102.

148. Alvarez-Dardet C, Belda J, Pena M, Nolasaco A. Outbreak of asthma associated with soybean dust. N Engl J Med 1989; 321:1127–1128 (letter).

149. Lee DK, ed. Environmental factors in respiratory disease. New York, Academic Press, 1972, pp 1–252.

150. Samet JM, Marbury MC, Spengler JD. Health effects and sources of indoor pollution. Part 1. Am Rev Respir Dis 1987; 136:1486–1508.

151. Bates DV, Sizto R. Relationship between air pollution levels and hospital admissions in southern Ontario. Can J Public Health 1983; 74:117–122.

152. Bates DV, Baker-Anderson M, Sizto R. Asthma attack periodicity: a study of hospital emergency visits in Vancouver. Environ Res 1990; 51:51–70.

153. Wagner GR. Screening and Surveillance of Workers Exposed to Mineral Dusts. Geneva: World Health Organisation, 1996:1–68.

154. Sybbalo N. Occupational asthma in a developing country. Chest 1991; 99:528 (letter).

155. Gaddie J, Legge JS, Friend JAR, Reid TMS. Pulmonary hypersensitivity in prawn workers. Lancet 1980; 2:1350–1353.

156. Baur X, Konig G, Bencze K, Fruhmann G. Clinical symptoms and results of skin test, RAST and bronchial provocation test in thirty-three papain workers: evidence for strong immunogenic potency and clinically relevant "proteolytic effects of airborne papain." Clin Allergy 1982; 12:9–17.

157. Jyo T, Kohmoto K, Katsutani T, Otsuka T, Oka SD, Mitsui S. Hoya (sea-squirt) asthma. In: Occupational Asthma. London: Von Nostrand Reinhold, 1980:209–228.

158. Desjardins A, Malo JL, L'Archevêque J, Cartier A, McCants M, Lehrer SB. Occupational IgE-mediated sensitization and asthma due to clam and shrimp. J Allergy Clin Immunol 1995; 96:608–617.

159. Burge PS, Edge G, O'Brien IM, Harries MG, Hawkins R, Pepys J. Occupational asthma in a research centre breeding locusts. Clin Allergy 1980; 10:355–363.

160. Cockcroft A, McCarthy P, Edwards J, Andersson N. Allergy in laboratory animal workers. Lancet 1981; 1:827–830.

161. Gross NJ. Allergy to laboratory animals: epidemiologic, clinical, and physiologic aspects, and a trial of cromolyn in its management. J Allergy Clin Immunol 1980; 66:158–165.

162. Vandenplas O, Delwich JP, Evrard G, Aimont P, Brempt X van der, Jamart J, Delaunois L. Prevalence of occupational asthma due to latex among hospital personnel. Am J Respir Crit Care Med 1995; 151:54–60.

163. Burge PS, Edge G, Hawkins R, White V, Taylor AN. Occupational asthma in a factory making flux-cored solder containing colophony. Thorax 1981; 36:828–834.

164. Weill H, Salvaggio JE, Neilson A, Butcher B, Ziskind M. Respiratory effects of toluene diisocyanate manufacture: a multidisciplinary approach. Environ Health Perspect 1975; 11:101–108.

165. Malo JL, Cartier A, L'Archevêque J, Trudeau C, Courteau JP, Bhérer L. Prevalence of occupational asthma among workers exposed to eastern white cedar. Am J Respir Crit Care Med 1994; 150:1697–1701.

166. Reijula K, Haahtela T, Klaukka T, Rantanen J. Incidence of occupational asthma and persistent asthma in young adults has increased in Finland. Chest 1996; 110:58–61.

167. Blanc P. Occupational asthma in a national disability survey. Chest 1987; 92:613–617.

168. Timmer S, Rosenman K. Occurrence of occupational asthma. Chest 1993; 104:816–820.

169. Blanc PD, Cisternas M, Smith S, Yelin E. Occupational asthma in a community-based survey of adult asthma. Chest 1996; 109:56S–57S.

4

Genetics and Occupational Asthma

Anthony J. Newman Taylor
Imperial College School of Medicine at the National Heart and Lung Institute, London, England

INTRODUCTION

Many common diseases such as asthma and diabetes mellitus cluster in families. The risk of developing the disease, if a first-degree relative is affected, is 5–10%, greater than the prevalence of the disease in the population, but less than the 25% risk for a recessive and 50% risk for a dominant single-gene disorder. The familial clustering is not due to a single gene defect, but is the outcome of multiple genes (polygenic) and their interaction with the environment.

Genetic variation between individuals, such as differences in blood groups, are widespread in the population. Such variants, whose frequency is stable between generations, are known as *polymorphisms*. Polymorphisms are the basis of diversity within human populations and contribute not only to differences in characteristics such as height and blood pressure, but also to variation in the ability to resist infection and handle environmental challenges. Such challenges include the response to agents inhaled at work, both inorganic and organic. Differences between individuals in their responses are likely to be determined, at least in part, by the functional consequences of polymorphisms of relevant genes, and their interactions with each other.

The techniques of molecular genetics provide the opportunity to identify relevant genetic polymorphisms. However, it is important to appreciate that in a multifactorial disease such as occupational asthma, a single polymorphism, although increasing susceptibility to the development of asthma in those exposed to a particular agent, is unlikely to be sufficient alone, and may not even be necessary, to cause the disease. Polymorphic genes may increase susceptibility or resistance to a disease but do not determine it. The identification of a single polymorphic gene is therefore unlikely alone to provide the basis for a screening test for susceptibility to occupational asthma. Knowledge of the genes involved, the function of their protein products, and of their interaction with the relevant environmental influences does, however, have the potential to illuminate disease mechanisms of the disease at the molecular level and provide new opportunities to treat and prevent it.

THE IMPORTANCE OF WELL-DEFINED PHENOTYPES IN GENETIC STUDIES

The genetic constitution of an organism is its *genotype;* the physical expression of the genotype, as either an observable characteristic or protein product, is its *phenotype.* Mendel inferred the patterns of inheritance in sweet peas by studying the transmission of pairs of clearly contrasted physical characteristics (phenotypes) such as tallness versus shortness of the plant, green versus yellow, and round versus wrinkled seeds. Similar patterns of inheritance can be inferred for human diseases such as cystic fibrosis. In such Mendelian disorders, genotype and phenotype (the observable characteristics of the disease) correspond (one gene, one protein). In common diseases such as asthma and diabetes, this correspondence is not observed either because the same phenotype (e.g., asthma) is associated with different genotypes (genetic heterogeneity) or the same genotype is associated with different phenotypes, because of interaction with other genes, with environmental factors, or both.

Genetic studies of disease in humans require an unequivocal definition of phenotype. This implies diagnostic criteria that are comprehensive (i.e., high sensitivity with few false negatives) and exclusive (high specificity with few false positives) to minimize misclassification bias. Genetic studies of atopy and asthma have been considerably impeded by the lack of widely accepted diagnostic criteria. Asthma is usually defined as reversible airway narrowing whose characteristic symptoms are episodic wheeze and breathlessness. However, all that wheezes is not asthma and not all asthma wheezes; furthermore, cases of asthma may not have demonstrable reversibility at the time of testing. Another defining characteristic of asthma is airway hyperresponsiveness, an increased responsiveness of the airways to nonspecific provocative stimuli such as exercise, inhaled cold air, or histamine. Airway hyperresponsiveness, however, although sensitive, is not a specific characteristic of asthma, being found in some 15% of the population. These problems make a comprehensive and exclusive definition of asthma difficult. Similarly atopy, which was defined by Pepys as the propensity to make IgE antibody in response to allergens encountered in everyday life, has been identified by different investigators as one, or two, or more immediate skin test responses to common inhalant allergens, an elevated total IgE in serum, or the presence of specific IgE antibody in serum to one or more common inhalant allergens. In their genetic studies, Cookson and Hopkins decided on a comprehensive case definition that included one or more of any of these three (1); in contrast, others have focused on the inheritance of total IgE. These difficulties and differences in case definition have made genetic studies of asthma and atopy difficult both to undertake and to compare the findings of different studies.

GENETIC BASIS OF ASTHMA

Asthma and atopy show clear indications of genetic susceptibility: the frequency of disease in family members of cases is greater than in the population as a whole, and is greater in identical, monozygotic (MZ), than in nonidentical, dizygotic (DZ), twins.

Family Studies

Genetic susceptibility is suggested if a disease occurs in greater frequency in the family members of a case than in the general population. The relative risk (λR) is the risk of a disease for the relative of an affected individual divided by the risk (prevalence) of the disease in the general population. λo and λs are the ratios for offspring and sibs to the population prevalence. The size of λR is taken to indicate the degree of concordant inheritance of genetic factors in affected relative pairs.

First-degree relatives—parents, brothers, sisters, and children—have half their genes in common with the index case (or proband). Second-degree relatives—grandparents, aunts, uncles, nephews, and nieces—have one-quarter of their genes in common. The most commonly reported value is for λs, but sibs usually also share a common childhood environment and λs > 1 may reflect a shared environment as well as a shared inheritance. An increased frequency of disease in second-degree relatives may therefore be a more reliable indication of genetic influences although λR will be lower in second- than in first-degree relatives. The value of λs for cystic fibrosis is about 500, for insulin-dependent diabetes 15, and for schizophrenia 8.5. The value for asthma probably lies between 2 and 5.

Several family studies have provided evidence that asthma and associated atopic disease—eczema and hay fever—are more frequent in the relatives of asthmatics than in the relatives of matched controls. Sibbald estimated that the population frequency of asthma was between 5 and 10%. The probability of a child of an atopic asthmatic parent having asthma varied from 14% when one parent was affected to 29% when both parents were affected (2). The risk for the child of a nonatopic asthmatic parent was little greater than the population frequency. Atopy increased the risk of a child developing asthma some threefold. Similarly, Jenkins et al. found the risk of asthma and associated atopic diseases in 7-year-old Tasmanian children was greater when one or both parents were asthmatic than when neither was affected (3). The risk of having asthma was increased some 2.5 times when either parent had asthma and 6.7 times when both parents had asthma.

Twin Studies

Twin studies, which compare the concordance of disease in identical (MZ) twins, who are genetically identical, and nonidentical (DZ) twins, who, like other sibs, share half their genes, can better disentangle genetic from environmental influences than family studies. Assuming the effect of a shared familial environment is the same for MZ and DZ twins, the frequency of a disease with no genetic component will be similar in MZ and DZ twins. A disease influenced by genetic factors will be more frequent in MZ than DZ twins; the larger the difference, the more likely that genetic factors are important in the development of the disease. The results of twin studies of multifactorial diseases can be expressed as "hereditability"—the proportion of the total variation of the phenotype due to genetic factors.

Twin studies have consistently shown the concordance of asthma to be higher between MZ than DZ twins. In a study of 7000 Swedish twin pairs Edfors-Lub (4) found the concordance of asthma between MZ twins was 19% and of DZ twins was 4.8% giving an estimated hereditability of some 15%. More recent twin studies have reported higher estimates for the hereditability of asthma. Hopper et al. (5) estimated an hereditability of 50% in a study of 3808 Australian twins. Harris et al. (6) in a study of 5684 Norwegian twins found that the risk of developing asthma in twins whose cotwin had a history of asthma (as compared to those whose cotwin did not) was increased 18-fold in MZ twins and 2.3-fold in DZ twins.

Hanson et al. (7) studied MZ and DZ twins reared together and apart. They found a greater concordance for asthma and specific IgE (estimated by skin test and RAST) in

MZ than DZ twins both when reared together and apart. Although the number of twins in the study was relatively small, the implications of its findings are considerable, suggesting a substantial genetic influence on the development of specific IgE and asthma, with little contribution from familial environment shared in childhood.

Twin studies indicate that asthma has an inherited component, but do not identify its mode of inheritance. This is usually addressed by segregation analysis in family studies in which the recurrence of asthma is determined in terms of the degree of genetic relatedness to the index case (or proband). Families studied may be nuclear (which include only first-degree relatives of the probands) or extended (which include more distant relatives and usually encompass three or more generations).

The results of such studies have been conflicting. Some have suggested that asthma is inherited as an autosomal dominant characteristic with incomplete penetrance; i.e., a single gene is responsible for asthma but not all who inherit it develop asthma (8,9). Cookson and Hopkins found that 90% of atopic asthmatics had an atopic parent and suggested a dominant mode of inheritance for atopy (1).

Others have suggested the inheritance of asthma is polygenic (10) implying asthma is the outcome of an interaction between several genes. In part these apparently striking different findings reflect differences in methods of ascertainment and phenotype definition, but probably also reflect considerable heterogeneity in the inheritance of atopy and asthma.

MOLECULAR GENETICS

Modern molecular techniques have provided the opportunity to disentangle the difficulties in genetic analysis of complex traits caused by factors such as genetic heterogeneity and polygenic inheritance. These studies are allowing identification of the genes that contribute to the development of multifactorial diseases such as asthma. The ultimate purpose of such investigations is to determine the protein products of the relevant genes, their functions, and how these differ from the protein products of those not at increased risk of disease. Understanding the biochemical basis of diseases such as diabetes, schizophrenia, and asthma should offer insights of therapeutic and preventive value.

Two complementary approaches have been taken: *genetic linkage* and investigation of *candidate genes*.

Genetic Linkage

The opportunity for human genetic linkage studies has been provided by recognition of the naturally occurring variation in human DNA sequences (on average individuals differ every 200–500 base pairs) and the identification of a large number of polymorphic markers spaced at short intervals along human chromosomes.

Genetic linkage is based on the simple principle that the closer the marker polymorphism to the gene of interest, the less likely is separation at meiosis and the more likely they are to be coinherited (linked). The genetic locus of a particular disease can be identified by the frequency of the coinheritance of the disease with a marker of known chromosomal location. If the genetic marker and the disease are unlinked (on a separate chromosome or far apart on the same chromosome), they are as likely to cosegregate as not, and the recombination fraction will be 50%, or 0.5. If the marker and disease locus are on the same chromosome, the shorter the distance between them, the less likely is crossing over during meiosis, the more likely are they to be inherited together and the fewer the recombinants. The recombination fraction will fall from 50% (reflecting independent assortment) toward ○ (reflecting tight linkage).

Initial linkage studies are undertaken in families with the disease, looking for cosegregation of a marker of known chromosomal location with the disease. Because of the large number of markers examined in a genome screen, any suggestive linkage needs to be replicated with more refined linkage mapping to identify a "candidate gene." DNA sequencing of the candidate gene allows identification of variations in the coding sequence (polymorphisms). Finally, population studies that investigate the degree of association between the polymorphism and the disease of interest allow estimation of the prevalence of the polymorphism and its contribution to disease frequency and severity.

This was the approach taken by the Oxford group in their investigation of the genetic basis of atopy. Having observed that 90% of atopic asthmatics had an atopic parent (1), a result they interpreted as indicating dominant inheritance, they undertook a linkage analysis within nuclear and extended families. They found significant linkage between a marker on chromosome 11q and atopy (11) (broadly defined as one or more skin prick test reactions, or specific IgE to common inhalant allergens, or an elevated serum total IgE), which they confirmed in a subsequent study of other Oxford families (12). Linkage was found to be primarily through maternal chromosomes (13). Because of its known location on chromosome 11q and plausible relevance to atopy, they postulated the β chain of the high-affinity IgE receptor (Fc ϵR 1-β) was the candidate gene (14). Subsequent sequence analysis identified two separate polymorphisms—Leu 181 and Leu 183—present either separately or together (15).

They subsequently studied a random population sample of the town of Busselton, in western Australia, and found the prevalence of the Leu 181/183 polymorphism was some 4.5%. All 13 children who had inherited the polymorphism from their mother were atopic and all but one had hay fever or asthma or both. In contrast, none of the eight who inherited the gene from their father was atopic, confirming maternal transmission of gene expression (16). A number of other studies failed to replicate these results (17,18), which was probably a reflection of the genetic heterogenicity of atopy and asthma.

Chromosome 5q has also been extensively investigated as it contains several candidate genes relevant to asthma and atopy. These include the IL-4 gene cluster, which contains IL-3, IL-4, IL-5, IL-9, IL-13, and GM-CSF, the β_2 adrenoceptor gene, and the corticosteroid receptor gene. Marsh and colleagues studied 170 individuals from 11 Amish families in the United States and found significant linkage with total IgE for five markers within the 5q 31.1 region but not for three markers lying just outside this region (19). Postma and colleagues studied the children and grandchildren of 84 Dutch probands with asthma. They found coinheritance of increased levels of total IgE with airway hyperresponsiveness and linkage of airway hyperresponsiveness with several markers on chromosome 5q (20).

These studies suggest polymorphisms of candidate genes on chromosome 5q are probably contributing to the development of asthma and atopy, but in the absence of defined polymorphisms it is difficult to estimate their prevalence in the population and the size of their contribution to the development or severity of disease.

Candidate Genes—MHC Proteins

The second parallel approach, applicable when the biochemical basis of the disease is understood, is to seek polymorphisms of the genes encoding for proteins of known function, which may be relevant to disease mechanism. The considerable knowledge of the cellular and molecular mechanisms of asthma, both the TH2 lymphocyte response and associated eosinophilic bronchitis, provides a remarkable array of plausible candidate genes. Investigations reported to date, particularly those relevant to occupational asthma, have investigated the association of asthma and specific IgE antibody with the highly polymorphic genes encoding the major histocompatibility (MHC) proteins, also known in humans as human leukocyte antigens (HLA), which play a central role in the immune recognition of foreign proteins.

MHC molecules are expressed as heterodimers on the cell surface. Foreign peptides, derived from within the cell by the degradation of endogenous or exogenous proteins, are bound in the groove of the MHC molecule and are expressed as an MHC-peptide complex, which is recognized in a very specific way by the T-cell receptor (TCR) on the surface of T lymphocytes. This trimolecular complex of [MHC protein-foreign peptide (epitope), TCR] is at the center of immune recognition and response. MHC proteins are divided into two classes: MHC I and MHC II. MHC class I proteins (HLA -A, B, and C antigens in humans) are expressed on the surface of all cells; MHC class II (HLA-DR, DP, and DQ antigens in humans) proteins are expressed on the surface of antigen-presenting cells, such as dendritic cells, B lymphocytes, macrophages, and some epithelial cells. MCH class I proteins present endogenous peptides that are in the main recognized by CD8+ (cytotoxic) T lymphocytes; MHC class II proteins present exogenous peptides that are recognized by CD4+ (helper) T lymphocytes, although there are exceptions where class I–peptide complexes are "seen" by CD4+ cells and class II–peptides by CD8+ cells.

MHC proteins are encoded on the short arm of chromosome 6. HLA-A, B, and C each have one gene on each chromosome. HLA-DR has up to four genes and HLA-DP and DQ each have two genes encoding α and β chains, a total of 12 genes for the HLA system on each chromosome allowing a potential 24 different HLA types in any individual. HLA genes are also highly polymorphic with more than 200 variants of these 12 genes, which are numbered in sequence (e.g., HLA-A1, HLA-A2, HLA-A3, etc.) providing billions of potential combinations of the 200 genes, which are unique to each individual (other than identical twins, who share the same HLA type).

MHC proteins have evolved as a mechanism of self-defense against infective agents, which are themselves continually changing and adapting. HLA genes are reshuffled in each generation, and the constantly changing resistance this provides against infection has been proposed as the major evolutionary benefit of sex.

Because MHC proteins bind epitopes in the molecular groove (Bjorksten groove), created by the β-pleated sheet of the heterodimer, polymorphisms in the genome determine the capacity to bind specific epitopes and present them to T cells. Epitopes that are not presented will not activate (and therefore effectively bypass) the immune response.

Allergens and low-molecular-weight chemical haptens, which bind to host proteins, are taken up by dendritic cells and degraded into oligopeptides, which are bound in the groove of MHC II proteins, expressed on the cell surface, and recognized by CD4+ T lymphocytes possessing the relevant specific TCR. Variation in the immunological response to inhaled allergens and haptens may therefore be determined in part by differences in HLA type. For this reason, studies of the molecular genetics in occupational asthma have to date focused on searching for associations between MHC class II (HLA-DR, DP, and DQ) genes and the development of specific IgE antibody and asthma in those exposed to allergens and haptens in the workplace.

Before the advent of molecular techniques HLA typing was undertaken serologically. The ability to distinguish HLA types by molecular methods—probing with sequence specific oligonucleotides (SSOs) after amplification by polymerase chain reaction (PCR) or, more specifically, using sequence specific primers (SSPs)—has increased considerably the number of different HLA types recognized and the accuracy of their identification. In addition, knowledge of the amino acid sequence of different HLA molecules has allowed the identification of single amino acid substitutions in HLA molecules, which may be associated with susceptibility, or resistance, to a particular disease (see isocyanate-induced asthma and chronic beryllium disease below).

Studies of the associations of disease with a particular HLA haplotype have usually been made by comparing the frequency of the HLA haplotype in patients with the disease with the frequency in an appropriately matched referent group. The relative risk in the two groups can be expressed as an odds ratio and appropriate statistical tests applied. A significant association between the disease and HLA type may imply:

1. *Causal relationship.* The particular HLA type is a genetic determinant of the disease whose importance is reflected in the size of the odds ratio. An odds ratio in excess of 100 (e.g., ankylosing spondylitis and HLA-B27) implies this is a major genetic determinant of the disease. Odds ratios of this size are rare and weaker associations more usual. In these circumstances, the contribution of the particular HLA to the disease, although real, may be of less importance than other genes or environmental factors. The effect of multiple gene polymorphisms, however, can be cumulative.

2. *Linkage disequilibrium.* This occurs when two genes occur together more frequently than would be expected by chance because of lack of genetic recombination between loci. This is particularly likely to occur with HLA polymorphisms, which can confer a selective advantage against infectious disease. For example HLA-A1 and B8 occur more frequently than would be expected by chance in North Europeans, possibly because this combination conferred protection against plague. An HLA type that is associated with a disease may therefore only be a marker for a polymorphism of another gene with which it is in linkage disequilibrium.

3. *Confounding.* The association of the disease with HLA type reflects the association of HLA type with a particular ethnic or geographical group that differs between the disease group and the referent group. As an illuminating example of such confounding, Lander and Schork highlighted the association of HLA-A1 with the ability to use chopsticks in the population of San Francisco, a relationship more likely to reflect the higher prevalence of this polymorphism in Chinese than Caucasians than immunological determinism of agility in handling chopsticks (21). Referent groups need to be matched with the disease group or be capable of adjustment for factors that may confound HLA relationships, which include social, geographical, and ethnic background.

4. *Overestimating the high probability of a chance association in multiple comparisons.* The majority of studies that have explored associations between HLA types and disease have been "fishing expeditions" undertaken without a specific prior hypothesis. The probability of an association occurring by chance among the multiple comparisons made with different HLA types is predictably high. This problem can be overcome in one or both of at least two ways.

   a. Applying Bonferroni's correction: the p value of each test is multiplied by the number (λ) of comparisons made ($p' = \lambda p$). For example, for a p value = 0.02, where five comparisons have been made, applying Bonferroni's correction: $p' = 5 \times 0.02 = 0.1$.

   b. The results of the fishing expedition are regarded as hypothesis generating, from which a specific hypothesis, informed by the results of the initial study, may be tested in a subsequent hypothesis-testing study in a second independent population.

OCCUPATIONAL ASTHMA

Investigation of the genetic influences and of genetic-environmental interactions in the development of asthma and atopy in the general community is beset by considerable difficulties. The problems of phenotype definition have already been described. In addition, there have to date been few identified polymorphisms associated with atopy or asthma. There is also a lack of accurate measures of exposure to relevant allergens in defined populations, necessary to assess exposure-response relationships and, from these, genetic-environmental interactions.

Occupational asthma overcomes many of these hurdles. Unambiguous case definition (phenotype) can be made on the basis of inhalation tests (for asthma) or serological tests for specific IgE or skin prick responses (for immunological sensitization). The disease occurs in identifiable and circumscribed populations in well-defined and measurable circumstances of exposure.

The great majority of reported cases of occupational asthma fulfill the criteria for a specific hypersensitivity response, implying the development of an immunological reaction to the responsible initiating agent. For most of the causes of hypersensitivity-induced occupational asthma there is accompanying evidence of specific IgE antibody. This implies specific activation of TH2 lymphocytes with IL-4 and IL-5 generation. Specific IgE antibody has been identified for all high-molecular-weight proteins and for some low-molecular-weight chemicals (e.g., acid anhydrides, complex platinum salts, and reactive dyes). However, asthma caused by low-molecular-weight chemicals, such as isocyanates and plicatic acid, have been accompanied by specific IgE antibody, at best inconsistently, in a minority of cases. Examination of the airway mucosa in bronchial biopsies from patients with asthma induced by isocyanates and plicatic acid, however, has shown the presence of activated lymphocytes and eosinophils, a pattern of cellular infiltration characteristic of asthma.

HLA and High-Molecular-Weight Allergens

HLA association studies are likely to be most fruitful when studying immunological responses or diseases initiated by proteins with a limited number of epitopes. HLA molecules bind to and present single epitopes to T lymphocytes. Multiple epitopes are likely to be expressed by different HLA molecules diluting the strength of any individual HLA-epitope associations that may be important in disease aetiology.

In their studies of the relationship of HLA types with specific IgE to purified short ragweed pollen allergens, Marsh and colleagues found the strongest associations with the low-molecular-weight allergens—HLA-DR 2.2 with specific IgE to Amb a V (22) and HLA-DR5 and Amb a V1 (23). The associations with high-molecular-weight allergens were weaker, probably reflecting the greater epitope density on high-molecular-weight proteins.

Possibly for this reason the majority of published studies of HLA associations in occupational asthma have been investigations of low-molecular-weight chemical sensitizers, which act as haptens and are probably a constituent of the epitope, potentially minimizing the number of epitopes, and therefore different HLA molecules, engaged in the immune response.

The few studies of occupational asthma caused by high-molecular-weight allergens have not found strong relationships. Two HLA association studies have been reported for laboratory animal allergy. One study found the prevalence of HLA-DR4 and B15 in 27 cases of laboratory animal allergy was about double that of normal controls, and of those drawn from the same workforce (24). In the other study Kerwin et al. reported HLA restriction of human T-lymphocyte responses from nine mouse-allergic patients to Mus m 1 (25). There was an excess of HLA-DR4, HLA-DR11 and HLA-DRW17 in the nine cases as compared to 100 controls tested in the same laboratory. Both studies included only a small number of cases and the first investigated the association of HLA with specific IgE to a complex mixture of high-molecular-weight protein allergens present in rat urine. Both studies need replication in a larger patient population with purified proteins and peptide fragments.

HLA and Low-Molecular-Weight Chemical Sensitizers

Low-molecular-weight chemical haptens have, at least in theory, the advantage for HLA association studies that if the haptens are a constituent part of the "foreign" epitope, the potential for dilution of association by multiple epitopes is diminished. Certainly the majority of association studies of HLA with the development of specific IgE or asthma have been reported for cases caused by low-molecular-weight chemicals.

Acid Anhydrides

Young et al. reported an association between HLA-DR3 and the presence of specific IgE antibody to albumin conjugates of trimellitic anhydride (TMA) but not the closely related phthalic anhydride (PA) (26). The 30 cases were chosen from acid anhydride workers identified from factory surveys or from clinical referrals as having specific IgE antibody to TMA, PA, or tetrachlorophthalic anhydride (TCPA). Twenty-eight (93%) of the workers had rhinitis, asthma, or both. The 30 referents were matched on type and duration of acid anhydride exposure to have allowed an at least equal opportunity for them to have developed specific IgE to anhydrides. Referents did not have specific IgE (identified by skin prick test or RAST) to acid anhydrides or symptoms of rhinitis or asthma. Referents were also matched on atopy and smoking habit.

The frequency of HLA-DR3 in cases and referents exposed to the three anhydrides is shown in Table 1. After correction for multiple comparisons HLA-DR3 was found significantly more frequently in the cases of TMA sensitization with an odds ratio of 16. Cases of PA sensitization, however, were no more likely to be HLA-DR3 positive than their referents. The proportion of TCPA cases who were HLA-DR3 positive (5/7) was similar to that of TMA (8/11) but unfortunately no referents were obtained for comparison.

Table 1 HLA-DR3 Frequency in Cases and Referents Exposed to the Acid Anhydrides TMA, PA, and TCPA

Acid anhydride exposure	Cases DR3+	Referents DR3+	Odds ratio	p
TMA	8/11	2/14	16	<0.05
PA	2/12	2/14		
TCPA	5/7	0/0		
Total	15/30 (50%)	4/28 (14%)		

Source: Ref. 26.

Table 2 Isocyanate-Induced Asthma and HLA-DQB1 *0501 and *0503

	Isocyanate asthma	Referents	RR	p
HLA-DQB1	(56)	(32)		
*0501	1 (2%)	5 (16%)	0.14	<0.03
*0503	7 (13%)	0 (0)	9.8	<0.04

Source: Ref. 27.

The results of the study suggested HLA type to be important in determining the development of specific IgE to TMA, possibly TCPA, but not PA. The study, however, had no specific prior hypothesis and the association of specific IgE to TMA with HLA-DR3 requires testing in another population.

Isocyanates (and Beryllium)

Isocyanate-induced asthma differs from the great majority of cases of acid-anhydride-induced asthma in the lack of a consistent accompaniment of specific IgE antibody. Although the explanation for the lack of specific IgE antibody to isocyanates may be technical, it suggests a possible difference in the nature of the immunological response underlying the development of isocyanate-induced asthma. Nonetheless, the finding of activated lymphocytes and eosinophils in bronchial biopsies from cases suggests an immunological basis for the disease.

Bignon and colleagues investigated HLA specificity in isocyanate-induced asthma and found an association of disease with HLA-DQB*0503 and an inverse relationship with HLA-DQB*0501 (27) (Table 2). In a subsequent study Balboni and colleagues confirmed these results in another population of isocyanate workers and observed that the amino acid in position 57 of HLA-DQB1 was aspartic acid in HLA-DQB1* 0503 and valine in HLA-DQB1*0501 (28) (Table 3). These observations suggested that the amino acid in residue 57 of HLA-DQB1 could be an important determinant of susceptibility to isocyanate sensitivity in exposed workforces.

Table 3 Isocyanate-Induced Asthma and HLA-DQB
Asp 57

HLA BAsp-57 haplotypes	Isocyanate asthma	Referents
	30	138
Asp-57-pos. homozygotes	17 (57%)	44 (32%)
Asp-57-neg. heterozygotes	12 (40%)	73 (53%)
Asp-57-neg. homozygotes	1 (3%)	21 (15%)

Source: Ref. 28.

The importance of a specific amino acid substitution in an HLA molecule in determining the ability of an individual to present a hapten has also been suggested by Richeldi and colleagues in relation to chronic beryllium disease (CBD) (29). CBD, a disease very similar in its clinical manifestations to sarcoidosis, is characterized by the presence of hypersensitivity granulomata and proliferation of T lymphocytes from blood and bronchoalveolar lavage when incubated with beryllium salts. Richeldi et al. demonstrated a strong association between the presence of glutamic acid in position 69 of the $\beta1$ chain of the HLA-DPB1 molecule and development of chronic beryllium disease in exposed workers. Thirty-one of 32 (97%) cases of CBD were HLA-DPB1* Glu 69 positive as compared to 27% of the 44 referents without CBD.

Complex Platinum Salts (and Beryllium Again)

Complex platinum salts, of which ammonium hexachloroplatinate (ACP) is the most important, are essential intermediates in platinum refining. ACP is a potent cause of asthma, which is associated with an immediate skin prick test response in the majority of cases.

In a case-referent study of the male workforce of a platinum refinery in South Africa, Lympany et al. found an excess of HLA-DR3 and a deficit of HLA-DR6 in skin-test-positive cases as compared to referents, matched on intensity and duration of exposure and ethnic background (30). Stratifying those employed into "high"- and "low"-exposure jobs, the relative risk of a case being HLA-DR3 positive or HLA-DR6 negative was markedly greater in the low- than in the high-exposure groups.

These results suggest that in those occupationally exposed to ACP, genetic susceptibility is an important determinant of the development of sensitization, and although the absolute risk of becoming a case was greater in the more heavily exposed, in those who were HLA-DR3 positive or DR6 negative the relative risk of becoming sensitized to ACP was markedly greater in those who had experienced exposures to ACP.

The other study that has investigated genetic environmental interactions is that reported by Richeldi et al. of the risks of developing CBD in a factory workforce exposed to beryllium, in relation to both intensity of exposure (using job title as a surrogate measure) and HLA-DPB1 Glu-69 (31) (Table 4). Six of 127 (4.7%) of those exposed to beryllium developed CBD, the majority of cases (5/6) occurring among the machinists in the high-exposure group (c.0.9 $\mu g/m^3$). Five cases occurred in the 41 HLA-DPB1 Glu-69-positive individuals (12.2%) and one case in the 86 HLA-DPB1 Glu-69-negative individuals (1.2%), a 10-fold increased risk for HLA-DPB1 Glu-69-positive individuals. Because the number in the study population was small, it is difficult to interpret genetic-environ-

Table 4 Beryllium Exposure

	Machinist (0.9 $\mu g/m^3$)	Nonmachinist (0.3 $\mu g/m^3$)	Total
HLA-DPB1			
Glu-69-pos.	4/16 (25%)	1/25 (4%)	5/41 (12.2%)
HLA-DPB1			
Glu-69-pos.	1/31 (3.2%)	0/55 (0%)	1/86 (1.2%)
Total	5/47 (10.6%)	1/80 (1.3%)	6/127 (4.7%)

Source: Ref. 31.

mental interactions with confidence, only one case of CBD occurring in a nonmachinist, who was HLA-DPB1 Glu-69-positive. The results, however, indicate an exposure-response relationship overall and in the Glu-69-positive group. In contrast to the findings in the ACP population the relative risk of developing CBD in Glu-69-positive individuals was greater at higher levels of exposure to beryllium.

Implications of HLA Associations

These HLA associations have clear biological implications. They provide substantial evidence for specific immunological response in the development of occupational asthma initiated by low-molecular-weight chemical sensitizers. This is of particular importance for isocyanate-induced asthma, where the absence of demonstrable specific IgE antibody has led to suggestions that the disease is not immunologically mediated. The clear evidence for HLA association, taken with the finding of infiltration by activated lymphocytes and eosinophils in bronchial biopsies, provides coherent evidence for an immunological mechanism. In the case of acid anhydrides and complex platinum salts, where there is evidence for an exposure-response relationship, modified particularly by smoking but also by atopy, the association of sensitization with HLA type identifies a further and important risk factor, whose magnitude may by analogy with ACP vary with level of exposure.

Genetic markers such as HLA polymorphisms hold out the hope that they will allow identification of susceptible individuals. However, to date, as with asthma caused by agents such as laboratory animals and platinum salts and atopy, the association is not sufficiently strong to be used as a discriminatory preemployment tool. In the best-studied, and only replicated, example of HLA-DPB1 Glu-69 and CBD, although 25–30% of the beryllium-exposed population were Glu-69-positive and the disease was virtually limited to Glu-69-positive individuals, only 12% of Glu-69-positive individuals developed disease. More than 85% (36/41) of exposed individuals who were Glu-69-positive did not develop CBD, suggesting that while HLA type has an influence on the development of the disease, other genetic and environmental factors are at least as important. One of these, described above, was intensity of exposure to beryllium, but even among machinists (the high-exposure group) only 10% overall and 25% who were Glu-69-positive developed CBD (or, expressed in the language of the racetrack, the odds of developing CBD in Glu-69-positive individuals in the high-exposure group was 3:1 against). Accurate prediction of individuals at risk of developing allergic lung disease, including occupational asthma, will have to await the identification of other relevant genetic polymorphisms, knowledge of which will need to be integrated into an understanding of exposure-response relationships, their modification by environmental (e.g., tobacco smoking) factors, and by the possibly varying influence of genetic susceptibility at different levels of exposure.

REFERENCES

1. Cookson WOCM, Hopkins JM. Dominant inheritance of atopic immunoglobulin responsiveness. Lancet 1988; 1:86–88.
2. Sibbald B. Genetic basis of asthma. Semin Respir Med 1986; 7:307–315.
3. Jenkins MA, Hopper JL, Flander LB, Carlin JB, Giles GG. The associations between childhood asthma and atopy and parental asthma, hay fever and smoking. Paediatr Perinat Epidemiol 1993; 7:67–76.
4. Edfors-Lub ML. Allergy in 7000 twin pairs. Acta Allergol 1971; 26:249–285.

5. Hopper JL, Hannah MC, Macaskill GT, Matthews JD. Twin concordance for a binary trait. III. A bivariate analysis of hay fever and asthma. Genet Epidemiol 1990; 7:277–299.
6. Harris JR, Magnus P, Samuelsen SO, Tambs K. No evidence for effects of family environment on asthma. A retrospective study of Norwegian twins. Am J Respir Crit Care Med 1997; 156: 43–49.
7. Hanson B, McGue M, Rortman-Johnson B, Segal NL, Bouchard TJ, Blumenthal MN. Atopic and immunoglobulin E in twins reared apart and together. Am J Hum Genet 1991; 48:873–879.
8. Cooke RA, Vander Veer A. Human sensitization. J Immunol 1996; 1:201–305.
9. Schwarz M. Heredity in Bronchial Asthma. Copenhagen: Munksgaard Press, 1952.
10. Sibbald B, Horn MC, Brain EA, Gregg I. Genetic factors in childhood asthma. Thorax 1980; 35:671–674.
11. Cookson WOCM, Sharp PA, Faux JA, Hopkin JM. Linkage between immunoglobulin E responses underlying asthma and rhinitis and chromosome 11q. Lancet 1989; 1:1292–1295.
12. Young RP, Sharp PA, Lynch JR, et al. Confirmation of genetic linkage between atopic IgE responses and chromosome 11q 13. J Med Genet 1992; 29:236–238.
13. Cookson WOCM, Young RP, Sandford AJ. Maternal inheritance of atopic IgE responsiveness on chromosome 11. Lancet 1992; 340:381–384.
14. Sandford AJ, Shirakawa T, Moffatt MF, et al. Localization of atopy and β subunit of high affinity IgE receptor (FCER1) on chromosome 11q. Lancet 1993; 341:332–334.
15. Shirakawa T, Airong L, Dubowitz M, et al. Associations between atopy and variants of the β subunit of the high affinity immunoglobulin E receptor. Nature Genet 1994; 7:125–130.
16. Hall J, Faux J, Ryan G, Hopkin J, Le Souf P, Musk A, Cookson WO. FCER1-β polymorphisms and risk of atopy in a general population sample. Br Med J 1995; 311:776–779.
17. Lympany P, Welsh KI, Cochrane GM, Kenemy DM, Lee TH. Genetic analysis of the linkage between chromosome 11q and atopy. Clin Exp Allergy 1992; 22:1085–1092.
18. Rich SS, Roitman Johnson B, Greenberg M, Roberts S, Blumenthal MN. Genetic analysis of atopy in three large kindreds: no evidence of linkage to D11S 97. Clin Exp Allergy 1992; 22: 1070–1076.
19. Marsh DG, Neely JD, Breazeale DR, Ghosh B, et al. Linkage analysis of IL4 and other chromosome 5q 31.1 markers and total serum IgE concentrations. Science 1994; 264:1152–1156.
20. Postma DS, Bleeker ER, Alemung PJ, et al. Genetic susceptibility to asthma—bronchial hyperresponsivenes coinherited with a major gene for atopy. N Engl J Med 1995; 333:894–900.
21. Lander ES, Schork NJ. Genetic dissection of complex traits. Science 1994; 265:2037–2048.
22. Maesg DG, Hsy SH, Roebber M, et al. HLA-DW1: a genetic marker for hyman immune response to short ragweed pollen allergen Ra5.1. Response resulting primarily from natural antigenic exposure. J Exp Med 1982; 155:1439–1451.
23. Marsh DG, Friedhoff LR, Ehrhick-Kautzky E, Bias WB, Roebber M. Immune responsiveness to *Ambrosia artemisi-ifolia* (short ragweed) pollen allergen Amba V1(Rae 6) is associated with HLA-DR5 in allergic humans. Immunogenetics 1987; 26:230–236.
24. Low B, Sjostedt L, Willirs S. Laboratory animal allergy—possible association with HLA B15 and DR4. Tissue Antigens 1988; 32:224–226.
25. Kerwin EM, Freed JH, Dresback JK, Rosenwagger LJ. HLA DR4 DRW 11 (15) and DR 17 (3) function as restriction elements for Mus m 1 allergic human T cells. J Allergy Clin Immunol 1993; 91:235.
26. Young RP, Barker RD, Pile KD, Cookson WOCM, Newman Taylor AJ. The association of HLA DR3 with specific IgE to inhaled acid anhydrides. Am J Respir Crit Care Med 1995; 151:219–221.
27. Bignon JS, Aron L, Ju Y, et al. HLA Class II alleles in isocyanates induced asthma. Am J Respir Crit Care Med 1994; 149:71–75.
28. Balboni A, Baricoidi OR, Fabbri LM, Gandini E, Ciaecia A, Mapp CE. Association between toluene diisocyanate induced asthma and DQB1 markers: a possible role for aspartic acid at position 57 . Eur Respir J 1996; 9:207–210.

29. Richeldi L, Sorrentino R, Saltini C. HLA-DPB1 glutamate 69: a genetic marker of beryllium disease. Science 1993; 262:242.

30. Lympany PA, Haris JM, Dowdeswell R, Cullinan P, du Bois RM, Newman Taylor AJ. Interaction of HLA phenotype and smoking with exposure in sensitisation to complex platinum slats. Am J Respir Crit Care Med 1997; 155(4 part II):A135.

31. Richeldi L, Kreiss K, Mroz MM, Zhen B, Tartoni P, Saltini C. Interaction of genetic and exposure factors in the prevalence of berylliosis. Am J Ind Med 1997; 32:337–340.

5
Pathophysiology

Leonardo M. Fabbri, Piera Boschetto, and Gaetano Caramori
University of Ferrara, Ferrara, Italy

Cristina Elisabetta Mapp
University of Padova, Padova, Italy

INTRODUCTION

Much of the significant progress in elaborating the complex pathophysiological pathways of asthma within the past 30 years can be attributed to collaborative interdisciplinary contributions of physiologists, pathologists, and immunologists/allergists. These students of the disease now agree that inflammation is the common denominator among the other pathological hallmarks of asthma. The complex cascade of events associated with asthmatic inflammation has, to a large extent, been demonstrated by study of immunological or allergic asthma utilizing bronchoalveolar lavage and new immunohistochemical methods for processing biopsies and, more recently, induced sputum. Some of these findings have been made using the model of occupational asthma. None of these advances would have been possible without access to sophisticated immunohistological and molecular biological technology.

Clinical, functional, and pathological alterations in occupational asthma are similar to those found in nonoccupational asthma. Airway smooth muscle contraction and mucosal edema are probably the main causes of acute airflow obstruction. Chronic airflow obstruction may be due to increase of airway wall thickness caused by accumulation of inflammatory cells, edema, hypertrophy of airway smooth muscles, subepithelial fibrosis, obstruction of airway lumina by exudate and/or mucus, and changes of mechanical properties of airway wall. Airway hyperresponsiveness, i.e., an excessive reaction to bronchoconstrictor stimuli, is the hallmark of both occupational and nonoccupational asthma. The pathogenesis of this airway hyperresponsiveness, which is generally long-lasting and poorly reversible, remains unknown. By contrast, the transient increase of airway responsiveness observed during exacerbations of occupational asthma most often seems to be associated with an acute inflammatory reaction in the airways. The pathological alterations of the airways in occupational asthma are characterized by infiltration of the airway mucosa by inflammatory cells, including eosinophils, mast cells, activated lymphocytes. Subepithelial fibrosis is an end result of the inflammatory cascade that is rather specific for asthma. The relationship between these pathological alterations and the clinical and functional features of asthma is only partially understood. In particular, the mechanisms of "induction" or sensitization by which many allergenic occupational agents cause asthma

81

parallel the events of nonoccupational IgE-mediated asthma. Induction mechanisms have not been well defined for other "nonallergic" low-molecular-weight agents.

Although the pathogenetic basis of occupational asthma is closely interwoven with previous and current research of natural-occurring asthma, several cogent features of occupational asthma provide an optimal milieu for enhancing the global understanding of asthma in general. First, both immunological (i.e., extrinsic) and nonimmunological (i.e., intrinsic) asthma occur in occupational settings, and occasionally both forms of asthma may be concurrent. Thus, similarities and/or differences of pathogenetic mechanisms between these major categories of asthma may be directly observed. Second, in the case of immunologically induced asthma, immunopathogenesis can be investigated through various phases of the immune response: onset of sensitization, the latent period, the elicitation episode(s), and the effect of repetitive elicitation. Similarly, the roles of epithelial cell injury, microvascular leakage, reflex, and pharmacologically mediated mechanisms can be explored in a systematic way. Finally, etiological and/or inciting agents can be more easily identified and characterized for clinical diagnostic purposes. This advantage is particularly noteworthy for industrial chemicals, as contrasted to non-work-related chemicals, which often cannot be distinguished or measured. Taken together, these special attributes confer unique advantages on occupational asthma as an immunopathogenetic model for non-work-related asthma.

Most of what we know of the mechanisms of asthma has been obtained from studies of nonoccupational asthma, as unfortunately not as many mechanistic studies have been performed in occupational asthma. In this chapter, we will therefore describe pathophysiological mechanisms involved in both nonoccupational and occupational asthma. We will also analyze these mechanisms with special emphasis on what can be learned from the similarities and the dissimilarities between nonoccupational and occupational asthma.

PATHOPHYSIOLOGICAL MECHANISMS COMMON TO NONOCCUPATIONAL ASTHMA AND OCCUPATIONAL ASTHMA

Acute and Chronic Airway Narrowing

Airway narrowing may be due to airway smooth muscle contraction, airway edema, accumulation of fluid in the airway lumen, or loss of elastic support from lung parenchyma (1). Airway smooth muscle contraction and mucosal edema are probably the main causes of acute airflow obstruction, whereas late asthmatic reactions are caused by accumulation of inflammatory cells and exudate in the airway walls and lumen (2). The relative proportion of airflow obstruction due to each mechanism remains to be established.

If exposure continues after diagnosis, both nonoccupational and occupational asthma subside only in a minority of subjects. Rather, it persists or may even deteriorate, as measured by tests of airway hyperresponsiveness and/or chronic airflow limitation (3–8). Interestingly, about 10% of non-occupational adult asthmatics spontaneously recover from asthma in 25 years (9).

Chronic airflow obstruction may be due to increase of airway wall thickness due to accumulation of inflammatory cells, edema, increased thickness of smooth muscle (1,2), subepithelial fibrosis, airway wall remodelling (10,11), obstruction of the airway lumen by exudate and/or mucus (2), and changes of elastic properties of the airway walls and/or loss of the interdependence between the airways and the surrounding parenchyma (1,12). In most asthmatic patients the hypertrophy of airway smooth muscle is more pronounced in the central airways, but in a subgroup of patients it is extended to peripheral bronchioles (13). Recent studies show that persistence of occupational asthma is associated with long-term airway inflammation, suggesting that once triggered, the inflammatory process in the airways may continue even without further exposure (14–16).

Airway Hyperresponsiveness

The principal feature that distinguishes asthmatic from normal airways is an excessive response to bronchoconstrictor stimuli, resulting in airway narrowing that far exceeds that which can be induced by the same stimuli in normal airways. Airway hyperresponsiveness to either methacholine or histamine is the hallmark of both occupational (17,18) and nonoccupational asthma (19). In subjects with occupational asthma, the degree of airways responsiveness to methacholine or histamine is usually, but not invariably, increased (20,21). Figure 1 illustrates the variability of peak expiratory flow rate (PEFR) and PD_{meth20} in a representative subject sensitized to toluene diisocyanate (TDI). It is noteworthy that both parameters decrease after occupational exposure. Similarly, although airway hyperresponsiveness to methacholine or histamine may be normal prior to the diagnosis of occupational asthma in the laboratory, it usually increases (i.e., a decrease in PD_{meth20}) after a positive inhalation challenge with a sensitizing agent, particularly in subjects who develop a late asthmatic reaction (22,23). Clinical investigations indicate that the increase in hyperresponsiveness may begin as early as 2 h after challenge with either large- or

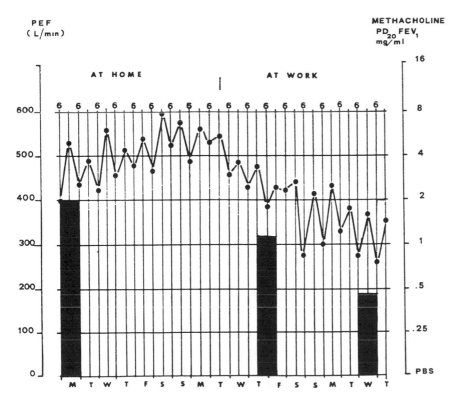

Figure 1   Daily variability of peak expiratory flow (PEF) and changes of $PD_{20}FEV_1$ in one subject with occupational asthma. Measurements were obtained during and after 1 week while the subject was at work and before, during, and after 1 week while the subject was not working.

small-molecular-weight sensitizing agents (24–26). The increase in airway responsiveness induced by sensitizing agents may last for days or even longer (6). Moreover, a decrease in PC_{meth20} may be the only residual effect of exposure to a sensitizing agent in a worker previously known to be sensitive to that agent (23). Taken together, these data suggest that airway hyperresponsiveness is one of the most important sequelae of occupational asthma even if its significance in nonoccupational asthma remains questionable (27,28). Indeed, Josephs et al. showed that variations in airway hyperresponsiveness does not parallel changes in asthma severity, and that it may not be a valuable marker of severity for monitoring of asthma (27).

Workers with occupational asthma often demonstrate airway hyperresponsiveness even when they are asymptomatic. Their airway hyperresponsiveness, present during asymptomatic stages of the disease, seems to be long-lasting and only partly or nonreversible even after treatment (4,6–8). The pathogenesis of such long-lasting, poorly reversible, nonspecific airway hyperresponsiveness in occupational asthma remains unknown. By contrast, the transient increase of airway hyperresponsiveness occurring during or after asthmatic reactions induced by a specific inhalation laboratory challenge seems to be associated with an acute inflammatory reaction in the airways (29,30). An exception to the association with inflammation is the report of Durham et al. (26), who observed increases in histamine-induced airway responsiveness 2–3 h after challenges with various occupational agents, prior to the main cellular inflammatory response in the airways. A similar observation had been reported after challenge with high-molecular-weight allergens (24,25).

Specific Airway Hyperresponsiveness to Allergens and Sensitizing Agents

The specific inhalation challenge is considered to be the gold standard for the confirmation of occupational asthma (31) (see Chapter 12). Inhalation challenges with occupational agents may cause early, progressive, dual, or late asthmatic reactions.

Dual, late, and even some early asthmatic reactions induced by sensitizing agents are associated with increased hyperresponsiveness to methacholine and/or histamine (22,24,25,32). Such increase of airway hyperresponsiveness seems to be specifically related to the response to the allergenic challenge because it is not observed in normal subjects or in nonsensitized asthmatic patients (22). The cellular and biochemical events responsible for the different types of reactions will be discussed in other sections of this chapter.

MECHANISMS OF OCCUPATIONAL ASTHMA

Similar to non-work-related asthma, the signals that initiate and perpetuate occupational asthma are highly variable depending on the agent and the extent of exposure. Large- and some small-molecular-weight substances typically induce Th2 cytokine/IgE-dependent allergic (atopic) asthma while some chemicals (e.g., polyisocyanates, plicatic acid) may induce asthma in nonatopic individuals through mechanisms which are independent of classic IgE-mediated pathways (see Chapter 30). In non-work-related asthma, it has been postulated that expression of Th2 cytokines, C-C chemokines, and IgE are similar in atopic and nonatopic forms of asthma (33–37). However, nonatopic asthma appears to have increased numbers of monocytes/macrophages, increased submucosal infiltration by CD68+ cells, and up-regulation of the granulocyte-macrophage colony-stimulating factor

(GM-CSF) receptors on CD68+ cells (38–40). Although these sophisticated similarities and dissimilarities have not yet been fully explored in occupational asthma, new data concerning the roles of genetic predisposition and immunological mechanisms in occupational asthma have been reported.

Genetic Aspects

Occupational asthma induced by high- and some small-molecular-weight agents is often mediated by the Th2 cytokine/IgE cascade and is more frequent in atopic subjects. Genetic research concerning atopic linkages with atopy have included reports of allelic polymorphisms associated with genes encoding the β-subunit of the high-affinity IgE receptor, regulatory cytokines [i.e., IL-3, IL-4, IL-5, IL-9, IL-10, IL-12 β-chain, IL-13, and GM-CSF], the β_2-adrenergic receptor, and the IL-4α receptor (41). In addition, weak associations between susceptibility or resistance to asthma occurring after exposure to large- and some small-molecular-weight agents (e.g., diisocyanates) and HLA class II and/or T cell receptor genes have been described (42–48). These are discussed extensively in Chapter 4. By contrast, an association between isocyanate-induced asthma and HLA class II genes was not found in 2 other studies (49,50). This discrepancy may reflect differences in diagnostic criteria for isocyanate-induced asthma and in control populations.

Immune Aspects

Basic Principles

Functionally, the immune system is separable into antibody and cellular arms. Specific humoral antibodies are produced and secreted by B cells, while T lymphocytes modulate B-cell function by helper and suppressor functions, modulate delayed hypersensitivity responses, and mediate several types of cellular cytotoxicity.

The initiation of the immune response is well established. A pivotal step in the generation of an immune response is the activation of T cells by recognition of antigen, which is presented on the surface of accessory cells (51–53). T cells can only recognize soluble antigens that have been processed by accessory (antigen-presenting) cells (i.e., macrophages, dendritic cells, B cells, and epithelial cells) in a groove of the major histocompatibility gene complex (MHC) molecule (52–55). Accessory cells have three major properties: (1) processing antigen; (2) facilitating the binding of processed antigen to intracytoplasmic MHC molecules, which subsequently migrate to and are expressed on their cell surfaces; and (3) elaborating and secreting IL-1, a major T-cell-stimulatory cytokine (Fig. 2). Helper CD4+ T cells recognize antigen bound to class II MHC molecules while suppressor/cytotoxic CD8+ cells recognize antigen bound to class I MHC molecules. Critical cells for airway sensitization are antigen-presenting cells, particularly dendritic cells present in the airway epithelium. These cells capture allergens through high (Fc$_\varepsilon$RI) or low (Fc$_\varepsilon$RII) affinity receptors, process them, and, after migrating to local lymph nodes, present selected peptide epitopes of these allergens in the groove of MHC class II surface molecules to the T-cell receptor of CD4+ T cells. High affinity IgE receptors (FC$_\varepsilon$RI) on lung dendritic cells may play a direct role in allergen uptake. The cytokine milieu may determine whether ThO cell differentiation is biased toward a Th1 or Th2 response with IL-12 production leading to Th1 and IL-4 to Th2 phenotypes, respectively. The presence of a co-stimulatory molecule (B7-2) on an APC interacting with CD28 as a second "signal" could bias CD4+ cells toward the Th2 phenotype.

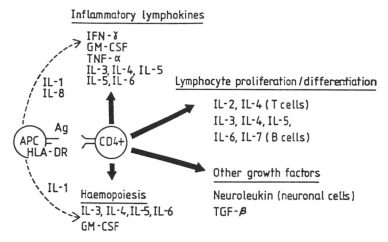

Figure 2 Current concept of the antigen presentation and the cascade of cellular events that follow the interaction between antigen-presenting cells and T cells.

In mice two distinct phenotypic subsets of CD4+ T lymphocytes have been characterized on the basis of their respective profiles of cytokine production: both secrete IL-3 and GM-CSF, but one subset, Th1, produces IL-2, which stimulates T-lymphocyte and macrophage proliferation, and interferon-γ (IFN-γ), which inhibits B-cell activation and IgE synthesis (56–58). Th1 cells are also believed to be responsible for delayed-type hypersensitivity reactions and IgG2 immune responses in mice. The other subset (Th2) produces and secretes IL-4, IL-5, IL-9, IL-10, and IL-13 but not IL-2 and IFN-γ, and supports IgE production (59,60). These cells are believed to be responsible for IgE-mediated type of hypersensitivity reactions. Direct phenotypic correlates of murine Th1 and Th2 CD4+ T lymphocytes have not yet been conclusively shown in humans. However, there is an increased proportion of functionally equivalent Th2-like lymphocytes, many of which also express CD30 surface protein, in peripheral blood and tissues of atopic subjects (58). As these cells secrete IL-4 and IL-5, it is postulated that they may play an important regulatory role in both IgE production and eosinophil recruitment/activation at the tissue level (56–60). In genetically susceptible individuals, antigen presentation to naive (ThO) CD4+ T cells shift them to a Th2-like cell with the capacity to secrete cytokines encoded by the IL-4/IL-5/IL-9/IL-13 gene cluster present in the long arm of chromosome 5. Isotype switching to specific IgE occurs when B-cell-processed allergen interacts with specific Th2-like T cells, a process promptly enhanced by accessory molecule amplifiers (CD40/CD40L and CD28/B7.2), which induce a high rate of secretion of IL-4 and IL-13 and subsequent downstream signaling via the STAT 6 transcription factor (61).

After activation by antigen, T lymphocytes secrete a number of cytokines that attract, activate, and promote growth and differentiation of other leukocytes (see Fig. 2). In this sense, activated CD4+ T cells are inflammatory cells in their own right as well as helper cells for production of humoral antibodies by B cells (56–58). The induction of allergen sensitization, followed by repeated exposure to the same allergen, is responsible for the amplification of the Th2-like response, with production and release of the inflammatory cytokines, particularly IL-3, IL-4, IL-5, IL-9, IL-13, GM-CSF, and β-chemokines responsible for the characteristic chronic eosinophilic airway inflammation present in asthma as well as IgE isotype switching as described above (62–66). In parallel, allergen may trigger airway inflammation through the crosslinking of surface IgE on mast cells, resulting in the release of inflammatory mediators that contribute to initiation and perpetuation of the inflammatory cascade through a separate pathway (57,58,66) (see Fig. 2). Thus, activated T cells could initiate and propagate allergic inflammation of the airways and thus participate directly in the pathological events responsible for asthma exacerbations.

Antibody-Dependent Hypersensitivity

Many occupational sensitizers, particularly high-molecular-weight proteins and vegetable gums, are believed to act through an IgE-mediated reaction (Fig. 3; see Chapter 7). According to this mechanism, inhaled allergenic agents crosslink specific IgE on the surface of mast cells, basophils, and probably macrophages, eosinophils, and platelets. High-molecular-weight agents act as complete antigens and are therefore capable of crosslinking surface-bound IgE. However, low-molecular-weight chemicals must first react with autologous or heterologous proteins to produce a complete allergen. The specific reaction between allergen and IgE gives rise to the cascade of events that is responsible for inflammatory cell activation with subsequent synthesis and/or release of a wide variety of preformed and newly formed inflammatory mediators, which then orchestrate the inflam-

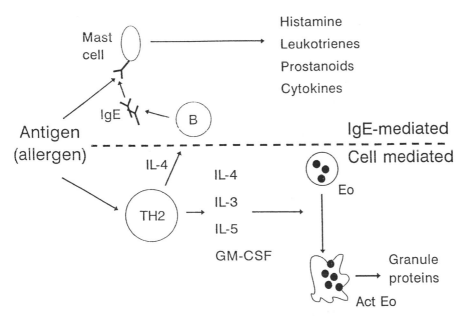

Figure 3 Inflammatory mechanisms in asthma. Activation of Th2 CD4+ T-LC by specific antigen (such as allergens) results in the secretion of cytokines, particularly IL-5, IL-4, IL-3, and GM-CSF, which induce specific eosinophil accumulation and activation (Eo, Act Eo). β Chemokines may also play a role. In parallel, allergens may trigger inflammatory processes through the cross-linking of surface IgE on mast cells, resulting in the release of mediators such as histamine and leukotrienes. The relative importance of these processes in asthmatic and allergic inflammation in different clinical settings remains to be determined. The two systems are interdependent in the sense that IL-4 derived from Th2 T-LC is essential for IgE switching by B-LC (B), and thus mast cell sensitization, whereas IL-4 release from IgE-triggered mast cells may further promote Th2 T-LC development. Th, T helper, IL, interleukin; GM-CSF, granulocyte macrophage colony-stimulating factor; IgE, immunoglobulin E.

matory reaction (67,68). Although other classes of antibodies have been hypothesized to have a role in asthma, substantive evidence for their participation is not available. The potential role of humoral antibody mechanics can be investigated in humans by in vivo skin tests and in vitro [e.g., radioallergosorbent (RAST), CAP®, Magic Lite®, Maxisop®, EAST®, or ELISA] tests (69,70) (see Chapter 7).

Antibody Studies in Occupational Asthma

Most occupational asthma studies have concentrated on antibody-mediated immunity. These consist of surveys using skin and/or in vitro antibody tests. Positive skin and specific immunoglobulin (IgE, IgG) tests have been shown to be present mainly in atopic subjects sensitized to high-molecular-weight proteins, vegetable gums, and polysaccharides (69), but also in some subjects sensitized to low-molecular-weight chemical agents (e.g., acid anhydride compounds, platinum salts, nickel, diisocyanates, plicatic acid) (71–74). Positive skin tests against animal allergens, cereal flours, egg white antigens, enzymes derived from animals and plants, coffee, castor beans, and other high-molecular-weight agents may be found both in symptomatic and in some asymptomatic exposed workers (75–78). However, positive skin or RAST tests may harbinger respiratory sensitization, and skin test–positive asymptomatic patients should be monitored carefully by routine tests of pulmonary function or airway hyperresponsiveness. Skin prick tests against some high-molecular-weight proteins (e.g., detergent enzymes, egg white antigens) are specific and/or sufficiently sensitive for the identification of occupational asthma in enzyme workers and egg processors (79,80). No special diagnostic or pathogenetic information is gained by the presence of specific IgG subclass antibodies (particularly the IgG4 reagin), which are equally distributed between exposed symptomatic and asymptomatic subjects (81,82).

Specific IgG antibodies are present in some subjects sensitized to diisocyanates, primarily in subjects with a positive inhalation challenge (73). However, specific IgG antibodies are also present in exposed workers with no history of asthma and negative inhalation challenges. Interestingly, despite the low proportion of diisocyanate-specific IgE serum antibody reactions, recent studies have revealed that when present, they are specific but not sensitive diagnostic markers for OA (73,83).

In contrast to the variability of immune responsiveness in diisocyanate-exposed workers, investigations of acid anhydride–induced asthma have revealed that IgE-mediated immune responses may play a major role in the development of asthma (90). This may be due to the fact that various compounds in this class of chemicals [phthalic anhydride (PA), trimellitic anhydride (TMA), himic anhydride (HA), hexahydrophthalic anhydride (HHPA), tetrachlorophthalic anhydride (TCPA), and methyl tetrahydrophthalic anhydride (MTHPA)] readily form highly allergenic epitopes after conjugation with body proteins. Cutaneous puncture tests with these reagents also have exhibited good diagnostic sensitivity (84). RAST cross-inhibition studies using sera of PA-, HHPA-, and HA-sensitized workers have demonstrated that antibody responses are heterogeneous. In some workers, specific IgE responses are directed primarily against the haptenic ligand (i.e., PA, HA) while in others IgE antibodies are directed against new antigenic determinants with no evidence of hapten specificity (85). Some TMA-exposed workers develop late respiratory and systemic symptoms that are associated with elevated serum specific IgG antibodies to TMA-HSA (86). A few workers exposed to high concentrations of TMA fumes develop pulmonary hemorrhage and hemolytic anemia in association with high levels of IgG antibody (presumably type 2–cytotoxicity-mediating antibody) to TMA-HSA (87–89).

A special role for IgE-mediated immunopathogenesis has been demonstrated in workers exposed to chlorinated platinum salts. These workers exhibit positive prick tests to very dilute concentrations of these salts (91–95). Specific IgE tests also correlate with clinical respiratory symptoms (94).

From the previous discussion, it is apparent that the presence of specific IgE antibodies may be highly diagnostic and prognostic in the case of high-molecular-weight allergens and some low-molecular-weight chemicals such as acid anhydrides and platinum salts. Under other circumstances, either specific IgE or IgG antibodies may be useful adjuncts in association with pulmonary function tests in following the evolutionary course of immunologically mediated asthma (90). Finally, when IgG antibodies (i.e., MDI) and in some cases IgE antibodies (i.e., plicatic acid) are present in both symptomatic and asymptomatic workers, their sole value may be as biological markers of exposure.

IgE-Independent Cellular Immune Responses in Occupational Asthma

IgE-dependent mechanisms may not explain all the manifestations of nonatopic (intrinsic) or some forms of chemical-induced occupational asthma (e.g., toluene diisocyanate, western red cedar). Thus, Walker et al. reported more pronounced activation of peripheral blood CD4+, CD8+, and memory T cells as well as high concentrations of IL-5, but not IL-4, in bronchoalveolar lavage fluid (BAL) of intrinsic asthmatic patients (96). Concordant with these results were the findings of Maestrelli et al., who observed that the majority of T-cell clones derived from patients with TDI-induced asthma were CD8+ and capable of producing IL-5 (97). Frew et al. demonstrated that plicatic acid stimulated T lymphocytes produced IL-5 and IFN-γ, a pattern that is compatible with a nonatopic profile but still capable of inducing an eosinophilic inflammatory response (98). Other examples of chemical-induced asthma associated with non-IgE-independent, cellular immune responses have been observed (99–101). Repetitive antigenic stimulation of diisocyanate asthmatic peripheral blood mononuclear cells in tissue culture revealed that these cells synthesized tumor necrosis factor alpha (TNF$_\alpha$), a non-IgE-dependent proinflammatory cytokine, and the C-C chemokine, mononuclear chemoattractant protein-1 (MCP-1), but not IL-4 or IL-5 (102). None of the above studies had addressed the possibility that local bronchial mucosal IgE-mediated processes could be involved in the absence of systemic IgE, as has been postulated to occur in nonoccupational intrinsic asthma (39). This pathogenetic possibility could be particularly germane in those occupational syndromes where systemic immune mechanisms have either not yet been (e.g., colophony, secondary and tertiary amines, vanadium) or may never be demonstrated (i.e., RADS).

Structure-Function Aspects of Low-Molecular-Weight Sensitizers

The role of halides in conferring allergenicity to chemicals such as platinum salts and chlorohexidine was first cited by Cleare et al. and Layton et al. (91,103). Other unique chemical structure-activity relationships of haptenic allergenicity have been studied extensively and revealed that chemical structure may determine the degree of IgE-mediated sensitization (104). These and other investigations have led to the development of a computer-assisted model of chemical structure as a basis of predicting human allergenicity in workers exposed to these compounds (105). Rodent animal models are also being explored as predictors of human sensitization (see Chapter 6).

PATHOLOGICAL FEATURES OF OCCUPATIONAL ASTHMA

There is overwhelming evidence, as demonstrated by sputum cellular histology, BAL, bronchial biopsies, surgical specimens, and postmortem lung tissue, that chronic inflammation is the hallmark of asthma and that variations of clinical activity of asthma are associated with the degree and type of airway inflammation (65,66,106–109). Identical findings occur in occupational asthma. Airway inflammation in all variants of asthma is thought to account for airway hyperresponsiveness and other sequelae that result in airway limitation.

The pathology of several patients who died as a direct consequence of occupational asthma was remarkably similar to postmortem changes of nonoccupational asthma (110,111). Thus, in one of these fatal cases associated with diisocyanate exposure, there was marked epithelial desquamation, an extensive layer of collagen beneath the true basement membrane, and massive infiltration of inflammatory cells, particularly eosinophils (110). In addition, the lungs showed edematous airways plugged by mucus, inflammatory cells, and exudate. However, this was an extremely severe stage of the disease, and it is unclear to what extent these postmortem findings reflect the pathology of occupational asthma in living patients, especially those evaluated during periods of remission between asthma attacks.

Quantitative structural analysis of bronchial biopsies obtained from patients with occupational asthma induced by TDI showed an increased number of inflammatory cells as compared to biopsies of normal control subjects (117). It was also noted that eosinophils were increased in mucosal and submucosal layers while mast cells were increased only in the epithelium. Both cell types showed evidence of degranulation. In the immunochemistry survey of these specimens, both eosinophils and lymphocytes showed evidence of activation (112) (Fig. 4).

Interestingly, the intercellular spaces between basal epithelial cells were increased. This morphological finding is consistent with an abnormality of intercellular adhesion, which keeps basilar cells attached to each other and to columnar cells, thereby preventing epithelial desquamation, a characteristic feature of asthma (111–113). Glycoprotein adhesion molecules are also known to modulate the migration of inflammatory cells through endothelial intercellular spaces. Biopsy specimens also revealed that the thickness of the basement membrane was increased in the reticular layer. This phenomenon has been demonstrated to be due to the deposition of interstitial crosslinked collagens (types I, III, and V) produced by myofibroblasts (15,16,116) and not deposition of collagen IV, which is one of the specific components of the "true" basement membrane. This is true in both nonoccupational and occupational asthma (10,11,115,117). Similar results have been obtained in bronchial biopsies obtained from subjects sensitized to western red cedar (118). Somewhat different results have been obtained in biopsies from subjects who developed the reactive airways dysfunction syndrome after acute exposure to irritants: the airway epithelium is extensively damaged, the submucosa is infiltrated predominantly by mononuclear cells, and, more importantly, the subepithelial fibrosis is more evident with a thickness of the reticular layer of the basement membrane that can reach 30–40 μm (119) compared to 6–15 μm reported in isocyanate asthma and 3–8 μm in normal subjects (15,16,116) (see Chapter 30).

Although cessation of exposure is not always associated with clinical improvement of occupational asthma, there may be improvement at the histopathological level, as suggested by a decrease of the number of inflammatory cells in the airway mucosa, and by the reversal of the subepithelial fibrosis present at the time of diagnosis (14,16). Deposition

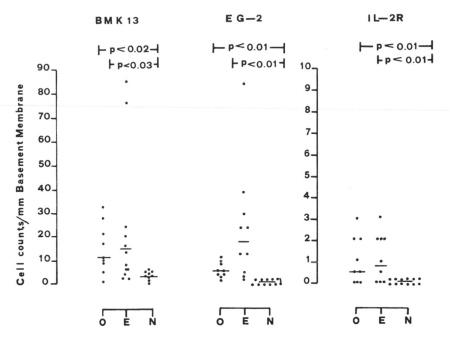

Figure 4 Cells expressing major basic protein (MBP, labeled with the antibody BMK 13), eosinophil cationic protein (labeled with the antibody EG-2), and CD25 (IL-2 receptor-bearing cells) in the bronchial submucosa, expressed as the number of positive cells per millimeter of basement membrane. Median values are represented by the horizontal bars: (O) occupational; (E) extrinsic; and (N) normal nonatopic controls.

of collagen beneath the bronchial epithelium has been described in young patients with mild atopic asthma (120), and even shortly after an allergen inhalation challenge (121), indicating that it may be an early change and not necessarily dependent on severe irreversible chronic asthma. This hypothesis is supported by the observation that subepithelial collagen thickening is reversible after cessation of exposure to occupational insults (15,16), and also after treatment with inhaled steroids (122).

A correlation between indices of airway inflammation, as assessed by inflammatory cell counts and/or activation status and severity of asthma, has been reported (19). This concept has recently been challenged taking into account the several studies showing either a weak or no correlation between airway hyperresponsiveness and inflammation (123). A weak, but significant correlation between the thickness of the reticular layer of the basement membrane and the severity of asthma has been reported (124), suggesting a cardinal role of subepithelial fibrosis, one of the features of airway remodeling, as a contributor to progressive disease. These findings were similar to previous reports of cessation of workplace exposure in which reduction of subepithelial fibrosis and airway inflammation were associated with reduction of disease severity (15,16). Improvement after cessation of exposure was associated not only with a decrease in inflammatory cells in the airway mucosa but also, and more consistently, a decrease in the thickness of the basement membrane reticular layer (15,16). Interestingly, the decrease in thickness of the basement membrane reticular layer was also associated with a decrease in the number of fibroblasts in the submucosa. Similar results have also been obtained after steroid therapy of nonoccupational asthma (122,125).

Pathogenesis of Asthma Exacerbations

Exacerbations are important features of chronic asthma and account for a major portion of medical care in emergency departments and hospitals in developed countries. They are usually associated with increased variability of peak flow, decreased forced expiratory flows and, in more severe patients, acute respiratory failure with marked abnormalities of ventilation/perfusion and blood gases (126).

The chain of events of acute airway inflammation and subsequent exacerbation of asthma can be hypothesized as follows: allergen, chemical sensitizers, viruses or other irritant stimuli activate immunocompetent, and/or other resident cells of the airways (e.g., mast cells, macrophages, bronchial epithelium) which release a cascade of pro-inflammatory mediators, cytokines, and chemokines that mobilize inflammatory cells from the bone marrow and circulation. While mild exacerbations of asthma are associated with sputum eosinophils (127) and mixtures of sputum eosinophils and neutrophils, severe asthma exacerbations are associated predominantly with sputum neutrophils and increased IL-8 in sputum (181). Similarly, sudden asthma death is associated with marked neutrophil infiltration in the airways and the lung (182). In addition, arterial blood concentrations of the most potent neutrophil chemoattractant, leukotriene B4 (LTB4), correlate with the severity of asthma exacerbations and are reduced by glucocorticoids, further suggesting the importance of neutrophils in severe asthma exacerbations (128). Since spontaneous exacerbations of occupational asthma have not been properly examined and described, most of the current information about the inflammatory milieu in the foregoing discussion is derived from bronchoprovocation studies which may not always reflect progressive changes which occur during the natural course of asthma.

The Phases of Airway Inflammation in Asthmatic Reactions

Early asthmatic reactions induced by allergens or occupational sensitizing agents are probably associated with smooth muscle contraction and/or edema induced by inflammatory mediators, but they are often not associated with an abundant inflammatory response (129,130); on the other hand, late asthmatic reactions induced by the same stimuli are associated with a prolific influx of inflammatory cells, which may release the inflammatory mediators responsible for the characteristic features of asthma (Fig. 5). Bronchoalveolar lavage samples obtained during various time intervals of late asthmatic reactions demonstrate a significant increase of neutrophils and/or eosinophils after exposure to TDI and plicatic acid, respectively (29,131). Histamine, prostanoids, leukotrienes, and other inflammatory mediators have also been measured in bronchoalveolar lavage fluid during early asthmatic reactions induced by occupational and nonoccupational agents (129,130,132).

The source and nature of the chemotactic factors responsible for leukocyte infiltration in the airways are not known. However, metabolites of the lipoxygenase pathway of arachidonic acid have been identified in lavage supernatants obtained during asthma attacks induced by occupational agents (e.g., LTB4 after TDI challenge), which may be responsible for at least part of this chemotactic activity (133). BAL fluid obtained during asthmatic reactions induced by plicatic acid contain clumps of ciliated epithelial cells, which are probably the end result of epithelial desquamation (132). Since columnar epithelial cells adhere both to themselves and to basal cells and/or basement membrane, epithelial cell desquamation and inflammatory cell infiltration imply changes of adherence properties of the cells (134).

Histamine and leukotriene E4 (LTE4) are increased in BAL fluids sampled during early asthmatic reactions by plicatic acid (132). Urinary LTE4 is increased during early,

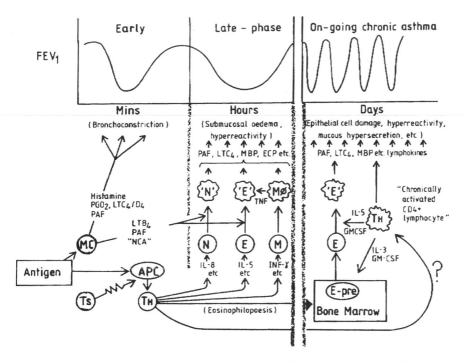

Figure 5 Diagram of the current concepts of the relationship between asthmatic reactions, chronic ongoing asthma, and airway inflammation. Antigen or sensitizing agents may react either directly with antigen-presenting cells (APC) and/or with IgE present on cells that have receptors for IgE on their surface (most likely mast cells, but also probably macrophages, eosinophils, and platelets) and trigger the release of mediators causing directly or through the recruitment of other cells the pathological changes responsible for the development of asthmatic reactions.

but not late, asthmatic reactions induced by various occupational agents including diisocyanates in workers with occupational asthma (135). Taken together, these results suggest the importance of sulfidopeptide leukotrienes in asthmatic reactions (136,137) and the potential diagnostic utility of measuring urinary leukotriene metabolites as an index of airway inflammation of asthma in general and occupational asthma in particular.

Recruitment of Inflammatory Cells into Asthmatic Airways

Circulating leukocytes are recruited to sites of tissue inflammation via a multistep mechanism involving the sequential interaction of cell adhesion molecules (CAMs) present on the surfaces of leukocytes and endothelial cells lining the postcapillary venules. Leukocyte recruitment occurs in three broad steps: rolling, firm adhesion, and transendothelial migration; the first is mainly caused by selectins, the second and the third mainly by the interaction of cell adhesion molecules with integrins (138,139) (Fig. 6).

The recruitment of inflammatory cells into the airway mucosa is initiated by the effect of rapidly acting mediators (e.g., histamine, leukotrienes) that up-regulate P-selectin on the surface of endothelial cells. The interaction of P-selectin with lectins present on the surface of leukocytes causes the rolling of leukocytes on endothelial cells, which is the first step of leukocyte migraion. This is followed by additional expression of adhesion

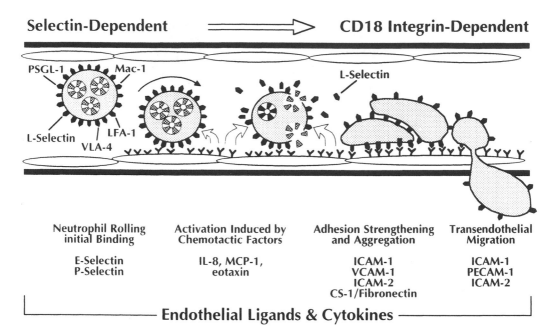

Figure 6 Schematic representation of the multistep paradigm of leukocyte recruitment to inflamed airway. ICAM, intercellular adhesion molecule; VCAM-1, vascular cell adhesion molecule 1; PECAM-1, platelet endothelial cell adhesion molecule 1; IL, interleukin; MCP-1, monocyte chemoattractant protein 1; VLA, very late antigen.

molecules such as E-selectin, intercellular adhesion molecule 1 (ICAM-1), and vascular cell adhesion molecule 1 (VCAM-1), which interact with integrins expressed on rolling leukocytes, resulting in cell adhesion, activation, and transendothelial migration (139).

Several inflammatory mediators participate in this complex process. Because of the consistent finding of eosinophils in asthmatic airways, the mechanisms of eosinophil recruitment and activation have been intensively investigated. The C-C chemokines [i.e., chemoattractant cytokines: RANTES (regulated upon activation, normal T cell expressed and secreted), MCP-3 (monocyte chemotactic protein-3); and the highly potent eotaxin (140)] are chemoattractants mainly responsible for eosinophil migration through the airway wall. The chief activities of cytokines such as IL-5 and GM-CSF are upon eosinophilic activation, chemokinesis, and prolongation of tissue survival (141,142). They also have modest effects on eosinophilic migration.

The main target of asthmatic inflammation is believed to be the airway epithelium. The eosinophilic proteins eosinophil cationic protein (ECP) and major basic protein (MBP), as well as metalloendoproteases (MMPs), produced and released by different inflammatory cells, are involved in the disruption of the airway epithelium that seems to represent the first step of airway wall remodeling. In fact, the disruption of the epithelium is associated with the release of a range of growth and matrix degradation factors that are responsible for tissue injury and repair. This process is responsible for one of the most characteristic features of asthma pathology, subepithelial fibrosis. In fact, proteolytic destruction of the epithelial basement membrane and simultaneous stimulation of submucosal myofibroblasts lead to the production, release, and deposition of collagen I, III and V in the lamina reticularis of the basement membrane, which is characteristically thickened in asthma (115,116).

Cellular Components of Airway Inflammation

The chronic airway inflammation that characterizes asthma and its functional and clinical manifestations are most likely caused by complex interactions among inflammatory cells, structural cells, and nerves. The paracrine interaction between the various cells and nerves takes place through the synthesis and release of proinflammatory mediators and cytokines of different chemical structure. Among these cells T lymphocytes appear to orchestrate the inflammatory process (57,58). Eosinophils, mast cells, epithelial cells, and neutrophils appear to be the main effector cells that cause the characteristic manifestations of asthma through the release of their respective inflammatory mediators (i.e., smooth muscle contraction, mucus hypersecretion, plasma exudation with bronchial wall edema, and epithelial damage) (Fig. 7).

T Lymphocytes

There is increasing evidence that T lymphocytes are central participants in asthma and the bronchial inflammatory process because they produce key cytokines that may modulate the activity of other inflammatory and structural cells (57,58).

The morphometric analysis of peripheral airways and BAL in asthmatic patients have consistently demonstrated the presence of activated T lymphocytes. Also, most studies have demonstrated that both the number of T lymphocytes and the expression of their

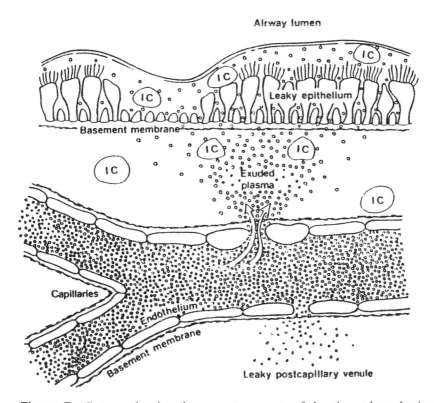

Figure 7   Cartoon showing the current concepts of the site and mechanism of airway microvascular leakage occurring in asthma. Macromolecules leak from the vascular bed at the level of the postcapillary venules, through gaps formed between endothelial cells, and water follows through an osmotic mechanism.

activation markers (e.g., HLA-DR, CD25) correlate with the clinical severity of asthma (58,143–145).

After activation by antigen, T lymphocytes secrete a number of lymphokines that attract, activate, and promote the growth and the differentiation of other leukocytes. As discussed earlier, murine T-helper (Th) clones may be subdivided on the basis of their Th1 and Th2 cytokine profiles (59,60). In vivo studies in humans confirm the existence of functionally distinct subsets of CD4+ T lymphocytes, although Th1 and Th2 phenotypic markers have not been clearly established and there is a large proportion of Th0 cells, which have an intermediate cytokine profile (58,60).

Early studies had suggested a distinct profile of T cells in atopic and nonatopic asthma, with CD4+ Th cells producing IL-3, IL-4, IL-5, and GM-CSF in atopic asthma, and mainly CD8+ suppressor/cytotoxic cells, producing IL-2, IL-3, IL-5, and GM-CSF, but not IL-4, in nonatopic asthma (59,60,96,146,147). However, as previously mentioned, more recent mRNA and protein product studies in bronchial biopsy specimens suggest that there are more similarities than differences between atopic and nonatopic asthmatics (33–37).

In addition to their role as helper cells for the production of humoral antibodies by B cells, activated CD4+ lymphocytes may be considered as inflammatory cells. Activated T cells secrete interleukin-8 (IL-8), which is a chemoattractant cytokine for polymorpho-nuclear leukocytes. They are also an important source of GM-CSF and IL-5. GM-CSF is important in eosinophil development and activation and plays a significant role in the amplification of eosinophilic inflammation. IL-5 appears to be specific in promoting the development, adhesion, chemokinesis, and activation of eosinophils, and it is the predominant eosinophil-active cytokine present in BAL fluids during allergen-induced, late-phase inflammation (141–147).

Activated T cells may therefore initiate and propagate allergic inflammation in the airways and participate directly in the events responsible for asthma exacerbations. Although, a number of other cells also produce IL-3, IL-4, IL-5, GM-CSF, and other relevant cytokines, there is now compelling evidence that both activated lymphocytes and eosinophils are present in asthma of diverse severity and etiology (i.e., IgE-mediated, intrinsic, and occupational) (142,151).

Regarding CD8+ T cells, different subsets participate directly in B-cell suppressor function or act as cytotoxic cells for exogeneous and endogenous antigens (51,52). Interestingly, the development of chronic inflammation in asthma is associated with the infiltration by both CD4+ and CD8+ cells (148), and T-cell clones obtained from bronchial biopsies of nonatopic subjects with isocyanate-induced asthma are mainly CD8+ (97).

B Lymphocytes

In asthma, and more specifically in atopic asthma, B lymphocytes are required for both antigen presentation and isotype switching to specific IgE synthesis. Since IgE-mediated mechanisms play a major role in both nonoccupational and occupational asthma by initiating and maintaining bronchial inflammation, mRNA and protein products derived from B cells (ε germ-like gene transcripts, mRNA encoding the heavy chain of IgE, total IgE, and specific IgE), as well as increased numbers of B lymphocytes expressing CD20+ and high-affinity IgE receptors ($Fc_\varepsilon RI$), could represent markers of airway inflammation (39,149).

Eosinophilic Granulocytes

The most characteristic feature of asthmatic inflammation is a significant increase of eosinophils (117,142,145,150–153), which further increases during exacerbations (126). An increase in the number of eosinophils may also be found in the peripheral venous blood (151,154). The absolute number of peripheral blood eosinophils is slightly, but significantly, correlated with the severity of asthma, as reflected by the degree of airway responsiveness and/or decrease of FEV_1 (142,155). The number of eosinophils increases in BAL and decreases in peripheral blood during late asthmatic reactions (LAR) induced by allergens (130,142,156,157). Eosinophils can damage airway epithelium, stimulate mucus secretion, and contribute to airway smooth muscle contraction and edema of airway mucosa (142). Indeed, eosinophils produce a variety of inflammatory mediators that may contribute further to asthmatic inflammation. These include eicosanoids, proteins, proteases, cytokines, chemokines, growth factors, neuropeptides, and oxygen metabolites.

Mast Cells

Similar to basophils, mast cell membranes have $Fc_\varepsilon RI$ receptors for IgE. The crosslinking of two IgE molecules with specific allergen triggers mast cell activation, with degranulation and release of inflammatory mediators. Rapidly acting mediators such as histamine, prostanoids (e.g., PGD2), leukotrienes (e.g., LTC4, LTD4, and LTE4), and proteases are mainly responsible for the acute manifestations of asthma, such as acute bronchoconstriction, airway wall edema due to microvascular leakage, mucus secretion, and initial leukocyte recruitment.

The number of mast cells has been reported to be increased in the airway mucosa of asthmatics in some (117,158), but not other, studies (144,159). Tryptase, a more specific indicator of mast cell activation, is also found in lavage samples immediately after antigen exposure (160). High levels of histamine, tryptase, and prostaglandin D2 have been shown in samples of BAL in asthmatic patients (160–162). In some studies of asthmatic patients, tryptase concentration within airways could be correlated with histamine airway hyperresponsiveness but other studies did not confirm this relationship (160,163–165). Collectively, these data demonstrate the active participation of mast cell mediators in type I asthmatic responses. In addition to their role in type I immune response, mast cells may also participate in chronic immune responses inasmuch as they produce a variety of preformed and newly generated proinflammatory cytokines that may be involved in asthma.

Neutrophilic Granulocytes

Both human and animal studies suggest that long term airway hyperresponsiveness which persists between asthmatic exacerbations is associated with mild airway inflammation, characterized by increase and activation of lymphocytes, mast cells, eosinophils and possibly macrophages, but not neutrophils. Also, while several studies have shown a correlation between the number of eosinophils, mast cells, and/or epithelial cells in BAL and asthma severity indices, only a few studies have reported such a relationship with neutrophils. Based on these observations, it would appear that neutrophils are not involved in the chronic airway inflammation associated with mild to moderate, stable asthma. It remains to be demonstrated whether they may be involved in severe asthma (166).

By contrast, there is substantial evidence, particularly in humans, that neutrophils may be involved in exacerbations of asthma, particularly in the early stages of sudden and severe asthma exacerbations. Also, the predominant involvement of neutrophils in some types of asthma exacerbations (i.e., induced by allergens, viral infections, or occupational sensitizers) suggests that different triggers of asthma may induce airway inflammation through different mechanisms (166).

Epithelial Cells

The airway epithelium is both an initial target and an initial effector cell in asthma (65,134,167). Increased expression of MHC class II and ICAM-1 in the airway epithelium of asthmatics has been reported. Airways epithelial cells of asthmatic subjects may produce increased amounts of inflammatory mediators, including interleukin-1β (IL-1β) IL-6, IL-8, TNFα, GM-CSF, C-C chemokines (e.g., MCP-1, eotaxin, and RANTES), endothelins, neuropeptides, fibronectin, oxygen metabolites, and eicosanoids such as LTB4, thromboxane A_2, and 15-hydroxyeicosatetranoic acid (15-HETE) (65,167). Bronchial epithelium of asthmatic patients also has both high (Fc$_e$RI) and low Fc$_e$RII affinity receptors and therefore may be triggered directly by an IgE-dependent stimulus (168).

Alveolar Macrophages and Mucosal Monocytes

There are data to suggest that alveolar macrophages and mucosal macrophage/monocytes are involved in the inflammatory process of asthmatic airways. In the bronchial submucosa there are increased numbers of activated macrophages. Many of them are monocytes recently recruited to the airways (169). Activated macrophages may produce a variety of inflammatory mediators. Usually macrophages in the lungs of normal subjects secrete powerful suppressive mediators to limit the proliferative potential of T-lymphocyte activation in the lower airways, thus maintaining local immunological homeostasis (170,171). However, in asthma alveolar macrophages exhibit both an enhanced capacity to release proinflammatory cytokines [e.g., IL-1β, IL-6] ,TNFα, GM-CSF, and macrophage inflammatory protein-1α (MIP-1α) and a reduced capacity to produce anti-inflammatory mediators (i.e., IL-10) (171).

Reflex Mechanisms and Neurogenic Inflammation

The innervation system of the airways is much more complex than was previously believed. In addition to the classic cholinergic and adrenergic mechanisms, nonadrenergic, noncholinergic (NANC) neural pathways have been described in human airways (172). The demonstration that an extensive network of nerve fibers contain potent peptides, in addition to classic neurotransmitters, has revived interest concerning the possible involvement of neurogenic inflammatory mechanisms in the pathogenesis of asthma (109).

Substance P (SP), neurokinin A (NKA), neurokinin B (NKB), calcitonin gene-related peptide (CGRP), and vasoactive intestinal peptide (VIP) are the chief neuropeptides that could be involved in the pathophysiology of asthma. Vasointestinal peptide has been localized in cholinergic nerves of the airways where it may act as a contransmitter with acetylcholine. It may therefore function as a counterbalancing bronchodilator to cholinergic bronchoconstriction. In addition to causing vagally mediated reflex bronchoconstriction, several irritants may stimulate sensory nerves (i.e., the nonmyelinated sensory C-fiber endings) to release SP and other related tachykinins, which have the remarkable ability to affect multiple cells in the airways, thereby provoking responses referred to as neurogenic inflammation (109,173).

Neurogenic inflammation and release of neuropeptides are well-established amplifying mechanisms in rodent models of airway inflammation and asthma. However, evidence that the same mechanisms are operative in human asthma is much less convincing.

Many neuropeptides, particularly NKA (174), SP, and CGRP, are localized in airway nerves and may participate in airway inflammation by causing or amplifying plasma exudation, mucus secretion, recruitment, and activation of inflammatory cells. Other neuropeptides (e.g., VIP), may exert the opposite effect and modulate asthmatic inflammation (109).

Neuropeptides elicit most of the characteristic features of asthma (i.e., cough, mucus secretion, smooth muscle contraction, plasma extravasation, and neutrophil adhesion). Neutral endopeptidase (NEP), an enzyme present on the surface of the cells containing receptors for neuropeptides, limits the concentration of neuropeptides that reach the receptors of the cell's surface by cleaving and inactivating them. This interaction modulates and inhibits neurogenic inflammation (109,173).

The neuropeptide found in highest concentration is VIP. It is found in efferent nerves of human lung and functions as a neurotransmitter of NANC inhibitory nerves. Although a primary defect of NANC innervation seems unlikely, airway inflammation may trigger a functional defect in this system. In asthmatic airways, inflammatory cells such as eosinophils, neutrophils, and mast cells may release a variety of peptidases (e.g., tryptase), which could inactivate VIP. The consequent, unchecked reflex cholinergic bronchoconstriction could contribute to the development of airway hyperresponsiveness associated with airway inflammation. However, local production of nitric oxide appears to be the main inhibitory mechanism of neurally mediated bronchoconstriction (175).

A striking increase of SP-like immunoreactive nerves, and a decrease of VIP+ nerves has been reported in the airways of asthmatics in some studies (176,177), but not confirmed in others (178,179). The effects of tachykinins and tachykinin antagonists in humans have not yet convincingly shown that neurogenic inflammation plays a significant role in airway inflammation in asthma (109).

Several nonspecific workplace stimuli (i.e., sulfur dioxide, dust, cold air) may trigger reflex bronchoconstriction by stimulating the sensory receptors in the airways. This physiological defense mechanism may trigger bronchoconstriction in both normal and asthmatic subjects.

Toluene diisocyanate has been shown to stimulate the release of both SP and CGRP. It also inhibits neutral endopeptidase in experimental animals and in vitro preparations (180). Thus, occupational stimuli that activate the "efferent" function of capsaicin-sensitive nerves and/or inhibit neutral endopeptidases could trigger neurogenic inflammation and precipitate asthma. Although this mechanism of action of isocyanates has been demonstrated in rats and guinea pigs (180), it has not been shown in man, and particularly in subjects with occupational asthma induced by isocyanates, probably because of the lack of specific antagonists.

Epithelial Disruption

Destruction and denudation of airway epithelium are important intermediate consequences in the pathophysiology of asthma. Damaged epithelium may generate arachidonic acid metabolic products such as 8,15-HETE neutrophil chemotactic factor (134,167). It has also been shown that epithelial-derived relaxant factor may modulate the bronchoconstricting effects of many exogenous and endogenous bronchoconstrictor substances (134). Widespread epithelial damage would result in deprivation of this regulating mechanism. Desquamation of the airway epithelium exposes afferent nerve endings, which are more readily stimulated to release SP and other neurotachykinins, the end results of which have been discussed. If epithelial repair processes are delayed by excessive exposure to an environmental irritant or allergen, altered epithelial function could persist even after cessation of exposure.

Airway Microvascular Leakage

There is an increased concentration of albumin in the supernatant of BAL fluid obtained during late asthmatic reactions induced by occupational agents (e.g., isocyanates and plicatic acid) compared to the concentration of albumin present in atopic asthmatic patients after early asthmatic reactions or in normal subjects (19,29,131). It has been suggested that the increased concentration of albumin in lavage supernatants reflects microvascular leakage and mucosal edema (2) (Fig. 7). Macromolecules of albumin leak between gaps of endothelial cells in postcapillary venules. They cross both endothelial and epithelial basement membranes and then accumulate in airway lumina. This process of plasma exudation is associated with significant movement of water, which causes mucosal edema and accumulation of exudate in the airway lumen (2). Airway edema and exudate in airway lumina have been observed in a subject with occupational asthma who died after exposure to the sensitizing agent at work (110). It is therefore apparent that both the increased concentration of albumin and cellular exudate occurring during asthmatic reactions induced by occupational agents provide further compelling evidence that an acute inflammatory reaction of the airways is a conditio sine qua non for active asthmatic reactions.

CONCLUSIONS

Occupational asthma induced by high-molecular-weight compounds and by some low-molecular-weight occupational sensitizers (e.g., anhydrides, platinum halide salts) shares many characteristics with IgE-mediated asthma. In both, the responsible agent is known, and the predisposition of atopic subjects, the clinical presentation, the inhalation challenge in the laboratory, and the response to antiasthma drugs are remarkably similar. By contrast, many workers with occupational asthma induced by some low-molecular-weight occupational agents, particularly toluene diisocyanate and plicatic acid, show no evidence of an IgE-mediated mechanism, and atopy is not a risk factor. The pathology of the airway mucosa of atopic, nonatopic, and all the variants of occupational asthma is remarkably similar, suggesting similar terminal pathogenetic events for asthma independent of cause. However, immunological mechanisms of occupational asthma may have distinctive pathways with IgE-mediated mechanisms more likely to be relevant for asthma induced by high-molecular-weight and some low-molecular-weight (e.g., acid anhydrides, platinum halide salts), and cellular immune–mediated mechanisms for occupational asthma induced by other low-molecular-weight occupational sensitizers (e.g., toluene diisocyanates and western red cedar).

Because most of the inducing occupational agents can be identified as either immunogens, allergens, or irritants, occupational asthma is an ideal model for nonoccupational asthma. The occupational venue enables long-term studies of the consequences of airways obstruction and bronchial hyperresponsiveness. Since diagnostic bronchial challenge is required more often in occupational asthma, there are increased opportunities for investigation of local, humoral, and cellular immune responses, airways microvascular leakage, pharmacological inducers, irritant effects, and neurogenic inflammation.

ACKNOWLEDGMENTS

This work was supported by MURST (Grants 60% and 40%), Consorzio Ferrararicerche, Azienda Ospedaliera Sant'Anna, Ferrara; and European Community (Biomed 2 Research Project "ENFUMOSA," Contract BMH4-CT96-1471).

REFERENCES

1. Wiggs B, Moreno R, James A, Hogg JC, Parè PD. A model of the mechanics of airway narrowing in asthma. In: Kaliner MA, Barnes PJ, Persson CGA, eds. Asthma: Its Pathology and Treatment. New York: Marcel Dekker, 1991:73–101.
2. Persson CGA. Microvascular-epithelial exudation of bulk plasma in airway defense, disease and repair. In: Holgate ST, Busse WW, eds. Inflammatory Mechanisms in Asthma. New York: Marcel Dekker, 1998:Chapter 26.
3. Chan-Yeung M, Grzybowsky S. Prognosis in occupational asthma. Thorax 1985; 40:241–243.
4. Allard C, Cartier A, Ghezzo H, Malo JL. Occupational asthma due to various agents. Absence of clinical and functional improvement at an interval of four or more years after cessation of exposure. Chest 1989; 96:1046–1049.
5. Cote J, Kennedy S, Chan-Yeung M. Outcome of patients with cedar asthma with continuous exposure. Am Rev Respir Dis 1990; 141:373–376.
6. Mapp CE, Chiesura-Corona P, De Marzo N, Fabbri LM. Persistent asthma due to isocyanates: a follow-up study of subjects with occupational asthma due to toluene diisocyanate. Am Rev Respir Dis 1988; 137:1326–1329.
7. Vedal S, Enarson DA, Chan H, Ochnio J, Tse KS, Chan-Yeung M. A longitudinal study of the occurrence of bronchial hyperresponsiveness in western red cedar workers. Am Rev Respir Dis 1988; 137:651–655.
8. Banks DE, Rando RJ, Barkman HW Jr. Persistence of toluene diisocyanate-induced asthma despite negligible workplace exposures. Chest 1991; 97:121–125.
9. Panhuysen CIM, Vong JM, Koeter GH, Schouten JP, van Altena R, Bleecker ER, Postma D. Adult patients may outgrow their asthma. A 25-year follow-up study. Am J Respir Crit Care Med 1997; 155:1267–1272.
10. Redington AE, Howarth PH. Airway wall remodeling in asthma. Thorax 1997; 52:310–312.
11. Redington AE, Sime PJ, Howarth PH, Holgate ST. Fibroblasts and the extracellular matrix in asthma. In: Holgate ST, Busse WW, eds. Inflammatory Mechanisms in Asthma. New York: Marcel Dekker, 1998:Chapter 21.
12. Macklem PT. Mechanical factors determining bronchoconstriction. Eur Respir J 1989; 2(Suppl 6):516s–519s.
13. Ebina M, Yaegashi H, Chiba R, et al. Hyperreactive sites in the airway tree of asthmatic patients revealed by thickening of bronchial muscles: a morphometric study. Am Rev Respir Dis 1990; 141:1327–1332.
14. Paggiaro PL, Paoletti P, Bacci E, et al. Eosinophils in bronchoalveolar lavage (BAL) of patients with toluene diisocyanate (TDI) asthma after cessation of work. Chest 1990; 98:536–542.
15. Saetta M, Maestrelli P, Di Stefano A, De Marzo N, Milani GF, Pivirotto F, Mapp CE, Fabbri LM. Effect of cessation of exposure to toluene diisocyanate (TDI) on bronchial mucosa of subjects with TDI-induced asthma. Am Rev Respir Dis 1992; 145:169–174.
16. Saetta M, Maestrelli P, Turato G, Mapp CE, Milani G, Pivirotto F, Fabbri LM, Stefano A. Airway wall remodeling after cessation of exposure to isocyanates in sensitized asthmatic subjects. Am J Respir Crit Care Med 1995; 151:489–494.
17. Chan-Yeung M, Malo JL. Occupational asthma. N Engl J Med 1995; 333:107–112.
18. Venables KM, Chan-Yeung M. Occupational asthma. Lancet 1997; 349:1465–1469.

19. O'Byrne PM. Mechanisms of airway hyperresponsiveness. In: Holgate ST, Busse WW, eds. Inflammatory Mechanisms in Asthma. New York: Marcel Dekker, 1998:Chapter 34.

20. Hargreave FE, Ramsdale EH, Pugsley SO. Occupational asthma without bronchial hyperresponsiveness. Am Rev Respir Dis 1984; 130:513–515.

21. Mapp CE, Dal Vecchio L, Boschetto P, De Marzo N, Fabbri LM. Toluene diisocyanate–induced asthma without airway hyperresponsiveness. Eur J Respir Dis 1986; 68:89–95.

22. Mapp CE, Di Giacomo R, Broseghini C, et al. Late but not early asthmatic reactions induced by toluene diisocyanate (TDI) are associated with increased airway responsiveness to methacholine. Eur J Respir Dis 1986; 69:276–284.

23. Cartier A, L'Archeveque J, Malo JL. Exposure to a sensitizing occupational agent can cause a long-lasting increase in bronchial responsiveness to histamine in the absence of significant changes in airway caliber. J Allergy Clin Immunol 1986; 78:1185–1189.

24. Thorpe JE, Steinberg D, Bernstein IL, Murlas CG. Bronchial reactivity increases soon after the immediate response in dual responding asthmatics. Chest 1987; 91:21–25.

25. Steinberg DR, Bernstein DI, Thorpe J, Bernstein IL, Murlas CG. Prednisone pretreatment leads to histaminic airways hypersensitivity soon after resolution of the immediate allergic response. Chest 1989; 95:314–319.

26. Durham SR, Graneck BJ, Hawkins R, Newman-Taylor AJ. The temporal relationship between increases in airway responsiveness to histamine and late asthmatic responses induced by occupational agents. J Allergy Clin Immunol 1987; 79:398–406.

27. Josephs LK, Gregg I, Mullee MA, Holgate ST. Nonspecific bronchial reactivity and its relationship to the clinical expression of asthma. A longitudinal study. Am Rev Respir Dis 1989; 140:350–357.

28. Postma DS, Kerstjens HAM. Characteristics of airway hyperresponsiveness in asthma and chronic obstructive pulmonary disease. Am J Respir Crit Care Med 1998; 158:S187–S192.

29. Lam S, LeRiche J, Phillips D, Chan-Yeung M. Cellular and protein changes in bronchial lavage fluid after late asthmatic reactions in patients with red cedar asthma. J Allergy Clin Immunol 1987; 80:44–50.

30. Chan-Yeung, M, Leriche J, McLean L, Lam S. Comparison of cellular and protein changes in bronchial lavage fluid of symptomatic and asymptomatic patients with red cedar asthma on follow-up examination. Clin Allergy 1988; 18:359–365.

31. Vandenplas O, Malo JL. Inhalation challenges with agents causing occupational asthma. Eur Respir J 1997; 10:2612–2629.

32. Malo JL, L'Archeveque J, Cartier A. Significant changes in nonspecific bronchial responsiveness after isolated immediate bronchospastic reactions caused by isocyanates but not after a late reaction caused by plicatic acid. J Allergy Clin Immunol 1989; 83:159–165.

33. Humbert M, Durham SR, Ying S, et al. IL-4 and IL-5 mRNA and protein in bronchial biopsies from patients with atopic and non-atopic evidence against "intrinsic" asthma being a distinct immunopathological entity. Am J Respir Crit Care Med 1996; 154:1497–1504.

34. Humbert M, Ying S, Corrigan C, et al. Bronchial mucosal expression of the genes encoding CC-chemokines RANTES and MCP-3 in symptomatic atopic and nonatopic asthmatics: relationship to the eosinophil-active cytokines IL-5, GM-CSF and IL-3. Am J Respir Cell Med Biol 1997; 16:1–8.

35. Ying S, Humbert M, Barkans J, et al. Expression of IL-4 and IL-5 mRNA and protein product by CD4+ and CD8+ T cells, eosinophils and mast cells in bronchial biopsies obtained from atopic and nonatopic (intrinsic) asthmatics. J Immunol 1997; 158:3539–3534.

36. Humbert M, Durham SR, Kimmitt P, et al. Elevated expression of mRNA encoding interleukin-13 in the bronchial mucosa of atopic and non-atopic subjects with asthma. J Allergy Clin Immunol 1997; 99:657–665.

37. Humbert M, Corrigan CJ, Durham SR, Kimmitt P, Till SJ, Kay AB. Relationship between interleukin-4 and interleukin-5 mRNA expression and disease severity in atopic asthma. Am J Respir Crit Care Med 1997; 156:704–708.

38. Bentley AM, Menz G, Storz C, et al. Identification of T lymphocytes, macrophages, and

activated eosinophils in the bronchial mucosa in intrinsic asthma: relationship to symptoms and bronchial responsiveness. Am Rev Respir Dis 1992; 146:500–506.

39. Humbert M, Grant JA, Taborda-Barata L, et al. High affinity IgE receptor (Fc$_e$RI)-bearing cells in bronchial biopsies from atopic and non-atopic asthma. Am J Respir Crit Care Med 1996; 153:1931–1937.

40. Kotsimbos ATC, Humbert M, Minshall E, et al. Upregulation of αGM-CSF-receptor in non-atopic but not in atopic asthma. J Allergy Clin Immunol 1997; 99:666–672.

41. Cookson WOCM. Genetic aspects of atopic allergy. In: Van Hage Hamsten M, Wickman M, eds. 30 years with IgE. Copenhagen: Munksgaard, 1998:13–18.

42. Mapp CE. Isocyanate-induced asthma. In: Banks DE, Parker JE, eds. Occupational Lung Disease. An International Perspective. London: Chapman & Hall, 1998:375–379.

43. Bignon JS, Aron Y, Ju LY, Kopferschmitt MC, Garnier R, Mapp C, Fabbri LM, Pauli G, Lockart A, Charron D, Swierczewski E. HLA class II alleles in isocyanate-induced asthma. Am J Respir Crit Care Med 1994; 149:71–75.

44. Balboni A, Baricordi OR, Fabbri LM, Gandini E, Ciaccia A, Mapp CE. Association between toluene diisocyanate induced asthma and DQB1 markers: a possible role for aspartic acid at position 57. Eur Respir J 1996; 9:207–210.

45. Young RP, Barker RD, Pile KD, Cookson OCM, Newman-Taylor AJ. The association of HLA-DR3 with specific IgE to inhaled acid anhydrides. Am J Respir Crit Care Med 1995; 151:219–221.

46. Home C, Quintana PJE, Keown PA, Dimitch-Ward H, Chan-Yeung M. Distribution of HLA class II DQB1 and DRB1 alleles in patients with occupational asthma due to western red cedar. Am J Respir Crit Care Med 1977; 155:A135.

47. Raulf-Heimsoth M, Chen M, Rihs HP, et al. Analysis of T-cell reactive regions and DLA-DR4 binding motifs on the latex allergen Hev b 1 (rubber elongation factor). Clin Exp Allergy 1998; 28:339–348.

48. Soriano JB, Ercilla G, Sunyer J, et al. HLA class II genes in soybean epidemic asthma patients. Am J Respir Crit Care Med 1997; 156:1394–1998.

49. Rihs H-P, Barbalho-Krolls T, Huber H, Baur X. No evidence for the influence of HLA class II in alleles in isocyanate-induced asthma. Am J Ind Med 1997; 32:522–527.

50. Bernstein JA, Munson J, Lummus ZL, Balakrishnan K, Leikauf G. T-cell receptor V beta gene segment expression in diisocyanate-induced occupational asthma. J Allergy Clin Immunol 1997; 99:245–250.

51. Mellmann I, Turley SJ, Steinman RM. Antigen processing for amateurs and professionals. Trends Cell Biol 1998; 8:231–237.

52. McWilliam AS, Holt PG. Immunobiology of dendritic cells in the respiratory tract: steady-state and inflammatory sentinels? Toxicol Lett 1998; 102–103:323–329.

53. Edgeworth JD, Lee TH, Grant VA. Antigen presentation in the asthmatic lung. In: Holgate ST, Busse WW, eds. Inflammatory Mechanisms in Asthma, New York: Marcel Dekker, 1998: Chapter 19.

54. Rossi GA, Sacco O, Balbi B, et al. Human ciliated bronchial epithelial cells: expression of the HLA-DR alpha antigens and of the HLA-DR alpha gene, modulation of the HLA-DR alpha antigens by gamma-interferon and antigen-presenting function in the mixed leukocyte reaction. Am J Respir Cell Mol Biol 1990; 3:431–439.

55. Roitt I, Brostoff J, Male D. Immunology. Fifth Ed. London, Mosby 19, 1998.

56. Kay AB, Frew AJ, Corrigan CJ, Robinson DS. The T-cell hypothesis of chronic asthma. In: Kay AB, ed. Allergy and Allergic Diseases. Oxford: Blackwell Science, 1997:1379–1394.

57. Kay AB. T-cell as orchestrators of the asthmatic response. Ciba Found Symp 1997; 206: 56–67.

58. Corrigan CJ. T cells in asthma. In Holgate ST, Busse WW, eds. Inflammatory Mechanisms in Asthma. New York: Marcel Dekker, 1998:Chapter 17.

59. Del Prete GF. Human Th1 and Th2 lymphocytes: their role in the pathophysiology of atopy. Allergy 1992; 47:450–455.

60. Krug N, Frew AJ. The Th2 cell in asthma: initial expectations yet to be realized. Clin Exp Allergy 1997; 27:142–150.
61. Monticelli S, DeMonte L, Vercelli D. Molecular regulation of IgE switching: let's walk hand in hand. In: Van Hage-Hamsten M, Wickman M, eds. 30 Years with IgE. Copenhagen: Munksgaard, 1998:9–11.
62. Teran LM, Davies DE. The chemokines: their potential role in allergic inflammation. Clin Exp Allergy 1996; 26:1005–1019.
63. Ryan JJ. Interleukin-4 and its receptor: essential mediators of the allergic response. J Allergy Clin Immunol 1997; 99:1–5.
64. Drazen JM, Arm JP, Austen KF. Sorting out the cytokines of asthma. J Exp Med 1996; 183: 1–5.
65. Holgate ST. Aetiology and pathogenesis of asthma. In: Kay AB, ed. Allergy and Allergic Diseases. Oxford: Blackwell Science, 1997:1366–1378.
66. Holgate ST. The cellular and mediator basis of asthma in relation to natural history. Lancet 1997; 350(Suppl 2):SII5–9.
67. Durham SR. Mechanisms of mucosal inflammation in the nose and lung. Clin Exp Allergy 1998; 28(Suppl 2):11–16.
68. Costa JJ, Galli SJ, Church MK. Mast cell cytokines in allergic inflammation. In: Holgate ST, Busse WW, eds. Inflammatory Mechanisms in Asthma. New York: Marcel Dekker, 1998.
69. Novey HS, Bernstein IL, Mihalas LS, Terr AI, Yunginger JW. Guidelines for the clinical evaluation of occupational asthma due to high molecular weight (HMW) allergens. J Allergy Clin Immunol 1989; 84:829–833.
70. Bindslev JC, Poulsen LK. In vitro diagnostic tests. In: Sampson HA, Simons E, Metcalfe DD, eds. Food Allergy, 2nd ed. London: Blackwell Scientific, 1996:137–150.
71. Maccia CA, Bernstein IL, Emmett EA, Brooks SM. In vitro demonstration of specific IgE in phthalic anhydride hypersensitivity. Am Rev Respir Dis 1976; 113:701–704.
72. Biagini RE, Bernstein IL, Gallagher JS, Moorman WJ, Brooks S, Gann PH. The diversity of reaginic immune responses to platinum and palladium metallic salts. J Allergy Clin Immunol 1985; 76:794–802.
73. Cartier A, Grammar L, Malo JL, et al. Specific serum antibodies against isocyanates: association with occupational asthma. J Allergy Clin Immunol 1989; 84:507–514.
74. Tse KS, Chan H, Chan-Yeung M. Specific IgE antibodies in workers with occupational asthma due to western red cedar. Clin Allergy 1982; 12:249–258.
75. Cartier A, Malo JL, Forest F, et al. Occupational asthma in snow crab processing workers. J Allergy Clin Immunol 1984; 74:261–269.
76. Mitchell CA, Gandevia B. Respiratory symptoms and skin reactivity in workers exposed to proteolytic enzymes in detergent industry. Am Rev Respir Dis 1971; 104:1–12.
77. Karr R. Bronchoprovocation studies in coffee worker's asthma. J Allergy Clin Immunol 1979; 64:650–654.
78. Davison AG, Britton MG, Forrester JA, Davies RJ, Hughes DTD. Asthma in merchant seamen and laboratory workers caused by allergy to castor oil beans: analysis of allergens. Clin Allergy 1983; 13:553–561.
79. Merget R, Stallfuss J, Wiewrodt R, et al. Diagnostic tests in enzyme allergy. J Allergy Clin Immunol 1993; 92:264–277.
80. Bernstein DI, Smith AB, Gallagher JS, et al. Clinical and immunologic studies among egg processing workers with occupational asthma. J Allergy Clin Immunol 1987; 80:791–797.
81. Tiikkainen U, Klockars M. Clinical significance of IgG subclass antibodies to wheat flour antigens in bakers. Allergy 1990; 45:497–504.
82. Popp W, Zwick H, Rauscher H. Short-term sensitizing antibodies in baker's asthma. Int Arch Allergy Appl Immunol 1988; 86:215–219.
83. Tee RD, Cullinan P, Welch J, Burge PS, Newman-Taylor AJ. Specific IgE to isocyanates: a useful diagnostic role in occupational asthma. J Allergy Clin Immunol 1998; 101:709–715.

84. Jielsen J, Welinder H, Skerfving S. Allergic airway disease caused by methyltetrahydro-phthalic anhydride in epoxy resin. Scand J Work Environ Health 1989; 15:154.

85. Bernstein DI, Gallagher JS, D'Souza L, et al. Heterogeneity of specific IgE response in workers sensitized to acid anhydride compounds. J Allergy Clin Immunol 1984; 74:794–801.

86. Zeiss CR, Wolkonsky P, Pruzansky JJ, et al. Clinical and immunologic evaluation of trimellitic anhydride workers in multiple industrial settings. J Allergy Clin Immunol 1982; 70:15.

87. Ahmad D, Morgan WKC, Patterson R, et al. Pulmonary haemorrhage and haemolytic anaemia due to trimellitic anhydride. Lancet 1979; 2:328–330.

88. Patterson R, Addington W, Banner AS, et al. Antihapten antibodies in workers exposed to trimellitic anhydride fumes: a potential immunopathogenetic mechanism for the trimellitic anhydride pulmonary disease-anemia syndrome. Am Rev Respir Dis 1979; 120:1259.

89. Turner SS, Pruzansky JJ, Patterson R, et al. Detection of antibodies in human serum using trimellityl-erythrocytes: direct and indirect haemagglutination and haemolysis. Clin Exp Immunol 1980; 39:470–476.

90. Venables KM, Topping MD, Nunn AJ, et al. Immunologic and functional consequences of chemical (tetrachlorophalic anhydride)-induced asthma after four years of avoidance of exposure. J Allergy Clin Immunol 1987; 80:212–218.

91. Cleare MJ, Hughes EJ, Jacoby B, Pepys J. Immediate (type I) allergic responses to platinum compounds. Clin Allergy 1976; 6:183–195.

92. Pepys J, Parish WE, Cromwell O, et al. Passive transfer in man and the monkey of type I allergy due to heat labile and heat stable antibody to complex salts of platinum. Clin Allergy 1979; 9:99–108.

93. Baker OB, Gann PH, Brooks SM, et al. Cross-sectional study of platinum salts sensitization among precious metals refinery workers. Am J Ind Med 1990; 18:653–664.

94. Biagini RE, Bernstein IL, Gallagher JS, et al. The diversity of reaginic immune responses to platinum and palladium metallic salts. J Allergy Clin Immunol 1985; 76:794.

95. Venables KM, Dally MB, Nunn AJ, et al. Smoking and occupational allergy in workers in a platinum refinery. BMJ 1989; 299:939–942.

96. Walker C, Bode E, Boer I, Hansel TT, Blaser K, Virchow JC Jr. Allergic and nonallergic asthmatics have distinct patterns of T cell activation and cytokine production in peripheral blood and bronchoalveolar lavage. Am Rev Respir Dis 1992; 146:109–115.

97. Maestrelli P, Del Prete GF, De Carli M, D'Elios MM, Saetta M, Di Stefano A, Mapp C, Romagnani S, Fabbri L. CD-8 T-cells producing interleukin-5 and interferon-gamma in bronchial mucosa of patients with asthma induced by toluene diisocyanate. Scand J Work Environ Health 1994; 20:376–381.

98. Frew A, Chang JH, Chan H, Quirce S, Noertjojo K, Keown P, Chan-Yeung M. T-lymphocyte responses to plicatic acid-human serum albumin conjugate in occupational asthma caused by western red cedar. J Allergy Clin Immunol 1998; 101(6 Pt 1):841–847.

99. Gallagher JS, Tse CST, Brooks S, Bernstein IL. Diverse profiles of immunoreactivity in toluene diisocyanate asthma. J Occup Med 1981; 23:610–616.

100. Herzog CH, Villiger B, Braun P. Nickel-specific T cell clones in asthma preferential use of V-beta 14 in T cell receptor beta chain: Third International Conference on Bronchoalveolar Lavage, Vienna, June 20–22, 1991. Eur Respir Rev 1991; 33s.

101. Kusaka Y, Nakano Y, Shirakawa T, Morimoto K. Lymphocyte transformation with cobalt in hard metal asthma. Ind Health 1989; 27:155–163.

102. Lummus ZI, Alam R, Bernstein JA, Bernstein DI. Diisocyanate Antigen-enhanced production of MCP-1, IL-8, and TNF-α by peripheral mononuclear cells of workers with occupational asthma. J Allergy Clin Immunol 1998; 102:265–274.

103. Layton GT, Stanworth DR, Amos HE. Factors influencing the immunogenicity of the hapten drug chlorhexidine in mice. II. The role of the carrier and adjuvants in the induction of IgE and IgG anti-hapten responses. Immunology 1986; 59:459–465.

104. Zhang XD, Litvall JL, Skerfving S, Welinder H. Antibody specificity to the chemical structures of organic acid anhydrides studied by in vitro and in vivo methods. Toxicology 1997; 118:223–232.

105. Karol MH, Graham C, Gealy R, Macina OT, Sussman N, Rosenkranz HS. Structure activity relationships and computer-assisted analysis of respiratory sensitization potential. Toxicol Lett 1996; 86:187–191.

106. Boushey HA, Fahy JV. Basic mechanisms of asthma. Environ Health Perspect 1995; 103(Suppl 6):S229–S233.

107. Holgate ST, Bradding P, Sampson AP. Leukotriene antagonists and synthesis inhibitors: new directions in asthma therapy. J Allergy Clin Immunol 1996; 98:1–13.

108. Li JT. Mechanisms of asthma. Curr Opin Pulm Med 1997; 3:10–16.

109. Barnes PJ. Airway neuropeptides and their role in asthma. In: Holgate ST, Busse WW, eds. Inflammatory Mechanisms in Asthma. New York: Marcel Dekker, 1998:Chapter 24.

110. Fabbri LM, Danieli D, Crescioli S, et al. Fatal asthma in a subject sensitized to toluene diisocyanate. Am Rev Respir Dis 1988; 137:1494–1498.

111. Saetta M, Rosina C, Di Stefano A, Thiene G, Fabbri LM. Quantitative structural analysis of peripheral airway and arteries in sudden fatal asthma. Am Rev Respir Dis 1991; 143: 138–143.

112. Bentley AM, Maestrelli P, Saetta M, Fabbri LM, Robinson DS, Bradley BL, Jeffery PK, Durham SR, Kay AB. Activated T-lymphocyte and eosinophils in the bronchial mucosa in isocyanate-induced asthma. J Allergy Clin Immunol 1992; 89:821–828.

113. Montefort S, Roberts JA, Beasley R, Holgate ST, Roche WR. The site of disruption of the bronchial epithelium in asthmatic and nonasthmatic subjects. Thorax 1992; 47:499–503.

114. Montefort S, Djukanovic R, Holgate ST, Roche WR. Ciliated cell damage in the bronchial epithelium of asthmatics and nonasthmatics. Clin Exp Allergy 1993; 23:185–189.

115. Roche WR, Beasley R, Williams JH, Holgate ST. Subepithelial fibrosis in the bronchi of asthmatics. Lancet 1989; 1:520–524.

116. Brewster CEP, Howarth PH, Djukanovic R, Wilson J, Holgate ST, Roche WR. Myofibroblasts and subepithelial fibrosis and bronchial asthma. Am J Respir Cell Mol Biol 1990; 3: 507–511.

117. Saetta M, Di Stefano A, Maestrelli P, et al. Airway mucosal inflammation in occupational asthma induced by toluene diisocyanate. Am Rev Respir Dis 1992; 145:160–168.

118. Frew AJ, Chan H, Lam S, Chan-Yeung M. Bronchial inflammation in occupational asthma due to western red cedar. Am J Respir Crit Care Med 1995; 151:340–344.

119. Gautrin D, Boulet L, Boutet M, et al. Is reactive airways dysfunction syndrome (RADS) a variant of occupational asthma? J Allergy Clin Immunol 1994; 93:12–22.

120. Beasley R, Roche WR, Roberts JA, Holgate ST. Cellular events in the bronchi in mild asthma and after bronchial provocation. Am Rev Respir Dis 1989; 139:806–817.

121. Gizycki MJ, Adelroth E, Rogers AV, O'Byrne PM, Jeffery PK. Myofibroblasts involvement in the allergen-induced late response in mild atopic asthma. Am J Respir Cell Mol Biol 1997; 16:664–673.

122. Trigg CJ, Manolitsas ND, Wang J, Calderon MA, McAulay A, Jordan SE, Herdman MJ, Jhalli N, Duddle JM, Hamilton SA, Devalia JL, Davies RJ. Placebo-controlled immunopathologic study of four months of inhaled corticosteroids in asthma. Am J Respir Crit Care Med 1994; 150:17–22.

123. Crimi E, Spanevello A, Neri M, et al. Dissociation between airway inflammation and airway hyperresponsiveness in allergic asthma. Am J Resp Crit Care Med 1998; 157:4–9.

124. Chetta A, Foresi A, Del Donno M, Consigli GF, Bertorelli G, Pesci A, Barbee RA, Olivieri D. Bronchial responsiveness to distilled water and methacholine and its relationship to inflammation and remodeling of the airways in asthma. Am J Respir Crit Care Med 1996; 153: 910–917.

125. Olivieri A, Chetta A, Del Donno M, Bertorelli G, Casalini A, Pesci A, Testi R, Foresi A. Effect of short-term treatment with low-dose inhaled fluticasone propionate on airway inflammation and remodeling in mild asthma: a placebo-controlled study. Am J Respir Crit Care Med 1997; 155(6):1864–1871.
126. Fabbri LM, Beghe B, Caramori G, et al. Similarities and discrepancies between exacerbations of asthma and chronic obstructive pulmonary diseases. Thorax 1998; 53:803–808.
127. McIvor RA, Pizzichini E, Turner MO, et al. Potential masking effects of salmeterol on airway inflammation in asthma. Am J Resp Crit Care Med 1998; 158(3):924–930.
128. Shindo K, Fukumura M, Miyakawa K. Leukotriene B4 (LTB4) levels in the arterial blood of asthmatic patients and the effect of prednisolone. Eur Resp J 1995; 8:605–610.
129. Peters SP, Shaver JR, Zangrilli JG, Fish JE. Airways responses to antigen in asthmatic and nonasthmatic subjects. In: Holgate ST, Busse WW, eds. Inflammatory Mechanisms in Asthma. New York: Marcel Dekker, 1998:Chapter 7.
130. Sheth KK, Lemanske RF. The early and late asthmatic reaction to allergen. In: Holgate ST, Busse WW, eds. Inflammatory Mechanisms in Asthma. New York: Marcel Dekker, 1998: Chapter 34.
131. Fabbri LM, Boschetto P, Zocca E, et al. Bronchoalveolar neutrophilia during late asthmatic reactions induced by toluene diisocyanate (TDI). Am Rev Respir Dis 1987; 136:36–42.
132. Chan-Yeung M, Chan H, Tse KS, Salari H, Lam S. Histamine and leukotrienes release in bronchoalveolar lavage fluid during plicatic acid induced bronchoconstriction. J Allergy Clin Immunol 1989; 84:762–768.
133. Zocca E, Fabbri LM, Boschetto P, et al. Leukotriene B4 and late asthmatic reactions induced by toluene diisocyanate. J Appl Physiol 1990; 68:1576–1589.
134. White SR, Leff AR. Epithelium as a target. In: Holgate ST, Busse WW, eds. Inflammatory Mechanisms in Asthma. New York: Marcel Dekker, 1998:Chapter 23.
135. Manning PJ, Rokach J, Malo J, et al. Urinary leukotriene E4 levels during early and late asthmatic responses. J Allergy Clin Immunol 1990; 86:211–220.
136. O'Byrne PM. Leukotrienes in the pathogenesis of asthma. Chest 1997; 111(Suppl 3): 27S–34S.
137. Dahlen SE. Leukotrienes. In: Holgate ST, Busse WW, eds. Inflammatory Mechanisms in Asthma. New York: Marcel Dekker, 1998:Chapter 18.
138. Bell FP, Bennet B, Manning AM. Leukocyte-endothelial adhesion. In: Holgate ST, Busse WW, eds. Inflammatory Mechanisms in Asthma. New York: Marcel Dekker, 1998: Chapter 28.
139. DeLisser HM, Albelda SM. The function of cell adhesion molecules in lung inflammation: more questions than answers. Am J Respir Cell Mol Biol 1998; 19(4):533–536.
140. Lamkhioued B, Renzi PM, Abi-Younes S, Garcia-Zepada EA, Allakhverdi Z, Ghaffar O, Rothenberg MD, Luster AD, Hamid Q. Increased expression of eotaxin in the bronchoalveolar lavage and airways of asthmatics contributes to the chemotaxis of eosinophils to the site of inflammation. J Immunol 1997; 159:4593–4601.
141. Lee NA, Lee JJ. Asthma: does IL-5 have a more provocative role? Am J Respir Cell Mol Biol 1997; 16:497–500.
142. Kumar A, Busse WW. Eosinophils in asthma. In: Holgate ST, Busse WW, eds. Inflammatory Mechanisms in Asthma. New York: Marcel Dekker, 1998:Chapter 13.
143. Azzawi M, Bradley B, Jeffery PK, Frew AJ, Wardlaw AJ, Assoufi B, Collins JV, Durham SR, Knowles GK, Kay AB. Identification of activated T lymphocytes and eosinophils in bronchial biopsies in stable atopic asthma. Am Rev Respir Dis 1990; 142:1407–1413.
144. Djukanovic R, Wilson JW, Britten KM, Wilson SJ, Walls AF, Richo WR, Howarth PH, Holgate ST. Quantification of mast cells and eosinophils in the bronchial mucosa of symptomatic atopic asthmatics and healthy control subjects using immunohistochemistry. Am Rev Respir Dis 1990; 142:863–871.

145. Bentley AM, Menz G, Storz CHR, Robinson DS, Bradley B, Jeffery PK, Durham SR, Kay
      AB. Identification of T lymphocytes, macrophages, and activated eosinophils in the bronchial
      mucosa in intrinsic asthma: relationship to symptoms and bronchial hyperresponsiveness. Am
      Rev Respir Dis 1992; 146:500–506.
146. Robinson DS, Hamid Q, Ying S, Tsicopoulos A, Barkans J, Bentley AM, Corrigan C, Durham
      SR, Kay AB. Predominant Th2 like bronchoalveolar T-lymphocyte population in atopic
      asthma. N Engl J Med 1992; 326:298–304.
147. Bentley AM, Meng Q, Robinson DS, et al. Increases in activated T-lymphocytes, eosinophils,
      and cytokine mRNA expression for interleukin-5 and granulocyte/macrophage colony-stim-
      ulating factor in bronchial biopsies after allergen inhalation challenge in atopic asthmatics.
      Am J Respir Cell Mol Biol 1993; 8:35–42.
148. Stanciu LA, Shute J, Promwong C, Holgate ST, Djukanovich R. Increased levels of IL-4 in
      CD8+ve T cells in atopic asthma. J Allergy Clin Immunol 1997; 100:373–378.
149. Kidney JC, Wong AG, Efthimiads A, Morris MM, Sears MR, Dolovich J, Hargreave FE.
      Elevated B cells in asputum of asthmatics. Close correlation with neutrophils. Am J Respir
      Crit Care Med 1996; 153(2):540–544.
150. Humbert M. Pro-eosinophilic cytokines in asthma. Clin Exp Allergy 1996; 26:123–127.
151. Bousquet J, Chanez P, Lacoste JY, Barneon G, Ghavanian N, Enander I, Venge P, Ahlstedt
      S, Simony-Lafontaine J, Godard P, Michel F-B. Eosinophilic inflammation in asthma. N Engl
      J Med 1990; 323:1033–1039.
152. Gleich GJ. Eosinophil granule proteins and bronchial asthma. Allergol Int 1996; 45:35–44.
153. Laitinen LA, Laitinen A, Haahtela T. A comparative study of the effects of an inhaled cor-
      ticosteroid, budesonide, and a beta2-agonist, terbutaline, on airway inflammation in newly
      diagnosed asthma: a randomized, double-blind, parallel-group controlled trial. J Allergy Clin
      Immunol 1992; 90:32–42.
154. Durham SR, Loegering DA, Dunnette S, Gleich GJ, Kay AB. Blood eosinophils and eosin-
      ophil-derived proteins in allergic asthma. J Allergy Clin Immunol 1989; 84 I:931–993.
155. Durham SR, Kay AB. Eosinophils, bronchial hyperreactivity and late-phase asthmatic reac-
      tions. Clin Allergy 1985; 15:411–418.
156. DeMonchy GR, Kauffman HF, Venge P, et al. Bronchoalveolar eosinophilia following
      allergen-induced late asthmatic reactions. Am Rev Respir Dis. 1985; 131:373–376.
157. O'Byrne PM, Dolovich J, Hargreave FE. Late asthmatic responses. State-of-the-art. Am Rev
      Respir Dis 1987; 136:740–751.
158. Pesci A, Foresi A, Bertorelli G, Chetta A, Olivieri D. Histochemical characteristics and de-
      granulation of mast cells in epithelium and lamina propria of bronchial biopsies from asth-
      matic and normal subjects. Am Rev Respir Dis 1993; 147:684–689.
159. Jeffery PK, Wardlaw AJ, Nelson FC, Collins JV, Kay AB. Bronchial biopsies in asthma. Am
      Rev Respir Dis 1989; 140:1745–1753.
160. Calhoun WJ, Jarjour NN, Gleich GJ, Schartz LB, Busse WW. Effect of nedocromil sodium
      pretreatment on the immediate and late responses of the airway to segmental antigen chal-
      lenge. J Allergy Clin Immunol 1996; 98(2):S46–S50, S64–S66.
161. Casale TB, Wood D, Richardson HB, Trapp S, Metzger WJ, Zavala D, Hunninghake GW.
      Elevated bronchoalveolar lavage fluid histamine levels in allergic asthmatics are associated
      with methacoline bronchial hyperresponsiveness. J Clin Invest 1987; 79(4):1197–1203.
162. Liu MC, Bleecker ER, Lichtenstein LM, Kagey-Sobotka A, Niv Y, McLemore TL, Permutt
      S, Proud D, Hubbard WC. Evidence for elevated levels of histamine, prostaglandin D2, and
      other bronchoconstricting prostaglandins in the airways of subjects with mild asthma. Am
      Rev Respir Dis 1990; 142(1):126–132.
163. Broide DH, Gleich GJ, Cuomo AJ, Coburn DA, Federman EC, Schwartz LB, Wasserman SI.
      Evidence of ongoing mast cell and eosinophil degranulation in symptomatic asthma airway.
      J Allergy Clin Immunol 1991; 88(4):637–648.
164. Bosso JV, Schwartz LB, Stevenson DD. Tryptase and histamine release during aspirin-
      induced respiratory reactions. J Allergy Clin Immunol 1991; 88/6:830–837.

165. Bousquet J, Chanez P, Lacoste JY, Enander I, Venge P, Peterson C, Ahlstedt S, Michel FB, Godard P. Indirect evidence of bronchial inflammation assessed by titration of inflammatory mediators in BAL fluid of patients with asthma. J Allergy Clin Immunol 1991; 88(4): 649–660.

166. Fabbri LM, Boschetto P, Caramori G, Maestrelli P. Neutrophils and asthma. In: Holgate ST, Busse WW, eds. Inflammatory Mechanisms in Asthma. New York: Marcel Dekker, 1998: Chapter 15.

167. Knobil K, Jacoby DB. Mediator functions and epithelial cells. In: Holgate ST, Busse WW, eds. Inflammatory Mechanisms in Asthma. New York: Marcel Dekker, 1998:Chapter 22.

168. Campbell AM, Vachier I, Chanez P, Vignola AM, Lebel B, Kochan J, Godard P, Bousquet J. Expression of the high-affinity receptor for IgE on bronchial epithelial cells of asthmatics. Am J Respir Cell Mol Biol 1998; 19:92–97.

169. Daftary SS, Calhoun WJ, Jarjour NN. Macrophages and macrophage diversity in asthma. In: Holgate ST, Busse WW, eds. Inflammatory Mechanisms in Asthma. New York: Marcel Dekker, 1998:Chapter 18.

170. Poulter LW, Janossy G, Power C, Sreenan S, Burke C. Immunological/physiological relationships in asthma: potential regulation by lung macrophages. Immunol Today 1994; 15: 258–261.

171. John M, Lim S, Seybold J, Jose P, Robichaud A, O'Connor B, Barnes PJ, Chung KF. Inhaled corticosteroids increase interleukin-10 but reduce macrophage inflammatory protein-1α, granulocyte-macrophage colony-stimulating factor, and interferon-γ release from alveolar macrophages in asthma. Am J Respir Crit Care Med 1998; 157:256–262.

172. Barnes PJ, Baraniuk JN, Belvisi M. Neuropeptides in the respiratory tract. Part II. Am Rev Respir Dis 1991; 144:11391–1399.

173. Nadel JA. Neutral endopeptidase modulates neurogenic inflammation. Eur Respir J 1991; 4: 745–754.

174. Heaney LG, Cross LJ, McGarvey LP, Buchanan KD, Ennis M, Shaw C. Neurokinin A is the predominant tachykinin in human bronchoalveolar lavage fluid in normal and asthmatic subjects. Thorax 1998; 53:357–362.

175. Barnes PJ. NO or no NO in asthma? Thorax 1996; 51:218–220.

176. Ollerenshaw SL, Jarvis D, Woolcock AJ, Sullivan CE, Scheibner T. Absence of immunoreactive vasoactive intestinal polypeptide in tissue from the lungs of patients with asthma. N Engl J Med 1991; 320:1244–1248.

177. Ollerenshaw SL, Jarvis D, Sullivan CE, Woolcock AJ. Substance P immunoreactive nerves from asthmatics and nonasthmatics. Eur Respir J 1991; 4:673–682.

178. Lilly CM, Bai TR, Shore SA, Hall AE, Drazen JM. Neuropeptide content of lungs from asthmatic and nonasthmatic patients. Am J Respir Crit Care Med 1995; 151:548–553.

179. Howarth PH, Springall DR, Redington AE, Djukanovic R, Holgate ST, Polak JM. Neuropeptide-containing nerves in endobronchial biopsies from asthmatic and nonasthmatic subjects. Am J Respir Cell Mol Biol 1995; 13:288–296.

180. Mapp C, Lucchini RE, Miotto D, Chitano P, Jovine L, Saetta M, Maestrelli P, Springall DR, Polak J, Fabbri LM. Immunization and challenge with toluene diisocyanate decrease tachykinin and calcitonin gene-related peptide immunoreactivity in guinea pig central airways. Am J Respir Crit Care Med 1998; 158:263–269.

181. Fahy JV, Kim KW, Liu J, Boushey HA. Prominent neutrophilic inflammation in sputum from subjects with asthma exacerbation. J Allergy Clin Immunol 1995; 94:843–852.

182. Sur S, Crotty TB, Kephart GM, Hyma BA, Colby TV, Reed CE, Hunt LW, Gleich GJ. Sudden-onset fatal asthma: a distinct entity with few eosinophils and relatively more neutrophils in the airway submucosa? Am Rev Respir Dis 1993; 148:713–719.

6

Animal Models of Occupational Asthma

Katherine Sarlo
The Procter & Gamble Company, Cincinnati, Ohio

Meryl Karol
University of Pittsburgh, Pittsburgh, Pennsylvania

INTRODUCTION

The prevalence of occupational asthma has been reported to range from 2% to 15% of the workforce (1). A wide variety of compounds have been shown to cause occupational allergy and asthma. These materials may be high-molecular-weight (HMW) compounds, such as proteins, or low-molecular-weight (LMW) compounds, such as reactive chemicals. Respiratory allergic reactions in humans are caused by IgE-mediated antibody responses. Other types of immune mechanisms may play a role in responses to LMW chemicals. The mechanisms of allergy/asthma mediated by allergic antibody reactions are fairly well understood. Therefore, the development and use of animal models as predictive tools has enjoyed some success with certain protein allergens. The mechanism of occupational allergy and asthma to many of the LMW-reactive chemicals is poorly understood. It is generally believed to be mediated by lymphocytes that contribute to airway inflammation.

Animal models can be used to enhance our understanding of causes and mechanisms involved in occupational asthma and allergy. Animal models, however, should be interpreted with caution in that experimental findings may not be directly applicable to human asthma. An ideal model would demonstrate the primary characteristics of the disease, i.e., allergic antibody, airway inflammation, and hyperresponsiveness for allergic asthma or persistent airway inflammation and hyperresponsiveness for nonallergic asthma. Models differ with regard to: animal species, route of administration of antigen, protocol used for induction and elicitation of responses, and the type of response measured. Guinea pigs, rats, and mice have been used to study allergy and asthma. Murine models offer advantages for immunological investigations since the cellular and humoral immunological components of mice have been well studied and gene transfer and deletion models are possible for mechanistic studies. Asthma investigations have centered on the inflammatory reaction occurring in the respiratory tract since the inflammatory cells (eosinophils, lymphocytes, and mast cells) have been implicated in the pathophysiology of the disease. Investigations into allergic asthma have also focused on production of allergic antibody and its relationship to the inflammatory response in the airways.

Although numerous models have been developed to study asthma, only a few have been used in hazard identification and risk assessment for occupational disease. This chapter provides a brief overview of these models and describes how they are used or can be used as predictive tests for risk assessment of proteins and LMW chemicals as respiratory allergens and asthmagens.

GUINEA PIG MODELS FOR OCCUPATIONAL RESPIRATORY ALLERGY AND ASTHMA

The guinea pig has been used as an animal model for respiratory allergy and anaphylaxis for many decades (2). Guinea pigs exhibit pulmonary responses upon exposure to histamine and experience both immediate-onset and late-onset reactions upon exposure to allergens (3,4). They have also been used to study the pathogenesis of antigen-induced rhinitis (5,6). Airway hyperreactivity can be demonstrated in the guinea pig (7). Eosinophilic influx, one hallmark of asthma in humans, occurs in the guinea pig (8,9). Agents that block eosinophilic influx also block allergen-stimulated airway hyperreactivity in the guinea pig (10,11). The role of neurotransmitters (substance P, tachykinins), leukotrienes, prostaglandins, thromboxanes (TxB, TxA2) and histamine in the development of bronchoconstriction, rhinitis, and airway hyperreactivity has been studied in this species as well as the relationship between nitric oxide production and changes in antigen-induced airway resistance (12).

The major homocytotropic antibody in the guinea pig is IgG_1, which is associated with respiratory symptoms and eosinophilic inflammatory responses after exposure to allergen. Eosinophilia has been demonstrated in the respiratory tract (3) as well as in the peritoneal cavity and skin (13) of guinea pigs. Guinea pigs may also produce IgE antibody in small amounts after allergen exposure (14), but the level of allergen-specific IgE is generally lower than that of IgG_1. Guinea pig IgE can be detected in a 4–7-day passive cutaneous anaphylaxis (PCA) test and will cause the same type of hypersensitivity responses as IgG_1 antibody. The presence of IgE antibodies to ovalbumin has been associated with late-onset pulmonary reactions in the guinea pig. The relationship between IgG_1 antibody and IgE antibody and the development of pulmonary reactivity is not fully understood in this species. Guinea pigs respond to a wide range of protein and chemical allergens, and dose-dependent allergic antibody and pulmonary responses can be shown to occur upon exposure to a variety of allergens. In addition, its docile nature and small size make the guinea pig a good species for the examination of allergic responses.

Guinea Pig Models of Occupational Allergy to Proteins

Several guinea pig models have been developed to understand mechanisms of respiratory allergy to protein and many investigators have used ovalbumin as a protein allergen to develop these models (15–17). However, only a few models have been developed using proteins known to be occupational allergens. One example is the guinea pig model developed to study occupational allergy induced by detergent enzymes.

Exposure and sensitization of guinea pigs to detergent enzymes has occurred primarily through the respiratory tract via inhalation or intratracheal instillation. Intradermal injection has also been used as a route for sensitization. A general protocol for sensitizing guinea pigs to protein aerosols was developed by Karol and colleagues (17) and was used successfully to sensitize animals to the detergent enzyme subtilisin (18,19). The presence of subtilisin-specific antibody indicated immunological sensitization whereas the presence of immediate-onset or late-onset pulmonary symptoms (visual observation of labored breathing and/or the use of plethysmography to measure changes in breathing rate and pattern) indicated pulmonary sensitization. An elevation of core body temperature (febrile response) accompanied late-onset pulmonary responses (20). These investigators showed that animals exposed to atmospheres of 150 μg of subtilisin protein/m^3 for 15 min/day for 5 consecutive days generated enzyme-specific allergic antibody and developed immediate-onset and late-onset pulmonary responses when reexposed to the enzyme aerosol. Animals exposed to lower concentrations (8 or 41 μg of subtilisin protein/m^3) did not experience pulmonary symptoms, but did develop low levels of antibody to subtilisin.

The guinea pig intratracheal (GPIT) test was devised originally as an alternative to inhalation tests for the assessment of enzymes as occupational allergens (21). Subtilisin (Alcalase®) was used as the model allergen since a threshold limit value (TLV) has been established for this protein (22). In addition, a wealth of human data pertaining to antibody and pulmonary responses to this enzyme in the exposed workforce exists (23–25) and provides a basis for comparing responses in humans to those in the guinea pig.

The response (allergic antibody and immediate-onset pulmonary symptoms) to weekly instillations of Alcalase protein in the GPIT test was comparable with the response to weekly inhalation exposures to Alcalase in the guinea pig (21). This model has been used to assess the allergenic potency of new enzymes by comparison with Alcalase (26). Allergenic potency is defined by the dose of enzyme protein needed to induce allergic antibody titers similar to those obtained with Alcalase protein. The antibody titers are measured at several time points during the 10–12 weeks of the GPIT test. New enzymes can be assessed as more potent, less potent, or equipotent to Alcalase. This information has been used to develop operational exposure guidelines to protect workers against developing allergic antibody to new enzymes. Prospective evaluation of skin prick test responses among workers exposed to various enzymes showed that these guidelines were protective, thus supporting the use of the GPIT test as a predictive tool. In addition, this model has been used to examine allergic responses to mixtures of detergent enzymes (27). The data from these studies showed that protease enzymes act as adjuvants and enhance allergic responses to other proteins. Exposure guidelines for enzyme mixtures must take into account the adjuvant activity of the protease enzyme.

Finally, a guinea pig injection model has also been developed for comparison of the allergenic potency of new enzymes to that of Alcalase (28). Guinea pigs receive intradermal injections of enzyme over several weeks and enzyme-specific serum allergic antibody and tissue-fixed allergic antibody are assessed. Pulmonary symptoms were not measured in this model. The number of animals developing antibody to a new enzyme was compared with the number of animals developing antibody to the reference enzyme Alcalase. The difference in the response rate is used to assign potency to the new enzyme with this information being used to develop operational exposure guidelines for the manufacturing facilities. The ranking of new enzymes as compared to Alcalase with this injection model was very similar to that obtained with the intratracheal model (L. Blaikie, personal communication, 1997).

Guinea Pig Models of Occupational Allergy/Asthma to Chemicals

LMW chemicals are generally too small to be recognized by the immune system. When these chemicals bind in vivo to a larger carrier molecule (usually protein), this chemical-carrier conjugate may be recognized by the immune system. An immunological response specific to the chemical or to new antigenic determinants formed by the combination of chemical to carrier molecule can develop and mediate respiratory responsiveness to the chemical. Clinically, not all individuals with pulmonary symptoms to a specific chemical have demonstrable specific allergic antibody to the chemical. This situation is common among workers with occupational asthma to toluene diisocyanate (TDI) (29,30). Therefore, other unidentified immune or nonimmune mechanisms may play a role in respiratory responses to certain chemicals. This makes it difficult to develop predictive animal models for asthmagenic/allergenic chemicals, and one animal model may not be sufficient to study all chemicals or be a predictive tool for risk assessment.

Several guinea pig models rely on the development of chemical specific allergic antibody following exposure to free chemical or chemical-protein conjugate. In animal models, a homologous protein such as guinea pig serum albumin (GPA) is the common carrier protein used to develop the conjugate (31,32). Work done by Jin et al. (33) showed that GPA was one of several proteins in bronchoalveolar lavage fluid adducted with TDI after animals were exposed by inhalation to TDI atmospheres. Since nonimmune or poorly understood immune mechanisms may play a role in occupational allergy and asthma to certain chemicals, some of the animal models rely on pulmonary symptoms, profile of mediator release, and so forth, as a measure of reactivity to the chemical. Symptoms may be elicited from these animals by exposure to atmospheres of free chemical or chemical-carrier conjugate. In certain cases, pulmonary sensitivity could only be demonstrated by exposure to chemical-carrier conjugates and not to the chemical alone (reviewed in 32).

Guinea pigs were initially used to understand the mechanism of TDI-induced occupational asthma. These animals made IgG_1 and IgE antibody to TDI or hexamethylene diisocyanate (HDI) following parenteral injection with TDI or HDI protein conjugates (34). Early work by Karol et al. (35) showed that inhalation exposure to a monofunctional isocyante (*p*-tolyl isocyanate)-conjugate induced allergic antibody and respiratory reactivity specific to the hapten. Continued development of this inhalation model by Karol (36) examined immune and pulmonary responses to TDI. Karol found that inhalation exposure (3 hr/day for 5 days) to levels of TDI vapor of 120 ppb and higher led to antibody and pulmonary reactivity to the chemical. Increased concentrations of TDI vapor that led to an increase in antibody titer did not always correlate with the severity of pulmonary responses to this chemical. Using the Karol model, Kuang and colleagues (37) showed that the threshold for IgE production, pulmonary reactivity, and histamine release from lung mast cells following TDI exposure was between 20 and 200 ppb, confirming Karol's original observations of a threshold near 120 ppb. The TLV for TDI is 36 $\mu g/m^3$, or 0.005 ppm, a value that falls below the threshold range identified in the guinea pig (22).

The clinical experience with TDI indicates that many cases of occupational asthma cannot be linked with allergic antibody to TDI. Data suggest that other mechanisms consistent with an immune mechanism and rooted in an inflammatory response may be responsible for this asthma. Work in guinea pigs support this mechanism for TDI asthma. Kalubi, et al. (38) exposed guinea pigs to 5% TDI via intranasal application over a period of several weeks. They found an increase in substance P and CGRP immunoreactive fibers in the nasal mucosa along with an increase in substance P and CGRP mRNA in the trigeminal ganglia. Secretion of these neuropeptides lead to increased vasodilation and mucous secretion. Depletion of capsaicin-sensitive afferent nerves also prevented pulmonary hyperreactivity to TDI (39) providing further support for a mechanism of neural inflammation. Erjefalt and Persson (40) showed that repeated application of TDI to guinea pig tracheobronchial tissue led to an increase in plasma extravasation. Karol et al. (41) showed that TDI formed adducts in the apical regions of the epithelium of the nares, trachea, bronchi, and bronchioles suggesting that TDI could cause epithelial injury leading to changes in permeability and greater access to airway receptors. Finally, intradermal injection of guinea pigs with TDI followed by inhalation challenge induced allergic antibody to TDI, an increase in blood eosinophils, an increase in mast cells and eosinophils in the submucosa of central and peripheral airways, and an infiltration of CD4+ T lymphocytes into the airways supporting an inflammatory process involving T cells and eosinophils in TDI asthma (42).

Other investigators have used the Karol inhalation model to examine immune and pulmonary responses to TDI and other chemical allergens in an attempt to develop a predictive tool for risk assessment. Other chemicals tested in this model include diphenylmethane diisocyanate (MDI) (43), trimeric hexamethylene diisocyanate (Des-N) (44), trimellitic anhydride (TMA) (44,45), phthalic anhydride (PA) (31,46), procion yellow mx4r (45), and reactive black B dye (31). All of the investigators were able to reproduce Karol's TDI experience, which points to the robustness of the model.

Pulmonary reactivity (measured by changes in breathing rate and pattern) was detected in animals exposed to the isocyanates and the anhydrides (with the exception of Des-N) and challenged with the appropriate chemical-protein conjugate. Pulmonary responses were also elicited by challenge with free chemical from animals exposed to TDI, MDI, and TMA. No pulmonary reactivity was elicited from animals exposed to the dyes and challenged with either dye-protein conjugate or free dye. Animals sensitized and challenged with phthalic anhydride displayed lung pathology that was consistent with the hemorrhagic responses sometimes observed with TMA allergy (46). Also, specific allergic IgG$_1$ antibody (measured by PCA) and specific IgG antibody (measured by ELISA) were found to each chemical. Generally, as the exposure concentration of the chemical was increased, there was an increase in the amount of antibody produced. In addition, the number of animals responding with allergic antibody production increased with increased exposure. Animals with pulmonary reactivity had antibody to the chemical; however, not all animals demonstrating allergic antibody experienced pulmonary responses.

The exposure conditions needed to induce an immune response may be different from those required to elicit pulmonary reactions. In one inhalation study of TDI, the investigators found that animals exposed to 0.02 ppm TDI did not make antibody to this chemical but animals exposed to concentrations of greater than 0.2 ppm did make TDI-specific antibody (47). When sensitized animals were challenged with 0.02 ppm TDI, animals with antibody to the chemical experienced immediate-onset pulmonary symptoms. There was no relationship between antibody titer and the pulmonary response. This study showed that pulmonary symptoms could be elicited in sensitized animals by an exposure concentration that does not induce antibody production. Experiences with TDI and other chemicals demonstrate that an understanding of exposure conditions associated with antibody production versus elicitation of symptoms can be important when establishing occupational exposure guidelines designed to prevent either sensitization or symptoms in a workforce.

Several guinea pig injection models have been developed as an approach to quickly and cheaply assess whether or not a chemical is immunogenic and allergenic. Some of the models were also developed as a way to quickly sensitize animals to assess pulmonary reactions upon inhalation challenge with chemical. These models include intradermal injections (44,48), intraperitoneal injection (34), or subcutaneous injection (31) with free chemical or chemical-protein conjugate. Most investigators have used anhydrides (TMA, PA) and isocyanates (TDI, MDI) as model chemicals. Animals generate specific allergic antibodies (detected by ELISA or PCA) to these chemicals. In the intradermal model, animals received one to three injections of the highest tolerated dose of chemical to sensitize (44,48–50) whereas the subcutaneous injection model relied on injection of three to four doses of chemical over time, making it possible to compare dose-response curves among chemicals (31). Pulmonary reactivity, measured as changes in breathing rate, were also noted after inhalation challenge with free chemical in the intradermal models. However, high concentrations of chemical, i.e., up to 36 mg/m^3 MDI, 50 mg/m^3 TMA, and 52 mg/m^3 PA were needed to elicit such reactions. Pauluhn (51,52) has shown that the amount of chemical needed to elicit pulmonary reactions in guinea pigs is often an irritating concentration, confounding specific airway responses. However, an increase in sensitivity to acetylcholine challenge, along with an increase in eosinophils in lungs and lung-associated lymph nodes, was often found in those animals sensitized to the chemical. This information may be applicable to protect workers from developing pulmonary symptoms upon exposure to reactive chemicals.

Other investigators have used injection of guinea pigs and rats to understand the relationship between the structure of chemicals and antibody formation (53,54). Using antibody reactivity and inhibition in an ELISA and PCA test along with airway provocation measuring changes in resistance and plasma extravasation with dye, these investigators found that for acid anhydrides, the ring structure, the position of double bonds, and addition of methyl groups were important to immunogenicity. Such studies are important since the development of structure-activity models can be used as a first line of assessment of chemicals as potential occupational allergens and asthmagens (55).

Several studies have examined antibody and pulmonary responses of guinea pigs after dermal exposure to various isocyanates. One or two dermal applications of 25% or 100% TDI led to the generation of TDI-specific allergic antibody and one-third of the animals experienced pulmonary reactions upon inhalation exposure to TDI or TDI-GPA conjugate (56). When animals were exposed to a single, 6 hr occluded application of 10%, 30%, or 100% MDI, a dose-dependent increase in the number of animals with antibody to MDI was noted (49). In addition, pulmonary reactivity was noted in about one-fourth of the animals exposed to atmospheres containing between 25.9 and 36.4 mg/m^3 MDI. Investigators have had mixed success with inducing antibody and pulmonary responses in animals exposed to MDI via the inhalation route (43,49). It is possible that for certain chemicals, dermal exposure can be a relevant exposure route for sensitization of the respiratory tract.

Other variations of guinea pig injection models have been used by several investigators to examine antibody, pulmonary, and neurogenic responses to chemical allergens. In one model, guinea pigs received an intramuscular injection of TMA conjugated to carrier protein (57) and several weeks later, animals were exposed to 130 mg/m^3 TMA dust. These animals experienced significant changes in lung pathology (most notably hemorrhage) consistent with one of the TMA syndromes described by Zeiss et al. (58,59). The same investigators found that these animals produced both IgG$_1$ and IgE antibody to TMA and developed airway hyperreactivity accompanied by eosinophilic influx (60).

In a similar model used by Arakawa et al. (61,62) and Hayes et al. (63,64), animals injected with TMA and challenged by intratracheal instillation of TMA-GPA conjugate experienced a significant increase in airway resistance, extravasation of Evans blue dye into the airways, airway hyperreactivity, and an influx of eosiniphils into the subepithelium of the airways. The IgG$_1$ antibody titer did not correlate with increased airway resistance, but did correlate with extravasation. Treatment of the animals with an antihistamine alleviated changes in airway resistance, but had no effect on extravasation. Rather, treatment of animals with capsaicin and hexamethonium (to block release of neurogenic mediators) alleviated the extravasation, but had no effect on airway resistance. These findings suggest that pulmonary reactions to chemical allergens, like TMA, may be mediated by different mechanisms, and that antibody responses may correlate with some of these mechanisms.

MURINE MODELS OF ALLERGY TO PROTEINS

The murine ovalbumin (OVA) model has been used to study the pulmonary inflammation typical of asthma. It involves systemic sensitization to antigen and repeated aerosol challenge. An adjuvant-free protocol is used. Repeated inhalation challenge results in epithelial damage, decreased lung function, and chronic inflammation of the lungs. The severity of the changes increases with repetitive OVA challenge.

Variations of the basic protocol have been used to distinguish key events linking the early and late-onset phases of asthma. The early phase is due to release of airway-constricting mediators by mast cells in response to cross-linkage of their FcɛR1 receptors.

Acute inflammation of the lung was produced upon the i.p. administration of ovalbumin and inhalation challenge (65–67). Lungs appeared densely infiltrated with CD4+ T cells and eosinophils.

Airway hyperreactivity (AHR) is measured after inhalation challenge with OVA by exposing animals to methacholine. Typically, an aerosol of methacholine (30 mM) is delivered for 60 sec and the respiratory breathing pattern is noted. Evidence for the involvement of interferon-γ (IFN-γ) in development of AHR was obtained. Treatment of the mice with antibodies to IFN-γ completely prevented development of AHR (68). The antibodies had no effect on the lung eosinophilia suggesting differential regulation of AHR and eosinophilia in this animal model. The model also demonstrates high levels of OVA-specific IgE in the serum.

Murine models have been developed to address the late-phase response. Models that demonstrate the numerous cardinal features of the response include: airway hyperreactivity (69), eosinophilic lung inflammation (70), increase in TH2 cytokine expression (71), mucin accumulation in the airspace (72), and increased circulating IgE (73).

Murine models (as well as rat models) are appropriate for addressing the genetic influence on allergic lung disease. Genomes of mice and rats are being characterized, and manipulation of genes is emerging as a method to study pathology and toxicology of asthma. For example, a transgenic mouse model has been developed that constitutively expresses IL-4 selectively in the lung (74). Another mouse model that is deficient in p-selectin shows reduced hyperresponsiveness to methacholine (75) as do B-cell-deficient mice (76).

The major allergic antibody in the mouse is IgE although IgG_1 antibody can drive type I allergic/anaphylactic responses in this species (76–80). Different inbred strains of mice will also respond to proteins differently. It has been recognized for many years that the robustness of the allergic antibody response to proteins such as bovine gamma globulin, ovalbumin, or ovamucoid varies with the strain (81–83). Therefore, the choice of strain can be important when developing mouse models to assess occupational allergy to proteins. Having said this, investigators are using mice to study the development of allergic responses to occupational protein allergens. A mouse intranasal model (MINT) for assessing enzymes as respiratory allergens was developed by Robinson et al. (84). In this model, BDF1 mice receive intranasal instillations of enzyme protein and the amount of enzyme-specific IgG_1 antibody in sera is measured by ELISA. These animals will also generate enzyme-specific IgE antibody. Since IgG_1 antibody and IgE antibody are regulated by a TH2/IL-4 pathway (85) and since additional animals (rat PCA) are needed to measure the

IgE antibody, the IgG_1 antibody is used as a "surrogate" for the IgE antibody. Like the guinea pig models for protein occupational allergy, the mouse model will rank new enzymes as more potent, less potent, or equipotent to the benchmark enzyme Alcalase (86). These assessments mirror those obtained in the guinea pig, which in turn are associated with skin prick test responses in workers. So far, the MINT has the potential to be a predictive tool for risk assessment of protein respiratory allergens.

Other investigators have used intraperitoneal injection of the Balb/c mouse as an approach to develop a predictive test for protein allergens (87). In this model, animals are injected with OVA or bovine albumin. The investigators postulate that OVA is a good allergen in humans and the immune response is driven by TH2 cells. They also postulate that bovine albumin is a poor allergen in humans and the immune response is driven by TH1 cells. By evaluating TH1 versus TH2 responses in the mouse (e.g., cytokines, antibody subclasses), then such an approach can be used to predict which proteins can cause occupational allergy in humans. Whether this approach will be successful must wait the test of time.

Mouse Models for Chemically Induced Asthma

An epicutaneous model has demonstrated that contact allergens and respiratory allergens produce different patterns of cytokine production in draining lymph nodes (88). Contact allergens stimulate predominantly TH1 cytokines (IFN-γ) whereas TDI and TMA stimulate TH2-type cytokines, such as IL-4.

Topical administration of chemicals has been shown to lead to pulmonary inflammation and airway hyperreactivity (89). Balb/c mice were sensitized by application of a 0.5% picryl chloride solution to the shaved abdomen, thorax, and four feet. One week later, animals were challenged by intranasal administration of a solution of picryl sulfonic acid. The pulmonary inflammation was characterized by mononuclear cells around the airways and vasculature. Lung function was measured in anesthetized, but spontaneously breathing mice, as pulmonary resistance and dynamic compliance (90). Airway hyperreactivity was determined by ex vivo challenge of the trachea to carbachol or serotonin. These studies indicated a delayed-type hypersensitivity reaction (occurring 2 hr after challenge) in the lungs, characterized by tracheal hyperreactivity and altered lung function. The response was reproduced in naïve animals following transfer of T cells. It is also dependent upon mast cells, since reduced hyperresponsiveness and fewer arachadonic acid metabolites were observed in mast cell-deficient mice.

Studies have been undertaken in a mouse model to determine the response to a recognized cause of occupational asthma, TDI. The model was also examined to determine whether it could distinguish chemicals having the potential to cause respiratory sensitization from those that cause dermal sensitivity (91). Balb/c mice were sensitized by epicutaneous exposure to 0.5% TDI or dinitrochlorobenzene (DNCB), and challenged 8 days later by intranasal administration of DNB sulfonic acid or *p*-toluene sulfonic acid. Mononuclear inflammatory reactions around the pulmonary vasculature, but not around the airways, were noted with both chemicals. Only the TDI-exposed animals demonstrated antigen-specific IgG antibody. Total serum IgE was not increased in this group, but was actually lower than in control or DNCB-exposed animals. These findings indicate that a single challenge with the chemical allergen was insufficient to elicit an airway inflammatory reaction in the sensitized animals and suggest that measurement of hapten-specific IgG may distinguish chemicals that cause respiratory sensitivity from those able to cause dermal sensitivity.

A mouse inhalation model to study airway responses to sensitizing chemicals has been developed (92) but has been used with only a few chemicals, such as dinitrochlorobenzene and picryl chloride.

An intrabronchial mouse model of TDI asthma has been reported. The model exposes only pulmonary tissue to a chemical allergen, thus avoiding exposure of the gastrointestinal tract and the upper airways (93) and eliminating the need to generate chemical atmospheres. The model has the advantage of delivery of the chemical allergen, in reactive form, to a designated site in the respiratory tract. The chemical in corn oil is delivered to the left lung lobe through a cannulae (Fig. 1). Animals are challenged 15 days later by delivery of the chemical to the same location in the lung. The response to challenge is measured 24 hr later. It consisted of eosinophilic pulmonary inflammation around the airways and vasculature. Since the same response was seen in animals that were sensitized but not challenged, it was concluded that the inflammation was due to the initial TDI

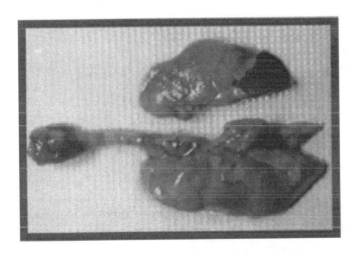

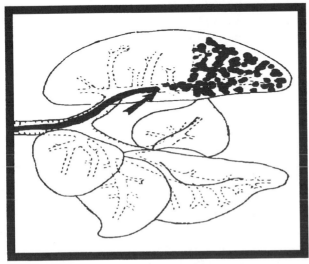

Figure 1 Instillation of antigen into bronchus. Antigen is directed into the left lobe by correct positioning of the cannula. (Adapted from Ref. 93.)

exposure. Moreover, the degree and localization of the inflammation were not affected by the challenge exposure. Immunostaining of lung sections, using an antibody specific to TDI, indicated that the chemical was localized largely to the epithelium of the airways and present only in the lung that had received the chemical. IgG antibodies to TDI were detected in the circulation but titers did not correspond with the degree of pulmonary inflammation.

RAT MODELS

Brown Norway Rat

The inbred Brown Norway (BN) rat has been found to produce IgE antibody readily and thus has become useful as an animal model of asthma (94). Sensitization routes have varied. One model utilizes subcutaneous administration of OVA precipitated in aluminum hydroxide gel. At the same time, animals also receive heat-killed *Bordetella pertussis* i.p. (95). Serum IgE increases for 14 days, and then remains stable. Inhalation challenge is performed at 2 weeks and airflow is monitored. An increase in airway resistance is indicative of a response. A large number of late-onset responses are seen, frequently following early responses. The mean time of response is 7 hr following challenge and the mean duration of late response is 90 min. No increase in airway hyperresponsiveness to methacholine was noted. The IgE response did not correlate with the magnitude of either the early or late response. The early response was blunted by repeated challenge, but the late response was not (96). Nagase et al. (97) showed that the early airway response in the BN rat was dependent upon the production of 5-hydroxytryptamine (5-HT) and leukotriene D4 (LTD4) since pretreatment with antagonists blocked changes in airway resistance upon challenge with OVA. Investigators have also used OVA in the BN rat model to understand the pathophysiology of asthma in this species. Taylor and colleagues (98) have shown that inhalation challenge of OVA-sensitized BN rats leads to a significant increase in lung permeability (plasma extravasation) and eosinophil accumulation into the alveolar spaces. Lung edema and cell infiltrates were observed 24–72 hr after challenge. Pretreatment with antibody to ICAM-1 and/or alpha-4-integrin blocked eosinophil accumulation in the lung but had no effect on microvascular leakage and lung edema.

BN rats were used to develop a model of TMA-induced occupational asthma. Rats were given single or multiple exposures at several concentrations of TMA dust. Challenge was also with dust. The model was characterized by an allergic inflammation. Animals developed a delayed influx of eosinophils into the lung, and TMA-specific IgG and IgE antibodies (99). Continued work with this model showed that TMA-sensitized BN rats, challenged via inhalation with TMA-rat albumin conjugate, had airway hyperresponsiveness 24 hr postchallenge along with some damage to airway epithelium (100). Repeated challenges with the conjugate led to airway hyperreactivity and damage to epithelium but did not cause eosinophilia in lung. Eosinophil infiltration was associated with a single inhalation challenge with conjugate, which did not cause significant airway hyperreactivity.

Topical exposure of BN rats to TMA or the contact allergen oxazolone led to the production of IgG antibody to both chemicals (101). IgE antibody was produced to TMA only. Cytokine production from cells obtained from the draining lymph nodes showed a TH1 pattern (IFN-γ) for oxazolone and a TH2 pattern (IL-4 and IL-5) for TMA. Like the mouse, the BN rat can discern between a contact chemical allergen and a chemical respiratory allergen via production of IgE antibody and divergent cytokine expression. This approach in the rat, as well as in the mouse, may have utility as a screen for the potential of chemicals to be contact or respiratory allergens.

Wistar rats have also been used to develop a model of respiratory hypersensitivity due to chemical exposure (102). The chemical is administered via inhalation for 1–2 weeks. Histological examination of the lung tissue following exposure to phenyl isocyanate revealed many key features of chronic asthma including goblet cell hyperplasia, eosinophilia of the airways, smooth muscle hypertrophy, and mucus plugs and cellular debris in the airway lumen. Decreased forced expiratory flow was noted as was airway hyperreactivity to acetylcholine.

A rat bioassay for pulmonary hypersensitivity has been proposed (102). Animals are given nose-only inhalation exposure of a nonirritating concentration of test chemical for 1–2 weeks. Endpoints to be monitored include lung function testing, as well as biochemical and morphological signs of effects.

SUMMARY

The various animal models described have been used to understand the nature of occupational allergy and asthma. Some have been developed as risk assessment tools to determine whether HMW compounds, such as proteins, and LMW compounds, such as reactive chemicals, are respiratory allergens/asthmagens. For proteins, one can assume that exposure of sufficient magnitude, duration, and/or frequency can lead to recognition by the immune system and induce the production of allergic antibody in some individuals. Therefore, the risk assessment process addresses how to protect workers from developing antibodies and eventually symptoms to these materials. In the detergent industry, guinea pig and mouse models are used to assess enzymes as allergens and the information from the models is used to establish protective exposure guidelines (21,26,27,84,86).

Assessment of chemicals as allergens and/or asthmagens is more difficult. The mechanism of asthma and/or allergy to chemicals is poorly understood and it is difficult to develop animal models as tools for risk assessment. Computational models may prove helpful (55). Animal models rely on production of antibody or differential expression of TH2 versus TH1 cytokines. Other models rely on elicitation of symptoms. No single model may work for all chemicals. It has been suggested that one can compare the potential of an unknown chemical to be an allergen/asthmagen to known chemical allergens/asthmagens in various animal models (31,32,103,104). Information gained from these models can be used to set protective exposure guidelines. Confirmation of the adequacy of these guidelines would need to be done by extensive monitoring of the exposed workforce.

REFERENCES

1. Chan-Yeung M. Occupational asthma. Chest 1990; 98:148s–161s.
2. Ratner B, Jackson HC, Gruehl HL. Respiratory anaphylaxis: sensitization, shock, bronchial asthma and death induced in the guinea pig by nasal inhalation of dry horse dander. Am J Dis Child 1927; 34:23–52.
3. Griffith-Johnson, DA, Jin R, Karol MH. The role of purified IgG_1 in pulmonary hypersensitivity responses of the guinea pig. J Toxicol Environ Health 1993; 40:117–127.
4. Karol MH, Stadler J, Underhill D, Alarie Y. Monitoring delayed onset pulmonary hypersensitivity in guinea pigs. Toxicol and Appl Pharmacol 1981; 61:277–285.

5. Ishida M, Amesara R, Ukai K, Sakakura Y. Antigen induced allergic rhinitis model in the guinea pig. Ann Allergy 1994; 72:240–244.

6. Yasui K, Asanuma F, Furue Y, Arimura A. Involvement of thromboxane A-2 in antigen induced nasal blockage in guinea pigs. Int Arch Allergy Immunol 1997; 112:400–405.

7. Griffith-Johnson DA, Karol MH. Validation of a non-invasive technique to assess development of airway hyperreactivity in animal models of immunologic pulmonary hypersensitivity. Toxicology 1991; 65:283–294.

8. Lapa e Silva JR, Bachelet CM, Pretolani M, Baker D, Scheper RJ, Vargaftig BB. Immunopathologic alterations in the bronchi of immunized guinea pigs. Am J Respir Cell Mol Biol 1993; 9:44–53.

9. Lapa e Silva JR, Pretolani M, Bachelet CM, Baker D, Scheper RJ, Vargaftig BB. Emergence of T lymphocytes, eosinophils and dendritic cells in the bronchi of actively sensitized guinea pigs after antigenic challenge. Brazil J Med Biol Res 1994; 27:1653–1658.

10. Pretolani M, Ruffie C, Lapa e Silva JR, Joseph D, Lobb RR, Vargaftig BB. Antibody to very late activation antigen 4 prevents antigen induced bronchial hyperreactivity and cellular infiltration in the guinea pig airways. J Exp Med 1994; 180:795–805.

11. van Oosterhout AJM, van Ark I, Folkerts G, van der Linde HJ, Savelkoul HFJ, Verheyen ACKP, Nijkamp FP. Antibody to interleukin 5 inhibits virus induced airway hyperresponsiveness to histamine in guinea pigs. Am J Respir Crit Care Med 1995; 151:177–183.

12. Mehta S, Lilly CM, Rollenhagen JE, Haley KJ, Asano K, Drazen J. Acute and chronic effects of allergic airway inflammation on pulmonary nitric oxide production. Amer J Physiol 1997; 272:L124–L131.

13. Parish WE. Eosinophilia: cutaneous eosinophilia in guinea pigs mediated by passive anaphylaxis with IgG_1 or reagin, and antigen-antibody complexes: its relation to neutrophils and mast cells. Immunology 1972; 23:19–34.

14. Dobson C, Morseth DJ, Soulsby JL. Immunoglobulin E-type antibodies induced by *Ascaris suum* infections in guinea pigs. J Immunol 1971; 106:128–133.

15. Dunn CJ, Elliott GA, Oostveen JA, Richards IM. Development of a prolonged eosinophil-rich inflammatory leukocyte infiltration in the guinea pig asthmatic response to ovalbumin inhalation. Am Rev Respir Dis 1988; 137:541–547.

16. Karol MH, Hillebrand J, Thorne PT. Characteristics of weekly pulmonary hypersensitivity responses elicited in guinea pigs by inhalation of ovalbumin aerosols. Toxicol Appl Pharmacol 1989; 100:234–246.

17. Karol MH, Stadler J, Mangreni CM. Immunotoxicologic evaluation of the respiratory system: animal models for immediate and delayed-onset pulmonary hypersensitivity. Fund Appl Toxicol 1985; 5:459–472.

18. Thorne PT, Hillebrand J, Magreni C, Riley EJ, Karol MH. Experimental sensitization to subtilisin: production of immediate and late onset pulmonary reactions. Toxicol Appl Pharmacol 1986; 86:112–123.

19. Hillibrand J, Thorne PT, Karol MH. Experimental sensitization to subtilisin: production of specific antibodies following inhalation exposure of guinea pigs. Toxicol Appl Pharmacol 1987; 89:449–456.

20. Thorne PT, Karol MH. Association of fever with late onset pulmonary hypersensitivity responses in the guinea pig. Toxicol Appl Pharmacol 1989; 100:247–258.

21. Ritz HL, Evans BLB, Bruce RD, Fletcher ER, Fisher GL, Sarlo K. Respiratory and immunological responses of guinea pigs to enzyme containing detergents: a comparison of intratracheal and inhalation modes of exposure. Fund Appl Toxicol 1993; 21:31–37.

22. Threshold Limit Values and Biological Exposure Indices. Cincinnati: American Conference of Governmental Industrial Hygienists. 1997:36, 38.

23. Juniper CP, How MJ, Goodwin BFJ, Kinshott AK. *Bacillus subtilis* enzymes: a seven year clinical epidemiological and immunological study of an industrial allergen. J Soc Occup Med 1977; 27:3–12.

24. Flood DFS, Blofeld RE, Bruce CF, Hewitt JI, Juniper CP, Roberts DM. Lung function, atopy, specific hypersensitivity and smoking of workers in the enzyme detergent industry over 11 years. Br J Ind Med 1985; 42:43–50.

25. Sarlo K, Clark ED, Ryan CR, Bernstein DI. ELISA for human IgE antibody to subtilisin A (Alcalase): correlation with RAST and skin test results with occupationally exposed individuals. J Allergy Clin Immunol 1990; 86:393–399.

26. Sarlo K, Fletcher ER, Gaines WG, Ritz HL. Respiratory allergenicity of detergent enzymes in the guinea pig intratracheal test: association with sensitization of occupationally exposed individuals. Fund Appl Toxicol 1997; 38:44–52.

27. Sarlo K, Ritz HL, Fletcher ER, Schrotel K, Clark ED. Proteolytic detergent enzymes enhance the allergic antibody responses of guinea pigs to nonproteolytic detergent enzymes in a mixture: implications for occupational exposure. J Allergy Clin Immunol 1997; 100:480–487.

28. Blaikie L, Basketter DA, Morrow T. Experience with a guinea pig model for the assessment of respiratory allergens. Hum Exp Toxicol 1994; 9:743.

29. Karol MH, Jin R. Mechanisms of immunotoxicity to isocyanates. Chem Res Toxicol 1991; 4:503–509.

30. Karol MH, Tollerud DJ, Cambell TP, Fabbri L, Maestrelli P, Saetta M, Mapp CE. Predictive value of airway hyperresponsiveness and circulating IgE for identifying types of responses to TDI inhalation challenge. Am J Respir Crit Care Med 1994; 149:611–615.

31. Sarlo K, Clark ED, A tier approach for evaluating the respiratory allergenicity of low molecular weight chemicals. Fund Appl Toxicol 1992; 18:107–114.

32. Sarlo K, Karol MH. Guinea pig predictive tests for respiratory allergy. In: Dean JH, Luster MI, Munson AE, Kimber I, eds. Immunotoxicology and Immunopharmacology. New York: Raven Press, 1994:703–720.

33. Jin R, Day BW, Karol MH. TDI protein adducts in the bronchoalveolar lavage of guinea pigs exposed to vapors of the chemical. Chem Res Toxicol 1993; 6:906–912.

34. Chen SE, Bernstein IL. The guinea pig model of diisocyanate sensitization: immunological studies. J Allergy Clin Immunol 1982; 70:383–392.

35. Karol MH, Ioset HH, Riley EJ, Alarie YC. Hapten-specific respiratory hypersensitivity in the guinea pig. Am Ind Hyg Assoc J 1978; 39:546–556.

36. Karol MH. Concentration dependent immunologic response to TDI following inhalation exposure. Toxicol Appl Pharmacol 1983; 68:229–241.

37. Kuang J, Aoyama K, Ueda A. Experimental study on respiratory sensitivity to inhaled toluene diisocyanate. Arch Toxicol 1993; 67:373–378.

38. Kalubi B, Takeda N, Irifune M, Ogino S, Abe Y, Hong SL, Yamano M, Matsuhaga T, Tohyama M. Nasal mucosa sensitization with TDI increases preprotachykinin A and prepro CGRP mRNAs in guinea pig trigeminal ganglion neurons. Brain Res 1992; 576:287–296.

39. Baur X, Marek W, Ammon J, Czuppon AB, Marczynski B, Raulfheimsoth M, Roemmelt H, Fruhmann G. Respiratory and other hazards of isocyanates. Int Arch Occup Environ Health 1994; 66:141–152.

40. Erjefalt I, Persson CGA. Increased sensitivity to TDI in airways previously exposed to low doses of TDI. Clin Exp Allergy 1992; 22:854–862.

41. Karol MH, Jin RZ, Lantz RC. Immunochemical detection of TDI adducts in pulmonary tissue of guinea pigs following inhalation exposure. Inh Toxicol 1997; 9:63–83.

42. Mapp CE, Lapa e Silva JR, Lucchini RE, Chitano P, Rado V, Saetta M, Pretolani M, Karol MH, Maestrelli P, Fabbri LM. Inflammatory events in the blood and airways of guinea pigs immunized to TDI. Am J Respir Crit Care Med 1996; 154:201–208.

43. Karol MH, Thorne PS. Pulmonary hypersensitivity and hyperreactivity: implications for assessing allergic responses. In: Gardner DE, Crapo JD, Massaro EJ, eds. Toxicology of the Lung New York: Raven Press, 1988:427–448.

44. Pauluhn J, Eben A. Validation of a non-invasive technique to assess immediate or delayed onset airway hypersensitivity in guinea pigs. J Appl Toxicol 1991; 11:423–431.

45. Botham PA, Hext PM, Rattray NJ, Walsh ST, Woodcock DR. Sensitization of guinea pigs by inhalation exposure to low molecular weight chemicals. Toxicol Lett 1988; 41:159–173.

46. Sarlo K, Clark ED, Ferguson J, Zeiss CR, Hatoum N. Induction of type I hypersensitivity in guinea pigs after inhalation of phthalic anhydride. J Allergy Clin Immunol 1994; 94:747–756.

47. Aoyama K, Huang J, Ueda A, Matsushita T. Provocation of respiratory allergy in guinea pigs following inhalation of free toluene diisocyanate. Arch Environ Contam Toxicol 1994; 26:403–407.

48. Botham PA, Rattray NJ, Woodcock DR, Walsh ST, Hext PM. The induction of respiratory allergy in guinea pigs following intradermal injection of TMA: a comparison with the response to DNCB. Toxicol Lett 1989; 47:25–39.

49. Rattray NJ, Botham PA, Hext PM, Woodcock DR, Fielding I, Dearman RJ, Kimber I. Induction of respiratory hypersensitivity to MDI in guinea pigs: influence of route of exposure. Toxicology 1994; 88:15–30.

50. Blaikie L, Morrow T, Wilson AP, Hext P, Hartop PJ, Rattray NJ, Woodcock D, Botham PA. A two-centre study for the evaluation and validation of an animal model for the assessment of the potential of small molecular weight chemicals to cause respiratory allergy. Toxicology, 1995; 96:37–50.

51. Pauluhn J. Assessment of chemicals for their potential to induce respiratory allergy in guinea pigs: a comparison of different routes of induction and confounding effects due to pulmonary hyperreactivity. Toxicol In Vitro 1994; 8:981–985.

52. Pauluhn J, Mohr U. Assessment of respiratory hypersensitivity in guinea pigs sensitized to MDI and challenged with MDI, acetylcholine or MDI-albumin conjugate. Toxicology 1994; 92:53–74.

53. Welinder H, Zhang X, Gustavsson C, Bjork B, Skerfving S. Structure activity relationships of organic acid anhydrides as antigens in an animal model. Toxicology 1995; 103:127–136.

54. Zhang X, Lotvall J, Skerfving S, Welinder H. Antibody specificity to the chemical structures of organic acid anhydrides studied by in vitro and in vivo methods. Toxicology 1997; 118:223–232.

55. Graham C, Rosenkranz HS, Karol MH. Structure-activity model of chemicals that cause human respiratory sensitization. Regul Toxicol Pharm 1997; 26:296–306.

56. Karol MH, Hauth BA, Riley EJ, Mangreni CM. Dermal contact with TDI produces respiratory tract hypersensitivity in guinea pigs. Toxicol Appl Pharmacol 1981; 58:221–230.

57. Tao Y, Sugiura T, Nakamura H, Kido M, Tanaka I, Kuriona A. Experimental lung injury induced by TMA inhalation in guinea pigs. Int Arch Allergy Appl Immunol 1991; 96:119–127.

58. Zeiss CR, Patterson R, Pruzansky JJ, Miller M, Rosenberg M, Levitz D. TMA induced airway syndromes: clinical and immunological studies. J Allergy Clin Immunol 1977; 60:96–103.

59. Zeiss CR, Wolkonsky P, Chacon R, Tuntland AP, Levitz D, Pruzansky JJ, Patterson R. Syndromes in workers exposed to TMA: a longitudinal clinical and immunological study. Ann Intern Med 1983; 98:8–12.

60. Obata H, Tao Y, Kido M, Nagata N, Tanaka I, Kuroiwa A. Guinea pig model of immunologic asthma induced by inhalation of TMA. Am Rev Respir Dis 1992; 146:1553–1558.

61. Arakawa H, Lotvall J, Kawikova I, Tee R, Hayes J, Lofdahl CG, Newman Taylor AJ, Skoogh BE. Airway allergy to trimellitic anhydride in guinea pigs: different time courses of IgG_1 titer and airway responses to allergen challenge. J Allergy Clin Immunol, 1993; 92:425–434.

62. Arakawa H, Lotvall J, Linden A, Kawikova I, Lofdahl CG, Skoogh BE. Role of eicosanoids in airflow obstruction and airway plasma exudation induced by TMA-conjugate in guinea pigs 3 and 8 weeks after sensitization. Clin Exp Allery 1994; 24:582–589.

63. Hayes JP, Daniel R, Tee R, Barnes PJ, Chung KF, Newman Taylor AJ. Specific immunological and bronchopulmonary responses following intradermal sensitization to free TMA in the guinea pig. Clin Exp Allergy 1992; 22:694–700.

64. Hayes JP, Han-Pin K, Rohde JAL, Newman Taylor AJ, Barnes PJ, Fan-Chung K, Rogers DF. Neurogenic goblet cell secretion and bronchoconstriction in guinea pigs sensitized to trimellitic anhydride. Euro J Pharmacol Environ Toxicol Pharmacol Sect 1995; 292:127–134.

65. Gavett SH, Chen X, Finkelman F, Wills-Karp M. Depletion of murine CD4+ T lymphocytes prevents antigen-induced hyperreactivity and pulmonary eosinophilia. Am J Respir Cell Mol Biol 1994; 10:587.

66. Hessel EM, Van Oosterhout AJM, Hofstra CL, De Bie JJ, Garssen J, Van Loveren H, Verheyen AKCP, Savelkoul HFJ, Nijkamp FP. Bronchoconstriction and airway hyper-responsiveness after ovalbumin inhalation in sensitized mice. Eur J Pharmacol 1995; 293: 401–412.

67. Lukacs NW, Strieter RM, Shaklee CL, Chensue SW, Kunkel SL. Macrophage inflammatory protein-1α influences eosinophil recruitment in antigen-specific airway inflammation. Eur J Immunol 1995; 25:245.

68. Hessel EM, Van Oosterhout AJM, Van Ark I, Van Esch B, Hofman G, Van Loveren H, Savelkoul HFJ, Nijkamp FP. Development of airway hyperresponsiveness is dependent on interferon-γ and independent of eosinophil infiltration. Am J Respir Cell Mol Biol 1997; 16: 325–334.

69. Kline JN, Waldschmidt TJ, Businga TR, Lemish JE, Weinstock JV, Thorne PS, Krieg AM. Modulation of airway inflammation by CpG oligodeoxynucleotides in a murine model of asthma. J Immunol 1998; 160:2555–2559.

70. Zhang Y, Rogers KH, Lewis DB. B$_2$-microglobulin-dependent T cells are dispensable for allergen-induced T helper 2 responses. J Exp Med 1996; 184:1507–1512.

71. Corry DB, Folkesson HG, Warnock ML, Erle DJ, Matthay MA, Wiener-Kronish JP, Locksley RM. Interleukin 4, but not interleukin 5 or eosinophils, is required in a murine model of acute airway hyperreactivity. J Exp Med 1996; 183:109–117.

72. Henderson WR, Lewis DB, Albert RK, Zhang Y, Lamm WJE, Chiang GKS, Jones F, Eriksen P, Tien Y-T, Jonas M, Chi EY. The importance of leukotrienes in airway inflammation in a mouse model of asthma. J Exp Med 1996; 184:1483–1494.

73. Renz H. T cell receptor-Vb repertoire in allergen-specific sensitization and increased airway responsiveness. Allergy 1995; 50(Suppl 25):15–19.

74. Rankin JA, Picarella DE, Geba GP, Temann UA, Prasad B, DiCosmo B, Tarallo A, Stripp B, Whitsett J, Flavell RA. Phenotypic and physiologic characterization of transgenic mice expressing interleukin 4 in the lung: lymphocytic and eosinophilic inflammation without airway hyperreactivity. Proc Natl Acad Sci USA 1996; 93:7821–7825.

75. De Sanctis GT, Wolyniec WW, Green FHY, Qin S, Jiao A, Finn PW, Noonan T, Joetham AA, Gelfand E, Doerschuk CM, Drazen JM. Reduction of allergic airway responses in P-selectin deficient mice. J Appl Physiol 1997; 83:681–687.

76. Hamelmann E, Vella AT, Oshiba A, Kappler JW, Marrack P, Gelfand EW. Allergic airway sensitization induces T cell activation but not airway hyperresponsiveness in B cell–deficient mice. Proc Natl Acad Sci USA 1997; 94:1350–1355.

77. Nussenzweig RS, Merryman C, Benacerraf C. Electrophoretic separation and properties of mouse antihapten antibody involved in passive cutaneouis anaphylaxis and passive hemolysis. J Exp Med 1964; 120:315–328

78. Faccione S, deSiqueira ALP, Jancar S, Russo M, Barbuto JAM, Mariano M. A novel murine model of late-phase reaction of immediate hypersensitivity. Mediat Inflamm 1997; 6:127–133.

79. Miyajima I, Dombrowicz D, Martin TR, Ravetch JV, Kinet JP, Gali SJ. Systemic anaphylaxis in the mouse can be mediated largely through IgG$_1$ and Fc gamma RIII—assessment of cardiopulmonary changes, mast cell degranulation and death associated with active IgE- or IgG$_1$-dependent passive anaphylaxis. J Clin Invest 1997; 99:901–914.

80. Mehlop PD, vandeRijn M, Goldberg AB, Brewer JP, Kurup VP, Martin TR, Oettgen HC Allergen-induced bronchial hyperreactivity and eosinophilic inflammation occur in the absence of IgE in a mouse model of asthma. Proc Natl Acad Sci USA 1997; 94:1344–1349.

81. Vaz NM, Levine BB. Immune responsiveness of inbred mice to repeated low doses of antigen: relationship to H-2 type. Science 1970; 168:852–854.

82. Vaz NM, Vaz EM, Levine BB. Relationship between H-2 genotype and immune responsiveness to low doses of ovalbumin in the mouse. J Immunol 1970; 104:572–580.

83. Vaz NM, Philips-Quagliata JM, Levine BB, Vaz EM. H-2 linked genetic control of immune responsiveness to ovalbumin and ovamucoid. J Exp Med 1971; 134:1335–1348.

84. Robinson MK, Babcock LS, Horn PA, Kawabata TT. Specific antibody responses to subtilisin Carlsberg (Alcalase) in mice: development of an intranasal exposure model. Fund Appl Toxicol 1996; 34:15–24.

85. Purkeson JM, Isakson PC. IL5 provides a signal that is required in addition to IL4 for isotype switching to IgG_1 and IgE. J Exp Med 1992; 175:973–982.

86. Robinson MK, Horn PA, Kawabata TT, Babcock LS, Fletcher ER, Sarlo, K. Use of the mouse intranasal test to determine the allergenic potency of detergent enzymes: comparison to the guinea pig intratracheal test. Toxicol Sci, 1998; 43:39–46.

87. Hilton J, Dearman RJ, Sattar N, Basketter DA, Kimber I. Characteristics of antibody responses induced in mice by protein allergens. Food Chem Toxicol 1997; 35:1209–1218.

88. Dearman RJ, Moussavi A, Kemeny DM, Kimber I. Contribution of CD4+ and CD8+ T lymphocyte subsets to the cytokine secretion patterns induced in mice during sensitization to contact and respiratory chemical allergens. Immunology 1996; 89:502–510.

89. Garssen J, Nijkamp FP, Wagenaar SS, Zwrt A, Askenase PW, Van Loveren H. Regulation of delayed-type hypersensitivity-like response in the mouse lung, determined with histological procedures: serotonin, T-cell suppressor-inducer factor and high antigen dose tolerance regulate the magnitude of T-cell dependent inflammatory reactions. Immunology 1989; 68:51–58.

90. Garssen J, Nijkamp FP, Van Vugt E, Van Der Vliet H, Van Loveren H. T cell-derived antigen binding molecules play a role in the induction of airway hyperresponsiveness. Am J Respir Crit Care Med 1994; 150:1528–1538.

91. Satoh T, Kramarik JA, Tollerud DJ, Karol MH. A murine model for assessing the respiratory hypersensitivity potential of chemical allergens. Toxicol Lett 1995; 78:57–66.

92. Garssen J, Nijkamp FP, Van der Vliet H, Van Loveren H. T-cell mediated induction of airway hyperreactivity in mice. Am Rev Respir Dis 1991; 144:931–938.

93. Ebino K, Kramarik J, Lemus R, Karol MH. A mouse model for study of localized toluene diisocyanate (TDI) adducts following intrabronchial administration of the chemical: inflammation and antibody production. Inhal Toxicol 1998; 10:503–529.

94. Waserman S, Xu LJ, Olivenstein R, Renzi PM, Martin JG. Association between late allergic bronchoconstriction in the rat and allergen-stimulated lymphocyte proliferation. Am J Respir Crit Care Med 1995; 151:470–474.

95. Eidelman DH, Bellofiore S, Martin JG. Late airway responses to antigen challenge in sensitized inbred rats. Am Rev Respir Dis 1988; 137:1033–1037.

96. Waserman S, Olivenstein R, Renzi PM, Xu LJ, Martin JG. The relationship between late asthmatic responses and antigen-specific immunoglobulin. J Allergy Clin Immunol 1992; 90:661–669.

97. Nagase T, Dallaire MJ, Ludwig MS. Airway and tissue behavoir during early responses in sensitized rats: role of 5-HT and LTD4. J Appl Physiol 1996; 80:583–590.

98. Taylor BM, Kolbasa KP, Chin JE, Richards IM, Fleming WE, Gruffin RL, Fidler SF, Sun FF. Roles of adhesion molecules ICAM-1 and alpha-4 integrin in antigen-induced changes in microvascular permeability associated with lung inflammation in sensitized Brown Norway rats. Am J Respir Cell Mol Biol 1997; 17:757–766.

99. Andius P, Arakawa H, Molne J, Pillerits T, Skoogh B-E, Lotvall J. Inflammatory responses in skin and airways after allergen challenge in Brown Norway rats sensitized to trimellitic anhydride. Allergy 1996; 51:556–562.

100. Cui ZH, Sjostrand M, Pullerits T, Andius P, Skoogh BE, Lotvall J. Bronchial hyperresponsiveness, epithelial damage and airway eosiniphilia after single and repeated allergen exposure in a rat model of anhydride-induced asthma. Allergy 1997; 52:739–746.

101. Vento KL, Dearman RJ, Kimber I, Basketter DA, Coleman JW. Selectivity of IgE responses, mast cell sensitization and cytokine expression in the immune response of Brown Norway rats to chemical allergen. Cell Immunol 1996; 172:246–253.

102. Pauluhn J. Predictive testing for respiratory sensitization. Toxicol Lett 1996; 86:177–186.

103. Briatico-Vangosa G, Braun CLJ, Cookman GR, Hoffman T, Kimber I, Loveless SE, Morrow T, Pauluhn J, Sorensen T, Niessen HJ. Respiratory allergy: hazard identification and risk assessment. Fund Appl Toxicol 1994; 23:145–158.

104. Selgrade MK, Zeiss CR, Karol MH, Sarlo K, Kimber I, Tepper JS, Henry MC. Workshop on the status of test methods for assessing potential mechanisms of chemicals to induce respiratory allergic reactions. Inhal Toxicol 1994; 6:303–319.

7
Natural History of Occupational Asthma

Moira Chan-Yeung
Vancouver General Hospital and University of British Columbia, Vancouver, British Columbia, Canada

Jean-Luc Malo
Université de Montréal and Sacré-Coeur Hospital, Montréal, Quebec, Canada

INTRODUCTION

Although asthma has been recognized since the time of Hippocrates (460–370 B.C.) (1) and major advances in the pharmacological treatment have been achieved during the past two decades, the underlying pathogenetic mechanism(s) is still not fully understood. Since the study of the natural history of a disease often provides insight into the understanding of the pathogenetic mechanisms, a review of the natural history of asthma is useful.

The progression from a normal state to the development of asthma or occupational asthma (OA) on exposure to allergens or sensitizing chemicals is illustrated in Figure 1. There have been many prospective studies to examine the natural history of childhood-onset asthma from birth, as discussed below. However, such studies for adult-onset asthma, or "intrinsic asthma," is virtually impossible as it is not possible to predict which agent is responsible and to measure them. Although retrospective information can be obtained from these individuals who have already developed adult-onset asthma, it is difficult to establish causal relationship. The predisposing host factors for adult-onset asthma are not clear although it has been hypothesized that some type of IgE-related reaction may be the primary step in the inflammatory cascade even in nonatopic subjects.

Occupational asthma provides an excellent model to study the natural history of adult-onset asthma. Information can be gathered on the baseline immunological status, lung function, nonspecific bronchial hyperresponsiveness (NSBH), and genetic status before employment in high-risk industries. Regular follow-up examinations can be carried out for early detection of development of sensitization and asthma. Furthermore, environmental monitoring of exposure can be done to establish dose-response relationship.

NATURAL HISTORY OF NONOCCUPATIONAL ASTHMA

Age of Onset

Asthma can be divided into two clinical types, childhood onset and adult onset, with different clinical features (2). Childhood-onset asthma is usually associated with a history

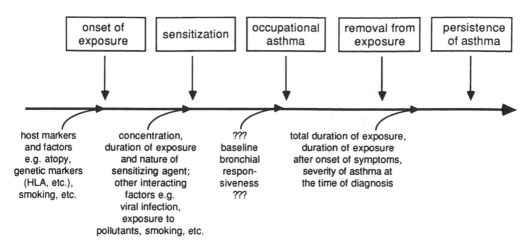

Figure 1   Natural history of occupational asthma.

of infantile eczema, hay fever, or allergic rhinitis often together with a family history of these conditions. These patients usually show positive immediate skin reactivity to a number of common allergens. They have eosinophilia and increased serum-specific IgE antibodies. In adult-onset asthma there is usually no clear relation with atopy and eosinophilia is often more marked; the condition is usually persistent and requires long-term corticosteroid therapy.

Burrows (3), in his study of children with asthma in Tucson, Arizona, found that the condition began very early in life. Very few new cases were diagnosed during adolescence. Among individuals with asthma first diagnosed after the age of 40, a high proportion had preceding respiratory symptoms, and many had frank spirometric abnormalities. The author suggested that the majority of patients with adult-onset asthma had the condition during the first few years of life or during early adulthood. These findings have been confirmed by others (4–6). It is not uncommon for asthma to develop after the age of 65 with an age-adjusted incidence of 95/100,000 [95% confidence interval, 76–115/100,000 (7)].

Irrespective of the age of onset, asthma is characterized by the presence of nonspecific bronchial hyperresponsiveness (NSBH), although this is not unique to asthma. Both host and environmental risk factors are important in the pathogenesis of asthma.

Host Risk Factors

Atopy, NSBH, age, and gender are important host factors. The influence of age on asthma has been discussed in the previous section. Clinical and epidemiological studies have shown that asthma occurring early in life tends to affect boys (8–10) while asthma occurring later in life tends to be more common in women (10–12). The reason for this gender difference is not clear. It could be due to smaller airway diameter in young boys compared to girls during the first 18 months of life and hormonal differences in later years (13). Gender differences in occupational asthma have not been explored since industries tend to employ mostly either men (e.g., foundries) or women (nursing) depending on the nature of employment.

Atopy is probably the single most important host factor in childhood asthma. The prevalence of atopy in subjects with asthma varies from 23 to 80% depending on the age of the population and how asthma and atopy are defined (14). This association is particularly strong in childhood-onset asthma. It has been known for many years that diseases such as asthma, hay fever, and eczema tend to run in families. In many families these diseases occur in successive generations (15). However, a consistent mode of inheritance was not identified. Atopy is strongly associated with NSBH. However, some individuals may have atopy but not NSBH while others have NSBH but not atopy. This discrepancy has led to the hypothesis that NSBH is a separately inherited phenotypic trait. The genetics of asthma and NSBH have been discussed in a previous chapter.

Environmental Risk Factors

Several environmental factors can induce asthma. Some induce attacks of asthma associated with an increase in NSBH, while others induce asthma without associated NSBH. Exercise and exposure to cold air induce asthma attacks without increasing the degree of NSBH. On the other hand, exposure to allergens or chemicals following sensitization may induce a prolonged and pronounced increase in NSBH. An accidental exposure to a high dose of chemicals, gases, or fumes has been found to be associated with a prolonged increase in NSBH in some subjects in reactive airways dysfunction syndrome (16). Such exposure occurs not uncommonly in occupational settings.

Allergens

Sensitization to indoor aeroallergens is more important than to outdoor aeroallergens in asthma particularly in temperate climates where people spend much of their time indoors. Exposure to house dust mite is responsible for asthma in children in many parts of the world where humidity is high (17). In other parts of the world where house dust mite allergens are not prevalent, as in central Canada, sensitization to domestic pets may play an important role in childhood asthma (18). In inner cities, sensitization to cockroaches is an important risk factor for hospitalization for asthma (19).

Exposure to allergens, either in the laboratory (20) or under natural conditions (21,22), results in increase in NSBH often large in magnitude and frequently persisting for several days or longer. Some subjects allergic to pollen show a seasonal increase in NSBH and a decrease in NSBH at the end of the season (22). In others, persistence of NSBH occurs despite reduction in allergen exposure.

The majority of subjects with allergic-type asthma are sensitized to multiple common environmental allergens. Sensitization to multiple allergens is uncommon in OA.

Infection

Viral infection may cause acute exacerbation of asthma or act as a cofactor in the development of asthma. Empey and co-workers (23) showed that NSBH was increased in subjects with colds compared to normal controls. Human peripheral leukocytes, when incubated with influenza A and adenovirus in vitro, showed enhanced antigen-dependent histamine release (24). During acute illness due to human rhinovirus, basophil histamine release resulting from antigen stimulation was also found to be increased (25). These observations suggest that respiratory viral infections may cause NSBH by enhancing airway inflammation (26). There have been many studies showing that infants with a family history of atopy had a higher risk for development of asthma after bronchiolitis due to respiratory syncytial virus infection (27–29).

Not all infections predispose to the development of asthma. A study of Japanese children showed that those with a positive tuberculin skin test had a much lower prevalence of asthma and allergies compared to those with a negative skin test (30). Young Italian military recruits who were serology positive for hepatitis A virus had a lower prevalence of asthma and allergies compared to those who were seronegative (31). It is postulated that these infections may induce IFN-γ production, which inhibits the expansion of TH2 lymphocytes. The latter are responsible for the production of interleukin-4 cytokines necessary for IgE synthesis (31).

The role of viral or bacterial infection in OA is not clear. Many patients with OA at the onset of their illness complain that they have a persistent "cold." It is difficult to know whether the symptoms of a "cold" are due to a viral infection or due to sensitization to the occupational agent.

Environmental Tobacco Smoke and Active Smoke

Cross-sectional studies have consistently showed a detrimental effect of parental smoking on asthma severity in children (32,33). Murray and Morrison (33) found impressive differences in asthma severity and the degree of NSBH in children whose mother smoked compared to those whose mother did not smoke. There are now several longitudinal studies of birth cohorts demonstrating the association between maternal smoking and a significant higher risk for the development of asthma in children (34–36). The effects of active smoking on asthma are less well studied. A few studies have shown that women, not men, who smoked had a higher prevalence of asthma compared to nonsmokers (37–38).

In the occupational setting, current smokers have been found to be at a higher risk of developing sensitization to high-molecular-weight agents while nonsmokers have been found to be at a higher risk for developing asthma due to low-molecular-weight compounds.

Air Pollution

Air pollution is associated with acute exacerbations of asthma. Ozone, nitrogen dioxide, and particulates have all been implicated (39–40). The relationship between asthma exacerbations and sulfur dioxide level is less clear; while the Nashville pollution studies (42,43) found an association, studies in New York City failed to demonstrate such a relationship (41,44). Bates and co-workers (45) found a significant correlation with SO_2 levels on the same day and a lag response 24 and 48 hr later with hospital emergency room visits by asthmatics in Vancouver. Particulates less than 10 micron (PM10) are associated with emergency room visits for acute asthma in a dose-response manner (46). While all investigators agree that air pollutants aggravate asthma, there is no conclusive evidence that air pollution is responsible for the increased prevalence of asthma in developed countries.

Outcome

While there are many studies of the natural history of asthma in childhood (9,10,47–55), longitudinal studies of adult-onset asthma are scarce (7,56). Most of the studies have shown that asthma symptoms in children persist into adulthood in 30–80% of cases (9,10,47–55). Even in the absence of asthma symptoms, airflow obstruction and increased NSBH were found in some patients (57–59). Risk factors associated with persistence of asthma into adulthood include early onset of symptoms (47,60), severity of the disease (8,61), and low lung function and a marked degree of NSBH (7,58). While epidemiological studies suggest that the presence of allergic eczema or rhinitis with asthma has a negative effect on asthma prognosis (62,63), the results of clinical studies are inconclusive. Some clinical studies have shown a negative effect (9,64) while others showed no relationship (10,53). The prognosis of asthma for women is worse than it is for men (65,66).

Panhuysen et al. (67) conducted a follow-up study 25 years later on 181 adult asthmatic patients who were 13–44 years of age at the time of diagnosis between 1962 and 1970. They found that the disease improved in a substantial number of symptomatic asthmatics; a small subset may even outgrow their asthma in adulthood. Gender and atopy did not influence the outcome of the disease. The authors attributed the good prognosis to early intervention leading to a better outcome. In patients who developed asthma for the first time after the age of 65, there was no reduction in survival. However, there was considerable morbidity in terms of emergency room visits and hospital admissions in these patients (67).

There has been considerable interest in the possibility that asthma may represent an important risk for chronic airflow obstruction in later life. Studies of longitudinal decline in lung function in patients with asthma are difficult to conduct and interpret because of the variable nature of the disorder and the large influence of medications on lung function. Most cross-sectional studies in adults showed that lung function in patients with asthma was lower than predicted. Table 1 shows lung function decline in patients with asthma in several longitudinal studies (53,64–72). The results of these studies suggest that the mild form of asthma may be associated with a normal rate of decline in lung function. More severe forms of asthma may be associated with a more rapid decline in lung function and some degree of chronic airflow obstruction. Smoking appears to play an important role, but it is often not possible to separate asthma and chronic bronchitis in middle-aged or elderly smokers with wheeze and chronic airflow obstruction.

NATURAL HISTORY OF OCCUPATIONAL ASTHMA

Onset

The latent period between the onset of exposure and the onset of symptoms is highly variable. The majority of patients develop asthma within the first 1–2 years of exposure. A recent study has shown that sensitization to low-molecular-weight agents requires a shorter interval than sensitization to high-molecular-weight compounds (Fig. 2). The duration of exposure prior to onset of symptoms in patients with occupational asthma due to western red cedar, diisocyanates, and high-molecular-weight agents was analyzed. These

Table 1 Decline in Lung Function in Asthmatics

		n	Years of follow-up	Excess ΔFEV_1^a/year
Schacter et al.	(68)	73	6	18 ml/year
Fletcher et al.	(69)	17	8	22 ml/year
Buist and Vollmer.	(70)	35	10	No consistent difference
Peat et al.	(71)	92	18	15 ml/year
Ulrik and Lange.	(72)	177 male	5	39 ml/year
		219 female	5	11 ml/year

[a]Excess ΔFEV_1 = ΔFEV_1 greater than controls.

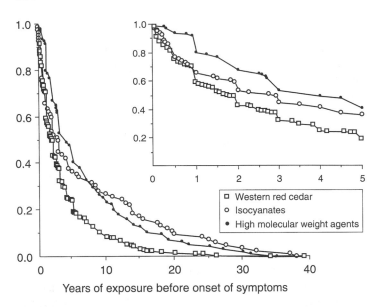

Years of exposure before onset of symptoms

Figure 2   Occupational agents and latency period among patients with occupational asthma.

patients had their diagnosis confirmed by objective tests. Approximately 40% of patients exposed to western red cedar and diisocyanates (low-molecular-weight agents), developed symptoms within the first year after exposure started, while only 18% of patients exposed to high-molecular-weight agents developed asthma during this period ($p < 0.001$). A small proportion (10%) of patients develop asthma after 10 years of exposure. It is not known what factors initiate the onset of symptoms in these patients.

Host and Environmental Determinants of Occupational Asthma

Once an individual enters a high-risk industry, both host and environmental factors are important in determining whether occupational asthma develops. Both the intensity and timing of exposure are important. It is now possible to quantify airborne proteins with immunological methods using personal samplers. Studies have shown that there is a positive correlation between the level of exposure and/or the duration of exposure and the likelihood of developing asthma among workers in bakeries (73,74) and in sawmills (75). An association has been found between work-related symptoms and exposure intensity to animal proteins in workers exposed to laboratory rats (76). On the other hand, exposure to high concentrations encountered in sudden spills may be a factor in isocyanate-induced asthma.

Atopy is an important host risk factor for sensitization to high-molecular-weight compounds although its predictive value is low. Smoking has been shown to be the single most important risk factor for sensitization to platinum salt among refinery workers (77). Among workers exposed to tetrachlorophthalate anhydride, smoking appears to interact with atopy and predisposes to sensitization (78). The role of HLA class II antigens in occupational asthma due to low-molecular-weight compounds has already been discussed in previous chapters.

Outcome of Patients Removed from Exposure

Patients with pneumoconiosis such as asbestosis and silicosis often have permanent, irreversible damage to their lungs. The fact that occupational asthma can lead to permanent disability remained unsuspected until the late 1970s. It was taken for granted for a long time that removing patients with occupational asthma from exposure to the offending agent would lead to a cure. Several retrospective studies, summarized in Table 2, have refuted this dogma and demonstrated that the majority of patients with occupational asthma failed to recover years after removal from exposure. These findings have altered our perspective on the natural history of asthma. Using this analogy, one can postulate that patients who develop nonoccupational allergic asthma may have permanent asthma even though the sensitizing agent has been eliminated.

Chan-Yeung first published evidence that subjects with occupational asthma can be left with permanent symptoms, airflow limitation, and NSBH after removal from exposure (79). Thirty-eight subjects with occupational asthma caused by western red cedar were studied after they left exposure for at least 6 months. Although the majority (71%) became asymptomatic and had normal airway caliber at the follow-up visit, every subject was left with bronchial hyperresponsiveness. These findings were confirmed in a subsequent study carried out on a larger number of subjects and followed for a longer period, 3 1/2 years (80). They also found that those who remained in the same job experienced a worsening in their asthma symptoms and an increase in NSBH (81). Several factors of prognostic significance were identified: age, total duration of exposure, duration of exposure after onset of symptoms. The investigators concluded that early diagnosis and removal from exposure were essential in ensuring recovery.

Burge extended these observations to occupational asthma caused by colophony (82). Only two of the 20 workers who left work became symptom free after an interval varying from 1 to 4 years. Thirteen of these 20 subjects had normal bronchial responsiveness. Only one of the seven workers who remained exposed had normal bronchial responsiveness at the time of follow-up. These findings suggest that NSBH was the result rather than the cause of occupational asthma. Hudson and co-workers assessed 63 workers exposed

Table 2 Retrospective Evidence for the Persistence of Symptoms and Bronchial Hyperresponsiveness After Removal from the Offending Agent

Agent	n	Duration of follow-up (years)	Persistence of symptoms (%)	NSBH (%)		Ref.
Red cedar	38	0.5–4	29	38/38	(100%)	79
Red cedar	75	1–9	49	25/33	(76%)	80
Colophony	20	1.3–3.8	90	7/20	(35%)	82
Snow-crab	31	0.5–2	61	28/31	(90%)	83
Snow-crab	31	4.8–6	100	26/31	(84%)	84
Various	32	0.5–4	93	31/32	(97%)	83
Isocyanates	12	1–3	66	7/12	(58%)	86
Isocyanates	50	>4	82	12/19	(63%)	87
Isocyanates	20	0.5–4	50	9/12	(75%)	88
Isocyanates	22	1	77	17/22	(77%)	89
Various	28	4–11	100	25/26	(96%)	90

to various high- and low-molecular-weight agents more than 6 months after they had left work (83). Only three of 31 workers had a normal level of bronchial responsiveness at the time of follow-up. Improvement was found only in subjects exposed to snow-crab and not to other agents. By studying a sample of 31 snow-crab workers at three separate intervals after they had left work (1, 2 1/2, and 5 years), Malo and co-workers were able to show that the improvement of bronchial caliber and responsiveness reached a plateau approximately 1 year and 2 years, respectively, after the workers left exposure (84) (Fig.

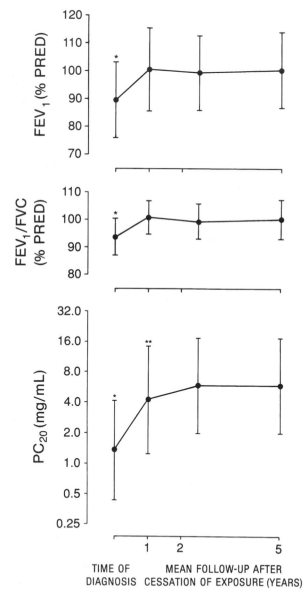

Figure 3 FEV_1, FEV_1/FVC, and PC_{20} (mg/ml) and duration after removal from exposure in patients with snow-crab-induced asthma, showing more rapid improvement in FEV_1 and FEV_1/FVC and a slower improvement in PC_{20}.

3). Levels of specific IgE to crab antigens (meat and boiling water) decreased progressively without reaching a plateau, confirming earlier reports that the half-life for disappearance of specific IgE antibodies could be prolonged as in the case of another occupational agent, phthallic anhydride (85).

Persistence of asthmatic symptoms after removal from exposure to isocyanates was confirmed in several studies (86–89). Allard and co-workers showed no improvement in symptoms, airway caliber, or NSBH in 28 subjects exposed to various agents at two mean intervals of 2 and 6 years (90). Only three subjects had improvement in NSBH at one or the other of the two follow-up visits.

The above studies and others demonstrated that the majority of patients with OA may improve but do not recover completely after the cessation of exposure; they worsen if exposure continues. The duration of exposure and the duration of symptoms are important prognostic factors. Thus, early diagnosis and removal from exposure are recommended.

There is a histological basis to the persistence of symptoms and NSBH in patients with OA. Patients who failed to recover from western red cedar asthma had higher total cell count and eosinophils in bronchoalveolar lavage fluid than those who recovered completely after removal from exposure (91). Saetta and co-workers have documented improvement in bronchial inflammation (diminution of mast cells and lymphocytes) and airway wall remodeling (reduction in the thickness of subepithelial fibrosis and the number of subepithelial fibroblasts) in patients with TDI-induced asthma after the cessation of exposure (92).

The reasons for the persistence of NSBH after removal from exposure are not known. The persistence of NSBH could be the result of airway remodeling with subepithelial fibrosis and from chronic airway inflammation. The latter could be due to a number of possibilities: (1) continuous exposure to the responsible agent in the environment even though the subject is not at work; for example, there is cross-reactivity between the latex antigen and a number of foods such as kiwi and avocado; this may be responsible for symptoms in health care workers with latex-induced asthma (93); (2) the development of an "autoimmune" process when agents such as isocyanates may combine with a body protein and remain in the airways or the persistence of a protein adduct (94); (3) genetic susceptibility that predisposes the individuals to the development and the persistence of asthma; (4) sensitization to other environmental allergens as a result of development of asthma (95). None of these hypotheses have been proven.

Two clinical trials have explored the possibility of "curing" subjects with OA with inhaled steroids after removal from the workplace. Maestrelli and co-workers documented a fourfold improvement in PC_{20} in the treated group after 5 months (96). Malo and co-workers also showed improvement in various clinical and functional parameters (97). Although no case of cure from asthma was documented, their results indicated that early initiation of inhaled steroids yielded greater improvement than later initiation (1 year after the cessation of exposure).

Outcome of Patients with Continuous Exposure

There have been case reports of subjects with OA who died while working and exposed to the same agent (98–100). Most studies have shown that subjects with OA deteriorate if they continue in the same job (81,86). In a study by Côté and co-workers (81), 48 subjects with western red cedar asthma confirmed by specific challenge testing were reassessed from 1 to 13 (mean 6.5) years after the initial examination. Using criteria based on four parameters (PC_{20}, FEV_1, asthma symptom score, and antiasthma medication requirement), the investigators found that only 10% of subjects improved, 62.5% remained stable, and 37.5% deteriorated. None of the subjects recovered. Measures to reduce dust exposure, including change from daily to intermittent exposure or job relocation to a less dusty area or use of respiratory protective devices (paper mask, twin-cartridge respirator, air-purifying respirator), did not influence the outcome with the exception of the use of a twin-cartridge respirator.

No data are available on the use of immunotherapy with extracts of high-molecular-weight occupational allergens to allow the subject to continue to work. Such a modality seems unlikely to be helpful since continuous exposure has not led to the development of immunity and improvement of symptoms. The efficacy of inhaled steroids in the treatment of subjects with OA who opt to remain in the same job for financial reasons is not known. As fatality has been reported, every effort should be made to remove such subjects from further exposure.

Occupational Asthma as a Model to Study the Natural History of Asthma

Several prospective studies have been carried out in several industries to study the natural history of OA (74,76). An example of the natural history of NSBH due to sensitization to snow-crab is illustrated in Figure 4. In this subject, development of NSBH occurred after only 8 days of exposure but took 1 year to return to normal. In two prospective surveys conducted in workers exposed to laboratory animals and flour, respectively, Cullinan and co-workers have demonstrated that atopy and exposure intensity are significant determinants of specific sensitization (74,76). However, the subjects in these two studies had been

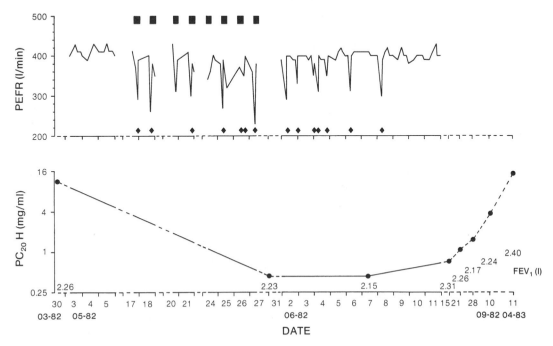

Figure 4 Change in PEF and PC_{20} in a patient with snow-crab-induced asthma, showing a rapid development of NSBH after a short period of exposure and a much slower improvement in NSBH after cessation of exposure.

Table 3 Prevalence and Incidence of IgE Sensitization and of Occupational Asthma in Apprentices 6–12 Months After Starting Exposure in the Relevant Program

	Animal facilities	Bakery	Dental hygiene	All
Prevalence	75/413	11/222	1/122	69/757
(preexposure)	(13.8%)	(5.0%)	(0.8%)	(9%)
Incidence of immediate	44/378	8/153	3/106	55/637
skin sensitization	(11.6%)	(5.2%)	(2.8%)	(9%)
Incidence of	20/376	1/152	3/106	24/634
occupational asthma	(5.3%)	(0.7%)	(2.8%)	(3.8%)

exposed to these specific agents before the surveys. Gautrin and co-workers (101) have conducted a prospective study on 769 apprentices entering study programs as animal health technicians, dental hygienists, and bakers. They found that 14%, 5%, and 0.8% of the apprentices had immediate skin reactivity to animal-derived allergens, flour, and latex, respectively, before entering the programs. In 637 subjects seen on the first follow-up visit at 6–12 months after entry into the cohort, 9% showed new immunological sensitization and NSBH (Table 3). Specific sensitization was associated with atopic status, work-related symptoms, and NSBH.

Since there is no difference between occupational high-molecular-weight allergens and common inhalant allergens in inducing host response, studies of the natural history of OA due to high-molecular-weight allergens will likely reflect the origin and progression of nonoccupational allergic asthma. Studies of the natural history of OA due to low-molecular-weight compounds and/or irritant-induced asthma will be very useful in our understanding of adult-onset, or intrinsic, asthma.

REFERENCES

1. Peterson WF. Hippocratic Wisdom. Springfield, IL: Charles C. Thomas, 1946:223.
2. Rackeman FM. A working classification of asthma. Am J Med 1947; 3:601–606.
3. Burrows B. The natural history of asthma. J Allergy Clin Immunol 1987; 30:373–377.
4. Peckhman C, Butler N. A national study of asthma in childhood. J Epidemiol Commun Health 1978; 32:79–85.
5. Anderson HR, Bland JM, Patel S, Peckham C. The natural history of asthma in childhood. J Epidemiol Commun Health 1986; 40:121–129.
6. Bronnimann S, Burrows B. A prospective study of the natural history of asthma. Remission and relapse rates. Chest 1986; 90:480–484.
7. Bauer BA, Reed CE, Yunginger JW, Wollan PC, Silverstein MD. Incidence and outcomes of asthma in the elderly. A population-based study in Rochester, Minnesota. Chest 1997; 111: 303–310.
8. Roorda R, Gerritsen J, van Aalderen W, Schouten J, Veltman J, Weiss S, Knol K. Risk factors for the persistence of respiratory symptoms in childhood asthma. Am Rev Respir Dis 1993; 148:1490–1495.
9. Roorda RJ, Gerritsen J, van Aalderen WMC, Schoute JP, Veltma JC, Weiss ST. Follow up of asthma from childhood to adulthood: influence of potential childhood risk factors on the outcome of pulmonary function ad bronchial responsiveness in adulthood. J Allergy Clin Immunol 1994; 93:575–584.

10. Gerritsen J, Koeter GH, Postma DS, Schouten JP, Knol K. Prognosis of asthma from childhood to adulthood. Am Rev Respir Dis 1989; 140:1325–1330.

11. Ryssing E. Continued follow up investigation concerning the fate of 298 asthmatic children. Acta Paediatr (Uppsala) 1959; 48:255–260.

12. Martin AJ, McLennan LA, Landau LI, Phelan PD. The natural history of childhood asthma to adult life. Br Med J 1980; 280:1397–1400.

13. Weller HH, van der Staeten M, Vermeulen A, Orie NGM. Hormonal pattern in bronchial asthma. Scand J Respir Dis 1969; 49:163–184.

14. Weiss ST, Speizer FE. The epidemiology of asthma: risk factors and natural history. Weiss EB, Segal MS, Stein M, eds. In: Bronchial Asthma: Mechanism and Therapeutics. Boston: Little, Brown, 1985:14–23.

15. Cooke RA, VanderVeer A. Human sensitization. J Immunol 1916; 1:201–305.

16. Brooks SM, Weiss MA, Bernstein IL. Reactive airways dysfunction syndrome. Chest 1985; 88:376–383.

17. Sporik R, Chapman M, Platts-Mills T. House dust mite exposure as a cause of asthma. Clin Exp Allergy 1992; 22:897–906.

18. Sporik R, Rose G, Muller M, Claytor D, Price G, Ingram J, Sussman J, Honsinger R, Platts-Mills T. Allergen sensitization of children with wheeze and bronchial hyperreactivity (BHR) resident at high altitude. Am Rev Respir Dis 1993; 147:A458.

19. Rosenstreich DL. The role of cockroach allergy and exposure to cockroach allergen in causing morbidity among inner-city children with asthma. N Engl J Med 1997; 336:1356–1363.

20. Cockcroft DW, Ruffin RE, Dolovich J, Hargreave FE. Allergen induced increase in nonallergic bronchial reactivity. Clin Allergy 1977; 7:503–508.

21. Boulet L-P, Cartier A, Thomson NC, Roberts RS, Dolovich J, Hargreave FE. Asthma and increases in nonallergic bronchial responsiveness from seasonal pollen exposure. J Allergy Clin Immunol 1983; 71:399–406.

22. Sotomayor H, Badier M, Vervloet D, Orehek J. Seasonal increase of carbachol airway responsiveness in patients allergic to grass pollen. Am Rev Respir Dis 1984; 130:56–58.

23. Empey FW, Laitinen LA, Jacob L, Gold WM, Nadel JA. Mechanisms of bronchial hyperreactivity in normal subjects after upper respiratory tract infection. Am Rev Respir Dis 1976; 113:131–139.

24. Ida S, Hooks JJ, Siraganian RP, Notkin AL. Enhancement of IgE mediated histamine release from human basophils by viruses: role of interferon. J Exp Med 1977; 145:892.

25. Busse WW, Swenson CA, Borden EC, Treuhaft UW, Dick EC. Effect of influenza A virus on leukocyte histamine release. J Allergy Clin Immunol 1983; 71:382–388.

26. Busse W. The contribution of viral respiratory infections to the pathogenesis of airway hyperreactivity. Chest 1988; 93:1076–1082.

27. Pullan CR, Hey EN. Wheezing, asthma and pulmonary dysfunction 10 years after infection with respiratory syncytial virus in infancy. Br Med J 1982; 284:1665–1669.

28. Sly PD, Hibbert ME. Childhood asthma following hospitalization with acute viral bronchiolitis in infancy. Paediatr Pulmonol 1989; 7:153–158.

29. Hall CB, Hall WJ, Gala CL, MaGill FB, Leddy JP. Long term prospectic study in children after respiratory syncytial virus infection. J Paediatr 1984; 105:358–364.

30. Shirakawa T, Enomoto T, Shimazu S, Hopkin JM. The inverse association between tuberculin responses and atopic disorder. Science 1997; 275:77–79.

31. Matricardi PM, Rosmini F, Ferrigno L, Nisini R, Rapicetta M, Chionne P, Stroffolini T, Pasquini P, D'Amelio R. Cross sectional retrospective study of prevalence of atopy among Italian military students with antibodies against hepatitis A virus. Br Med J 1997; 314:999–1007.

32. Guyatt G, Newhouse MT. Are active and passive smoking harmful? Determining causation. Chest 1985; 88:445–451.

33. Murray AB, Morrison BJ. Passive smoking and the seasonal difference of severity of asthma in children. Chest 1988; 94:701–708.

34. Gortmarker SL, Walker DK, Jacobs FH, Ruch-Ross H. Parental smoking and the risk of childhood asthma. Am J Public Health 1982; 72:574–578.

35. Martinez F, Cline M, Burrows B. Increased incidence of asthma in children of smoking mothers. Pediatrics 1992; 89:21–26.

36. Weitman M, Gortmacher S, Walker DK, Sobol A. Maternal smoking and childhood asthma. Paediatrics 1990; 85:505–511.

37. Larsson L. Incidence of asthma in Swedish teenagers: relation to sex and smoking habits. Thorax 1994; 50:260–264.

38. Chan-Yeung M, Dimich-Ward H, Sears MR, Siersted HC, Becklake MR, Ernst P, Sweet L, Vantil L, Bowie D, Anthonisen NR, Tate RB, Manfreda J. The effects of smoking on asthma and chronic chest symptoms in Canada. Am J Crit Care Med 1996; 153:A256.

39. Whittemore AS, Korn EL. Asthma and air pollution in the Los Angeles area. Am J Public Health 1980; 70:687–696.

40. Lobowitz MD, Holberg CJ, Boyer B, Hayes C. Respiratory symptoms and peak flow associated with indoor and outdoor air pollutants in the southwest. J Air Pollut Control Assoc 1985; 35:1154–1158.

41. Goldstein IF, Dulberg E. Air pollution and asthma. Search for a relationship. J Air Pollut Control Assoc 1981; 31:370–376.

42. Zeidberg LD, Prindle RA, Landau E. The Nashville air pollution study. I. Sulphur dioxide and bronchial asthma. Am Rev Respir Dis 1961; 84:489–503.

43. Landau E. The Nashville air pollution study. Sulphur dioxide and bronchial asthma—a multivariate analysis. Int J Environ Stud 1971; 2:41–45.

44. Goldstein IF, Weinstein AL. Air pollution and asthma: effects of exposures to short term sulphur dioxide peaks. Environ Res 1986; 40:332–345.

45. Bates DV, Baker-Anderson M, Sizto R. Asthma attack periodicity: a study of hospital emergency visits in Vancouver. Environ Res 1990; 51:51–70.

46. Schwartz J, Slater D, Larson T, Pierson W, Koenig J. Particulate air pollution and hospital emergency room visits for asthma in Seattle. Am Rev Respir Dis 1993; 147:826–831.

47. Buffum WP, Settipane GA. Prognosis of asthma in childhood. Am J Dis Child 1966; 112:214–217.

48. Barr LW, Logan GB. Prognosis of children having asthma. Pediatrics 1964; 333:856–860.

49. Blair H. Natural history of childhood asthma: 20 year follow up. Arch Dis Child 1977; 52:613–619.

50. McNicol KN, Williams HB. Spectrum of asthma in children. I. Clinician physiological components. Br Med J 1973; 4:7–11.

51. Rackeman FM, Edwards MD. Asthma in children: a follow up study of 688 patients after an interval of twenty years. N Engl J Med 1952; 246:815–823.

52. Ogilvie AG. Asthma: a study in prognosis of 1000 patients. Thorax 1962; 17:183–189.

53. Martin AJ, Landau LI, Phelan PD. Lung function in young adults who had asthma in childhood. Am Rev Respir Dis 1980; 122:609–613.

54. Oswald H, Phelan PD, Laniga A, Hibbert M, Bowes G, Olinsky A. Outcome of childhood asthma in midadult life. Br Med J 1994; 309:95–96.

55. Godden DJ, Ross S, Abdalla M, McMurray D, Douglas A, Oldman D, et al. Outcome of wheeze in childhood. Symptoms and pulmonary function 25 years later. Am J Respir Crit Care Med 1994; 149:106–112.

56. Aberg N, Engstrom I. Natural history of allergic diseases in children. Acta Paediatr Scand 1990; 79:206–211.

57. Ferguson AC. Persistent airway obstruction in asymptomatic children with asthma with normal peak expiratory flow rates. J Allergy Clin Immunol 1988; 82:19–22.

58. Cooper DM, Cutz E, Levison H. Occult pulmonary abnormalities in asymptomatic asthmatic children. Chest 1977; 71:361–365.

59. Blackhall M. Ventilatory function in subjects with childhood asthma who have become symptom free. Arch Dis Child 1970; 45:363–366.

60. Kjellman K, Hesselmar B. Prognosis of asthma in children: a cohort study into adulthood. Acta Paediatr 1994; 93:854–861.

61. Gerritsen J, Koeter GH, de Monchy JGR, van Lookeren Campagne JG, Kol K. Changes in airway responsiveness to inhaled house dust from childhood to adulthood. J Allergy Clin Immunol 1990; 85:1083–1089.

62. Kaplan BA, Mascie-Taylor CGN. Predicting the duration of childhood asthma. J Asthma 1992; 29:39–48.

63. Strachan DP. The prevalence and natural history of wheezing in early childhood. J R Coll Gen Pract 1985; 35:182–184.

64. Mazon A, Nieto A, Nieto FJ, Menendez R, Boquete M, Brines J. Prognostic factors in childhood asthma: a logistic regression analysis. Ann Allergy 1994; 72:455–461.

65. Kelly WJW, Hudson I, Phelan PD, Pain MCF, Olinsky O. Childhood asthma in adult life: a further study at 28 years of age. Br Med J 1987; 294:1059–1062.

66. Jenkins MA, Hopper JL, Bowes G, Carlin JB, Flander LB, Giles GG. Factors in childhood as predictors of asthma in adult life. Br Med J 1994; 309:90–93.

67. Panhuysen CIM, Vonk JM, Koeter GH, Schouten JP, van Altena R, Bleecker ER, Postma DS. Adult patients may outgrow their asthma A 25 year follow up study. Am J Respir Crit Care Med 1997; 155:1267–1272.

68. Schachter NE, Doyle CA, Beck GJ. A prospective study of asthma in a rural community. Chest 1984; 85:623–630.

69. Fletcher C, Peto R, Tinker C, Speizer F. The Natural History of Chronic Bronchitis and Emphysema. New York: Oxford University Press, 1987:272.

70. Buist SA, Vollmer WM. Prospective investigations in asthma. Chest 1987; 91:119-S–125-S.

71. Peat JK, Woolcock AJ, Cullen K. Rate of decline in lung function in subjects with asthma. Eur J Respir Dis 1987; 70:171–179.

72. Ulrik CS, Lange P. Decline of lung function in adults with bronchial asthma. Am J Respir Crit Care Med 1994; 150:629–634.

73. Musk AW, Venables KM, Crook B, Nunn AJ, Hawkins R, Crook GDW, Graneek BJ, Tee RD, Farrer N, Johnson DA, Gordon DJ, Darbyshire JH, Newman Taylor AJ. Respiratory symptoms, lung function, and sensitization to flour in a British bakery. Br J Ind Med 1988; 46:636–642.

74. Cullinan P, Lowson D, Nieuwenhuijsen S, Sandiford C, Tee RD, Venables KM, McDonald JC, Newman Taylor AJ. Work-related symptoms, sensitization, and estimated exposure in workers not previously exposed to flour. Occup Environ Med 1994; 51:579–583.

75. Vedal S, Chan-Yeung M, Enarson D, Fera T, MacLean L, Tse KS, Langille R. Symptoms and pulmonary function in western red cedar workers related to duration of employment and dust exposure. Arch Environ Health 1986; 41:179–183.

76. Cullinan P, Lowson D, Nieuwenhuijsen S, Gordon S, Tee RD, Venables KM, McDonald JC, Newman Taylor AJ. Work-related symptoms, sensitization, and estimated exposure in workers not previously exposed to laboratory rats. Occup Environ Med 1994; 51:589–592.

77. Venables KM, Dally MB, Nunn, AJ, Stevens JF, Stephens R, Farrer N, Hunter JV, Stewart M, Hughes EG, Newman Taylor AJ. Smoking and occupational allergy in workers in a platinum refinery. Br Med J 1989; 299:939–942.

78. Topping MD, Venables KM, Luczynska CM, Howe W, Newman Taylor AJ. Specificity of the human IgE response to inhaled acid anhydrides. J Allergy Clin Immunol 1986; 77:834–842.

79. Chan-Yeung M. Fate of occupational asthma. A follow-up study of patients with occupational asthma due to western red cedar (*Thuja plicata*). Am Rev Respir Dis 1977; 116:1023–1029.

80. Chan-Yeung M, Lam S, Koerner S. Clinical features and natural history of occupational asthma due to western red cedar (*Thuja plicata*). Am J Med 1982; 72:411–415.

81. Côté J, Kennedy S, Chan-Yeung M. Outcome of patients with cedar asthma with continuous exposure. Am Rev Respir Dis 1990; 141:373–376.

82. Burge PS. Occupational asthma in electronics workers caused by colophony fumes: follow-up of affected workers. Thorax 1982; 37:348–353.

83. Hudson P, Cartier A, Pineau L, Lafrance M, St-Aubin JJ, Dubois JY, Malo JL. Follow-up of occupational asthma caused by crab and various agents. J Allergy Clin Immunol 1985; 76: 682–687.

84. Malo JL, Cartier A, Ghezzo H, Lafrance M, Mccants M, Lehrer SB. Patterns of improvement on spirometry, bronchial hyperresponsiveness, and specific IgE antibody levels after cessation of exposure in occupational asthma caused by snow-crab processing. Am Rev Respir Dis 1988; 138:807–812.

85. Venables KM, Topping MD, Nunn AJ, Howe W, Newman Taylor AJ. Immunologic and functional consequences of chemical (tetrachlorophthalic anhydride)–induced asthma after four years of avoidance of exposure. J Allergy Clin Immunol 1987; 80:212–218.

86. Paggiaro PL, Loi AM, Rossi O, Ferrante B, Pardi F, Roselli MG, Baschieri L. Follow-up study of patients with respiratory disease due to toluene diisocyanate (TDI). Clin Allergy 1984; 14:463–469.

87. Lozewicz S, Assoufi BK, Hawkins R, Newman Taylor AJ. Outcome of asthma induced by isocyanates. Br J Dis Chest 1987; 81:14–27.

88. Rosenberg N, Garnier R, Rousselin X, Mertz R, Gervais P. Clinical and socio-professional fate of isocyanate-induced asthma. Clin Allergy 1987; 17:55–61.

89. Mapp CE, Corona PC, Marzo N de, Fabbri L. Persistent asthma due to isocyanates. A follow-up study of subjects with occupational asthma due to toluene diisocyanate. Am Rev Respir Dis 1988; 137:1326–1329.

90. Allard C, Cartier A, Ghezzo H, Malo JL. Occupational asthma due to various agents. Absence of clinical and functional improvement at an interval of four or more years after cessation of exposure. Chest 1989; 96:1046–1049.

91. Chan-Yeung M, LeRiche J, Chan H, Lam S. Comparison of cellular and protein changes in bronchial lavage fluid of symptomatic and asymptomatic patients with red cedar asthma on follow-up examination. Clin Allergy 1988; 18:359–365.

92. Saetta M, Maestrelli P, Turato G, Mapp CE, Milani G, Pivirotto F, Fabbri LM, DiStefano A. Airway wall remodeling after cessation of exposure to isocyanates in sensitized asthmatic subjects. Am J Respir Crit Care Med 1995; 151:489–494.

93. Ahlroth M, Alenius H, Turjanmaa K, Makinen-Kiljunen S, Reunala T, Palosuo T. Cross-reacting allergens in natural ribber latex and avacado. J Allergy Clin Immunol 1995; 96:167–173.

94. Jin R, Day BW, Karol MH. Toluene diisocyanate protein adducts in the bronchoalveolar lavage of guinea pigs exposed to vapors of the chemical. Chem Res Toxicol 1993; 6:906–912.

95. Perfetti L, Hébert J, Lapalme Y, Ghezzo H, Gautrin D, Malo JL. Changes in IgE-mediated to ubiquitous inhalants after removal from or diminution of exposure to the agent causing occupational athma. Clin Exp Allergy 1998; 28:66–73.

96. Maestrelli P, Marzo N. De, Saetta M, Boscaro M, Fabbri LM, Mapp CE. Effects of inhaled beclomethasone on airway responsiveness in occupational asthma. Am Rev Respir Dis 1993; 148:407–412.

97. Malo JL, Cartier A, Côté J, Milot J, Leblanc C, Paquette L, Ghezzo H, Boulet LP. Influence of inhaled steroids on recovery from occupational asthma after cessation of exposure: an 18-month double-blind crossover study. Am J Respir Crit Care Med 1996; 153:953–960.

98. Fabbri LM, Danieli D, Crescioli S, Bevilacqua P, Meli S, Saetta M, Mapp CE. Fatal asthma in a subject sensitized to toluene diisocyanate. Am Rev Respir Dis 1988; 137:1494–1498.

99. Licitra C, Sarno N, Ioli F. Death due to asthma at workplace in a diphenylmethane diisocyanate. Respiration 1997; 64:111–113.

100. Erlich I. Fatal asthma in a baker: a case report. Am J Ind Med 1994; 26:799.

101. Gautrin D, Infante-Rivard C, Dao TV, Magnan-Larose M, Desjardins D, Malo JL. Specific IgE-dependent sensitization, atopy and bronchial hyperresponsiveness in apprentices starting exposure to protein-derived agents. Am J Respir Crit Care Med 1997; 155:1841–1847.

8

Clinical Assessment and Management of Occupational Asthma

David I. Bernstein
University of Cincinnati College of Medicine, Cincinnati, Ohio

INTRODUCTION

The initial assessment of an individual worker suspected of having occupational asthma (OA) should include a comprehensive occupational history, spirometry, and a search for potential causative agents in the workplace. Exposure assessment, which is discussed in other chapters, is an essential component of the overall evaluation of a patient suspected of OA. If appropriate, specific immunological tests can aid in confirming causation by an agent encountered at work. There are, however, distinct clinical approaches and physiological methods that must be applied specifically to the diagnosis of OA (1). Those methods and/or instruments that are particularly useful in the evaluation of OA will be reviewed in this chapter. Finally, a stepwise rational approach for clinical diagnosis of OA will be presented as a diagnostic algorithm.

THE OCCUPATIONAL HISTORY

A comprehensive and detailed occupational history is essential in all patients presenting with asthmatic symptoms. Because many clinicians are not attuned to occupational diseases, the diagnosis of OA can be delayed for months or years. A physician experienced in the evaluation of occupational diseases is more likely to inquire about current and previous employment, workplace exposure to sensitizing agents, and work-related respiratory symptoms. A cursory interview is less informative than a structured occupational history. Structured questionnaires are useful in supplementing the physician's nondirected interview. An outline of essential information is shown in Table 1. The Appendix (see p. 731) contains an itemized questionnaire developed conjointly by the University of Cincinnati Occupational Allergy Laboratory and the National Institute of Occupational Safety and Health (NIOSH). This instrument has been used in cross-sectional and longitudinal medical surveillance for capturing data pertaining to employment history, current and previous work exposure, work-related symptoms, and risk factors (2,3). By administering both an itemized questionnaire and an open-ended medical history, important data omissions can be prevented. If possible, the history should be taken by more than one

Table 1   Key Elements of the Occupational History in the Evaluation of Occupational Asthma

 I. Demographic information
   A. Identification and address
   B. Personal data including sex, race, and age
   C. Educational background and number of school years completed
 II. Employment History
   A. Current department and job description including dates begun, interrupted, and ended
   B. List all processes and substances used in the employee's work environment; a schematic diagram of the workplace is helpful to track other direct or indirect exposure emanating from various work stations
   C. List prior jobs at current workplace with description of job, duration, and identification of material used
   D. Work history describing employment preceding current workplace. Job descriptions and exposure history must be included
 III. Symptoms
   A. Categories
     1. Chest tightness, wheezing, cough, shortness of breath
     2. Nasal rhinorrhea, sneezing, lacrimation, ocular itching
     3. Systemic symptoms—fever, arthralgias, myalgias
   B. Duration of symptoms
   C. Duration of employment at current job prior to onset of symptoms
   D. Identify temporal pattern of symptoms in relationship to work
     1. Immediate onset beginning at work with resolution soon after coming home
     2. Delayed onset beginning 4–12 hr after starting work or after coming home
     3. Immediate onset followed by recovery with symptoms recurring 4–12 hr after initial work exposure
   E. Improvement away from work
 IV. Identify potential risk factors
   A. Current smoking status and candidate number of pack-years
   B. Asthmatic symptoms preceding current work exposure
   C. Atopic status
     1. History of seasonal nasal or ocular symptom
     2. Familial history of atopic disease
     3. Confirmation by percutaneous testing to a panel of common aeroallergens
   D. History of accidental exposures to substances (e.g., heated gas fumes or chemical spills)

experienced physician to be certain that there is concordance with regard to the clinical diagnosis.

Employment History

The employment history must be detailed and comprehensive (see table 1). All details of the worker's job must be documented. All substances to which there is either direct or indirect exposure at work must be listed. Identification of generic chemical names and exact constituents of raw materials at work can be facilitated by obtaining material safety data sheets (MSDS) from employers or their suppliers. All aspects of work processes must be thoroughly reviewed to identify jobs or tasks that could be associated with ambient exposure to aerosols, dusts, or fumes. Processes in adjacent work areas must be reviewed, as indirect exposure to a substance could be significant. All preceding jobs should be listed to determine if there could have been prior exposure (and possibly sensitization) to agents similar or identical to those to which the worker is currently exposed. It is important to document both the duration and nature of exposure to all agents currently or previously encountered at work. This includes information about accidental spills and toxic exposure(s) to chemicals, fumes, or smoke that can initiate OA.

Medical History

The medical history should include possible upper and lower respiratory tract symptoms and determine whether or not they are work-related. Ocular symptoms (lacrimation, itching, or burning) and nasal complaints (sneezing, rhinorrhea, and nasal congestion) that precede or concur with asthmatic symptoms are characteristic of IgE-mediated disorders, which are most often due to high-molecular-weight natural allergens. Lower respiratory symptoms include cough, shortness of breath, chest tightness, and wheezing. Cough may be an initial symptom at work preceding the onset of wheezing or dyspnea. For each symptom, the examining physician should inquire about duration, time of onset after the beginning of the work shift, and resolution of symptoms on weekends or vacations. It should also be determined whether each reported symptom occurs in relationship to exposure to a specific substance(s) at work.

The duration of the ''latency period'' in the workplace prior to the onset of asthmatic symptoms should be quantified. A latency period is characteristic of IgE-mediated occupational asthma as well as asthma caused by certain reactive chemical substances for which immune mechanisms have not been defined (e.g., diisocyanates). Ocular burning, nasal stuffiness, rhinorrhea, and cough, occurring in a large proportion of the workforce in the absence of a latency period, is consistent with a respiratory irritant response. Typically, irritant symptoms quickly resolve after the worker leaves the workplace.

Several characteristic patterns of asthmatic responses have been recognized. These include: isolated early asthmatic responses (EAR); isolated late asthmatic responses (LAR); and dual-phase asthmatic responses (4). Dual (EAR and LAR) and isolated EARs are characteristic of IgE-mediated respiratory sensitization to low-molecular-weight (LMW) or high-molecular-weight (HMW) allergens but can also occur in the absence of a demonstrable immunological mechanism (5). An isolated LAR beginning after 4–12 hr at work is commonly associated with OA caused by LMW compounds (e.g., red cedar, diisocyanates).

Resolution of respiratory symptoms on weekends or vacations is characteristic of either occupational asthma or a nonspecific irritant response. Moderate and severe occupational asthma in its advanced stages is characterized by continuous daytime and nocturnal asthmatic symptoms, which often persist on weekends or on vacation reflecting an increase in nonspecific bronchial hyperresponsiveness. Asthma may continue for months or years after cessation of workplace exposure (6,34). Thus, the absence of symptomatic improvement following complete restriction from work exposure does not exclude a diagnosis of OA.

Finally, the medical history should seek to elicit information that identifies risk factors. Smoking has been identified as a risk factor for OA in laboratory animal workers and snow-crab workers (7,8). In contrast, nonsmoking red cedar sawmill workers are far more likely to develop OA than their smoking colleagues (9). Positive skin prick tests to panels of common aeroallergens are used to define atopy. In general, atopic workers are at greater risk than nonatopic for development of IgE-mediated OA caused by natural allergens such as laboratory animal, latex, or enzyme proteins (10,11). Atopic status is not a risk factor for OA due to reactive chemicals (3). However, Venables et al. reported that smoking and atopy are coassociated with elevated serum specific IgE antibody levels to TCPA-HSA among acid-anhydride-exposed workers (12).

In workers with preexisting asthma, work-related bronchospasm can be triggered by chemical irritants (e.g., SO_2, chlorine gas) or physical stimuli in the workplace (cold air). However, preexisting airway hyperresponsiveness has not been proven as a risk factor for development of OA due to specific causative agents (9).

The physical examination is rarely helpful in evaluating OA unless wheezing can be auscultated during or after the work shift. In many cases of OA, the chest examination is normal. Therefore, the absence of wheezing should not deter the clinician from aggressively evaluating workers reporting asthmatic symptoms. Auscultation of inspiratory crackles should cause prompt consideration of occupational pneumoconiosis, hypersensitivity pneumonitis, or congestive heart failure. In such cases, a chest X-ray is useful for excluding nonasthmatic cardiopulmonary diseases.

IMMUNOLOGICAL ASSESSMENT

Because immunological mechanisms are important in the pathogenesis of many cases of OA, measurement of immunological responses to suspected allergens can sometimes be useful in establishing a diagnosis. The immunological evaluation of occupational asthma is reviewed extensively in another chapter. In vivo skin testing and in vitro immunological methods readily detect specific IgE responses to HMW protein antigens in workers with OA but may also be detected in nonasthmatic workers. In vitro RAST or ELISA methods possess equivalent sensitivity for detecting serum-specific IgE responses (13). In general, in vitro assays of specific IgE are less sensitive but more specific than in vivo cutaneous testing in identification of cases of OA confirmed by specific bronchoprovocation testing (SBPT) (14). A positive skin prick test to a suspect antigen indicates the presence of IgE-mediated sensitization but is not in itself diagnostic.

The sensitivity and specificity of a skin prick test reagent must be evaluated against a diagnostic gold standard for OA, such as the SBPT (15). In a group of enzyme workers presenting with positive histories of OA (i.e., the pretest probability of OA was high), a positive skin prick test exhibited excellent sensitivity and specificity in identifying persons with OA confirmed by SBPT (14).

Skin testing can be useful for screening workers with possible sensitization to certain reactive chemicals. Although not generally available, acid anhydride skin test antigens can be prepared by in vitro conjugation of an acid anhydride with a protein carrier [e.g., human serum albumin (HSA)] (16). However, the sensitivity and specificity of these antigens have not been defined. Cartier et al. reported elevated serum-specific IgE and/or specific IgG responses to diisocyanate-HSA antigens in 72% of workers in whom the diagnosis of OA was confirmed by SBPT (17). The specificity of the test was 78%. In contrast to TDI and MDI, serum-specific IgE to HDI-HSA achieved 47% sensitivity and 95% specificity in identifying diisocyanate-challenge-positive subjects (17). Thus, serological testing for specific antibodies could be a specific, albeit insensitive, diagnostic marker of HDI-induced OA. In platinum-refining workers, skin prick testing with hexachloroplatinate salt solutions was shown to lack adequate diagnostic sensitivity and specificity for identifying those in whom OA was confirmed by SBPT (18). Although positive skin prick tests to MDI-HSA and HDI-HSA have been demonstrated in rare cases, cutaneous reactivity to diisocyanate-HSA antigens is not detectable in most workers with OA (3).

Before testing for immunological responses to chemicals, appropriate antigens must be prepared and fully characterized to determine the number of chemical ligands bound to each protein carrier molecule (16). Newly prepared reagents should be evaluated for in vitro and in vivo immunological reactivity in groups of sensitized and nonsensitized individuals. Skin test reagents should be evaluated at various dilutions to identify possible irritant concentrations. Nonspecific direct histamine-releasing effects have been observed with chloroplatinate salts (20). Measurements of serum-specific IgG_4 antibodies to occupational antigens have not been demonstrated to be diagnostically useful. Elevations in serum-specific IgG responses to reactive chemical protein conjugates may reflect exposure rather than clinical sensitization (21).

EVALUATION OF OCCUPATIONAL ASTHMA WITH LUNG FUNCTION STUDIES

The use of physiological tests of lung function in the assessment of OA is extensively discussed elsewhere. Baseline spirometry, which may reveal the presence of reversible airway obstruction, is not adequate for confirming a diagnosis. Spirometric measurements can be performed before and after the work shift. Ideally, these should be performed over an entire work week and during known exposure to the suspect causative substance(s). There is no guarantee that substantial exposure to a suspect agent will occur on any particular work day. Therefore, it is ideal to monitor exposure concentrations concurrent with measurements of lung function.

Cross-shift spirometry is an insensitive method for documentation of work-related asthma (22). When present, an intrashift change in FEV_1 of 10% or greater is considered significant. It is ideal to collect multiple measurements of lung function, which can best be accomplished by self-monitoring of serial peak expiratory flow rates (PEFR) (9). Workers are instructed on the proper use of these inexpensive devices. It is recommended that PEFRs be performed daily every 2–3 hr, for 2 weeks while at work and for an additional 2–3 week-period when away from work. Since the PEFR measurement is an effort-dependent maneuver, careful supervision and monitoring are required. Falsification of data can be prevented by concurrent use of compact computerized devices that store values and recording times (23).

Methods of analysis and interpretation of PEFR data are reviewed extensively in another chapter. Global evaluation of the PEFR records by an experienced clinician is the best method for interpreting peak flow records (24). The presence of significant diurnal variability in PEFR ($\geq$20%) detected on days at work but not on days away from work is consistent with OA. Figure 1 illustrates how this method was used successfully in a raw-egg-processing worker who reported work-related asthmatic symptoms and had positive skin prick tests to egg white proteins (25). There was greater than 20% variability in PEFRs on days when there was exposure to aerosolized liquid egg at work, compared to days away from the work environment. Differences in diurnal variability between work and home may not always be apparent in workers with OA, who may develop chronic persistent asthma for as long as months or years after terminating work exposure. Because PEFR variability correlates with airway responsiveness, histamine or methacholine inhalation tests may be used to validate abnormal serial PEFR studies (26). Methacholine or histamine PC_{20} should be determined on the last day of a work week and repeated 2–3 weeks after restriction from the work environment. In red cedar workers where plicatic acid bronchial challenge was used as the gold standard for diagnosis of OA, serial meth-

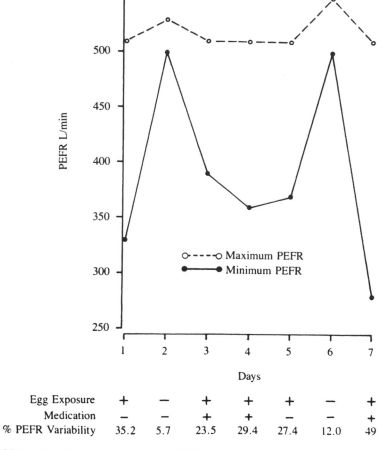

Egg Exposure	+	−	+	+	+	−	+
Medication	−	−	+	+	−	−	+
% PEFR Variability	35.2	5.7	23.5	29.4	27.4	12.0	49

Figure 1 The percentage of variability of PEFR (maximum PEFR value — minimum PEFR value/ mean PEFR value for 24 hr × 100) in an egg-processing worker with asthmatic symptoms at work and resolution of symptoms away from work.

acholine testing performed at work and repeated 7–10 days away from work did not provide additional diagnostic sensitivity over that obtained from serial PEFR studies (27).

   Usually, OA can be confirmed by data obtained from the physician-administered history combined with serial measurements of lung function (e.g., PEFR). A positive skin prick test or elevated serum specific IgE response to a workplace antigen is useful in confirming the identity of a causative agent. If there is diagnostic uncertainty regarding the diagnosis of OA, specific bronchial provocation testing should be considered. Indications and methods for SBPT with occupational agents are discussed in other chapters. There are three types of specific bronchial provocation tests: (1) workplace challenge, which involves closely supervised monitoring of lung function (e.g., FEV_1) during and away from work exposure to the suspect substance(s); (2) laboratory challenge, involving serial measurements of FEV_1 during simulation of a job or work task; and (3) specific bronchial provocation testing in the laboratory, where exposure to a challenge substance is generated and monitored closely (1,4). Each of these approaches has advantages and disadvantages. During a workplace challenge where there are multiple substances in a given work environment, it may be impossible to identify the exact causative agent. Simulation of the work activity in a closed, well-ventilated chamber does not allow precise control of exposure to the test substance. A controlled specific bronchial provocation test offers relative safety in that aerosols, fumes, or powdered agents can be generated in a closed chamber and the amount of exposure can be regulated and closely monitored. Ideally, exposure to the test substance can be generated safely at subirritant or subtoxic levels equivalent or below permissible exposure limits (PEL) in the workplace. Whichever method is selected, lung function must be monitored on a nonexposure control day. Specific challenge tests must be performed in a specialized center and by trained, experienced personnel.

DIFFERENTIAL DIAGNOSIS

A number of conditions must be considered in the differential diagnosis of OA. A worker with preexisting asthma may exhibit bronchoconstriction triggered by nonspecific stimuli, including chemical irritants, smoke, or physical factors (e.g., cold air). Therefore, it is important to determine whether symptoms are due to aggravation at work of preexisting asthma or airway hyperresponsiveness.

The reactive airway dysfunction syndrome (RADS), as originally described by Brooks et al., is a form of OA characterized by increased nonspecific airway reactivity and lower respiratory symptoms which begin within minutes or hours after high-level inhalational exposure to toxic agents (e.g., ammonia, acidic fumes, smoke, spray paint) (28). Symptoms of cough, wheezing, and/or dyspnea begin shortly after accidental exposure to the causative substance(s). Pathological features found in bronchial biopsies of RADS cases are often indistinguishable from asthma.

Bronchiolitis obliterans, a fibrotic obliterative disease of the terminal bronchioles and small airways, may follow exposure to toxic irritants, gases, or fumes (29). Affected individuals exhibit pulmonary infiltrates, evidence of airway obstruction, as well as diffusion abnormalities. Occasionally, nonasthmatic pulmonary diseases such as pneumoconioses or hypersensitivity pneumonitis can be mistaken for OA. Therefore, a chest roentgenogram and complete pulmonary function testing including lung volumes and diffusion capacity should be performed in all workers suspected of having other occupational pulmonary disorders. Metal fume fever is a nonasthmatic condition in welders of galvanized steel. In this disorder, systemic flu-like symptoms, fever, and myalgias accompanied by dyspnea and cough continue for 24–48 hr after inhalation of zinc oxide fumes. Clinical effects could be mediated by release of lung cytokines including tumor necrosis factor (30). This syndrome must be distinguished from occupational asthma, which has also been described in galvanized steel welders (31). The organic dust toxic syndrome (ODTS) presumably is caused by release of endotoxin or mycotoxin from microorganisms in grain or humidifiers.

GENERAL APPROACH TO THE CLINICAL ASSESSMENT OF OCCUPATIONAL ASTHMA

The clinical assessment of workers suspected of having OA should be approached in a stepwise fashion. A comprehensive evaluation begins with a detailed medical and occupational history. Elicitation of detailed information pertaining to substances and processes in the workplace is crucial. If single or multiple causative agents are suspected, the cli-

Table 2 Stepwise Approach to the Assessment of Occupational Asthma

1. Obtain a medical and occupational history.
2. Suspect an occupational etiology.
3. Research all suspect agents by searching the medical literature and compendiums provided in this book.
4. Visit the workplace to characterize the nature of the exposure (optional).
5. Instruct the worker not to leave his or her job until a diagnostic evaluation at work is completed. This does not apply to workers with severe occupational asthma in whom further exposure is deemed unsafe.
6. Follow specific steps in the diagnosis algorithm (Fig. 2) to confirm or exclude a diagnosis of OA. Referral to a specialist may be necessary.
7. Once a diagnosis of OA is confirmed, institute measures to reduce or eliminate exposure to the causative agent(s).

nician should pursue a thorough review of the medical literature and other data sources. As a resource, the editors of this book have provided compendia of recognized causes of OA and a NIOSH database listing occupations and related substances encountered in each job (see Chapt. 35). It may be necessary to visit the plant or worksite and confer with industrial hygienists and safety personnel about the worker's exposure.

It should be emphasized that the most important and useful data for diagnosis of OA are derived from physiological studies performed while the worker is still in the workplace. Such studies may include methacholine inhalation testing, serial recording of peak expiratory flow rates, and a workplace challenge study at the worksite. Therefore, it is essential that a worker remain at work until the OA evaluation is completed. This recommendation does not apply to those with severe asthmatic symptoms that are consistently triggered at work who should be restricted from further exposure. Once OA has been confirmed, the essential treatment is restriction or removal of the worker from further exposure to the causative substance (see Table 2).

GUIDELINES FOR THE DIAGNOSIS OF OCCUPATIONAL ASTHMA

Due to the complexity of modern work environments and the multitude of agents that are encountered by a worker, it can be very difficult to make a specific diagnosis of OA. A physician's diagnosis based on history alone is subjective and therefore must be confirmed in an objective manner. OA due to an HMW allergen encountered in the work environment is established when there is: (1) a history of work-related asthmatic symptoms associated with exposure to a substance known to cause OA; (2) demonstration of significant decrements in lung function at work and improvement away from work; (3) a positive methacholine test at work; and (4) evidence of specific IgE-mediated sensitization to the suspect agent. The existence of a latency period ranging between months and years prior to the onset of symptoms is also supportive of the diagnosis. Thus, the presence of supportive historical and physiological findings together with a positive skin prick test is adequate for making a specific diagnosis of OA due to a HMW allergen (32). Specific bronchoprovocation testing may be considered in cases where there is uncertainty and where objective demonstration of bronchial sensitivity may be necessary to determine whether a worker must be restricted from exposure to the causative substance (1).

A logical stepwise diagnostic algorithm for OA is described in Figure 2. The diagnostic algorithm can be applied only in those workers who remain at work during the entire course of the evaluation. Two decision pathways are presented in the algorithm. The first approach describes serial evaluation of lung function in the workplace whereas the second approach employs controlled specific inhalation testing in the laboratory. The physician's history is of utmost importance in identifying possible asthmatic responses at work. If a HMW or LMW allergen is suspected (and if test reagents are available), skin testing or in vitro serological assays for IgE antibody should be performed to confirm allergic sensitization. A methacholine test is performed in all workers with asthmatic symptoms at the end of the last working day of the week and after the worker has been exposed at work for at least 2 consecutive weeks. As shown in Figure 2, a normal methacholine test ($PC_{20} > 10$ mg/ml) excludes current asthma (and OA). On the other hand, a positive methacholine test ($PC_{20} \leq 10$ mg/ml) is a nonspecific result, and should prompt further evaluation by serial monitoring of lung function at work. Serial PEFR or FEV_1 monitoring for 1–2 weeks at work and at least 2 weeks away from work is recommended. OA can be diagnosed in workers with a positive methacholine study ($PC_{20} \leq 10$ mg/ml) and serial PEFR data plots compatible with OA. Alternatively, a workplace challenge or laboratory challenge test can be performed. A positive workplace challenge test confirms OA, whereas a negative test is indicative of non-OA. If there is no consistent improvement in the PEFR studies away from work, the worker most likely has nonoccupational asthma. It has been recognized that workers do not accurately record or report their PEFR readings obtained with portable devices (e.g., Wright meter) (33). Therefore, whenever possible, an electronic device should be used that records and stores PEFR or FEV_1 values on a memory chip.

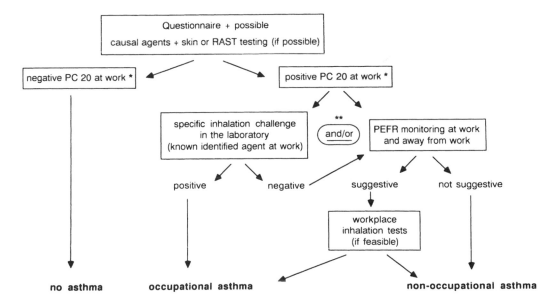

* assessed at the end of a working day and after a minimal period of 2 weeks at work.

** the choice depends on the facilities of the investigation center.

Figure 2 A diagnostic algorithm to be used to confirm or exclude a diagnosis of occupational asthma. These guidelines are to be used in workers who remain exposed at work during the course of the assessment.

As shown in Figure 2, an alternate approach for evaluation of a worker with a positive methacholine test at work is specific inhalation testing in the laboratory. A positive SBPT performed in a controlled fashion in the laboratory is diagnostic of OA, obviating the need for serial PEFR monitoring or a workplace challenge test. A negative laboratory SBPT does not exclude a diagnosis of OA. A negative result could be attributable to underestimation of the level or duration of exposure to the agent that is necessary to elicit an asthmatic reaction. A negative result could also be due to incorrect identification of the causative agent. In such cases, PEFR monitoring is subsequently performed for 2 weeks at work and 2 weeks away from work. Serial PEFR studies that are not consistent with OA would confirm a negative specific inhalation test and definitively exclude OA. If PEFR results are suggestive of OA even after a negative specific laboratory challenge, a closely supervised workplace challenge test should be performed to further confirm OA. The methods for lung physiological tests as well as their indications, advantages, and limitations are reviewed in other chapters.

CLINICAL MANAGEMENT

After a diagnosis of OA is established, treatment options are limited. As already mentioned, restriction from exposure to causative agents is essential and usually effective. Longitudinal studies of worker groups with confirmed OA induced by diisocyanates and red cedar wood dust indicate that an early diagnosis relative to the onset of asthma symptoms followed by prompt interventions (i.e., exposure cessation) results in favorable outcomes manifested by clinical improvement in asthma (3,6,34). In red cedar workers with OA, early recognition of symptoms and a preserved FEV_1 were favorable prognostic variables. Thus, an early diagnosis of OA followed by termination of further exposure is likely to prevent persistent morbidity and disability due to chronic asthma and even asthma mortality. Anecdotal reports of work-related asthma deaths have been reported among symptomatic diisocyanate and bakery workers who remained in the workplace, further emphasizing the folly of allowing sensitized workers with OA to remain in a hazardous work environment (35–37).

After a diagnosis of OA has been confirmed, the employer is required by the American Disabilities Act to institute a needed accommodation. This may involve interventions that prevent exposure to levels that are less than the TLV recommended by NIOSH and the ACGIH. Accommodating an employee with work-related asthma may involve use of protective equipment (i.e., respirators) during short-term unavoidable exposures. Once an exposure restriction has been implemented, all workers with OA who continue to work in the same workplace should undergo periodic medical evaluations. Subsequent evidence of deterioration in asthma symptoms or lung function should prompt complete removal from the workplace followed by medical surveillance. Pharmacotherapy with antiasthmatic drugs should not be considered a suitable alternative to elimination of workplace exposure to the causative substance. The effects of pharmacotherapy in workers with occupational asthma have been evaluated. Pretreatment with beclomethasone inhibits the late-phase asthmatic response after controlled diisocyanate challenge (38). On the other hand, cromolyn was found to have no effect on either the immediate or late-phase responses to diisocyanate challenge. It is unlikely that inhaled or oral corticosteroids have long-term efficacy in the amelioration of OA in workers who are exposed to diisocyanates.

Once workers with OA are sensitized to diisocyanates, minute subthreshold doses can elicit bronchoconstriction. Thus, it may be impossible to prevent OA symptoms via modification of ambient exposure to diisocyanates. Similarly, Venables and Newman-Taylor have demonstrated that early- and late-phase asthmatic reactions are elicited in sensitized acid anhydride workers at ambient levels of tetrachlorophthalic anhydride (TCPA) that are below 100 mg/m^3 (39). These and other data suggest that certain individuals sensitized to TCPA cannot continue to work safely in an environment where there was low-level exposure to acid anhydrides (40).

Industrial hygiene measures that successfully decrease ambient trimellitic anhydride (TMA) exposure in an epoxy-resins-manufacturing facility have resulted in symptomatic improvement among workers with the late respiratory systemic syndrome (41). It is likely that strict environmental controls in terms of ideal ventilation systems and respiratory equipment can reduce the incidence of OA but seldom can these completely prevent development of OA.

Immunomodulation has not been investigated extensively as a treatment modality for occupational asthma. Wahn and Siraganian reported improvement in allergic respiratory symptoms among laboratory animal workers receiving immunotherapy with purified rodent proteins (42). Immunotherapy with a well-characterized epidermal cat allergen has been demonstrated to decrease symptoms and modify asthmatic responses after cat allergen inhalation challenge (43). The latter treatment could be applied to veterinary workers.

CONCLUSIONS

Approaches used for clinical assessment and confirmation of OA have been nonuniform. There is a need for a validated occupational asthma questionnaire. Immunological studies may be useful adjunctive tests but alone do not confirm a diagnosis of OA even in the presence of a positive history. Therefore, a logical stepwise algorithmic approach is recommended to confirm OA, which includes methacholine testing at work, serial monitoring of lung function, and (if necessary) specific inhalation testing. Longitudinal studies and evaluation of outcome are required to evaluate the validity of this approach.

REFERENCES

1. Cartier A, Bernstein IL, Burge PS, Cohn JR, Fabbri LM, Hargreave FE, Malo J-L, McKay RT, Salvaggio JE. Guidelines for bronchoprovocation on the investigation of occupational asthma. Report of the Subcommittee on Bronchoprovocation for Occupational Asthma. J Allergy Clin Immunol 1989; 84(5)(Suppl):823–829.
2. Smith AB, Castellan RM, Lewis D, Matte T. Guidelines for the epidemiologic assessment of occupational asthma. J Allergy Clin Immunol 1989; 84:794–805.
3. Bernstein DI, Korbee I, Stauder T, Bernstein JA, Bernstein IL. The low prevalence of occupational asthma and antibody dependent sensitization to MDI in a plant engineered for minimal exposure to diisocyanates. J Allergy Clin Immunol 1993; 92:387.
4. Pepys J, Hutchcroft BJ. Bronchial provocation tests in etiology diagnosis and analysis of asthma. Am Rev Respir Dis 1975; 112:829–859.
5. Burge PS. Occupational asthma in electronics workers caused by colophony fumes; followup of affected workers. Thorax 1982; 37:438–442.
6. Chan-Yeung M, Maclean L, Paggiaro PL. Follow-up study of 232 patients with occupational asthma caused by western red cedar (*Thuja plicata*). J Allergy Clin Immunol 1987; 79:792–796.
7. Venables KM, Upton JL, Hawkins ER, Tee RD, Longbottom JL, Newman Taylor AJ. Smoking, atopy and laboratory animal allergy. Br J Ind Med 1988; 45:667–671.

8. Cartier A, Malo J-L, Forest F, LaFrance M, Pineau L, St-Aubin JJ, Dubois JY. Occupational asthma in snow crab processing workers. J Allergy Clin Immunol 1984; 74:261–269.
9. Chan-Yeung M. Occupational asthma. Chest 1990; 98:1485–1615.
10. Sjostedt L, Willers S. Predisposing factors in laboratory animal allergy: a study of atopy and environmental factors. Am J Ind Med 1989; 16:199–208.
11. Liss GM, Sussman GL, Seal K, et al. Latex allergy: epidemiology study of 1951 hospital workers. Occup Environ Med 1997; 54:335–342.
12. Venables KM, Topping MD, Howe W, Lucznska CM, Hawkin R, Newman Taylor AJ. Interaction of smoking and atopy in producing specific IgE against a hapten protein conjugate. Br Med J 1985; 290:201–206.
13. Sarlo K, Carl ED, Ryan CA, Bernstein DI. ELISA for human IgE antibody to subtilisin A (Alcalase): correlation with RAST and skin test results with occupationally exposed individuals. J Allergy Clin Immunol 1990; 86:393–399.
14. Merget R, Stollfuss J, Wiewrodt R, et al. Diagnostic tests in enzyme allergy. J Allergy Clin Immunol 1993; 92:264–277.
15. Vandenplas O, Delwich JP, Evrard G, Aimont P, van der Brempt X, Jamart J, Delaunois L. Prevalence of occupational asthma due to latex among hospital personnel. Am J Respir Crit Care Med 1995; 151:54–60.
16. Bernstein DI, Zeiss CR. Guidelines for preparation and characterization of chemical-protein conjugate antigens. J Allergy Clin Immunol 1989; 84(5):820–822.
17. Cartier A, Grammar L, Malo J-L, et al. Specific serum antibodies against isocyanate association with occupational asthma. J Allergy Clin Immunol 1989; 84:507–514.
18. Merget R, Schultze-Werninghaus G, Bode F, et al. Quantitative skin prick and bronchial provocation tests with platinum salt. Br J Ind Med 1991; 48(12):830–837.
19. Liss GM, Bernstein DI, Moller DR, Gallagher JS, Stephenson RL, Bernstein IL, et al. Pulmonary and immunologic evaluation of foundry workers exposed to methylene diphenol diisocyanate (MDI). J Allergy Clin Immunol 1989; 82:55–61.
20. Parrot JL, Hebert R, Saindell A, Ruff F. Platinum and platinosis. Allergy and histamine release due to some platinum salts. Arch Environ Health 1969; 919:685–691.
21. Lushniak BD, Reh CM, Bernstein DI, Gallagher JS. Indirect assessment of 4,4-diphenylmethane diisocyanate (MDI) exposure by evaluation of specific humoral immune responses to MDI conjugated to human serum albumin (HSA). Am J Ind Med 1998; 33:471–477.
22. Burge PS. Single and serial measurements of lung function in the diagnosis of occupational asthma. Eur J Respir Dis 1982; 63(Suppl 123):47–59.
23. Quirce S, Contreras G, Dybuncio A, Chan-Yeung M. Peak expiratory flow monitoring is not a reliable method establishing the diagnosis of occupational asthma. Am J Respir Crit Care Med 1995; 152:1100–1102.
24. Moscato G, Godnic-Cvar J, Maestrelli P. Statement on self-monitoring of peak expiratory flow rates in the investigation of occupational asthma. J Allergy Clin Immunol 1995; 96:295–301.
25. Bernstein DI, Smith AB, Moller DR, Aw TC, Moller DR, London M, Koop S, Carson G. Clinical and immunological studies among egg-processing workers with occupational asthma. J Allergy Clin Immunol 1987; 80:791–797.
26. Cartier A, Pineau L, Malo J-L. Monitoring of maximum expiratory peak flow rates and histamine inhalation tests in the investigation of occupational asthma. Clin Allergy 1984; 14:193–196.
27. Cote J, Kennedy S, Chan-Yeung M. Sensitivity and specificity of PC_{20} and peak expiratory flow rate in red cedar asthma. J Allergy Clin Immunol 1990; 85:592–598.
28. Brooks SM, Weiss MA, Bernstein IL. Reactive airways dysfunction syndrome (RADS). Chest 1985; 88:376–384.
29. Epler GR, Colby TV. The spectrum of bronchiolitis obliterans. Chest 1983; 83:161–162.
30. Boushey HA, Wong H, Wintermeyer SF, Bernstein MS. Cytokines in metal fume fever. Am Rev Respir Dis 1993; 147(1):134–138.
31. Malo J-L, Cartier A. Occupational asthma due to fumes of galvanized metal. Chest 1987; 92:375–377.

32. Bardy JD, Malo J-L, Seguin P, Ghezzo H, Desjardins J, Dolovich J, Cartier A. Occupational asthma and IgE sensitization in a pharmaceutical company processing psyllium. Am Rev Respir Dis 1987; 13(5):1033–1038.

33. Malo J-L, Trudeau C, Ghezzo H, et al. Do subjects investigated for occupational asthma through serial peak expiratory flow measurements falsify their results? J Allergy Clin Immunol 1995; 96:601–607.

34. Moller DR, Brooks SM, McKay RT, et al. Chronic asthma due to toluene diisocyanate (TDI). Chest 1986; 90:494–499.

35. Erlich I. Fatal asthma in a baker: a case report. Am J Ind Med 1994; 26:799.

36. Fabbri LM, et al. Fatal asthma in a subject sensitized to toluene diisocyanate. Am Rev Respir Dis 1988; 137:1494.

37. Licitra C, Sarno N, Ioli F. Death due to asthma at workplace in a diphenylmethane diisocyanate subject. Respiration 1997; 64(1):111–113.

38. Mapp C, Boschetto P, Dal Vecchio L, Crescioli S, De Marzo N, Paleari D, Fabbri LM. Protective effect of anti-asthmatic drugs on late asthmatic reactions and increased airway responsiveness (induced by toluene diisocyanate) in sensitized subjects. Am Rev Respir Dis 1990; 136:1403–1407.

39. Venables KM, Newman Taylor AJ. Exposure-response relationships in asthma caused by tetrachlorophthalic anhydride. J Allergy Clin Immunol 1990; 85:55–58.

40. Grammar LC, Shaughnessy MA, Henderson J, Zeiss CR, Kavich DE, Collins MJ, Pecis KM, Kenamore BD. A clinical and immunologic study of workers with trimellitic anhydride induced immunologic lung disease after transfer to low exposure jobs. Am Rev Respir Dis 1993; 148: 54.

41. Bernstein DI, Zeiss CR, Wolkonsky P, Levitz D, Roberts M, Patterson R. The relationship of airborne trimellitic anhydride concentrations to trimellitic anhydride induced symptoms and immune responses. J Allergy Clin Immunol 1983; 72:709–714.

42. Wahn U, Siraganian RP. Efficacy of specificity of immunotherapy with laboratory animal allergen extracts. J Allergy Clin Immunol 1980; 65:413–421.

43. Ohman JL, Findlay SR, Leiterman M. Immunotherapy in cat induced asthma. Double blind trial with evaluation of in vivo and in vitro responses. J Allergy Clin Immunol 1984; 74: 230–239.

9

Immunological Evaluation of Occupational Asthma

Leslie C. Grammer and Roy Patterson
Northwestern University Medical School, Chicago, Illinois

INTRODUCTION

The immunological evaluation of occupational asthma is similar to that of nonoccupational asthma. However, in the case of occupational asthma, identification of the etiological agent is especially important because the particular etiological agent may affect treatment, job placement, and even worker's compensation. Further, if the sole cause of the asthma is an occupational exposure, elimination of exposure would result in a potential cure for the asthma. Finally, in a sensitized worker, a fatality could occur with high-level, accidental exposure.

The requisites for the diagnosis of asthma due to an occupational allergen are essentially identical to those for the diagnosis of asthma due to a nonoccupational allergen such as cat dander. First, the patient's signs, symptoms, and pulmonary functions must be compatible with occupational asthma due to a given etiological agent. In addition, immunological tests must demonstrate that the patient has an immunological response to the given etiological agent. It must be appreciated that an immunological response to an agent, in and of itself, is not sufficient evidence for the diagnosis of allergic occupational asthma due to that agent. The immunological response to an agent simply means that prior immunizing exposure to the agent has occurred. The diagnosis of allergic occupational asthma requires a compatible clinical picture and physiological evidence of work-related airways obstruction in addition to the immunological response. Occupational asthma should be diagnostically approached as outlined in another chapter with the immunological findings being corroborative, not diagnostic.

TYPES OF IMMUNE RESPONSE

Mechanisms of hypersensitivity responses can be classified according to the classic Gell and Coombs nomenclature (1) with modifications proposed by Janeway and Travers (2) and further extensions by Kay (3). Types I–III are initiated by allergen and antibody interaction while type IV is initiated by allergen and T-cell surface receptor interaction. Type I is immediate, IgE-dependent anaphylactic hypersensitivity that accounts for immediate-phase allergic reactions. Type II reactions can be subdivided into type IIa, or

159

antibody-mediated cytotoxic responses, and type IIb, or cell-stimulating responses. Type III is immune complex or Arthus response such as occurs in serum sickness and probably contributes to the immunopathogenesis of hypersensitivity pneumonitis

Type IV reactions involving sensitized T cells reacting with allergen can be divided into three subtypes. Type IVa$_1$ is classic delayed-type hypersensitivity involving sensitized CD4+ type 1 T cells, which mediate contact dermatitis and tuberculin reactions. Type IVa$_2$ is cell-mediated eosinophilic hypersensitivity due to sensitized CD4+ type 2 T cells, which account for the late phase of IgE-mediated allergic reactions. There is increasing evidence for functional subsets of CD8+ cells. Tc1-type CD8+ cells provide tissue injury via cytoxic T cells while Tc2-type CD8+ cells produce IL-4 and IL-5 resulting in eosinophilic inflammation (3). There is also evidence that CD8+ Tc2-type cells may be the initiating cell in some type IVa$_2$ cell-mediated eosinophilic hypersensitivity reactions (4). Type IVb is cytotoxic T-cell injury mediated by CD8+ Tc1-type cytotoxic T cells.

Most high-molecular-weight occupational allergens and many low-molecular-weight allergens are believed to mediate asthma, at least in part, by a type I IgE-dependent mechanism resulting in immediate-type symptoms. Allergens, both occupational and non-occupational, are well known to also be associated with a late-phase response. Biopsy of bronchi, nasal mucosa, or skin during the late-phase reaction reveals eosinophilic-cell-mediated hypersensivity, a type IVa$_2$ reaction, and a preponderance of cells expressing mRNA for TH2-type cytokines (5,6).

The pathogenesis of some occupational asthma caused by low-molecular-weight allergens, in particular diisocyanates, is less clear. Humoral mechanisms do not appear to be operative. From bronchial biopsy studies and analysis of bronchoalveolar lavage, CD8+, IL-5, and IFN-producing cells and other activated cells appear to be of some importance (7,8). Perhaps this could represent a cellular immunological response mediated by CD8+ Tc2-type cells.

ANTIGENS (ALLERGENS)

Proteins (Complete Antigens)

Whenever a patient's symptoms are respiratory, a careful occupational history should be elicited to determine whether exposure to known workplace allergen(s) has occurred. This is especially true if the symptoms are consistent with asthma as 2–15% of asthma in industrialized countries is reported to be occupational in origin (9,10).

Asthma has been described to be due to a variety of protein antigens from plant and animal sources. A listing of examples of several such agents is provided in Table 1. Enzymes used in a variety of pharmaceutical and food-manufacturing processes are examples of such proteins: pancreatic enzymes (50), hog trypsin (35), *Bacillus subtilis* enzymes (13,14), papain (47). Proteins extracted from insect scales have been associated with asthma in numerous occupations: mealworms in bait handlers (40), locusts in insect control personnel (38), mites in grain workers (42). Asthma has also been described to be due to the inhalation of many different food products: wheat flour (15,17,63), buckwheat flour (16), coffee beans (23), garlic (30), and mushroom (43).

Chemicals (Haptens, Incomplete Antigens)

Low-molecular-weight, reactive chemicals can also act as allergens when the chemical is coupled to appropriate carrier molecules such as autologous human proteins; a complete hapten-carrier antigen is then formed. The antigenic determinant may be the hapten or it

Table 1 Examples of Etiological Agents of Occupational Asthma

Agent	Skin test	Immunoassay	Broncho-provocation	Ref.
Arthropods	+	+	+	11
Azodicarbonamide	+	+	+	12
B. subtilis enzymes	+	+	+	13,14
Buckwheat	+	+	+	15,16
Carmine dye	+	+	+	17
Castor bean	+	+	ND	18
Chloramine-T	+	+	+	19
Chromate	+	+	+	20,21
Clam	+	+	+	22
Coffee bean	+	+	+	23
Coriander (nutmeg shell and paprika)	+	+	+	24
Diazonium tetrafluroborate (DTFB)	ND	+	ND	25
Dimethylethanolamine	ND	ND	+	26
Dyes, textile	+	+	+	27
Egg	+	+	+	28,64
Fennel seed	+	+	+	29
Garlic	+	+	+	30
Grasshoppers	+	+	+	31
Hexamethylene diisocyanate (HDI)	ND	+	+	32
Hexahydrophthlic anhydride (HHPA)	+	+	ND	33,34
Hog trypsin	+	+	+	35
Laboratory animals	+	+	ND	36
Latex	+	+	+	37
Locusts	+	+	ND	38
Maple wood dust	+	+	+	39
Mealworm	+	+	+	40
Diphenylmethane diisocyanate (MDI)	+	+	+	32,41,65
Mite (red spider mite)	+	+	+	42
Mushroom	+	ND	+	43
Nickel	+	+	+	21,44,45,46
Papain	+	+	+	47
Pancreatic extract	+	ND	+	48
Penicillin	+	ND	+	49
Penicillamine	+	+	+	50
Phthalic and tetrachlorophthalic anhydride (PA, TCPA)	+	+	+	51,52
PA	+	+	+	51,53
Platinum	+	+	+	54,55
Protease bromelain	+	+	+	56
Senna	+	+	+	57
Shrimp	+	+	+	22
Spiramycin	+	+	+	58
Toluene diisocyanate (TDI)	ND	+	+	59,60
Trimellitic anhydride (TMA)	+	+	+	61
Wheat flour components	+	+	+	15,62,63

may be a new antigenic determinant formed by the chemical reaction between the hapten and the carrier protein molecule. A listing of examples of such agents can be found in Table 1 in addition to complete protein antigens.

A number of pharmaceuticals have been described to cause asthma: penicillin (49), penicillamine (50), spiramycin (58). Metal-processing-plant workers can develop occupational asthma caused by chromate (20,21), nickel (21,44–46), and platinum (54,55). Acid anhydrides used in curing of epoxy resins, plasticizers, and anticorrosive coatings have been reported to cause several immunological respiratory diseases including occupational asthma; these include trimellitic anhydride (TMA) (61), phthalic anhydride (PA) (51–53), hexahydrophthalic anhydride (HHPA) (33,34), and tetrachlorophthalic anhydride (TCPA) (51–53).

Polyisocyanates are reactive chemicals used in the manufacture of paints, surface coatings, and polyurethane foams; several have been reported to cause occupational asthma: methylene diphenyldiisocyanate (MDI) (41), hexamethylene diisocyanate (HDI) (32), and toluene diisocyanate TDI (59,60). Polyisocyanates are somewhat unusual occupational sensitizers in that most all workers with positive specific inhalation challenge tests do not have positive skin tests or in vitro tests for diisocyanate-HSA serum-specific IgE. This also occurs in western red cedar workers.

IMMUNOPATHOGENESIS

Most immunological causes of immediate-type occupational asthma appear to be due to a type I hypersensitivity reaction. It is becoming quite apparent that type I reactions are not simply a matter of crosslinking IgE on mast cells and basophils with subsequent release of preformed and newly synthesized mediators. First, the high-affinity IgE receptor is not confined to mast cells and basophils (66,67). Moreover, the low-affinity IgE receptor, CD23, found on several cells including monocytes and a subset of T cells appears to be functionally significant (68,69). Finally, while IgE affected workers mediated occupational asthma clearly has an immediate component, many also have a late-phase response after specific inhalation challenge that may occur alone (isolated late-phase asthma) or preceded by an early asthmatic reaction (dual-phase response) (70). Whether the late-phase response is a result of the action of newly formed mediators or is a cell-mediated hypersensitivity or both is not entirely clear at present. Biopsy data suggest that this might represent type IVa_2 cell-mediated hypersensitivity (71).

The immunopathogenesis of some forms of occupational asthma, such as that due to isocyanates, remains elusive. Diisocyanate asthma has many characteristics consistent with an immunological mediation: there is almost always a latency period; the bronchial biopsies of affected workers look identical to extrinsic asthma (72); in addition, there is a reported association with certain MHC class II alleles (73). CD8+, IL-5-producing cells, eosinophils, eosinophil cationic protein (ECP), and peripheral mononuclear cells capable of producing histamine-releasing factors (HRF) and chemokine (MCP-1) in response to specific antigen stimulation have all been described and may contribute to the pathogenesis of diisocyanate asthma (7,8,74).

PREPARATION AND CHARACTERIZATION OF TEST REAGENTS
Proteins

Ideally, test reagents used in the diagnosis of occupational asthma should be standardized extracts of known allergen content (75). At this point, efforts to produce such reagents (e.g., natural rubber latex skin test reagents) are underway but are in very early stages. There are no commercially available standard occupational extracts or reference sera.

For an extract to be standardized, the following should be identified: allergen source, extraction procedure, and biochemical composition. The allergen source should be collected fresh, be well identified, and be free of foreign substances (e.g., endotoxin). Aspects of the extraction procedure such as temperature, extraction medium, time, and filtration should be noted.

A wide variety of procedures exist for determination of biochemical composition. Among the properties that are appropriate to assess are quantitation of total protein content, molecular weight distribution, isoelectric points of individual components, and immunological or allergenic composition. Protein content can be assessed by a variety of techniques including the biuret method (76) and the triketohydrinene hydrate assay (77). Molecular weight determination can be determined by column chromatography using any of a variety of gels. Isoelectric points can be ascertained by isoelectric focusing (78). Immunological or allergenic composition can be assessed using a variety of in vitro or in vivo immunoassays: immunoelectrophoresis (79), immunoblotting (80), RAST inhibition (81), leukocyte histamine release (82), and quantitative cutaneous endpoint titration (83).

Ideally, reference preparations should be available in lyophilized form; they could be used to standardize other preparations or as diagnostic reagents in occupational asthma patients. In addition, it is essential to have reference sera from patients with known occupational asthma due to given etiological agents because these sera are required as positive controls in immunoassays.

Chemical-Protein Conjugates

Low-molecular-weight chemicals are not complete antigens and therefore are generally conjugated to a carrier protein for immunodiagnostic tests (84). There are several exceptions to this general rule. Platinum salts and chloramine T represent two occupational situations in which unconjugated chemicals (haptens) can be used as reliable reagents for detection of immediate-type hypersensitivity responses in the skin (19,54). In the case of platinum hexachloroplatinate, prick test reactivity has been observed at concentrations of unconjugated salt as low as 10^{-9} g/ml (54,55). Only reagent-grade chemicals should be used for preparation of hapten-protein conjugates. A commonly used protein is human serum albumin (HSA). Other proteins including ovalbumin have been used (85). The preparation of the conjugate including buffer, quantity of protein, quantity of chemical, time, and temperature should be noted. It is, of course, imperative to ascertain whether chemical linkage has actually occurred, and if so, the ratio of chemical ligands per protein carrier molecule. It is well known that antigenicity and immunogenicity vary with epitope density.

Spectrophotometric analysis can be used for aromatic compounds (86). Free amino group analysis (87) is useful for chemicals that bind to carrier amines. For other conjugates, gas chromatography (88) or mass spectroscopy (84) may be required. It is obligatory that the degree of ligand binding to protein carriers be determined by one of the above methods. Under- or oversubstitution of ligand can result in either false-negative or false-positive tests.

As with protein antigens described above, protein content and immunological or allergenic composition should be ascertained. Protein content can be assayed as described above. Allergenic or immunological composition is generally determined by immunoassay using sera from workers with occupational asthma due to a given chemical. As described for protein antigens above, availability of standardized, lyophilized extracts and reference serum pools from patients with known occupational asthma due to a given chemical would be useful for optimization of immunodiagnosis of occupational asthma.

CLINICAL IMMUNOLOGICAL TESTS

In Vivo Tests

Two types of cutaneous tests are generally used to assess immediate-type reactivity: the prick test and the intradermal test (83). Prick testing is always performed first. A drop of antigen solution is placed on the skin, which is gently pricked with a needle.

The prick test is the least sensitive and safest method at a standard concentration of antigen. Positive and negative control tests using histamine and saline, respectively, should also be performed. When the prick test is negative, a more sensitive test, the intradermal test, can be used. It is performed by intradermal injection of 0.02–0.03 ml of an appropriate concentration of antigen solution. The prick test concentration is generally 1–10 mg/ml, approximately 10,000 allergy units (AU)/ml, while the intradermal is generally 50- to 1000-fold less concentrated. To determine a nonirritating dose of a new antigen, it is often useful to titrate the solution beginning with a very dilute solution on normal, non-atopic individuals. Table 1 lists many occupational allergens for which positive skin testing has been reported. However, none of the above agents in Table 1 have yet been assessed by rigorous bioequivalency protocols.

In Vitro Tests

Numerous in vitro tests have been reported for the estimation of serum-specific IgE directed against occupational allergens. As discussed above, it is important that the antigen used in immunoassays be allergenic and well characterized. Procedures for standardization and quality control of immunoassays are well described (81). A commonly utilized technique is the radioallergosorbent test (RAST) in which the allergen is coupled to a solid phase. The allergen-coated solid phase is incubated sequentially with the patient's serum and radiolabeled antihuman IgE. The number of counts bound is proportionate to the amount of specific IgE in the patient's serum. Another commonly utilized immunoassay is the enzyme-linked immunosorbent assay (ELISA) (89), which is similar to RAST except that the antihuman IgE is conjugated to alkaline phosphatase, which catalyzes a colorimetric change that is proportional to the amount of specific IgE in the serum. In both assays false-positives can occur with high serum levels of total IgE due to nonspecific binding, and false-negatives can occur due to interference from specific antibody of an isotype other than IgE. Other immunoassays have also been reported. Table 1 lists many occupational allergens for which in vitro immunoassays have been reported.

The ELISA assay is also used for demonstrating the presence of IgG antibodies. Although the significance of IgG antibodies in many occupational diseases is not always evident, the presence of these antibodies should be interpreted with the following principles in mind. IgG antibodies, presumptively cytotoxic, have been reported in association with hemolytic anemia and pulmonary hemorrhage experienced by a few workers exposed to trimellitic anhydride (90). This same antibody isotype may also be found in some workers who experience late systemic symptoms after exposure to trimellitic anhydride. In other cross-sectional studies of occupational asthma, the presence of IgG antibodies may only be indicative of a biological marker of exposure (91). Finally, there is a possibility that

IgG antibodies could function as classic protective antibodies and prevent exposed workers from developing IgE-mediated clinical sensitivity. High titers of IgG antibody can be demonstrated by precipitin assays, although these tests are useful diagnostic aids for hypersensitivity pneumonitis but not asthma (92). Some investigations of immunologically mediated occupational asthma have also measured total antibody (90). This technique is a modification of the Farr method in which radiolabeled antigen is incubated with a suspected serum. If antibodies are present, the labeled antigen will react with all isotypic classes of specific antibodies in the serum. Final measurement is accomplished by immunoprecipitation, which can be accomplished with either 50% saturated ammonium sulfate or a specific polyclonal isotypic (usually anti-IgG) antibody.

In at least one example of occupational asthma total IgE may have diagnostic potential. Skin reactivity to chlorinated platinum salts is associated with increased symptoms and elevated total serum IgE (55). Although the increase in total serum IgE in this case is partially due to platinum-specific IgE antibodies, there is suggestive evidence that platinum salts also act as nonspecific adjuvants and may, in fact, boost the total amount of IgE presumably to other naturally occurring antigens or allergens through a noncognate immunological mechanism (93).

Cellular components of the immune system express a variety of receptors, adhesion molecules and other cell surface markers that can be identified by monoclonal antibodies directed against them. Many of these are identified as clusters of differentiation (CD) markers, enumerated CD1–CD130 (94). Using flow cytometry technology, cell populations can be identified. T-cell activation has been identified in patients with severe asthma (95). Lymphocyte stimulation in vitro has been correlated with events in vivo when antigen interacts with sensitized T cells (96). Cytokines or activation markers such as CD69 can be measured after antigen stimulation (97). The latter techniques are not routine diagnostic tests, but may be useful in immunopathogenetic investigation of occupational asthma. Also, in situ hybridization methods are available for tissue localization of lymphocyte-derived cytokines and/or their respective mRNAs. Monoclonal antibodies against several T-cell activation markers (e.g., CD25 for CD4+ lymphocytes; CD38 for CD8+ lymphocytes) are also being used as immunohistological reagents.

Local immune responses in the bronchi may not correlate with either humoral antibodies or sensitized peripheral blood lymphocytes. These potentially confusing diagnostic problems need to be resolved by future study comparing specific antigenic responses of cells obtained from bronchial lavage fluids and bronchial biopsies to peripheral immune reactions.

The limitations and risks of skin testing are reasonably well recognized because of the use of these techniques for decades. As much or even more caution must be used by the physician responsible for interpreting in vitro test results for occupational allergens, especially those detecting immune responses to low-molecular-weight chemicals. If these tests are performed with unreliable reagents or without appropriate positive and negative controls as discussed above, false-positive results may be obtained. Moreover, even under optimal test conditions, their ranges of sensitivity and specificity may not suffice for routine use as screening or diagnostic tests. The misapplication or misuse of immunological techniques applied to occupational asthma may have adverse effects on workers or industry.

Both skin and in vitro tests should be used in conjunction with other diagnostic modalities for the proper diagnosis of occupational asthma. For example, in the case of high-molecular-weight allergens, a positive prick skin and/or RAST test combined with a positive PC_{20} test will establish a clear-cut clinical diagnosis in many cases. On the other hand, both the specificity and sensitivity of immunological tests are not nearly as satis-factory in the case of low-molecular-weight antigens.

It is also noteworthy that both skin and in vitro tests of IgE-mediated sensitivity will diminish over time when workers are removed from further exposure. In the case of tetrachlorophthalic anhydride, 50% reduction of specific IgE has been observed 1 year after cessation of work exposure (52). Significant reduction of IgE diagnostic tests occurred about 20 months after sensitized workers were removed from further exposure in the snow-crab-processing industry (98). Therefore, it is ill-advised to rely on results of tests in workers with remote exposure to causative agents.

PREVENTION

Primary prevention is the most desirable goal; minimizing exposure to sensitizing agents is the obvious example of this approach. Currently there are no preemployment immu-nological tests that have been shown to be very useful in predicting occupational asthma. Even if there were, it is not likely that they would be mandatory because they would likely be deemed discriminatory. However, voluntary testing with appropriate explanation of risks and benefits might be useful. An example of a potentially useful test would be HLA-DR, DQ typing, as there are reported associations between certain MHC class II alleles and occupational asthma due to TDI (73) and TMA (99).

Secondary prevention by early detection is another approach. In studies of TMA-exposed workers, development of antibody has been shown to be predictive of develop-ment of occupational asthma (100–102). Reduction of exposure, as determined by indus-trial hygiene data, has been associated with reduced prevalence of specific antibody positivity and of disease. Methodologies involving in vivo and in vitro immunological surveillance have been and will continue to be useful in secondary prevention of disease in workers with exposure to other occupational allergens. For example, careful monitoring of enzyme detergent workers who exhibit recent onset positive prick tests by longitudinal respiratory questionnaires and pulmonary function tests has greatly diminished the overall prevalence of occupational asthma in this industry (103).

SUMMARY

The immunological evaluation of occupational asthma is similar to that of nonoccupational asthma. In general, type I or IgE-mediated mechanisms have correlated best with clinically active occupational diseases. Although the precise role of cell-mediated mechanisms is unclear, several manifestations of cellular immune responses, both CD4 + and CD8+, have been reported in occupational asthma. Prick tests and several in vitro antibody tests may be used to corroborate the diagnosis of occupational asthma caused by high-molec-ular-weight-allergens, but the specificity and sensitivity of these tests for occupational asthma induced by low-molecular-weight antigens are not as reliable. Serial immunological tests are useful adjuncts for early detection and prevention of occupational asthma.

ACKNOWLEDGMENT

This work was supported by the Ernest S. Bazley Grant to Northwestern Memorial Hos-pital and Northwestern University Medical School.

REFERENCES

1. Coombs RRA, Gell PGH. The classification of allergic reactions responsible for clinical hypersensitivity and disease. In: Gell PGH, Coombs RRA, Lachman PJ, eds. Clinical Aspects of Immunology, 3rd ed. Oxford: Blackwell Scientific Publications, 1975:761–781.
2. Janeway C, Travers P. Immunobiology, 2nd ed. London: Garland Press, 1995:Chapter 11.
3. Kay AB. Concepts of allergy and hypersensitivity. In: Kay AB, ed. Allergy and Allergic Disease. Oxford: Blackwell Science, 1997:23–35.
4. Salgame P, Abrams JS, Clayberger C, Goldstein H, Convit J, Modlin RL, Bloom BR. Differing lymphokine profiles of functional subsets of human CD4 and CD8 T cell clones. Science 1991; 254(5029):279–282.
5. Azzawi M, Bradley B, Jeffery PK, Frew, AJ Wardlaw, Wardlaw AJ, Knowles G, Assoufi B, Collins JV, Durham S, Kay AB. Identification of activated T lymphocytes and eosinophils in bronchial biopsies in stable atopic asthma. Am Rev Respir Dis 1990; 142:1410–1413.
6. Ying S, Durham SR, Corrigan CJ, Hamid Q, Kay AB. Phenotype of cells expressing mRNA for Th2-type (interleukin-4 and interleukin-5) cytokines in bronchoalveolar lavage and bronchial biopsies from atopic asthmatics and normal control subjects. Am J Respir Cell Mol Biol 1995; 12:477–487.
7. Maestrelli P, Del Prete GF, De Carli M, D'Elios MM, Saetta M, Di Stefano A, Mapp CE, Romagnani S, Fabbri LM. CD8 T-cell clones producing interleukin-5 and interferon-gamma in bronchial mucosa of patients with asthma induced by toluene diisocyanate. Scand J Work Environ Health 1994; 20:376–381.
8. Maestrilli P, diStefano A, Occari P, Turato G, Milani G, Pivirotto F, Mapp CE, Fabbri LM, Saetta M. Cytokines in the airway mucosa of subjects with asthma induced by toluene diisocyanate. Am J Respir Crit Care Med 1995; 151:607–612.
9. Kobayashi D. Different aspects of occupational asthma in Japan. In: Frazier CA, ed. Occupational Asthma. New York: Van Nostrand-Rheinhold, 1980:229–243.
10. Meredith S. Reported incidence of occupational asthma in the United Kingdom. J Epidemiol Commun Health 1993; 47:459–463.
11. Cipolla C, Lugo G, Sassi C, Bonfiglioli R, Maini S, Tommasini MG, Raffi GB. A new risk of occupational disease: allergic asthma and rhinoconjunctivitis in persons working with beneficial arthropods. Int Arch Occup Environ Health 1996; 68:133–135.
12. Kobayashi S. Occupational asthma due to inhalation of pharmacologicao dust and other chemical agents with some reference to other occupational asthma in Japan. In: Yamamaura Y, Frick OL, Hariuchi Y, eds. Allergology. Amsterdam: Excerpta Medica, 1974:124.
13. Slavin RG, Lewis CR. Sensitivity to additives in laundry detergent workers. J Allergy Clin Immunol 1971; 48:262–266.
14. Pepys J, Wells ID, D'Souza MF, Greenberg M. Clinical and immunologic responses to enzymes of *Bacillus subtilis* in factory workers and consumers. Clin Allergy 1973; 3:143–160.
15. Sutton R, Skerritt JH, Baldo BA, Wrigley CW. The diversity of allergens involved in baker's asthma. Clin Allergy 1984; 14:93–107.
16. Park HS, Nahm DH. Buckwheat flour hypersensitivity: an occupational asthma in a noodle maker. Clin Exp Allergy 1996; 26:423–427.
17. Quirce S, Cuevas M, Olaguibel JM, Tabar AI. Occupational asthma and immunologic responses induced by inhaled carmine among employees at a factory making natural dyes. J Allergy Clin Immunol 1994; 93:44–52.
18. Thorpe SC, Kemeny DM, Panzani RC, McGurl B, Lord M. Allergy to castor bean II. Identification of the major allergens in castor bean seeds. J Allergy Clin Immunol 1988; 82:67–72.
19. Blasco A, Joral A, Fuente R, Rodriguez M, Garcia A, Dominguez A. Bronchial asthma due to sensitization to chloramine-T. J Invest Allergol Clin Immunol 1992; 2:167–170.
20. Card WI. A case of asthma sensitivity to chromates. Lancet 1935; 2:1348–1349.
21. Novey HS, Habib M, Wells ID. Asthma and OigE antibodies induced by chromium and nickel salts. J Allergy Clin Immunol 1983; 72:407–412.

22. Desjardins A, Malo JL, L'Archeveque, Cartier A, McCants M, Lehrer SB. Occupational IgE-mediated sensitization and asthma caused by clam and shrimp. J Allergy Clin Immunol 1995; 96:608–617.

23. Karr RM. Bronchoprovocation studies in coffee worker's asthma. J Allergy Immunol 1995; 64(6 pt 2):650–654.

24. Sastre J, Olmo M, Novalvos A, Ibanezz D, Lahoz C. Occupational asthma due to different spices. Allergy 1996; 51:117–120.

25. Luczynskaa CM, Hutchcroft BJ, Harrison MA, Dornan JD, Topping MD. Occupational asthma and specific IgE to a diazonium salt intermediate used in the polymer industry. J Allergy Clin Immunol 1990; 85:1076–1082.

26. Vallieres M, Cockcroft DW, Taylor DM, Dolovich J, Hargreave FE. Dimethyl ethanolamine–induced asthma. Am Rev Respir Dis 1977; 115:867–871.

27. Nilsson R, Nordlinder R, Wass U, Meding B, Belin L. Asthma, rhinitis, and dermatitis in workers exposed to reactive dyes. Br J Ind Med 1993; 50:65–70.

28. Bernstein JA, Kraut A, Bernstein DI, Warrington R, Bolin T, Warren CP, Bernstein IL. Occupational asthma induced by inhaled egg lysozyme. Chest 1993; 103:532–535.

29. Schwartz HJ, Jones RT, Rojas AR, Squillace DL, Yunginger JW. Occupational allergic rhinoconjunctivitis and asthma due to fennel seed. Ann Allergy Asthma Immunol 1997; 78:37–40.

30. Lemiere C, Cartier A, Lehrer SB, Malo JL. Occupational asthma caused by aromatic herbs. Allergy 1996; 51:647–649.

31. Soparkar GR, Patel PC, Cockcroft DW. Inhalant atopic sensitivity to grasshoppers in research laboratories. J Allergy Clin Immunol 1993; 92:61–65.

32. Grammer LC, Harris KE, Malo JL, Cartier A, Patterson R. The use of an immunoassay index for antibodies against isocyanate human protein conjugates and application to human isocyanate disease. J Allergy Clin Immunol 1990; 86:94–98.

33. Moller DR, Gallagher JS, Bernstein DI, Wilcox TG, Burroughs HE, Bernstein IL. Detection of IgE mediated respiratory sensitization in workers exposed to hexahydrophthalic anhydride. J Allergy Clin Immunol 1985; 75:665–672.

34. Grammer LC, Shaughnessy MA, Lowenthal M, Yarnold PR. Risk factors for immunologically mediated respiratory disease from hexahydrophthalic anhydride. J Occup Environ Med 1994; 36:642–646.

35. Colten HR, Polakoff PL, Weinstein SF, Strider DJ. Immediate hypersensitivity to hog trypsin resulting from industrial exposure. N Engl J Med 1975; 292:1050–1053.

36. Newill CA, Eggleston PA, Prenger VL, Fish JE, Diamond EL, Wei Q, Evans RE. Prospective study of occupational asthma. J Allergy Clin Immunol 1995; 95:707–715.

37. Brugnami G, Marabini A, Siracusa A, Abbritti G. Work related late asthmatic response induced by latex allergy. J Allergy Clin Immunol 1995; 96:457–464.

38. Burge PS, Edge G, O'Brien IM, Harries MG, Hawkins R, Pepys J. Occupational asthma in a research center breeding locusts. Clin Allergy 1980; 10:355–363.

39. Reijula K, Kujala V, Latvala J. Sauna builder's asthma caused by obeche (African maple) dust. Thorax 1994; 49:622–623.

40. Bernstein DI, Gallagher JS, Bernstein IL. Meal worm asthma: clinical and immunologic studies. J Allergy Clin Immunol 1983; 72:475–480.

41. Littorin M, Truedsson L, Welinder H, Skarping G, Martensson U, Sjoholm AG. Acute respiratory disorder, rhinoconjunctivitis and fever associated with the pyrolysis of polyurethane derived from diphenylmethane diisocyanste. Scand J Work Environ Health 1994; 20:216–222.

42. Delgado J, Gomez E, Palma JL, Gonzalez J, Monteseirin FJ, Martinez A, Martinez J, Conde J. Occupational rhinoconjunctivitis and asthma caused by *Tetranychus urticae* (red spider mite). A case report. Clin Exp Allergy 1994; 24(5):477–480.

43. Symington IS, Kerr JW, McLean DA. (1981) Type I allergy in mushroom soup processors. Clin Allergy 1981; 11:43–47.

44. Block GT, Yeung M. Asthma induced by nickel. JAMA 1982; 247:1600–1602.

45. McConnell LH, Fink JN, Schlueter DP, Schmidt MG. Asthma caused by nickel sensitivity. Ann Intern Med 1973; 78:888–890.

46. Malo JL, Cartier A, Doepner M, Nieboer E, Evans S, Dolovich J. Occupational asthma caused by nickel sulfate. J Allergy Clin Immunol 1982; 69:55–59.

47. Novey HS, Keenan WJ, Fairshter RD, Wells ID, Wilson AI, Culver BD. Pulmonary disease in workers exposed to papain: clinicophysiological and immunological studies. Clin Allergy 1980; 10: 721–731.

48. Hill D. Pancreatic extract lung sensitivity. Med J Aust 1975; 2:553–555.

49. Davies RJ, Hendrick DJ, Pepys J. Asthma due to inhaled chemical agents: ampicillin, benzyl penicillin, 6 amino penicillamic acid and related substances. Clin Allergy 1974; 4:227–247.

50. Lagier F, Cartier A, Dolovich J, Malo JL. Occupational asthma in a pharmaceutical worker exposed to penicillamine. Thorax 1989; 44:157–158.

51. Grammer LC, Harris KE, Chandler MJ, Flaherty D, Patterson R. Establishing clinical and immunologic criteria for diagnosis of occupational immunologic lung disease with phthalic anhydride and tetrachlorophthalic anhydride exposures as a model. J Occup Med 1987; 29: 806–811.

52. Venables KM, Topping MD, Nunn AJ, Howe W, Newman Taylor AJ. Immunological and functional consequences of clinical tetrachlorophthalic anhydride induced asthma after four years of avoidance of exposure. J Allergy Clin Immunol 1987; 80:212–218.

53. Maccia CA, Bernstein IL, Emmett EA, Brooks SM. In vitro demonstration of specific IgE in phthalic anhydride hypersensitivity. Am Rev Respir Dis 1976; 113:701–704.

54. Cromwell O, Pepys J, Parish WE, Hughes EG. Specific IgE antibodies to plantinum salts in sensitized workers. Clin Alllergy 1979; 9:109–117.

55. Biagini RE, Bernstein IL, Gallagher JS, Moorman WJ, Brooks S, Gann PH. The diversity of reaginic immune responses to platinum and palladium metallic salts. J Allergy Clin Immunol 1985; 76:794.

56. Gailhofer G, Wilders-Trusching M, Smolle J, Ludvan M. Asthma caused by bromelain: an occupational allergy. Clin Allergy 1988; 18:445–450.

57. Helin T, Makinen-Kiljunen S. Occupational asthma and rhinoconjunctivitis caused by senna. Allergy 1996; 51:181–4.

58. Davies RJ, Pepys J. Asthma due to inhaled chemical agents. The macrolide antibiotic spiramycin. Clin Allergy 1975; 1:99–107.

59. Butcher BT, O'Neil CE, Reed MA, Salvaggio JE. Radioallergosorbent testing of toluene diisocyanate-reactive individuals using p-tolyl isocyanate antigen. J Allergy Clin Immunol 1980; 66:213–216.

60. Butcher BT, O'Neil CE, Reed MA, Salvaggio JE. Inhalation challenge and pharmacologic studies of toluene dissocyanate (TDI) sensitive workers. J Allergy Clin Immunol 1979; 64: 146–152.

61. Zeiss CR, Levitz D, Chacon R, Wolkonsky P, Patterson R, Pruzansky JJ. Quantitation and new antigenic determinant (NAD) specificity of antibodies induced by inhalation of trimellitic anhydride in man. Int Arch Allergy Appl Immunol 1980; 61:380–388.

62. Block G, Tse KS, Kijeck K, Chan H, Chan-Yeung M. Baker's asthma. Clinical and immunological studies. Clin Allergy 1983; 13:359–370.

63. Houba R, Heederik DJ, Doekes G, van Run PE. (1996) Exposure-sensitization relationship for alpha amylase in the baking industry. Am J Respir Crit Care Med 1996; 154:130–136.

64. Bernstein DI, Smith HB, Moller DI, Gallagher JS, Tar-Ching AW, London M, Kopp S, Carson G. Clinical and immunologic studies among egg-processing workers with occupational asthma. J Allergy Clin Immunol 1987; 80:791–797.

65. Liss GM, Bernstein DI, Moller DI, Gallagher JS, Stephenson RL, Bernstein IL. Pulmonary and immunologic evaluation of foundry workers exposed to methylene diphenyldiisocyanate (MDI). J Allergy Clin Immunol 1988; 82:51–61.

66. Wang B, Rieger A, Kilgus O, Ochiai K, Maurer D, Fodinger D, Kinet JP., Stingl G. Epidermal Langerhans cells from normal human skin bind monomeric IgE via Fc epsilon RI. J Exp Med 1992; 175:1353–1365.

67. Grant JA, Humbert M, Taborda-Barata L, Sihra BS, Kon OM, Rajakulasingam K, Durham SR, Kay AB. High-affinity IgE receptor Fc epsilon RI expression in allergic reactions. Int Arch Allergy Immunol 1997; 113(1–3):376–378.

68. Suemura M, Kikutani H, Barsumian EL, Hattori Y, Kishimoto S, Sato R, Maeda A, Nakamura H, Owaki H, Hardy RR. Monoclonal anti-Fc epsilon receptor antibodies with different specificities and studies on the expression of Fc epsilon receptors on human B and T cells. J Immunol 1986; 137(4):1214–1220.

69. Borish L, Mascali JJ, Rosenwasser LJ. IgE-dependent cytokine production by human peripheral blood mononuclear phagocytes. J Immunol 1991; 146:63–67.

70. Perrin B, Cartier A, Ghezzo H, Grammer L, Harris K, Chan H, Chan-Yeung M, Malo JL. Reassessment of the temporal patterns of bronchial obstruction after exposure to occupational sensitizing agents. J Allergy Clin Immunol 1991; 87(3):630–639.

71. Robinson DS, Hamid Q, Ying S, Tsicopoulos A, Barkans J, Bentley AM, Corrigan C, Durham SR, Kay AB. Predominant TH2-like bronchoalveolar T-lymphocyte population in atopic asthma. N Engl J Med 1992; 326(5):298–304.

72. Saetta M, Maestrelli P, Turato G, Mapp CE, Milani G, Pivirotto F, Fabbri LM, DiStefano A. Airway wall remodeling after cessation of exposure to isocyanates in sensitized asthmatic subjects. Am J Respir Crit Care Med 1995; 151(2 Pt 1):489–494.

73. Bignon JS, Aron Y, Ju LY, Kopferschmitt MC, Garnier R, Mapp C, Fabbri LM, Pauli G, Lockhart A, Charron D. HLA Class II allelles in isocyanate-induced asthma. Am J Respir Crit Care Med 1994; 149(1):71–75.

74. Lummus ZL, Alam R, Bernstein JA, Bernstein DI. Characterization of histamine releasing factors in diisocyanate-induced occupational asthma. Toxicology 1996; 111(1–3):191–206.

75. Bush RK, Kagen SL. Guidelines for the preparation and characterization of high molecular weight allergens used for the diagnosis of occupational lung disease. J Allergy Clin Immunol 1989; 84:814–819.

76. Kabat EA, Mayer MM. Experimental Immunochemistry. Springfield, IL: Charles C Thomas, 1967;559–565.

77. Richman PG, Cissell DS. Total protein in the ninhydri method. In: Methods of the Laboratory of Allergenic Products. Bethesda, MD: US Food and Drug Administration, 1984.

78. Moulds JM. Genetic typing of the complement system. In: Rose NR, de Macario EC, Folds JD, Lane HC, Nakamura RM, eds. Manual of Clinical Laboratoary Immunology. Washington DC: American Society of Microbiology, 1987:203–207.

79. Price JA, Longbottom JL. Allergy to rabbits. I. Specificity and non-specificity of RAST and crossed-radioimmunoelectrophoresis due to presence of light chains in rabbit allergenic extracts. Allergy 1986; 41:603–612.

80. Thorpe SC, Kemeny DM, Panzaani RC, McGurl B, Lord M. Allergy to castor bean. II. Identification of the major allergens in castor bean seeds. J Allergy Clin Immunol 1988; 82:67–72.

81. Hamilton RG, Adkinson NF. Immunologic tests for diagnosis and management of human allergic disease: total and allergen-specific IgE and allergen-specific IgG. In: Rose NR, de Macario EC, Folds JD, Lane HC, Nakamura RM, eds. Manual of Clinical Laboratory Immunology. Washington DC: American Society for Microbiology, 1997:881–892.

82. Schroeder JT, Kagey-Sobotka A. Assay methods for measurement of mediators and markers of allergic inflamation. In: Rose NR, de Macario EC, Folds JD, Lane HC, Nakamura RM, eds. Manual of Clinical Laboratory Immunology. Washington, DC: American Society for Microbiology, 1997:899–907.

83. Norman PS, Peebles RS. In vivo diagnostic allergy testing methods. In: Rose NR, de Macario EC, Folds JD, Lane HC, Nakamura RM, eds. Manual of Clinical Laboratory Immunology. Washington, DC: American Society for Microbiology, 1997:875–880.

84. Bernstein DI, Zeiss CR. Guidelines for preparation and characterization of chemical-protein conjugate antigens. J Allergy Clin Immunol 1989; 84:820–822.

85. Patterson R, Roberts M, Zeiss CR, Pruzansky JJ. Human antibodies against trimellityl pro-

teins: comparison of specificities of IgG, IgA and IgE classes. Int Arch Allergy Appl Immunol 1981; 66:332–340.

86. Zeiss PR, Patterson R, Pruzansky JJ, Miller MM, Rosenberg M, Levitz D. Trimellitic anhydride (TMA) induced airway syndromes: clinical and immunologic studies. J Allergy Clin Immunol 1977; 60:96–103.

87. Snyder SL, Sobocinski PZ. An improved 2,4,6-trinitrobenzinesulfonic acid method for the determination of amines. Ann Biochem 1975; 64:284–288.

88. Bernstein DI, Gallagher JS, D'Souza L, Bernstein IL. Heterogeneity of specific IgE responses in workers sensitized to acid anhydride compounds. J Allergy Clin Immunol 1984; 74:258–260.

89. Carpenter AB. Enzyme-linked immunoassays. In: Rose NR, de Macario EC, Folds JD, Lane HC, Nakamura RM, eds. Manual of Clinical Laboratory Immunology. Washington, DC: American Society for Microbiology, 1997:20–29.

90. Zeiss CR, Patterson R, Pruzansky JJ, Miller MM, Rosenberg M, Levitz D. Trimellitic anhydride-induced airway syndromes: clinical and immunologic studies. J Allergy Clin Immunol 1977; 60:96–103.

91. Lushniak BD, Reh CM, Gallagher JS, et al. Indirect assessment of MDI exposure by evaluation of specific humoral immune responses to MDI conjugated to human serum albumin. J Occup Med (in press).

92. Walker CL, Grammer LC, Shaughnessy MA, Duffy M, Stoltzfus VD, Patterson R. Diphenylmethane diisocyanate hypersensitivity pneumonitis: a serologic evaluation. J Occup Med 1989; 31:315–319.

93. Murdoch RD, Pepys J. Enhancement of antibody production by mercury and platinum metal halide salts. Kinetics of total and ovalbumin-specific IgE synthesis. Int Arch Allergy Appl Immunol 1986; 80:405–411.

94. Schlossman SF, Boumsell L, Gilks W, Harlan JM, Kishimoto T, Morimoto C, Ritz J, Shaw S, Silverstein RL, Springer TA. CD antigens 1993. Immunol Today 1994; 15(3):98–99.

95. Corrigan CJ, Kay AB. CD4 T lymphocyte activation in acute severe asthma. Relationship to disease severity and atopic status. Am Rev Respir Dis 1990; 141:970–977.

96. Adelman DC. Functional assessment of mononuclear cells. Immunol Clin North Am 1994; 14:241–263.

97. Lopez-Cabrera M, Santis AG, Fernandez-Ruiz R, Esch F, Sanchez-Mateos P, Sanchez-Madrid F. Molecular cloning, expression, and chromosomal localization of the human earliest lymphocyte activation antigen AIM/CD69, a new member of the C-type animal lectin superfamily of signal transmitting receptors. J Exp Med 1993; 178:537–547.

98. Malo JL, Cartier A, Ghezzo H, Lafrance M, McCants M, Lehrer SB. Patterns of improvement on spirometry, bronchial hyperresponsiveness and specific IgE antibody levels after cessation of exposure in occupational asthma caused by snow-crab processing. Am Rev Respir Dis 1988; 138:807–812.

99. Young RP, Barker RD, Pile KD, Cookson WOCM, Newman Taylor AJ. The association of HLA-DR3 with specific IgE to inhaled acid anhydrides. Am J Respir Crit Care Med 1995; 151:219–221.

100. Boxer MB, Grammer L, Harris KE, Roach DE, Patterson R. Six-year clinical and immunologic follow-up of workers exposed to trimellitic anhydride. J Allergy Clin Immunol 1987; 80:147–152.

101. Zeiss CR, Mitchell JH, Van Peenen, PFD, Harris J, Levitz D. A twelve-year clinical and immunologic evaluation of workers involved in the manufacture of trimellitic anhydride (TMA). Allergy Proc 1990; 11:71–76.

102. Grammer LC, Shaughnessy MA, Hogan MB, Berggruen SM, Watkins DM, Yarnold PR. Value of antibody level in diagnosing anhydride-induced immunologic respiratory disease. J Lab Clin Med 1995; 125:650–653.

103. Juniper CP, Roberts DM. Enzyme asthma: 14 years' clinical experience of a recently described disease. J Soc Occup Med 1984; 34:127–132.

10

Nonspecific Bronchial Hyperresponsiveness

Anthony Johnson
Royal Prince Alfred Hospital, Sydney, Australia

Moira Chan-Yeung
Vancouver General Hospital and University of British Columbia, Vancouver, British Columbia, Canada

INTRODUCTION

Asthma is characterized by nonspecific bronchial hyperresponsiveness (NSBH), an abnormality of the airways that allows the bronchi to narrow too much and too easily to a range of agents (1). Most of these stimuli are nonspecific and affect all asthmatics. Specific responses to known allergens can be demonstrated only in asthmatics sensitized to a particular agent. Specific inhalational challenge tests are discussed elsewhere. NSBH can be evaluated using a number of stimuli including adenosine, serotonin, bradykinin, prostaglandin D_2 and $F2_a$, leukotrienes, β-adrenergic blocking agents, cold air, hyperventilation, and hypoosmolar and hyperosmolar stimuli. In the laboratory, the most frequently used stimuli to detect NSBH are histamine and methacholine. NSBH is not confined to asthma, it may be found in other conditions, for example chronic obstructive pulmonary disease (COPD) (2), atopic rhinitis, or in asymptomatic individuals.

HISTORY

It has been known for a long time that histamine and methacholine induce bronchoconstriction. In the late 1920s and early 1930s, Weiss and co-workers (3) demonstrated histamine-induced bronchoconstriction in asthmatics and in normals. Starr and co-workers reported the precipitation of asthmatic attacks in asthmatics by acetyl-beta-methyl choline in the early 1930s (4,5). Curry reported the effect of intravenous, intramuscular, and aerosolized histamine and methacholine on the respiratory tract in normals, allergic subjects, and asthmatics in the 1940s (6,7). The measurement of NSBH as a diagnostic test for asthma was originated by Tiffeneau in the 1950s (8). However, it was not widely used in clinical settings until the 1970s in Europe and in North America (9–11). The standardizing of the methacholine or histamine challenge test by a number of investigators (12–15) has enabled the measurement of NSBH not only in clinical settings but also in epidemiological studies.

MEASUREMENT OF NSBH

Histamine and methacholine challenges are the most commonly performed in the laboratory and will be discussed here. The change in lung function caused by progressively increasing doses or concentrations of provoking agent is recorded. The provoking agent may be administered in two ways, either by a timed period of tidal breathing of aerosols of known concentration (15) or by controlled inhalation of discrete doses, for example the rapid method of Yan et al. (16). The time between dosages is 1 min for the Yan method (16) and about 5 min for most others (14,15). The response is usually measured as the percentage change in FEV_1 from baseline. This is then plotted against the log of concentration or dose. The dose plotted may be either cumulative or noncumulative. Doubling doses of histamine at 1 min intervals produce a cumulative effect whereas when histamine or methacholine is being given in doubling doses at 5 min intervals, there is no significant cumulative effect. The position of the resulting curve indicates the sensitivity of the airways to the provoking agent. The result is usually reported as the dose or concentration that causes a 20% fall in FEV_1, $PD_{20}FEV_1$ or $PC_{20}FEV_1$, respectively. If airway conductance is used as the measure of lung function, the dose causing a 35–50% fall in conductance is used ($PD_{35}SG_{AW}$ or $PD_{50}SG_{AW}$). Values for $PD_{20}FEV_1$ or $PC_{20}FEV_1$ are repeatable to within 1.5–2 doubling doses (17,18). Results from the tidal breathing method are usually reported as $PC_{20}FEV_1$. In adults, histamine and methacholine appear to be equipotent in asthmatics (19) but probably not in patients with COPD (20). The dose-response curve in asthmatics is characterized by a shift to the left and an increased maximal response (21) (Fig. 1).

Measurements of bronchial responsiveness are log-normally distributed (22) in the population. An arbitrary cutoff must therefore be selected in defining an abnormal test, for example, a $PD_{20}FEV_1$ of 3.9–7.8 μmol or a $PC_{20}FEV_1$ of 8–16 mg/ml. Cutpoints have been selected to be highly sensitive, including all asthmatics, but have moderate specificity.

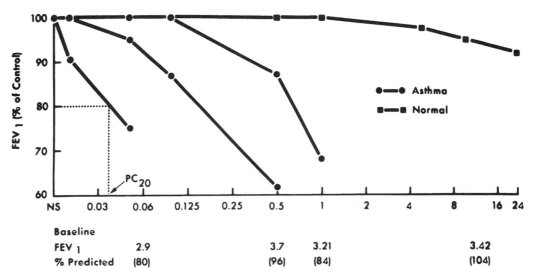

Figure 1   Methacholine dose-response curves in a normal subject and three asthmatic patients. FEV_1 after each inhalation expressed as a percentage of the control value is shown on the vertical axis. (From Ref. 28.)

In population samples the prevalence of asthma is usually <10%. When NSBH is measured in such samples, because of its high sensitivity but moderate specificity, it has a high negative predictive value for symptoms (99–100%) but a low positive predictive value (25–35%) (23).

FACTORS AFFECTING MEASUREMENT

Technical factors may influence measurement of NSBH; the most important is nebulizer output. The nebulizer's output should be calibrated regularly at 2–3 month intervals.

Many subject factors may also influence measurement of NSBH. Perhaps the most important is prechallenge FEV_1 (24). Other factors include recent exposure to allergens (25–27) or occupational sensitizers (28–31), time of day, recent respiratory infection, acute exacerbations of asthma, and posture. H_1 inhibitors block the effect of histamine, and anticholinergic drugs the effect of methacholine. All bronchodilators inhibit the effects of histamine and methacholine (32). The drugs should be withheld for an appropriate length of time before the challenge tests (Table 1).

It has been recommended that methacholine or histamine challenge test should not be done with a baseline FEV_1 below 70% of predicted (33). Challenge can be done at levels below this (34), but the results are difficult to interpret.

OTHER METHODS OF MEASURING NSBH

Isocapnic hyperventilation of cold air and exercise at room temperature also measure NSBH. These methods have the advantage of using natural stimuli, not being dependent on particle deposition or nebulization, and being easy to perform. Children as young as 5 years can perform isocapnic ventilation of cold air (35). There are, however, some dis-

Table 1 Factors and Drugs Affecting Bronchial Responsiveness

Factor	Recommended interval
Cigarette smoke	2 hr
Upper and lower respiratory tract infection	6 weeks
Vaccination with live attenuated influenza virus	3–6 weeks
Specific antigen exposure with late asthmatic reaction	1 week or longer
Occupational sensitizers	Several months

Drug	Recommended duration of withholding drug
Aerosols	
β_2-adrenergic agonist	12 hr
Anticholinergic	12 hr
Oral medications	
β_2-adrenergic agonist	12 hr
Theophyllines	48 hr
H_1-receptor antagonists	48 hr
Corticosteroids	—

advantages; some adults are unable to perform the necessary hyperventilation (35–37). In comparison to methacholine or histamine tests, exercise tests and isocapnic hyperventilation of cold air are less well standardized and require subject cooperation and relatively expensive equipment. Some investigators found a close correlation between histamine or methacholine and isocapnic hyperventilation of cold air (38,39), but others failed to do so (40,41). Although there is a correlation between histamine or methacholine and exercise challenge (42–44), some individuals can be more responsive to one stimulus than the other, probably reflecting different mechanisms of action of different stimuli. In general, isocapnic hyperventilation and exercise challenge tests are less sensitive than methacholine or histamine for the detection of NSBH (32).

Challenges using hypertonic saline or distilled water (fog), although less sensitive than histamine or methacholine challenges, are reportedly highly specific in diagnosing current asthma (45–47). There is good concordance between response to hypertonic saline and exercise-induced asthma (46). Hypertonic saline does not act directly on bronchial smooth muscle but causes airway narrowing by indirect means, and treatment with anti-inflammatory therapy inhibits the response to hypertonic saline, suggesting it may provide an index of airway inflammation (48). Its specificity is also an advantage in epidemiological studies. Distilled water challenge has been shown to be more specific but less sensitive than methacholine challenge for the diagnosis of occupational asthma caused by low-molecular-weight agents (confirmed by specific inhalational challenge) (49,50). Hypertonic saline challenge has been used successfully in epidemiological studies of workers (51). Recently, an osmotic challenge method using a dry powder preparation of mannitol delivered via an inhaler device has been described (52).

PATHOPHYSIOLOGY

Reduced airway caliber, increased bronchial contractility, altered permeability of the bronchial mucosa, humoral and cellular mediators, and dysfunctional neural regulation are important in the pathogenesis of bronchial hyperresponsiveness. It is beyond the scope of this chapter to review these in detail.

A gene governing NSBH has been located near a major locus on chromosome 5q that regulates serum IgE levels in Dutch families (53). Evidence for linkage of the asthma phenotype to this region has also been obtained in the same families (54).

INTERPRETATION OF RESULTS

NSBH is identifiable in almost all subjects with current symptomatic asthma. Mild NSBH is measurable in some subjects with rhinitis but no chest symptoms and in some asymptomatic individuals (55,56). Measurement of NSBH is helpful when correlated with symptoms. In subjects with atypical chest symptoms and normal spirometry, finding NSBH increases the likelihood of asthma. In a subject with current chest symptoms the absence of NSBH virtually excludes the diagnosis of asthma (provided there is no other reason for the lack of NSBH such as high-dose corticosteroids). NSBH cannot be used to distinguish asthma from COPD in subjects with a mild decrease in FEV_1 and symptoms that do not clearly suggest asthma or COPD. However, a dose-response curve to methacholine is helpful. If there is a plateau, and the PD_{20} FEV_1 is more than 4.0 µmol, it is unlikely to be asthma (2).

Serial measurement of NSBH may be helpful in assessing asthma treatment but usually offers no advantage over traditional means of following therapy such as symptoms, need for bronchodilators, and serial peak flow measurements (57).

OCCUPATIONAL ASTHMA AND NSBH

General Considerations

Lam and co-workers (28) studied NSBH in a series of patients with occupational asthma due to a variety of agents. They found that symptomatic patients with occupational asthma had evidence of NSBH at the time of diagnosis. Patients who left exposure and became asymptomatic had a much smaller degree of NSBH. In a subgroup of patients with occupational asthma due to western red cedar, they were able to observe a progressive increase in PC_{20} from the time of diagnosis with increasing duration away from work. Since then many other studies have confirmed these findings in patients with occupational asthma due to isocyanates (29), colophony (58), snow-crab processing (59), and other agents (60). Occupational asthma without NSBH has been described (61) but is almost only present in subjects who have been removed from the relevant exposure. When subjects return to the workplace for at least 2 weeks, NSBH can then be documented.

Onset of NSBH

It has been controversial whether NSBH was a predisposing risk factor for occupational asthma or developed with the symptoms of occupational asthma. There are now several studies showing the development of NSBH coincides with the onset of occupational asthma in workers in both low- and high-molecular-weight allergens.

In a study of four western red cedar workers NSBH developed in parallel with the development of asthma and was not present in any of the workers beforehand (62). In laboratory animal workers (63), the development of chest symptoms was associated with an increase in NSBH after 18 months of exposure and correlated with intensity of exposure. The level of preemployment NSBH did not predict sensitization.

Vedal et al. (64) followed a cohort of western red cedar workers longitudinally. The development of NSBH was associated with a decrease in pulmonary function, whereas loss of NSBH corresponded to improvement in pulmonary function. They were unable to determine whether the change in NSBH was due to changes in airway caliber or whether both were caused by another factor. They hypothesized that variability in NSBH may identify a group of workers at risk for developing more symptoms and lower levels of lung function, as well as persistent NSBH with continued exposure to western red cedar dust. Persistent NSBH was associated with higher estimated dust exposure.

NSBH may have prognostic significance. In a study of cases of occupational asthma due to western red cedar (65) more marked NSBH to methacholine at the time of diagnosis was associated with the persistence of symptoms at follow-up.

NSBH After Exposure Has Ceased

After exposure to the sensitizing agent has ceased, NSBH may improve; with ongoing exposure, it is likely to deteriorate. In a study of snow-crab workers with occupational asthma NSBH significantly improved by the first follow-up assessment at a mean of 12.8 months after the subjects left work (59). The plateau for improvement in NSBH occurred at about 2 years. These authors had found no significant change in NSBH in subjects with occupational asthma from a variety of agents, on average 5.8 years (range 4.3–10.9 years) after the cessation of exposure (66). If subjects are followed for a long period there may be improvement. In a recent report of 48 subjects examined 8.9 years on average after ceasing exposure, there was significant improvement in NSBH when compared to another group of subjects who had ceased exposure for less than 5 years (67).

At the occupational asthma clinic at Vancouver General Hospital, 490 subjects have been diagnosed with western red cedar asthma by specific challenge test since 1970. A total of 293 have had at least one follow-up visit with a PC_{20} measurement and exposure status recorded. Of these, 81 continued exposure without interruption, 65 permanently ceased exposure within 12 months of diagnosis, and the remainder either ceased exposure more than 12 months after diagnosis or continued intermittent exposure. The mean PC_{20} at diagnosis and for successive time periods for those subjects who ceased exposure permanently within 12 months of diagnosis ($n = 65$) are shown in Figure 2. The median duration of follow-up was 4 years (range <1–21.9 years). The mean PC_{20} for the time period 1–2 years away from exposure was significantly higher than the value at diagnosis ($p < 0.01$, ANOVA). There was no further increase in mean PC_{20} values after this. In those who continued exposure without interruption ($n = 81$), the median duration of follow-up was 3 years (range <1–21.1 years). There was no significant change in PC_{20} during this period of follow-up ($p = 0.5$) (Fig. 2).

The prognosis for improvement in NSBH in platinum-sensitized subjects after exposure has ceased appears to be poor; symptoms may improve despite NSBH remaining unchanged. In a group of platinum workers with occupational asthma and an immediate-type asthmatic reaction on specific challenge there was no change in NSBH after removal from exposure for an average of 19 months (range 1–77 months) despite 29% ceasing to have asthmatic symptoms (68).

In a group of patients with isocyanate-induced asthma, NSBH did not change during follow-up in most subjects despite specific challenges becoming negative (69). Persistence of NSBH after the cessation of exposure has also been reported in occupational asthma secondary to other agents (70,71). No association has been found between changes in NSBH and changes in specific challenge tests after exposure has ceased (72).

The probability of NSBH returning to normal after exposure has ceased appears to depend on the degree of airflow obstruction, the degree of NSBH, and the dose and duration of exposure to the offending agent at the time of diagnosis (29,64,65,73). When the diagnosis is made early after the onset of symptoms and further exposure is avoided completely, the chances of NSBH returning to normal are higher. After removal from exposure, treatment with inhaled beclomethasone for 5 months has been shown to significantly improve NSBH in toluene diisocyanate-induced asthma in a placebo-controlled trial (74).

After returning to normal, NSBH may recur in conjunction with symptoms of asthma on reexposure to the offending agent (75).

NSBH and Specific Challenge Tests

The induction of a late or dual asthmatic reaction with a specific challenge test is associated with an increase in NSBH. In toluene diisocyanate asthma it has been observed that late and dual, but not early, asthmatic reactions are associated with a transient increase of bronchial responsiveness (76). This has also been demonstrated in subjects with asthma due to western red cedar (28). The increase in NSBH after challenge with a specific

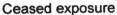

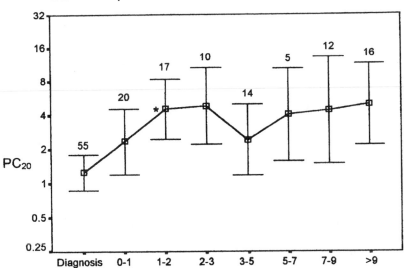

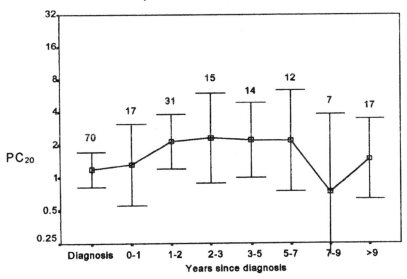

Figure 2 Mean PC_{20} mg/ml methacholine (±2 SEM, log scale) of patients with occupational asthma caused by western red cedar who continued exposure ($n = 81$) without interruption or permanently ceased exposure within 12 months of diagnosis ($n = 65$). The diagnosis was confirmed by specific challenge in all cases. The mean PC_{20} at diagnosis and for successive time periods are shown. *The mean PC_{20} for the time period $1-2$ years was significantly higher than the value at diagnosis ($p < 0.01$, ANOVA) in the group who ceased exposure; there was no significant change in those who continued exposure. Numerical values with each error bar are the number of measurements available for each time period.

sensitizer may last for a short period, 2–3 days, or for a prolonged period, up to 4 weeks (31,77).

Late asthmatic reactions have been demonstrated, generally, to increase bronchial responsiveness and are believed to respond poorly to inhaled bronchodilator. However, this has recently been shown to be variable. In a retrospective review of specific challenge tests (78), 57/101 (56%) subjects with late reactions and 24/63 (38%) subjects with isolated immediate reactions demonstrated a twofold or greater change in PC_{20} from baseline. These authors also found that subjects with late asthmatic reactions responded well to β-agonists by inhalation.

The relationship between the specific responsiveness to plicatic acid and NSBH was explored by Lam and associates (79). The specific responsiveness to plicatic acid was defined as the percentage decrease in FEV_1 per milligram of plicatic acid nebulized during inhalation challenge test and the NSBH was expressed as PC_{20} mg/ml methacholine. These authors found a direct correlation between the degree of NSBH and the degree of specific responsiveness to plicatic acid (Fig. 3). Since skin test cannot be used to determine the initial concentration of occupational chemical sensitizers in specific inhalation challenge tests, NSBH should be determined. The higher the degree of NSBH, the lower the initial concentration of chemical sensitizer that should be used.

The increase in NSBH after a specific inhalation challenge in the absence of significant change in the FEV_1 can be an early and sensitive marker of bronchial response to occupational agents, especially in subjects removed from workplace exposure for a long time. It is an indicator that subjects will respond to the specific agent at the next or subsequent dose (80).

NSBH and Reactive Airways Dysfunction Syndrome

Reactive airways dysfunction syndrome (RADS) (81), or irritant-induced asthma, occurs after an acute exposure to high concentrations of an irritant. Respiratory symptoms develop acutely. One of the main characteristics of the syndrome is the development of NSBH, which persists after the acute inhalation. In one report, persistence of NSBH was found up to 13 years after the initial episode (82).

ROLE IN CLINICAL OCCUPATIONAL ASTHMA

The measurement of NSBH has been found to be useful in the following clinical settings.

Diagnosis of Asthma

Detecting NSBH is useful when the diagnosis of asthma has not been confirmed or when a patient describes symptoms of cough, chest tightness, and dyspnea that cannot be ascribed to other causes. Also, because wheezing is a symptom of other disorders, inhalation challenge tests can be useful in defining its cause when reversible airflow obstruction has not been documented. Cockcroft and co-workers (83) performed histamine challenge tests on 500 randomly selected university students. They concluded that a PC_{20} greater than 8 mg/ml virtually rules out current symptomatic asthma, a PC_{20} below 1 mg/ml is diagnostic of current symptomatic asthma, whereas values between 1 and 8 mg/ml are borderline.

A normal NSBH does not exclude the diagnosis of occupational asthma particularly when the subjects are being tested after they have been away from work for a period of

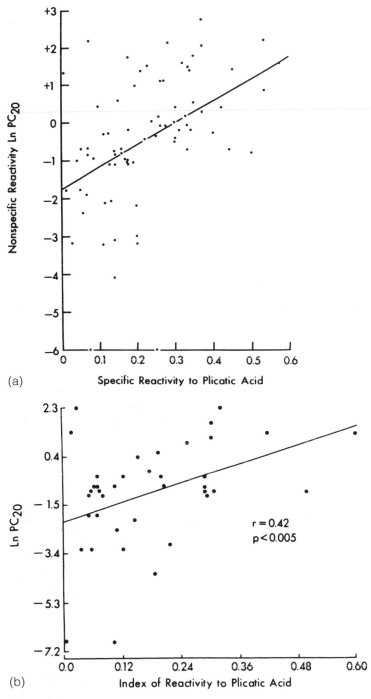

Figure 3 (a) Relationship between the severity of LAR to plicatic acid and methacholine PC_{20}. The severity of the reaction to plicatic acid was expressed by the ratio of the amount of plicatic acid nebulized to the maximal fall in FEV_1 from the baseline. Logarithmic value (Ln) of methacholine PC_{20} is shown on the Y-axis. (b) Relationship between the severity of the early reaction of DAR to plicatic acid and methacholine PC_{20}.

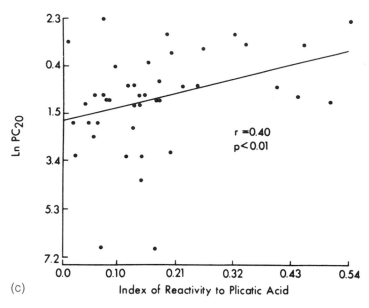

Figure 3 (Continued)   (c) Relationship between the severity of the late reaction of DAR to plicatic acid and the methacholine PC_{20}. (From Ref. 79.)

time (84). In patients with early occupational asthma, NSBH can return to normal within a short period of time without exposure, as short as 2 or 3 days (77). Even though the subject may not have NSBH beforehand, specific inhalation challenge test with the offending agent can induce bronchoconstriction associated with the induction of NSBH (84,85).

Assessment of Work-Relatedness

Specific challenge testing with the offending agent is an excellent way to determine the work relationship of asthma when the agent is known and inhalation challenge test is feasible. However, in many instances, the agent responsible for asthma is unknown and the subject may be exposed to multiple sensitizers in the workplace. In these situations, prolonged recording of the peak expiratory flow rates over a period of several weeks when the patient is working and when off work has been found to be very useful in demonstrating the work-relatedness of the asthma (86,87). Occupational exposure usually induces a gradual fall in the peak expiratory flow rates and withdrawal from exposure results in a gradual improvement in the peak expiratory flow rates. Since the patient is asked to monitor his/her peak expiratory flow rate, this test is not considered objective enough by some investigators because of the possibility of malingering. Serial measurements of NSBH in addition to prolonged recording of peak expiratory flow rates have been recommended (Fig. 4). Significant changes in NSBH do not occur when subjects with nonoccupational asthma are exposed to particulates (88). Similarly, exposure to low levels of irritant gases such as sulfur dioxide (89), ozone (89,90), and nitrogen dioxide (91) produces only transient and small changes in NSBH in both healthy and asthmatic subjects.

While it is much easier to demonstrate an increase in NSBH when the patient is exposed to the allergen or chemical sensitizer in the workplace, it is not as easy to demonstrate a decrease in NSBH when the patient is away from work as it may take a long

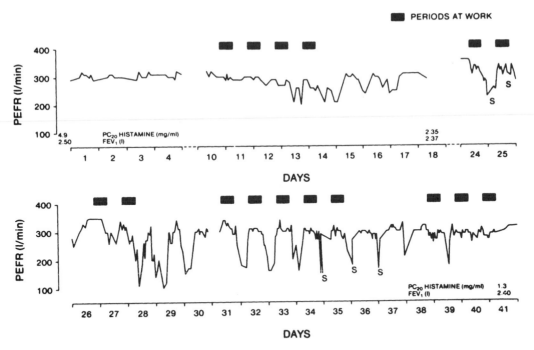

Figure 4 Serial daily changes in PEFRs demonstrating significant fluctuations on return to work without recovery on weekends. PC_{20} results and baseline FEV_1 are presented. S = inhaled salbutamol (200 μg) used. (From Ref. 120.)

time before NSBH improves (28). A period of observation longer than a weekend is usually necessary. In a study of western red cedar workers with the results of a specific challenge test as the gold standard, the sensitivity and specificity of changes in PC_{20} alone for the diagnosis of occupational asthma were 62% and 78%, respectively (87). The addition of NSBH measurement did not improve the diagnostic accuracy of PEFR alone. Perrin et al. (92) confirmed this finding in a group of patients with occupational asthma due to other agents. Nevertheless, the demonstration of appropriate changes in NSBH together with changes in peak expiratory flow rates confirms the work relationship.

Determination of Initial and Subsequent Doses of Occupational Agents for Specific Challenge Tests

Specific challenge tests, although very useful in establishing work-relatedness of asthma, have to be performed with care to avoid the induction of anaphylaxis or a severe attack of asthma. When the occupational agent is a high-molecular-weight allergen and an extract is available for skin tests, it is easy to determine the initial concentration of the occupational allergen to use for specific challenge tests. Cockcroft and co-workers (93) recommended that the initial concentration of high-molecular-weight allergen to use for inhalation challenge test should be 3–4 doubling dilutions below the predicted allergen PC_{20} (the dose of allergen that induces a 20% fall in FEV_1). The allergen PC_{20} is predicted from the formula Log_{10} allergen $PC_{20} = 0.68\ Log_{10}\ (PC_{20} \times SS)$ where SS = skin sensitivity, which is defined as the lowest allergen dilution that gives a wheal 2 mm in diameter (the mean of two perpendicular measurements on each of the two duplicate prick tests). However, when the occupational agent is a low-molecular-weight compound, such as isocyanate and plicatic acid, skin tests cannot be used as they are usually negative. In these circumstances, measurement of NSBH is essential before specific challenge test. Patients with a high degree of NSBH should be challenged very cautiously by starting at a very low concentration of the specific agent to avoid severe reactions.

Inhalation challenge tests with low-molecular-weight agents induce isolated late asthmatic reaction frequently. Specific challenge tests with isocyanates are time consuming. To avoid serious reactions, the duration of exposure or the nonirritative concentration (5–20 ppb) is usually increased stepwise over several days. When no airflow obstruction is detected at 8 hr after the specific challenge, it is useful to determine the level of NSBH. If the PC_{20} decreases in the absence of airflow obstruction, one can expect the patient to react to the next dose (either increased concentration or increased duration of exposure) of the specific agent the following day. If the PC_{20} fails to change at 8 hr, a higher dose of the agent can be given the following day. The measurement of NSBH has increased the safety of the specific challenge test.

Assessment of Respiratory Impairment/Disability in Occupational Asthma

NSBH has been found to correlate with various aspects of the assessment of the severity of asthma including diurnal variation of peak flow rates (94), asthma severity score (95), and the minimum medication requirement necessary to achieve control of symptoms (96). Measurement of the degree of NSBH may add another dimension in the objective assessment of respiratory impairment in occupational asthma (97,98). The rationale for applying measurement of NSBH in the assessment of respiratory impairment will be discussed in detail in another chapter.

MEASUREMENT OF NSBH IN EPIDEMIOLOGICAL STUDIES

Methacholine, histamine, hypertonic saline, and isocapnic hyperventilation of cold air have been used successfully in field studies (99). It is more difficult to control some of the technical factors in isocapnic hyperventilation of cold air such as inspired air temperature, humidity, and minute ventilation. For these reasons histamine and methacholine have been most widely utilized.

Some protocols used in the laboratory take 45–60 min; therefore, shortened protocols are needed when studying large populations. Such protocols have been developed. Yan et al. (16) described a rapid method using hand-held nebulizers to administer eight different doses of histamine. The entire test takes 15 min and the results correlate well with those obtained from the dosimeter technique. Other shortened techniques have been described and validated (51,100–102).

In population studies most subjects will not respond to a nonspecific challenge with a drop in FEV_1 of 20% or more, which means that a lot of data is censored if only PC_{20} is used as an outcome. Other methods have been developed that enable a value to be calculated in all subjects, such as dose-response curves to methacholine. The simplest is the two-point slope, obtained by joining the first and last points of the dose-response curve. Mathematical models may be fitted to such curves but extrapolation of dose-response curves should be avoided (103).

The prevalence of NSBH found in different populations varies. This is related to different methods of measurement of NSBH, differing definitions, and a difference in the true prevalence of NSBH. The prevalence of NSBH is highest in the newborn, decreases to its lowest level between age 20 and 30 years, and then increases again with aging (104).

Of relevance to occupational asthma is the prevalence of NSBH in adults. Some randomly sampled population surveys are available. In Bussellton, Australia, the prevalence of bronchial hyperresponsiveness in adults was found to be 11.4% (105). In a random sample of adults aged 18–65 years in England, the prevalence of NSBH to histamine was 14% (106). A study in The Netherlands (107) found that the prevalence of NSBH was 22–28% in adults but used a higher dose of histamine and a lower threshold to define NSBH than the above studies. In the European Community Respiratory Health Survey (ECRHS), surveys with similar protocols with randomly selected adults (aged 20–44 years) from the population were conducted in various European nations, Australia, and New Zealand (108). NSBH was defined as a 20% drop in FEV_1 during methacholine challenge. A cumulative dose of up to 2 mg of methacholine was used. In East Germany, the prevalence of NSBH was 27.6% in females and 13.2% in males (109). This sex difference disappeared after allowing for FEV_1 (109). In Hamburg, West Germany, the prevalence was 30.1% in females and 15.9% in males, giving an overall prevalence of 22.6% (95% CI 20.1–25.3%). In New Zealand, the overall prevalence of NSBH was 33% (110). In Canada, a study was done with a protocol adapted from the ECRHS in six communities (111); the prevalence of NSBH varied from 13 to 29%. It is apparent that there is substantial variation in the population prevalence of NSBH.

NSBH alone is not a good predictor of asthma symptoms in epidemiological studies. Typically it has been found to have a high negative predictive value (99–100%) but a low positive predictive value (25–35%) (23). In the Canadian study, of those with NSBH 41.6% denied wheeze in the last 12 months and 66.7% denied ever having asthma. Of those reporting wheeze in the last 12 months only 27.8% had NSBH. Of those reporting ever having asthma, diagnosed by a doctor, 41.2% had current NSBH.

Atopic subjects without a history of asthma have a higher prevalence of NSBH than nonatopic subjects (105,112–115). In population-based studies, the relationship between atopy and NSBH depends on age (115). Among young adults, there is an association between immediate skin test reactivity and NSBH. This association disappears in older age groups. One possible reason is the decrease in prevalence of atopy with age and the occurrence of other causes of NSBH in older age groups, such as COPD.

A universally accepted definition of asthma for epidemiology is not available. The use of questionnaire data alone is subjective and subject to a wide variety of cultural, psychological, and sociological influences (116). Measurement of NSBH in epidemiological studies adds some objective data. The combination of symptoms with NSBH has been found to be very useful in epidemiological settings. Wheeze in the last 12 months and NSBH identifies a group with clinically important asthma (117). Malo and Cartier (118), in a study of 51 subjects exposed to spiramycin, found that a combination of history of asthma and presence of NSBH ($PC_{20} \leq 16$ mg/ml) or a decrease in NSBH after a period off work correctly identified all three subjects subsequently shown to have occupational asthma by specific challenge tests. They suggested that it is one of the more useful tests in screening subjects with possible occupational asthma because it provides objective information and may detect subjects who deny their symptoms.

In workforce surveys attempting to detect cases of occupational asthma NSBH has been used as a screening procedure. In industries involving exposure to low-molecular-weight allergens, current workers with NSBH are referred for further evaluation, including specific challenge tests (119). In industries with high-molecular-weight exposures, workers with NSBH or positive skin tests to the suspected agent are investigated further (119). Owing to the high sensitivity of NSBH in the diagnosis of asthma, cases are unlikely to be missed using this approach.

SUMMARY

Standardized, safe, and rapid methods of assessment of NSBH are now available. NSBH is a useful tool in the clinical assessment of occupational asthma, particularly in confirming the diagnosis of asthma when symptoms are atypical. NSBH develops in parallel with the development of occupational asthma and often persists after exposure to the sensitizing agent has ceased. In epidemiological studies, NSBH in combination with symptoms is useful in identifying asthma in populations.

REFERENCES

1. Woolcock AJ. What is bronchial hyperresponsiveness from the clinical standpoint? In: Page C, Gardiner P, eds. Airway Hyperresponsiveness: Is It Really Important for Asthma? Oxford: Blackwell Scientific Publications, 1993.
2. Woolcock AJ, Anderson SD, Peat JK, Du Toit JI, Zhang YG, Smith CM, Salome CM. Characteristics of bronchial hyperresponsiveness in chronic obstructive pulmonary disease and in asthma. Am Rev Respir Dis 1991; 143(6):1438–1443.
3. Weiss S, Robb GP, Ellis LE. The systemic effects of histamine in man with special reference to the responses of the cardiovascular system. Arch Intern Med 1932; 49:360–396.
4. Starr IJ, Elsom KA, Reisinger JA, Richards AN. Acetyl-beta-methyl cholin. I. The action on normal persons: with a note on the action of the ethyl ether of beta-methyl cholin. Am J Med Sci 1933; 186:313.
5. Starr IJ. Acetyl-beta-methyl cholin. III. Its action on paroxysmal tachycardia and peripheral vascular disease with a discussion of its action in other conditions. Am J Med Sci 1933; 186: 330.
6. Curry JJ. The action of histamine on the respiratory tract in normal and asthmatic subjects. J Clin Invest 1946; 25:785–791.
7. Curry JJ. Comparitive action of mecholyl chloride and histamine. J Clin Invest 1947; 26: 430–438.
8. Tiffeneau R. Hypersensibilitie cholinergo-histaminique pulmonaire de l'asthmatique. Acta Allergol 1958; 5(Suppl):187–221.
9. Herxheimer H. Bronchial obstruction induced by allergens, histamine and acetyl-beta-methylcholine chloride. Int Arch Allergy 1951; 2:27–39.
10. Parker CD, Bilbo RE, Reed CE. Methacholine aerosol as test for bronchial asthma. Arch Intern Med 1965; 115:452–458.
11. de Vries K, Goei JT, Booy-Noord H, Orie NGM. Changes during 24 hours in the lung function and histamine hyperreactivity of the bronchial tree in asthmatic and bronchitic patients. Int Arch Allergy 1962; 20:93–101.
12. Hargreave FE, Ryan A, Thomson NCO, Byrne PM, Latimer K, Juniper EF, Dolovich J. Bronchial responsiveness to histamine or methacholine in asthma: measurement and clinical significance. J Allergy Clin Immunol 1981; 68:347–355.
13. Ryan G, Dolovich MB, Roberts RJ, Frith PA, Juniper EF, Hargreave FE, Newhouse MT. Standardization of inhalation provocation tests: two techniques of aerosol generation and inhalation compared. Am Rev Respir Dis 1981; 123:195–199.

14. Chai H, Farr R, Froehlich LA, Matheson DA, McLean JA, Rosenthal RR, Sheffer AL, Spector SL, Townley RG. Standardization of bronchial inhalation challenge procedures. J Allergy Clin Immunol 1975; 56:323–327.

15. Cockcroft DW, Killian DN, Mellon JJA, Hargreave FE. Bronchial reactivity to inhaled histamine: a method and clinical survey. Clin Allergy 1977; 7:235–243.

16. Yan K, Salome C, Woolcock AJ. Rapid method for measurement of bronchial responsiveness. Thorax 1983; 38(10):760–765.

17. Chinn S, Britton JR, Burney PG, Tattersfield AE, Papacosta AO. Estimation and repeatability of the response to inhaled histamine in a community survey. Thorax 1987; 42(1):45–52.

18. Peat JK, Salome CM, Bauman A, Toelle BG, Wachinger SL, Woolcock AJ. Repeatability of histamine bronchial challenge and comparability with methacholine bronchial challenge in a population of Australian schoolchildren. Am Rev Respir Dis 1991; 144(2):338–343.

19. Salome CM, Schoeffel RE, Woolcock AJ. Comparison of bronchial reactivity to histamine and methacholine in asthmatics. Clin Allergy 1980; 10(5):541–546.

20. Du Toit JI, Woolcock AJ, Salome CM, Sundrum R, Black JL. Characteristics of bronchial hyperresponsiveness in smokers with chronic air-flow limitation. Am Rev Respir Dis 1986; 134(3):498–501.

21. Woolcock AJ, Salome C, Yan K. The shape of the dose-response curve to histamine in asthmatics and normal subjects. Am Rev Respir Dis 1984; 130:71–75.

22. Peat JK, Unger WR, Combe D. Measuring changes in logarithmic data, with special reference to bronchial responsiveness. J Clin Epidemiol 1994; 47(10):1099–1108.

23. Backer V. Bronchial hyperresponsiveness in children and adolescents. Danish Med Bull 1995; 42(5):397–409.

24. Ulrik CS. Bronchial responsiveness to inhaled histamine in both adults with intrinsic and extrinsic asthma: the importance of prechallenge forced expiratory volume in 1 second. J Allergy Clin Immunol 1993; 91(1 Pt 1):120–126.

25. van der Heide S, de Monchy JG, de Vries K, Bruggink TM, Kauffman HF. Seasonal variation in airway hyperresponsiveness and natural exposure to house dust mite allergens in patients with asthma. J Allergy Clin Immunol 1994; 93(2):470–475.

26. Cartier A, Thomson NC, Frith PA, Roberts R, Hargreave FE. Allergen-induced increase in bronchial responsiveness to histamine: relationship to the late asthmatic response and change in airway caliber. J Allergy Clin Immunol 1982; 70(3):170–177.

27. Cockcroft DW, Ruffin RE, Dolovich J, Hargreave FE. Allergen-induced increase in non-allergic bronchial reactivity. Clin Allergy 1977; 7(6):503–513.

28. Lam S, Wong R, Yeung M. Nonspecific bronchial reactivity in occupational asthma. J Allergy Clin Immunol 1979; 63(1):28–34.

29. Mapp CE, Corona PC, De MN, Fabbri L. Persistent asthma due to isocyanates. A follow-up study of subjects with occupational asthma due to toluene diisocyanate (TDI). Am Rev Respir Dis 1988; 137(6):1326–1329.

30. Chan-Yeung M. Occupational asthma. Chest 1990; 98(Suppl):148S–161S.

31. Cartier A, L'Archeveque J, Malo JL. Exposure to a sensitizing occupational agent can cause a long-lasting increase in bronchial responsiveness to histamine in the absence of significant changes in airway caliber. J Allergy Clin Immunol 1986; 78(6):1185–1189.

32. Hargreave FE, Dolovich J, Boulet LP. Inhalation provocation tests. Semin Respir Med 1983; 4:224–236.

33. AAAAI. Diagnosis and evaluation in "Practice parameters for the diagnosis and treatment of asthma." J Allergy Clin Immunol 1995; 96(5 part 2):737–738.

34. Martin RJ, Wanger JS, Irvin CG, Bucher Bartelson B, Cherniack RM, and ACRN. Methacholine challenge testing: safety of low starting FEV_1. Chest 1977; 112(1):53–56.

35. Weiss ST, Tager IB, Weiss JW, Munoz A, Speizer FE, Ingram RH Jr. The epidemiology of airways responsiveness in a population sample of adults and children. Am Rev Respir Dis 1984; 129:898–902.

36. Scarf SM, Heimer D, Waters M. Bronchial challenge with room temperature isocapnic hyperventilation. Chest 1985; 88:686–693.

37. Desjardins A, de Luca S, Cartier AL, L'Archevêque J, Ghezzo H, Malo JL. Nonspecific bronchial hyperresponsiveness to inhaled histamine and hyperventilation of cold dry air in subjects with respiratory symptoms of uncertain etiology. Am Rev Respir Dis 1988; 137: 1020–1025.

38. O'Byrne PM, Ryan G, Morris M, McCormack D, Jones NL, Morse JLC, Hargreave FE. Asthma induced by cold air and its relation to nonspecific bronchial responsiveness to methacholine. Am Rev Respir Dis 1982; 125:281–285.

39. Weiss JW, Rossing TH, McFadden ER, Ingram RH. Relationship between bronchial responsiveness to hyperventilation with cold air and methacholine in asthma. J Allergy Clin Immunol 1983; 72:140–144.

40. Neijens HJ, Hofkamp M, Degenhart HJ, Kerrebijn KF. Bronchial responsiveness as a function of inhaled histamine and the methods of measurement. Bull Eur Physiopathol Respir 1982; 18:427–438.

41. Tessier P, Ghezzo H, L'Archevêque J, Cartier A, Malo JL. Shape of the dose response curve to cold air inhalation in normal and asthmatic subjects. Am Rev Respir Dis 1987; 136:1418–1423.

42. Chatham M, Bleecker ER, Smith PL, Rosenthal RR, Mason P, Norman PS. A comparison of histamine, methacholine, and exercise airway reactivity in normal and asthmatic subjects. Am Rev Respir Dis 1982; 126:235–240.

43. Eggleston PA. A comparison of the asthmatic response to methacholine and exercise. J Allergy Clin Immunol 1979; 63:104–110.

44. Anderton RC, Cuff MT, Frith PA, Cockcroft DW, Morse JLC, Jones NL, Hargreave FE. Bronchial responsiveness to inhaled histamine and exercise. J Allergy Clin Immunol 1979; 63:315–320.

45. Anderson SD, Smith CM. Osmotic challenges in the assessment of bronchial hyperresponsiveness. Am Rev Respir Dis 1991; 143(3 Pt 2).

46. Smith CM, Anderson SD. Inhalational challenge using hypertonic saline in asthmatic subjects: a comparison with responses to hypernoea, methacholine and water. Eur Respir J 1990; 3(2): 144–151.

47. Makker HK, Holgate ST. Relation of the hypertonic saline responsiveness of the airways to exercise-induced asthma symptom severity and to histamine or methacholine reactivity. Thorax 1993; 48(2):142–147.

48. Anderson S, Gibson P. Use of aerosols of hypertonic saline and distilled water (fog). Barnes P, Grunstein M, Leff A, Woolcock A, eds. Asthma. Philadelphia: Lippincott-Raven, 1997: 1135–1149.

49. Dellabianca A, Omodeo P, Colli MC, Bianchi P, Scibilia J, Moscato G. Bronchial responsiveness to ultrasonic "fog" in occupational asthma due to low molecular weight chemicals. Ann Allergy Asthma Immunol 1996; 77(5):378–384.

50. Moscato G, Dellabianca A, Corsico A, Biscaldi G, Gherson G, Vinci G. Bronchial responsiveness to ultrasonic fog in occupational asthma due to toluene diisocyanate. Chest 1993; 104(4):1127–1132.

51. Rabone SJ, Phoon WO, Anderson SD, Wan KC, Seneviratne M, Gutierrez L, Brannan J. Hypertonic saline challenge in an adult epidemiological survey. Occup Med 1996; 46(3): 177–185.

52. Anderson SD, Brannon J, Spring J, Spalding N, Rodwell LT, Chan K, Gonda I, Walsh A, Clark A. A new method for bronchial-provocation testing in asthmatic subjects using a dry powder of mannitol. Am J Respir Crit Care Med 1997; 156:758–765.

53. Postma DS, Bleecker ER, Amelung PJ, Holroyd KJ, Xu J, Panhuysen CI, Meyers DA, Levitt RC. Genetic susceptibility to asthma–bronchial hyperresponsiveness coinherited with a major gene for atopy. N Engl J Med 1995; 333(14):894–900.

54. Panhuysen CIM, Levitt RC, Postma DS, Xu J, Amelung PJ, Holroyd KJ, van Altena R, Koater GH, Meyers DA, Bleecker ER. Evidence for a susceptibility locus for asthma mapping to chromosome 5q. J Invest Med 1995; 43(Suppl):281A.

55. Varpela E, Laitinen LA, Keskinen H, Korhola O. Asthma, allergy and bronchial hyper-reactivity to histamine in patients with bronchiectasis. Clin Allergy 1978; 8(3):273–280.

56. Laitinen LA, Haahtela T, Kava T, Laitinen A. Non-specific bronchial reactivity and ultrastructure of the airway epithelium in patients with sarcoidosis and allergic alveolitis. Eur J Respir Dis 1983; 131(Suppl):267–284.

57. Cockcroft D. Airway responsiveness. Barnes P, Grunstein M, Leff A, Woolcock A, eds. In: Asthma. Philadelphia: Lippincott-Raven, 1997:1253–1266.

58. Burge PS. Occupational asthma in electronics workers caused by colophony fumes: follow-up of affected workers. Thorax 1982; 37(5):348–353.

59. Malo JL, Cartier A, Ghezzo H, Lafrance M, McCants M, Lehrer SB. Patterns of improvement in spirometry, bronchial hyperresponsiveness, and specific IgE antibody levels after cessation of exposure in occupational asthma caused by snow-crab processing. Am Rev Respir Dis 1988; 138(4):807–812.

60. Graneek BJ, Durham SR, Newman Taylor AJ. Late asthmatic reactions and changes in histamine responsiveness provoked by occupational agents. Bull Eur Physiopathol Respir 1987; 23(6):577–581.

61. Mapp CE, Dal VL, Boschetto P, De MN, Fabbri LM. Toluene diisocyanate-induced asthma without airway hyperresponsiveness. Eur J Respir Dis 1986; 68(2):89–95.

62. Chan-Yeung M, Desjardins A. Bronchial hyperresponsiveness and level of exposure in occupational asthma due to western red cedar (*Thuja plicata*). Serial observations before and after development of symptoms. Am Rev Respir Dis 1992; 146(6):1606–1609.

63. Renstrom A, Malmberg P, Larsson K, Larsson PH, Sundblad BM. Allergic sensitization is associated with increased bronchial responsiveness: a prospective study of allergy to laboratory animals. Eur Respir J 1995; 8(9):1514–1519.

64. Vedal S, Enarson DA, Chan H, Ochnio J, Tse KS, Chan-Yeung M. A longitudinal study of the occurrence of bronchial hyperresponsiveness in western red cedar workers. Am Rev Respir Dis 1988; 137(3):651–655.

65. Chan-Yeung M, Lam S, Koener S. Clinical features and natural history of occupational asthma due to western red cedar (*Thuja plicata*). Am J Med 1982; 72(3):411–415.

66. Allard C, Cartier A, Ghezzo H, Malo JL. Occupational asthma due to various agents. Absence of clinical and functional improvement at an interval of four or more years after cessation of exposure. Chest 1989; 96(5):1046–1049.

67. Perfetti L, Cartier A, Ghezzo H, Gautrin D, Malo J-L. Follow-up of occupational asthma after removal from or dimunition of exposure to the responsible agent: revelence of the length of the interval from cessation of exposure. Chest 1998 (in press).

68. Merget R, Reineke M, Rueckmann A, Bergmann EM, Schultze-Werninghaus G. Nonspecific and specific bronchial responsiveness in occupational asthma caused by platinum salts after allergen avoidance. Am J Respir Crit Care Med 1994; 150(4):1146–1149.

69. Paggiaro PL, Vagaggini B, Dente FL, Bacci E, Bancalari L, Carrara M, Di FA, Giannini D, Giuntini C. Bronchial hyperresponsiveness and toluene diisocyanate. Long-term change in sensitized asthmatic subjects. Chest 1993; 103(4):1123–1128.

70. Pisati G, Zedda S. Outcome of occupational asthma due to cobalt hypersensitivity. Sci Total Environ 1994; 150(1–3):167–171.

71. Saric M, Marelja J. Bronchial hyperreactivity in potroom workers and prognosis after stopping exposure. Br J Ind Med 1991; 48(10):653–655.

72. Lemiere C, Cartier A, Dolovich J, Chan-Yeung M, Grammer L, Ghezzo H, L'Archeveque J, Malo JL. Outcome of specific bronchial responsiveness to occupational agents after removal from exposure. Am J Respir Crit Care Med 1996; 154(2 Pt 1):329–333.

73. Chan-Yeung M, MacLean L, Paggiaro PL. Follow-up study of 232 patients with occupational asthma caused by western red cedar (*Thuja plicata*). J Allergy Clin Immunol 1987; 79(5): 792–796.

74. Maestrelli P, De MN, Saetta M, Boscaro M, Fabbri LM, Mapp CE. Effects of inhaled beclomethasone on airway responsiveness in occupational asthma. Placebo-controlled study of subjects sensitized to toluene diisocyanate. Am Rev Respir Dis 1993; 148(2):407–412.

75. Banks DE, Rando RJ. Recurrent asthma induced by toluene diisocyanate. Thorax 1988; 43(8): 660–662.

76. Fabbri LM, Picotti G, Mapp CE. Late asthmatic reactions, airway inflammation and chronic asthma in TDI sensitized subjects. Eur Respir J 1991; 13(Suppl)(2).

77. Cockcroft DW, Mink JT. Isocyanate-induced asthma in an automobile spray painter. Can Med Assoc J 1979; 121(5):602–604.

78. Malo JL, Ghezzo H, L'Archeveque J, Cartier A. Late asthmatic reactions to occupational sensitizing agents: frequency of changes in nonspecific bronchial responsiveness and of response to inhaled beta 2-adrenergic agent. J Allergy Clin Immunol 1990; 85(5):834–842.

79. Lam S, Tan F, Chan H, Chan-Yeung M. Relationship between types of asthmatic reaction, nonspecific bronchial reactivity, and specific IgE antibodies in patients with red cedar asthma. J Allergy Clin Immunol 1983; 72(2):134–139.

80. Vandenplas O, Delwiche JP, Jamart J, Van de Weyer R. Increase in non-specific bronchial hyperresponsiveness as an early marker of bronchial response to occupational agents during specific inhalation challenges. Thorax 1996; 51(5):472–478.

81. Brooks SM, Weiss MA, Bernstein IL. Reactive airways dysfunction syndrome (RADS). Persistent asthma syndrome after high level irritant exposures. Chest 1985; 88(3):376–384.

82. Piirila PL, Nordman H, Korhonen OS, Winblad I. A thirteen-year follow-up of respiratory effects of acute exposure to sulfur dioxide. Scand J Work Environ Health 1996; 22(3):191–196.

83. Cockcroft DW, Murdock KY, Berscheid BA, Gore BP. Sensitivity and specificity of histamine PC_{20} determination in a random selection of young college students. J Allergy Clin Immunol 1992; 89(1 Pt 1):23–30.

84. Hargreave FE, Ramsdale EH, Pugsley SO. Occupational asthma without bronchial hyperresponsiveness. Am Rev Respir Dis 1984; 130(3):513–515.

85. Smith AB, Brooks SM, Blanchard J, Bernstein IL, Gallagher J. Absence of airway hyperreactivity to methacholine in a worker sensitized to toluene diisocyanate (TDI). J Occup Med 1980; 22(5):327–331.

86. Burge PS. Single and serial measurements of lung function in the diagnosis of occupational asthma. Eur J Respir Dis 1982; 123(Suppl):47–59.

87. Cote J, Kennedy S, Chan-Yeung M. Sensitivity and specificity of PC_{20} and peak expiratory flow rate in cedar asthma. J Allergy Clin Immunol 1990; 85(3):592–598.

88. De Luca S, Caire N, Cloutier Y, Cartier A, Ghezzo H, Malo JL. Acute exposure to sawdust does not alter airway calibre and responsiveness to histamine in asthmatic subjects. Eur Respir J 1988; 1(6):540–546.

89. Kulle TJ, Kerr HD, Farrell BP, Sauder LR, Bermel MS. Pulmonary function and bronchial reactivity in human subjects with exposure to ozone and respirable sulfuric acid aerosol. Am Rev Respir Dis 1982; 126(6):996–1000.

90. McDonnell WF, Horstman DH, Abdul-Salaam S, House DE. Reproducibility of individual responses to ozone exposure. Am Rev Respir Dis 1985; 131(1):36–40.

91. Koenig JQ, Covert DS, Morgan MS, Horike M, Horike N, Marshall SG, Pierson WE. Acute effects of 0.12 ppm ozone or 0.12 ppm nitrogen dioxide on pulmonary function in healthy and asthmatic adolescents. Am Rev Respir Dis 1985; 132(3):648–651.

92. Perrin B, Malo JL, L'Archeveque J, Ghezzo H, Lagier F, Cartier A. Comparison of monitoring of peak expiratory flow rates and bronchial responsiveness with specific inhalation challenge in occupational asthma. Am Rev Respir Dis 1990; 141:A79.

93. Cockcroft DW, Murdock KY, Kirby J, Hargreave F. Prediction of airway responsiveness to allergen from skin sensitivity to allergen and airway responsiveness to histamine. Am Rev Respir Dis 1987; 135(1):264–267.

94. Ryan G, Latimer KM, Dolovich J, Hargreave FE. Bronchial responsiveness to histamine: relationship to diurnal variation of peak flow rate, improvement after bronchodilator, and airway calibre. Thorax 1982; 37(6):423–429.

95. Makino S. Clinical significance of bronchial sensitivity to acetylcholine and histamine in bronchial asthma. J Allergy 1966; 38(3):127–142.

96. Juniper EF, Frith PA, Hargreave FE. Airway responsiveness to histamine and methacholine: relationship to minimum treatment to control symptoms of asthma. Thorax 1981; 36(8):575–579.

97. Chan-Yeung M, Becklake M, Bleeker ER, Fish JE, Malo J-L, Rosenstock L, Samet J. Impairment of men and women for work: some scientific issues and evaluation. Am Rev Respir Dis 1987; 136(4):1052–1054.

98. American Thoracic Society. Guidelines for the evaluation of impairment/disability in patients with asthma. Am J Respir Crit Care Med 1993; 147(4):1056–1061.

99. Riedler J, Reade T, Dalton M, Holst D, Robertson C. Hypertonic saline challenge in an epidemiologic survey of asthma in children. Am J Respir Crit Care Med 1994; 150(6 Pt 1): 1632–1639.

100. Hendrick DJ, Fabbri LM, Hughes JM, Banks DE, Barkman HW Jr, Connolly MJ, Jones RN, Weill H. Modification of the methacholine inhalation test and its epidemiologic use in polyurethane workers. Am Rev Respir Dis 1986; 133(4):600–604.

101. Chatham M, Bleecker ER, Norman P, Smith PL, Mason P. A screening test for airways reactivity. An abbreviated methacholine inhalation challenge. Chest 1982; 82(1):15–18.

102. Sparrow D, O'Connor G, Colton T, Barry CL, Weiss ST. The relationship of nonspecific bronchial responsiveness to the occurrence of respiratory symptoms and decreased levels of pulmonary function. The Normative Aging Study. Am Rev Respir Dis 1987; 135(6):1255–1260.

103. Verlato G, Cerveri I, Villani A, Pasquetto M, Ferrari M, Fanfulla F, Zanolin E, Rijcken B, de M R. Evaluation of methacholine dose-response curves by linear and exponential mathematical models: goodness-of-fit and validity of extrapolation. Eur Respir J 1996; 9(3):506–511.

104. Horsley JR, Sterling IJ, Waters WE, Howell JB. How common is increased airway reactivity amongst the elderly? Gerontology 1993; 39(1):38–48.

105. Woolcock AJ, Peat JK, Salome CM, Yan K, Anderson SD, Schoeffel RE, McCowage G, Killalea T. Prevalence of bronchial hyperresponsiveness and asthma in a rural adult population. Thorax 1987; 42(5):361–368.

106. Burney PG, Britton JR, Chinn S, Tattersfield AE, Papacosta AO, Kelson MC, Anderson F, Corfield DR. Descriptive epidemiology of bronchial reactivity in an adult population: results from a community study. Thorax 1987; 42(1):38–44.

107. Rijcken B, Schouten JP, Weiss ST, Meinesz AF, de Vries K, van der Lende R. The distribution of bronchial responsiveness to histamine in symptomatic and in asymptomatic subjects. A population-based analysis of various indices of responsiveness. Am Rev Respir Dis 1989; 140(3):615–623.

108. Burney PG, Luczynska C, Chinn S, Jarvis D. The European Community Respiratory Health Survey. Eur Respir J 1994; 7(5):954–960.

109. Wassmer G, Jorres RA, Heinrich J, Wjst M, Reitmeir P, Wichmann HE. The association between baseline lung function and bronchial responsiveness to methacholine. Eur J Med Res 1997; 2(2):47–54.

110. Fishwick D, Pearce N, D'Souza W, Lewis S, Town I, Armstrong R, Kogevinas M, Crane J. Occupational asthma in New Zealanders: a population based study. Occup Environ Med 1997; 54(5):301–306.

111. Manfreda J, Chan-Yeung M, Dimich-Ward H, Sears M, Sierstead H, MR B, Ernst P, Sweet L, VanTil L, Bowie D, Anthonisen N, Tate R. Prevalence of asthma in Canada. Am J Respir Crit Care Med 1996; 153:A432.

112. Townley RG, Ryo UY, Kolotkin BM, Kang B. Bronchial sensitivity to methacholine in current and former asthmatic and allergic rhinitis patients and control subjects. J Allergy Clin Immunol 1975; 56(6):429–442.

113. Enarson DA, Chan-Yeung M, Tabona M, Kus J, Vedal S, Lam S. Predictors of bronchial hyperexcitability in grainhandlers. Chest 1985; 87(4):452–455.

114. Kennedy SM, Burrows B, Vedal S, Enarson DA, Chan-Yeung M. Methacholine responsiveness among working populations. Relationship to smoking and airway caliber. Am Rev Respir Dis 1990; 142(6 Pt 1):1377–1383.

115. Sparrow D, Weiss S. Background. In: Sparrow D, Weiss S, eds. Airway Responsiveness and Atopy in the Development of Chronic Lung Disease. New York: Raven Press, 1989:1–19.

116. Burney P, Chinn S. Developing a new questionnaire for measuring the prevalence and distribution of asthma. Chest 1987; 91(Suppl)(6):79S–83S.

117. Toelle BG, Peat JK, Salome CM, Mellis CM, Woolcock AJ. Toward a definition of asthma for epidemiology. Am Rev Respir Dis 1992; 146(3):633–637.

118. Malo JL, Cartier A. Occupational asthma in workers of a pharmaceutical company processing spiramycin. Thorax 1988; 43(5):371–377.

119. Malo JL, Cartier A, L'Archeveque J, Trudeau C, Courteau JP, Bherer L. Prevalence of occupational asthma among workers exposed to eastern white cedar. Am J Respir Crit Care Med 1994; 150(6 Pt 1):1697–1701.

120. Cartier A, Chan H, Malo J-L, Pineau L, Tse KS, Chan-Yeung M. Occupational asthma due to eastern white cedar (*Thuja occidentalis*) with demonstration that plicatic acid is present in this wood dust and is the causal agent. J Allergy Clin Immunol 1986; 77:639–645.

11
Physiological Assessment: Serial Measurements of Lung Function

Sherwood Burge
Birmingham Heartlands Hospital, Birmingham, England

Gianna Moscato
Salvatore Maugeri Foundation, Institute for Rehabilitation and Care,
Medical Center of Pavia, Pavia, Italy

INTRODUCTION

The diagnosis of occupational asthma can usually be made from a history of the relationship of symptoms to work exposures. Physiological measurements aim to confirm the medical history. Supervised measurements of lung function can be carried out before and after a work shift or at regular intervals during employment as part of medical surveillance. If measurements are to be made before and after work and on days away from work, the only practical means is for workers to make their own measurements. Until recently the only portable measuring devices available measured peak expiratory flow. Portable devices measuring FEV_1 have recently become available using turbines, pressure transducers, and pneumotachographs. This chapter reviews the use of lung function testing in the diagnosis of occupational asthma, particularly the use of serial measurements of peak flow at home and at work.

DIURNAL VARIATION IN AIRWAYS CALIBER

The spontaneous diurnal variation in airways caliber is fundamental to the understanding of physiological measurements of lung function in relationship to work. A spontaneous diurnal rhythm (for instance in peak flow) can be demonstrated in the majority of the normal population, which is exaggerated in asthma (1). The lowest readings are usually around the time of waking; there is then improvement for 6–8 hr followed by a subsequent decline until sleeping, with a further decline overnight. The trigger for the diurnal variation appears to be sleep stage. Airway caliber is reduced during periods of rapid-eye-movement sleep, particularly during narrative dreams. Any reaction at work will be superimposed on this diurnal variation. The relationship between work and sleep can be altered substantially by shift work. Most day workers and workers on early shifts (for instance 06:00–14:00 hr) wake shortly before going to work. The first few hours at work will therefore coincide with the period of improving lung function. The effect of an immediate reaction is then to blunt the rise in peak flow rather than to cause any fall (2). Workers on afternoon shifts (for instance 14:00–22:00 hr) usually wake substantially before going to work and go to sleep shortly after returning from work. This results in the occupational exposure coinciding with the decreasing phase of lung function. Immediate reactions are usually more obvious on such shifts. The pattern of sleep in night workers is very variable and usually changes between days at work and days away from work. Some workers have long periods without sleep and some sleep more than once per 24 hr. As each period of sleep is usually associated with a "morning dip," the patterns of reaction can then be complex. The diurnal variation usually resets itself within 24 hr of a change in sleep pattern (for instance, working nights) unlike the diurnal variations of cortisol and adrenaline, which take longer to reset.

BEFORE AND AFTER SHIFT MEASUREMENTS

There have been many attempts to document occupational asthma from before and after shift measurements. They are surprisingly difficult to carry out, i.e., to make the first reading before any work exposure and the last reading at the end of work exposure. Great care is needed to prevent indirect work exposure, for instance during clocking on, changing, and so forth, which often involves walking through an area of exposure. Most studies have looked at the whole workforce and tried to document changes between different exposure groups. The changes seen are usually exceedingly small (in the order of 100–200 ml over an 8-hr shift) and are rarely standardized for the time of waking (3–9). It has often been impossible to differentiate those with and without occupational asthma from these measurements. In a study of electronics workers exposed to colophony, FEV_1 fell by more than 10% in 16/48 cases and 2/43 controls (10). In a similar study of pharmaceutical manufacturers exposed to psyllium, 3/5 with occupational asthma and 7/13 without occupational asthma had similar changes (11); and 0/3 with occupational asthma due to spiramycin had a 10% postshift fall in FEV_1 (12).

LONGITUDINAL MEASUREMENTS OF LUNG FUNCTION

Many surveillance schedules require measurements of lung function serially in workers exposed to occupational allergens such as isocyanates; these records are rarely standardized for time of day or recent exposure. The assumption is made that workers whose lung function falls between measurements are those developing occupational asthma. In practice the intrasubject variability over periods of months is large, such that changes of at least 500 ml are seen in workers without sensitization. Figure 1 shows supervised measurements of FEV_1 made 6–9 months apart in workers exposed to isocyanates. There are workers with a fall of at least 20% (also some with a rise of at least 20%) between the two measurements. The distribution of the results is normal; the outliers represent the tails of the normal distribution. This type of surveillance provides a good measure of the mean change in FEV_1. It is good for studying longitudinal decline in a group, but is a poor method of picking out individuals developing symptoms, for which a surveillance questionnaire is much better. There is some evidence that there is an accelerated loss of FEV_1 in a number of jobs with exposure to occupational allergens in those without occupational asthma. These serial measurements should form the best means of detecting such an accelerated loss. However, the methods of calculating declines are not yet standardized.

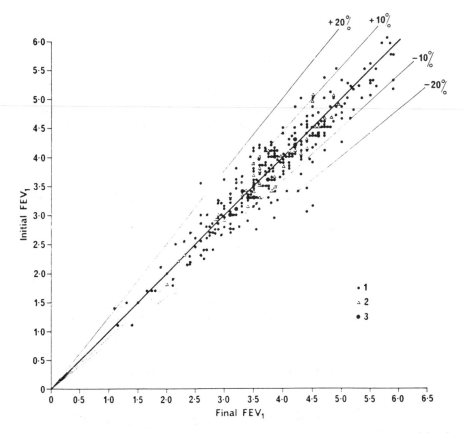

Figure 1 Printing workers exposed to isocyanates in the printing inks and laminating adhesives had measurements of FEV_1 twice 6–9 months apart as part of a surveillance scheme. The initial and final reading for each worker are compared. In five workers FEV_1 has declined more than 20% between the two measurements (and two have improved by more than 20%). The plot shows a normal distribution of results, and not a bimodal distribution, which would be needed to identify workers with occupational asthma from such records. Thirteen workers challenged positive for isocyanates in the factory; the two with the largest falls on this plot had negative isocyanate challenges as expected.

Different results are obtained if a regression line is calculated for each individual through a series of readings with subsequent meaning of the regression lines, compared with declines that are calculated by using the mean measure at each time interval.

PATTERNS OF ASTHMA IN THE WORKPLACE

The response to occupational allergens was first documented with bronchial provocation testing following single exposures of short duration. Immediate, late, dual, or recurrent reactions may follow a single exposure. In the work situation exposure usually continues for 8 hr or more every day of the week. The descriptions of the patterns of response to these types of exposure awaited the development of portable peak flow meters, as lung function measurements are needed throughout the working day and in the evening at home as well as on days away from work for their elucidation (13–15). With regular daily exposure the pattern of response depends principally on the rate of recovery. The following patterns can be recognized.

Hourly Patterns

The response to exposure using hour-by-hour records depends on the relationship between the time of exposure to the occupational allergen and the individual worker's underlying diurnal variation.

Immediate Reactions

Immediate reactions start within an hour of coming to work. They usually progress hour by hour at work. They may show an improvement during a period away from work during the midday break and usually improve shortly after leaving work. Lung function often returns to normal by the following morning (Fig. 2).

Late Reactions

On a morning shift the reactions frequently do not start until leaving work. They progress in the evening after work and often wake the workers from sleep. Lung function mea-

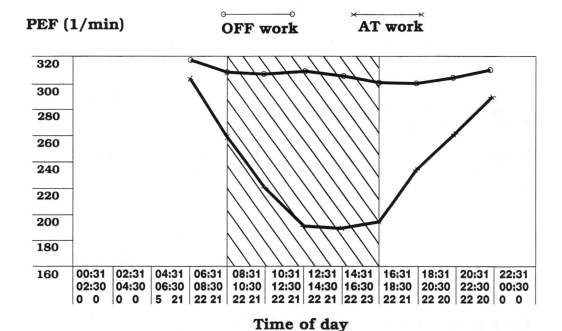

Figure 2 Mean hourly PEF from the OASYS plotter. Each line represents the mean of all days away from work (top line), and all days working a 08:00–16:00 hr shift. The period at work is hatched. The bottom set of figures represents the number of individual readings that make up the mean reading at each time point (days away from work on the left, at work on the right). There is an immediate fall in PEF within 1 hr of arriving at work, with improvement on leaving in the evening. The record was made by a hard-metal grinder who used two machines, one using coolant oil containing colophony, and the other dry grinding. Contaminants in the cooling oil, the colophony in the coolant, and cobalt in the hard metal were all possible causes of his occupational asthma.

surements on leaving work are often better than on arriving at work, and many workers say they are not worse at work (but are much better on days away from work). Recovery is rarely complete by the following morning and reactions usually progress from day to day.

The Flat Reaction

After repeated exposures deterioration usually ceases and the stage of relatively fixed airways obstruction is reached with little diurnal variation and little obvious reaction to work exposure. It may take many days away from work for such reactions to resolve. Workers are often identified as having fixed airways obstruction at this stage, which develops commonly with regular exposure to agents such as isocyanates and wood dusts. Similar changes are seen in workers on early shifts with immediate reactions, where the decline due to work is equivalent to the increase that would have occurred if there had been no work exposure.

The occupational exposure is rarely the only provoker of asthma in a sensitized worker. Once occupational asthma develops, reactions usually occur to other nonspecific stimuli, particularly to exercise and infection. If travel to and from work requires exercise (for instance, on a bicycle), reactions to exercise may be superimposed on those due to work exposures.

Diurnal Variation in Peak Flow

Asthma is traditionally associated with increased diurnal variation. There is, however, no standard method of calculating diurnal variation, and no clear distinction between asthma and normality. Asthma by definition is a variable condition, so a normal diurnal variation does not exclude the diagnosis. Population studies have generally shown that the diurnal variation is best expressed as the daily maximum minus the daily minimum divided by the daily mean. This calculation has problems when subjects with reduced peak flow are studied, as the random and systematic variations in the measurements account for increasing percentages as the mean peak flow decreases. When the mean peak flow is below predicted, the diurnal variation is best expressed as a percentage of the predicted value. In patients with chronic obstructive airways disease this method is least correlated with absolute peak flow (16). An increased diurnal variation is usually seen in those with immediate and late reactions, but is usually lost in those with flat reactions. Increased diurnal variation (for instance, a diurnal variation in peak flow > 20%) is not always seen in workers with occupational asthma but can often be demonstrated by taking the worker away from exposure for a number of days. In other situations, very small deteriorations at work occur with low diurnal variation. This may be due to a number of situations including an irritant effect superimposed on a predominantly nonasthmatic airflow obstruction, very low levels of exposure in a sensitized asthmatic wearing good respiratory protection, or during the flat reaction in a sensitized worker with severe occupational exposure. They can only be differentiated by removing the worker from exposure.

The diurnal variation in lung function can be studied by trying to fit a cosine wave to the observed data, and performing tests to see if the data conform to this pattern (1). A 24-hr cosinor analysis can be done on the majority of peak flow records from normal subjects and asthmatics. From the analysis the amplitude and time of the peak (acrophase) and mesor (a measure of the mean) can be calculated. A study in electronic workers with colophony occupation asthma showed that the amplitude decreased from 29% to 19%

comparing the 5-day workweek with 5-day periods off work; the acrophase was at 15:24 hr away from work and 11:44 hr at work; and treatment with cromoglycate or corticosteroids postponed the acrophase by about 90 min. It should be possible to fit cosinor rhythms to whole workweeks; this has, however, proved less successful (2). The ability to fit symmetrical cosine waves depends on the number of readings available per 24 hr; the fewer the readings, the better the statistical fit. The discrepancy is due to the actual asymmetry of the rise and fall, which is lost with fewer readings.

Day-by-Day Reactions

The patterns of reaction that can be readily identified are as follows:

Equivalent Daily Deterioration

In this situation the deterioration each day is similar with each day of exposure (Fig. 3). Recovery is usually rapid on days away from work and is usually complete before the next day's exposure. Such reactions are common with laboratory animal workers and with colophony. Variations of this with low diurnal variation are associated with the flat hourly pattern.

Progressive Daily Deterioration

This may take several days of exposure before becoming readily identifiable. It is usually associated with incomplete recovery the following morning and frequently with nocturnal wakening. It is common with wood dust and isocyanates among others. The pattern from week to week depends on whether recovery is complete during rest days or not. If a 2-day rest period occurs, recovery taking up to 3 days is compatible with repeated patterns on a week-by-week basis. If recovery takes 3 days, the first day at work is usually better than the days away from work, with deterioration occurring subsequently. If recovery takes more than 3 days with a 2-day break, then the next work period starts from a lower baseline, so deterioration may occur week by week.

First Day Worst and Midweek Deterioration

There are a few situations where deterioration is maximal on the first day with subsequent recovery despite continuing exposure. This situation is classically seen in byssinosis and is also seen in other situations where microbial aerosols are found, such as aerosols from used coolant oils and from humidifiers in ventilation systems (17,18). However, in all these situations, some workers have progressive daily deterioration, the usual pattern when hypersensitivity is the cause, probably implying that different individuals can react to the same agent in different ways. In a small study of workers with occupational asthma in a building with a contaminated humidifier in the air-conditioning system, positive skin prick tests to an extract from the humidifier were seen only in workers with progressive daily deterioration (18). A variant of first-day deterioration is deterioration that progresses for the first 2–3 days after work and then improves despite continuing exposure. It probably has the same underlying mechanism and implies the development of tolerance to repeated exposures, such as may occur within endotoxin.

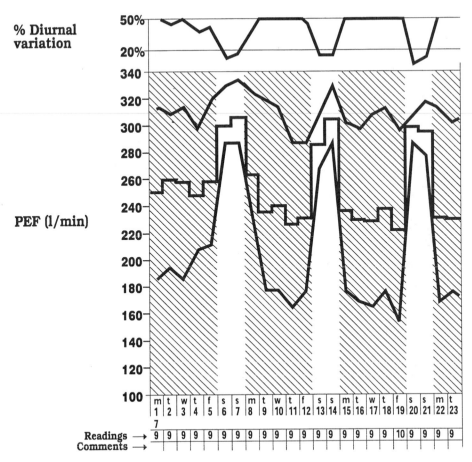

Figure 3   Daily PEF pattern from the OASYS plotter in the same worker shown in Figure 2. The upper panel shows the daily diurnal variation in PEF. The central panel shows daily maximum (top line), mean (middle line), and minimum (bottom line) PEF. The days at work have a shaded background, the days away from work a clear background. There is equivalent deterioration on each workday with recovery on days away from work, which is usually greater on the second day away from work. Below the day and date at the foot of the plot are the number of readings making up each day's mean (9–10 in this case showing 2-hourly readings). The record shows clear occupational asthma. Cobalt was shown to be the cause by finding a positive prick test to cobalt chloride, a positive immediate reaction on specific challenge testing, and finding high levels of urinary cobalt following a day at work (23.5 μg/L).

Measurements Before, During, and Following a Longer Period Off Work

When exposures are irregular, or the changes in mean PEF are small, or in other situations where the plots are equivocal, measurements either side of a 2-week period away from exposure are often helpful (Fig. 4).

PORTABLE MEASURING DEVICES IN OCCUPATIONAL ASTHMA

The ideal device should be robust, small, and light, should be easy to calibrate, be stable over a period of weeks, have a linear response and should include a logging device to

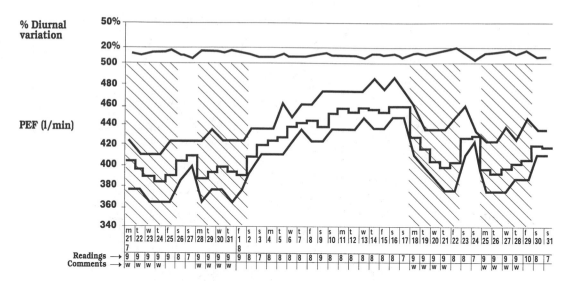

Figure 4   Daily maximum, mean, and minimum PEF from the OASYS plotter. The record shows two workweeks with diurnal variation within the normal range, and mean PEF about 15 L/min lower on workdays. The significance of these small changes is made clearer during a 16-day period off work, when the mean PEF is 75 L/min higher than at work. The deterioration is much larger on the first week back at work. (The "w" in the comments line at the foot of the plot shows that the first measurement of the day is not within 1 hr of waking, a situation that sometimes leads to underestimation of the diurnal variation). He was indirectly exposed to the isocyanate MDI in a factory molding parts of car doors, which were the likely cause for his occupational asthma despite a negative RAST to MDI-HSA conjugates.

record at least the time, date, and measurement of lung function. It should also be able to make an assessment of the adequacy of the quality of the expiratory maneuver. At present such a device does not exist, although several companies have products that fulfill some of these requirements. Meters with turbines measure FEV_1 more reliably than peak flow, meters with pneumotachographs often loose calibration during a 4-week period away with a patient, and do not perform well when cold (for instance when kept in a car in a cold winter). In practice it is difficult to obtain reliable repeated measurements of vital capacity, as this causes substantial discomfort at the end of even one day's reading. There is some evidence that the readings are about 30 L/min lower when unsupervised (19), and that some workers improve in the first few days of a record due to a learning effect. Workers should be trained in peak flow measurement, should make at least three readings on each occasion and record the maximum. The best two readings should be within 20 L/min of each other or further readings should be made.

Peak flow measurement was chosen for serial patient measurement because of the availability of portable meters, rather than because of any physiological advantage of PEF over FEV_1. Portable logging FEV_1 meters are now available giving a choice of parameter for measurement. Studies comparing PEF with FEV_1 are compounded by the different methods of measuring each. The original Wright peak flow meter, and those modeled on it (the Mini-Wright, Vitalograph, and Ferraris meters) have all been found to be nonlinear when calibrated with a computer-controlled syringe that delivers air in the form of a forced expiration (20). The meters overread by about 70 L/min at about 300 L/min and underread at flows greater than 600 L/min. The consequence depends on the range of PEF recorded by the individual, with the greatest increases in diurnal variation in those whose readings are around 300 L/min. This nonlinearity has been corrected in the meters used in some countries, particularly North America. Some peak flow meters (e.g., the Assess) are unable to record high flows; the analysis is flawed if the worker can exceed the maximum value of the meter (21).

There is no reason why the percentage change in PEF should be the same as the percentage change in FEV_1. The PEF is mainly a measure of the large airways, whereas the FEV_1 has a greater component derived from the small airways. There is some evidence that the FEV_1 is more sensitive at detecting late rather than early asthmatic reactions following bronchial provocation testing (22). A comparison of FEV_1 and PEF measured with a Mini-Wright or Assess meter showed a poor correlation. The median fall in FEV_1 (27%) was greater than the median fall in PEF (17%), following challenges selected to have a >15% fall in FEV_1 (23). Another study found that the differences were similar in challenges affecting predominantly large airways and those induced by allergen affecting all airways (24). Two studies have compared FEV_1 and PEF using the same instrument away from the hospital. Using the Micromedical diarycard (with a turbine) the diurnal variation was the same for PEF (12.95%) and FEV_1 (12.13%). The turbine does not have the same error profile as the Wright meter (25). Serial measurements of PEF and FEV_1 were obtained from the VMX (using a pressure transducer) and analyzed for occupational effect by experts. The sensitivity was 60% when the PEF plots were used and 50% when the FEV_1 plots were used. The specificity was 91% for both sets when compared with specific provocation tests (26). On current evidence both PEF and FEV_1 are suitable for unsupervised monitoring; PEF should be linearized before analysis if a nonlinear meter is being used.

FREQUENCY OF MEASUREMENT

Serial PEF measurements were originally described following hourly readings from waking to sleeping in workers keeping records over many weeks (13,14). In most situations they can conveniently be done 2-hourly rather than hourly. However, if the records are carried out less frequently than this, there may be one or no readings during the work period, and immediate reactions at work may be missed; they are also more susceptible to isolated low readings (e.g., following exercise) and are more variable (27). Expert interpretation of occupational effect using 4-hourly rather than 2-hourly readings decreased the sensitivity from 73% to 61% when compared with specific challenges (28). Measurements made 4-hourly are optimal for the calculation of diurnal variation; fewer readings tend to underestimate the changes, more frequent readings do not increase precision (29). It is important to make the first reading on waking, including on rest days, and to strive for reproducibility (it is my practice to make at least three readings, the highest two to be within 20 L/min on each occasion). The full method for performing these tests has been described (30).

ASSESSMENT OF SERIAL PEAK FLOW RECORDS

Initial attempts were made to analyze these records statistically. An analysis of variance using the model Glim 3 was performed on each record separately. Estimates with their standard errors were derived from the effects of (1) work exposure or rest day, (2) treatment, and (3) hour of the day (from waking). F tests were performed separately on the work-type effect. As this was a nonorthogonal analysis, the factor being assessed was run after the other factors. For work type the effects of treatment and time of day preceded the assessment of work effect. Table 1 shows the number of records showing a significantly positive F test in groups of workers exposed to either colophony in the electronics industry or isocyanates in the printing of flexible packaging, who also had occupational type challenges (31). The statistical analysis was clear when the visual inspection of the record was clear. It had a number of substantial limitations. When treatment was being taken, treatment was often increased on days at work. Running the effect of treatment before the effect of work reduced the significance of the work effect. This particularly applied to the colophony-exposed workers, who mostly recovered quickly after leaving work. The isocyanate workers frequently took a long time to recover away from work. The statistical analysis depended substantially on the number of days recording away from work as the first few days away from work were frequently worse than the days at work. The statistical results were often positive in those with negative challenges, mostly in workers where the differences between work days and rest days were extremely small in absolute terms but were consistent in statistical terms. This sometimes resulted because of a lower reading on waking in workers who were getting up earlier on work days than on rest days. It is clear from these results that the statistical analysis will have to be more sophisticated.

Rule-based systems establish criteria for a work effect, for example the number of times a given decrease in PEF occurs on work and rest days. Although some success has been reported (32–34), there are two problems with this approach. Basing diagnosis on a specific percentage fall in PEF will produce bias against those with a low peak flow for other reasons, such as smokers but also workers in certain industries, for example those exposed to oil mist who tend to have a low peak flow only recovering after an extended time away from work (17). Criteria based on percentage falls in PEF are again very dependent on the accuracy and linearity of the peak flow meters used. Some studies have used more sophisticated statistical methods. Henneberger et al. (35) used t-tests to compare the mean peak flow and mean diurnal variation of work days versus rest days. Compared with the visual interpretation of the record by three experts, mean peak flow had a sensitivity of 86% and specificity of 71%; for the diurnal variation, sensitivity was 43% and specificity 86%. The number of subjects, however, was small, the method of plotting the peak flow was not stated, and two types of peak flow meter were used. Perrin et al. (36) used a number of statistical indices but found none as satisfactory as visual interpretation

Table 1   Results of Analysis of Variance, the Significance of the Work Effect Is Tested After Adjusting for Treatment and Time-of-Day Effects[a]

	Bronchial provocation test result	
Significant F tests for work effect	Positive	Negative
Colophony exposure—no treatment	15/15	2/6
Colophony exposure with steroid or DSCG treatment	6/15	—
Isocyanate exposure	5/6	5/8

[a]The number of records showing a significantly positive F test in groups of workers exposed to either colophony in the electronics industry or isocyanates in the printing of flexible packaging, who also had occupational-type challenges.

of the record. The Italian working group on peak flow measurement also used several indices of daily and day-to-day variability (24). They found that the mean peak flow, the coefficient of variation, and the maximum amplitude were all statistically different on days at work compared with days away from work for those with occupational asthma but not for those with nonoccupational asthma. The same group later commented using the same indices that peak flow monitoring allowed the detection only of typical cases of occupational asthma (37).

PLOTTING OF SERIAL RECORDS

Peak flow records are usually plotted serially predominantly to document the response to treatment, i.e., to look for progressive change over time. Occupational records plotted in this way are difficult to interpret unless the changes are obvious. The differences related to work exposure can be seen more easily by plotting the daily maximum, mean, and minimum peak flow as illustrated in Figures 3 and 4. Days at work are differentiated from days away from work by background shading. To maximize the difference between days at and away from work, the workday starts with the first reading at work and finishes with the last reading before work the following day. In this way the morning dip is included with the previous day. It is important to include a waking value in each day's plot, and to make sure that records are made on waking on days away from work, as a delay after waking can increase the peak flow and occasionally produce artificial improvement on restdays (38). Workers changing shifts are more complicated. Those starting work say at 14:00 hr would have the 14:00-hr reading as the first reading of that workday, which would continue to 13:00 hr the next day, even if it was a restday.

The original analyses of these records were designed to be specific, rather than sensitive. The criteria for a positive record were identified deterioration in at least 3/4 workweeks and improvement in at least 3/4 periods off work. For those with long time periods (taking more than 3 days to improve away from work), two periods of deterioration and one period of improvement (or vice versa) were required (Fig. 4). The sensitivity and specificity of peak flow records assessed in this way are shown in Table 2. The records have acceptable sensitivity when no prophylactic treatment is being taken, but have a serious lack of sensitivity when corticosteroids of cromoglycate are being used regularly. In these circumstances the changes in peak flow are much smaller; sometimes a larger-than-usual exposure is required to result in a breakthrough of the asthma. The difficult

Table 2 Sensitivity and Specificity of Visual Assessments of Plotted PEF Records and Specific Provocation Testing, Compared with a Diagnosis Based on the Subsequent Course of the Disease with Prolonged Follow-up[a]

	Isocyanate exposure		Colophony exposure	
	Sensitivity	Specificity	Sensitivity	Specificity
Specific challenge	82	100	100	67
Serial PEF; no prophylaxis	100	80	77	100
Serial PEF; on steroids or cromoglycate			44	—

[a]Subjective assessments required changes related to work/rest on >75% of periods.

records to assess are those showing small absolute changes, or changes that are irregular. It is likely that the above criteria for a positive record can be relaxed without lack of specificity. Recent guidelines have suggested, as the ideal period of peak flow self-monitoring, three working periods separated by periods away from work with at least one of the periods off work longer than 1 week (39). In general, it is up to the physician to indicate the duration and the sequence of periods at work and off work, considering that periods at work should be prolonged enough to permit a careful evaluation of the pattern of response and to avoid negative results due to a lack of exposure to the suspected offending agent(s), particularly when exposure is intermittent. In any case, the period at work should be stopped when a significant pattern of occupational asthma is observed, as in this case there is no need to maintain exposure (40). Periods off work should be prolonged enough to allow for recovery, the start of which could be delayed and take a long time to complete (15). It is obviously important that a worker uses the same peak flow meter for all readings in one record and for subsequent records (41).

Recent work has shown again that visual inspection of the records is more helpful than statistical testing (36,42). Perrin and co-workers (36) prospectively studied 61 subjects with suspected occupational asthma with serial peak flow readings, methacholine responsiveness before and after a period off work, and specific bronchial provocation testing. They took the specific provocation test as the gold standard (this is not always fully sensitive and specific), and compared the peak flow record as assessed by three people, and as analyzed statistically. They excluded seven peak flow records that were regarded as inadequate for making firm conclusions. The sensitivity and specificity of their analyses are shown in Table 3. Subjective assessment of the records achieved 87% sensitivity (by undefined criteria) and 84% specificity. A 3.2-fold change in methacholine while off work was 48% sensitive and 64% specific while the best statistical analysis achieved 76% sensitivity and 58% specificity. Agreement between readers is important but not always appreciated. In studies to date looking at relatively clear-cut cases Liss and Tarlo (34), for example, quoted agreement as measured by a kappa score of 0.62–0.83 for interreader agreement, while Malo et al. (28) quoted intrareader agreement as 83–100%.

Expert interpretation requires experts, who do not always agree and are not always consistent in their interpretation. To overcome these problems computer-based pattern recognition systems have been developed for the identification of work effects in serial peak

Table 3 Sensitivity and Specificity of Measures Taken from Serial Plots of Peak Flow, and Measurements of Methacholine Reactivity Before and After a Period of at Least Two Weeks Off Work, Compared with Specific Bronchial Provocation Tests, Used as the Gold Standard[a]

	Sensitivity	Specificity
Visual inspection of peak flow plot	87%	84%
Methacholine PC_{20} > 3.2-fold change	43%	65%
Mean peak flow lower at work	76%	58%
Maximum peak flow lower at work	44%	81%
Minimum peak flow lower at work	57%	81%
Three workdays with mean peak flow >2 SD of values away from work	52%	22%

[a]The work period was 2 weeks unless obvious deterioration occurred earlier.
Source: Results from the Montreal group (Perrin et al., 1990).

flow records. Unlike the human experts, these techniques have the advantage of complete repeatability. All start from the plot of daily maximum, mean, and minimum and are modeled on expert interpretation unrelated to the final diagnosis. They are designed to detect an occupational effect rather than occupational asthma. The analyses split the record up into a series of overlapping elements containing either a period at work, a period away from work, and a period at work (a work-rest-work complex), or its counterpart, a rest-work-rest complex. Discriminant analysis has been developed to mimic the effects of an expert, and tested against a wide range of workers records. OASYS-2, one such system, has a sensitivity of 69% and a specificity of 94% when applied to records from workers with a final diagnosis made independently of the peak flow record (43). A neural net version with increased sensitivity is under development (44).

The interpretation of equivocal records can be enhanced by including measurements of nonspecific bronchial responsiveness before and after a 2-week period away from exposure (45,46), or after removal from exposure (47). A fourfold increase in the dose of histamine or methacholine required to drop the FEV_1 by 20% after a period without exposure increases the probability of occupational asthma. Failure to show an improvement in nonspecific reactivity, or measurements within the normal range at work, are, however, both relatively frequent in workers with genuine occupational asthma (48).

It is unclear as yet whether these records can differentiate between irritant and allergic asthmatic reactions, largely owing to the problem of differentiating between these types of mechanisms using other criteria. There are some workers who have quite large day-by-day changes at work, with very low diurnal variations throughout. It seems unlikely that smooth muscle constriction in the bronchi is a prominent feature in this type of reaction. Large diurnal variations can certainly be due to nonallergic mechanisms, for instance, the classic asthmatic reaction to exercise. Identification of patterns of reactions from serial peak flow records does allow the separation of reactions into different groups suitable for mechanistic evaluation.

CONFOUNDING FACTORS

The control for confounding factors is fundamental before meaningful analysis of work effect can take place. Varying treatment is the most difficult to control for and is best eliminated by making the PEF record on the same treatment throughout. The effect of bronchodilator use can be minimized by making readings before inhalation. Without control some individuals will increase treatment in anticipation of, or following, deterioration at work, thereby minimizing any change in PEF. If less treatment is taken on days away from work, the maximum PEF may be lower; this, combined with an increase in the minimum daily PEF on the same days, should alert the reporter to the problem (49). Periods on and off corticosteroids need analyzing separately. Respiratory infections are the most serious, as they can cause large changes in PEF. If the worker takes time off with the infection, it appears that the period away from work is worse than the period at work. A worker may be more susceptible (owing to the effects of the infection) or less susceptible (owing to the effects of treatment) to the effects of the working environment for some time after the acute infection. Upper respiratory tract infections can produce effects as large as those due to work, with a maximum mean fall in PEF of around 20%, lasting for an average of 7 days (50). The most appropriate solution is to remove that part of a record affected by respiratory infection. There can be problems with differentiating between respiratory infection and occupational rhinitis when symptoms alone are used. Previously normal workers who develop occupational asthma also wheeze with nonspecific triggers such as exercise, perfumes, cold air, and so forth, causing the PEF to drop. Provided the record is long enough, it is unlikely that confounding will occur. The possible exception is exercise, which may be a fundamental part of some jobs, in which case it may be impossible to separate the effects of sensitization and exercise from PEF records alone.

Exposure to the offending agent is usually not measured and likely to vary from day to day. Days when exposure is known not to occur should be analyzed as days away from exposure. Varying daily exposure is likely to be a major determinant of the inconsistent work effects seen in some records.

PRACTICAL ASPECTS

Performing records suitable for analysis involves repeated and usually unsupervised exposures to a work environment that may be causing occupational asthma. It is clearly not suitable for workers with anaphylactic-type reactions, for whom carefully controlled bronchial provocation testing with suitable minute levels of exposure is more appropriate if a specific diagnosis is required. Serial peak flow measurement requires commitment from workers and is difficult to achieve in some workplaces where full respiratory protection is required. It is usually possible to make recordings on waking, on arrival at work, during each formal rest period at work, on leaving work, at home after work, and on retiring to bed. Such records are unlikely to be evenly spaced in time; this probably does not matter provided that there are at least six readings per day (although it provides a problem for spectral analysis) (51). It is best to aim for 2-hourly readings, particularly in those with mild reactions or those whose peak flow pattern is chaotic. After very minimal instruction adequate records are produced by about 50% in the occupational setting. After further instruction about 80% produce adequate records (41). Most workers who fail to keep an adequate record transcribed manually also fail to produce adequate records with a logging meter. Some workers keep much better records on workdays than restdays. Restday records are often the most important, as there are usually fewer of them. Some workers seem to take amazingly few days off work. In these workers records over annual holidays are often required.

Records may be compounded by workers making up readings, or recording them inaccurately. Twenty-one subjects, eight of whom had occupational asthma, were asked to keep 2-hourly measurements of PEF with a VMX meter (fairly bulky), for a mean of 36 days. There was some entry for 80% of the possible 2-hourly measurements; of these 69% were recorded by hand and logged by the meter, 3% logged but not hand-recorded, and 28% recorded by hand and not logged (and probably invented) (52). The hand record differed from the logged record by more than 20 L/min for 11% of readings, and the timing differed by more than 1 hr for 29% of the readings. Those seeking compensation kept records less satisfactorily. Similar results were obtained in a study of 13 workers investigated for occupational asthma; 11% of recordings had different values between the manual and logged readings, 13% had differences in timing, and 20% had manual readings that were not logged. The subjects were asked to keep six readings a day for an average of 23 days; there was a logged entry for 97% of the required times (53). The records from these two studies were pooled for an assessment of expert interpretation. Experts found it easier to agree about the interpretation of the hand records rather than the logged records, but also diagnosed occupational asthma more often from the hand records. Records from the less compliant were more difficult to interpret (52). Some have interpreted the inaccuracy of the hand over the logged record as invalidating the diagnosis of occupational asthma using this method (53). The sensitivities of the assessments ranging from 69 to 100% and the specificities ranging from 84 to 100% described above include the presumably prefabricated and mistimed readings, suggesting that the method is robust enough to cope with these inaccuracies.

THE FUTURE

Self-recorded lung function always lacks credibility to the skeptic. Logging meters overcome some of the problems. Such meters should record all blows and provide quality control in real time so that the worker knows whether further blows are required. The meters should obviously be technically satisfactory and linear. In our experience compliance with logging meters is often less than with conventional peak flow meters. Logging meters are heavier, and some are quite complicated. Many require a FEV_1 maneuver, which can be more difficult. We have tried to incorporate the waking sleeping and starting and stopping work markers into such data loggers with very limited success, mainly due to the inability to edit the input, which needs to be timed by the worker rather than the data logger (unlike their use for registering symptoms in drug trials).

Further work is needed on the analysis of long periods off work. If significant improvement occurs during a 2–4-week period off work, with deterioration on return to work, occupational asthma is likely whatever the rest of the record shows. It is possible that further analysis of the diurnal variation changes and average hourly plots may produce further insights. It is unclear whether irritant reactions can be distinguished from those due to hypersensitivity; further work is needed to elucidate this.

CONCLUSION

Serial peak expiratory flow rate monitoring is a valid tool for confirming the relationship between occupational exposure and symptoms of asthma. It is feasible in nonspecialized centers, and it is simple and safe to perform; nevertheless, it is time consuming and requires patient collaboration and honesty. Efforts should be made to improve this means by designing cheap instruments that can assess the reliability of the measurement, and by further ameliorating methods for the analysis of records. The sensitivity rates of peak flow monitoring show that there is a variable percentage of false-negative results, so a stable peak flow should not completely exclude the presence of occupational or work-related asthma. However, even in the case of a pattern of peak flow monitoring indicative of a positive relationship between occupational exposure and symptoms, peak flow monitoring cannot relate symptoms to a specific agent. Therefore, it is not proper for etiological diagnosis, except in those cases of occupational asthma where there is a clear demonstration of specific sensitization (i.e., strongly positive for IgE antibody) to agents present at work.

REFERENCES

1. Hetzel MR, Clark TJH. Comparison of normal and asthmatic circadian rhythms in peak expiratory flow rate. Thorax 1980; 35:732–738.

2. Randem B, Smolensky MH, Hsi B, Albright D, Burge PS. Field survey of circadian rhythm in PEF of electronics workers suffering from colophony-induced asthma. Chronobiol Int 1987; 4:263–271.

3. do Pico GA, Reddan W, Anderson S, Flaherty D, Smally E. Acute effects of grain dust exposure during a work shift. Am Rev Respir Dis 1983; 128:399–404.

4. Enarson DA, Vedal S, Chan-Yeung M. Fate of grainhandlers with bronchial hyperreactivity. Clin Invest Med 1988; 11:193–197.

5. Gee JB, Morgan WKC. A 10 year follow-up study of a group of workers exposed to isocyanates. J Occup Med 1985; 27:15–18.

6. Krumpe PE, Finley TN, Martinez N. The search for expiratory obstruction in meat wrappers studied on the job. Am Rev Respir Dis 1979; 119:611–618.

7. Liss GM, Bernstein DI, Moller DR, Gallagher JS, Stephenson RL, Bernstein IL. Pulmonary and immunologic evaluation of foundry workers exposed to methylene diphenyldiisocyanate (MDI). J Allergy Clin Immunol 1988; 82:55–61.

8. Moller DR, Gallagher JS, Bernstein DI, Wilcox TG, Burroughs HE, Bernstein IL. Detection of IgE mediated respiratory sensitisation in workers exposed to hexahydrophthalic anhydride. J Allergy Clin Immunol 1985; 75:663–672.

9. Orford RR, Wilson JT. Epidemiologic and immunologic studies in processors of the king crab. Am J Ind Med 1985; 7:155–169.

10. Burge PS, Perks WH, O'Brien IM, Burge A, Hawkins R, Brown D, et al. Occupational asthma in an electronics factory; a case control study to evaluate aetiological factors. Thorax 1979; 34:300–307.

11. Bardy J-D, Malo J-L, Seguin P, Ghezzo H, Desjardins J, Dolovich J, et al. Occupational asthma and IgE sensitisation in a pharmaceutical company processing psyllium. Am Rev Respir Dis 1987; 135:1033–1038.

12. Malo J-L, Cartier A. Occupational asthma in workers of a pharmaceutical company processing spiramycin. Thorax 1988; 43:371–377.

13. Burge PS, O'Brien IM, Harries MG. Peak flow rate records in the diagnosis of occupational asthma due to colophony. Thorax 1979; 34:308–316.

14. Burge PS, O'Brien IM, Harries MG. Peak flow rate records in the diagnosis of occupational asthma due to isocyanates. Thorax 1979; 34:317–323.

15. Burge PS. Single and serial measurements of lung function in the diagnosis of occupational asthma. Eur J Respir Dis 1982; 123(Suppl):47–59.

16. Weir DC, Burge PS. Measures of reversibility in response to bronchodilators in chronic airflow obstruction: relation to airway calibre. Thorax 1991; 46:43–45.

17. Robertson AS, Weir DC, Burge PS. Occupational asthma due to oil mists. Thorax 1988; 43: 200–205.

18. Burge PS, Finnegan M, Horsfield N, Emery D, Austwick P, Davies PS, et al. Occupational asthma in a factory with a contaminated humidifier. Thorax 1985; 40:248–254.

19. Gannon PFG, Dickinson S, Hitchings D, Burge PS. Quality of self recorded peak expiratory flow. Thorax 1993; 48:1062

20. Miller MR, Dickinson SA, Hitchings DJ. The accuracy of portable peak flow meters. Thorax 1992; 47:904–909.

21. Shapiro SM, Hendler JM, Ogirala RG, Aldrich TK, Shapiro MB. An evaluation of the accuracy of Assess and MiniWright peak flowmeters. Chest 1991; 99:358–362.

22. Berube D, Cartier A, L'Archeveque J, Ghezzo H, Malo J-L. Comparison of peak expiratory flow rate and FEV_1 in assessing bronchomotor tone after challenges with occupational sensitizers. Chest 1991; 99:831–836.

23. Giannini D, Paggiaro PL, Moscato G, Gherson G, Bacci E, Bancalari L, et al. Comparison between peak expiratory flow and forced expiratory volume in one second (FEV_1) during bronchoconstriction induced by different stimuli. J Asthma 1997; 34:105–111.

24. Paggiaro PL, Moscato G, Giannini D, di Pede F, Bertoletti R, Bacci E, et al. The Italian working group on the use of peak expiratory flow rate (PEFR) in asthma. Eur Respir Rev 1993; 3:438–443.

25. Bright P, Burge PS. Comparison of mean daily diurnal variation in PEF and FEV_1. Am J Respir Crit Care Med 1997; 155:A137.

26. Leroyer C, Perfetti L, Trudeau C, Ghezzo H, Chan-Yeung M, Malo J. Comparison of PEF and FEV_1 monitoring with specific inhalation challenge in the diagnosis of occupational asthma. Am J Respir Crit Care Med 1997; 155:A137

27. Blainey AD, Ollier S, Cundell D, Smith RE, Davies RJ. Occupational asthma in a hairdressing salon. Thorax 1986; 41:42–50.

28. Malo JL, Cote J, Cartier A, Boulet LP, L'Archeveque J, Chan-Yeung M. How many times per day should peak expiratory flow rates be assessed when investigating occupational asthma? Thorax 1993; 48:1211–1217.

29. Gannon PFG, Newton DT, Pantin CFA, Burge PS. The effect of the number of peak expiratory flow readings per day on the estimation of diurnal variation. Thorax 1998; 53:790–792.

30. Bright P, Burge PS. The diagnosis of occupational asthma from serial measurements of lung function at and away from work. Thorax 1996; 51:857–863.

31. Burge PS. Prolonged and frequent recording of peak expiratory flow rate in workers with suspected occupational asthma due to colophony or isocyanate fumes. MSc thesis, London School of Hygiene, 1978.

32. Smith AB, Bernstein DI, Aw T-C, Gallagher JS, London M, Kopp S, et al. Occupational asthma from inhaled egg protein. Am J Ind Med 1987; 12:205–218.

33. Cartier A, Bernstein IL, Burge PS, Cohn JR, Fabbri LM, Hargreave FE, et al. Guidelines for bronchoprovocation on the investigation of occupational asthma. J Allergy Clin Immunol 1989; 84:823–829.

34. Liss GM, Tarlo SM. Peak expiratory flow rates in possible occupational asthma. Chest 1991; 100:63–69.

35. Henneberger PK, Stanbury MJ, Trimbath LS, Kipen HM. The use of portable peak flow meters in the surveillance of occupational asthma. Chest 1991; 100:1515–1521.

36. Perrin B, Lagier F, L'Archeveque J, Cartier A, Boulet LP, Cote J, et al. Occupational asthma: validity of monitoring of peak expiratory flow rates and non-allergic bronchial responsiveness as compared to specific inhalation challenge. Eur Respir J 1992; 5:40–48.

37. Giannini D, di Pede F, Moscato G, Bacci E, Carletti A, Carrara M, et al. Sensitivity of peak flow monitoring to detect occupational asthma in relationship with specific bronchial challenge. Eur Respir J 1994; 7:312s

38. Venables KM, Davison AG, Browne K, Newman Taylor AJ. Pseudo-occupational asthma. Thorax 1989; 44:760–761.

39. Subcommittee on "Occupational Allergy" of the European Academy of Allergology and Clinical Immunology. Guidelines for the diagnosis of occupational asthma. Clin Exp Allergy 1992; 22:103–108.

40. Moscato G, Godnic-Cvar J, Maestrelli P. Statement on self-monitoring of peak expiratory flows in the investigation of occupational asthma. Subcommittee on Occupational Allergy of European Academy of Allergy and Clinical Immunology. J Allergy Clin Immunol 1995; 96:295–301.

41. Gannon PFG, Newton DT, Burgess DCL, Burge PS. Interpretation of serial peak expiratory flow records for workers in an electroplating factory. Eur Respir J 1992; 5(Suppl 15):403s.

42. Cote J, Kennedy S, Chan-Yeung M. Sensitivity and specificity of PC_{20} and peak expiratory flow rate in cedar asthma. J Allergy Clin Immunol 1990; 85:592–598.

43. Gannon PFG, Newton DT, Belcher J, Pantin CF, Burge PS. Development of OASYS-2: a system for the analysis of serial measurement of peak expiratory flow in workers with suspected occupational asthma. Thorax 1996; 51:484–489.

44. Bright P, Burge PS. Computer assisted interpretation of occupational peak flow plots; OASYS-N. Eur Respir J 1995; 8:220s.

45. Cartier A, Pineau L, Malo J-L. Monitoring of maximum expiratory peak flow rates and histamine inhalation tests in the investigation of occupational asthma. Clin Allergy 1984; 14:193–196.

46. Kongerud J, Soyseth V, Burge PS. Serial measurements of peak expiratory flow and responsiveness to methacholine in the diagnosis of aluminium potroom asthma. Thorax 1992; 47: 292–297.

47. Malo J-L, Cartier A, Ghezzo H, Lafrance M, McCants M, Lehrer SB. Patterns of improvement in spirometry, bronchial hyperresponsiveness, and specific IgE antibody levels after cessation of exposure in occupational asthma caused by snow-crab processing. Am Rev Respir Dis 1988; 138:807–812.

48. Burge PS. Non-specific hyperreactivity in workers exposed to toluene diisocyanate, diphenyl methane diisocyanate and colophony. Eur J Respir Dis 1982; 63(suppl.123):91–96.

49. Burge PS. Single and serial measurements of lung function in the diagnosis of occupational asthma. Eur J Respir Dis 1982; 63 (suppl.123):47–59.

50. O'Brien C, Bright P, Nicholson C, Burge PS. Patterns of peak expiratory flow response to upper respiratory tract infections in asthmatics. Eur Respir J 1995; 8 suppl 19:272.

51. Belcher J, Hampton JS, Tunicliffe Wilson G. Parameterisation of continuous time autoregressive models for irregularly sampled time series data. Appl Statist 1993.

52. Malo JL, Cartier A, Ghezzo H, Chan-Yeung M. Compliance with peak expiratory flow readings affects the within- and between-reader reproducibility of interpretation of graphs in subjects investigated for occupational asthma. J Allergy Clin Immunol 1996; 98:1132–1134.

53. Quirce S, Contreras G, Dybuncio A, Chan-Yeung M. Peak expiratory flow monitoring is not a reliable method for establishing the diagnosis of occupational asthma. Am J Respir Crit Care Med 1995; 152:1100–1102.

12

Occupational Challenge Tests

André Cartier and Jean-Luc Malo
Université de Montréal and Sacré-Coeur Hospital, Montréal, Quebec, Canada

HISTORICAL BACKGROUND

It is reported that Charles Blackley was the first researcher to do inhalation challenges using common allergens (1). In 1952, Herxheimer documented the occurrence of late reactions, which have been the subject of numerous studies in the last few years as they are related to the development of bronchial inflammation and the "eosinophilic bronchitis" characteristic of asthma (2). The occurrence of these late reactions after exposure to common allergens was later confirmed by other investigators (3). Based on the work of Colldahl in Stockholm (4), Citron and Pepys described dual reactions in the case of other immunologically mediated bronchoalveolar reactions such as allergic bronchopulmonary aspergillosis (5), farmers' lung (6), and bird fancier's lung (7). In 1970, Pepys suggested the use of specific inhalation tests in the investigation of occupational asthma (OA). As Pepys wrote in a letter:

> The next development was in occupational asthma. We did not know how to test by aerosol inhalation with agents such as TDI, etc. or with potentially irritant or extremely potent allergens such as the platinum salts. The answer to this was the patient with severe asthma clearly related to his work. He made the boats for the Oxford and Cambridge boat race and used a two-part polyurethane/TDI marine varnish. As soon as I heard this, he was asked to provide these two separate materials which are mixed together prior to use. The first day, he painted on a slab of wood with the polyurethane with no effect, whereas the mixture tested in the same way the next day elicited asthmatic reactions. This was the answer to the problem and the origin of simulated "occupational type" provocation tests, in other words a piece, and usually a very, very small piece of real life as a highly analytical, precise and reproducible form of testing. There can be no objections to this if carried out properly since it is no different from the work exposure.

Originally, these tests were carried out in the corridors of the Brompton hospital with people walking about. A well-ventilated cubicle in a room was later made available. A series of reports were published beginning in 1972, dealing with dusts, powders, fumes, gaseous emanations, and aerosols (8–11). For these tests, subjects were asked to reproduce their usual work in a small cubicle under close supervision and with functional assessment. A summary of the proposals for the tests was later published (12). At that time, occupational challenge tests (OCT) in the laboratory were the only objective way to confirm that asthma was caused by an agent that was present in the workplace. Since then, other means, such as the monitoring of peak expiratory flows (PEF) at work and away from work (13,14), have been proposed. Several summary publications and statements give general guidelines for the investigation of OA (15–20). For most investigators, OIC, either in the laboratory or at the workplace, is still the gold standard against which other means should be compared. There are reviews on the use of these tests in the investigation of OA (21,22) and guidelines have been issued by the American Academy of Allergy and Clinical Immunology (23) and the European Respiratory Society (24).

PURPOSE AND JUSTIFICATION FOR THE TESTS

Asthma is now the most common of the respiratory ailments as determined by sentinel-based studies (25,26) and medicolegal statistics (27,28). Approximately 5% of all cases of asthma can be attributed to the workplace (29). The purpose of the tests is to confirm that the asthma is caused by a product present in the workplace so that both employee and employer can be properly advised. This aim is in keeping with the definition of OA. Indeed, OA is defined as a type of asthma causally related to exposure to an agent present at the workplace. The importance of distinguishing between a "causal" and an "irritant" mechanism has been outlined (30).

Long-term exposure to a causal agent in subjects with asthma or OA can be harmful, whereas there is no evidence that this is true of "irritant" agents such as pollutants (NO_2, SO_2, ozone), cold air, particles, and so forth, especially if exposure concentration limits are observed. Diagnosing OA through OCT can be done in the context of a medicolegal investigation, although these tests should not be carried out solely to settle medicolegal claims. However, if an asthmatic condition persists and the worker has been exposed to a possible causal agent at work, provision should be made to confirm the diagnosis as long-term sequelae can be compensated in some countries.

As a clear distinction should be made between an irritant reaction and OA defined as asthma caused by an agent at work, it is important to insure that the bronchospastic reaction is nonirritant but is the result of sensitization to this agent. This is particularly relevant in the case of immediate bronchospastic reactions. The time of maximum reaction and the pattern of recovery from an immediate bronchospastic reaction caused by a sensitizer and an irritant such as exercise or cold air are very similar, with a maximum reaction 5–20 minutes after exposure and recovery in the first hour (31,32). Although this is debated, it is unlikely that exposure to an irritant product would cause an isolated late reaction or even a dual reaction (immediate and late reaction).

In our opinion, a history of exposure to an agent that has previously been shown to cause OA or a history of work-related increases in asthma symptoms, the presence of specific antibodies, or the presence of asthma or bronchial hyperresponsiveness is insufficient, alone or combined, to make the diagnosis of OA likely or very likely, particularly if these are considered in combination and in a stepwise manner (33). However, OCT represents the test that confirms the diagnosis. This statement is based on several arguments detailed in an earlier chapter. First, the closed questionnaire used for epidemiological assessments of OA is a sensitive, but not specific, tool for detecting OA, as is demonstrated in Table 1. Only 13–52% of those with a history suggestive of OA were shown to have OA using objective investigation (including specific inhalation challenges). In our clinical experience, based on the prospective assessment of 162 subjects referred for possible OA for whom objective assessment (OCT, monitoring of PEF, and PC_{20}) was performed, a clinical questionnaire administered by chest physicians trained in OA did not have a suf-

Table 1 Comparison of Results of Questionnaire and Objective Investigation in the Assessment of Occupational Asthma

Agent/workplace	Number of workers	Number of workers with a questionnaire suggestive of OA	Number of workers with OA (% of those with a history suggestive of OA)	Reference
Snow-crab/processing plants	303	64	33 (52%)	67
Isocyanates/paint shop	48	14	6 (43%)	83
Psyllium/pharmaceutical company	130	39	5 (13%)	35
Spiramycin/pharmaceutical company	51	12	3 (25%)	104
Psyllium/nurses	193	20	8 (40%)	41
Guar gum/carpet company	162	37	3 (8%)	42

Legend: OA = occupational asthma

ficient positive (63%) or negative predictive value (83%) to be used as a diagnostic tool (34). The presence or absence of typical symptoms such as improvement at weekends or during vacations was not a satisfactory index for the presence of OA.

Immunological sensitization does not mean that the subject has OA, as discussed in another chapter. The presence of specific antibodies is generally too sensitive in the case of an IgE-mediated phenomenon (35). For polypolyisocyanates, the presence or absence of specific IgG antibodies is not sensitive or specific enough for making a diagnosis of OA (36). Assessing bronchial responsiveness to pharmacological agents at work or away from work may demonstrate that a worker has bronchial responsiveness; but it does not prove that he or she has asthma or OA. As for immunological testing, this test is more useful in excluding the diagnosis of work-related asthma. Changes in bronchial responsiveness between periods at work and off work may, however, be useful in some instances (37) although this is not the rule (38).

Finally, the combination of the presence of immediate skin reactivity to an allergen and increased bronchial responsiveness does not necessarily prove that the subject will develop an asthmatic reaction when exposed to this agent. A close relationship was found (r^2 value close to 0.8) (39,40) but in some subjects (about 20%, as might have been expected from the relationship observed for common allergens) with skin reactivity to psyllium or guar gum and bronchial hyperresponsiveness we were unable to cause significant bronchial obstruction after exposure to the specific agent (41,42). Monitoring PEF at work and away from work, alone or combined with the assessment of nonspecific bronchial hyperresponsiveness, is an interesting tool, which is discussed below.

Screening programs for OA in high-risk workplaces should rely on several means. However, OCT should still be considered as the confirmatory step. OCT can also be used to assess the efficacy of preventive measures. The bronchial response to latex gloves with a low protein content has been assessed using OCT in health-care workers (43). Combining OCT with quantitative assessment of airborne agents could help to determine the level that elicits reactions in already sensitized subjects, and results used as a guide to establish permissible exposure levels at work. The efficacy of protective devices can be assessed in a similar way. OCT are often discussed on ethical grounds. Pepys once said: "One of the primary obligations of the clinician in asthma, as in any other disease, is to make a precise etiologic diagnosis. This is particularly relevant to allergic disorders, in which avoidance of the causative agent may terminate or reduce the disorder. . . . Failure to do the tests (OCT) could be regarded as an act of omission" (12). The possibility of inducing sensitization is sometimes raised as an ethical question, but it can be argued that the usual workplace exposure is much more prolonged than that found in an OCT context.

In conclusion, OCT represent an important tool to confirm the diagnosis of OA, identify new agents responsible for asthma, identify the agent responsible for asthma when there are multiple possible agents in the workplace, and for research purposes (see below). When they are available in a specialized center, they should be preferred to other means to confirm work-related asthma.

PERFORMING THE TEST

Since 1980, more than 1500 subjects have undergone such challenges at Sacre-Coeur Hospital. OCT are potentially dangerous as they can cause severe, life-threatening asthmatic reactions. They should therefore be carried out in specialized centers by trained personnel under the close supervision of physicians who have expertise in this field. The tests can be performed on an outpatient basis. Subjects come to the hospital laboratory in the morning and leave in the late afternoon. If the induced airway obstruction is still present at the end of the day, the physician should insure that the subject responds to an inhaled beta-2 adrenergic agent before he or she is discharged. The subject should know how to use an inhaled beta-2 adrenergic agent at home whenever needed and should have rapid access to medical treatment if needed. If the response to bronchodilator at the end of the day is insufficient, the subject should be kept in hospital for further observation and the asthmatic reaction treated accordingly with bronchodilators and steroids, if required.

Stability of Asthma and Need for Medication

As shown in Table 2, it is important to first ensure that the asthmatic is in a reasonably steady state. This is done by monitoring airway caliber on a control day with no exposure. FEV_1 fluctuations should be less than 10% throughout an observation period of 8 h. Ideally, all bronchodilator and anti-inflammatory medications should be withheld before the challenge. However, this is often not possible in moderate to severe asthmatic subjects where large fluctuations in FEV_1 can occur spontaneously. Short-acting, inhaled beta-2 adrenergic agents should be stopped at least 8 h before the challenge whereas long-acting beta-2 adrenergic agents and sustained-release theophylline preparations should be withheld at least 48 h before the challenge. However, some subjects may require continuous use of theophylline and beta-2 adrenergic preparations if their asthma proves too unstable. This also applies to anti-inflammatory medications such as sodium cromoglycate and inhaled steroids. If a subject takes these drugs to control asthma, the total dose should be administered at the end of each challenge day, but no sooner than 8 h before the next challenge. Challenges in subjects on antiasthma medication performed in this way have elicited positive reactions.

Table 2 Scheme for Performing Specific Inhalation Challenges on the Control Days

Day 1: Control day

aim: make sure asthma is stable

prerequisite: stop inhaled beta-2 adrenergic agent 8 hours, oral sustained-release theophylline 48 hours before, inhaled or oral antiinflammatory preparation in the morning of the test

procedure:
1. baseline spirometry, oral temperature, WBC and serum
2. FEV_1 every 10 minutes in the first hour, every 30 minutes for the second hour and hourly for 7–8 hours; oral temperature hourly
3. PC_{20} at the end of the day
4. PEFR monitoring in the evening at home

If: Baseline $FEV_1 < 2$ L and/or FEV_1 fluctuations > 10%, improve asthma treatment and postpone tests

Day 2: Control day of exposure

aim: make sure subjects do not react to a control agent

prerequisite: same as for Day 1 + baseline FEV_1 is ±10% of baseline FEV_1 on Day 1

procedure:
exposure for 30–120 minutes to a control agent (examples: lactose if the causal agent is flour, other wooddust if it is a wooddust, diluent of isocyanates, etc.); same monitoring as for day 1; no PC_{20} at the end of the day.

If: changes in $FEV_1 > 10\%$, same management as for Day 1

Functional Tests

FEV_1

The FEV_1 is still regarded as the gold standard for assessing airway caliber for nonspecific and specific inhalation challenges. It has the advantage of being easy to perform both for the technician and for the subject. It also requires only portable and relatively inexpensive instruments. From a physiological point of view, it reflects the presence of large and small airway obstruction. However, it is effort-dependent and requires a satisfactory collaboration from the subject. It is also influenced by volume history (i.e. the inspiratory manoeuvre from tidal volume breathing to total lung capacity), which can provoke bronchodilatation. This has been described both for nonspecific challenges using pharmacological agents (44–46) and for hyperventilation of unconditioned air (47,48). This effect also occurs with allergen challenges (49). Forced expiratory maneuvers can cause bronchoconstriction in subjects with enhanced bronchial responsiveness (50).

Baseline FEV_1 should be equal to or greater than 2 L for reasons of safety and proper interpretation of the test. Fluctuations in FEV_1 on the control day should not exceed 10% (Table 2). To be considered positive, investigators generally require a fall of 20% or more in FEV_1 at the time of an immediate reaction with progressive recovery in the first hour, or a sustained fall in FEV_1 of at least 20% in the case of nonimmediate reactions provided such changes are absent on the day of exposure to the control product.

Other Functional Tests

Other tests have been proposed. PEF can be obtained with cheaper apparatus and has a reproducibility that is little less than FEV_1. However, this test is even more effort-dependent than the FEV_1 and we have recently shown that it is less sensitive to detect a reaction (51). Forced expiratory flow rates in the middle half of the forced vital capacity (FEF25–75%) and flow rates derived from the lower half of the expiratory flow-volume curve, which are not effort-dependent, have also been proposed; however, these tests have poor reproducibility and the interpretation of what constitutes significant changes is questionable. Tests not requiring maximum inspiratory breathing maneuvers for assessing airway resistance/conductance in a body plethysmograph or using the oscillometry methodology have been proposed as well. However, the relative advantage of these tests because they are not affected by breathing maneuver is greatly counterbalanced by the fact that they have a less satisfactory reproducibility in a challenge situation (52). They also require more expensive and cumbersome equipment.

Assessment of Nonspecific Bronchial Responsiveness

Assessment of nonspecific bronchial responsiveness using pharmacological agents such as histamine or methacholine should be carried out at the end of the control day (see Table 2). It is useful to assess the level of bronchial responsiveness of the airways before the test as this is one of the predictors of a response to a specific agent (53–55). A negative pharmacological test does not exclude the possibility of OA; indeed, some workers may have ended exposure a long time prior to testing and show brisk changes in airway responsiveness after exposure to a specific agent (56–58). It also indicates whether a longer exposure should be considered. It has been demonstrated that changes in nonspecific bronchial responsiveness can occur when no significant changes in spirometry occurred; a longer exposure to the suspected agent can later reveal the bronchospastic reaction (59). Vandenplas and co-workers identified five subjects who failed to react to an occupational agent in terms of changes in FEV_1 but had changes in responsiveness to histamine at the end of the day. They reacted to the agent when exposure was prolonged on subsequent days (60).

An increase in nonallergic bronchial responsiveness classically occurs after late reactions but not after immediate asthmatic reactions (54). However, this is not constant (61). Indeed, we showed that 41/101 (41%) subjects with late reactions and 11/63 (17%) subjects with isolated immediate reactions demonstrated a 3.2-fold or greater change in the provocative concentration of histamine or methacholine causing a 20% fall in FEV_1 (PC_{20}) from baseline (63). There was a marked overlap between the changes in PC_{20} for those with immediate and late reactions.

Other Assessments

Although the subject is discharged at the end of the day, he or she can continue measuring PEF during the evening of the test or during the night whenever required. This will enable the investigator to know on the following day whether airway obstruction occurred after the subject left the hospital. However, when changes in FEV_1 are less than 10% at 8 hr after the end of exposure test, in our experience, significant changes in PEF later in the evening or at night do not occur.

Oral temperature is recorded hourly to document any possible hypersensitivity pneumonitis that can accompany asthmatic reactions in some instances (62). In an analysis of 317 subjects who had positive reactions to occupational agents, we showed that 5% of reactions were accompanied by fever; these occurred with late reactions and they were accompanied by blood neutrophilia (63). Blood is drawn at the beginning and end of the first day and at the same time intervals or the following morning (which is even more sensitive) (64) when challenges are positive. The occurrence of eosinophilia or leukocytosis can then be demonstrated. The serum can also be stored for immunological tests (specific IgE and/or IgG) when applicable.

Duration and Schedule of Exposure and Monitoring Spirometry

Spirometry should be assessed for at least 8 h, i.e., every 10 min for the first hour, every 30 min for the second hour, and then hourly. After a control day to ensure functional stability, subjects should be exposed to a control substance (lactose in the case of an agent in powder form such as flours, pharmaceutical products, etc.) or a control vapor, aerosol, or fume. In the specific case of polyisocyanates, this can be the chemical normally mixed with isocyanate in the two- or three-system component (see Table 2).

The duration and intensity of the initial exposure to the suspected offending agent should be dictated by clinical history; if there is any indication of a severe immediate reaction, short exposure under controlled conditions should be considered. The level of bronchial obstruction and responsiveness should also help in determining the duration and level of the initial exposure. We would normally start exposure to isocyanates for 5 min (total duration) on the first exposure day if the PC_{20} is ≥ 0.25 mg/ml but for only 1 min if it is lower. The principle is to draw a dose-response curve by increasing the duration and/or concentration of exposure. In our experience, it is always preferable to start with the following durations: 1 breath, 10 sec, 30 sec, 1 min, 5 min etc. (Table 3). For agents likely to cause immediate reactions such as high-molecular-weight agents (flour, psyllium, animal danders, etc.), the increase in duration of exposure can be progressive until an immediate reaction occurs. For agents likely to cause isolated late reactions, such as western red cedar and polyisocyanates, a total initial exposure of 1–5 min (depending on the history and level of nonspecific responsiveness) done progressively as for high-molecular-weight agents should be considered for the first day of exposure, increasing it to 15–30 min and then up to 2 h the following 2 days. This gradual increase in exposure intervals can be modified especially if there is evidence that the onset of an asthmatic reaction has been induced by monitoring PC_{20} at the end of the day.

It has been shown that it is neither the concentration nor the duration of exposure per se but the dose (i.e., concentration $\times$ duration of exposure) (65) that determines the magnitude of the asthmatic reaction.

METHODOLOGY

Nature of the Agent

Water-Soluble, High-Molecular-Weight Allergens

Some antigens, such as flour (66) or snow-crab extracts (67), can be diluted in water and the concentration assessed. These testing solutions should be compared and assayed under conditions recommended for commercial allergenic extracts. Materials are prepared by extraction into phenolated saline solution. The preferred technique of assuring stabilization is to use lyophilized extracts, which are reconstituted with phenolated saline diluent prior to use. All reconstituted extracts should be stored at 4°C, and allergy extracts diluted to 1:1000 or higher should be discarded after 1 month. The concentration of allergy extracts

Table 3   Scheme for Performing Specific Inhalation Challenge Tests to the Possible Causal Agent

---

Active day(s): Day 3 and subsequent days

aim: verify if subjects show a significant reaction (changes in $FEV_1 \geq 20\%$) after exposure to the suspected agent

prerequisite: same as for Day 2

procedure: progressive exposure with in-between functional assessments *high molecular weight agent*, IgE mediated mechanism, expect immediate reaction: progressive exposure: one breath, 10 sec, 20 sec, 30 sec, 2 min, 5 min, 30 min, etc. for a total of 2 hours; *low molecular weight agent*: exposure for one breath, 10 sec, 20 sec, 30 sec (total one min) on the first day, 1, 2, and 2 min (total = 5 min) on the second day, 5, 10 and 15 min (total = 30 min) on the third day and 15, 15, 30, 30 and 30 min (total = 2 hours) on the last day; assess FEV_1 immediately and 10 min after each exposure period; if changes <10%, continue with the proposed protocol; if changes >10%, repeat a similar period of exposure as the previous one; if changes ≥20%, stop exposure

---

$\downarrow$

If positive reaction: repeat PC_{20} at the end of the day or in the following morning provided FEV_1 is back to baseline; if significantly lower than on Day 1, treat with antiinflammatory preparation; repeat PC_{20} until it is back to baseline;

If *late reaction*: administer inhaled beta-2 adrenergic agent; if FEV_1 back to ±10% baseline 15–20 minutes later, discharge with advise to subject that he (she) may require inhaled beta-2 adrenergic agent in the evening or night; if FEV_1 not back to baseline, administer oral steroids and discharge; see the subject on the following day to make sure FEV_1 is back to baseline; follow-up required if not;

If *negative test*, repeat PC_{20} at the end of the day; if no significant change, no further exposure; if significantly lower PC_{20}, increase duration of exposure to a maximum of 4 hours on the following day.

---

to be used for aerosolized bronchial challenges is expressed as either weight per volume (w/v) or protein nitrogen units per milliliter (PNU/ml). In some cases it may be desirable to determine biological allergen activity (allergy units).

Before OCT is attempted with these solutions, a skin prick test should be done to assess the threshold concentration, which is expressed as that dilution of test allergen that gives a 3-mm wheal. The first inhalational test dose should be threefold dilutions below the calculated skin dose. As for common allergens, the idea is to assess the concentration of the occupational sensitizer required to give a 20% fall in FEV_1 for suspected immediate reactions by determining the PC_{20} and the wheal diameter of the allergen with skin prick testing (39,40).

Test aerosols may be administered by continuous aerosol generation and tidal breathing or individual breaths drawn from a hand-operated nebulizer. The output of the nebulizer, which is the principal technical determinant of the response, should be assessed as for nonspecific inhalation challenges. When either the intermittent (68) or continuous (69) aerosol generation methods are used, doses of allergens can be expressed in inhalation units. One inhalation unit equals one breath of 1/5000 w/v dilution of one breath of 100 PNU/ml (a protein solution with 1 μg protein nitrogen/ml). In the intermittent method, the subject inhales five breaths of allergen solution beginning with the most dilute and proceeding to the most concentrated (1:100 or 5000 PNU/ml) (68). FEV_1 is measured immediately and 10 min after each dose challenge. The test proceeds in this manner until there has been at least a 20% fall in FEV_1 from baseline or when the most concentrated dose has been nebulized.

The results of aerosolized provocation tests are expressed on log-linear paper, the dose of allergen being plotted on the logarithmic abscisssa and the FEV_1 response in linear units on the ordinate. As for pharmacological agents, sensitivity to the allergen is determined by the provocation dose causing a 20% fall in FEV_1 (PD_{20}).

Agents in Powder or Dust Form

It was originally suggested by Pepys and Hutchcroft (12) that these agents be tipped from one tray to another in a challenge room that is well ventilated and preventing against contamination of the laboratory and sensitization of the personnel. Models of well-ventilated rooms have been proposed by others (70). However, this method does not allow for monitoring of the concentration of particles in the air. There should be provision to keep the levels of dust below the threshold limit value, short-term exposure limit (TLV-STEL) set by the American Conference for Governmental Industrial Hygienists (ACGIH). An apparatus that makes exposure to steady and low concentrations of particles possible and permits monitoring of the diameter of the particles has been developed (71–73) (Fig. 1). It is important that a significant percentage of particles be <10 μ (respirable dusts). Dose-response curves can be obtained by increasing the duration or concentration of exposure (Fig. 2). This apparatus has the advantage of making the procedure safe, as subjects are exposed to low levels of dusts in a progressive way. It can furthermore distinguish satisfactorily between irritant and sensitizing reactions; irritant reactions are unlikely to occur if TLV-STEL concentrations are used. This apparatus can be used for different types of dust: flour, sawdust (including western red cedar), pharmaceutical powders, guar gum, and so forth. There is no contamination of the air in the room where the apparatus is located. If the test is negative after 2 hr of exposure using this apparatus, we would perform the test in the realistic way as proposed by Pepys and Hutchcroft (12) for 2 hr to ensure that the test is negative.

Polypolyisocyanates

On the control day (second day of the challenge tests), the isocyanate subjects are exposed to the control chemical (the chemical that is usually mixed with polyisocyanates) for a total of 15 min in a challenge room. For hexamethylene diisocyanate (HDI), the most frequently used isocyanate incorporated into paints for cars, airplanes, and so forth, the control chemical is an enamel containing aromatic hydrocarbons, ketones, aliphatic, and ether ester; for diphenylmethane diisocyanate (MDI), used in making molds and in the plastics industry, various aromatic hydrocarbons and fluorocarbons are used. For toluene diisocyanate (TDI), used mainly in the preparation of foam, we use a commercial preparation made of polyol (99%) and aliphatic amine (1%) as the diluent. On the third and subsequent days if required, subjects are exposed to polyisocyanates in one of the following ways: (1) for TDI, approximatively 100 ml of pure commercial TDI (80% 2,4-TDI and 20% 2,6-TDI) is deposited in a small cup, (2) for HDI, the commercial preparation

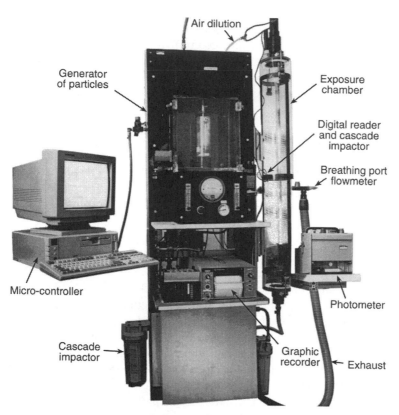

Figure 1 Closed-circuit apparatus for inhalation challenges in the specific case of dry particles. The components are: (1) generation device for dry aerosol; (2) photometer from which concentration is derived; (3) exposure chamber; (4) self-control computerized feedback (left end side).

the subject is exposed to at work (from 20% to 75% of HDI/HDI biuret, depending on the product), is nebulized with the diluent (1:3 concentration) using a nebulizer; (3) for MDI, the commercial preparation containing 40%–50% MDI and 50%–60% polymethylene polyphenyl isocyanate is heated in a metal cup to approximatively 80C. On the isocyanate challenge day(s), subjects are asked to remain in the challenge room for progressively longer periods of time: one breath, 15 and 45 sec for a total of 1 min on the first day (if the PC_{20} is ≤ 0.25 mg/ml and/or there is a history of an important reaction), 1 min, 2 min, and 2 min for a total of 5 min on the second day (this can be done on the first day if the PC_{20} is >0.25 mg/ml and there is no clinical history pointing to a severe reaction on exposure), and total periods varying from 15 to 120 min on subsequent days.

Challenges with isocyanates and other agents in vapor, powder, or gas form have so far been performed in relatively large challenge rooms (74). These rooms are well ventilated with a circuit near the ceiling. By controlling the ventilation in the room, the technician can stabilize the concentration of isocyanates in the challenge room (which is monitored continuously with a MDA-7100 or a GMD monitor) and keep it below 20 ppb (TLV-STEL). The technician has a direct view of the monitor's digital reading. Humidity is kept at 50% in the challenge room (the reading of isocyanates by the MDA 7100 monitor is affected by humidity) and there is a ventilator in the challenge room to homogenize the isocyanate in the air. An improved closed-circuit mixing chamber was designed in con-

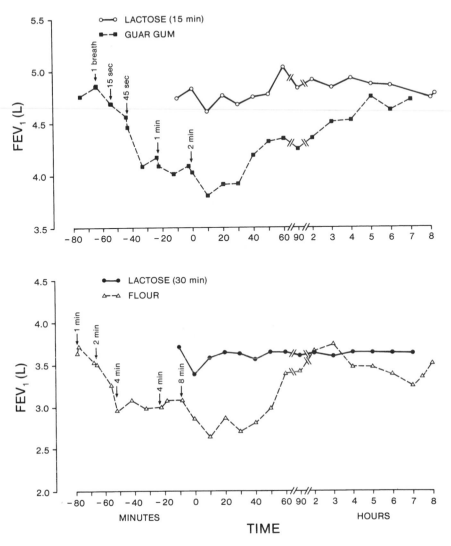

Figure 2 Examples of dose-response curves for two subjects with guar gum (top panel) and flour (lower panel) for consecutive exposures (shown) on the same day. The falls in FEV$_1$ are progressive. "0" time corresponds to the end of last exposure. FEV$_1$ forced expiratory volume in one second. (From Ref. 71 with permission.)

junction with engineer Yves Cloutier of the Institut de Recherche en Santé et Sécurité du Travail du Québec (IRSST) for polyisocyanates and other agents (Fig. 3) (75). This circuit is similar to what is described above for agents in powder or dust form. Isocyanate can be generated in vapor and aerosol. Continuous recording of the isocyanates is possible and concentrations can be kept stable at ±2 ppb. Preset levels of isocyanates are generated by adjusting the airflow to a small receptacle containing the isocyanate, which can be heated if needed (in the case of HDI or MDI). The isocyanate is inhaled through an orofacial mask in the middle of an exposure tube. The expelled air is filtered through charcoal. A similar procedure can be used for other agents that exist in vapor form such as formaldehyde (76) and glutaraldehyde.

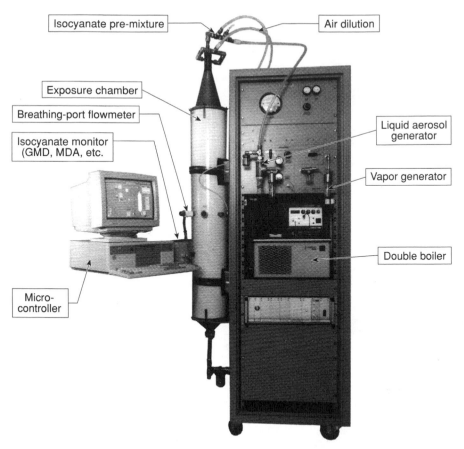

Figure 3 Closed-circuit apparatus for inhalation challenges with isocyanates. GMD: GMD Systems Inc. Pittsburgh; MDA: MDA Scientific, Glenview, IL. Similar apparatuses exist for dry aerosols (dusts and particles) (Fig. 1) and other vapors besides isocyanates (formaldehyde, glutaraldehyde).

In summary, challenge rooms have evolved from the one originally proposed by Pepys and co-workers to more sophisticated versions still based on relatively large chambers and, more recently, to small, closed-circuit chambers, which presents the advantage of a more precise and stable generation of the agent.

Duration of Exposure

It remains unknown how long a subject should be exposed to a product before the test is considered negative. It is our experience that subjects have to be exposed for up to 2 hr before the test can be considered negative. We have even documented cases where subjects had to be exposed for 4 hr (77). However, in general, an asthmatic reaction can be documented after exposure for a maximum of 2 hr; this was the case in 14 of 15 subjects in whom specific inhalation challenges were repeated 2 years or more after cessation of exposure (78). When there is a negative test, subjects have to return to the workplace where PEF is serially monitored. This may happen when subjects have been away from work for too long (79,80). OCT are then repeated in the laboratory if returning to work provokes an exacerbation of asthma accompanied by changes in PEF. The test is then repeated in the laboratory if returning to work provokes an exacerbation of asthma.

PATTERNS OF REACTION

In clinical practice, specific inhalation challenges are generally considered positive when there is a sustained fall in FEV_1 of 20% or more from prechallenge value in the absence of significant (10%) changes after exposure to a control product. Typical patterns of reaction have been summarized by Pepys and Hutchcroft (81). Figure 4 illustrates these reactions.

The immediate reaction is characterized by a brisk onset at a maximum of 10–20 min after exposure ends and lasting 1–2 hr. These reactions respond well to bronchodilator therapy. These reactions are assumed to be harmless as they cause no inflammation, but they can actually be the most dangerous because they can be unpredictable, particularly in subjects for whom skin testing with the suspected agent is not possible. By contrast, late reactions are the cause of airway inflammation but are easy to manage; there is plenty of time to intervene (see below). When the history is highly suggestive of severe acute reactions and greatly enhanced bronchial responsiveness ($PC_{20} \leq 0.25$ mg/ml), it is im-

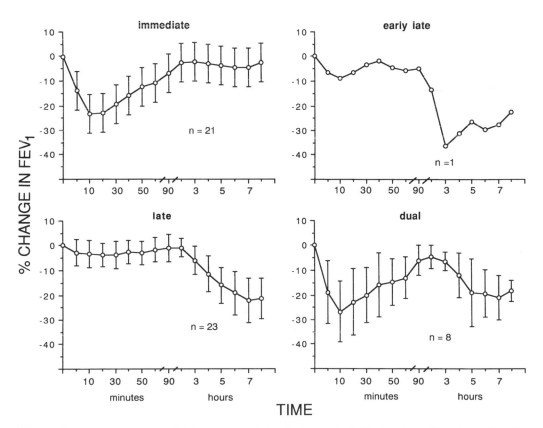

Figure 4 Mean ± SD or individual values of the % change in FEV_1 (on the ordinate) as a function of time since exposure (on the abscissa) for the four typical patterns of reactions (see text for definition). The number of subjects for each pattern is shown.

portant to start inhalation challenge test with a very low concentration and for only one breath. In this instance, an indwelling intravenous catheter should be placed for immediate administration of bronchodilators and a beta-2 adrenergic solution be ready for inhalation with oxygen.

Late reactions develop slowly and progressively either 1–2 hr ("early late") or 4–8 h (late) after exposure. They may be accompanied by fever [this being documented in approximately 5% of cases (63)] and general malaise. Unlike immediate reactions, they cause eosinophilia (82). If they are accompanied by fever, this may be accompanied by leukocytosis (63). Contrary to popular belief, they generally respond well to inhaled beta-2 adrenergic agents. We showed that in 99 subjects with late reactions, changes in $FEV_1 > 20\%$ occurred in 78% of them after administration of albuterol; in 66%, FEV_1 returned to >90% baseline. These findings were confirmed in a double-blind, placebo-controlled, prospective study in 22 subjects with late reactions in whom we also showed that the duration of the bronchodilator effect was equivalent to what can be observed with common asthma (63). In the event of a late reaction, an inhaled beta-2 adrenergic agent should be administered and confirmation that the FEV_1 is ≥90% baseline should be shown before the subject is discharged. The patient should receive precise instructions on how relapsing bronchoconstriction monitored at home with portable instruments assessing PEF and/or FEV_1 should be managed after leaving the laboratory. Anti-inflammatory preparations (inhaled or oral depending on the severity of the reaction) can be given for 2 weeks. Bronchial responsiveness to methacholine or histamine can then be reassessed, making sure it is back to baseline.

Dual reactions are a combination of immediate and late reactions. Atypical reactions principally after exposure to polyisocyanates have been reported (83,84). In a group of 23 subjects who had positive reactions to isocyanates, it was found that 30% had atypical reactions (85) (Fig. 5). They were mainly of the progressive type (starting within minutes after exposure ended, progressing to a maximum 7–8 hr later). A previously unrecognized "square-waved" reaction (no recovery between the immediate and late components of the reaction) was also described. "Progressive recovery" patterns were also seen where subjects had maximum bronchoconstriction immediately after exposure, but functional recovery took 7–8 hr.

COMPARISON WITH OTHER MEANS

The specificity and sensitivity of serial monitoring of PEF in confirming a diagnosis of OA were originally studied by Burge and colleagues by comparing them with the history and the effect of subsequent exposure at work (13). The gold standard in this study was not the specific inhalation challenge. These investigators found PEF to have an overall sensitivity of 77% and a specificity of 100% in 29 workers examined for OA, 22 of whom had positive specific inhalation challenges after exposure to colophony. The same group found the test to be 83% sensitive and 100% specific in 23 workers exposed to isocyanates, 11 of whom had had positive specific inhalation challenges (14). Direct comparison between specific inhalation challenges and PEF showed that sensitivity varied from 81% to 86% and specificity from 74% to 86% (38,86) in the diagnosis of OA. Table 4 lists the advantages and disadvantages of OCT as compared with PEF monitoring in the investigation of OA. These factors have been discussed and a statement on PEF monitoring in OA has been published (87). Even though PEF can be performed easily for periods at work and away from work, their interpretation should be made by experts who generally

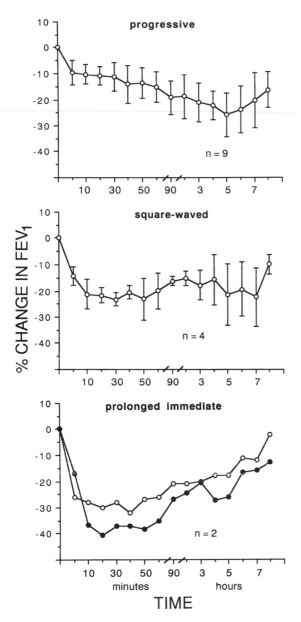

Figure 5 Mean ± SD or individual values of the % change in FEV$_1$ (on the ordinate) as a function of time since exposure (on the abscissa) for the three atypical patterns of reactions (see text for definition). The number of subjects for each pattern is shown.

show a satisfactory between-reader reproducibility (88,89). Results can be falsified (90,91) and compliance affects the interpretation of results (89). In our opinion OCT should be carried out first in subjects exposed to a known agent at work if facilities are available and if there are experts who can perform and interpret the tests. If the test is negative and the subject has a history of acute and severe reaction at work, provision should be made to send a technician to monitor FEV$_1$ after progressive and cautious increase in duration

Table 4 Advantages and Disadvantages of PEF Monitoring and Specific Inhalation Challenges in the Individual Investigation of Occupational Asthma

	PEF monitoring	Specific inhalation challenges
Advantages	Easy to do; inexpensive equipment.	Direct control of the subject and of the environment.
Disadvantages	Difficult to interpret especially in more severe asthmatics; can be falsified; lack of understanding by the subject; impossible in illiterate subjects.	Expensive equipment; can be done on only a few subjects at a time; reserved to highly specialized centers; exposure that is too short or to the wrong agent may result in falsely negative results.

of exposure at work (79,92). If this is not possible or if no reaction occurs on the first day of exposure, monitoring of PEF should be done until a significant fall occurs. OCT can then be repeated with a monitoring of FEV_1.

PITFALLS

Even if OCT are the gold standard, there may be instances in which false-positive or false-negative tests occur.

Reasons for a False-Positive Test

With immediate reactions, it is sometimes difficult to distinguish between an "irritant" and a reaction similar to that which could occur after exposure to a proper sensitizing agent. Indeed, the pattern of reaction in terms of peak effect and recovery is similar to what has been described for nonspecific reactions such as exercise and hyperventilation (31,32). The use of a control "irritant" substance (lactose for powders, the varnish usually mixed with polyisocyanates, etc.) is suggested as well as using an apparatus that gives information on the concentration and diameter of the particles and polyisocyanates. False-positive late reactions can also be observed in subjects in an unstable clinical state. This is why subjects should always be observed on a control day to make sure that they are in a stable clinical state.

Reasons for a False-Negative Test

There are several reasons for a false-negative test. First, subjects can be exposed to the wrong agent. In an interesting case reported by Carroll and co-workers; a subject became sensitized to a product used in a nearby plant rather than to the agent worked with (93). More often, subjects may well have been away from work for too long (79,80), although such instances seem rare (78). If the OCT is negative in the laboratory, provisions should be made to return the subject to his normal workplace while serial monitoring of PEF is done. As soon as changes in PEF or bronchial responsiveness is demonstrated, OCT should be repeated in the laboratory.

Dangers

OCT should only be done in specialized centers with the facilities for administering bronchodilators and intubation quickly if needed. When OCT are done with care (see pattern of reaction with safety measures above), severe reactions are rare. Inhalation challenge tests have been performed in more than 1500 subjects at the Sacre-Coeur Hospital of Montréal in the past 10 years. A severe reaction requiring intubation happened only once, at a time apparatuses described above were not available (94). The subject was a nurse exposed to psyllium. She was exposed to it for 1 min; we were not aware at the time that this preparation is highly volatile. The subject developed severe, immediate bronchoconstriction. She required intubation for 3 hr after which functional recovery was complete. In a subject with a history of acute reactions or increased bronchial responsiveness, an i.v. should be made ready beforehand and an appropriate beta-2 adrenergic agent in solution ready for inhalation.

As mentioned above, OCT can be done at the workplace. Although this is not ideal because there is no control over exposure (at times, the exposure is intermittent and the worker may well not be exposed to the sensitizing agent if it is unknown; at other times, he or she may be exposed to very high levels) and it may be difficult to exclude an irritant reaction, which is sometimes the only way to document an asthmatic reaction.

OCCUPATIONAL INHALATION CHALLENGES IN THE CASE OF ALVEOLITIS

On occasion, exposure to an occupational agent can cause alveolitis or hypersensitivity pneumonitis. Cases of alveolitis after exposure to polyisocyanates have been described by several authors (62,95–97). Criteria for defining a positive "alveolar" reaction have been described by Hendrick and co-workers (98). These include a body temperature >37.2C, an increase in circulating neutrophils of 2500/mm^3 or more, and a fall in forced vital capacity of 15% or more. Diffusing capacity and changes in lung subdivisions proved to be too insensitive to be useful. These tests can be performed in the laboratory or at the workplace, and the value of other tools (chest examination and radiograph, in vitro tests for cell-mediated immunity, bronchoalveolar lavage, lung biopsy, therapeutic trial) have been reviewed elsewhere (99).

OCCUPATIONAL INHALATION CHALLENGES WITH OCCUPATIONAL AGENTS AS A RESEARCH TOOL

OCT may lead to interesting observations on the pathophysiology of asthma. Fabbri and co-workers have shown that both neutrophils and eosinophils were involved in late asthmatic reactions caused by polyisocyanates, as demonstrated by bronchoalveolar lavage at different time intervals after exposure (100). The same group of investigators later showed that only beclomethasone was effective in preventing changes in bronchial responsiveness following exposure to isocyanates (101). Lam and co-workers have demonstrated an increase in eosinophils in the bronchoalveolar lavage after late reactions caused by plicatic acid (102). Urinary leukotrienes were shown in the case of immediate reactions to common and occupational agents (103). Multiple studies summarized elsewhere have evaluated the efficacy of antiasthma drugs in suppressing asthmatic reactions following exposure to occupational agents (81). OCT can therefore be useful in improving our understanding of the pathophysiology of asthma.

CONCLUSION

It is our opinion that OCT in investigating OA should still be regarded as the gold standard for confirming the diagnosis. Since the proposal of these tests by Pepys in the 1970s, attempts have been made to improve the methodology of the test from a functional and exposure point of view. These efforts are aimed at offering a more precise diagnosis of OA and more appropriate advice to the employee and employer. These tests can also be helpful as a research tool because human asthma is a better model than various types of bronchial hyperresponsiveness that have been induced in animals.

ACKNOWLEDGMENT

The authors would like to thank Katherine Tallman for reviewing the manuscript.

REFERENCES

1. Aas K. The Bronchial Provocation Test. Springfield, IL: Charles C Thomas Publisher, 1975.
2. Herxheimer H. The late bronchial reaction in induced asthma. Int Arch Allergy Appl Immunol 1952; 3:323–328.
3. Dominjon-Monnier F, Carton J, Guibert L, Burtin P, Brille D, Kourilsky R. Èpreuves ventilatoires aux extraits de moisissures atmosphériques. Rev Franç Mal Respir 1962; 2:191–202.
4. Colldahl H. A study of provocation test on patients with bronchial asthma. Acta Allergol 1952; 5:133–142.
5. Pepys J, Riddell RW, Citron KM, Clayton YM, Short EI. Clinical and immunologic significance of aspergillus fumigatus in the sputum. Am Rev Respir Dis 1959; 80:167.
6. Pepys J, Jenkins PA. Precipitin (F.L.H.) test in farmer's lung. Thorax 1965; 20:21–35.
7. Hargreave FE, Pepys J, Longbottom JL, Wraith DG. Bird breeder's (fancier's) lung. Lancet 1966; 1:445–449.
8. Pickering CAC, Batten JC, Pepys J. Asthma due to inhaled wood dusts—western red cedar and iroko. Clin Allergy 1972; 2:213–218.
9. Pepys J, Pickering CAC, Terry DJ. Asthma due to inhaled chemical agents—tolylene diisocyanate. Clin Allergy 1972; 2:225–236.
10. Pickering CAC. Inhalation tests with chemical allergens: complex salts of platinum. Proc R Soc Med 1972; 65:272–274.
11. Davies RJ, Hendrick DJ, Pepys J. Asthma due to inhaled chemical agents:ampicillin, bensyl penicillin, 6 amino penicillanic acid and related substances. Clin Allergy 1974; 4:227–247.
12. Pepys J, Hutchcroft BJ. Bronchial provocation tests in etiologic diagnosis and analysis of asthma. Am Rev Respir Dis 1975; 112:829–859.
13. Burge PS, O'Brien IM, Harries MG. Peak flow rate records in the diagnosis of occupational asthma due to colophony. Thorax 1979; 34:308–316.
14. Burge PS, O'Brien IM, Harries MG. Peak flow rate records in the diagnosis of occupational asthma due to isocyanates. Thorax 1979; 34:317–323.
15. Chan-Yeung M, Lam S. Occupational asthma. Am Rev Respir Dis 1986; 133:686–703.

16. Pauli G, Bessot JC, Dietemann-Molard A. L'asthme professionnel: investigations et principales étiologies. [Occupational asthma: investigations and aetiological factors.] Bull Eur Physiopathol Respir 1986; 22:399–425.

17. Chan-Yeung M, Malo JL. Occupational asthma. Chest 1987; 91:130S-136S.

18. Chan-Yeung M. Occupational asthma update. Chest 1988; 93:407–411.

19. Bernstein DI, Cohn JR. Guidelines for the diagnosis and evaluation of occupational immunologic lung disease: preface. J Allergy Clin Immunol 1989; 84:791–793.

20. Ad Hoc Committee on Occupational Asthma of the Standards Committee Canadian Thoracic Society. Occupational asthma: recommendations for diagnosis, management and assessment of impairment. Can Med Assoc J 1989; 140:1029–1032.

21. Spector SL. Provocative Challenge Procedures: Bronchial, Oral, Nasal and Exercise. Boca Raton, FL: CRC Press, 1983.

22. Malo JL, Cartier A. Bronchoprovocation testing. In: Harber P, Schenker MB, Balmes JR, eds. Occupational and Environmental Respiratory Disease. St. Louis: Mosby Yearbook, 1996: 55–66.

23. Cartier A, Bernstein IL, Burge PS, Cohn JR, Fabbri LM, Hargreave FE, Malo JL, McKay RT, Salvaggio JE. Guidelines for bronchoprovocation on the investigation of occupational asthma. Report of the subcommittee on bronchoprovocation for occupational asthma. J Allergy Clin Immunol 1989; 84:823–829.

24. Sterk PJ, Fabbri LM, Quanjer PH, Cockcroft DW, O'Byrne PM, Anderson SD, Juniper EF, Malo JL. Airway responsiveness. Standardized challenge testing with pharmacological, physical and sensitizing stimuli in adults. Report working party standardization of lung function tests European Community for Steel and Coal. Official statement of the European Respiratory Society. Eur Respir J 1993; 6(Suppl 16):53–83.

25. Ross DJ, Sallie BA, McDonald JC. SWORD'94: surveillance of work-related and occupational respiratory disease in the UK. Occup Med 1996; 45:175–178.

26. Contreras GR, Rousseau R, Chan-Yeung M. Occupational respiratory diseases in British Columbia, Canada in 1991. Occup Environ Med 1994; 51:710–712.

27. Lagier F, Cartier A, Malo JL. Statistiques médico-légales sur l'asthme professionnel au Québec de 1986 and 1988. [Medico-legal statistics on occupational asthma in Quebec between 1986 and 1988.] Rev Mal Respir 1990; 7:337–341.

28. Reijula K, Patterson R. Occupational allergies in Finland in 1981–91. Allergy Proc 1994; 15:163–168.

29. Kogevinas M, Anto JM, Soriano JB, Tobias A, Burney P. The Spanish Group of the European Asthma Study. The risk of asthma attributable to occupational exposures: a population-based study in Spain. Am J Respir Crit Care Med 1996; 154:137–143.

30. Dolovich J, Hargreave FE. The asthma syndrome: inciters, inducers, and host characteristics. Thorax 1981; 36:641–644.

31. Godfrey S, Silverman M, Anderson SD, Konig P. Exercise-induced asthma. Br J Dis Chest 1975; 69:1–39.

32. Malo JL, Cartier A, L'Archevêque J, Ghezzo H, Martin RR. Kinetics of the recovery from bronchial obstruction due to hyperventilation of cold air in asthmatic subjects. Eur Respir J 1988; 1:384–388.

33. Chan-Yeung M, Malo JL. Occupational asthma. N Engl J Med 1995; 333:107–112.

34. Malo JL, Ghezzo H, L'Archevêque J, Lagier F, Perrin B, Cartier A. Is the clinical history a satisfactory means of diagnosing occupational asthma? Am Rev Respir Dis 1991; 143:528–532.

35. Bardy JD, Malo JL, Saguin P, Ghezzo H, Desjardins J, Dolovich J, Cartier A. Occupational asthma and IgE sensitization in a pharmaceutical company processing psyllium. Am Rev Respir Dis 1987; 135:1033–1038.

36. Cartier A, Grammer L, Malo JL, Lagier F, Ghezzo H, Harris K, Patterson R. Specific serum antibodies against isocyanates: association with occupational asthma. J Allergy Clin Immunol 1989; 84:507–514.

37. Hargreave FE, Ramsdale EH, Pugsley SO. Occupational asthma without bronchial hyperresponsiveness. Am Rev Respir Dis 1984; 130:513–515.

38. Perrin B, Lagier F, L'Archevêque J, Cartier A, Boulet LP, Cata J, Malo JL. Occupational asthma: validity of monitoring of peak expiratory flow rates and non-allergic bronchial responsiveness as compared to specific inhalation challenge. Eur Respir J 1992; 5:40–48.

39. Cockcroft DW, Ruffin RE, Frith PA, Cartier A, Juniper EF, Dolovich J, Hargreave FE. Determinants of allergen-induced asthma: dose of allergen, circulating IgE antibody concentration, and bronchial responsiveness to inhaled histamine. Am Rev Respir Dis 1979; 120:1053–1058.

40. Cockcroft DW, Murdock KY, Kirby J, Hargreave F. Prediction of airway responsiveness to allergen from skin sensitivity to allergen and airway responsiveness to histamine. Am Rev Respir Dis 1987; 135:264–267.

41. Malo JL, Cartier A, L'Archevêque J, Ghezzo H, Lagier F, Trudeau C, Dolovich J. Prevalence of occupational asthma and immunologic sensitization to psyllium among health personnel in chronic care hospitals. Am Rev Respir Dis 1990; 142:1359–1366.

42. Malo JL, Cartier A, L'Archevêque J, Ghezzo H, Soucy F, Somers J, Dolovich J. Prevalence of occupational asthma and immunological sensitization to guar gum among employees at a carpet-manufacturing plant. J Allergy Clin Immunol 1990; 86:562–569.

43. Vandenplas O, Delwiche JP, Depelchin S, Sibille Y, Weyer R Vande, Delaunois L. Latex gloves with a lower protein content reduce bronchial reactions in subjects with occupational asthma caused by latex. Am J Respir Crit Care Med 1995; 151:887–891.

44. Nadel JA, Tierney DF. Effect of a previous deep inspiration on airway resistance in man. J Appl Physiol 1961; 16:717–719.

45. Fish JE, Kelly JF. Measurements of responsiveness in bronchoprovocation testing. J Allergy Clin Immunol 1979; 64:592–596.

46. Sestier M, Pineau L, Cartier A, Martin RR, Malo JL. Bronchial responsiveness to methacholine and effects of respiratory manoeuvres. J Appl Physiol 1984; 56:122–128.

47. Lim TK, Pride NB, Jr RH Ingram. Effects of volume history during spontaneous and acutely induced air-flow obstruction in asthma. Am Rev Respir Dis 1987; 135:591–596.

48. Malo JL, L'Archevêque J, Cartier A. Comparative effects of volume history on bronchoconstriction induced by hyperventilation and methacholine in asthmatic subjects. Eur Respir J 1990; 3:639–643.

49. Fish JE, Ankin MG, Kelly JF, Peterman VI. Comparison of responses to pollen extract in subjects with allergic asthma and nonasthmatic subjects with allergic rhinitis. J Allergy Clin Immunol 1980; 65:154–161.

50. Gayrard P, Orehek J, Grimaud CH, Charpin J. Mechanisms of the bronchoconstrictor effects of deep inspiration in asthmatic patients. Thorax 1979; 34:234–240.

51. Bérubé D, Cartier A, L'Archevêque J, Ghezzo H, Malo JL. Comparison of peak expiratory flow rate and FEV_1 in assessing bronchomotor tone after challenges with occupational sensitizers. Chest 1991; 99:831–836.

52. Dehaut P, Rachiele A, Martin RR, Malo JL. Histamine dose-response curves in asthma: reproducibility and sensitivity of different indices to assess response. Thorax 1983; 38:516–522.

53. Killian D, Cockcroft DW, Hargreave FE, Dolovich J. Factors in allergen-induced asthma: relevance of the intensity of the airways allergic reaction and non-specific bronchial reactivity. Clin Allergy 1976; 6:219–225.

54. Cartier A, Thomson NC, Frith PA, Roberts R, Hargreave FE. Allergen-induced increase in bronchial responsiveness to histamine: relationship to the late asthmatic response and change in airway caliber. J Allergy Clin Immunol 1982; 70:170–177.

55. Lam S, Tan F, Chan G, Chan-Yeung M. Relationship between types of asthmatic reaction, nonspecific bronchial reactivity, and specific IgE antibodies in patients with red cedar asthma. J Allergy Clin Immunol 1983; 72:134–139.

56. Banks DE, Jr HW Barkman, Butcher BT, Hammad YY, Rando RJ, Glindmeyer HW, Jones RN, Weill H. Absence of hyperresponsiveness to methacholine in a worker with methylene diphenyl diisocyanate (MDI)-induced asthma. Chest 1986; 89:389–393.

57. Mapp CE, Vecchio L Dal, Boschetto P, Marzo N De, Fabbri LM. Toluene diisocyanate-induced asthma without airway hyperresponsiveness. Eur J Respir Dis 1986; 68:89–95.

58. Hargreave FE, Ramsdale EH, Pugsley SO. Occupational asthma without bronchial hyperresponsiveness. Am Rev Respir Dis 1984; 130:513–515.

59. Cartier A, L'Archeveque J, Malo JL. Exposure to a sensitizing occupational agent can cause a long-lasting increase in bronchial responsiveness to histamine in the absence of significant changes in airway caliber. J Allergy Clin Immunol 1986; 78:1185–1189.

60. Vandenplas O, Delwiche JP, Jamart J, Weyer R Van de. Increase in non-specific bronchial hyperresponsiveness as an early marker of bronchial response to occupational agents during specific inhalation challenges. Thorax 1996; 51:472–478.

61. Malo JL, Ghezzo H, L'Archeveque J, Cartier A. Late asthmatic reactions to occupational sensitizing agents: frequency of changes in nonspecific bronchial responsiveness and of response to inhaled beta-2 adrenergic agent. J Allergy Clin Immunol 1990; 85:834–842.

62. Malo JL, Ouimet G, Cartier A, Levitz D, Zeiss R. Combined alveolitis and asthma due to hexamethylene diisocyanate (HDI), with demonstration of crossed respiratory and immunologic reactivities to diphenylmethane diisocyanate (MDI). J Allergy Clin Immunol 1983; 72:413–419.

63. Lemire C, Gautrin D, Trudeau C, Ghezzo H, Desjardins A, Cartier A, Malo JL. Fever and leucocytosis accompanying asthmatic reactions due to occupational agents: frequency and associated factors. Eur Respir J 1996; 9:517–523.

64. Durham SR, Kay AB. Eosinophils, bronchial hyperreactivity and late-phase asthmatic reactions. Clin Allergy 1985; 15:411–418.

65. Vandenplas O, Cartier A, Ghezzo H, Cloutier Y, Malo JL. Response to isocyanates: effect of concentration, duration of exposure, and dose. Am Rev Respir Dis 1993; 147:1287–1290.

66. Block G, Tse KS, Kijek K, Chan H, Chan-Yeung M. Baker's asthma. Clin Allergy 1983; 13:359–370.

67. Cartier A, Malo JL, Ghezzo H, McCants M, Lehrer SB. IgE sensitization in snow crab-processing workers. J Allergy Clin Immunol 1986; 78:344–348.

68. Chai H, Farr RS, Froehlich LA, Mathison DA, McLean JA, Rosenthal RR, Sheffer AL, Spector SL, Townley RG. Standardization of bronchial inhalation challenge procedures. J Allergy Clin Immunol 1975; 56:323–327.

69. Cockcroft DW, Killian DN, Mellon JJA, Hargreave FE. Bronchial reactivity to inhaled histamine: a method and clinical survey. Clin Allergy 1977; 7:235–243.

70. Salvaggio JE, Butcher BT, O'Neil CE. Occupational asthma due to chemical agents. J Allergy Clin Immunol 1986; 78:1053–1058.

71. Cloutier Y, Lagier F, Lemieux R, Blais MC, St-Arnaud C, Cartier A, Malo JL. New methodology for specific inhalation challenges with occupational agents in powder form. Eur Respir J 1989; 2:769–777.

72. Cloutier Y, Malo JL. Update on an exposure system for particles in the diagnosis of occupational asthma. Eur Respir J 1992; 5:887–890.

73. Cloutier Y, Lagier F, Cartier A, Malo JL. Validation of an exposure system to particles for the diagnosis of occupational asthma. Chest 1992; 102:402–407.

74. Butcher BT. Inhalation challenge testing with toluene diisocyanate. J Allergy Clin Immunol 1979; 64:655–657.

75. Vandenplas O, Malo JL, Cartier A, Perreault G, Cloutier Y. Closed-circuit methodology for inhalation challenge tests with isocyanates. Am Rev Respir Dis 1991; 145:582–587.

76. Lemire C, Cloutier Y, Perrault G, Drolet D, Cartier A, Malo JL. Closed-circuit apparatus for specific inhalation challenges with an occupational agent, formaldehyde, in vapor form. Chest 1996; 109:1631–1635.

77. Cartier A, Chan H, Malo JL, Pineau L, Tse KS, Chan-Yeung M. Occupational asthma caused by eastern white cedar (*Thuja occidentalis*) with demonstration that plicatic acid is present in this wood dust and is the causal agent. J Allergy Clin Immunol 1986; 77:639–645.

78. Lemière C, Cartier A, Dolovich J, Chan-Yeung M, Grammer L, Ghezzo H, L'Archevêque J, Malo JL. Outcome of specific bronchial responsiveness to occupational agents after removal from exposure. Am J Respir Crit Care Med 1996; 154:329–333.

79. Cartier A, Malo JL, Forest F, Lafrance M, Pineau L, St-Aubin JJ, Dubois JY. Occupational asthma in snow crab-processing workers. J Allergy Clin Immunol 1984; 74:261–269.

80. Butcher BT, O'Neil CE, Reed MA, Salvaggio JE, Weill H. Development and loss of toluene diisocyanate reactivity: immunologic, pharmacologic, and provocative challenge studies. J Allergy Clin Immunol 1982; 70:231–235.

81. Pepys J, Hutchcroft BJ. Bronchial provocation tests in etiologic diagnosis and analysis of asthma. Am Rev Respir Dis 1975; 112:829–859.

82. Durham SR, Kay AB. Eosinophils, bronchial hyperreactivity and late-phase asthmatic reactions. Clin Allergy 1985; 15:411–418.

83. Séguin P, Allard A, Cartier A, Malo JL. Prevalence of occupational asthma in spray painters exposed to several types of isocyanates, including polymethylene polyphenylisocyanates. J Occup Med 1987; 29:340–344.

84. Zammit-Tabona M, Sherkin M, Kijek K, Chan H, Chan-Yeung M. Asthma caused by diphenylmethane diisocyanate in foundry workers. Clinical, bronchial provocation, and immunologic studies. Am Rev Respir Dis 1983; 128:226–230.

85. Perrin B, Cartier A, Ghezzo H, Grammer L, Harris K, Chan H, Chan-Yeung M, Malo JL. Reassessment of the temporal patterns of bronchial obstruction after exposure to occupational sensitizing agents. J Allergy Clin Immunol 1991; 87:630–639.

86. Côté J, Kennedy S, Chan-Yeung M. Sensitivity and specificity of PC_{20} and peak expiratory flow rate in cedar asthma. J Allergy Clin Immunol 1990; 85:592–598.

87. Moscato G, Godnic-Cvar J, Maestrelli P, Malo JL, Burge PS, Coifman R. Statement on self-monitoring of peak expiratory flows in the investigation of occupational asthma. J Allergy Clin Immunol 1995; 96:295–301.

88. Venables KM, Burge P Sherwood, Davison AG, Newman Taylor AJ. Peak flow rate records in surveys: reproducibility of observers' reports. Thorax 1984; 39:828–832.

89. Malo JL, Cartier A, Ghezzo H, Chan-Yeung M. Compliance with peak expiratory flow readings affects the within- and between-reader reproducibility of interpretation of graphs in subjects investigated for occupational asthma. J Allergy Clin Immunol 1996; 98:1132–1134.

90. Malo JL, Trudeau C, Ghezzo H, L'Archevêque J, Cartier A. Do subjects investigated for occupational asthma through serial PEF measurements falsify their results? J Allergy Clin Immunol 1995; 96:601–607.

91. Quirce S, Contreras G, Dybuncio A, Chan-Yeung M. Peak expiratory flow monitoring is not a reliable method for establishing the diagnosis of occupational asthma. Am J Respir Crit Care Med 1995; 152:1100–1102.

92. Malo JL, Cartier A, Boulet LP. Occupational asthma in sawmills of eastern Canada and United States. J Allergy Clin Immunol 1986; 78:392–398.

93. Carroll KB, Secombe CJP, Pepys J. Asthma due to non-occupational exposure to toluene (tolylene) diisocyanate. Clin Allergy 1976; 6:99–104.

94. Cartier A, Malo JL, Dolovich J. Occupational asthma in nurses handling psyllium. Clin Allergy 1987; 17:1–6.

95. Charles J, Bernstein A, Jones B. Hypersensitivity pneumonitis after exposure to isocyanates. Thorax 1976; 31:127–136.

96. Fink JN, Schlueter DP. Bathtub refinisher's lung: an unusual response to toluene diisocyanate. Am Rev Respir Dis 1978; 118:955–959.

97. Baur X, Dewair M, Rommelt H. Acute airway obstruction followed by hypersensitivity pneumonitis in an isocyanate (MDI) worker. J Occup Med 1984; 26(4):285–287.

98. Hendrick DJ, Marshall R, Faux JA, Krall JM. Positive ''alveolar'' responses to antigen inhalation provocation tests: their validity and recognition. Thorax 1980; 35:415–427.

99. Richerson HB, Bernstein IL, Fink JN, Hunninghake GW, Novey HS, Reed CE, Salvaggio JE, Schuyler MR, Schwartz HJ, Stechschulte DJ. Guidelines for the clinical evaluation of hypersensitivity pneumonitis. J Allergy Clin Immunol 1989; 84:839–844.

100. Fabbri LM, Boschetto P, Zocca E, Milani G, Pivirotto F, Plebani M, Burlina A, Licata B, Mapp CE. Bronchoalveolar neutrophilia during late asthmatic reactions induced by toluene diisocyanate. Am Rev Respir Dis 1987; 136:36–42.

101. Mapp C, Boschetto P, Vecchio L Dal, Crescioli S, Marzo N De, Paleari D, Fabbri LM. Protective effect of antiasthma drugs on late asthmatic reactions and increased airway responsiveness induced by toluene diisocyanate in sensitized subjects. Am Rev Respir Dis 1987; 136:1403–1407.

102. Lam S, LeRiche J, Phillips D, Chan-Yeung M. Cellular and protein changes in bronchial lavage fluid after late asthmatic reaction in patients with red cedar asthma. J Allergy Clin Immunol 1987; 80:44–50.

103. Manning PJ, Rokach J, Malo J-L, Ethier D, Cartier A, Girard Y, Charleson S, O'Byrne PM. Urinary leukotriene E4 levels during early and late asthmatic responses. J Allergy Clin Immunol 1990; 86:211–220.

13

Environmental Monitoring of Protein Aeroallergens

Charles E. Reed, Mark C. Swanson, and James T. Li
Mayo Clinic, Rochester, Minnesota

INTRODUCTION

The general principles of industrial hygiene apply in all respects to occupational allergens, just as they do for any airborne toxic agent. Differences in application of these general principles to occupational asthma arise from the requirement for specialized sampling and assay techniques and from the fact that only some workers are affected by the illness. Workers unfortunate enough to develop lung hypersensitivity to airborne antigens become ill upon exposure to very small concentrations of the agent, concentrations that have no effect on other workers. The methods of identifying the offending agents and the individual patients affected by occupational asthma are considered in other chapters. This chapter will discuss the methods of air sampling and immunochemical assay, the principles for devising means of reducing the concentration of the allergen in the air, and the procedures for follow-up monitoring to assure that the measures undertaken to control exposure continue to be effective.

PURPOSE OF AIR SAMPLING

Confirmation of Exposure as Cause of Disease

Identification of an occupation as being the source of occupational asthma has historically started with workers' or physicians' suspicions that asthma symptoms are temporally related to some occupation that uses a material that is a known or possible allergen. This suspicion is usually followed up by an epidemiological survey of the workers that includes symptom diaries, spirometry, serial peak flow measurements, and skin or RAST tests for IgE antibody to the allergen. For investigation of individual cases, inhalation challenge tests are often added to confirm that the material that evoked IgE antibody actually can cause an asthmatic response (1,2). A valuable additional, but often unused, link in the chain of evidence that a suspected allergen is the cause of occupational asthma is measurement of the allergen in the air at the worksite. Knowledge of the concentration encountered at work also allows correlation of the response of the worker to the inhalational challenge test in the laboratory to the exposure at work.

Investigation of a Plant

Where Occupational Asthma Exists

Planning a specific sampling protocol depends on the objectives appropriate to the stage of the investigation and management of the problem. In the initial phase of investigation of a plant or process suspected of being the source of occupational asthma, it is useful to confirm that the putative allergen does actually become airborne and to determine its approximate concentration at various locations within the plant. Often the manufacturing equipment, operation, or activity responsible for aerosolization of the allergen is self-evident, but there are other circumstances in which a closer evaluation of the situation through personal work-shift or task sampling will localize the time and place of the exposure and permit design of more precise and cost-effective control measures.

Monitoring the Worksite

After changes to reduce the exposure have been made, a schedule of periodic air sampling is desirable to assure that the changes have been successful in achieving the goals. When the control strategy depends upon scheduled housekeeping, cleaning, or equipment maintenance, periodic monitoring is useful to assure that the program has not lapsed.

Investigating the Spread of Allergen from the Plant to the Community

Cases of asthma from castor bean allergy have occurred in residents living downwind from castor-bean-processing plants in Ohio, South Africa, France, and Brazil (3–5). These observations suggest that allergen can escape the confines of the plant and affect nearby residents. More serious epidemics of asthma occurred during the 1980s in Barcelona, Spain (6,7). On epidemic days as many as 100 patients sought treatment for acute, severe asthma at hospitals in Barcelona. Several patients died. Epidemiological investigation identified a point source of the epidemic in the harbor on days when soybeans were being unloaded at a soybean-processing plant and weather conditions favored a slow drift of dust from the harbor over the populous part of the city. The affected patients had IgE antibody to soybean dust. On the epidemic days high concentrations of soybean sterols and a low-molecular-weight glycopeptide allergen from soybean hulls were found in the air over the city (8,41). After equipment was installed to control dust emission, the epidemics ceased and allergen was present in the air in only low concentrations. Unfortunately, the control became flawed, and the epidemics have recurred.

Individuals who live near grain elevators or cotton mills have developed asthma suspected of being due to allergy to these dusts, but this situation has not yet been fully investigated.

Establishment of Risk Levels

A final purpose of measurement of occupational allergens is to establish risk levels in the working environment (9). Two separate levels are needed: the level that sensitizes initially and the level that provokes symptoms in workers already sensitized. The first level seems to be at least an order of magnitude higher than the second. For some substances occasional very high concentrations that occur during accidental spills seem to be the main source of initial sensitization. This goal of determining threshold limit values (TLV) (10) is an obvious ideal for the future, but the situation is more complicated than the usual determination of a TLV for a toxic material because the concentration that provokes asthma in sensitized workers varies over at least two orders of magnitude. Two independent host factors account for this variability, the amount of specific IgE antibody and the degree of airway hyperresponsiveness to methacholine or histamine. Within this range of individual variability between patients, accumulation of data from a variety of occupations allows preliminary estimates of the minimum aeroallergen concentrations required to sensitize ($100-1000$ ng/m^3) and provoke symptoms (10 ng/m^3 or less). Certainly in situations where a purified allergen is aerosolized, such as enzymes, these concentration ranges will no doubt be too liberal by as much as an order of magnitude.

Immunochemical assays for specific allergens are much more sensitive than the assays for protein and should become the norm. The TLV for subtilisins (60 ng/m^3) was set because of analytical limitation and not clinical observation. This analytical limit no longer suffices and considerable thought and further study must be given to the exposure-response relationships involved with occupational asthma.

PROTOCOLS FOR MONITORING OCCUPATIONAL EXPOSURE

Monitoring Health of Exposed Workers

As in all aerobiological model systems, the health impact upon affected workers is itself a reflection of the quality of ambient air in the workplace. Thus, occurrence of frequent acute episodes of asthma or progression to chronic airways obstruction in certain worker populations should be a direct signal that environmental control is not optimal. Under certain conditions it is possible to monitor both old and newly hired employees by skin and in vitro antibody tests. If atmospheric exposure conditions have been optimally modified to prevent sensitization, previously nonsensitive and newly hired workers' tests will remain negative. For this purpose, properly performed skin prick tests are more sensitive than serological (RAST) tests, but either is appropriate. Recently, it has also been suggested that the appearance of specific IgG antibodies could be a sensitive indicator of exposure (although not of disease).

Monitoring the Air at the Worksite

A schedule of air sampling at the place of maximum concentration should be established to assure that the control measures are effective when they are installed and continue to be effective during production or regular operation. This is particularly important when control depends upon proper housekeeping and equipment maintenance. The optimum sampling procedure will vary with the particular circumstances. It may include area or personal sampling and may be periodic or continuous. The concentration of any allergen can be measured in the air provided a reliable reference standard of the allergen and a specific antiserum are available (Table 1).

METHODS

The principles for measuring the amount of protein allergens in the air are the same as those for measuring any chemical substance. Only the method of the assay differs. If it is desired to quantify the amount of viable microorganisms in the air, either culture techniques or counting particles deposited on a microscope slide using morphological criteria

Table 1   Occupational Aeroallergens for Which
Immunochemical Assays Have Been Developed

Chilled water air-conditioner-humidifier slime
   Textile manufacturing plants, office buildings
Micro-organisms
   Aspergillus fumigatus dairy barns
Thermophilic actinomycetes—dairy barns
Enzymes
   Esperase-detergent packaging
   Papain-meat packing
   Bromelin-clinical laboratory
Insects (39,40)
   Honey bee, honey-packing houses
   Blowflies
   Cockroaches
Mites
   Storage mites—dairy barns, grain dust
Animal derived
   Rats, mice, guinea pig—laboratory animal quarters
   Cows—dairy barns
   Parakeets—bird breeder rooms
   Hen's egg protein—egg-processing plants
Plant derived
   Ragweed—dairy bum
   Grass
   Soybean—grain dust
   Tomato pollen—greenhouse
Natural rubber latex
Flour

for identification are preferred. These techniques not only are very sensitive, but also allow taxonomic classification (11). The following section will describe methods for quantifying nonviable amorphous proteins (12–15). First, however, one additional point should be mentioned. Many occupations involve exposure to complex dusts that contain concentrations of endotoxin sufficient to cause acute febrile illness (16). Many of these workers develop acute and chronic airway obstruction that could be considered a form of asthma. It is possible to measure endotoxin in the air at such worksites using a *Limulus* amebolysates assay (17).

Air-Sampling Equipment

Depending on the concentration of an airborne allergen, the volume of air that will allow sufficient concentrations of allergen to be collected for accurate analysis may vary from 0.5 m^3 to 1000 m^3. Since flow rates generally are fixed on most sampling devices, the run times are varied to accommodate the required collection volume. Longer sampling periods have the disadvantage of lessened ability to correlate temporal changes in concentration with specific activities that generate exposure (Fig. 1A).

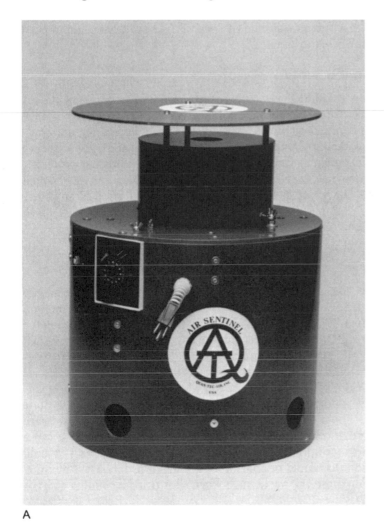

A

Figure 1 (A) Automated sampler for unattended collection of serial air samples on a programmed schedule. Flow rate = 1 l/sec; 110 VAC (Quan-Tec-Air, Rochester, MN).

Fig. continues

Area Sampling

Properly located area samplers operated at flow rates of 1–3 L/sec provide samples large enough to quantify allergens present in sufficient amounts to be clinically significant. Area sampling is a suitable way to provide information about the general presence or absence of exposure and to confirm the identity of the allergen. In addition, area sampling allows comparison of different parts of the plant and changes in concentration over time in the same location. Being relatively simple and unobtrusive, it is suitable for long-term monitoring of the success of control measures. Automated samplers are available with programmable filter-changing devices to simplify collection of sequential samples and avoid overloading the filter (Fig. 1).

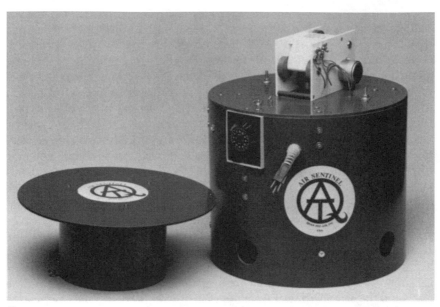

B

Figure 1   (B) A view of the sampler's cassette, which holds the filter medium and takes up samples as they are completed.

Particle Sizing

The behavior of aerosol particles inhaled into the lung depends upon their aerodynamic properties, which in turn depend upon their size, density, and shape (18). Deposition of particles along the airways is not only determined by these aerodynamic properties, but is also influenced by the rate of airflow and patterns of respiration. For example, during nasal breathing particles of 20 μm aerodynamic diameter and larger (such as pollen grains) are virtually all removed on the turbinates. Only about half of particles 5 μm and smaller pass through the nose to the thoracic airways. Particles with aerodynamic diameter less than 10 μm are considered "respirable." Aerodynamic diameter, or "mean mass aerodynamic diameter," is calculated from the particles' terminal settling velocity by comparison with spheres of unit density and is a function of the shape, size, and density of the aerosol particles. Aerosols generated by nebulizers for therapy and aerosols used experimentally to study deposition and clearance are more or less unit density spheres, but occupational dusts often have complex fibrous shapes and may form irregular, noncompact aggregates. Thus, their behavior is not determined solely by their size or density. Particles can deposit in the airways in four ways: sedimentation, inertial impaction, interception, and diffusion. Sedimentation by gravity depends upon the density and diameter of the particles, and for particles that are more or less spherical, sedimentation is the chief means of deposition in large airways. Inertial impaction occurs when the direction of the airstream is changed by curving or branching. The particles tend to follow the original path of the airstream and deposit on the epithelium through inertia. In the airways inertial impaction is the chief means of deposition in the nose and is important in the central airways where flow rates are high. Interception is an important mechanism of deposition of fibrous particles and other particles of irregular shape. Long fibers less than 3 μm in diameter and as long as 200 μm tend to stay oriented longitudinally in the airstream and can penetrate

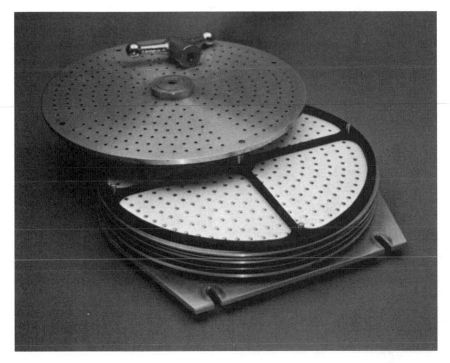

Figure 2 Model GMW 65000 Andersen cascade impaction particle sizing head for collection of particles in discrete size ranges (Andersen Samplers, Atlanta, GA).

deeply into the lung. Alveolar deposition of asbestos fibers is an example. Diffusion, the chief way gases react with the airways, is responsible for deposition of submicrometer-sized particles. Most particles of this size are expelled in the expired air, however. Thus, it is often of interest to determine the particle size and aerodynamic behavior of allergenic aerosols. Anderson cascade impaction heads for high-volume samplers are available for this purpose (Fig. 2). Figure 3 illustrates the morphology of particles separated by this device after several hours of operation in a rat animal care room. Note especially the filaments, presumably rat hairs, that have penetrated to the final stage with spherical particles smaller than the diameter of the fiber. The amount of allergen or medication carried in a droplet of 5 μm is 1000-fold more than that in a droplet 10 times smaller, 0.5 μm, so it is more valuable to know the total amount of allergen in various aerodynamic sizes than the number of particles.

Personal Sampling

Equipment that samples the air in the personal breathing zone is useful for defining the particular tasks in the job that are associated with heavy, and therefore dangerous, exposure (Fig. 4).

Such sampling also allows evaluation of the success of changes in the manufacturing equipment, ventilation, air filtration, and job performance at particular sites or tasks. Either area sampling or personal sampling allows estimation of time-weighted average of exposure. It is not yet established, however, whether brief, heavy exposures are more likely to cause disease than prolonged, light exposures, so it is not clear whether time-weighted

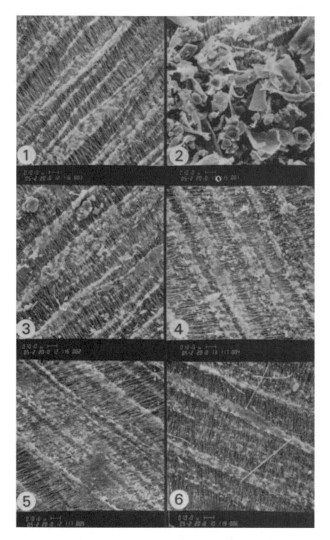

Figure 3 Scanning electron photomicrographs (×500) of PTFE media supporting sized particles from different mean mass aerodynamic diameter size ranges: (1) unexposed; (2) >9.4; (3) 9.4–4.5; (4) 4.5–2.7; (5) 2.7–1.6; (6) <1.6 μm. Note the fibers (probably hair) collected along with particles <1.6 μm. These fibers have oriented themselves in such a way as to attain a mean mass aerodynamic diameter similar to small particles.

averages carry the same biological significance for allergen exposure that they do for toxin exposure.

Filter Medium and Sample Preparation

Proper filter medium is essential for success. The filter should offer low resistance to the air being sampled and yet have efficient retention of respirable particles. It should not denature the protein; it should not adsorb the allergen, but permit high yields of recovery; and it should allow (Figs. 3 and 4) extraction of the allergen in small volumes (1 ml or

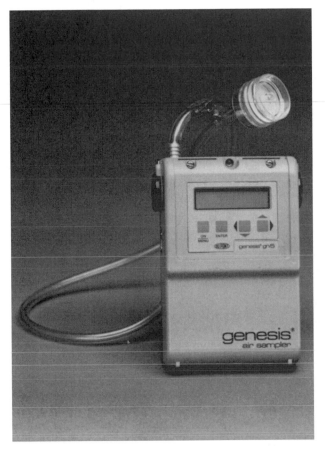

Figure 4 Battery-powered, portable air sampler for collection of personal breathing zone samples. The pump is typically worn on the hip. Flow rate: 1–5 L/min (E.I. DuPont de Nemours & Co., Kenneth Square, PA).

less) so that concentration of the extract is not needed. Concentration not only adds to the cost of the assay but may cause loss of allergen through denaturation or adsorption. Poly-tetrafluoroethylene (PTFE, or Teflon) has proven to be the most satisfactory filter medium (Quan-Tec-Air, Rochester, MN). During the process of development and validation of an assay for a new allergen, it is desirable to determine the stability of the allergen on the filter and the efficiency of the extraction procedure.

Although rigorous determinations have been done for only a few allergens, it appears that exposed dry filters can be stored for several months at $-20°C$ without significant loss of allergen. After extraction many allergens are unstable in aqueous solutions, partly because of inherent instability, and partly because of enzymatic activity of proteases in the solution. Lyophilization is an appropriate means of stabilizing some extracts, but many allergens are denatured by freeze drying. We have found it most practical to perform the extraction of the PTFE filter membranes in a 50% glycerin buffer and then to store the extract at $-20°C$. Of course, the reference standards for subsequent assays should also be prepared in the 50% glycerin buffer.

Radioimmunoassay

Allergen Reference Standards

A desirable goal for expressing allergen concentrations would be a purified protein standard for each allergen in question and monoclonal antibodies to the allergen. Unfortunately, this goal is at present unrealistic, so it is necessary to settle for less rigorous reference preparations. Choice of a working standard depends upon the circumstances. If the allergen is a single protein such as papain, the standard may be a purified protein and the results can be expressed in mass units. More often the exposure involves complex dusts such as humidifier sludge, grain dust, or rat urine, which are mixtures of many allergenic molecules from several different microbial, plant, or animal sources. In such cases it is necessary to prepare a reference extract of the crude material that is used or generated as a result of the occupation and is likely to be the source of the allergen exposure (19–22). It is also useful to confirm that this material has the relevant allergens by immunoblotting because many sources contain a complex mixture of allergens. Results of the assay can be expressed in terms of the protein content of this extract or in terms of some arbitrary unit assigned to the reference preparation. Such assays are internally consistent within a single experiment, and if the reference preparation is reasonably stable, the results are consistent over the shelf life of the reference preparation. For consistency between laboratories it is desirable for investigators to exchange reagents and work toward establishment of internationally accepted reference standards. If the particular exposure is widespread affecting many workers in many plants, it may be cost-effective to identify and isolate the responsible molecule(s) and to prepare monoclonal antibodies, both for the purpose of allergen standardization and for the purpose of assay reproducibility.

Antibody Source

Several kinds of antibodies are suitable for radioimmunoassay. When they are available, two monoclonal antibodies directed to different epitopes on an allergenic molecule are the most suitable. One antibody serves as a capture antibody; the other after radioiodination serves as detecting antibody. A high-titer polyclonal animal or human antiserum can also be adapted to a two-site assay or can be used for inhibition assays. For the two-site assay the whole serum can serve as the capture antibody, and the affinity-purified antibody from it serves as the detection antibody. In monoclonal systems unfractionated mouse ascites fluid serves well for capture antibody, but the detection antibody should be purified by a protein A column. One advantage of the monoclonal system is that the antibody is available in unlimited amounts as long as the clone is maintained. An advantage of the animal or human IgG system over the human IgE system is that the serum can be diluted 100- or 1000-fold, so a reasonable-sized serum collection will suffice for many assays. The antibody remains stable for several years stored at −70°C.

For some applications it is best to employ human IgE antibody. It may be the only antiserum available and has the advantage of assuring that the substance causing the disease is being measured when the identity of the allergenic molecules is uncertain or the dust contains a complex mixture of allergens. If a human IgE system is adopted for the study, it is desirable to obtain a large pool, at least 500 ml from each of 5–10 donors, to assure sufficient antibody to complete the entire project.

Two-Site Assays

For most applications we have found the two-site assay to be the simplest to perform and the most sensitive (Fig. 5). It has the additional advantage over inhibition assays of being

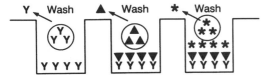

2-Site Radioimmunoassay

Y Antibodies (antigen specific)

▲ Antigens (allergens)

* Radioisotopic tracers
(labeled purified antibodies)

Figure 5 Two-site radioimmunoassay for airborne allergens. (Left) A capture antibody (monoclonal if available, or polyclonal animal or human IgG antibody) to the allergen is absorbed non-specifically to plastic microliter plates. (Center) Either known amounts of the allergen standard or the unknown sample is added. Allergen binds to the antibody. (Right) A radiodinated antibody (either a monoclonal antibody to a second epitope on the allergen molecule or affinity-purified polyclonal IgG) is added and binds to a second site on the allergen. The amount of radioactivity is a measure of the amount of allergen.

accurate over a several-log range of protein concentrations. Thus, it is usually not necessary to perform a preliminary assay to determine the appropriate sample dilution. The assay is performed in microliter wells that have been designed to adsorb proteins efficiently. We use Immulon II or Immulon IV Removawell strips (Dynatech Labs, Alexandria, VA). The serum or ascites fluid containing the polyclonal or monoclonal capture antibody is diluted in 20–200 mM carbonate buffer at pH 9.2 and 100 μl added to wells of the microliter plate, which is then incubated overnight at room temperature in a humid chamber and the wells washed. The appropriate antibody dilution must be determined for each new assay system to provide conditions of substantial antibody excess.

The albumin and other nonspecific proteins in the serum or ascites fluid usually suffice to block all protein-binding sites on the plate, but this needs to be confirmed experimentally for each system. The second step is to add 100 μl of the air sample extract, an internal standard, and dilutions of the reference standard antigen preparation. After a second overnight incubation and washing, the radioiodinated detection antibody is added. After the third incubation, the wells are washed, separated, and counted. The incubations are performed in a humid chamber at room temperature.

In addition to two-site monoclonal assays and polyclonal assays using affinity-purified antibody, it is possible to use an animal polyclonal antiserum for capture and a human IgE-antibody-containing serum for detection. The amount of IgE antibody bound to the plate in this sandwich assay is measured with radiolabeled anti-IgE.

The results are calculated using a log-logit transformed least-squares regression equation. In graphic terms, the x-axis is designated $\log_{10}$ of the antigen concentration. The y-axis is designated $\log_{10}$ of the percent of the maximum of the total counts bound, where

$$y = \mathrm{Ln} \ - \ \frac{\text{binding/binding}_{(max)}}{1 \ - \ \text{binding/binding}_{(max)}}$$

Concentrations of the unknown are then interpolated from the standard regression curve (23).

Inhibition Assays

Inhibition assays are used when only a single antibody is available. The first step is to prepare a solid-phase allergen. Although cyanogen-activated paper discs, microcrystalline cellulose, or Sepharose can be used to prepare the solid phase, we have found the Immulon wells described above to be more convenient, reproducible, and sensitive. The optimum adsorption conditions of protein concentration and buffer strength and pH must be determined for each new allergen system. After the allergen has been adsorbed, the remaining protein-binding sites on the well must be blocked with an inert protein such as human albumin. Then the concentration of antiserum needed for maximum antibody binding should be determined for each serum pool. It is important that the amount of allergen on the plate be in considerable excess and oriented properly so that sufficient antibody is bound to give a strong signal. A reference curve of inhibition by serial doubling dilutions of the reference allergen standard is constructed, and the results of individual samples are calculated along with an internal standard.

After the details of the assay conditions have been established, fresh antigen-coated plates should be prepared for each batch of assays. Fifty microliters of the air sample extract (or internal standard or dilutions of the reference allergen extract to construct the standard curve) and 50 μl of antiserum are added to duplicate wells. After overnight incubation in a humid chamber at room temperature, the wells are washed and the radioiodinated detection reagent added. For IgG antibody this reagent can be a monoclonal antibody to the gamma chain or *staphylococcus* protein A; for IgE it is an affinity-purified rabbit antibody to the epsilon chain. After the final incubation and washing, the wells are counted. If the allergen concentration falls outside the range of the inhibition assay, it should be repeated with appropriate dilutions of the sample. The results are calculated using a log-linear transformation where the *x*-axis is designated log of the antigen concentration and the *y*-axis percent inhibition. Percent inhibition is defined as counts bound when the antigen standard or unknown is mixed with the antibody pool subtracted from counts bound by the antibody pool alone, divided by the counts bound by the antibody pool, all multiplied by 100.

Modification for ELISA

If solid-phase, enzyme-linked assays are desired, the Immulon plate assays described above can be modified by coupling the detecting antibody to an enzyme instead of labeling it with radioiodine. After the final incubation the color substrate is added, the color developed for an appropriate time, and the reaction terminated. The results are read in a spectrophotometric plate reader. Careful attention to the temperature and duration of the color development step is critical for reproducible results.

Amplification Procedures

The sensitivity for both radioimmunoassay and enzyme-linked assay can be increased severalfold by amplifying the detection step with biotin-avidin. The detection antibody is biotinylated instead of iodinated, and the final detection reagent is radioiodinated or enzyme-conjugated streptavidin. This amplification of sensitivity may be useful for personal sampling studies in which only small air volumes can be collected.

Quality Control

Although all the usual laboratory quality control procedures apply, some are particularly worth mentioning. The air samplers must be calibrated and the flow rate determined under the actual conditions of operation. Because calculation of the results is based on the volume of air drawn through the sampler, it is also of the utmost importance that the duration of the sampling period be accurately recorded. Precise records of extraction volumes as well as test volumes for air samples are required for proper dilution and aliquot factors to be used for final calculations of allergen per cubic meter of air. Because degradation of the reagents can lead to serious error in results, appropriate controls must be used in every assay. For samples batched together in a single assay, an internal standard is included to demonstrate consistent assay performance with respect to previous assays. For samples taken over extended periods and groups of them assayed in several assays, control standards are needed for the assay performance and accuracy of the assay from time to time with respect to sample quantification.

MEASUREMENTS TO CONTROL EXPOSURE TO OCCUPATIONAL ALLERGENS

The aim of controlling exposure is, of course, to reduce the concentration of the allergen in the air below the level that causes disease. In principle, two levels of allergen need to be considered: the level that initiates the sensitization in the first place and the level that elicits reactions in already sensitized subjects. Unfortunately, reliable information about either of these levels is still unavailable for most allergens, but it appears that in general, sensitizing levels are considerably higher and that occasional very high levels (for example, spills of toluene diisocyanate) are particularly likely to sensitize. After sensitization has occurred, much lower allergen levels can elicit reactions. For diisocyanates and similar chemicals, the eliciting level is of the order of $1-30$ ng/m^3 (9). From what we know about protein allergens, they appear to fall in this same order of magnitude. Therefore, the goal of allergen abatement is to control both the occasional peak concentrations and the usual steady-state concentration. Preventing spills or other accidental reasons for occasional high concentrations is usually a matter of following proper operating procedures and of design and proper maintenance of the manufacturing, cleaning, and air-handling equipment.

The steady-state concentration of any indoor air pollutant is determined by ratio between the rate of production of the pollutant and the rate of its removal (24). The general mass balance equation describing the ratio is:

$$C_{ss} = \frac{Pq_vC_o + S}{E_vQ_v + NE_dQ_d}$$

C_{ss} represents steady-state concentration; the numerator represents the rate of generation of allergen, the denominator the rate of removal. PC_vC_o is the outdoor source term; P is an empirically derived penetration factor, which for respirable-sized particles can be assumed to be 1. Q_v equals ventilation rate; C_o is outdoor concentration. For most occupational allergens the outdoor source term is zero. S is indoor source substance generation rate. It has two components: de novo generation into the air and resuspension of settled allergen from dust. E_vQ_v, is removal by ventilation. E_v is ventilation efficiency, calculated from the ratio of the concentration in the exhaust air to concentration in the occupied space divided by a mixing factor. In spaces where air is recirculated and mixing is good, E_v can reasonably be assumed to be 1. Q_v is ventilation rate. K is natural decay rate (settling for particulates). NE_dQ_d is removal rate by air cleaning; N is cleaner removal efficiency; E_d is device ventilation efficiency analogous to E_v; and Q_d is device flow rate. Reduction in steady-state concentrations can be achieved by three different strategies: (1) prevent or reduce aerosolization at the source, (2) increase ventilation and air filtration, and (3) use personal respiratory protective equipment. Choice of one of these strategies or of a combination of them depends on the particular situation.

Prevent Aerosolization of the Allergen at the Source

From the above considerations it is apparent that the most desirable means of controlling exposure is to eliminate the antigen at the source. Sometimes it is possible to substitute a nonallergenic material, or it may be possible to substitute a less volatile chemical, for example, MDI for TDI in polyurethane processes. Sometimes the source of the allergen is some contaminating agent that can be removed. For example, an outbreak of hypersensitivity pneumonitis occurred among employees of nylon-manufacturing plants who worked in areas supplied by air from a chilled water cooling and humidification system (14). They and most of their fellow workers developed antibody to antigens extracted from the slime growing in the water reservoirs of this system. Inhalation challenge with these antigen preparations reproduced an acute episode of the disease (25). A number of engineering changes were made, including carefully controlled chlorination of the water. The slime was eradicated. Airborne concentrations of the slime antigens declined rather slowly because of considerable residual material in inaccessible ducts, but eventually the concentration inside the plant was reduced and the goal of keeping indoor levels lower than those outdoors was achieved. Parenthetically, these antigens that arise from a variety of organisms are ubiquitous, being detectable in low concentrations in outdoor air, stagnant water, and soil. After these changes were effected, no new cases of hypersensitivity pneumonitis developed, and newly hired workers did not develop antibody, although the original workers' antibody levels declined very slowly. From these observations it is possible to estimate roughly the minimum allergen concentrations required to sensitize ($100-1000$ ng/m^3) and to elicit symptoms ($1-10$ ng/ml). Eradication of the source was possible in this and similar cases because the antigen was not necessary to the purpose of the plant (26).

When the allergen is an integral part of the product, such as *Bacillus subtilis* enzyme in the detergent industry (27), eradication is not an option, and other means of reducing the amount of airborne allergen must be sought. In one instance, to reduce the concentration of the enzyme, the process used the enzyme encapsulated in granular form to reduce dust generation, and although it was not possible to eliminate the allergen from the air entirely, concentrations were reduced (28). However, measurable amounts remained in submicrometer-sized particles, and a few cases of occupational asthma occurred in employees who continue to work in a well-controlled environment. Newly hired workers may develop positive skin tests to the enzyme. This instance of occupational asthma illustrates the difficulty of determining threshold limit values for allergens because of the wide variation among individuals of the concentration that elicits sensitization and provoke symptoms.

Sometimes the allergen is a component of the product. This is the case with natural rubber proteins associated with powdered latex examination gloves. Health care environments using powdered latex gloves will likely have measurable concentrations of natural rubber allergens in the air. The measured concentrations vary up to 1000-fold. This is a situation where the source can be eliminated, modified, or selected. The allergens are carried on cornstarch particles and become airborne during donning and removal of the gloves. Allergic sensitization to these rubber proteins has been recognized in significant numbers of health care workers who developed sinusitis and asthma. Concentrations in 10 medical center worksites where rubber gloves were frequently used ranged from 13 to 121 ng/m^3 and in areas where rubber gloves were seldom or never used ranged from 0.3 to 1.8 ng/m^3. Concentrations in operating suites ranged from 53 to 208 ng/m^3. Personal breathing zone concentrations for health care workers in high rubber glove use areas ranged from 8 to 974 ng/m^3. Aeroallergen concentrations in nine dental offices, all using powdered gloves, ranged from 2 to 52 ng/m^3 (29). Particle sizing for natural rubber allergens demonstrated allergen distribution throughout all particle sizes, but predominantly in particles greater than 7 microns, mass median aerodynamic diameter. Although most of the allergen is carried on large particles, the amount of allergen that is carried on smaller particles is sufficient to provoke asthma and lower respiratory symptoms in sensitized individuals. The use of powder-free gloves is an obvious solution to eliminate airborne exposure. Measurement of allergen content in latex gloves and selecting low-allergen gloves for use is another option (30).

Improve Ventilation and Air Filtration

In some occupations the source of allergen generation cannot be controlled. One example is laboratory animal handling, where the source is the animal itself, chiefly the urine (31,32). In this occupation, ventilation and filtration techniques are the only ones that are feasible. Our measurements indicate that male mice, rats, and guinea pigs shed very large amounts of urinary allergens into the air, about 2, 20, and 200 ng/min per animal, respectively.

In a typical rat care room housing 250–300 rats with ventilation above the recommended ventilation rate of 15 changes of air per hour, we found the concentration of rat urinary protein allergen to range around 200 ng/m^3. In a room with only 30 animals and relatively low concentrations of allergen, doubling the air-exchange ratio by recirculating air through high-efficiency particle absolute filter (HEPA) reduced the concentration in half. But in a similar room with 300 animals, the HEPA filter had a negligible effect because the total allergen production rate was so high, about 6 g/min. To effectively reduce the steady-state allergen concentration in such a room required increasing the filtration with laminar flow, HEPA-filtered isolation cages (Fig. 6) to 172 changes of air per hour. This is about 100 times the air-exchange rate in most homes and offices. Particle sizing using the Andersen impaction head allowed assessment of the distribution of allergens in

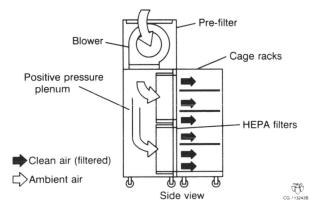

Figure 6 Schematic design of a laminar flow, HEPA-filtered small animal isolation racking system (Forma Scientific, Mallinckrodt, Marietta, OH).

particles of defined size ranges. Allergen was found in all particle size ranges (see Fig. 3) (32). Sampling with a different device yielded similar results (33).

Area air sampling is useful for confirmation and identification of possible air quality problems, but sometimes the data may mislead the investigator as to actual individual exposure during particular tasks. Even when an indoor environment can be defined and steady-state air concentrations measured, an individual's exposure within that work environment may vary considerably. Studies involving animal handlers, both laboratory technicians and animal care workers, have illustrated this point very well. Area samples were taken in animal housing rooms and personal samples were taken during full work shifts and during discrete tasks that were 15 min–1 1/2 hr in duration (Fig. 6). The personal samples included times in the animal rooms exclusively as well as times outside these confines. In general, time-weighted average exposures calculated from the area and full shift samples indicate similar values. However, discrete task samples frequently indicate much heavier exposures, up to an order of magnitude or more. When monitoring a worker performing a specific duty, important information is obtained regarding procedures, task-related equipment, and actual task performance simply by the personal exposure an individual receives. From this information recommendations about procedural changes and equipment changes or modifications can be made objectively and with confidence. For example, this was the case when some workers emptied the bedding into open, unvented garbage cans and received substantial exposure, while others used HEPA-filtered waste disposal stations and their exposures were below limits of detection (Fig. 7).

Individual Protection Equipment

It appears that it will rarely be feasible to reduce allergen by increasing ventilation or air filtration rates in most occupations to ambient levels that will not elicit symptoms in sensitized workers. Instead, workers can use individual protective equipment (34). Masks or laminar flow helmets have been reported to reduce allergic symptoms and anecdotally are useful in many situations (Fig. 8). Also, it is possible to provide work stations with airflow characteristics that minimize exposure during specific tasks. In theory, at least, full protective equipment with an outside air supply could be useful but does not seem a practical solution.

In summary, the principles of dealing with working environments where occupational respiratory disease occurs are no different when the disease is asthma than they are when the disease is pneumonoconiosis or any other respiratory illness. Choice of abatement strategies depends upon the particular process, the physical structure of the equipment, and the rate of aerosolization of the allergen. When feasible, primary effort should be placed on preventing aerosolization. Increased ventilation and air filtration are feasible only when allergen production rate is low or localized to areas where exhaust fans can remove the allergen before it reaches the workers' breathing zone. Masks or other personal respiratory protective equipment may be useful in circumstances of unavoidable exposure.

ILLUSTRATIONS OF APPLICATION

We have mentioned several applications above, but two additional examples illustrate other points. Employee exposure to the enzyme papain in a meat-portioning facility caused allergic symptoms and asthma in some workers. In this case, a single, relatively pure and defined protein was the aeroallergen of interest. For this purpose a commercially available

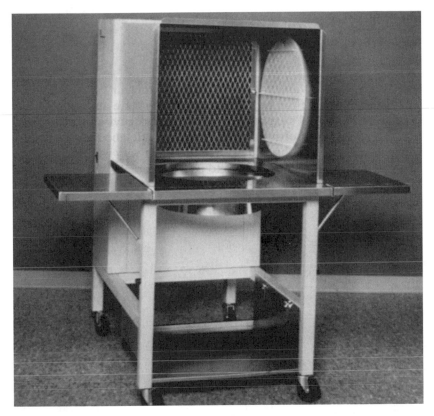

Figure 7 HEPA-filtered waste disposal station found effective at reducing animal allergen exposure of animal caretakers (Forma Scientific, Mallinckrodt, Marietta, OH).

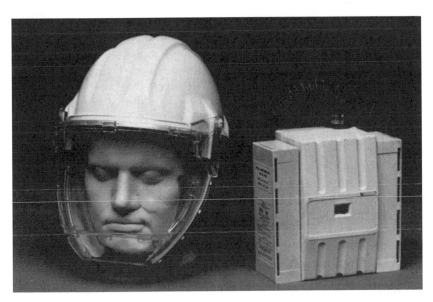

Figure 8 HEPA-filtered laminar flow helmet for protection against airborne particulates which include allergens (Racal Airstream, Frederick, MD).

rabbit antibody specific for papain proved useful. This polyclonal antibody was adsorbed to the surface of plastic rnicrotiter wells and used as a capture antibody. The specific antibodies were isolated by affinity column chromatography and radiolabeled for papain detection in a two-site sandwich assay. The approach yielded a specific, highly sensitive assay for papain capable of measuring picogram quantities of the enzyme. This allowed personal air samples to be collected and effective measurement of papain exposure during discrete tasks. Although most personal exposures were in hundreds of nanograms per cubic meter, some ranged upward well into micrograms per cubic meter of air. Area air samples demonstrated low-nanogram to microgram quantities of papain and on the whole indicated widespread distribution of the enzyme throughout the plant. Task sampling effectively identified personnel and certain tasks as the main sources of allergen dispersion. Interestingly, one of the most effective exposure control measures was frequent changing of work clothing (35).

Another example illustrates the problem more than the solution. Workers in plants where raw eggs are processed into liquid or powdered egg products may develop asthma from allergy to inhaled egg white protein (36,37). These plants process 1.5 million eggs a day. In a continuous operation the eggs are cracked, the shells blown away, and the whites separated from the yolk. Liquid whole egg or the separated egg white and yolk are pumped to refrigerated storage. Subsequently, the liquid is pumped through high-pressure spray nozzles into a drying oven. The dried product is picked up by a vacuum and transported to a cyclone separator, sifted, and packaged. Workers are exposed to aerosolized liquid egg products in the transfer and breaker rooms and to powdered egg yellow or white dust in the packaging room. Immunoassay of air samples in such a plant showed extraordinarily high levels of egg protein, hundreds of micrograms per cubic meter of air for ovalbumin, ovomucoid, and lysozyme (38). In this application, quantification of separate and specific egg white components is possible from a simple air sample. Worker's sera containing specific IgE are used in inhibition assays allowing quantification of many individual egg protein components making up a total airborne allergen load rarely ever seen. The concentrations of these egg proteins are so high that an air sample taken in a worker's bedroom demonstrated a level of 50 ng/m^3 of ovalbumin. This allergen was carried home on the worker's clothing. Concentrations of various allergens in other work environments are listed in Table 2. In egg-processing plants appropriate means of reducing exposure have not yet been devised. The plants supply filtered air to the breaking and packaging rooms to maintain positive pressure in accordance with U. S. Department of Agriculture guidelines. Total dust levels are often in accord with accepted values for nontoxic nuisance dusts, but are clearly much too high for a potent allergen. Even increasing ventilation 10-fold is not likely to be able to keep up with this extraordinary source. Major changes in the design of the egg cracking and transferring equipment will be required to prevent aerosolization of the egg proteins into the working environment.

SUMMARY

New immunological methods have been developed for measuring ambient exposure to protein allergens. When applied to the workplace setting, such methods have been utilized to monitor exposure to occupational allergens in a variety of industries. Further studies are required to determine the exposure-response relationships between ambient allergen exposure levels and the occurrence of occupational asthma. Although not currently available, data generated from future studies may allow establishment of allowable exposure

Table 2 Maximum Concentrations of Aeroallergens in Various Locations

Agent	Approximate concentration	Location
Micropolyspora faeni	2700 μg/m^3	Dairy barn during bedding chopping
Thermoactinomyces vulgaris	187 μg/m^3	Dairy barn during bedding chopping
Aspergillus fumigatus	1.2 μg/m^3	Quiet dairy barn in winter
Loliun perennae	0.085 μg/m^3	Quiet dairy barn in winter
Lepidoglyphus destructor (storage mite)	12 μg/m^3	Quiet dairy barn in winter
Mus musculua urinary protein	0.06 μg/m^3	Animal quarters
Rattus norvegicus urinary	1.2 μg/m^3	Animal quarters
Guinea pig urinary protein	17 μg/m^3	Animal quarters
Bos domesticus epithelium	16 μg/m^3	Quiet dairy barn in winter
Egg albumin	360 μg/m^3	Egg-processing plant
Papain	5 μg/m^3	Meat-processing plant
Esperase	0.18 μg/m^3	Detergent-packing plant
Humidifier slime protein	15 μg/m^3	Nylon-production plant
Natural rubber protein (latex)	1 μg/m^3	Surgical suite

limits that prevent respiratory sensitization in workers. In addition, such methods allow evaluation of the efficacy of industrial hygiene or process modification measures aimed at reducing airborne exposure to a sensitizing substance.

ACKNOWLEDGMENTS

This work was supported by NIAID #AI21255, Mayo Clinic and Foundation, and Minnesota Lung Foundation.

REFERENCES

1. Novey HS, Bernstein IL, Mihalas LS, Terr AI, Yunginger JW. Guidelines for the clinical evaluation of occupational asthma due to high molecular weight (HMW) allergens. Report of the Subcommittee on the Clinical Evaluation of Occupational Asthma due to HMW Allergens. J Allergy Clin Immunol 1989; 84(5 Pt 2):829–833.
2. Bush RK, Kagen SL. Guidelines for the preparation and characterization of high molecular weight allergens used for the diagnosis of occupational lung disease. Report of the Subcommittee on Preparation and Characterization of High Molecular Weight Allergens. J. Allergy Clin Immunol 1989; 84(5 Pt 2):814–819.
3. Figley KD, Elrod, RH. Endemic asthma due to castor bean dust. JAMA 1928; 90:79–82.
4. Ordman D. An outbreak of bronchial asthma in South Africa, affecting more than 200 persons, caused by castor bean dust from an oil-processing factory. Int Arch Allergy Appl Immunol 1955; 7:10–24.
5. Mendes E, Ulhoa Cintra A. Collective asthma, simulating an epidemic, provoked by castor-bean dust. J Allergy 1954; 25:253–259.

6. Anto J M, Sunyer J. Asthma Collaborative Group of Barcelona. A point-source asthma outbreak. Lancet 1986; 1:900–903.

7. Anto JM, Sunyer J, Rodriquez-Rosin R, Searey-Cervera M, Vasquez L. Community outbreaks of asthma and the toxic epidemiological committee associated with the inhalation of soybean dust. N Engl J Med 1989; 320:1097–1102.

8. Anto JM, Grimalt J, Aceves M, Reed CE. Outbreak of asthma associated with soybean dust. N Engl J Med 1990; 321:1128 (letter).

9. NIOSH. Criteria for a recommended standard. Occupational exposure to diisocyanates. U. S. Department of Health, Education and Welfare. Public Health Service. Centers for Disease Control. DHEW (NIOSH) publication, 1978; 78–215.

10. Threshold Limit Values and Biological Exposure Indices for 1987–1988. SCGIH, Cincinnati, OH: American Conference of Governmental Industrial Hygienists, 1987.

11. Solomon WR. Airborne microbial allergens: Impact and risk assessment. Toxicol Ind Health 1990; 6:309–324.

12. Swanson MC, Agarwal MK, Reed CE. An immunochemical approach to indoor acroallergen quantitation with a new volumetric air sampler. Studies with mite, roach, cat, mouse and guinea pig antigens. J Allergy Clin Immunol 1985; 76:724–729.

13. Reed CE, Swanson MC, Agarwal MK, Yunginger JW. Allergens that cause asthma. Identification and quantification. Chest 1985; 87:40S–44S.

14. Reed CE, Swanson MC, Lopez M, Ford AM, Major J, Witmer WB, Valdes TB. Measurement of IgG antibody and airborne antigen to control an industrial outbreak of hypersensitivity pneumonitis. J Occup Med 1983: 25:207–210.

15. Campbell AR, Swanson MC, Reed CE, May JJ, Pratt DS. Aeroallergens in dairy barns near Cooperstown, NY and Rochester, MN. Am Rev Respir Dis 1989; 140:317–320.

16. James AL, Zimmerman MJ, El H, Ryan G, Musk AW. Exposure to grain dust and changes in lung function. Br J Ind Med 1990; 47:466–472.

17. Milton DK, Gere RJ, Feldman HA, Greaves IA. Endotoxin measurement: aerosol sampling and application of a new limulus method. Am Ind Hyg Assoc J 1990; 51:331–337.

18. Parkes WR. Occupational Lung Disorders, 2nd ed. London: Butterworths 1982:42–53.

19. Schroeckenstein DC, Meier-Davis S, Yunginger JW, Bush RK. Allergens involved in occupational asthma caused by baby's breath (*Gypsophila paniculata*). J Allergy Clin Immunol 1990; 86:189–193.

20. Sutton R, Skerritt JH, Baldo BA, Wrigley CW. The diversity of allergens involved in bakers' asthma. Clin Allergy 1984; 14:93–107.

21. Davison AG, Britton MG, Foffester J A, Davies R J, Hughes DT. Asthma in merchant seamen and laboratory workers caused by allergy to castor beans: analysis of allergens. Clin Allergy 1983; 13:553–561.

22. Baur X, Weiss W, Sauer W, Fruhmann G, Kimm KW, Ulmer WT, Mezger VA, Woitowitz HJ, Steurich FK. Backmiittel als Mitursache des Backerasthmas. Deutsch Med Wochenschr 1988; 113:1275–1278.

23. Rodbard D, Hutt DM. Statistical analysis of radioimmunoassay and immunoradiometric (labeled antibody) assays: a generalized weighted, iterative, least squares method for logistic curve filling. In: Symposium on Radioimmunoassays and Related Procedures in Medicine. Vienna: International Atomic Energy Agency, 1984:165–192.

24. Offermann FJ, Girman JR, Sextro RG. Recent advances in health sciences and technology. In: Indoor Air, Vol. 1, Proceedings of the 3rd International Conference on Indoor Air Quality and Climate, 1984:257–261.

25. Stricker WE, Layton JE, Homburger HA, Katzmann JA, Swanson MC, Hyatt RE, Reed CE. Immunologic response to aerosols of affinity-purified antigen in hypersensitivity pneumonitis. J Allergy Clin Immunol 1986; 78:411–416.

26. Woodard ED, Friedlander B, Lesher RJ, Font W, Kinsey R, Hearne FT. Outbreak of hypersensitivity pneumonitis in an industrial setting. JAMA 1988; 259:1965–1969.

27. Agarwal MK, Ingram JW, Dunnette S, Gleich GJ. Immunochemical quantitation of an airborne proteolytic enzyme, esperase TM, in a consumer products factory. Am Ind Hyg Assoc J 1986; 47:136–143.

28. Liss GM, Kominsky JR, Gallagher JS, Melius J, Brooks SM, Bernstein IL. Failure of enzyme encapsulation to prevent sensitization of workers in the dry bleach industry. J Allergy Clin Immunol 1984; 73:348–355.

29. Swanson MC, Yunginger JW, Reed CE. Immunochemical quantification of airborne natural rubber allergen in medical and dental office buildings. In: Ventilation and Indoor Air Quality in Hospitals. Kleuver Academic Publishers, 1996: 251–262.

30. Yunginger JW, Jones RT, Fransway AF, Kelso JM, Warner MA, Hunt LW. Extractable latex allergens and proteins in disposable medical gloves and other rubber products. J Allergy Clin Immunol 1994; 93:836–840.

31. Newman Taylor AJ, Longbottom JL, Pepys J. Respiratory allergy to urine proteins of rats and mice. Lancet 1977; 2:847–849.

32. Swanson MC, Campbell AR, O'Hollaren MT, Reed CE. Role of ventilation, air filtration and allergen production rate in determining concentrate ons of rat allergens in the air of animal quarters. Am Rev Respir Dis 1991; 141:1578–1581.

33. Platts-Mills TAE, Heyman P, Longbottom J L, Wilkins SR. Airborne allergens associated with asthma: particle size carrying dust niite and rat allergens measured with a cascade impactor. J Allergy Clin Immunol 1986; 77:850–857.

34. Muller-Wening D, Repp H. Investigation on the protective value of breathing masks in farmer's lung using an inhalation provocation test. Chest 1989; 95:100–105.

35. Swanson MC, Boiano JM, Galson SK, Grauvogel LW, Reed CE. Immunochemical quantification and particle size distribution of airborne papain in a meat portioning facility. J Am Ind Hyg Assoc 1992; 53(1):1–5.

36. Smith AB, Bernstein DI, Tar-Ching AW, Gallagher JS, London M, Kopp S, Carson GA. Occupational asthma from inhaled egg protein. Am J Ind Med 1987; 12:205–218.

37. Bernstein DI, Smith AB, Moller DR, Gallagher JS, Tar-Ching AW, London M, Kopp S, Carson G. Clinical and immunologic studies among egg-processing workers with occupational asthma. J Allergy Clin Immunol 1987; 80:791–797.

38. Halverson PC, Swanson MC, Reed CE. Occupational asthma in egg crackers is associated with extraordinarily high airborne egg allergen conoentrations. J Allergy Clin Imunol 1988; 81:321.

39. Lee RD, Gordon DJ, Lacey J, Nunn AJ, Brown M, Newman Taylor AJ. Occupational allergy to the common house fly (*Musca domestica*): use of immunologic response to identify atmospheric allergen. J Allergy Clin Immunol 1985; 76:826–831.

40. Ostrom NK, Swanson MC, Agarwal MK, Yunginger, JW. Occupational allergy to honeybee-body dust in a honey processing plant. J Allergy Clin Immunol 1986; 77:736–740.

41. Rodrigo MJ, Morell F, Helm RM, Swanson M, Greife A, Anto JM, Sunyer J, Reed CE. Identification and partial characterization of the soybean-dust allergens involved in the Barcelona asthma epidemic. J Allergy Clin Immunol 1990; 85:778–784.

14

Environmental Monitoring of Chemical Agents

Jacques Lesage and Guy Perrault
Research Institute in Occupational Health and Safety, Montréal, Quebec, Canada

INTRODUCTION

The fact that asthmatic reactions may be induced and elicited by low and, on occasion, extremely low concentrations of a given substance has given occupational asthma its own place in industrial hygiene, where the classic notions of time-weighted average exposure (TWA), short-term exposure (STEL), and ceiling limits have been treated as more or less irrelevant. In the case of occupational asthma, emphasis has been put on identification of the causative agents and subsequent hygiene control so that subjects with occupational asthma are no longer exposed to the causal agent (1–3).

The rapid increase in new cases of occupational asthma (4,5) and in the number of agents causing asthma over the past few decades (6) has provided the impetus for establishing methods to quantify worker exposure. First, there is justification for verifying whether workers are exposed to a specific agent in the workplace. Second, surveillance and prevention of exposure are required to ensure that workers do not develop occupational asthma and that workers with occupational asthma are no longer exposed to the causal agent or are only exposed to a much lower concentration (7–9). Third, laboratory or workplace confirmation of occupational asthma is relevant for medical or medicolegal reasons. In all these instances, it is important to obtain information on the nature and concentrations of the agent(s) (10,11).

Occupational asthma agents are generally classified as low- and high-molecular-weight agents. The latter generally cause sensitization through immunological sensitization. The mechanism of occupational asthma caused by low-molecular-weight agents, which are a growing cause of work-related asthma, is usually unknown. Two main approaches have been adopted for exposure assessment: immunoassays (12–15) and chemical assays. This chapter will be devoted to the assessment of exposure to low-molecular-weight asthma agents by chemical assays in both the air and in biological matrices.

MONITORING METHODS

This section will briefly review the main analytical methods used in industrial hygiene to identify and evaluate the presence of chemicals in workplaces. For asthma prevention, the main route of absorption of chemicals is by inhalation, which emphasizes methods of determination of the concentration of chemicals in the air or a few possibilities of biological monitoring of exposure. Each method includes a sampling and an analytical protocol. Most methods can be used for personal monitoring or area sampling. The main sampling and instrumental techniques will be described briefly and separately. However, all these techniques have to be used in accordance with an environmental sampling strategy that takes into account factors related to the nature and toxicology of the suspected contaminants and the characteristics of the worksite. Since asthma induction by skin absorption has been mentioned in a few scientific articles (16,17), the sampling and characterization of chemicals on surfaces will also be mentioned.

Sampling Techniques

The first point to consider before choosing a sampling technique is the route of absorption of the chemicals into the human body, namely inhalation, absorption through the skin, or ingestion. In the case of asthma, the main and well-documented route of absorption is by inhalation. Consequently, the sampling and analysis of air samples will constitute a large part of this section. Surface sampling will be briefly mentioned in the prevention of absorption through the skin. Finally, for special cases, biological monitoring of exposure will be mentioned as a means of obtaining an overall evaluation of the dose absorbed by the worker, through different possible routes.

Air

The first steps in analyzing an air sample are to collect the pollutant in such a way as to be able to carry it to the laboratory for further characterization and to determine the volume of air from which this pollutant was obtained. In industrial hygiene and environmental analysis, several sampling techniques are used in most cases where a direct- or continuous-reading instrument is not available or not adaptable to the sampling strategy.

In ambient air, a chemical pollutant can be present as a gas, vapor, or aerosol (mist or dust). Sampling of gases is routinely done in plastic, teflon, or aluminum bags filled by a pump. The flow and time of operation of the pump provide the volume of air necessary to calculate the concentration in parts per million (ppm) or milligrams (mg) per cubic meter of air. These bags are then sent to the laboratory for qualitative or quantitative analysis. A variety of solid containers made of glass, plastic, or metals are also available. These containers can be filled by flushing them with the air to be collected if they are provided with an inlet and an outlet valve, or by placing the container under vacuum and filling it by opening only one valve equipped with a flow controller (18). Sampling in bags or containers is limited to the sampling of stable gaseous products that do not chemically react with, physically diffuse through, or adsorb on the bag or the container material.

Sampling of volatile organic compounds as vapors or gases is usually performed by adsorption of the compounds on a solid sorbent such as activated charcoal, tenax, silica gel, XAD-2, and so forth. These adsorbents are chosen on the basis of their adsorption efficiency for a given compound or mixture of compounds and their ease of desorption by a suitable solvent before the analysis. Solid sorbents can be used with an active or a passive sampling train.

In active sampling, the solid adsorbent is generally placed in a glass tube and retained at the inlet and the outlet of the tube by a fiberglass wool or polyurethane plug. This tube is then connected to a pump to draw a known quantity of air through the tube. The sample adsorbed on the sorbent is then sent to a laboratory to be desorbed and analyzed.

In passive sampling, the solid sorbent is placed in a cup and kept in place by a layer of material permeable to organic vapors. The sampling is then the result of the diffusion of the sample from the air, where it is at a certain concentration, to the inside of the passive sampler, where it is at a much lower concentration. It is then captured on the solid sorbent, and the entire sampling train (badge) is sent to the laboratory for analysis (Fig. 1). The sampling rate constant of a passive sampler has to be predetermined in a generation chamber with the known air concentration of the given organic compounds. This predetermined value is then combined with the sampling duration to obtain the air volume.

Bubblers (or impingers) containing liquid are being used less and less for sampling vapors and aerosols. Bubblers are made of glass, plastic, or teflon, and filled with an absorbing liquid to capture the sample. Spillproof versions are available for personal sampling, are well accepted by the workers. The bubbler is connected to a pump to draw a measured volume of air through the solvent. The pollutant is dissolved in the solvent, and the entire impinger or bubbler is sent to the laboratory for analysis (Fig. 2).

Aerosols, mists, or dusts are often sampled on filters (or membranes) composed of teflon, mixed cellulose esters, polyvinyl chloride, fiberglass, silver, and other materials. Filters are available in various pore sizes and are selected on the basis of the application. The choice of the filter is dictated by the requirements of the analytical methods. For sampling, the filter is placed in a plastic cassette of 37-mm, 25-mm, or 13-mm diameter. The cassette containing the filter is then connected to a pump to aspirate the air through the filter on which the dust or mist will be collected. The cassette is then sent to the laboratory for analysis. For most cases of asthma prevention, sampling for inhalable dust (19) (Fig. 3) (also referred to incorrectly as total dust) (20) is recommended for collecting

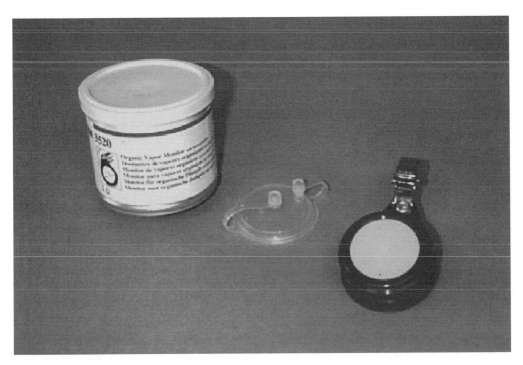

Figure 1 Passive sampler (badge). The sampling is the result of the diffusion of the sample from the air to the inside of the badge.

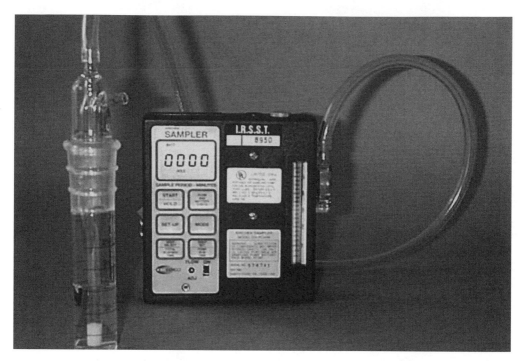

Figure 2   Sampling train with an impinger to collect vapors and aerosols in an absorbing liquid.

the portion of the aerosol that can be inhaled by the worker and can be deposited anywhere in the respiratory tract. In the absence of wind, inhalable dust can be collected at a flow rate of 2 L/min in a filter cassette having an opening of at least 15 mm. Respirable dust, the portion of the aerosol that can be deposited in the gas-exchange region of the lung, including the respiratory alveoles, bronchioles, and associated ducts, can be sampled through a cyclone (median cut-size aerodynamic diameter: 4 μm) with a filter cassette (Fig. 4).

Surface

To prevent skin absorption, two surface sampling techniques can be used to detect possible contamination of work surfaces by chemical agents. The first technique consists of placing the substance to be identified in contact with a selectively reacting compound. The product resulting from the reaction between both chemical substances should develop a coloration visible by the human eye. This technique has been used mainly for the detection of heavy metals, amines, or isocyanates. This technique has limitations in terms of specificity and quantitative evaluation but offers the advantages of an immediate on-site response to allow screening or immediate correction to avoid skin contamination with active agents. The second technique is a wipe test with an adsorbent material to collect the chemicals present on the work surface. The adsorbent material is then sent to the laboratory for identification and quantitative analysis.

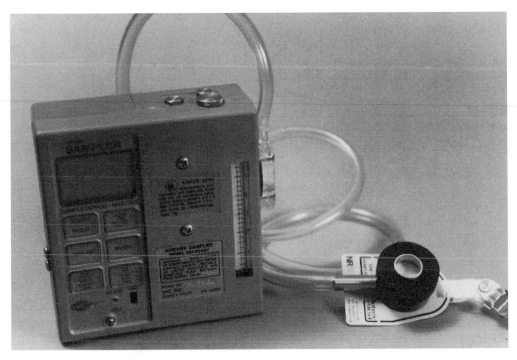

Figure 3 Sampling train for the collection of inhalable dust with the NR-701 personal dust sampler designed by the Instituted Occupational Medicine in Edinburgh, Scotland.

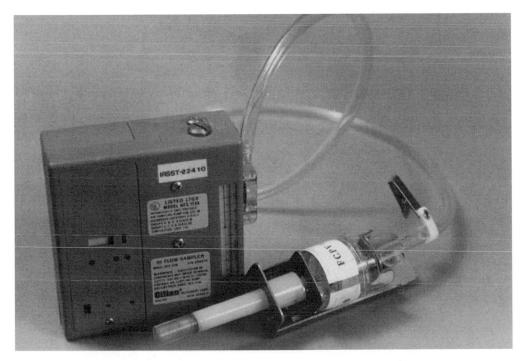

Figure 4 Respirable dust can be sampled through a cyclone (median cut-size aerodynamic diameter 4 μm) with a filter cassette.

Biological Monitoring of Exposure

The biological monitoring of exposure is a measure of the contaminant itself, or one of its metabolites, or any other biological parameter in a biological matrix (mainly blood, urine, and exhaled air). It gives an evaluation of the "internal dose" that has been absorbed by an individual worker, taking into account the characteristics of his job, the process, his individual parameters (age, sex, body mass, etc.), as well as the various routes of absorption, mainly by inhalation and through the skin.

All samples of urine or blood for biological monitoring of exposure must be collected by qualified medical personnel using state-of-the-art precautions to protect the worker and ensure the quality of the sample. For each contaminant, the sampling protocol has to take into account the requirements of the analytical technique, the integrity of the sample, and the sampling time. Results can be interpreted when the relationship between the internal dose and the biological effects has been established, which has not been done for many contaminants. In asthma, metabolites of isocyanates are being studied for the biological monitoring of exposure (see below).

Analytical Techniques

Gas Chromatography

Gas chromatography (GC) is essentially an analytical technique to achieve the chromatographic separation of mixtures of organic compounds in the gas phase and the quantitative assessment of each constituent. The instrumental protocol starts with the injection of a minute sample of a gas or a vapor into an inert gas flow. This injected gas or vapor is carried by the flow of inert gas to a chromatographic column on which it will be separated into its different constituents. In brief, chromatographic separation depends on the boiling point or vapor pressure of each organic compound and the type of adsorbents in the chromatographic column. At the end of the column, the sample is carried by the gas flow to a detector that should have a response proportional to the concentration of the sample. Many different types of detectors can be chosen for their sensitivity, specificity, or generality of application. Each constituent of the sample is identified by comparing its retention time (time from the injection of the sample to the response of the detector) to the retention time of a pure standard. Rather complex mixtures can be efficiently and rapidly analyzed using this instrumental technique.

Samples for GC analysis are generally collected in aluminum bags or on solid sorbents. GC can be used as a direct-reading instrument to monitor the concentration of a pure organic compound or well-identified mixtures of two or three organic compounds in a generation chamber. Portable instruments are available for use in the field by qualified technicians.

High-Performance Liquid Chromatography

Approximately 85% of all organic compounds cannot be analyzed by GC either because of their extremely low volatility or their high thermolability. In these cases, high-performance liquid chromatography (HPLC) is often used.

In HPLC, a liquid sample (a pure compound or a solution) is injected into the flow of a carrier liquid to be transported through a chromatographic column. Mixtures of organic compounds are separated by the diffusion of the analyte from the eluting solvent to the column's solid adsorbent. Each separated component is then detected by an appropriate detector giving a response that is proportional to the concentration of each compound. As in GC, each constituent of a mixture can be identified by comparing its retention time to the retention time of a reference compound. A choice of eluting solvents, chromatographic columns, and more or less specific detectors can be adapted to various analytical protocols.

For HPLC analysis, air samples are usually collected on solid sorbents, impingers, or filters. The requirement of injecting the sample as a liquid limits the practical use of HPLC to laboratory analysis of samples collected in workplaces or in generation chambers.

Atomic Absorption Spectrophotometry

Atomic absorption spectrophotometry (AAS) is essentially a quantitative analytical technique for metallic atoms. In occupational asthma, it can be particularly useful in the analysis of metallic atoms such as Pb, Cu, Zn, Cd, Ni, Cr, Co, and so forth. The principle of the analytical technique is the absorption of light with wavelengths specific to the emission spectra of the vaporized atom. The intensity of this absorption can be measured by a photometric detector or a spectrophotometer.

Air samples for atomic absorption spectrophotometry are usually collected as fumes, dusts, or mists on a filter or a membrane. The filter is then digested by appropriate acids to destroy the filter material and dissolve the collected fumes or dusts. The resulting solution is vaporized into a flame or another heating device (graphite furnace) and irradiated by light of appropriate wavelength from a hollow cathode lamp.

AAS has good sensitivity and specificity, but it analyzes only one element at a time or a given number of elements (six to eight) in sequence. The results are given as the total metallic atoms contained in the sample without speciation of derivatives or oxidation states. For applications where a multielement technique is required, inductively coupled plasma (ICP) is recommended.

Spectrometry

Spectrometry covers a wide range of analytical techniques based on the principle of the interaction of electromagnetic radiation with matter. In the electromagnetic radiation spectrum, the ranges of ultraviolet (UV), visible, and infrared radiation are of special interest in the analysis of low-molecular-weight compounds in air. Techniques operating in the visible range of electromagnetic radiation are routinely used in clinical as well as environmental laboratories mainly because of their wide applicability resulting from the transformation of the sample to colored derivatives and the simplicity of the instrumentation, resulting in low cost and ease of operation. The formation of colored derivatives is often used for identification of surface contamination.

A spectrometer's operating principle is based on the absorption, by the sample, of electromagnetic radiation of specific wavelengths from a light source, which is usually a tungsten lamp in the visible range. The absorption of light, which is measured and quantified by an appropriate detector such as a phototube, is proportional to the concentration of the analyte (Beer's law).

Generally, air samples for analysis by visible spectrometry are collected in impingers containing a solution of the derivative necessary for direct preparation of the colored compound that will be quantified. Direct-reading instruments using this technique have been developed for the analysis of a given analyte in a small volume of a derivatizing solution or on treated paper tapes.

Infrared Spectrophotometry

The basic principle of infrared spectrophotometry (IR) is identical to the absorption of electromagnetic radiation in visible spectrometry, except that the source's range of electromagnetic radiation is in the infrared region between 400 and 4000 cm^{-1} wave numbers. IR is mainly used to characterize pollutants but can be effective in quantifying concentrations. The IR absorption of light at certain wave numbers is specific to the presence of functional groups in the molecules, such as ketones, esters, alcohols, isocyanates, organic acids, anhydrides, amines, alkanes, alkenes, alkynes, and so forth. This provides useful information in the characterization of families of contaminants, and in identifying pure compounds especially for a region of the absorption spectrum containing many discrete absorption lines, which are said to be the fingerprint of each organic compound. The intensity of absorption at a given wave number can be used to quantify specifically a pure pollutant or a pollutant in a mixture of other organic compounds that do not contain the functional group absorbing the IR radiation.

Analysis by IR can be performed on solids, liquids, or gases as long as they are transparent to IR radiation or suited for reflectance (solid sample), giving the technique a wide range of applicability. Gaseous samples can be monitored continuously in the atmosphere or in a generation chamber. Field instruments are available and routinely used in the field by industrial hygienists (Fig. 5).

Ion Chromatography

Ion chromatography (IC) is similar to HPLC and separates, by chromatography, mixtures carried by a liquid flow. IC, however, is particularly useful for analyzing inorganic ions, cations, or anions in solution (usually in water).

In this case, the analyte solution is injected into the liquid flow and is transported through an ion-exchange column where the various ions are separated. The separated

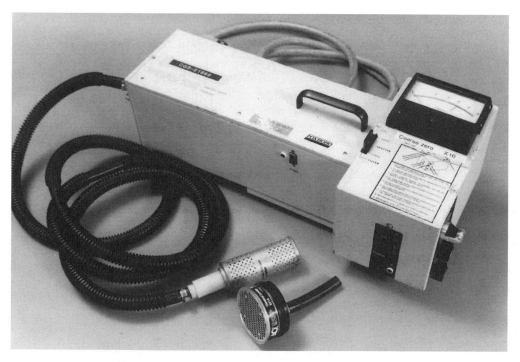

Figure 5 Example of an infrared direct-reading instrument (Miran 103) that can be used in the field or in a chamber.

constituents in solution are then treated in a suppressor and converted into strong acids or bases, which are detected and quantified by a conductivity or electrochemical cell.

In preparation for the IC technique, air samples are collected in impingers, on filters or solid sorbents. As with HPLC, this technique is limited from a practical standpoint to the laboratory analysis of samples collected in the field or in generation chambers.

Mass Spectrometry

Mass spectrometry (MS) is used to identify and quantify components of complex mixtures. Its principle consists of ionizing the sample in a source, of fractionating molecular ions, and of analyzing specific molecular or fractionated ions in a magnetic field. This technique is often coupled with a gas chromatograph (GC/MS) or an HPLC (HPLC/MS) to identify the components of a complex mixture that are separated by GC or HPLC before being introduced into the source of the MS. The information generated by MS is equivalent to a fingerprint of an unknown sample, allowing the sample to be identified without using a reference compound. The technique has been developed for gaseous, liquid, or solid samples. Recently, new techniques consist of a double mass analyzer separated by a collision cell. These techniques referred to as MS/MS or as a double mass spectrometer improve the specificity and sensitivity of mass spectrometry applied to the measure of a component in a complex matrix. Some sophisticated installations can perform continuous monitoring in the field or in a generation chamber.

Other Methods

X-ray diffractometry has applications for the identification and quantification of dust constituents. It is limited, however, to crystalline compounds such as some metallic oxides. Polarized light microscopy can be used for the identification of solid compounds (guar gum).

EXPOSURE EVALUATION STRATEGY AS RELATED TO OCCUPATIONAL ASTHMA

A variety of exposure limit values have been developed by different organizations or national regulatory agencies to protect workers from the toxicological effects of uncontrolled exposure to chemical contaminants. The Threshold Limit Values (TLV) proposed by the American Conference of Government Industrial Hygienists (ACGIH) have gained worldwide recognition for their quality and their acquisition by consensus. In the ACGIH list of TLVs, long-term exposure to low concentrations of contaminants resulting in chronic toxicological consequences has led to the notion of time-weighted average (TWA) values, below which no health effect should be suffered by a normal worker exposed for 8 working hours, 5 days a week, over his lifetime. Acute exposure to relatively high concentrations of a contaminant for a short period of time causing immediate toxicological reactions, such as irritation, chronic or irreversible tissue damage, or narcosis, is prevented by the observance of short-term exposure limits (STEL) or ceiling limits.

Most of these thresholds can be scientifically supported by or extrapolated from animal or in vitro toxicological tests. A few have been proven by epidemiological studies. However, these exposure limits are often suspected of being inadequate in the prevention of occupational asthma where individual susceptibility could play an important role in the sensitizing process. It could then be assumed that the protection of a sensitized worker against a given agent would require the observance of a much lower exposure limit than for unaffected workers. Conversely, it could be argued that there is a certain exposure limit that prevents most workers from becoming sensitized. This existence of a sensitizing threshold has not yet been scientifically proven, but the risk of developing occupational asthma has been shown to be related to the degree of exposure (21,22), even though studies continue to clarify the contribution of the duration of exposure (3), individual susceptibility (23), and routes of absorption.

EXAMPLES OF EVALUATION OF EXPOSURE TO SPECIFIC SENSITIZING AGENTS

Isocyanates

Analytical methods to determine air concentrations of diisocyanates have been extensively reviewed by Dharmarajan et al. (24), Brown et al. (25), and Lesage and Perrault (26). Most methods (Table 1) have been developed for impinger sampling and subsequently modified for sampling on adsorbent tubes or filters impregnated with a derivative reagent. Analytical methods are, in general, spectometry for determining all isocyanate groups, and HPLC with ultraviolet detector for specific analysis of a given diisocyanate molecule such as 2,4-toluene diisocyanate. Recently, a new analytical method using HPLC/mass spectometry gives a better sensitivity and specificity in the diisocyanate and polyisocyanate determination (27). Aliphatic compounds and cycloalkanes, e.g., hexamethylene diisocyanate (HDI) and methylene bis(4-cyclohexylisocyanate) (HMDI), can be detected by the ultraviolet spectroscopy detector only after derivatization with a UV-absorbing compound such as 9-(N-methyl aminomethyl) anthracene (Table 1).

A few recent publications have presented efforts to achieve lower limits of detection by optimizing the derivatization reaction to make the resulting compound sensitive to a

Table 1 Sampling and Analysis of Diisocyanates in the Air

Method	Sampling techniques	Analytical techniques	Limit of detection (μg/m$_3$)
2,4-Dinitro fluorobenzene	Impinger (HCl/dimethyl sulfoxide)	Visible spectrometry	13
Marcali[a] N-(1-naphthyl)-ethylene-diamine	Impinger (HCl/acetic acid)	Ultraviolet spectrometry	75
9-(N-Methylamino-methyl) anthracene	Impinger (toluene) or solid sorbent	HPLC ultraviolet	1
1-(2-Methoxyphenyl) piperazine	Impinger (toluene) or solid sorbent	HPLC ultraviolet	5
N-(4-Nitrobenzyl) propylamine	Impinger (toluene) or solid sorbent	HPLC ultraviolet	4.4
Tryptamine (28)	Impinger (2,2,4-trimethyl pentane)	HPLC ultraviolet	5
1-(2-Pyridyl) piperazine	Impinger (toluene) or solid sorbent	HPLC ultraviolet	2.3

[a]Limited to aromatic diisocyanates.

specific detector such as the electron capture detector of a gas chromatograph, or the fluorescence or the mass spectrometry detector of an HPLC. Dalene et al. (29) have reported a limit of detection (LOD) of 0.5–0.8 μg/m^3, respectively, for TDI and MDI using HPLC/ultraviolet, and a lower limit of 0.1 μg/m^3 by HPLC/mass spectrometry for 1,6-hexamethylene diisocyanate. The same group of researchers (29) has published an LOD of 0.1 μg/m^3 for 2,4- and 2,6-toluene diisocyanate with the electrochemical detector of an HPLC. Simon and Moulut (30) and Schmidtke and Seifert (31) have adapted the 1-(2-methoxyphenyl) piperazine method to tube sampling. Simon has added the quantification of isocyanate prepolymers to the methods, and Schmidtke has attained an LOD of 1 ng/m^3 with the electrochemical detector. Other groups are working on the development of new derivative agents such as 1-(9-anthracenylmethyl) piperazine (MAP) (32,33).

Lesage et al. (34,35) have reported an LOD of 1 μg/m^3 with a double-filter cassette for separating and trapping isocyanate monomers and oligomers before their analysis by HPLC. This group has also developed, using the same sampler, an analytical method with an HPLC coupled to a double mass spectrometer. The LOD observed is 0.05 μg/m^3 for HDI. The double-filter cassette also has the possibility of separating the aerosol into its liquid (mist) and gaseous phases. Other techniques have been suggested for achieving this separation (36,37).

Biological monitoring of exposure has been tested using albumin adducts in plasma (38) and their corresponding diamine in plasma and urine (39). In their present stage, these researches are still not applicable to the monitoring of worker exposure to isocyanates.

Two types of direct-reading instruments are commercially available. Their main characteristics are summarized in Table 2. These instruments are suitable for monitoring diisocyanate concentrations in a generation chamber or at a worksite where the diisocyanates have been identified by another technique. It is also recommended that the effect of humidity and of other air pollutants on instrument response be considered (Figs. 6,7). A coated piezoelectric detector (40) with a range of detection of 3–24 ppb could be promising for application in a direct-reading instrument.

In summary, many sampling and analytical methods are now available to determine the concentrations of diisocyanates in the air with the sensitivity required for detecting low-concentration or short-duration exposures. Research is continuing to further improve the limit of detection. Direct-reading instruments are also available to monitor exposure to monomer diisocyanates. The applicability of these instruments to different diisocyanates can still be improved as well as their response to simple interferences such as humidity. Research efforts are now devoted to the representative sampling of mists containing isocyanate monomers and oligomers and to the analysis of polyisocyanate prepolymers (Fig. 8). Blocked diisocyanates that are liberated by physical (such as temperature) or chemical (such as humidity) reactions could result in the presence of the blocked isocyanate moiety in the air and, eventually, the blocking agent. The characterization and reactivity of blocked

Table 2 Diisocyanate Determination by Direct-Reading Instruments

Instrument	Analytical technique	Limit of detection (ppm)	Response time
Impregnated paper tape	Visible spectrometry	0.002	2–5 min
Gas cell	Infrared spectrometry	0.03	Continuous

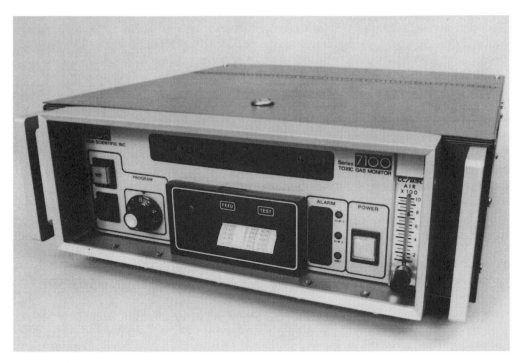

Figure 6 Example of a direct-reading instrument (MDA 7100) for continuous monitoring of isocyanates.

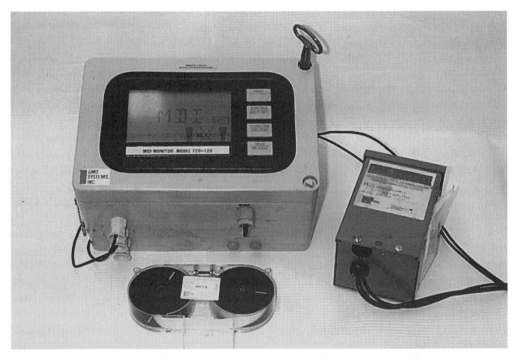

Figure 7 Example of a direct-reading instrument (GMD RIS) for continuous monitoring of isocyanates.

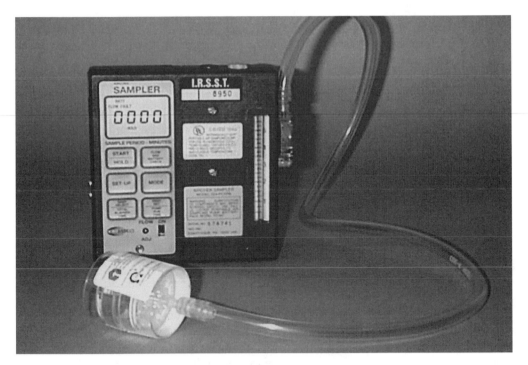

Figure 8 A sampling cassette (ISO-CHEK) designed to collect diisocyanates as a vapor and aerosol fraction. A first teflon filter collects the isocyanates that are present in the air as aerosols, while a second pretreated glass-fiber filter traps all vapor isocyanates.

diisocyanates and blocking agents in the air in relation to their sensitizing potential have still to be studied.

For surfaces contaminated by isocyanate, a wipe test has been developed by CLI Colorimetric Laboratories Inc. under the trade name of SWYPE. This product can be used for surface and skin contamination detection to identify exposures that contribute to dermal absorption. Work is continuing to increase the specificity and sensitivity of this technique.

Acid Anhydrides

Methods for sampling and analysis of hexahydrophthalic anhydride, phthalic anhydride, trimellitic anhydride, maleic anhydride, and methyltetrahydrophthalic anhydride have been described (41–43). The air concentration of anhydrides is often determined by sampling a known volume of air through a cellulose membrane filter to trap the organic aerosol. The anhydride is then hydrolyzed to the corresponding diacid, extracted with an aqueous ammonia solution, and analyzed by an HPLC with a UV detector (44). The limit of detection has been reported as being 1 mg/m^3 for a sampling volume of 100 L. A method developed for hexahydrophthalic anhydride (42) and methyltetrahydrophthalic anhydride (43) uses a sorbent tube or a bubbler for collecting the sample, and gas chromatography with flame ionization detector for the analysis. The limit of detection is then 10 μg/m^3 for a 20-L sample. For maleic, phthalic, and trimellitic anhydride, the Occupational Safety and Health Administration (OSHA) has recommended sampling on two glass fiber filters coated with veratrylamine/di-*n*-octylphthalate and analysis by HPLC/UV (44). NIOSH has recommended a gas chromatographic method for trimellitic anhydride after sampling on a PVC filter and an HPLC/UV method for maleic anhydride after collection in a bubbler (45). The gas chromatography method should be adaptable to most organic anhydrides that can be volatilized without decomposition.

Biological monitoring of exposure by analyzing hexahydrophthalic acid in urine has been described (46,47).

A direct-reading instrument for monitoring organic anhydride concentrations in a generation chamber could be based on infrared spectrophotometry but has not been described in the scientific literature. Dedicated gas chromatographs could be set up for monitoring organic anhydrides with sufficiently high vapor pressure.

Formaldehyde and Other Aldehydes

Various methods have been used to determine the concentration of formaldehyde and other aldehydes in the air. The subject was reviewed in 1985 by Kennedy et al. (48), who listed the chromotropic acid, pararosaniline, 2,4-dinitro phenylhydrazine (2,4-DNPH), 3-methyl-2-benzothiazolinone hydrazone (MBTH), Girard T reagent, hydrazine, and *N*-benzylethanolamine (BEA) methods. Most of these methods have been adapted to sampling with impingers (bubblers), adsorbent tubes, or passive samplers. Table 3 summarizes the reported performance of each method. The interferences given in this table refer to the application as a colorimetric technique. The pararosaniline, 2,4-DNPH, and BEA have been adapted to analytical techniques such as GC and HPLC to improve their specificity. OSHA (49) and NIOSH (50) recommend sampling on an XAD-2 sorbent tube coated with 2-(hydroxymethyl)piperidine (HMP) and analysis by GC or GC/MS. The 2-(hydroxymethyl)piperidine reacts with formaldehyde to form an oxazolidine derivative similar to that in the BEA method. Further studies on the development and validation of sampling and analytical methods applicable to the determination of many aldehydes simultaneously present in a work environment are still required.

Formaldehyde can also be released from textiles or wood. A method has been developed for formaldehyde on dust that requires the sampling of inhalable dust on a filter, extraction, derivatization with 2,4-DNPH, and analysis by HPLC (51).

Vairavamurthy et al. have reviewed the determination of aldehydes in the atmospheric environment (52). They cite methods similar to the ones already mentioned for the work environment and some direct-reading instruments. However, these direct-reading

Table 3 Analytical Methods for Formaldehyde in the Air

Method	Sampling volume (L)	Limit of detection (mg/m^3)	Interference
Chromotropic acid	60	0.025	Phenol and alcohols
Pararosaniline[a]	60	0.030	Aldehydes
2,4-DNPH[a]	30	0.002	Aldehydes and ketones
Girard T	18	0.300	Aldehydes
MBTH[a]	250	0.008	Aldehydes and ketones
Hydrazine	30	0.010	Specific by polarography
BEA	38	0.050	Specific by gas chromatography
2-(hydroxymethyl)piperidine	10	0.300	Specific by gas chromatography

[a]Colorimetric method.

spectroscopic instruments require long optical paths and are not easily applicable in a work environment. Another family of instruments uses colorimetric methods for quasi-continuous monitoring of formaldehyde (53). These instruments have the same problems with interference as other colorimetric techniques. A last family of instruments can be used in well-controlled atmospheres such as a generation chamber; these instruments are based on IR or UV spectroscopy (52). A direct-reading passive badge for glutaraldehyde monitoring has been described (54).

In summary, the analytical techniques for formaldehyde are well developed and are adaptable to a wide range of air concentrations. Many of these methods are adaptable to the analysis of other aldehydes, but methods for other aldehydes have not reached the same level of development as those for formaldehyde. Direct-reading instruments for the work environment are available and easy to use but are plagued with many types of interference. However, it should be remembered that formaldehyde and other aldehydes are often used as indicators (tracers) of worker exposure to complex mixtures of decomposed organic products of combustion or high-temperature uses. These exposures are extremely complex, containing hundreds of products, many of which could be asthma-inducing agents. A proper strategy will have to be developed for a rational approach to the analysis of these mixtures before their sensitization properties are examined.

Amines

The analytical techniques reported in the past 15 years use gas or liquid chromatography for the analysis of airborne volatile amines sometimes collected in impingers, but as often as possible in sorbent tubes or on treated filters. Table 4 summarizes the most recent publications on the analysis of aliphatic amines in the air, and Table 5, those for aromatic amines.

It is clear that many different analytical methods for analyzing amines in the air have been published. In general, the low limits of detection required by the application to occupational asthma are attainable only with methods in which the amine group is derivatized by attaching a moiety that is very sensitive to the detector of the analytical technique. The derivatization technique is not as easy, however, in the case of tertiary amines.

Table 4 Sampling and Analysis of Aliphatic Amines in the Air

Method	Sampling	Analysis	Sampling volume (L)	Limit of detection (mg/m^3)
Underivatized[a] (56,57,58)	Silica gel adsorbent	GC	20	0.1
Polymeric anhydride[b] (59,60,61)	Silica gel adsorbent	HPLC		1 μg
Naphthyl isothiocyanate[b] (62,63,64)	Adsorbent or filter	HPLC	15	0.01
m-Toluyl chloride[b]	Silica gel adsorbent	HPLC	60	0.1
	H$_3$PO$_3$-coated annular denuder	HPLC	30	0.001

[a]Primary, secondary, and tertiary amines.
[b]Primary and secondary amines.

Table 5 Sampling and Analysis of Aromatic Amines in the Air

Method	Sampling	Analysis	Sampling volume (L)	Limit of detection (mg/m^3)
Underivatized[a]	Silica gel adsorbent (65)	GC	3–150[c]	1.3–9[c,d]
	Filters and adsorbent tube (66)	GC	500	0.005–0.080[c]
Acetic anhydride[b] (67)	Acid-coated glass-fiber filter	HPLC	200	1.8–4.5[c,d]
Pentafluoropropionic anhydride[b] (68)	Acid-coated glass-fiber filter	GC/MS	500	0.001
Heptafluorobutyryl chloride[b] (69)	HCl bubbler	GC	1	0.0002

[a]Primary, secondary, and tertiary amines.
[b]Primary amines.
[c]Depending on the given amine.
[d]Low values in the working range.

Their methods are limited to the straight application of GC or HPLC with a specific nitrogen detector or a detector sensitive to quaternary amines for analysis by ion chromatography, but such methods have not yet been validated. Further studies are required before biological monitoring of exposure by measurement of adduct formation can be considered as a tool in human studies (55).

Colophony and Fluxes

This natural complex pine resin is largely composed of acidic resins of which abietic acid is the main constituent. Colophony can be used in two different applications, depending on whether it is heated below (as in paint and varnish application) or above its decomposition temperature of about 200°C (as in welding).

A method has been published for analyzing abietic acid and dehydroabietic acid in technical products (70). In this paper, reference is made to other methods such as gas chromatography and HPLC in effluents, shellac, and tall oil. However, measurements of abietic acid concentrations in the air when colophony is used do not seem to have been published.

In soldering or other similar uses, colophony is heated to high temperature and partly decomposed into fumes containing CO, CO_2, methane, ethylene, methanol, isopropyl alcohol, ketones, aldehydes, hydrocarbons, and terpenes. Historically, because of the complexity of the mixture, formaldehyde has been used as a tracer to monitor the exposure even though it had been shown (71) to be a minor component of the soldering fumes. Obviously, such results should not be used to extrapolate on a dose-effect relationship with formaldeyde. Sampling of total fumes with determination of their concentration by gravimetry could be used for an overall evaluation of all fumes and dust produced during soldering. This method, while relatively simple and economical, is uninformative due to its lack of specificity and its high limit of detection.

Metals

The concentration of airborne metals or inorganic metallic compounds is usually determined by sampling inhalable dust on a filter and analyzing its metallic content by AAS, ICP, or a variety of other techniques. For metals that have been reported as causing sensitization (Pt, Co, W, Ni, and Cr), industrial hygiene samples are collected on mixed cellulose ester filters and analyzed by atomic emission spectroscopy (AAS) or inductively coupled plasma atomic emission spectroscopy (ICP). By AAS, the limit of detection has been reported as being 0.011 mg/m^3 for a 180-L sampling volume (72), and by ICP, 0.005 mg/m^3 for a 500-L sampling volume (73). Because of the variation in carcinogenicity of some of their derivatives, Cr and Ni are often analyzed by analytical methods that can specify the state of oxidation of the metallic elements, such as sampling on filter, and analysis by colorimetry or by ion chromatography. However, there is no published information on the variation in sensitization potency of different derivatives of Cr and Ni.

Other Substances

In industrial hygiene, the sampling and analytical methods for other substances are well developed and could be used for occupational asthma studies. Inorganic acids can be sampled on silica gel tubes and analyzed by ion chromatography. Fibers can be collected on filters, identified, and analyzed by transmission electron microscopy. Cutting oils such as mineral oils could be sampled on filters and analyzed by IR spectrometry. Soluble metal-working fluids could be subjected to sampling and analysis of the amines or nitroso derivatives that they may contain. However, compounds such as azobisformamide, chloramine T, ammonium persulfate, diazonium salts, and dyes would require extensive efforts in analytical method development.

CONCLUSION

Although not exhaustive, this review of chemical monitoring of agents that induce occupational asthma emphasizes the progress being made in developing highly sensitive detection methods for certain compounds such as diisocyanates, formaldehyde, and anhydrides. When a low-molecular-weight compound is identified or suspected as an asthma agent, it is possible to develop analytical methods that will meet the stringent requirements of low concentration detectability and short exposure duration applicable to the evaluation of occupational asthma. Analytical methods covering a wider range of applications than the routinely used methods validated for industrial hygiene, and sampling strategies adapted to establish dose-effect relationships for sensitization and taking into account individual susceptibilities, should improve the prevention of occupational asthma. The monitoring of some families of compounds such as amines and aldehydes (other than formaldehyde) has not been significantly improved during the last 5 years.

The monitoring of chemical agents by direct-reading instruments is achievable in generation chambers used to perform specific bronchoprovocation of individuals. In this application, the atmosphere to be tested should have been chemically predefined, which allows the use of specialized instruments tailored to the specific requirements of the provocation test underway. Direct-reading instruments have to be used with caution on worksites because of the variability of the environment and the complexity of the matrices from other pollutants, which can cause interferences.

Biological monitoring of exposure and early indicators of lesion (not covered in this chapter) suggests future surveillance of global exposure of workers. But these tests have still not been validated for use in managing asthma prevention.

REFERENCES

1. Bernstein L. Occupational asthma. Clin Chest Med 1981; 2(2):255–272.
2. Parkes WR. Occupational Lung Disorders, 3rd ed., Oxford: Butterworth-Heinemann, 1994: 717.
3. Chan-Yeung M, Malo J-L. Occupational asthma. N Engl J Med 1995; 333:107–112.
4. Malo J-L. Compensation for occupational asthma in Quebec. Chest 1990; 98:236S–239S.
5. Nordman H. Occupational asthma—time for prevention. Scand J. Environ Health 1994; 20(special issue):108–115.
6. Chan-Yeung M, Malo J-L. Aetiological agents in occupational asthma. Eur Respir J 1994; 7: 346–371.
7. Reports of the Working Groups. Workshop on environmental and occupational asthma. Chest 1990; 98:240S–250S.
8. Reports by the Special Interest Group on Occupational Allergy of the British Society of Allergy and Clinical Immunology. Priorities for the understanding and managing of occupational allergy: a Delphi consensus. Clin Exp Allergy 1993; 23:634–637.
9. National Institute for Occupational Safety and Health (NIOSH). National Occupational Research Agenda. Asthma and Chronic Obstructive Pulmonary Disease 1996:10–11.
10. Bush RK. Occupational asthma from vegetable gums. J Allergy Clin Immunol 1990; 86: 443–444 (editorial).
11. Cloutier Y, Lagier F, Lemieux R, Blais, M-C, Cartier A, Malo J-L. Improved methodology for specific inhalation challenges with occupational agents in powder form. Eur Respir J 1989; 2: 769–777.
12. Reed EC, Swanson MC, Yuginger JW. Measurements of allergen concentration in the air as an aid in controlling exposure to aeroallergens. J Allergy Clin Immunol 1986; 78:1028–1030.
13. Newman Taylor A, Tee, RD. Environmental and occupational asthma. Exposure assessment Chest 1990; 98:209S–211S.
14. Grammer LC, Shaughnessy MA, Henderson J, Zeiss CR, Kavich DE, Collins, MJ, Pecis, KM, Kenamore BD. A clinical and immunologic study of workers with trimellitic-anhydride-induced immunologic lung disease after transfer to low exposure jobs. Am Rev Respir Dis 1993; 148:54–57.
15. Cullinan P, Lowson D, Nieuwenhuijsen, MJ, Sandiford C, Tee RD, Venables KM, McDonald JC, Newman Taylor AJ. Work related symptoms, sensitisation, and estimated exposure in workers not previously exposed to flour. Occup Environ Med 1994; 51:579–583.
16. Rattray NJ, Botham BA, Hext PM, Woodcock DR, Fielding I, Dearman RJ, Kimber I. Induction of respiratory hypersensitivity to diphenylmethane-4,4′diisocyanyate (MDI) in guinea pigs. Influence of route of exposure. Toxicology 1994; 88:15–30.
17. Piirila P, Estlander T, Keskinen, II, Jolanki R, Laakkonen A, Pfaffi P, Tupasela O, Tupparainen M, Nordman II. Occupational asthma caused by triglycidyl isocyanurate (TGIC) Clin Exp Allergy 1997; 25:510–514.
18. Simon A, Farant J-P. Personal communication.
19. American Conference of Governmental Industrial Hygienists (ACGIH). Particle Size-Selective Sampling in the Workplace, Cincinnati, Ohio, 1985:4.
20. American Conference of Governmental Industrial Hygienists (ACGIH). 1996 TLVs® and BEIs®. Cincinnati, OH, 1996.
21. Bernstein JA. Overview of diisocyanate occupational asthma. Toxicology 1996; 111:181–189.
22. Baur X. Occupational asthma due to isocyanates. Lung 1996; 174:23–30.

23. Yokokta K, Johyama Y, Yamaguchi K, Fujiki Y, Takeshita T, Morimoto K. Study on allergic rhinitis in workers exposed to methyltetrahydrophthalic anhydride. Environ Health Prev Med 1996; 1:133–135.

24. Dharmarajan V, Lingg RD, Booth KS, Hackathorn DR. Recent developments in the sampling and analysis of isocyanates in air. ASTM Special Technical Publication #957, Philadelphia, 1987:190–202.

25. Brown RH, Ellwood PA, Groves JA, Robertson SM. New Methods for the Determination of Airborne Isocyanates. London: Occupational Hygiene Laboratory, Health and Safety Executive, 1987:1–8.

26. Lesage J, Perrault G. Caractérisation physique et chimique de l'exposition des travailleurs aux isocyanates. Annexe au rapport de recherche. Institut de recherche en santé et en sécurité du travail, Montréal, Canada, 1989.

27. Lesage J, Ostiguy C, René L, Gaudette F, Nguyen P, Tra HV. New analytical method for the determination of ppt levels of isocyanates in workplace by triple quadruple mass spectrometry. Am Ind Hyg Conf Exh, Dallas, TX, May 1997.

28. Weh SW, Gaind VS. Application of tryptamine as a derivatizing agent for the determination of airborne isocyanates. Part 5. Investigation of tryptamine-coated XAD-2 personal sampler for airborne isocyanates in workplaces. Analyst 1992; 117:9–12.

29. Dalene M, Mathiasson L, Skarping G, Sango C, Sandstrom JF. Trace analysis of airborne aromatic isocyanates and related aminoisocyanates and diamines using high-performance liquid chromatography with utraviolet and electrochemical detection. Chromatography 1988; 20:469–481.

30. Simon P, Moulut O. Separation of the urea piperazine derivatives of polyisocyanate monomers and prepolymers by normal phase chromatography. J Liq Chromatogr 1988; 11:2071–2089.

31. Schmidtke F, Seifert B. A highly sensitive high-performance liquid chromatographic procedure for the determination of isocyanates in air. Fresenius J Anal Chem 1990; 336:647–654.

32. Streicher RP, Arnold JE, Ernst MK, Cooper CV. Development of a novel derivatization reagent for the sampling and analysis of total isocyanate groups in air and comparison of its performance with that of several established reagents. Am Ind Hyg Assoc J 1996; 57:905–913.

33. Rudzinski WE, Norman S, Dahlquist B, Greebon KW, Richardson A, Locke K, Thomas T. Evaluation of 1-(9-anthracenylmethyl) piperazine for the analysis of isocyanates in spray-painting operations. Am Ind Hyg Assoc J 1996; 57:914–917.

34. Lesage J, Goyer N, Desjardins F, Vincent J-Y, Perrault G. Workers' exposure to isocyanates. Am Ind Hyg Assoc J 1992; 53:146–153.

35. Lesage J, Perrault G. Sampling Device and Method for Its Use. U.S. patent #4,961,916; October 9, 1990, Canadian patent #1299114, July 21, 1992.

36. Rando, RJ, Poovey HG. Dichotomous sampling of vapor and aerosol of methylene-bis-(phenylisocyanate) [MDI] with an annular diffusional denuder. Am Ind Hyg Assoc J 1994; 55: 716–721.

37. Streicher RP, Kennedy ER, Lorberau CD. Strategies for the simultaneous collection of vapours and aerosols with emphasis on isocyanate sampling. Analyst 1994; 119:89–97.

38. Lind P, Dalane M, Lindstrom V, Grubb, A, Skarping G. Albumin adducts in plasma from workers exposed to toluene diisocyanate. Analyst 1997; 122:151–154.

39. Dalene M, Skarping G, Lind P. Workers exposed to thermal degradation products of TDI- and MDI-based polyurethane: Biomonitoring of 2,4-TDA, 2,6-TDA, and 4,4′-MDA in hydrolyzed urine and plasma. Am Ind Hyg Assoc J 1997; 58:587–591.

40. de Andrade JF, Fatibello-Filho O, Suleiman AA, Guilbault GG. A coated piezoelectric crystal sensor for the determination of 2,4-toluene diisocyanate in air. Anal Let 1989; 22:2601–2611.

41. National Institute for Occupational Safety and Health (NIOSH). Manual of Analytical Methods, 2nd ed. Cincinnati, OH. Vol. 3, Method S179, 1977.

42. Jönsson B, Welinder H, Skarping G. Determination of hexahydrophthalic anhydride in air using gas chromatography. J Chromatogr 1991; 558:247–256.

43. Welinder H, Gustavsson C. Methyltetrahydrophthalic anhydride in air—sampling and analysis. Ann Occup Hyg 1992; 36:189–197.

44. Occupational Safety and Health Administration. Chemical Data for Workplace Sampling and Analysis: OSHA's Chemical Information File, IMIS 1618, 1996.

45. National Institute for Occupational Safety and Health (NIOSH). Manual of Analytical Methods, 3rd ed, Cincinnati, OH, 1994.

46. Jönsson B, Skarping G. Method for the biological monitoring of hexahydrophthalic anhydride by the determination of hexahydrophthalic acid in urine using gas chromatography and selected-ion monitoring. J Chromatogr 1991; 572:117–131.

47. Jönsson B, Welinder H, Hansson C, Ståhlbom B. Occupational exposure to hexahydrophthalic anhydride: air analysis, percutaneous absorption, and biological monitoring. Int Arch Occup Environ Health 1993; 65:43–47.

48. Kennedy ER, Teass AW, Gagnon YT. Industrial hygiene sampling and analytical methods for formaldehyde. In: Tureski V, ed., Formaldehyde: Analytical Chemistry and Technology, Washington, DC: American Chemical Society, 1985.

49. Occupational Safety and Health Administration. Chemical Data for Workplace Sampling and Analysis: OSHA's Chemical Information File, Method OSHA 52, 1996.

50. National Institute for Occupational Safety and Health (NIOSH). Manual of Analytical Methods, 3rd ed., Method 2541, Cincinnati, OH, 1994.

51. National Institute for Occupational Safety and Health (NIOSH). Manual of Analytical Methods, 3rd ed., Method 5700, Cincinnati, OH, 1994.

52. Vairavamurthy A, Roberts JM, Newman L. Methods for determination of low molecular weight carbonyl compounds in the atmosphere: a review. Atmospher Environ 1992; 26A:1965–1993.

53. American Conference of Governmental Industrial Hygienists (ACGIH). Air Sampling Instruments for Evaluation of Atmospheric Contaminants. 7th ed, ACGIH, Cincinnati, OH. 1989: 549–573.

54. Kirollos KS, Mihaylov GM, Chapman KB. Direct-read, passive, glutaraldehyde STEL monitoring system. U.S. Patent 5364593, 1994.

55. Wilson PM, La DK, Froines JR. Hemoglobin and DNA adduct formation in Fischer-344 rats exposed to 2,4- and 4,6-toluene diamine. Arch Toxicol 1996; 70:591–598.

56. Blome H, Hennig M. Dosage des amines aliphatiques et aromatiques dans l'air. Cahier de notes domcumentaries de l'Institut national de recherche en sécuirté N.D. 1572, 1984:122–186.

57. Andersson B, Andersson K. Air sampling of N-methylmorpholine on solid sorbent and determination by capillary gas chromatography and a nitrogen-phosphorus detector. Anal Chem 1986; 58:1527–1529.

58. National Institute for Occupational Safety and Health (NIOSH). Manual of Analytical Methods, 3rd ed., Method 2010 Cincinnati, OH, 1994.

59. Chou T-Y, Colgan T, Kao DM, Krull IA. Pre-chromatographic derivatization of primary and secondary amines with a polymeric anhydride for improved high-performance liquid chromatographic detection. J Chromatogr 1986; 367:335–344.

60. Gao CX, Krull IS, Trainor UM. Determination of volatile amines in air by on-line solid-phase high-performance liquid chromatography with ultraviolet and fluorescence detection. J Chromtogr 1989; 463:192–200.

61. Jedrzejczak K, Gaind VS. Polymers with reactive functions as sampling and derivatizing agents. Part 1. Effective sampling and simultaneous derivatization of an airborne amine. Analyst 1990; 115:1359–1362.

62. Levin J-O, Andersson K, Fängmark I, Hallgren C. Determination of gaseous and particulate polyamines in air using sorbent and filter coated with naphthylisothiocyanate. Appl Ind Hyg 1989; 4:98–100.

63. Levin J-O, Lindhal R, Andersson K, Hallgren C. High-performance liquid chromatographic determination of diethylamine in air using diffusive sampling and thiourea formation. Chemosphere 1989: 18:2121–2129.

64. Levin J-O, Andersson K, Hallgren C. Determination of monoethanolamine and diethanolamine in air. Ann Occup Hyg 1989; 33:175–180.

65. National Institute for Occupational Safety and Health (NIOSH). Manual of Analytical Methods, 3rd ed., Method 2002, Cincinnati, OH, 1994.

66. Otson R, Leach JM, Chung TK. Sampling of airborne aromatic amines. Anal Chem 1987; 50: 58–62.

67. Gunderson EC, Anderson CC. A sampling and analytical method for airborne m-phenylene-diamine (MPDA) and 4,4'-methylenedianiline (MDA). Am Ind Hyg Assoc J 1988; 49:531–538.

68. Roussel R, Gaboury A, Larivière. Aromatic amines in the workplace of an aluminum smelter. In: Rooy EL, ed. Light Metals. Minerals, Metals and Materials Society, Warrendale, PA, 1991: 503–507.

69. Meddle DW, Smith AF. Field method for the determination of aromatic primary amines in air. Part I. Generation of standard atmospheres of amines. Analyst 1981; 106:1082–1087.

70. Ehrin E, Karlberg A-T. Detection of rosin (colophony) components in technical products using an HPLC technique. Contact Derm 1990; 23:359–366.

71. Cassebras M, Rolin A. Fils à souder à flux incorporé. Nuisances chimiques lors de la mise en oeuvre. Cahier des notes documentaires de l'Institut National de Recherche en Sécurité (France). ND 1492, 1984; 116–184.

72. Institut de recherche en santé et en sécurité du travail (IRSST). Méthodes analytiques. Méthodes 2-2 (Co), Méthodes 3-1 (Cr), Méthodes 10-2 (Ni), Montréal, Canada, 1990.

73. National Institute for Occupational Safety and Health (NIOSH). Manual of Analytical Methods, 4th ed., Elements by ICP. Method 7300, Cincinnati, OH, 1994.

15
Medicolegal and Compensation Aspects

I. Leonard Bernstein
University of Cincinnati College of Medicine, Cincinnati, Ohio

Helena Keskinen
Finnish Institute of Occupational Health, Helsinki, Finland

Jean-Luc Malo
Université de Montréal and Sacré-Coeur Hospital, Montréal, Quebec, Canada

BACKGROUND

As a prelude to a discussion of compensation issues specifically concerned with occupational asthma, it is useful to review how occupational diseases per se evolved from the preeminence of injury as a raison d'être for workers' disability and compensation. The concept of protecting workers from the consequences of occupational disease—as contrasted to occupational injury—is a relatively recent development among industrial countries. In the late nineteenth century, middle European countries, starting with Switzerland, Germany, and Austria, began to compensate workers for work-related injuries (1). Similar legislation appeared in Britain in the first decade of the twentieth century. In the United States, workers' compensation legislation was under the purview of individual states, thereby resulting in a heterogeneity of disease definitions, covered diseases, exposure criteria, and other inconsistencies that still exist. Apart from three separate federal systems administered under the Federal Coal Mine Health and Safety Act of 1969, the Longshoreman's and Harbor Worker's Compensation Act, and the Federal Employees Compensation Act, there are no uniform governmental standards in the United States to guide individual state compensation disability programs. The first compensation laws adopted by individual states restricted compensation to those diseases caused by accidental injuries. These were modeled after the original British Workers' Compensation Statue of 1897. Massachusetts was the first state to extend legislation allowing for the compensation of "nontraumatic" occupational diseases. In 1920, New York State adopted the first schedule of compensable occupational diseases (2,3). California rapidly followed suit, and by the early 1930s, most states had passed workers' compensation laws concerning occupational diseases, although few of these provided broad coverage for many of the occupational diseases then being reported.

The principle underlying workers' compensation is that of a "no-fault insurance system" in which employees waive their common law right to sue their employers for damages in exchange for income, medical benefits, and rehabilitation services paid for by private or state government insurers (4). The impetus for compensation coverage of respiratory diseases was heightened in the early 1930s by the large number of claims for dust-induced diseases, particularly silicosis (1). In that economically depressed era, many large suits were being awarded through the common law tort system. Coincidentally, the public was alerted to a major industrial disease calamity, which occurred when hundreds of workers succumbed to fatal doses of inhaled silica dust in a tunneling project at Gauley Bridge, West Virginia (4,5). These events catalyzed lobbying by both employers and unions for legislative compensation relief in several states, which subsequently culminated in special workers' compensation legislation dealing specifically with pneumoconiotic disease ("dust funds") (6). Although there subsequently was considerable variability in the recognition of other types of occupationally induced lung disease from state to state, by 1978 every state in the United States had provided workers' compensation for disability resulting from this category of disease (4). Thus the thrust of workers' compensation disease legislation was focused primarily on dust-induced entities such as silicosis and asbestosis as well as respiratory conditions due to toxic agents. The possibility that occupational asthma might also require special legislative attention had not yet surfaced in most states.

As occupational diseases were gradually incorporated into the matrix of industrial compensation, it became apparent—in contrast to occupational injuries—that the legislative approach to such problems would be greatly influenced by special circumstances leading to the illness (1). For conditions such as asthma, specific etiological factors cannot always be demonstrated, and multiple-factor causality (e.g., interactions with atopy, cigarette smoking) frequently complicated the situation. To address these issues, special schedules or tables of specific diseases, occupations, and etiological agents were established by Euro-Canadian compensation agencies as well as several states in the United States. Since such lists were deemed to be overly restrictive and were generally not amended in a timely manner when new scientific evidence mandated a change, all states eventually abandoned the use of scheduling for occupational diseases. Even with the adoption of regulations that permit claims for all occupational disease, potential claimants still face problems in seeking compensation for their work-related illness.

When diagnostic approaches are inaccurate or recognition of the work-relatedness of a presenting condition by the medical community is poor, occupational disease may not be identified and therefore not reported (7). On the other hand, ignorance about appropriate diagnostic techniques necessary to confirm a disease may result in unwarranted claims. "Pragmatic" interactions of socioeconomic and political stresses may result in restriction of the scope of coverage or the clinical recognition of a particular occupational disease (8). The following definition of occupational disease used by the Nebraska compensation system contains many elements in common with other state definitions: "The term 'occupational disease' shall mean only a disease which is due to causes and conditions which are characteristic of and peculiar to a particular trade, occupation, process or employment, and shall exclude all ordinary diseases of life to which the general public are exposed" (2).

Aggravation or acceleration of preexisting conditions add to the complexity of what constitutes an occupational disease. If a disease is rare and is due to a claimant's allergy in combination with workplace exposures, a disease will usually be held to be work-related if "the increased exposure occasioned by employment in fact brought on the disease" (2). Placing time limitations on occupational diseases may overlook certain diseases (e.g., asbestos-induced mesothelioma), which develop only after a lengthy latency period. Many state laws also stipulate that the worker must have been on the job for a "somewhat extended period." Finally, the definition of an occupational disease often includes a minimum exposure rule in an attempt to exclude the frequently confounding variable of a concurrent "ordinary life disease." Many of the above issues impact on the diagnosis of occupational asthma and will be discussed in greater detail in the following section.

CURRENT STATE OF THE COMPENSATION SYSTEM FOR ASTHMA IN THE UNITED STATES

Regulations and policies governing compensation for occupational asthma vary from state to state. Reliable prevalence and incidence statistics are not available for most states. This is due chiefly to the varied manner in which workers' compensation programs define occupational asthma and the fact that most states do not keep accurate statistics of asthma as a distinct disease entity. The majority of states employ the American National Standards Institute (ANSI) nature of disease coding as specified by the supplementary data system (SDS) of disease reporting, as instituted by the United States Department of Labor. Under this coding system, asthma is included with a number of other unrelated diseases such as influenza, bronchitis, emphysema, and pneumonia. Currently, ANSI specifies two codes for asthma embedded within broad classes of disease: (1) systemic poisoning (from inhalation, ingestion, etc.) (code 274), and (2) conditions of the respiratory system (code 572). Thirty-one states maintain workers' compensation claims in machine-readable format that would permit retrieval of asthma data if there were a single code for that condition (6). With appropriate coding, compensation claims have proven to be a valuable tool for occupational disease surveillance (9,10). Secondary data sources such as death certificates and hospital discharge summaries have not served as reliable sources of disability induced by occupational asthma (6,11,12).

A retrospective analysis of the 1978 Social Security Disability Survey yielded interesting data about the contribution of workplace exposures to the prevalence of asthma in adults (13). In this study, an affirmative response to the question "Was this condition caused by bad working conditions, such as noise, heat, or smoke?" met the case definition of work-relatedness for any given disease. This question was asked for each identified condition in the survey so as not to create bias and the questionnaire elicited information concerning the respondent's occupational history. The presence of asthma coupled with an affirmative answer to the question quoted above was accepted as occupationally related asthma for the epidemiological purpose of this study. Seventy-two (1.2%) of 6063 respondents, or 15.4% of all those with asthma, attributed their asthmatic symptoms to workplace exposures. These subjects were older and included more men, cigarette smokers, and former smokers. The relative risk for occupationally attributed asthma was elevated among industrial and agricultural workers as compared to white-collar and service occupations. Analysis of disability benefit status among various cohorts of this survey did not indicate that this method of analysis introduced major reporting bias. It was therefore concluded that the high prevalence of occupationally self-attributed asthma in this study was a valid observation.

Annual prevalence data of occupational asthma derived from workers' compensation claims are just beginning to appear from several states that are collating occupational asthma cases from Doctors' First Report Forms or that are participating in the Sentinel Event Notification System for Occupational Risks (SENSOR) instituted by NIOSH in 1987 (Table 1) (12,14,15). Wisconsin, New York and Colorado participated in SENSOR from 1987–1992. Massachusetts, Michigan and New Jersey have been in the program from 1987 to the present while California has been a participant since 1992. Although there is considerable variation among states reporting these data, it is interesting that the number of reported cases of occupational asthma and RADS has exceeded the total number of dust diseases of the lungs in the United States, as self-reported by respondents in the 1988 National Health Interview Survey (16). The occupational asthma database contained in Table 1 illustrates how difficult it is to make interstate comparisons. Asthma case data for California are based on Doctors' First Reports of Occupational Injury of Illness Forms. In

Table 1 Number of Cases of Occupational Asthma (OA) and Reactive Airways Dysfunction (RADS)* by State–California, Massachusetts, Michigan, and New Jersey SENSOR Work-Related Asthma Programs, 1988–1997

	Sensor states							
	California[†]		Massachusetts[§]		Michigan[¶]		New Jersey**	
Year	OA	RADS	OA	RADS	OA	RADS	OA	RADS
1988	—	—	—	—	30		27	
1989	—	—	—	—	55		25	
1990	—	—	—	—	122		31	
1991	—	—	—	—	84		38	
1992	—	—	—	—	118	113	20	70
1993	93		45		144		27	
1994	76		39		124		19	
1995	79	39	37	24	91		20	
1996	90		[48]		108		23	
1997	[38]		[50]		[69]		[7]	
Subtotals	376 + 39		219 + 24		945 + 113		237 + 70	
Totals	415		243		1058		367	

—indicates no case counts available for the specified year.

[ ]indicates data are incomplete for the specified years.

*This table includes provisional surveillance data as of June 1998. Data for 1997 are incomplete. The occupational asthma cases included in this table represent occupational asthma and RADS cases that are identified by the state-based SENSOR asthma programs. They do not include work-aggravated asthma (preexisting asthma that has been exacerbated by exposures encountered in the workplace).

[†]California data are based on Doctor's First Reports of Occupational Injury or Illness (DFR). From 1993–1997, there were a total of 1,442 asthma cases identified through DFRs. However, only about half of all of the DFR asthma cases identified from 1993–1997 could be interviewed to determine their case classification status.

[§]Massachusetts data are based on physician reports and cases identified through hospital discharge data. Potential cases from hospital discharge data have primary or secondary discharge diagnoses coded to ICD–9 493 (asthma) and report Workers' Compensation as the expected payer or ICD–9 506 (respiratory conditions due to chemical fumes and vapors) regardless of who the expected payer is. Data from 1996–1997 are preliminary and have not yet been edited for duplicates.

[¶]Michigan data are based on physician reports, hospital discharge information, Workers' compensation claims, information obtained from regulatory agencies (the Mine Safety and Health Administration and the Occupational Safety and Health Administration), and index case follow-up investigations where co-workers of the index case are administered a symptoms questionnaire that is reviewed by a physician. Co-workers with symptoms suggestive of work-related asthma are sent letters by the surveillance program informing them of their questionnaire findings and encouraging them to seek medical evaluation of their symptoms. Hospital discharge data are searched for the same criteria as used by New Jersey and Massachusetts. Data from 1997 are incomplete.

**New Jersey data are based on physician reports and hospital discharge data. Hospital discharge data are searched for the same criteria as used by Michigan and Massachusetts. In addition, 63 reports of work-related asthma for this time period are still undergoing evaluation and therefore these potential cases are pending case classification assignment.

Table 2 Most Frequently Reported Agents Associated with
New Onset Occupational Asthma and RADS in All Four
SENSOR States, 1993–1995*

Agents	Number of cases
Air Pollutants, indoor	67
Chemicals, NOS**	56
Lubricants, NOS	55
Mineral and Organic dust, NOS	45
Cleaning Materials, NOS	43
Toluene diisocyanate	41
Smoke, NOS	40
Solvents, NOS	37
Diisocyanates, NOS	34
Formaldehyde	32
Welding fumes, stainless steel	31
Methylene diisocyanate	24
Latex, natural rubber	24
Paint	22

*The information in Tables 1 and 2 was kindly supplied by the fol-
lowing agencies and professionals:
  California SENSOR WRA program: Robert Harrison, M.D., M.P.H.
  and Jennifer Flattery, M.P.H.
  Massachusetts SENSOR WRA program: Catharine Tumpowsky,
  M.P.H. and Letitia Davis, Sc.D.
  Michigan SENSOR WRA program: Kenneth D. Rosenman, M.D.,
  Mary Jo Reilly, M.S., and Doug Kalinowski, C.I.H.
  New Jersey SENSOR WRA program: Martha Stanbury, M.S.P.H.,
  Donald Schill, C.I.H., and David Valiante, C.I.H.
  From CDC/NIOSH: Ruth Ann Jajosky, D.M.D., M.P.H.
**NOS - not otherwise specified

Massachusetts and New Jersey, workers' compensation cases are based upon physician
reports and hospital discharge data. The data shown for Michigan are based on physician
reports, hospital discharge information, worker's compensation claims, regulatory agency
information and index case followup investigations. Table 2 is a compilation of the most
frequently reported agents associated with new onset asthma as reported by the four current
SENSOR programs (California, Massachusetts, Michigan and New Jersey) from 1993–
1995. Although the SENSOR system was not designed to be a comprehensive surveillance
system, it has led to reports of previously unrecognized causes of occupational asthma
(17). Moreover, the use of surveillance data may have been instrumental in detection of
additional symptomatic coworkers and inadequate work practices. The goal of the current
four state SENSOR program is to develop a prototypic surveillance system which could
be used as a model for other states and territories (17).

DEFINING DISEASE/ASSESSING DISABILITY

Many of the key problems associated with the definition of occupational disease also apply
to occupational asthma (1). Multiple causality, the difficulty of diagnosis, the dilemma of

preexistent asthma being aggravated by workplace stimuli, the persistence of occupational asthma after leaving the workplace, and the variability in legal adjudication of occupational asthma in the United States are issues that will be addressed in this section.

Multiple Causality

Etiological factors are not always readily identifiable, especially by nonoccupationally trained, primary care practitioners. In some cases, even when materials are determined to be probable suspects, their intrinsic hazardous properties may preclude further objective testing. The question of multiple-factor causality is a major problem in defining occupational asthma. It is well known that cigarette smoking is an additive factor in certain types of occupational asthma but that it does not pose a risk factor in others. Moreover, in certain industries, concurrent exposure to known asthma stimuli (e.g., platinum salts and chlorine gas) may enhance the development of clinical asthma (18). Workplace temperature and the amount of exercise required during a job may also affect both the onset and severity of asthma.

The Difficulty of Diagnosis

It is acknowledged that the diagnosis of occupational asthma may be difficult, especially for the untrained, primary care practitioner. Since, by definition, asthma typically presents with episodic and reversible clinical manifestations, a worker's physical examination and objective tests may be completely normal after he is away from work for a few days. Physicians may not be aware that skin and serological tests can assist in the diagnosis in certain situations. If the diagnostic evaluation is limited to inadequate objective criteria, the correct diagnosis will not be made. Conversely, skin or laboratory tests may be improperly interpreted and a diagnosis of work-related asthma made, when in reality another condition is responsible for the presenting signs and symptoms.

Preexistent and Persistent Asthma

Preexisting asthma may be aggravated by conditions or substances at work. Aggravation of asthma must clearly be distinguished from chronic, low-level exposure to specific sensitizers in the workplace or from the reactive airways dysfunction syndrome (RADS) secondary to acute toxic exposures to nonsensitizing irritants such as gases and chemicals (17). Whether it is appropriate to include aggravation of preexisting asthma in the disease category of occupational asthma is largely unsettled in the United States. Some states (e.g., Pennsylvania, Michigan, and New York) clearly allow aggravation of preexistent asthma as a compensable condition, but many states do not (4). However, under most circumstances, if aggravating stimuli are asthmogenic, it must be ascertained that they are peculiar to the workplace and not commonplace in the nonwork environment (1). In addition, a worker who is aware of preexisting asthma induced by known environmental insults (e.g., pollen) should not knowingly attempt to work under conditions that would predictably involve increased exposure to prior known allergens (19). Some states impose specified time limitations on occupational diseases [i.e., a worker would have to be exposed to a substance in a certain worksite for a given period of time; or at the other end of the spectrum, a claim would not be considered timely if there was a long latency period between initial exposure and first onset of symptoms (4)]. Either situation could be unfair to a worker who develops occupationally induced airways obstruction and bronchial hyperresponsiveness. In the case of irritant-induced asthma (RADS), only a short, brief exposure is required and this could conceivably occur on the first or second day of work. On the other hand, it is not uncommon for bakers to work for many years before they actually develop symptoms due to one or more ingredients in flour. Another confounding variable is the increasing recognition that certain forms of occupational asthma, including RADS, may continue unabated for many years after cessation of exposure (20–25). Thus, the failure to improve or revert to normal status after the worker has been removed from the workplace is no longer a valid reason for a determination that the asthma was non-occupational (26).

Legal Adjudication of Occupational Asthma in the United States

While many states in the past have sought to limit the scope of compensation coverage for dust and respiratory diseases, restrictive regulations have not yet affected the diagnosis of occupational asthma. Some states still make it possible to include asthmatic disease under injury provisions (1). However, disputed questions of occupational asthma including formidable ones of diagnosis, causality, and disability are usually decided by litigation in an adversarial proceeding (4). Evidence from lay and expert witnesses is presented to adjudicators appointed by the compensation board. Since asthma may often be related to nonworkplace life exposures, tobacco smoking, and numerous irritants, it is estimated that 90% of these claims are litigated, often without success. Thus, of 242 workers' compensation claims filed for illnesses involving the respiratory system in the state of Washington for the period 1984–1988, 87 (36%) were rejected. This rate of rejection was higher than the average rate of rejection both for occupational diseases (18%) and for occupational injuries (4%). Those disease categories with the highest rates of rejection were those with the least well-developed diagnostic guidelines such as mental disorders (79%), and neoplasia (67%) (25). In some states the success of this litigation often depends upon objective proof of causation, which in the case of occupational asthma may require controlled bronchial challenges. However, other factors such as the experience of the diagnosing physician with the rules of the compensation system may be a factor in the success of the claim (27).

Once a claim is allowed, complete medical care is provided and medical expenses are paid by either the self-insured employer or the state compensation fund for workers qualified under the respective programs (4). In most states, workers' compensation wage replacement equals two-thirds of workers' predisability wages but no more than a maximum determined from the statewide average weekly wage for the duration of disability. Compensation is provided for proven objective disability, not for impairment. Providing less than complete compensation of wage loss is felt to serve as an incentive for healthy workers to avoid workplace injury and disease and for diseased workers to return to work, if at all possible. A particularly troubling feature of workers' compensation for occupational diseases in general is the small proportion (5%) of individuals who have a severe disability that resulted from a job-related exposure and rely on this system for benefits. According to a nationwide survey of disabled and nondisabled adults whose disability was the result of a job-related disease, the four primary sources of support were social security (53%), pensions (21%), veterans' benefits (17%), and public welfare (16%). It appears that the "safety net" in the United States may be social security, pension, and welfare systems (28). Rehabilitation and retraining programs are integral components of all state industrial programs. In the case of asthma, rehabilitation must be carried out with the goal of providing an environment free of future exposure to specific allergens and nonspecific aggravating agents.

THE INTERNATIONAL PERSPECTIVE

Reliance upon schedules or lists of covered diseases distinguishes workers' compensation systems in the United States from those in some industrialized countries in Europe (and some provinces in Canada) where compensation is allowed for all occupationally related diseases (1). In those countries relying upon schedules, if a claimant develops a disease within the scope of an approved schedule, there is a strong presumption that compensation will be allowed. On the other hand, if a worker claims for a disease not on the list, the presumption against compensation for that disease usually directs the worker to seek other sources of social assistance. In the United Kingdom and France, schedules are also used. Illustrations of representative lists of agents/exposures associated with occupational asthma in the United Kingdom and France are shown in Table 3 (29,30). Although the use of such restrictive lists of covered exposures may at first glance appear to be a harsh method of dealing with the socioeconomic hardships of an occupational disease, most of the countries in western Europe and provinces in Canada have well-developed secondary sources of health and disability insurance that compensate at levels comparable to those if industrial compensation were allowed. To assure an even-handed approach when compensation is based upon restrictive lists of diseases, it is essential that these lists be upgraded at frequent intervals to accommodate the rapid pace of medical advancement in the field of occupational asthma. Inequalities in such systems could arise if, despite evolving medical evidence, legislative upgradings fail to materialize due to sociopolitical forces. However, as mentioned above, the great equalizer of these compensation systems outside the United

Table 3   Agents Causing Occupational Asthma in the United Kingdom and France

---

United Kingdom
1. Platinum salts
2. Isocyanates
3. Epoxy resins
4. Colophony fumes
5. Proteolytic enzymes
6. Laboratory animals and insects
7. Grain (or flour dust)
8.[a] Miscellaneous

France
1. Aromatic amines (no. 13)
2. Phosphates, pyrophosphates, thiophophates (no. 34)
3. Tropical woods (no. 47)
4. Aromatic and alicyclic amines (no. 49)
5. Phenylhydrazine (no. 50)
6. Isocyanates (no. 62)
7. Enzymes (no. 63)

---

[a]Any occupational agent can be included if objective proof of causality is determined. *Source*: Ref. 29,30.

States appears to be that sick and disabled workers have readily available alternative benefits (e.g., national health insurance, etc.) that may be equal to or only slightly less than workers' benefits (1). While these safety nets provide for greater opportunity for "full" compensation for the disabled worker, the true costs of occupational disease to industry are shifted to other insurance schemes. Questions of compensation faced by adjudication of industrial claims are less dramatic and compelling when an alternative compensation system is so readily available. In general, the experiences thus far in such countries suggest that when there are no disincentives to contesting a worker's claim, the incidence of occupational disease claims is not necessarily higher than in privately insured systems, particularly in regard to serious claims (1). For example, recent incidence data of occupational disease claims from Germany (Table 4) demonstrated that 5–6% of all suspected cases were ultimately compensated for the period 1985 through 1987 regardless of whether the origin of the problem was allergic or irritative.

Apart from the generally agreed upon use of specific lists for the presumptive diagnosis of occupational asthma, compensation systems outside the United States have considerable heterogeneity (1). Many of the international compensation systems have been discussed in a recent review and are summarized in Table 5 (31). In France, workers with occupational diseases have been compensated since 1919. Two official lists exist, one for farms and one for general employers. There is a table for each work-related disease, which includes a list of symptoms, an indication of workplaces where subjects may be exposed, and the minimum exposure. Compensation is awarded only if the symptoms and workplace are listed in the table. If a worker has a proven but unlisted occupational disease, for which compensation is not allowed, a claim must be made through a judicial procedure. This is a rare occurrence, due to the complexity of the legal process. The listing system does not recognize all occupational diseases because they cannot be updated at regular intervals (30). In Belgium, compensation of occupational diseases is completely separated from that due to accidents in the workplace. The Belgian system removes the controversy between employers and workers over complex questions of etiology, diagnosis, and preexisting conditions by totally separating the financing of compensation and payment of benefits. Although asthma is not on the Belgian schedule of occupational illnesses, it is treated as an occupational disease when it occurs in workers having exposures to certain hazards appearing in the schedule. However, some of these cases, such as exposure to flax, are conditioned by minimum exposure. Denmark now has a "mixed" private and state insurance system. Although compensation for asthma is usually linked to specified occupations or exposure, it is also recognized that disability may occur as a result of exposure to substances not on the current schedule. The Danish system is almost completely nonadversarial because there are ample social alternatives for workers with illnesses that are

Table 4 Comparison of Allergic versus Irritative Occupational Asthma in Germany, 1985–1987

	Suspected		Compensated	
	Allergic	Irritative	Allergic	Irritative
1985	2414	703	147	44
1986	3349	883	166	49
1987	3393	1136	219	41

Source: Ref. 42.

Table 5 Review of Systems and Compensation for Occupational Asthma in Various Countries

	Who administers?	Who pays?	Is occupational asthma compensated?	Who examines cases?	How is the diagnosis made?	No. of cases (year)	Permanent disability allocated?
Australia	Cases handled by court	Private insurers	Yes	Specialist	Multiple means	?	Yes
Belgium	National agency	Employers	Yes	Board of specialists	Multiple means	?	Yes
Brazil	National agency	Employers (15 days) and government (afterward)	Yes	Physician designated by the national agency	Multiple means	?	Yes
Bulgaria	National agency	Employers	Yes	Board of specialists	Multiple means	?	Yes
Canada	Provincial agencies	Employers	Yes	Variable (provinces)	Variable (provinces)	~100 (Quebec)	Yes (Quebec) Variable (others)
Finland	National agency	Employers	Yes	Chest physician	Multiple means	352(1991)	Yes
France	Regional agency	Employers	Yes	Social Security practitioners	Multiple means	456(1985)	Yes

Italy	National agency	Employers	Yes	Decision made with specific expertise	Clinical	? Up to 550 in 1989	Yes
New Zealand	National	Employers	Yes	Agency physician and claimant's MD	Variable	?	Yes
Norway	National agency and private insurance	Employers *private insurers	Yes	Claimant's physician	Multiple means	52	Yes
Romania	National agency	Employers	Yes	Board of specialists	Multiple means	?	Yes
South Africa	National agency	Employers and private insurers	Yes	Medical advisory panels (to come)	Clinical	?	Provinces not necessarily applied
South Korea	National agency	Employers	Yes	Specialists	Multiple means	?	No
Spain	Government agency	Employers	Yes	Board of specialists	Multiple means	146 (1990)	Yes
The Netherlands	No specific system	Employers and employees	No official acceptance	Board of chest physicians	Multiple means	? (under-reporting)	No
United Kingdom	Governmental agency	General taxation	Yes	Career specialists for assessing occupational diseases	Variable	293 cases examined (Year 1991)	Yes ("prescribed disease provisions")
United States	No-fault insurance system	Employers	Yes	Variable (states)	Variable (states)	?	?

not compensable. The Workers' Compensation program has been completely abolished in the Netherlands. If a worker is unable to return to work within 1 year, or his disability limits his ability to earn income, he is entitled to disablement insurance, which continues until he has been fully cured, dies, or reaches the age of 65, at which time other pension arrangements supervene. How this broad and permissive program affects claims for occupational asthma is not yet clear.

In Finland all employees are insured in private insurance companies against occupational diseases. Of the self-employed workers, agricultural workers are entitled to compensation for an occupational disease. Voluntary insurance can be taken by other self-employed workers. An occupational disease is defined as "a disease caused mainly by a physical factor, a chemical substance or a biological agent encountered in the work done under contract of employment or as 'agricultural entrepreneur.'" The diagnosis "requires such medical examination where there is sufficient knowledge on exposure in the work and where in the case of occupational diseases, a specialist in the field is in charge." A disease is to be deemed as occupational when the factor "is present in a person's work to such an extent that its exposure effect is sufficient to cause the disease in question, unless it is stated that the disease has been clearly caused by exposure outside work." Table 6 lists covered diseases under various Finnish ordinances. The diagnosis of occupational asthma in Finland is carried out by lung specialists in the central or university hospitals where the workers are usually sent by the plant physician. The Finnish Institute of Occupational Health (FIOH) can also be consulted. The approximate annual number of new cases of occupational asthma reported to the Register of Occupational Diseases has been 400 (32). About 20% of these have been investigated at FIOH. A diagnosis of occupational asthma is made in about every third person investigated at FIOH for this suspected disease. When an occupational disease is suspected by a physician familiar with the exposure at the workplace, the insurance company is obligated to pay for the necessary diagnostic investigation. If the disease is accepted as occupational, the patient is entitled to several types of compensation, which are better than those obtained from national health insurance for a nonoccupational disease. This policy, combined with the fact that the investigations are free of charge, may create an increased incentive for the worker to claim occupational disease. Future costs of the disease, including medications, doctor's fees, travel expenses, reeducation as well as sick leave compensation, are totally paid. When the worker is

Table 6   Agents Listed as Causes of Occupational Asthma in Finland (Ordinance On Occupational Diseases, 1988)

Cobalt, chromium, and nickel and their compounds
Diisocyanates
Amines
Formaldehyde
Organic acid anhydrides
Antibiotics
Plastics and synthetic resins and the substances and intermediates involved in their production
Organic dusts (flours, grain, wood dusts and materials, animal epithelia, excretions and other
   exposures of animal origin, dusts of natural fibers and enzymes, natural resins, natural rubber)
Reactive and dispersion dyes
Moulds and other biologically active substances

Source: Ref. 32.

transferred to another, more suitable job without harmful exposure, but with a lower salary, the difference is largely compensated. If an occupational disease causes a permanent disability of more than 10%, a lump sum estimated to cover the harm caused by the disease is additionally paid according to the extent of the disability. When the occupational disease causes total disability, the pension granted will be higher (85% of the former salary) than that awarded for nonoccupational disability (60%). According to the statistics supplied to the Register of Occupational Diseases by insurance companies, about 80% of the claims for occupational asthma are accepted and compensated (Table 7). A Finnish statistical review of occupational diseases is compiled every year. A synopsis in English is available (32).

Several Canadian compensation programs have eliminated the adversarial approach to etiology and diagnosis. In all provinces, these issues are assigned to professionals representing neither the plaintiff nor the defendant (31). Thus, each case is decided solely on the merits of the exposure conditions and objective evidence of the disease. Prior experience with a similar administrative system had been gained in Quebec. Suspected cases of occupational asthma are referred for further investigation to specialists working in facilities devoted to such evaluations. However, the Quebec definition of occupational asthma is limited to specific sensitizing products, which are listed in Table 8 (33). Irritating agents are not considered to be compensable causes of occupational asthma if they aggravate preexisting asthma. However, there is sufficient latitude for compensation of workers with RADS or asthma occurring after exposure to certain nonsensitizers (e.g., colophony, vanadium, or pot-room asthma).

Occupational claims comparing changes in number of claims in Quebec from 1977 to 1997 (Table 9) suggest that there has been a marked increase in asthma claims compared to claims for both asbestosis and silicosis. Table 10 also shows the extent and distribution of compensation in Quebec as compared to other respiratory compensation claims. These data clearly reveal that asthma now is a significant cause of respiratory disease claims in Quebec. The most likely explanation for this appears to be improved detection and diagnosis because all suspected cases of occupational asthma are referred to highly trained specialists for sophisticated evaluations, which usually include immunological testing and challenge procedures where indicated. However, it is also possible that there has been a real increase in the frequency of asthma.

Determination of compensation costs in the Canadian provinces is based on a two-tier system (33). The first level provides for income replacement indemnity and complete costs for rehabilitation. Since many patients with occupational asthma are young, rehabilitation is mandatory. This process generally lasts 1–2 years. The second tier is based

Table 7 Occupational Asthma, Number of Claims and Accepted and Compensated Cases in 1990–1992 in Finland (Workforce 2.07 million)

	Reports to the register	Accepted
1990	375	285 (76%)
1991	352	314 (89%)
1992	380	297 (78%)

Source: Statistics of the Union of Accident Insurance Companies and the Accident Insurance for Agriculture.

Table 8 Etiological Agents of
Occupational Asthma, Total for Years
1988–1997 (10 Years), Quebec
Workers' Compensation Board

Isocyanates	149
Flour	99
Wood dust	56
Metals	39
Seafoods	38
Epoxy, glues, resins	37
Cereals	31
Laboratory animals	26
Drugs	22
Latex	18
Hairdressing	11
Guar gum	8
Chicken feathers	8
Coffee	4
Photographic products	2
Insects	2
Metabisulfite	2
Formaldehyde	2
Others	16
Total	570

Cases generally confirmed by specific inhalation challenges.
Source: Data obtained thanks to the medical
office of the WCB (Dr. Monique Rioux).

Table 9 New Cases of Compensated Occupational Lung Diseases in Quebec, 1997 and
1988–1997

Diagnosis	Year											
	1977	1987	1988	1989	1990	1991	1992	1993	1994	1995	1996	1997
Asthma	6	97	79	54	58	70	51	61	59	40	59	48
Asbestos-related	43	36	77	57	53	76	66	61	71	70	113	84
Silicosis	36	62	40	31	42	45	25	38	27	18	26	24
Total of all occupational lung diseases	—	—	230	203	249	234	171	198	189	157	220	172

Cases of asthma are most often confirmed by specific inhalation challenges; asbestos-related lung diseases
include asbestosis, mesothelioma, and bronchial carcinoma.
Source: Data obtained thanks to the medical offices of the WCB (Dr. Monique Rioux).

Table 10 Extent and Distribution of Compensation in Quebec

Diagnosis	New claims	Reassessments[a]	Total
Occupational asthma	81	89	170
Asbestosis	30	111	141
Silicosis	36	103	139
Cancer	46	38	84
Occupational bronchitis	15	8	23
Other	20	37	57

[a]Permanent disability is assessed 2 years after diagnosis is made and the worker removed from exposure.
Source: Ref. 31.

on permanent disability indemnity. The criteria used for determination of permanent disability are baseline bronchial obstruction, the degree of bronchial hyperresponsiveness, and the need for medication. There is consensus among occupational asthma experts that all three of these components are essential to determine an acceptable profile of disability (29,33–36).

It is possible that removal of the adversarial status for compensation of occupational disease may be a disincentive for employers' responsibilities for assuring healthy and safe workplaces. This is particularly germane to workplaces representing a clearly excessive risk for occupational asthma, where the need for remedial industrial engineering and more intensive medical surveillance is absolutely compelling. Unfortunately, a meta-analysis addressing this issue under adversarial and nonadversarial compensation systems has not yet been accomplished.

RECOMMENDATIONS FOR THE FUTURE

Based on the increased volume of medical research and literature concerning occupational asthma, it has been predicted that asthma will surpass pneumoconiosis as the leading cause of respiratory disability in workers (19,37). In 1989 a program for the surveillance of work-related and occupational respiratory disease (SWORD) was established in the United Kingdom. With chest and occupational physicians as the reporting units, 554 cases of occupational asthma were identified in the first year of the SWORD project as compared to 322 cases of pneumoconiosis (38). These data have since been extended to include irritant-induced asthma occurring after inhalation accidents (39). These now comprise 10% of all reported occupational lung diseases. Data being assessed in the United States by the SENSOR project states suggest that a similar shift may have already occurred in some localities (Table 2). Confirmation of this trend will not be possible by analysis of current statistical data collected by compensation systems in individual states because asthma is classified with a miscellaneous group of unrelated pulmonary problems. However, workers' compensation claims could constitute a significant database for detection, surveillance, and prevention of workplace asthma provided individual states, provinces, and nations reach agreement about defining, classifying, and coding occupational asthma.

All would agree that occupational asthma is characterized by reversible narrowing of the lower airways with varying degrees of airway hyperresponsiveness induced by exposure to work-related substances. However, there is still considerable controversy about

Table 11   Surveillance Guidelines for State Health Departments: Occupational Asthma

---

Reporting guidelines

State health departments should encourage providers to report all suspected or diagnosed cases of occupational asthma. These should include persons with:

a. A physician diagnosis of asthma
   and
b. An association between symptoms of asthma and work

State health departments should collect appropriate clinical, epidemiological, and workplace information on reported cases to set priorities for workplace investigations.

Surveillance case definition

a. A physician diagnosis of asthma[a]
   and
b. An association between symptoms of asthma and work[b] and any one of the following:
   1. Workplace exposure to an agent or process previously associated with occupational asthma[c]
      or
   2. Significant work-related changes in forced expiratory volume in 1 sec (FEV_1) or peak expiratory flow rate (PEFR)
      or
   3. Significant work-related changes in airways responsiveness as measured by nonspecific inhalation challenge[d]
      or
   4. Positive response to inhalation provocation testing with agent to which patient is exposed at work. Inhalation provocation testing with workplace substances is potentially dangerous and should be performed by experienced personnel in a hospital setting where resuscitation facilities are available and where frequent observations can be made over a sufficient time period to monitor for delayed reactions.

---

[a]Asthma is a clinical syndrome characterized by increased responsiveness of the tracheobronchial tree to a variety of stimuli. Symptoms of asthma include episodic wheezing, chest tightness, and dyspnea, or recurrent attacks of "bronchitis" with cough, sputum production, and rhinitis. The primary physiological manifestation of wirways hyperresponsiveness is variable or reversible airflow obstruction, which may be demonstrated by significant changes in the forced expiratory volume in 1 sec (FEV_1) or peak expiratory flow rate (PEFR). Airflow changes can occur spontaneously, with treatment, with a precipitating exposure, or with diagnostic maneuvers, such as nonspecific inhalation challenge.

[b]Patterns of association can vary. The following examples are patterns that may suggest an occupational etiology: symptoms of asthma develop after a worker starts a new job or after new materials are introduced on the job (a substantial period of time may elapse between initial exposure and development of symptoms); symptoms develop within minutes of specific activities or exposures at work; delayed symptoms occur several hours after exposure, during the evenings of workdays; symptoms occur several hours after exposure, during the evenings of workdays; symptoms occur less frequently or not at all on days away from work and on vacations; symptoms occur more frequently on returning to work. Work-related changes in medication requirements may have similar patterns, also suggesting an occupational etiology.

[c]Many agents and processes have been associated with occupational asthma, and others continue to be recognized.

[d]Changes in nonspecific bronchial hyperreactivity can be measured by serial inhalation challenge testing with methacholine or histamine. Increased bronchial reactivity (manifested by reaction to lower concentrations of methacholine or histamine) following exposure and decreased bronchial reactivity after a period away from work are evidence of work-relatedness.

Source: Ref. 40.

whether such substances should be limited to sensitizing agents. Since many proven causes of asthma are due to nonsensitizing agents (e.g., polyvinyl chloride fumes, products of aluminum smelting) or accidental spills (RADS), it would seem unwise to restrict the definition to sensitizers. To resolve this issue there will have to be compromise on a subclassification of occupational asthma, which will encompass sensitizing, toxic irritating, and nontoxic irritating substances at work. In Germany, occupational asthma is distinguished as either allergic or irritative (see Table 4). If this system were universally adopted, it would then be possible to utilize Doctors' First Reports of occupational asthma, as is the case in California, where there appears to be an increasing trend of reported occupational asthma cases from 1983 to the present. Recognition of asthma as an occupational disease entity would also encourage standardized diagnostic coding and adoption of the International Classification of Disease (ICD) nomenclature. If these changes were incorporated into the reporting systems of various workers' compensation agencies, it would then be possible to compare and analyze outcome experiences, monitor trends, and target workplace inspections to prevent work-related asthma.

Implementation of these goals in the United States requires a concerted effort and cooperation among individual state health departments and bureaus of workers' compensation. Appropriate federal agencies, such as NIOSH and the Bureau of Labor Statistics, have an important role in standardizing disease definitions, coding, and reporting. NIOSH is currently attempting to initiate this process by the SENSOR program (12,14,15). One of the by-products of this program has been the development of a universally applicable surveillance case definition of occupational asthma. With validation and modification of this case definition, state health departments will begin to access reliable data concerning occupational asthma from primary or selected groups of health providers. A partially successful attempt has already been made to validate a proposed surveillance case definition of occupational asthma (40), and case definition modifications have been suggested. A subsequently revised surveillance case definition is presented in Table 11 (12). The use of a consistent case definition by all state workers' compensation boards coupled with consistent coding of occupational asthma claims will allow for a more accurate determination of the incidence and prevalence of this condition.

An interesting set of tentative principles for reforming disability legislation in the United States was proposed in 1981 by the Ad Hoc Committee on Disability Legislation of the American Thoracic Society Scientific Assembly on Environmental and Occupational Health (41). This committee suggested that respiratory disability should be determined by qualified professionals from the fields of law, education, economics, and the health sciences. Further, it recommended that decisions regarding causation should encompass all available scientific data, including the results of appropriate epidemiological studies. These features have already been incorporated into several Euro-Canadian models of workers' compensation for occupational asthma (33,42), but it appears that reform of current workers' compensation disability plans in the United States will be a more arduous process.

SUMMARY

Workers' compensation is a "no-fault insurance system" in which employees waive their common-law right to sue their employers for damages in exchange for income, medical benefits, and rehabilitation services paid for by private or state government insurers. Regulations and policies governing compensation for occupational asthma vary from state to state (43). This variation is due to different ways of defining occupational asthma. Annual workers' compensation claims for occupational asthma are increasing and outstripping pneumoconiosis claims in some states and countries. Many industrialized countries allow compensation for occupational asthma on the basis of schedules or lists of covered diseases. Future attempts to establish a uniform compensation system for occupational asthma will have to address multiple causality of asthma, difficulty of diagnosis, and methods to assess aggravating factors in the workplace.

REFERENCES

1. Barth PS, Hunt HA. Worker's Compensation and Work-Related Illnesses and Disease. Cambridge, MA: MIT Press, 1982.
2. Larson, A. Workers' Compensation Law: Cases, Materials and Text. New York: Matthew Bender & Company, 1990.
3. U.S. Chamber of Commerce. Analysis of Workers Compensation Laws. Washington, D.C., 1990.
4. Richman SI. Why change? A look at the current system of disability determination and workers' compensation for occupational lung disease. Ann Int Med 1982; 97:908–914.
5. Cherniak M. The Hawks Nest Incident: America's Worst Industrial Disaster. New Haven, CT: Yale University Press, 1986.
6. Muldoon JT, Wintermeyer LA, Eure JA, Fluortes L, Merchant JA, Van Lier SF, Richards, TB. Occupational disease surveillance data sources. Am J Pub Health 1987; 77:1006–1008.
7. Rosenstock L. Occupational medicine: Too long neglected. Ann Intern Med 1981; 95:774–776.
8. Rosenstock L, Hagopian A. Ethical dilemmas in providing health care to workers. Ann Intern Med 1987; 107:575–580.
9. Kleinman GD, Cant SM. Occupational disease surveillance in Washington. JOM 1978; 20:750–754.
10. Melius JM, Sestito JP, Seligman PJ. Occupational disease surveillance with existing data sources. AJPH 1989; 79(S):46–52.
11. Freund E, Seligman PJ, Chorba TL, Safford SK, Drachman JG, Hull HF. Mandatory reporting of occupational diseases by clinicians. JAMA 1989; 262:3041–3044.
12. Matte TD, Hoffman RE, Rosenman KD, Stanbury M. Surveillance of occupational asthma under the SENSOR model. Chest 1990; 98:173S–178S.
13. Blanc P. Occupational asthma in a national disability survey. Chest 1987; 92:613–617.
14. National Institute for Occupational Safety and Health. SENSOR: Sentinel Event Notification System for Occupational Risks: A Proposal. U.S. Dept. of Health and Human Services, Centers for Disease Control, Atlanta, GA, 1987.
15. Baker EL IV. Sentinel event notification system for occupational risks (SENSOR): The concept. AJPH 1989; 79:18–20.
16. U.S. Department of Health and Human Services, Public Health Service, Centers for Disease Control and Prevention, National Institute for Occupational Safety and Health, Work-Related Lung Disease Surveillance Report, 1994, Table 10-9, Other Lung Conditions, Morbidity, Morgantown, WV, 1994, 128.
17. Reilly MJ, Rosenman KD, Watt FC, Schill D, Stanbury M, Trimbath LS, Romero Jajosky, RA, Musgrave KJ, Castellan RM, Bang KM, and Ordin DL. Surveillance for Occupational Asthma—Michigan and New Jersey, 1988–1992, MMWR 1994; 43:SS-1, 9–17.
18. Bernstein DI and Bernstein IL. Occupational Asthma, Allergy Principles and Practice. Middleton E, Reed CE, Ellis EF, Adkinson NF, Yuninger JW, Busse WW, eds., St. Louis: Mosby Yearbook, Inc., 1998, 963–980.
19. Richman SI. Legal treatment of the asthmatic worker: A major problem for the nineties, J Occup Med 1990; 32:1027–1031.

20. Adams WG. Long-term effects on the health of men engaged in the manufacture of toluene diisocyanate, Br J Ind Med 1975; 32:72–78.

21. Moller DR, McKay RTK, Bernstein IL, and Brooks S. Long-term follow-up of workers with TDI asthma (abstract), Am Rev Respir Dis 1984; 129:(suppl)A159.

22. Paggiaro PL, Loi AM, Rossi O, Ferrante B, Pardi F, and Rosselli MG. Follow-up study of patients with respiratory disease due to toluene diisocyanate (TDI), Clin Allergy 1984; 14: 463–469.

23. Chan-Yeung M, Llam S, and Koerner S. Clinical features and natural history of occupational asthma due to western red cedar (Thuja plicata), Am J Med 1982; 72:411–415.

24. Burge PA. Occupational asthma in electronic workers caused by colophony fumes: Follow-up of affected workers, Thorax 1982; 37:348–353.

25. Hudson P, Cartier A, Pineau L, Lafrance M, St. Aubiad JJ, Dubois JY, and Malo JL. Follow-up of occupational asthma caused by snow crab and various agents, J Allergy Clin Immunol 1985; 76:682–688.

26. Lass N, Arion H, and Sahar J. Medico-legal aspects of occupational asthma, Ann Allergy 1971; 29:573–577.

27. Blessman JE. Differential Treatment of Occupational Disease versus Occupational Injury by Workers' Compensation in Washington State, JOM 1991; 33:121–126.

28. An Interim Report to Congress on Occupational Diseases, United States Department of Labor, Washington, D.C., 1980.

29. Hedrick DJ and Fabbri L. Compensating occupational asthma. Thorax 1981; 36:881–884.

30. Gervais P, Rosenberg N. Aspects médico-légaux internationaux de l'asthma professionnel. Rev Mal Respir 1988; 5:491–495.

31. Dewitte J-D, Chan-Yeung M, Malo J-L. Medicolegal and compensation aspects of occupational asthma. Eur Respir J 1994; 7:969–980.

32. Toikkanen J, Kauppinen T, Vaaranen V, Vasama M, Jolanki R. Occupational Diseases in Finland in 1993, Review 21. Finnish Institute of Occupational Health, Helsinki, Finland, 1994.

33. Malo J-L. Compensation for occupational asthma in Quebec. Chest 1990; 98:236S–239S.

34. Charpin J. Occupational asthma. In: Yamamura U, Frick OL, Horiuchi Y, et al., eds. Allergology. Amsterdam: Excerpta Medica, 1974:120–122.

35. Chan-Yeung M. Evaluation of impairment/disability in patients with occupational asthma. Am Rev Respir Dis 1987; 135:950–951.

36. Ad Hoc Committee on Occupational Asthma of the Standards Committee, Canadian Thoracic Society. Occupational asthma: recommendations for diagnosis, management and assessment of impairment. Can Med Assoc J 1989; 140:1029–1032.

37. Meredith S, Nordman H. Occupational asthma: measures of frequency from four countries. Thorax 1996; 51:435–440.

38. Meredith SK, Taylor VM, McDonald JC. Occupational respiratory disease in the United Kingdom 1989; a report to the British Thoracic Society and the Society of Occupational Medicine by the SWORD project group. Br J Ind Med 1991; 48:292–298.

39. Sallie B, Ross D, Meredith S, et al., SWORD '95. Surveillance of work-related and occupational respiratory disease in the UK. Occup Med 1994; 44:177–182.

40. Klees JE, Alexander M, Rempel D, Beckett W, Rubin R, Barnhard S, Balmes JJ. Evaluation of a proposed NIOSH surveillance case definition for occupational asthma. Chest 1990; 98: 212S–215S.

41. Ad Hoc Committee on Disability Legislation of the American Thoracic Society Scientific Assembly on Environmental and Occupational Health. Disability legislation for occupational lung disease. Am Thorac Soc News 1981; 29 (Summer).

42. Arbeitsmedizin, Sozialmedizin. Praventivmedizin (ASP) 1989; 24:97.

43. Centers for Disease Control. Occupational disease surveillance: occupational asthma. MMWR 1990; 39:119–123.

16

Evaluation of Impairment/Disability in Subjects with Occupational Asthma

Jean-Luc Malo
Université de Montréal and Sacré-Coeur Hospital, Montréal, Quebec, Canada

Paul Blanc
University of California–San Francisco, San Francisco, California

Moira Chan-Yeung
Vancouver General Hospital and University of British Columbia, Vancouver, British Columbia, Canada

INTRODUCTION

Asthma is a common chronic condition affecting disproportionately those of working age rather than older persons. It is a frequent cause of limitations and, specifically, disability in the workplace. Indeed, asthma is one of the leading medical conditions associated with limitation in the ability to work and work loss.

Based on 1992 National Health Interview Survey data, close to 2.6 million individuals in the United States reported asthma-related general activity limitations inside and outside the workplace (1). Among younger adults in the United States, an estimated 420,000 persons with asthma aged 18–44 years are limited by asthma in their ability to work, as are another 443,000 over age 45. In the 1978 Social Security Administration Survey of Disability and Work, 90% of those claiming severe limitation in work capacity due to asthma were out of the labor force, or 300,000 persons aged 18–44 (2). International data suggest that this issue is not peculiar to the United States (3–6). Moreover, the rising prevalence of asthma suggests that the problem is only likely to grow in the future (7–9).

On the individual case level, disability in asthma plays itself out in a complex series of consultations and evaluations in which the primary care provider or even the referral specialist may feel very much ill at ease. A shifting ground of physiological testing, subjective assessment of work capacity and activity limitation, psychosocial parameters reflecting both contributors to and the results of disability and handicap, and, finally, seemingly arcane medicolegal requirements all appear to combine, undermining even the most dedicated caregiver.

The goal of this chapter is to systematically address the key issues in the evaluation of impairment and the assessment of disability in persons with asthma.

DEFINITIONS

Clinicians often confuse the concepts of "impairment" and "disability." Yet it is critical that these commonly misused terms be clearly understood so that patients can be adequately evaluated and their health status assessed appropriately.

Impairment, in general terms, refers to a functional decrement. In lung diseases, functional impairment is quantified as a physiological deficit. There are multiple approaches to the physiological measurement of lung function, including assessments made at rest and during exercise. These assessment modalities (10–14) of functional impairment will be discussed more fully in the rest of the chapter. In conceptual terms, however, the physiological quantification of impairment is straightforward. It assumes an expectation of normal functional status, taking into account known demographic and anthropomorphic determinants. An observed deviation from that projected normal level quantifies the measured functional impairment.

Disability is another matter altogether. First, disability is inherently relative, rather than absolute. Second, and no less important, disability includes elements of both physician- and patient-assessed health status. It is important to recognize that both these assessments of disability are essentially qualitative, even if evaluators assign pseudoquantitative "ratings" as a summary disability measure.

Broadly defined, the concept of disability subsumes the compromised ability to perform activities or to fulfill duties over a wide spectrum of human endeavours including work, activities of daily living, and leisure pursuits (12,14–19). The specific concept of work disability, although more narrowly defined, is nonetheless a good focal point to illustrate the key elements that differentiate disability from impairment.

Work disability is most commonly defined in terms of compromised capacity for work. The relative nature of this capacity is quickly apparent. A person who develops exercise-induced asthma may become disabled from a job that requires frequent running up and down stairs, but that same person would not have become disabled from a more sedentary occupation. In either case, the physiological impairment quantified by exercise testing would be identical: only the disability is different. A parallel example would be that of symptom aggravation by cold air inhalation in a butcher whose job requires entering a cold storage meat locker many times each day. Even more clearly, a specific chemical sensitization is disabling in terms of any job duties directly involving contact with that material.

Work disability, assessed by either clinician or patient, does not necessarily equate with actual work status. The subjective nature of disability assessment is underscored by the observation that some individuals who report themselves subjectively as work-incapacitated are, in fact, employed. Many factors may come into play and may change over time such that disability status fluctuates without any substantial incremental change in quantitative impairment.

The structure and nature of employment itself, independent of physical demands or chemical exposures, may promote work disability. One example might be a highly structured, entry-level job where unanticipated work absences are poorly tolerated. This is particularly relevant to asthma, a condition marked by the rapid onset of exacerbations. An employee with asthma might very well become disabled due to work absences from such a job, but, with the same level of impairment, could have continued working as a self-employed, "telecommuting" consultant.

Although work disability in asthma is not easily quantifiable, it can be classified by varying criteria. These include complete work cessation associated with the condition, restrictions in work duties, change in job, increased days of work loss, or even limitation in work hours at the same job because of asthma (20,21). Similarly, disability outside of work can be defined over a range of criteria, from severe limitations in activities of daily living at one end of the spectrum to simply the avoidance of one specific leisure sport or activity, such as playing tennis.

Just as impairment does not equate with disability, so, too, neither of these constructs is synonymous with handicap. Handicap refers to the degree to which the individual adapts to impairment and disability. As a psychosocial concept, handicap is highly relevant to the care and well-being of persons challenged by disability. Because work is often central to self-identity, handicap in this arena can be particularly critical and should not be ignored in the context of a multidisciplinary team approach to asthma care. Nonetheless, a formal "assessment" of handicap is not generally part of either an occupational disability evaluation or even a more general assessment, for example, a comprehensive report submitted in support of a claim to the U.S. Social Security Administration.

GENERAL PRINCIPLES IN ASSESSMENT OF IMPAIRMENT AND EXISTING GUIDELINES

Impairment assessment of respiratory disease requires the establishment of a medical diagnosis and the evaluation of the degree of impairment arising from the disorder. The following procedures are recommended.

History and Physical Examination

It is generally agreed that the assessment of respiratory impairment should be guided by objective physiological tests and not determined by symptoms and physical findings alone. Nonetheless history and physical examination should be integral parts of the assessment. Dyspnea should not be used as the sole criterion for evaluation of impairment since individual response to a given degree of physiological abnormalities varies and is influenced by factors unrelated to the extent of lung disease, such as preoccupation with health, socioeconomic status, educational background, and physical fitness of the individual. Although there is some correlation between breathlessness and the degree of airflow obstruction in asthma (22), there are wide interindividual variations. Moreover, in asthma, dyspnea can be highly variable from time to time. Finally, although dyspnea is a symptom that is elicited in all types of respiratory conditions, others, such as coughing, chest tightness, and wheezing, are equally relevant in asthma as they reflect the degree of nonspecific bronchial hyperresponsiveness (NSBH), especially when these symptoms occur in certain circumstances such as after exercise or exposure to cold air or irritants.

Wheezing and decrease in breath sounds should be sought on physical examination. Reduction in breath sounds may reflect the degree of hyperinflation and air trapping, a common and sensitive physiological abnormality in asthma. In subjects with severe asthma, signs such as increased respiratory rate and the use of accessory muscles of respiration may be present.

Chest Radiograph

Chest radiographs are generally performed only to exclude other chest conditions in subjects with asthma. Chest radiographic findings correlate poorly with physiological changes in diseases with airflow limitation such as chronic bronchitis and asthma. For some subjects, especially those with a history of chronic smoking, a high-resolution computed-tomography scan might be indicated to exclude the possibility of concurrent emphysema.

Physiological Measurements

Lung function tests are pivotal in determining the nature and the degree of the physiological abnormality. They are essential in assessing whether or not impairment is present and in assessing its severity. The tests recommended by both the American Medical Association (AMA) and the American Thoracic Society (ATS) for impairment evaluation of respiratory disorders are spirometry and the measurement of diffusing capacity (11,12,13). Measurement of nonspecific bronchial hyperresponsiveness has been accepted as an integral part of evaluation for subjects with asthma in the 1993 ATS guidelines (13). It is usually recommended that the patient be evaluated after he or she has received ''optimum therapy'' or is in ''optimal health'' although no definition of optimal therapy or optimal health is given in these guidelines.

Spirometry

Spirometry is a well-standardized and simple test. ATS guidelines for spirometry include recommendations on equipment, methods of calibration, measurement of height, techniques of test performance (23), and strategies for interpretation for spirometric measurement (24). Adequate consistency, i.e., the two best values must be within 5% of each other, is required. Paradoxically, the inability to achieve adequate consistency may be an indicator of the presence of disease or it may represent poor technical or patient effort. Because poor reproducibility may represent disease, it may be necessary to present the data from several variable trials and comment on this factor rather than simply reject the results altogether (25). For impairment evaluation, only two parameters are specified in standard guidelines: forced expiratory volume in 1 sec (FEV_1) and forced vital capacity (FVC) and their ratio (12–15).

When airflow obstruction is present (FEV_1/FVC is below 75%), the measurements should be repeated after the administration of an inhaled bronchodilator. A significant increase is defined by the AMA criteria as a greater than 15% improvement in FEV_1 from the baseline level (10). However, the ATS recommends that an increase in FEV_1 or FVC of greater than 12% (increase of 200 ml or greater) from the baseline as the presence of airway reversibility suggestive of asthma (24). The postbronchodilator response is relevant to the assessment of respiratory impairment.

The widely accepted definition of normality, predicted value ±20%, is often used in impairment evaluation. The ATS, however, recommends defining abnormality as values outside 1.96× standard deviation (see the following section on normality of function) (24). It is important to choose the proper reference values taking into consideration age, gender, and height (24). Certain ethnic/racial groups such as the Hispanics, Asians, and blacks may have smaller lung volumes than whites of the same age and height. Frequently a 10–15% correction factor is applied, but there is no standard formula in this regard (24).

Measurement of Nonspecific Bronchial Hyperresponsiveness

NSBH is a hallmark of asthma. Much of the impairment in subjects with asthma is associated with the degree of NSBH, as discussed in the previous sections. Moreover, there is also a correlation between the severity of asthma as measured by the amount of medication required for the control of symptoms. The 1993 ATS guidelines for impairment evaluation in subjects with asthma include this measurement (13). Standardized protocols for methacholine and histamine challenge tests are recommended and these have been discussed in detail in another chapter. Since the degree of NSBH is correlated with the airway caliber, it is difficult to interpret the results of testing conducted on subjects with airflow obstruction (FEV$_1$ < 70% predicted) unless measurement of airway resistance could be carried out instead of FEV$_1$. The degree of bronchodilator response may be used as a surrogate measure of the degree of NSBH in these subjects (13). For subjects with FEV$_1$ between 70 to 80% of predicted, both bronchodilator response and methacholine or histamine challenge test could be used.

Exercise Tests

The ATS criteria state that the majority of patients do not require exercise testing in impairment evaluation (12) since there is a well-documented relationship between FEV$_1$, DLCO, oxygen consumption, and work capacity. By these criteria, subjects with no or mild impairment by these criteria should be able to perform all but the most unusually physically demanding of jobs. Conversely, patients with severe impairment are usually unable to perform almost any job. An exercise test is indicated only when there is reason to believe that routine lung function tests may have underestimated impairment. Exercise testing in such cases is used to determine whether a person is impaired and whether the impairment is due to a respiratory disorder. In subjects with asthma, exercise testing is sometimes indicated to assess bronchoconstriction in evaluation of impairment/disability in the performance of jobs requiring heavy exertion (12,13).

It is important to perform exercise testing properly. Maximal exercise rather than submaximal exercise test should be carried out. A completely normal exercise test provides strong evidence that abnormalities are not present. The test may indicate cardiac disease as a cause of dyspnea or physical deconditioning. The degree of abnormality can be measured by the maximal oxygen consumption (Vo$_2$ max) achieved during maximal exercise. Maximal exercise can be sustained at work for only a short period of time. It is generally assumed that a worker can perform a job comfortably at 40% of his Vo$_2$ max for a more prolonged period. Exercise testing can also indicate whether a subject is capable of doing a specific job that requires a certain Vo$_2$ max value.

Measurement of the Diffusing Capacity

Measurement of the diffusing capacity of the lung for carbon monoxide (DLCO) is a useful test in impairment evaluations in subjects with other types of lung diseases, but it is not useful in subjects with asthma. The test requires careful attention to detail standardization (26). The test result is dependent on hemoglobin concentration; results should be adjusted for hemoglobin concentration if the subject is anemic (27). Some authorities recommend that the blood carboxyhemoglobin be measured for adjustment of back diffusion in smokers because of high levels of carbon monoxide in the blood (28). However, it is simpler to ask the subject to refrain from smoking for 12 hr before the test.

Arterial Blood Gas

Measurements of oxygen and carbon dioxide tensions and pH level in arterial blood at rest are sometimes used in impairment evaluation (29). Many agencies consider arterial blood gas analysis to be an adjunct assessment. For example, the AMA guidelines do not incorporate it as a primary test.

CONTROVERSIAL ASPECTS OF IMPAIRMENT/DISABILITY EVALUATION

Normality of Lung Function Measurements

Although clear guidelines for maximal impairment (100%) are available, rating of partial impairment is difficult. This is partly due to difficulties of defining "normality" and of scaling between normality and total impairment.

The results of lung function tests are dependent on certain demographic characteristics, such as gender, age, height, and race. There are many prediction equations of reference populations but these are typically derived from white and nonsmoking population. Prediction equations vary for several reasons. These include: technical differences, differences in population selected for the study, and differences in mathematical models used to study the relationship between the predictors and lung function. For these reasons, one set of reference values is unlikely to be applicable to all laboratories.

There are also several means of comparing individual results with those of the reference population. The decision of where and how to draw the line between "normal" and "abnormal" pulmonary function is subject to disagreement. Lung function values may be expressed either as a percentage of the reference value, or as deviations from the reference values in terms of standard deviation or standard error. The use of 80% of the reference value as the demarcation between normal and abnormal lung function has been widely accepted. This method tends to overestimate the prevalence of abnormalities in an older individuals (30). The use of standard deviations from the mean or expected value, to define abnormality, was not generally used until recently when the ATS recommended the use of $1.96\times$ standard deviation defining the 95% confidence intervals. Harber and co-workers (30) utilized records of 900 respiratory disability applicants to estimate the direction and magnitude of the effect of choice of methods in determining normality on the overall number of persons who would be classified "impaired" and the manner in which personal characteristics (e.g., gender, race, height, and age) affect the likelihood of being classified "impaired." They found that while the choice of prediction equation had minor effects, the adjustment for race had more significant effects. Blacks were more likely to be considered impaired without race adjustment of the prediction equations.

Grading Impairment

As noted previously (see Definitions), impairment refers to a functional deficit. To the extent that such deficits can be based on well-delineated and expected normal physiological values, it may be logical to attempt quantification of impairment in numeric terms. On its face, this would appear consistent with the common practice of reporting pulmonary function data as a percentage of age-, height-, and gender-adjusted normal values. In practice, however, the quantification of impairment in asthma is far from straightforward. The American Medical Association (AMA) Guidelines for Evaluation of Permanent Impairment are often employed by practitioners as a primary source of guidance in matters related to impairment classification (Table 1) (10). Unfortunately, an overly simplistic approach to these criteria often leads evaluators astray, especially if lung function criteria alone are used to classify patients as having mild impairment (in AMA terminology, assigned a 10–25% "whole body impairment" value), moderate impairment (26–50%), or severe

Table 1 Classes of Respiratory Impairment

	Class 1 0% impairment of the whole person	Class 2 10–25% mild impairment of the whole person	Class 3 30–45% moderate impairment of the whole person	Class 4 50–100% severe impairment of the whole person
FVC, FEV$_1$, FEV$_1$/FVC (%) D$_{CO}$	FVC ≥ 80% of predicted, and FEV$_1$ ≥ 80% of predicted, and FEV$_1$/FVC ≥ 70% and D$_{CO}$ ≥ 80% of predicted	FVC between 60% and 79% of predicted, or FEV$_1$ between 60% and 79% of predicted, or FEV$_1$/FVC between 60% and 69%, or D$_{CO}$ between 60% and 79% of predicted	FVC between 51% and 59% of predicted, or FEV$_1$ between 41% and 59% of predicted, or FEV$_1$/FVC between 41% and 59%, or D$_{CO}$ between 41% and 59% of predicted	FVC ≤ 50% of predicted or FEV$_1$ ≤ 40% of predicted, or FEV$_1$/FVC ≤ 40%, or D$_{CO}$ ≤ 40% of predicted
	or	*or*	*or*	*or*
VO$_2$ max	>26 ml/(kg/min)	Between 20 and 25 ml/kg/ min	Between 15 and 20 ml/kg/ min	<15 ml/kg/min

FVC, forced vital capacity; FEV$_1$ forced expiratory volume in the first second; D$_{CO}$, diffusing capacity of carbon monoxide. The D$_{CO}$ is primarily of value for persons with restrictive lung disease in classes 2 and 3. If the FVC, FEV$_1$, and FEV$_1$/FVC ratio are normal and the D$_{CO}$ is between 41% and 79%, an exercise test is required. VO$_2$ max, or measured exercise capacity, is useful in assessing whether a person's complaint of dyspnea is a result of respiratory or other conditions. A person's cardiac and conditioning status must be considered in performing the test and in interpreting the results.

impairment (51–100%). Importantly, and often overlooked, the AMA guidelines themselves state explicitly, "Asthma presents a difficult problem in impairment evaluation because the results of pulmonary function studies may be normal or near normal between attacks" (10). In referring to asthma and other conditions in which impairment is "not readily quantifiable" the guidelines go on to say, "Impairments in persons with these conditions should be evaluated by physicians with expertise in lung disease, and the impairment estimate left to the physician's judgment." This caveat must be reiterated whenever asthma disability is graded, even semiquantitatively.

AMA guidelines have been strongly influenced by the official position statements on this subject by the American Thoracic Society (ATS). Reflective of a rapidly changing approach to this problem, the ATS adopted guidelines for evaluation of impairment/disability secondary to respiratory disease in 1982, but was compelled to extensively revise them only four years later, in 1986 (11,12). Finally, a specific set of guidelines for asthma was promulgated by the ATS in 1993 (13). Like previous guidelines, the asthma-specific document categorizes impairment ordinally and, as in previous ATS position papers, does not attempt to assign percentage impairment scores as in the AMA schema.

The key innovation in the ATS asthma guidelines (Table 2) is incorporation into the impairment classification of three distinct components: FEV_1, degree of airflow reversibility or NSBH, and, most importantly, medication reliance. In this schema, a person with normal airflow and a mild degree of bronchial hyperresponsiveness (PC_{20} 2–8 mg/ml), but requiring daily inhaled and systemic corticosteroids to achieve that level of function, would still be placed in impairment class II (0 being no impairment and V being maximal impairment) (13). This approach acknowledges the need to rely on more than one factor to categorize impairment, but is still limited in scope. In summary, grading impairment is an integrative process in which viewing the patient as a whole person remains paramount.

Assessing Work Disability

The medical evaluation process is geared to grade impairment, but not to quantify disability per se. Yet the information provided by the health care provider is typically used by public and private insurance adjusters to "rate" disability, for example within the U.S. workers' compensation system, which varies considerably from state to state or, internationally, through many national social security systems. Therefore, it is both appropriate and necessary for the health care provider to address, from a medical point of view, the patient's fitness for work of various kinds.

The most straightforward approach to the question of work fitness is to delineate those duties or requirements of work from which the person with asthma being evaluated should be restricted. The usual emphasis in published guidelines has been on work demands in terms of oxygen consumption, correlated in turn with the results of exercise testing in the individual case (10). This approach to work physiology may be problem-ridden on many counts, not the least of which is a lack of modern data on job-specific oxygen consumption demands. More important, however, is the irrelevance of this issue to most adults with asthma in the workplace.

In asthma, the critical work restrictions that impact on disability concern triggers for asthma exacerbation. This is most straightforward in the case of classic occupational asthma due to sensitization, to either larger- or small-molecular-weight substances. Although this will be discussed in greater length later, such triggers are particularly illustrative of the relationship between work restrictions and potential disability. The animal handler who has developed bronchospasm in response to rat antigens requires a work

Table 2 ATS Guidelines for Assessing Impairment/Disability in Asthma and Occupational Asthma

	Score					
	0	1	2	3	4	
FEV$_1$ (% predicted)	≥80	70–79	60–69	50–59	≤50	
Reversibility of airway obstruction or degree of bronchial responsiveness						
Reversibility						
% change in FEV$_1$	≤10	10–19	20–29	≥30		
PC$_{20}$ (mg/ml)	≥8	0.5–8	0.125–0.5	0.125		
Medication need						
Bronchodilators	None	Occasional	Daily	Daily		
Cromolyn	None	Occasional	Daily			
Inhaled steroid	None	Daily	Low dose daily (<800 μg)	High dose daily (>800 μg)	High dose daily (>800 μg)	
Systemic steroid	None		None	Occasional course (1–3 yr)	Daily	
Summary impairment/disability rating class						
Total score	0	1–3	4–6	7–9	10–11	
Impairment class	0	I	II	III	IV	Asthma not controlled V

restriction from all contact with rodents. This may clearly translate into work disability in terms of current duties, yet only the presence or absence of workplace accommodation with transfer to another job setting will determine whether or not job loss with that employer occurs. Disability from the standpoint of an insurance carrier occurs only in the latter circumstance. In the United States, the relatively recent Americans with Disabilities Act mandates that reasonable accommodations to employees with impairments be made. How this will impact employer responses to work restrictions in asthma remains largely untested (31,32).

Ongoing work aggravation or exacerbation of established asthma through nonspecific stimuli (irritant gases or vapours, nuisance dusts, temperature changes, or exercise-induced bronchospasm) often presents a real challenge in assessing appropriate work duty restrictions. For example, it is well established that sulfur dioxide, present in a number of industrial processes, induces bronchospasm in asthmatics at far lower concentrations that in persons without NSBH (33). Limited data suggest that chlorine gas may act similarly (34), while data for other irritants are far less clear-cut (35–37).

A work restriction excluding "all potential irritants and dusts" can be so broad as to preclude almost any potential accommodation, and would likely translate into complete work disability if implemented. Nonetheless, documented or suspected nonspecific asthma triggers should not be ignored when detailing work restrictions. This could certainly include exercise limitations in exercise-induced asthma, paralleling the approach to lifting restrictions applied in musculoskeletal injuries.

The evaluator may also play an important role in documenting that a particular restriction need not be applied, thus preventing disability in the face of a recognized impairment. This issue is particularly relevant to the evaluation of individuals for fitness to wear a respirator (38). Many occupations require medical clearance for the use of various levels of respiratory protection, typically needed by the worker only on a very sporadic basis. Historically, fixed cutoffs of impairment in terms of airflow as a percent predicted often have been invoked to preclude approval for respirator use. The net effect of such policies may be to inappropriately disable an employee from the job in question. A more rational approach would be to evaluate the employee's tolerance and performance with the respirator in place. If warranted, this might even include exercise testing while wearing the respirator.

Fitness for work, employability, and work disability are interrelated, but not synonymous. Although the health care provider is not the ultimate "rater" of disability, it is certainly within the purview of a comprehensive evaluation to comment on factors other than asthma that may impact on employment status. Obviously, other cardiopulmonary conditions are relevant, but so too are health conditions effecting other organ systems. This includes potential psychiatric diagnoses. Even an evaluator focused on the pulmonary system would be well served by a working familiarity with DSM-IV criteria for major diagnostic categories, especially for somatoform disorders that may involve respiratory symptoms (39). Psychosocial factors, especially education and prior job training, are also highly relevant to disability.

As the ATS noted in its position statement on asthma, "The rating of impairment is within the jurisdiction of a physician's expertise to quantitate. However, the determination of disability also requires consideration of many non-medical variables. Physicians have considerable knowledge about how impairment impacts their patients' lives. Therefore it is important for physicians to identify all the individual factors modifying the impact of impairment on their patients' lives for administrators who determine disability compensation'' (13). Assessing work disability is not quantitative, but it can and should be a systematic and rigorous process that addresses its inherent, multifactorial nature.

Asthma-Specific Quality of Life

Health-related quality of life (QOL) refers to the ways in which illnesses, especially chronic diseases, can impact on patient-perceived functioning and status. Several different validated questionnaire instruments have been used to assess the specific impact of asthma on QOL. One is a 20-item, asthma-specific QOL measure developed and validated by Woolcock (40). This brief battery includes breathlessness, mood, social, and ''concerns'' subscales. Another well-studied, asthma-specific QOL measure is the 32-question battery of Juniper and co-workers (41,42). Another asthma-specific scale from the United Kingdom is somewhat longer (43). There are also generic (not asthma-specific) batteries that assess health status in ways relevant to asthma QOL. For example, the SF-36 battery is the most widely accepted approach to measuring generic well-being, and it has been used in asthma (44). Although these instruments are important in assessing cohorts for epidemiological purposes, they have not typically been applied in individual assessments of impairment/disability.

IMPAIRMENT ASSESSMENT IN ASTHMA AND OCCUPATIONAL ASTHMA

General Principles

Upon establishment of the diagnosis of occupational asthma, the subject should be considered 100% impaired on a permanent basis for the job duties that caused the illness and for other jobs with exposure to the same causative agent. Relocation into new duties, either in the same worksite where he or she is no longer exposed even to low levels of the sensitizer or in a different workplace, or a program of rehabilitation learning a new trade is the ideal management strategy. Early ''retirement'' is a less attractive proposition.

Clinical parameters are helpful in the assessment of impairment. Symptoms (frequency, degree of limitation of activities, frequency of acute exacerbations) should be documented. Although the severity of symptoms should be considered in the assessment of impairment, symptomatology can be biased by the desire of obtaining financial compensation or the fear of losing one's livelihood. The type and frequency of medications required to control asthma as determined by the treating physician according to the recent guidelines for the treatment of asthma generally reflect the severity of asthma. Information on the compliance of the subjects in taking the prescribed medications should be obtained from the subject's primary care physician or specialist. The degree of impairment should also be supported by objective means such as measurement of spirometry and NSBH. The number of urgent care visits due to asthma acute exacerbations, by itself, may not reflect the severity of the disease. It may indicate that the disease is not being adequately controlled or there is poor access to routine health care. Exercise testing, measurement of lung volumes, and diffusing capacity are not helpful in assessing impairment due to asthma although they may be helpful in excluding other reasons for dyspnea or chest symptoms, whether occupationally or nonoccupationally related.

Timing of Evaluation

Subjects with occupational asthma are generally left with symptoms, airflow limitation, and NSBH after leaving exposure. Some improve with time even though they may not recover completely. Evaluation for permanent impairment should be carried out when the subject's asthma is under reasonably good control and the condition is stable. Although it has been shown that a plateau of improvement is achieved approximately 2 years after leaving exposure in snow-crab-induced asthma (45), such data are not available for other agents. In a more recent study of 99 subjects with occupational asthma, those who were reassessed more than 5 years after leaving exposure had better recovery than the group who had a shorter duration of follow-up (46). On the other hand, deterioration of asthma may also occur due to intercurrent respiratory infections. While evaluation of impairment should be carried out at 2 years after the cessation of exposure, periodic reevaluation after 2 years is desirable because of the changing nature of the disease. In many insurance systems, a finding of "permanent and stationary" status may be needed sooner than 2 years, but this should not preclude periodic reassessment.

Stability of Asthma

Subjects should be assessed at a time when the asthmatic condition is under reasonable control while on the lowest amount of medication. Assessment should be delayed when there has been a recent acute exacerbations requiring increased medication. It may be necessary to assess the stability of asthma by monitoring peak expiratory flow (PEF) for a period of time. Increased fluctuations in PEF are usually associated with a heightened degree of NSBH (47). Peak expiratory flow rate monitoring for assessment of occupational asthma and nonoccupational asthma has been plagued by the lack of patient compliance and possible falsification of data (48,49). Fortunately the use of computerized recorders obviates this issue. The criteria for appropriate asthma control and the method of achieving control should follow standard guidelines (50).

In a few patients with severe asthma, it is difficult to achieve completely good control even over a period of months. In this situation, evaluation for permanent impairment should be done even though the disease is only partly controlled.

Spirometry and Measurement of NSBH

These two parameters are recommended for impairment evaluation in patients with asthma. Baseline spirometry should be made before the subject would normally take the usual bronchodilator medication (theophylline, inhaled beta-2-agonist) but anti-inflammatory drug should be given as usual on the day of assessment. Although the ATS recommended the use of postbronchodilator FEV_1 and FVC for the grading of respiratory impairment (13), it is debatable whether such a recommendation reflects the actual impairment of the subject as these measurements represent the minimal values reached by the subject during his/her daily life and adequate compensation should consider the lowest function of the subject on reasonably good treatment. On the other hand, one can also argue that the postbronchodilator measurements reflect the real situation better particularly with the recent introduction of long acting beta-2-agonists, which lessen the degree of diurnal variation in lung function considerably. A marked degree of reversibility after the administration of an inhaled bronchodilator usually represents an inadequate control requiring adjustment of medication by the treating physician.

Measurement of NSBH should be carried out after bronchodilator medication have been withheld for periods as proposed by the special committee of the American Academy of Allergy, Asthma, and Clinical Immunology (51), i.e., 8 hr for short-acting inhaled beta-

2-agonists and 12 hr for sustained-release theophylline preparations and long-acting beta-2-agonists (51).

Proposed Grading of Impairment

Scales assessing impairment in occupational asthma should use three parameters: need for medication to control asthma, spirometry, and NSBH (52). In a similar way as scales have been proposed and used in respiratory impairment evaluation in pneumoconiosis, scales have been designed for asthma and occupational asthma using the above parameters (13). Table 2 shows the scaling system used by the ATS (13), which is modified from the one used in Quebec since 1984. It is possible that similar changes will be introduced in the next revision of the American Medical Association guidelines.

SUMMARY

In this chapter, we have underscored the importance of assessing permanent impairment and work disability in asthma. In occupational asthma, we have emphasized the importance of removal from the causative agent and that subjects with occupational asthma are often left with permanent asthma. In addition, subjects with work-related acute exacerbations of asthma should also be evaluated after control of the aggravating occupational factors. It is important to understand that the criteria used for other pulmonary diseases do not sufficiently address the actual impairment in the patient with asthma and that disease-specific impairment criteria be used in this condition. These criteria should include medication requirements, lung function, and the degree of NSBH. The assessment of impairment should take place when asthma is under reasonable control and when improvement is maximal. Reassessment may be required when the clinical status changes.

REFERENCES

1. LaPlante MP, Carlson D. Disability in the United States: Prevalence and Causes. Disability Statistics Rehabilitation Research and Training Center, Institute on Aging. San Francisco: University of California, July 1996.
2. Nagi S. An epidemiology of disability among adults in the U.S. Milbank Mem Fund Q Health Soc 1976; 54(4):439–467.
3. Mellis CM, Peat JK, Bauman AE, Woolcock, AJ. The cost of asthma in New South Wales. Med J Aust 1991; 155:522–528.
4. Sibbald B, Anderson HR, McGuigan S. Asthma and employment in young adults. Thorax 1992; 47:19–24.
5. McClellan VE, Garrett JE. Asthma and employment experience. NZ Med J 1990; 103:399–401.
6. Ignacio-Garcia JM, Gonzales-Santos P. Asthma self-management education program by home monitoring of peak expiratory flow. Am J Respir Crit Care Med 1995; 151:353–359.
7. Asthma—United States, 1980–1990. MMWR 1992; 41:733–735.
8. Gergen PJ, Weiss KB. The increasing problem of asthma in the United States. Am Rev Respir Dis 1992; 146:823–824.
9. Asthma mortality and hospitalization among children and young adults—United States, 1980–1993. MMWR 1996; 45:350–353.
10. Doege TC, Houston TP. In: Doege TC, Houston TP, eds. Guides to the Evaluation of Permanent Impairment, 4th ed. Chicago: American Medical Association, 1993:153–167.

11. American Thoracic Society. Evaluation of impairment/disability secondary to respiratory disease. Am Rev Respir Dis 1982; 126:945–951.

12. American Thoracic Society. Evaluation of impairment/disability secondary to respiratory disorders. Am Rev Respir Dis 1986; 133:1205–1209.

13. American Thoracic Society. Guidelines for the evaluation of impairment/disability in patients with asthma. Am Rev Respir Dis 1993; 147:1056–1061.

14. Balmes JR, Barnhart S. Evaluation of respiratory impairment/disability. In: Murray JF, Nadel JA, eds. Textbook of Respiratory Medicine, 2nd ed. Philadelphia: WB Saunders, 1994:920–942.

15. Haber L. Disabling effects of chronic disease and impairments. J Chronic Dis 1971; 24:469–487.

16. Berkowitz M, Johnson W, Murphy E. Public Policy Toward Disability. New York: Praeger, 1976.

17. Yelin E, Nevitt M, Epstein W. Toward an epidemiology of work disability. Milbank Q 1980; 58:386–415.

18. Yelin EH. Disability and the Displaced Worker. Brunswick, NJ: Rutgers University Press, 1992.

19. Institute of Medicine. Disability in America. Washington, DC: National Academy Press, 1991.

20. Blanc PD, Jones M, Besson C, Katz P, Yelin E. Work disability among adults with asthma. Chest 1993; 104:1371–1377.

21. Blanc PD, Cisternas M, Smith S, Yelin E. Asthma, employment status, and disability among adults treated by pulmonary and allergy specialists. Chest 1996; 109:688–696.

22. Boulet LP, Cournoyer I, Deschesnes F, LeBlanc P, Nouwen A. Perception of airflow obstruction and associated breathlessness in normal and asthmatic subjects: correlation with anxiety and bronchodilator needs. Thorax 1994; 49:965–970.

23. American Thoracic Society. Standardization of spirometry—1987 update. Am Rev Respir Dis 1987; 136:1285–1298.

24. American Thoracic Society. Lung function testing: selection of reference values and interpretation strategies. Am Rev Respir Dis 1991; 144:1202–1218.

25. Becklake MR. Epidemiology of spirometric test failure. Brit J Ind Med 1990; 47:73–74.

26. American Thoracic Society. Single breath carbon monoxide diffusing capacity (transfer factor): recommendations for a standard technique. Am Rev Respir Dis 1987; 136:1299–1307.

27. Dinakara P, Blumental WS, Johnston RF, Kauffman LA, Solnick PB. The effects of anaemia on pulmonary diffusing capacity with derivation of a corrected equation. Am Rev Respir Dis 1970; 102:965–969.

28. Sue DY, Oren A, Hansen JE, Wasserman K. Diffusing capacity for carbon monoxide as a prediction of gas exchange during exercise. N Engl J Med 1987; 316:301–306.

29. Morgan WKC, Zaldivar GL. Blood gas analysis as determinant of occupationally related disability. J Occup Med 1990; 135(5):440–443.

30. Harber P, Schnur R, Emery J, Brooks S, Ploy-Song-Sang Y. Statistical "biases" in respiratory disability determination. Am Rev Respir Dis 1992; 128:413–418.

31. West J. Social and policy context of the Americans with Disabilities Act of 1990. Milbank Q 1991; 69(Supp 1–2):3–24.

32. Harber P, Fedoruk MJ. Work placement and worker fitness: implications of the Americans with Disabilities Act for pulmonary medicine. Chest 1994; 105:1564–1571.

33. Sheppard D, Wong WS, Uehara CF, Nadel JA, Boushey HA. Lower threshold and greater bronchomotor responsiveness of asthmatic subjects to sulphur dioxide. Am Rev Respir Dis 1980; 122:873–878.

34. D'Alessandro A, Kuschner W, Wong H, Boushey HA, Blanc PD. Exaggerated responses to chlorine inhalation among persons with nonspecific airway hyperreactivity. Chest 1996; 109:331–337.

35. Aris RM, Tager I, Christian D, Kelly T, Balmes JR. Methacholine responsiveness is not associated with O_3-induced decreases in FEV_1. Chest 1995; 107:621–628.

36. Koenig JQ, Covert DS, Morgan MS, Horike M, Horike N, Pierson WE. Acute effects of 0.12 ppm ozone or 0.12 ppm nitrogen dioxide on pulmonary function in healthy and asthmatic adolescents. Am Rev Respir Dis 1985; 132:648–651.

37. Balmes JR. Asthma and air pollution. West J Med 1995; 163:372–373.

38. Harber P, Barnhart S, Boehlecke BA, Beckett WS, Gerrity T, McDiarmid MA, Nardbell E, Repsher L, Brousseau, L, Hodous TK, Utell MJ. Respiratory protection guidelines. Am J Repsir Crit Care Med 1996; 142:1153–1165.

39. Diagnostic and Statistical Manual of Mental Disorders: DSM-IV, 4th ed. Washington, DC: American Psychiatric Association, 1994.

40. Marks GB, Dunn SM, Woolcock AJ. A scale for the measurement of quality of life in asthma. J Clin Epidemiol 1992; 45:461–472.

41. Juniper EF, Guyatt GH, Ferrie PJ, Griffith LE. Measuring quality of life in asthma. Am Rev Respir Dis 1993; 147:832–838.

42. Juniper EF, Guyatt GH, Willan A, Griffith LE. Determining the minimal important change in a disease-specific quality of life questionnaire. J Clin Epidemol 1994; 47:81–87.

43. Hyland ME, Finnis S, Irvine SH. A scale for assessing quality of life in adult asthma sufferers. J Psychosom Res 1991; 35:99–110.

44. Bousquet J, Knani J, Dhivert H, Richard A, Chicoye A, Ware JEJR, Michel FB. Quality of life in asthma. I. Internal consistency and validity of the SF-36 questionnaire. Am J Respir Crit Care Med 1994; 149:371–375.

45. Malo JL, Cartier A, Ghezzo H, LaFrance M, McCants M, Lehrer SB. Patterns of improvement on spirometry, bronchial hyperresponsiveness, and specific IgE antibody levels after cessation of exposure in occupational asthma caused by snow-crab processing. Am Rev Respir Dis 1988; 38:807–812.

46. Perfetti L, Cartier A, Ghezzo H, Gautrin D, Malo J-L. Follow-up of occupational asthma after removal from or diminution of exposure of the responsible agent: relevance of the length of the interval after cessation of exposure. Chest 1998; 114:398–403.

47. Ryan G, Latimer KM, Dolovich J, Hargreave FE. Bronchial responsiveness to histamine: relationship to diurnal variation of peak flow rate, improvement after bronchodilator, and airway calibre. Thorax 1982; 37:423–429.

48. Quirce S, Contreras G, DyBuncio A, Chan-Yeung M. Brief communication: Peak expiratory flow monitoring is not a reliable method in establishing the diagnosis of occupational asthma. Am J Respir Crit Care Med 1995; 152:1100–1102.

49. Verschelden P, Cartier A, L'Archevêque J, Trudeau C, Malo J-L. Compliance with and accuracy of daily self-assessment of peak expiratory flows (PEF) in asthmatic subjects over a three month period. Eur Respir J 1996; 9:880–885.

50. Moscato G, Godnic-Cvar J, Maestrelli P, Malo J-L, Burge PS, Coifman R. Statement on self-monitoring of peak expiratory flows in the investigation of occupational asthma. J Allergy Clin Immunol 1995; 96:295–301.

51. Chai H, Farr RS, Froehlich LA, Mathison DA, McLean JA, Rosenthal RR, Sheffer AL, Spector SL, Townley RG. Standardization of bronchial inhalation challenge procedures. J Allergy Clin Immunol 1975; 56:323–327.

52. Diagnosis and Clarification in Global Strategy for asthma management and prevention. NHLBI/WHO workshop report. National Institutes of Health, 1995:47–61.

17

Surveillance and Prevention

David I. Bernstein
University of Cincinnati College of Medicine, Cincinnati, Ohio

Gary M. Liss
Ontario Ministry of Labour and University of Toronto, Toronto, Ontario, Canada

DEFINITIONS

Surveillance can be defined as the collection, analysis, and dissemination of information pertaining to individual disease occurrences and its consequences in terms of morbidity, disability, and death (1). Surveillance methods can be used to monitor the occurrence of occupational disease(s) for evaluating small or large populations. Medical surveillance has been defined as the serial performance of an observation or test used to detect evidence of a disease process that can be altered by appropriate intervention; it is a method of secondary prevention (2). Its goal is to detect workers with established disease early in its course and thereby ultimately prevent progression to moderate or even severe disease with increasing morbidity and disability (3); or to be followed by appropriate interventions to prevent further cases (2).

The purpose of a medical surveillance program is to periodically evaluate the health status of the entire workforce in relation to the work environment, with the following objectives: (1) to recognize changes in health among groups of workers whenever possible before clinically important adverse health outcomes occur in individuals; (2) to identify potentially hazardous working conditions using grouped health and environmental information; and (3) to evaluate the effectiveness of exposure controls through the ongoing collection and analysis of all relevant data. To assure adequate monitoring of the health of the workforce, the overall surveillance program should periodically evaluate medical data in relation to industrial hygiene and other quantitative and nonquantitative exposure information.

The ultimate benefit of public health surveillance is identification of sentinel health events, which could result in measures that reduce or prevent new cases. Rutstein et al. defined a sentinel health event as "a preventable disease, disability or untimely death whose occurrence serves as a warning signal that the quality of preventive and/or therapeutic medical care may need to be improved" (4). When applied to occupational asthma, preventive measures that address sentinel events might include modification of a work environment to reduce exposure to causative substances or exclusion of individuals presumed to be at high risk. Reduction of exposure could be achieved by process modification, ventilation, engineering innovations, and use of personal protective equipment (1).

315

MEDICAL SCREENING AND SURVEILLANCE

In contrast to public health surveillance, the major goal of medical surveillance programs for occupational asthma (OA) is to detect workers with a disease early in its course and then to institute measures to prevent progression to moderate or severe stages of the disease that are associated with greater morbidity and disability. This goal may be particularly relevant to OA for which there is evidence that early case detection after the initial onset of symptoms may result in a favorable prognosis (5). Although not proven, it is also possible that medical surveillance may prevent rare fatal acute asthmatic episodes that have been associated with exposure to certain causative agents (e.g., diisocyanates) (6–8).

Rationale for Medical Surveillance

In the past, the inclusion of medical surveillance programs has been recommended, particularly in the context of exposure to isocyanates (9). For example, in Canada and in the United Kingdom, inclusion of provisions for surveillance in regulations have been instituted without reference to their rationale or effectiveness (10,11). In the United Kingdom, health surveillance is mandated for exposed employees who have a reasonable likelihood of developing OA (11,12). Musk et al. concluded that serial measurement of the FEV_1 was a useful means of identifying acute and long-term effects of isocyanates and suggested that the effects of exposure in a workforce be monitored (13).

Recently, Brooks stated that "medical surveillance programs are the keystone for prevention and should identify individuals who are at increased risk of developing occupational asthma, as well as detect asthma at an early stage when intervention options are likely to be successful" (14). The 1989 Recommendations for Occupational Asthma issued by the Canadian Thoracic Society concluded that "there is really no evidence that periodic screening is worthwhile or that preemployment screening or measurement of airway responsiveness is justified" (15). A more recent consensus statement suggested that "routine surveillance be performed in all workers with exposure to agents known to cause asthma, and especially if cases of work-related asthma have occurred at a particular worksite" (16).

The main rationale for medical surveillance is the considerable *indirect* evidence that the prognosis in OA is improved by early detection followed by prompt removal from exposure (5,17,18). In other words, a short duration of symptoms before diagnosis, preserved lung function (FEV_1), and lesser degree of airway hyperresponsiveness at the time of diagnosis are indicators of less severe disease and predictors of more favorable outcomes of asthma severity after leaving the workplace (19,20). Consistent with this, screening programs are secondary prevention programs if it is assumed that early detection improves long-term prognosis and ultimately leads to primary prevention measures to control exposure to causative agents (21,22).

Despite this rationale underpinning recommendations in support of medical surveillance, the overall effectiveness of such programs has been assessed only rarely (22). Bernstein et al. described a medical surveillance program that was effective for early detection of workers with diisocyanate (MDI) asthma. In a 2-year longitudinal study, 243 foam workers with low-level exposure to MDI were surveyed with annual questionnaires, screening spirometry, and MDI-HSA specific antibodies (23). Methacholine testing and serial evaluations of PEFRs were used to confirm or rule out suspect cases of OA. Three new cases of OA were identified that had not been previously reported or recognized. One of the latter workers reported no respiratory symptoms and was initially identified by a decreased FEV_1 on screening spirometry. Once identified, asthma remitted in all three cases 1 year after diagnosis and after removal from further MDI exposure.

The only other published data evaluating the effectiveness of long-term medical surveillance programs for OA and outcomes in groups of workers who have undergone surveillance was recently reported by Tarlo et al. from Ontario, Canada (24). Tarlo et al. previously reviewed characteristics and outcomes in a large group of worker's compensation claims for OA (18) and observed a better outcome among those with isocyanate-induced asthma than among those with OA due to other causes. This population has since been further characterized to identify factors that may have accounted for this difference (24). The 136 of 235 claimants with OA due to isocyanates had a shorter duration of symptoms before diagnosis than those with OA due to other causes (2.0 years vs. 3.0 years; $p < 0.05$). Follow-up outcome at a mean interval of 1.9 years after initial assessment was better among those with isocyanate OA (73% cleared or improved vs. 56% with other causes of OA; $p < 0.05$). Under the isocyanate regulation in effect in Ontario since the mid-1980s, workplaces with exposure to isocyanates were required to provide 6-monthly (or at least twice-yearly) respiratory questionnaires as well as spirometry if indicated by the questionnaire. Workers with new symptoms considered related to work or with spirometry changes were referred for further evaluation.

It was found that 71 (52%) of those with OA claims associated with isocyanates had worked in plants known (based on Ministry of Labour records) to have had medical surveillance programs in place during the year of diagnosis (24). These patients had diagnoses that were confirmed earlier as reflected by a mean duration of disease of 1.7 ± 2.4 years after the onset of symptoms, compared to a mean disease duration of 2.7 ± 3.1 years after onset of symptoms in those working at plants that were not known to be in compliance with surveillance requirements ($p < 0.05$). The outcomes for the patients whose workplaces had surveillance measures in place were not statistically significantly different from those among patients at workplaces not under surveillance. However, worsening of asthma at follow-up was recorded for only 8% of those from plants with surveillance versus 18% of those without known surveillance, suggesting a trend to better outcomes among those plants under surveillance. It is not possible from this investigation to determine whether the earlier diagnosis was due to the increased awareness of isocyanate asthma by workers and health care providers associated with the presence of the program, or due to the program itself (questionnaire and/ or spirometry), or due to a combination of these factors. Furthermore, it is not known how many of the "cases" of occupational asthma were identified as a result of the surveillance activities per se, rather than being identified through clinical encounters outside of surveillance.

Medical Surveillance Methods

The screening tests used for the purpose of medical surveillance are discussed in other chapters. These methods would not differ considerably from those previously used in cross-sectional epidemiological studies of occupational asthma. A test used as a surveillance tool should possess several characteristics (25). The test should have simplicity and be easily performed by trained paramedical personnel. The test should be valid or measure the characteristic it is intended to measure and must be reliable or reproducible. The costs of a test should be weighed against the potential benefit for generating useful data and for improving outcomes. An optimal screening test must have good sensitivity or be able to detect most individuals with the disease; often such a test lacks adequate specificity for establishing a diagnosis of an occupational disease.

Questionnaires

The most widely utilized methods for medical screening and surveillance of OA have been itemized questionnaires. Such questionnaires should be administered on an annual or semi-annual basis with ancillary tests such as spirometry and, if appropriate, immunological studies (i.e., skin tests, specific antibody assays). Although many have been utilized, no single questionnaire has been widely adapted or validated for evaluation of OA. An itemized questionnaire has been used in medical surveillance of populations of egg-processing and diisocyanate workers to identify new cases of occupational asthma (see Appendix, page 731) (23,26). Malo et al. reported that diagnoses derived from an occupational questionnaire failed to correctly identify workers with OA in whom the diagnosis was confirmed by specific bronchoprovocation testing. It performed better in excluding, rather than confirming, the presence of OA (27). Brooks et al. devised a questionnaire to define the presence or absence of airway hyperresponsiveness; a symptoms score was based on the percentage of respiratory responses to a list of 22 commonly encountered irritants, which correlated ($r = 0.60$; $p < 0.002$) with methacholine PC_{20} (28). However, this questionnaire-derived irritant index has not yet been tested for medical surveillance of worker populations. Finally, Burge has recently proposed a surveillance questionnaire reproduced in the Appendix of this chapter (29).

Spirometry

Spirometry is another tool that has been extensively utilized in screening worker populations. The FEV_1 has been employed in a considerable number of cross-sectional studies because it is reproducible, has a low coefficient of variation, and is simple to perform. Cross-shift changes in FEV_1 performed in a random fashion lack the necessary sensitivity required for detecting occupational asthma (30). However, spirometric testing should be combined with a screening questionnaire in medical surveillance of worker populations (72). Workers concerned about job security issues may give spurious negative responses to queries pertaining to asthma; however, a decreased FEV_1 (or decline from baseline) or FEV_1/FVC ratio may alert the physician to evaluate an "asymptomatic" worker who could indeed have OA (23).

Tests of Nonspecific Bronchial Hyperresponsiveness (NSBH)

Tests of NSBH (e.g., the methacholine inhalation test) are impractical for screening entire worker populations owing to the nonspecificity of these tests. There is no convincing evidence that preemployment testing of NSBH can predict subsequent development of OA. However, in workers in whom the pretest probability of OA is high (i.e., workers with positive skin prick tests and/or a history compatible with OA), methacholine testing is very useful in evaluating individual workers for OA while they are still actively exposed and symptomatic at work. A negative methacholine test excludes asthma if performed at the end of the work shift and after a 2-week duration of work exposure to the putative causative agent during which time the worker is reporting asthma symptoms at work (31). A positive test warrants further evaluation to confirm OA with specific challenge testing or serial measurements of PEFR both at and away from work exposure. This approach has been used successfully in a 3-year surveillance study of MDI-exposed urethane foam workers (23). Methacholine testing was performed at work in all those reporting lower respiratory symptoms. None of those with negative methacholine tests exhibited work-related decrements in lung function or were subsequently diagnosed with OA over the subsequent 3 years of the survey. Positive methacholine tests were detected in all workers in whom the diagnosis of OA was subsequently confirmed based on serial monitoring of PEFR both at and away from work. Protocols for performing methacholine testing have been abbreviated, allowing these tests to be performed safely and expeditiously at the worksite (32).

Immunological Tests

Standardized antigens are not commercially available for evaluation of OA. When appropriate, detection of specific IgE by serological immunoassay or skin testing with occupational allergens may serve as useful screening tools. This may be particularly relevant for high-molecular-weight (HMW) proteinaceous allergens. Sensitivity of the skin prick test with protein allergens (e.g., natural enzymes, latex protein, and psyllium allergens) has been validated using specific inhalation testing as the gold standard for diagnosis of OA. These studies indicate that the prick test is an excellent tool for surveillance of IgE-mediated forms of OA because its sensitivity equals or approaches 100%. In vitro measurements of serum specific IgE (e.g., RAST) to natural protein allergens are approximately 20–40% less sensitive than the skin prick test in detecting allergic sensitization and, therefore, should not be considered as a suitable alternative to skin testing for medical surveillance of worker populations (33,34).

Serum-specific IgG to an occupational antigen can be used as an index of exposure in surveillance of worker populations. As shown in Figure 1, Biagini et al. studied a group

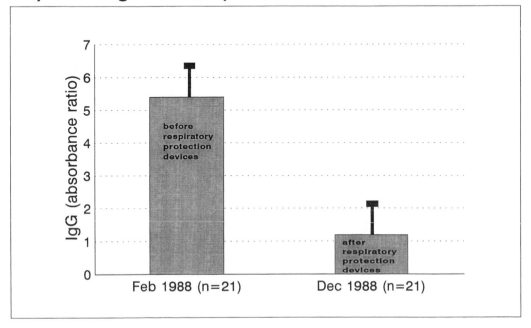

Figure 1 Mean serum-specific IgG responses to morphine-6-hemisuccinate-HSA antigen in narcotic manufacturing workers exposed to morphine before and after introduction of mandatory respiratory protection devices.

of legal-narcotics-manufacturing workers some of whom had respiratory symptoms associated with work exposure to morphine. Levels of specific IgG to morphine-6-hemisuccinate-human serum albumin (HSA), which were elevated on initial evaluation, diminished dramatically 10 months after institution of air-supplied respirators (35).

In a group of workers with IgE-mediated asthma caused by exposure to TMA, Grammar et al. followed TMA-HSA serum-specific IgE levels longitudinally in workers diagnosed with OA after moving from high to low TMA exposure areas of a plant. A rise in specific IgE correlated with persistent OA symptoms in a subgroup of workers, indicating that these workers had not been adequately restricted from exposure to TMA (36).

Within populations of detergent workers regularly exposed to microbial enzymes, there are high rates of prick test reactivity to *Aspergillus* or *Bacillus subtilis*–derived enzymes. Serial skin testing can be used to screen for new cases but also as a means to monitor sensitization rates among worker populations and thereby assess the effectiveness of industrial hygiene measures that are intended to reduce dermal and inhalational exposure to enzymes. A relationship has been identified between worker sensitization rates and levels of ambient enzyme exposure in various factories where microbial enzymes are utilized (37). Skin prick testing with HMW allergens at the beginning can be used to predict risk for development of clinical allergic responses. Laboratory animal workers presensitized to laboratory animals or common environmental allergens (i.e., atopic) are about 7 times more likely to develop occupational respiratory symptoms (38).

Recommendations

Should Medical Surveillance Be Conducted?

In 1994, Venables recommended the use of a questionnaire on work-related respiratory symptoms for use in screening programs for OA (21). She questioned whether it was possible for a screening program to detect cases of asthma at an early enough stage to reduce subsequent functional impairment and consequent disability. The answer to this question is not yet known.

However, there appears to be better evidence in support of medical surveillance compared to that which was available at the time of preparation of the 1989 Canadian guidelines (15), based on recent cohort analytical studies (23,24). The Canadian Thoracic Society Subcommittee recently revised its Guidelines for Occupational Asthma (39) and concluded that "the value of this is unproven, although OA in Ontario has been diagnosed earlier in companies with surveillance programs in place." The quality of evidence for this recommendation for medical surveillance was based on nonrandomized studies, and the category of strength of the evidence in favor of this recommendation was graded as moderate.

The need for validation of programs was emphasized by the ACCP consensus statement, which recommended that surveillance methods for occupational asthma need to be better defined, and that the methods require proper validation and testing (16). It was recommended that such surveillance programs should be assessed for efficacy in a prospective manner, and finally, that such programs should be confined to workers in high-risk industries.

Preventive Measures Should Be Linked to Surveillance

As pointed out by Balmes (2), it is recommended that those conducting the medical surveillance must be ready to respond to the results of surveillance with appropriate interventions to reduce or eliminate asthma-inducing exposures. Criteria for the effectiveness of screening programs in the workplace [i.e., with reference to groups (rather than individuals)] have been described (40,41). One obvious criterion is that identification of disease leads to measures that prevent additional cases; that is, the initial case may act as a sentinel health event. To the extent that such preventive measures take place, this increases the benefit (reduction of morbidity) that may follow from medical surveillance. On the other hand, workplace preventive measures should also be aimed at reducing the levels of exposures (i.e. primary prevention) (21,22).

Which Instruments Should Be Included?

There is not agreement on what instruments should be included in a medical surveillance program of OA. Again, it should be emphasized that these programs are to be applied to the entire exposed population, not as part of a confirmatory workup of suspected cases of OA. Venables (21) suggested that a short questionnaire would have advantages as a first-line screening tool for exposed workers, but that spirometry is insensitive; serial peak expiratory flow rate recordings (PEFR) are sensitive and specific but too labor intensive as a first-line screening tool. Bernstein echoed these findings and called for a stepwise plan for medical surveillance with initial questionnaire and, if appropriate, immunological tests such as skin testing, particularly if suspect causative agents are HMW natural allergens (3). Workers with positive questionnaire responses and/ or positive skin prick tests should be studied further. Balmes argued that spirometry with its reproducibility has a role and serial PEFR is an underutilized method for surveillance of OA (2). Spirometry may be worthwhile, particularly for workers affected with OA who present with false-negative questionnaires (23).

With respect to symptom questionnaires, a caveat to bear in mind is that, despite the allure of early detection, the validity of symptoms or questionnaires is limited: Stenton et al. found questionnaires (and spirometry) to have low sensitivity and specificity for detecting asthma (42). This is consistent with previous reports that the history is not a reliable indicator of asthma (43) or of OA (27). Most recently, Burge suggested that although symptoms alone are rarely diagnostic, symptoms are sufficiently sensitive for use in respiratory surveillance of OA (29). He proposed a sensitive, but nonspecific surveillance questionnaire (see Appendix).

Timing Considerations

Assuming that surveillance should be conducted, when is an appropriate interval after the start of employment to initiate surveillance? Malo et al. pointed out that for low-molecular-weight (LMW) sensitizers, the symptoms often appear early in the course of exposure (perhaps in the first year), so surveillance should be instituted relatively quickly or more often. As for HMW agents, work-related asthma symptoms may, on average, take longer to appear, so that surveillance efforts should be spread out over longer time intervals and initiated immediately after the onset of exposure (44).

PUBLIC HEALTH SURVEILLANCE

It is generally agreed that there are inadequate data pertaining to prevalence and incidence of a variety of occupational diseases (45). Effective surveillance programs, on the state and national level, are required so that public health strategies can be developed for OA.

Initial attempts at the state level have been limited to data from "mandatory" reporting of new cases by physicians. However, there has been limited education of physicians about these programs and, as a result, minimal compliance with their requirements. Reporting requirements lack uniformity from state to state (1). Worker's compensation records of claims made for occupational health problems have been more useful.

In the United States, the Occupational Safety and Health Act established the Occupational Safety and Health Administration (OSHA), which since 1970 has provided a standard reporting mechanism for collecting data of work-related injuries and diseases on a national level. Data from occupational injuries and diseases reported to OSHA can be reviewed in the annual survey of the Bureau of Labor Statistics (45).

A few countries have instituted systematic surveillance programs for occupational lung diseases. In 1989, a system for collecting data related to pulmonary disorders was established in Great Britain. This program, Surveillance of Work Related and Occupational Respiratory Disease (SWORD), is based on voluntary physician-reporting coordinated through two professional societies, the British Thoracic Society and the Society of Occupational Medicine (46). The stated objectives of this program are to: (1) monitor the frequency of disease; (2) recognize and investigate new problems; (3) provide feedback of information to participating physicians; and (4) initiate investigations of worker groups if required. A high initial participation rate was achieved by enrolling 80% of known chest physicians in the United Kingdom (46). During the first year of the SWORD program, 554 (26.4%) of 2101 total reported cases were classified as OA, exceeding the annual rates of other occupational respiratory diseases (e.g., pneumoconioses, allergic alveolitis, lung malignancies). Suspected causative agents included a variety of proteinaceous and chemical substances. Diisocyanates were the most frequently cited as suspect causes, representing 22% of all reported cases of OA. The annual incidence for asthma within the entire British work population was estimated at 22 cases per million.

The extended experience of SWORD through 1994 was recently reported; OA remained the predominant cause of occupational lung disorders. The majority of workers diagnosed with OA had failed to recover (47). A similar surveillance system based on physician reporting from Quebec revealed that OA was the most commonly reported occupational respiratory disorder (63%). The most frequently reported sensitizing agents were the isocyanates, flour, and wood dust. It was also recognized that 15% of cases had not been reported to the Worker's Compensation Board (48).

Despite the high initial participation rate by physicians, it was recognized that data derived from the SWORD project may underestimate the true incidence of the diseases. It is noteworthy that diagnoses were not confirmed by objective means, which could result in overestimation of the true incidence. In the United States, NIOSH has instituted the Sentinel Event Notification System for Occupational Risks (SENSOR), the aim of which is to identify and characterize new case reports of targeted occupational diseases (49). To date, this project has been tested in 10 states. The four components of SENSOR are: (1) selection of preventable work-related cases whose occurrence may serve as sentinel events; (2) identification and education of sentinel providers (e.g., physicians, nurses, and occupational clinics) likely to encounter the diseases targeted for study; (3) establishment of a regional surveillance center whose purpose is to analyze incoming data and to disseminate data back to sentinel providers; and (4) initiation of intervention strategies aimed at screening and educating worker populations identified to be at high risk. This surveillance program has established a broad case definition of occupational asthma, which includes: (1) a physician diagnosis of asthma; and (2) an association between work and exposure to a recognized causative agent, documented work-related changes in lung function, airway hyperresponsiveness, or a positive specific inhalation test (50,51).

A summary of SENSOR findings in the states of New Jersey and Michigan over the initial 5 years of the program identified 535 cases that met the case definition of OA; in Michigan the largest number of cases (40%) were in the automobile industry whereas greater numbers of cases (15%) in New Jersey were employed in chemical industries (52). The most frequent causal agents were diisocyanates (19% of all cases). Previously unrecognized causes of OA were identified. Follow-up industrial sampling detected suspect agents at levels below permissible limits but prompted institution of more comprehensive industrial hygiene measures. Continuation of the SENSOR program may provide a model for state-based surveillance of OA.

There is an obvious worldwide need for improvement in occupational disease surveillance. The goal of improving disease surveillance has been established as a NIOSH priority in the United States. In Finland, since 1995 the National Institute of Occupational Health has compiled annual statistics on occupational allergic diseases (both respiratory and cutaneous) that physicians are required to report (53). In that country there are adequate data to estimate the annual incidence of various forms of OA and hypersensitivity pneumonitis. The results of this survey showed that the most frequent cause of OA was cow epithelium affecting primarily dairy farmers followed by flour affecting bakers. In contrast to the SWORD data from the United Kingdom, diisocyanates were the eighth most frequent cause of OA in Finland. Thus, survey results from one country cannot be liberally applied to another. Annual statistics collected from 1987 to 1991 in the Finland survey demonstrated a trend showing an increase in the case incidence of OA. Such data are extremely useful in identifying potential problems among specific industries that could lead to targeted intervention strategies.

A consideration that has not received much attention is assessment of risk of inhabitants living adjacent to factories where agents known to cause OA could extend to the surrounding environment. Nuorteva et al. (54) performed a survey of nonworker inhabitants living in the vicinity of a polyurethane factory in Finland. No increased prevalence of asthma was found in the latter populations compared to control referent groups. Community outbreaks of acute asthma have been temporally associated with unloading of soybeans in a harbor adjacent to the city of Barcelona (55). Asthmatics admitted to emergency rooms during outbreaks exhibited significantly higher levels of serum-specific IgE to soybean antigens on days when soybeans were unloaded in the harbor in comparison to asthmatics seen on days when soybeans were not handled (56). Outbreaks were traced back to the point source, the harbor, from where grain-dust-bearing soybean allergens were blown and dispersed downwind to the city of Barcelona.

PREVENTION

General Considerations

The most effective means of primary prevention of OA is by reduction of environmental exposure to the causative substance(s). Broad categories of measures that can reduce exposure to a causative agent include: (1) substitution of a recognized harmful agent with one that is less harmful; (2) improved ventilation or automation of a process (e.g., robotics) so that human exposure is reduced or eliminated; (3) modification of the process or agent to reduce risk of sensitization; and (4) identification and exclusion of high-risk workers from potentially hazardous exposures. There is little, if any, information that precisely defines exposure levels that favor respiratory sensitization to HMW allergens or LMW substances. Development of immunochemical assays that can quantitate levels of airborne exposure to HMW allergens should eventually facilitate determination of exposure-response relationships in the workplace. At that time, permissible limits of exposure could be determined that might prevent respiratory sensitization and development of OA.

Environmental exposure-response data are available for a few substances, which could be applied to development of strategies for prevention of OA. Long-term spirometry studies performed in asymptomatic diisocyanate-exposed workers demonstrated that decrements in FEV_1 were associated with high cumulative TDI exposure in comparison to workers with lower cumulative exposure (57). These data supported proposed NIOSH standards of 5 ppb [8-hr time-weighted average (TWA)]. Although these results addressed the effects of chronic TDI exposure on changes in lung function, they may not be useful for establishing limits of TDI exposure levels that prevent development of OA. Omae studied 106 workers exposed for over 2 years to TDI at levels of 1 ppb (8-hr TWA). Decrements in lung function were not detected in TDI-exposed groups compared to non-exposed reference groups (58). However, eight workers in this group were identified with possible TDI asthma. Once a worker develops TDI asthma, TDI exposure can elicit bronchoconstriction at levels as low as 10 ppb (59,60).

It has been observed that the onset of TDI asthma is often preceded by an accidental chemical spill during which TDI is elevated above permissible exposure limits. Baur reported that 50% of workers with established TDI asthma experienced asthmatic responses after exposure to 10–20 ppb of TDI (60). Animal studies in guinea pigs have also shown that induction of TDI asthma is dose dependent and more likely to occur with short exposures above the accepted TLV (61). Based on the above studies, it is reasonable to recommend engineering modifications that maintain diisocyanate levels below the TWA of 5 ppb.

In western red cedar workers, larger decrements in lung function have been reported in those exposed to >2 mg/m^3 of wood dust (62). Phthalic anhydride (PA) causes IgE-mediated OA as well as mucosal irritant effects at higher levels (4–40 mg/m^3) (63). Once sensitization has been established, asthmatic responses can be elicited (both EAR and LAR) by inhalation of acid anhydride at concentrations less than 1.0 mg/m^3 (64). Because the exposure conditions required for induction of OA due to LMW agents are not known, the best approach may be to aim for reduction of exposure levels below that which is known to elicit asthmatic responses in workers with confirmed OA.

In a modern plant, it is possible that no-effect exposure levels could be achieved by means of process modifications. Preventive measures have been particularly effective in controlling sensitization among workers exposed to detergent enzymes (65). Following industrial hygiene measures aimed at reducing airborne enzyme levels, the number of workers transferred from production areas owing to medical reasons decreased by more than 50%. After institution of improved ventilation and enzyme encapsulation new cases of clinical sensitization have been recognized (66). Prevention of respiratory sensitization and symptoms have been successfully achieved when enzyme levels are maintained below the ACGIH guideline of 60 ng/m^3 for total enzyme dust exposure.

Consideration of Personal Risk Factors

Atopy and smoking status are risk factors that have been associated with the development of OA. As discussed, atopy clearly enhances the risk for sensitization to HMW occupational allergens. In the 1960s and 1970s, it was recognized that atopic detergent enzyme workers were at particular risk for IgE-mediated sensitization to *B. subtilis* enzymes. Approximately 85% of atopic and 35% of nonatopic workers exhibited skin prick test sensitivity to enzyme antigens. After atopic workers in the United Kingdom were excluded from working with enzymes, the overall sensitization rate fell to 20%. However, in North America, the presence of atopy cannot be used as an exclusion criterion for hiring but may be considered in assigning jobs or tasks to hired workers in which there is predictable exposure to protein allergens. The potential increased risk should be discussed as part of the preplacement, postjob offer interaction with the worker. In addition, newly hired asymptomatic workers entering a workplace may already have cutaneous sensitization to an occupational allergen (e.g., laboratory animal proteins) via a previous work exposure; such workers, if identified, should be restricted from significant inhalational exposure to such antigens (38). Certain HLA-D loci alleles are associated with relatively greater risk of OA caused by diisocyanates. However, gene typing lacks adequate sensitivity or specificity for inclusion in a medical surveillance program.

Respirators

Although substitution, engineering controls, ventilation, and process modifications are preferred control measures, personal protective appliances such as respirators may be recommended in certain circumstances, particularly for individual workers with jobs (e.g., maintenance) in which short-term exposure to high levels of a causative agent is unavoidable.

These measures should not be recommended for a worker with confirmed OA and should not be considered as a substitute for restrictions from exposure to the causative agent. A variety of respiratory devices are available. NIOSH, under authorization of the Federal Mine Safety and Health Act of 1977 and the Occupational Safety and Health Act of 1970, has established a program that tests, certifies, and approves commercially available protective breathing devices (67). Devices that have been evaluated and published in the NIOSH-certified equipment list include self-contained breathing apparatus such as gas masks designed for protection from toxic irritants and vapors (e.g., ammonia, acid gases, chlorine), supplied air respirators, protective devices for particulates, chemical cartridges approved for a variety of agents (e.g., ammonia, methylamine, chlorine, paints, lacquers, etc.), powered air respirators, and vinyl chloride respirators.

Selection of an appropriate respirator for protection from exposure to a particular agent should be decided based upon official NIOSH and OSHA recommendations. An excellent resource that summarizes such recommendations is contained in the *NIOSH Pocket Guide to Chemical Hazards* (68). This is an alphabetical listing of known carcinogens and toxic agents. Information is provided pertaining to chemical properties, exposure limits (TWA), adverse health effects, and recommendations for respirator selection. For example, the NIOSH respirator recommendations for TDI are either a self-contained breathing apparatus or air-supplied respirator with a full face piece operated in either pressure-demand or positive-pressure modes. Each respirator must be properly fitted to the wearer. Supervisory personnel must monitor the use of the respirator to make certain it is being worn properly. Medical surveillance must also be conducted to determine whether adequate protection is achieved by using the respirator.

In aluminum pot-room workers, use of helmet respirators resulted in a significant increase in PEFR measurements but not improvement in symptoms at work in comparison to periods when respirators were not in use (69). Rosenberg and Tuomi (70) evaluated levels of HDI inside and outside respiratory devices used by spray painters. Respirators with both gas filters or combined gas and particle filters were evaluated. Measurable levels of HDI were detected inside the respirators indicating that these devices are not always reliable in preventing HDI exposure. Respirators can be effective for preventing asthma symptoms in workers with established OA due to laboratory animals (71). Twin cartridge respirators have been reported to effectively prevent exposure to wood dust and clinical deterioration in red cedar workers with OA (72). However, there is generally poor compliance with the use of respirators, which are often cumbersome and uncomfortable. Thus, it is often impractical to recommend respirators as a primary prevention strategy for an entire workforce.

Once preventive measures have been initiated, medical surveillance programs such as those described earlier should be instituted to monitor the efficacy of modifications in production processes, ventilation, or worker procedures.

CONCLUSIONS

Although definitive evidence of their effectiveness is still required, there is now some evidence suggesting that cost-effective medical surveillance programs should be instituted in any workplace where agents known to cause OA are in use. More effective public health surveillance programs are required on a worldwide basis to identify new cases and perhaps new causes of OA. Although unproven, it is likely that more timely and accurate case identification will result in institution of preventive measures in work environments that could avert adverse clinical outcomes and prevent new cases of OA.

APPENDIX: OCCUPATIONAL ASTHMA SCREENING QUESTIONNAIRE

Since your last medical (or in the last 12 months for new starters)		
Have you had episodes of wheeze or chest tightness?	Yes	No
Have you taken any treatment for your chest?	Yes	No
Have you woken from sleep with cough or chest tightness?	Yes	No
Have you had any episodes of breathlessness?	Yes	No
Have you had any time off work with chest illness?	Yes	No
Have you developed chest tightness or breathlessness after exercise?	Yes	No
Have you developed difficulty breathing?	Yes	No
The following additional questions may be asked:		
Have you had irritation or watering of the eyes?	Yes	No
Have you had a stuffy nose?	Yes	No
Have you had soreness of the nose, lips, or mouth?	Yes	No
Have you had itching or irritation of the skin?	Yes	No

Any positive response should lead to a full history and investigation by a health professional with expertise in the diagnosis of OA. The questionnaire has been designed to be sensitive rather than specific.
Source: From Ref. 29.

REFERENCES

1. Freund E, Seligman PJ, Chorba TL, et al. Mandatory reporting of occupational diseases by clinicians. MMWR 1990; 39:19–23.
2. Balmes JR. Surveillance for occupational asthma. Occupational Medicine: State of the Art Reviews 1991; 6 (Jan-March):101–110.

3. Bernstein DI. Surveillance and prevention. In: Bernstein IL, Chan-Yeung M, Malo J-L, eds. Asthma in the Workplace. New York: Marcel Dekker, 1993:359–372.

4. Rutstein DD, Mullan RJ, Frazier TM, Halperin WE, Melius M, Sestito MS. Sentinel health events (occupational): a basis for physician recognition and public health surveillance. Am J Public Health 1983; 73:1054–1062.

5. Chan-Yeung M, MacLean L, Paggiaro PL. Follow-up study of 232 patients with occupational asthma caused by western red cedar *(Thuja plicata)*. J Allergy Clin Immunol 1987; 79:792–796.

6. Fabbri LM, Danieli D, Crescioli S, Bevilacqua P, Meli S, Saetta M, Mapp CE. Fatal asthma in a subject sensitized to toluene diisocyanate. Am Rev Respir Dis 1988; 137:1494–1498.

7. Carino M, Aliani M, Licitra C, Sarno N, Ioli F. Death due to asthma at workplace in a diphenylmethane diisocyanate–sensitized subject. Respiration 1997; 64:111–113.

8. Erlich I. Fatal asthma in a baker: a case report. Am J Ind Med 1994; 26:799.

9. National Institute for Occupational Safety and Health. Criteria for a Recommended Standard: Occupational Exposure to Diisocyanates. Cincinnati, OH: National Institute for Occupational Safety and Health, 1978 (DHEW publication no. 78–215).

10. Ontario Ministry of Labour. Regulation respecting isocyanates made under the Occupational Health and Safety Act, 1980. Revised Statutes of Ontario, 1983; Chapter 321, Ontario Regulation 455,80.

11. COSHH. Control of Substances Hazardous to Health Regulations 1988. SI 1657. London: HMO, 1988.

12. Smedly J, Coggon D. Health surveillance for hospital employees exposed to respiratory sensitizers. Occup Med 1996; 46:33–36.

13. Musk AW, Peters JM, Wegman DH. Isocyanates and respiratory disease: current status. Am J Ind Med 1988; 13:331–349.

14. Brooks SM. Occupational asthma. Toxicology Lett 1995; 82/83:39–45.

15. Ad Hoc Committee on Occupational Asthma of the Standards Committee, Canadian Thoracic Society. Occupational asthma: recommendations for diagnosis, management and assessment of impairment. Can Med Assoc J 1989; 140:1029–1032.

16. Chan-Yeung M, Brooks S, Alberts M, et al. ACCP Consensus Statement: Assessment of asthma in the workplace. Chest 1995; 108:1084–1117.

17. Hudson P, Cartier A, Pinea L, Laurence M, St Agin JJ, Dubois JY, Malo J-L. Follow-up of occupational asthma caused by crab and various agents. J Allergy Clin Immunol 1985; 76:262–268.

18. Tarlo SM, Liss G, Corey P, Broder I. Classification and outcome of occupational asthma claims in Ontario. Chest 1995; 107:634–641.

19. Chan-Yeung M. Occupational asthma. Chest 1990; 98(Suppl):148S–161S.

20. Chan-Yeung M. Occupational asthma—coming of age. J Occup Med Toxicol 1993; 2:230–266.

21. Venables KM. Prevention of occupational asthma. Eur Respir J 1994; 7:768–778.

22. Vandenplas O, Malo J-L, Saetta M, Mapp CE, Fabbri LM. Occupational asthma and extrinsic alveolitis due to isocyanates: current status and perspectives. Br J Ind Med 1993; 50:213–228.

23. Bernstein DI, Korbee L, Stauder T, Bernstein JA, Bernstein IL. The low prevalence of occupational asthma and antibody dependent sensitization to diphenylmethane diisocyanate (MDI) in a plant engineered for minimal exposure to diisocyanates. J Allergy Clin Immunol 1993; 92:387–396.

24. Tarlo SM, Banks D, Liss G, Broder I. Outcome determinants for isocyanate induced occupational asthma among compensation claimants. Occup Environ Med 1997; 54:756–761.

25. Cochrane AL. Validation of screeing procedures. Br Med Bull 1971; 27:3–8.

26. Smith AB, Bernstein DI, Tar-Ching AW, Gallagher JS, London M, Kopp S, Carson GA. Occupational asthma from inhaled egg protein. Am J Ind Med 1987; 213:205–218.

27. Malo J-L, Ghezzo H, L'Archeveque J, Lagier F, Perrin B, Cartier A. Is the clinical history a satisfactory means for diagnosing occupational asthma? Am Rev Respir Dis 1991; 143:528–532.

28. Brooks SM, Bernstein IL, Raghuprasad PK, Maccia CA, Mieckowski L. Assessment of airway hyperresponsiveness in chronic stable asthma. J Allergy Clin Immunol 1990; 85:17–26.

29. Burge S. Respiratory symptoms. Occup Med 1997; 47:55–56.

30. Burge PS. Problems in the diagnosis of occupational asthma. Br J Dis Chest 1987; 81:105–115.

31. Cockroft DW, Murdock KY, Berscheid BA, Gore BP. Sensitivity and specificity of histamine PC_{20} determination in a random selection of young college students. J Allergy Clin Immunol 1992; 89:23–30.

32. Hendrick DJ, Fabbri LM, Hughes JM, Banks DE, Barkman HW Jr, Connolly MJ, Jones RN, Weill H. Modification of the methacholine inhalation test and its epidemiologic use in polyurethane workers. Am Rev Respir Dis 1986; 133:600–604.

33. Bernstein DI, Bernstein IL, Gaines WG, Stauder T, Wilson ER. Characterization of skin prick testing responses for detecting sensitization to detergent enzymes at extreme dilutions. Inability of the RAST to detect lightly sensitized individuals. J Allergy Clin Immunol 1994; 94:498–507.

34. Merget R, Stollfuss J, Wierodt R, et al. Diagnostic tests in enzyme allergy. J Allergy Clin Immunol 1993; 92(2):264–277.

35. Biagini RE, Kincewicz SL, Henningsen GM, MacKenzie BA, Gallagher JS, Bernstein DI, Bernstein IL. Antibodies to morphine in workers exposed to opiates at a narcotics manufacturing facility and evidence for similar antibodies in heroin abusers. Life Sci 1990; 47(10):897–908.

36. Grammar LC, Shaughnessy MA, Henderson J. A clinical and immunologic study of workers with trimellitic anhydride induced immunologic lung disease after transfer to low exposure jobs. Am Rev Respir Dis 1993; 148:54.

37. Biological effects of proteolytic enzyme detergents. Thorax 1976; 31:621.

38. Botham PA, Lamb CT, Teasdale EL, Bonner SM, Tomenson JA. Allergy to laboratory animals: a follow up study of its incidence and of the influence of atopy and pre-existing sensitisation on its development. Occup Environ Med 1995; 52(2):129–133.

39. Tarlo SM, Boulet L-P, Cartier A, et al. Canadian thoracic guidelines for occupational asthma. Can Respir J 1998; 5(4):289–300.

40. Levy BS, Halperin WE. Screening for occupational disease. In: Levy BS, Wegman DH, eds. Occupational Health: Recognizing and Preventing Work-Related Disease, 2nd ed. Toronto: Little, Brown, 1988:75–86.

41. Halperin WE, et al. Medical screening in the workplace: proposed principles. J Occup Med 1986; 28:547–552.

42. Stenton SC, Beach JR Avery AJ, Hendrick DJ. The value of questionnaires and spirometry in asthma surveillance programs in the workplace. Occup Med 1993; 43:203–206.

43. Adelroth E, Hargreave FE, Ramsgate EH. Do physicians need objective measurements to diagnose asthma? Am Rev Respir Dis 1988; 134:704–707.

44. Malo J-L, Ghezzo J, D'Aquino C, L'Archeveque J, Cartier A, Chan-Yeung M. Natural history of occupational asthma: relevance of type of agent and other factors on the rate of development of symptoms in subjects with disease. J Allergy Clin Immunol 1992; 90:937–943.

45. Wegman DH, Froines JR. Surveillance needs for occupational health. Am J Public Health 1985; 75:1259–1261.

46. Meredith SK, Taylor VM, McDonald JC. Occupational respiratory disease in the United Kingdom 1989: a report to the British Thoracic Society and the Society of Occupational Medicine by the SWORD project group. Br J Ind Med 1989; 48:292–298.

47. Ross DJ, Sallie BA, McDonald JC. SWORD '94: surveillance of work-related and occupational respiratory disease in the UK. Occup Med 1995; 45(4):175–178.

48. Provencher S, Labreche FP, deGuire L. Physician based surveillance system for occupational respiratory diseases: the experience of PROPULSE, Quebec, Canada. Occup Environ Med 1997; 54(4):272–276.

49. Matte TD, Hoffman R, Rosenman KD. Surveillance of occupational asthma under the SENSOR model. Chest 1990; 98:735–1788.

50. Centers for Disease Control. Occupational disease surveillance: asthma. JAMA 1990; 263: 1613–1616.

51. Klees JE, Alexander M, Rempel D, Beckett W, Rubin R, Barnhart S, Balmes JR. Evaluation of a proposed NIOSH surveillance case definition for occupational asthma. Chest 1990; 98: 212S–215S.

52. Reilly MJ, Rosenman KD, Watt FC, Schill D, Stanbury M, Trimbath LS, Romero Jajosky RA, Musgrave KJ, Castellan RM, Bang KM, et al. Surveillance for occupational asthma—Michigan and New Jersey, 1988–1992. MMWR CDC Surveillance Summaries 1994; 43(1):9–17.

53. Frequencies of occupational allergic diseases and gender differences in Finland. Int Arch Occup Environ Health 1994; 66:111–116.

54. Nuorteva P, Assmuth T, Hahtela T, Ahti J, Kurnonen E, Nieminin T, Saarainen T, Seppala K, Veide P, Viholainen S. The prevalence of asthma among inhabitants in the vicinity of a polyurethane factor in Finland. Environ Res 1987; 34:308–316.

55. Anto JM, Sunyer J, Rodriguez-Roisin R, Suarez-Cervera M, Vazquez L. Toxicoepidemiologic committee. Community outbreaks of asthma associated with inhalation of soybean dust. N Engl J Med 1989; 320:1097–1102.

56. Sunyer J, Rodrigo M-J, Anto JM, Morell F. Clinical and Toxicological Committee. Case-control study of serum immunoglobulin-E antibodies reactive with soybean in epidemic asthma. Lancet 1989; 1(Jan 28):179–182.

57. Diem JE, Jones RN, Hendrick DJ, Glindmeyer HW, Dharmarajan V, Butcher BT, Salvaggio JE, Weill H. Five-year longitudinal study of workers employed in a new toluene diisocyanate manufacturing plant. Am Rev Respir Dis 1982; 126:420–428.

58. Omae K. Two-year observation of pulmonary function in workers exposed to low concentrations of toluene diisocyanate. Int Arch Occup Environ Health 1984; 55:1–12.

59. Moller DR, McKay RT, Bernstein IL, Brooks SM. Persistent airways disease caused by toluene diisocyanate. Am Rev Respir Dis 1986; 134:175–176.

60. Baur X. New aspects of isocyanate asthma. Lung 1990; (Suppl):606–613.

61. Stevens MA, Palmer R. The effects of toluene diisocyanate on certain laboratory animals. Proc R Soc Med 1970; 63:380–382.

62. Vedal S, Chan-Yeung M, Enarson D, Fera T, MacLean L, Tse KS, Langille R. Symptoms and pulmonary function in western red cedar workers related to duration of employment and dust exposure. Arch Environ Health 1986; 41:179–183.

63. Venables KM. Low molecular weight chemicals, hypersensitivity and direct toxicity: the acid anhydrides. Br J Ind Med 1988; 46:222–232.

64. Howe W, Venables KM, Topping MD, Dally MB, Hawkins R, Law JS, Newman Taylor AJ. Tetrachlorophthalic anhydride asthma: evidence for specific IgE antibody. J Allergy Clin Immunol 1983; 71:5–11.

65. Brown NM, Dolovich J., Witmeur O, Zachariae H, Pham QT, et al. Biological effects of proteolytic enzyme detergents. Thorax 1976; 31:621–634.

66. Liss GM, Kominsky JR, Gallagher JS, Melius J, Brooks SM, Bernstein IL. Failure of enzyme encapsulation to prevent sensitization of workers in the dry bleach industry. J Allergy Clin Immunol 1984; 73:348–355.

67. NIOSH Certified Equipment List. DHHS (NIOSH), 1995, Publication no. 91–105.

68. NIOSH Pocket Guide to Chemical Hazards. DHHS (NIOSH), 1990, Publication no. 90–117.

69. Kongerud J, Rambjor O. The influence of the helmet respirator on peak flow rate in aluminum potroom. Am Ind Hyg Assoc J 1991; 52:243–248.

70. Rosenberg C. Tuomi. T. Airborne isocyanates in polyurethane spray painting: determination and respiratory efficiency. Am Ind Hyg Assoc J 1984; 45:117–121.

71. Slovak AJM, Hill RN. Laboratory animal allergy: a clinical survey of an exposed population. Br J Ind Med 1981; 38:38–41.

72. Cote J, Kennedy S, Chan-Yeung M. Outcome of patients with cedar asthma with continuous exposure. Am Rev Respir Dis 1990; 141:373–376.

18

Upper Airways Involvement

David C. Christiani
Harvard School of Public Health and Massachusetts General Hospital, Harvard Medical School, Boston, Massachusetts

Jean-Luc Malo
Université de Montréal and Sacré-Coeur Hospital, Montréal, Quebec, Canada

DEFINITION

In the working environment exposures may result in inflammation of the upper airways: the nasal passages, nasopharynx, sinus, and larynx. For the purpose of this review, the nasal passages are emphasized because (1) the nose has a critical role in respiratory defenses and (2) a growing body of epidemiologic and clinical data is available on effects of airborne contaminants on the nose.

The nasal passage serves several critical functions. It is the first respiratory mucosa to encounter inhaled particles, gases, vapors, and fumes (1). It warms and humidifies inhaled air and filters large particles, including many allergens. It is the primary absorptive surface for water-soluble gases, such as sulfur dioxide. It removes substantial quantities of even less soluble gases, such as ozone. Obstruction of the nasal passages may result in a change from nasal to oral respiration. Oral breathing bypasses the filtering functions of the nose, increasing the hazard to the lower airways and the lung.

Rhinitis is defined as inflammation of the nasal mucosa, whether the result of a specific immune reaction or as a direct irritant effect. As for occupational asthma (OA), rhinitis can occur due to a "sensitizing" mechanism or following acute exposure to high concentrations of an irritant material.

EXPOSURES

A variety of occupational exposures have been associated with rhinitis. Experimental exposures to ozone have demonstrated neutrophilia in nasal lavagate (2). This observation was confirmed in studies of children exposed to ambient ozone (3). Exposure to fuel-oil ash among boilermakers resulted in a significant increase in nasal neutrophils among nonsmokers, but not smokers, although smokers had high baseline neutrophil concentrations (4). Agricultural exposures such as grain dust cause rhinitis and peripheral neutrophilia (6) and grain dust extracts and endotoxin result in upper and lower respiratory tract inflammation (7). Other agents and processes likely to cause occupational rhinitis include, but

331

are not limited to: livestock breeding; feed manufacture and handling; wood dust; cotton, flax, and hemp processing; silicate dust; pollens; gases (e.g., NO_x, NH_3, H_2S); insect parts; fungi and insecticides. Many agents inducing occupational asthma with a latency period, particularly those of the high-molecular-weight (protein-derived) type, can cause rhino-conjunctivitis symptoms (8). In the latter situation, both conditions, occupational asthma and occupational rhinitis, are IgE-mediated. Finally, a condition called by some authors reactive upper disease syndrome (RUDS), equivalent to reactive airway disease syndrome (RADS), can occur after exposure to high concentrations of irritant materials (9).

CLINICAL FEATURES

Intermittent or persistent rhinorrhea may be caused by a variety of clinical disorders including allergic rhinitis and irritant rhinitis. The evaluation of a patient with upper airway symptoms consists of a careful history and physical examination. The history is the simple most important tool for evaluation of the upper respiratory tract. Temporal patterns of irritation, congestion, rhirorrhea, or sneezing may suggest likely causes. A symptom diary may be useful to clarify these patterns. The history may also suggest concomitant reactive airways or asthma, such as paroxysmal cough, episodic chest tightness, exertional or nocturnal wheeze, or dyspnea.

Rhinitis caused by sensitization to airborne agents is characterized byrhinorrhea, sneezing, nasal obstruction, lacrimation, and occasionally, pharyngeal itching. Episodic symptoms are the hallmark of allergic rhinitis. In addition to the nasal symptoms, there may be conjunctival congestion and edema. Swelling of the nasal turbinates and mucosa with obstruction of the sinus ostia and eustachian tubes can precipitate secondary infections of the sinus and middle ear. The latter is more common in perennial (vs. seasonal) rhinitis. Washings, swabs, or biopsy of the mucosa will usually reveal eosinophils, but some polymorphonuclear leukocytes are usually present.

Irritant rhinitis is often found when sensitizers are not identified or may be caused by exposure to irritants in the working environment. Nasal washings and biopsy usually reveal a predominant PMN response. There is evidence that air pollutants can initiate allergic responses among atopic individuals (5).

If the history is strongly suggestive of a sensitized response, a referral for allergy skin tests is indicated. Another approach is to obtain a multiallergen radioallergosorbent test (RAST), with referral for skin testing if the RAST is positive.

ASSESSMENT OF NASAL RESPONSES

Nasal resistance varies by many factors such as nasal congestion, inflammation, or physiological state. A group of tests to measure nasal resistance and/or airway flow through the nose is called rhinomanometry. It is widely used for clinical purposes for the assessment of anatomical variation, quantification of therapeutic effect on nasal obstruction, and measurement of pathophysiological responses such as allergy. Rhinomanometry has also been applied to assess environmental and occupational factors causing the change of nasal flow or resistance. Resistance is expressed as the pressure difference divided by flow ($R = dP/V$), and both of them can be measured simultaneously. There are three major types of rhinomanometry: anterior active rhinomanometry, posterior active rhinomanometry, and passive rhinomanometry. "Active" tests are done while subjects voluntarily inhale or exhale through the manometer. "Passive" means that air is blown into the subject's nose. Anterior active rhinomanometry places the tube in the nostrils, and a posterior manometer is placed near the pharynx through the mouth. Manometry is useful and easy to perform, but there are some limitations, including the subject's degree of cooperation, collapse of alae, relatively high variability, and unsatisfactory correlation with symptoms. Manometry is sometimes not sensitive to pathology in some parts of the cavity. Acoustic rhinometry utilizes sound reflection to obtain the area-distance curve from the nostril through the nasal cavity. It is more accurate and reliable than manometry in measuring patency in terms of anatomical area, but it is based on assumptions that there is no turbulence, no viscous loss of acoustic energy, no influence by contralateral cavity, and that the walls are rigid. All of these assumptions are actually not true, limiting the interpretation. However, comparison between acoustic rhinometry and measurement by computed-tomography scan and by nasal model showed an excellent correlation. Another limitation is that it is inaccurate behind severe constriction.

Nasal peak-flow measurement is especially of interest because it can be used for repeated examinations, usually by the subject, many times a day during the workdays to detect early reversible signs (10). Expiratory flow has been measured in many studies, and recently inspiratory-flow measurement has been used in several studies with good results.

Development of acoustic rhinometry can reduce measurement variability and improve sensitivity (11–14). Other techniques that can be used in epidemiologic studies, such as nasal peak flow, can be performed serially throughout the working day (15–17) to detect early, reversible nasal airflow limitation.

BIOCHEMICAL MARKERS OF INFLAMMATORY AND IMMUNE RESPONSE

Nasal lavage has been used to collect secretions and assess the inflammatory response of the upper airway to allergens and irritants (2,5,18–22). The technique is simple, though not yet standardized. The most common method, briefly described, is: while seated, subjects tilt their heads backward at 45 degrees. With a needleless syringe, 5 ml of warm (37°C) sterile PBS (without calcium or magnesium) is instilled into the nostril. The saline is retained for 10 sec and then allowed to drain passively for 30 sec into a sterile specimen cup. The volume of lavage fluid recovered is recorded and used to adjust cell counts. Cells are counted on a hemocytometer and differential counts done on slides prepared by sytospin and stained with Wright-Giemsa. Although the method is not yet standardized, recent study indicates that intraindividual variability in PMN counts is less than interindividual variability, supporting utility for epidemiological studies (23). Nasal secretions can also be analyzed for biochemical components such as protein, albumin, histamine, IgE, antioxidants, and complement (23). The intraindividual variability and kinetics of these constituents in nasal fluid are as yet unknown. Although this type of challenge can be used with occupational challenges that can be diluted, it cannot be performed for occupational agents of the low-molecular-weight type, which are usually chemicals.

Inflammatory and immune responses of the upper airways are mostly studied to understand the pathophysiology of allergic and nonallergic rhinitis. Basic study methodology is to give a challenge by a specific antigen or nonspecific agent such as methacholine and then collect nasal secretions to analyze the cellular and biochemical components of the secretion.

In most of the recent studies, nasal lavage has been the mainstay of collecting nasal secretion to assess inflammatory and immune responses of the upper airway to allergen or irritants. Biochemical analysis of various mediators in nasal secretions and/or morphological analysis of cellular components are performed on the lavage fluid, after centrifugation, if needed. Brush method can be used mainly to harvest cells (24). Other techniques such as nasal blowing, smears, and imprints were also used to collect the specimen in some studies. Those methods are reviewed by Pipkorn and Karlsson (25).

Nasal secretions originate from several sources, such as transudated serum components including albumin and other proteins, locally synthesized proteins including enzymes and surface IgA, mucous glycoprotein derived from the glandular elements, and chemical mediators and other products from various cells including plasma cells, mast cells, basophils, and epithelial cells. Many studies assessed cellular or biochemical components of nasal lavage fluid before and after challenge test using methacholine or specific allergens (26,27).

Nasal challenge of sensitive individuals with antigen or cold dry air increases the levels of histamine, TAME-esterase activity, PGD2, and kinins in nasal lavage fluid (28). These mediators originate from the influx of activated cells such as eosinophils, neutrophils, mast cells, and basophils. Neutrophils represent the greatest number of infiltrating cells in the late-phase reaction.

The interpretation of the markers is well summarized by Koren and Devlin (21) and reproduced in Table 1.

Nasal lavage studies in subjects exposed to agricultural dusts are limited. One study reported elevated nasal PMN counts in farmers exposed to sorghum dust (28). Another study, a controlled human-exposure experiment, reported elevated lymphocytes in subjects exposed to dusts from corn and soybean as well as for endotoxin (29). In a recent study, we performed challenges in 15 subjects with OA (eight due to high-molecular-weight agents—flour and guar gum—and seven due to isocyanates) on two occasions, 2–4 weeks apart in a random fashion (30). On one occasion, subjects inhaled through the nose and on the other, through the mouth, using apparatuses that allow for exposing subjects to concentrations below the irritant levels and comparable to what is authorized in workplaces. The FEV_1 was monitored for up to 8 hr afterward and symptoms were documented with a standardized questionnaire on nasal synmptomatology, assessment of nasal resistance by rhinomanometry, and nasal lavage for examination of cells and mediators. We

Table 1 Biomarkers of NAL with Potential Use in Occupational Studies

Marker	Indication
PMNs	Inflammatory response
Protein, albumin	Permeability
Eosinophils, mast cells	Allergic response
Histamine, tryptase, kinins, PGD2, TAME-esterase, serotonin	Mast cell degranulation/allergic response
IgE	Allergic response
Eicosanoids, substance P, antioxidants, kallikrein, kinins cytokines, C5a, C3a	Inflammatory/allergic responses

PGD2, prostaglandin D2; TAME, *N*-alpha-*p*-tosyl-L-arginine methyl ester.
Source: Reproduced from Ref. 21.

showed that inhaling through the mouth and through the nose: (1) yielded similar asthmatic responses ($25 \pm 8\%$ and $22 \pm 10\%$ maximum changes in FEV_1); and (2) more than doubled the peak nasal symptoms and nasal resistance when comparing the maximum daily response with prechallenge results. This increase occurred on the days of inhalational challenges through the mouth and through the nose, this being explained by backflow of air into the upper airways on the day of challenge through the mouth. There were some significant, though low-magnitude, responses assessed by nasal lavage in terms of cells and mediators, again with no differences between the days of challenges through the mouth and through the nose. This study in which subjects were exposed to low concentrations of occupational agents therefore showed that inhaling occupational agents of high or low molecular weights, including isocyanates, whether through the mouth or nose: (1) results in a similar asthmatic response; (2) causes a significant nasal response in terms of symptoms and an increase in nasal resistance; and (3) causes some significant changes in inflammatory cells and mediators. Nasal challenge test has been shown by others to be useful in the diagnosis of rhinitis accompanying OA to flour (31). Gorski and co-workers (31) administered specific challenges through the nose by the nasal pool method in which a concentrated solution of flour is inserted into the nostril. In 100 subjects with OA and rhinitis caused by flour, the authors documented a significant increase in symptoms as well as in the cellular and mediator influx after the nasal challenge. As for nasal challenges performed with common inhalants, this study used concentrations that are more elevated than what occurs with natural exposure, therefore questioning the interpretation of findings. However, the authors found that 40 controls, either atopic subjects not sensitized to flour or healthy subjects, did not show significant changes after comparable challenges.

PATHOGENESIS

The nasal mucosa is covered by a mucosal blanket that moves by cilia posteriorly toward the pharynx carrying pollutants. Except for the olfactory cells, nasal epithelium is respiratory epithelium, which is identical to that of the lower respiratory tract. The nasal mucosa metabolizes certain chemicals such as formaldehyde and SO_2. Immune defenses of the nose consist of humoral immunity (IgA, IgE), cellular immunity involving machrophages and PMN, and other immunoreactive materials such as interferon, lactofevron, and lysozymes. Inhalation exposures can produce rhinitis by several mechanisms. Sensitization with the production of IgE specific for a substance can lead to symptoms on reexposure via mast cell degranulation and the release of inflammatory mediators. Respiratory irritants can lead to rhinitis through interaction with chemical irritant receptors in the airway, leading to the release of substance P from sensory nerves and neurogenic inflammation (29).

Dusts, fumes, and gases can exert several kinds of effects on the nasal mucosa, including irritation, increased airflow resistance, impairment of mucociliary clearance, impairment of defenses, inflammation, and direct cell damage (32).

Mucociliary abnormalities may result from many environmental exposures including dry air, acid aerosols, infection, and chemical gases such as NO_2 and SO_2. Mucociliary clearance can be measured either by radioisotope-labeled particles with a gamma camera, or by a very simple method called a saccharin test. The saccharin test measures the time of mucosal transport by placing a 0.5-mm piece of saccharin on the anterior inferior turbinate, 1 cm from the end. Normally, a sweet taste is detected within 30 min, with an average transit time of 6 mm/min.

OCCURRENCE

Allergic rhinitis requires prior sensitization to the offending agent(s). Sensitization to natural products occurs most commonly in the atopic portion of the population, estimated to be between 10 and 20% of the total population. This proportion of the agricultural workforce may therefore be expected to have a higher risk of becoming sensitive to organic dusts when suitably exposed. A recent survey of occupational rhinitis in Finland reported that 20% of all rhinitis cases were occupational, and the most common exposures were from agricultural environments: flour, wood dust, animal dander, and vegetable fibers (e.g., cotton) (33). Swedish surveys of pig and dairy farmers have reported irritation of eyes, nose, and throat to be in excess of 20% (34).

Precise estimates of occupational rhinitis and mucous membrane irritation of the eyes and throat are unknown, but are the most commonly observed symptoms in persons exposed to agricultural dusts, gases, vapors, and fumes (35). They are probably more common and more significant in subjects exposed to high-molecular-weight agents (8). Their precise frequency needs to be estimated not only by questionnaire but also by objective means of assessment.

NATURAL HISTORY

Upper airway symptoms will persist as long as exposure to the offending agent(s) continue(s). The natural history of the upper airway response to agricultural environment exposures is unknown. It is possible that such responses may be an early marker of lower airway responses (8,19). Upper airway symptoms precede the development of asthma symptoms in subjects in whom the diagnosis of OA is confirmed to high-molecular-weight agents (8). They seem to start occurring at the same time as asthmatic symptoms in subjects exposed to low-molecular-weight agents (8). The magnitude of symptoms is generally higher in subjects exposed to high-molecular-weight agents by comparison with those exposed to low-molecular-weight agents (8).

In the case of RUDS (9), symptoms are acute on the occasion of exposure to an irritant material. These are characterized by acute burning of the upper airways, followed by sneezing, secretions, and congestion. Anosmia or hyposmia may be a long-term consequence of such accidental inhalational exposures, especially if they are repeated.

MANAGEMENT

For allergen-associated rhinitis, consistent avoidance of the sensitizing agent is essential. Since asthma prognosis is related to duration of symptomatic exposure, it is likely that the same relationship holds true for occupational rhinitis, although this has yet to be established. Antihistamines are helpful for treatment of allergic symptoms and chronic rhinitis. Treatment for concomitant nasal congestion requires a decongestant. The sedating side effects of antihistamines may create a workplace hazard (35). Job duties should be reviewed to determine whether decreased alertness of motor coordination results in a hazardous condition. Newer antihistamines that minimize these side effects are available.

Nasal-inhaled corticosteroids are effective and will often obviate the need for antihistamines. They block the inflammatory cell influx that occurs in the late-phase IgE response also. Nasal cromalyn sodium is safe and effective in the management of seasonal and perennial rhinitis. The management of irritant rhinitis also requires avoidance of the known irritant or nonspecific (irritant) conditions that trigger symptoms in patients with chronic rhinitis (36). This approach may require adjustments in workplace ventilation or in work practices, even when environmental assessments find no evidence of increased concentrations of specific chemicals above permissible exposure limits. Medical removal may be indicated, though rarely, particularly if the symptoms are linked with other symptoms such as severe headache, visual disturbances, or neurological symptoms. It is our experience that subjects affected by rhinitis symptoms due to sensitization to a high-molecular-weight agent can continue working in the same environment provided there are no accompanying asthma symptoms and they take appropriate medications. These subjects should be followed more closely to make sure they do not develop asthma symptoms or bronchial hyperresponsiveness. Adequate respiratory protection may be temporarily effective, but is should not substitute for engineering, process, and administrative controls. One patient's mucosal reactions to a particular process or material may represent a sentinel event for future problems with other workers in that setting.

Other standard recommendations for medical management of upper airways disorders may be helpful. These may include elevation of head at night and nasal saline washes. Intranasal decongestants are not advised for chronic use because they may induce rhinitis medicamentosa, an iatrogenic nasal vasodilation and obstruction caused by overuse of topical sympathomimetics. A combination of oral antihistamines and oral decongestants may be helpful in the treatment of nonallergic nasal hyperreactivity characterized by increased secretions.

FUTURE RESEARCH

The development and application of new biological markers for upper airway responses to workplace exposures will help define the prevalence, distribution, and impact of upper airway disease in the workforce. There is a pressing need for standardization of techniques such as nasal lavage and nasal airflow measurements. Molecular techniques to detect early inflammatory responses need to be developed and evaluated.

In addition to development of techniques for evaluation of epidemiologic studies of upper airway responses, research must also focus on whether the upper airway responses to contaminants reflect or predict lower airway responses. Research should focus on whether conditions such as irritant rhinitis may be an early marker of chronic bronchitis and airflow obstruction. The methodology of nasal challenges with occupational agents, particularly low-molecular-weight agents that cannot be diluted in saline solutions, needs to be developed. Such a methodology would be very useful for diagnostic purposes in subjects with rhinitis but no asthmatic symptom.

REFERENCES

1. Witek TJ. The nose as a target for adverse effects from the environment: applying advances in nasal physiologic measurements and mechanisms. Am J Ind Med 1993; 24:649–657.

2. Graham D, Henderson F, House D. Neutrophil influx measured in nasal lavages of humans exposed to ozone. Arch Environ Health 1988; 43(3):229–233.

3. Frischer TM, Kuehr J, Pullwitt A, et al. Ambient ozone causes upper airways inflammation in children. Am Rev Respir Dis 1993; 148:961–964.

4. Hauser R, Elreedy S, Hoppin JA, Christiani DC. The upper airway response in workers exposed to fuel-oil ash: nasal lavage analysis. J Occup Environ Med 1995; 52:353–358.

5. Bascom R, Naclerio RM, Fitzgerald TK, et al. Effect of ozone inhalation on the response to nasal challenge with antigen of allergic subjects. Am Rev Respir Dis 1990; 142:594–601.

6. Von Essen S, O'Neill D, Robbins R. Grain sorghum dust inhalation at harvest causes nasal inflammation and peripheral blood neutrophilia. Am Rev Respir Dis 1993; 147(4):A528 (abstract).

7. Clapp WD, Thorne PS, Frees KL, et al. The effects of inhalation of grain dust extract and endotoxin on upper and lower airways. Chest 1993; 104(3):825–830.

8. Malo JL, Lemière C, Desjardins A, Cartier A. Prevalence and intensity of rhinoconjunctivitis in subjects with occupational asthma. Eur Respir J 1997; 10:1513–1515.

9. Meggs WJ. RADS and RUDS—the toxic induction of asthma and rhinitis. J Toxicol Clin Toxicol 1994; 32:487–501.

10. Cho SI, Hauser R, Christiani DC. Nasal inspiratory peak-flow assessment of epidemiologic utility. Chest 112:1547–1553.

11. Bridger GP, Proctor DF. Maximum nasal inspiratory flow and nasal resistance. Ann Otol Rhinol Laryngol 1970; 79:481–488.

12. Benson MK. Maximum nasal inspiratory flow rate: use it assessing the effect of pseudoephrine in vasomotor rhinitis. Eur J Clin Pharmacol 1970; 3:182–184.

13. Taylor G, MacNeil AR, Freed DLJ. Assessing degree of nasal patency by measuring peak expiratory flow-rate through the nose. J Allergy Clin Immunol 1973; 52:193–198.

14. Gleeson MJ, Youlten LJF, Shelton DM, Siodlak MZ, Eiser NM, Wengraf CL. Assessment of nasal airwaypatency: a comparison of four methods. Clin Otolaryngol 1986; 11:99–107.

15. Frolund L, Madsen F, Mygind N, Nielsen N, Svendsen U, Weeke B. Comparison between different techniques for measuring nasal patency in a group of unselected patients. Acta Otolaryngol 1987; 104:175–179.

16. Ahman M. Nasal peak flow-rate records in work-related nasal blockage. Acta Otolaryngol 1992; 112:839–844.

17. Toren K, Hagberg S, Brisman J, et al. Nasal inflammation in pulp mill workers exposed to lime dust—investigation before and after a reconstruction of the mill. Am J Respir Crit Care Med 1994; 149(4):A409 (abstract).

18. Koren HS, Hatch GE, Graham DE. Nasal lavage as a tool in assessing acute inflammation in response to inhaled pollutants. Toxicology 1990; 60:15–25.

19. Graham DE, Koren HS. Biomarkers of inflammation in ozone-exposed humans. Am Rev Respir Dis 1990; 142:152–156.

20. Bascom R, Kulle T, Kagey-Sobotka A, et al. Upper respiratory-track environmental tobacco smoke sensitivity. Am Rev Respir Dis 1991; 143:1304–1311.

21. Koren HS, Devlin RB. Human upper respiratory-track responses to inhaled pollutants with emphasis on nasal lavage. Ann NY Acad Sci 1992; 641:215–224.

22. Koren HS, Graham DE, Devlin RB. Exposure of humans to a volatile organic mixture. III. Inflammatory response. Arch Environ Health 1992; 47(1):39–44.

23. Hauser R, Garcia-Closas M, Kelsey K, Christiani DC. Variability of nasal lavage polymorphonuclear leukocyte counts in unexposed subjects: its potential utility for epidemiology. Arch Environ Health 1994; 49:267–272.

24. Pipkorn U, Karlsson G, Enerback L. A brush method to harvest cells from the nasal mucosa for microscopic and biochemical analysis. J Immunol Methods 1988a; 112:37–42.

25. Pipkorn U, Karlsson G. Methods for obtaining specimens from the nasal mucosa for morphological and biochemical analysis. Eur Respir J 1988; 1:856–862.

26. Shelhamer J, Marom Z, Michael K. The constituents of nasal secretion. Ear Nose Throat J 1984; 63:82–84.

27. Raphael GD, Druce HM, Baraniuk JN, et al. Pathophysiology of rhinitis. Am Rev Respir Dis 1988; 138:413–420.
28. Togias A, Naclerio RM, Proud D, et al. Studies on the allergic and nonallergic nasal inflammation. J Allergy Clin Immunol 1988; 81:782–790.
29. Clapp WD, Thorne PS, Frees KL, Zhang X, Lux CR, Schwartz DA. The effects of inhalation of grain dust extract and endotoxin on upper and lower airways. Chest 1993; 104:825–830.
30. Desrosiers M, Nguyen B, Ghezzo H, Leblanc C, Malo JL. Nasal response in subjects undergoing challenges by inhaling occupational agents causing asthma through the nose and mouth. Allergy (in press).
31. Gorski P, Krakowiak A, Pazdrak K, Palcynski C, Ruta U, Walusiak J. Nasal challenge test in the diagnosis of allergic respiratory diseases in subjects occupationally exposed to a high molecular allergen (flour). Occup Med 1998; 48:91–97.
32. Leopold DA. Pollution: the nose and sinuses. Otolaryngol Head Neck Surg 1992; 106:713–719.
33. Kanerva L and Vaheri E. Occupational rhinitis in Finland. Int Arch Occup Environ Health 1993; 64:565–568.
34. Rylander R, Essle N. Donham KJ. Bronchial reactivity among farmers. Am J Ind Med 1990; 17:66–69.
35. Meltzer EO. Antihistamine- and decongestant-induced performance decrements. J Occup Med 1990; 32:327–334.
36. Rosenhall L. Organic dust and lung disease: influence of atopy and smoking on symptoms. Am J Ind Med 1990; 17:130–131.

19
Occupational Urticaria

Boris D. Lushniak
National Institute of Occupational Safety and Health, Cincinnati, Ohio

C. G. Toby Mathias
Group Health Associates and University of Cincinnati Medical Center, Cincinnati, Ohio

INTRODUCTION

Many exposures in the workplace that can result in occupational asthma can also cause a variety of dermatological problems. These include irritant contact dermatitis, allergic contact dermatitis (Type IV delayed hypersensitivity), and urticaria (Type I immunologic and nonimmunologic). Urticaria will be discussed here because of its more direct association with occupational asthma, in terms of both clinical coexistence and mechanistic similarities.

Urticaria is defined as the transient appearance of elevated, erythematous pruritic wheals or serpiginous exanthem, usually surrounded by an area of erythema. In addition, areas of macular erythema or erythematous papules may also be present. These skin lesions appear and peak in minutes to hours after the etiological exposure and individual lesions usually disappear within 24 hours. Urticarial lesions usually involve the trunk and extremities, although they can involve any epidermal or mucosal surface. Large wheal formation, where the edema extends from the dermis into the subcutaneous tissue, is referred to as angioedema. This condition is more commonly seen in the more distensible tissues, such as the eyelids, lips, ear lobes, external genitalia, and mucous membranes.

Urticarial wheals result from local subcutaneous and intradermal leakage of plasma filtrate from postcapillary venules. The erythema and surrounding swelling result from locally increased blood flow. Biopsy specimens of urticarial lesions may exhibit only subtle microscopic changes. There may be evident subcutaneous or dermal edema, an increase in the number of mast cells, and a modest perivascular lymphocytic infiltrate, perhaps intermingled with cosinophils. Electron microscopy reveals mast cell and eosinophilic degranulation (1).

CLASSIFICATIONS OF URTICARIA

Urticarial lesions can be classified in one or more of the following categories based upon characteristic features:

1. Duration or chronicity—acute or chronic.

341

2. Clinical distribution of the lesions or the extra-dermal manifestations—localized, generalized, or systemic associated with rhinitis, conjunctivitis, asthma, or anaphylaxis.
3. Etiology—idiopathic or cause-specific.
4. Route of exposure—direct contact, inhalation, or ingestion.
5. Mechanism—nonimmunological, immunological, or idiopathic.

Acute urticaria ranges from a single episode of urticaria to recurrences lasting less than 6 weeks. Common causes of acute urticaria include insect bites or stings and food or drug allergies. Chronic urticaria occurs daily (or almost daily) over a period longer than 6 weeks. Food, drugs, and infections can also be causes of chronic urticaria. However, in the chronic form, the exact causative agents may never be identified. The majority of cases of urticaria remain idiopathic.

Occupational urticaria is a general etiological classification of urticaria. It is urticaria that is presumed or proven to be caused by exposure to one or more substances or physical agents in the workplace. Beyond this definitional idiosyncracy, occupational urticaria may fall into any of the other classifications of urticaria. It may be acute or chronic, may be localized, generalized, or associated with systemic manifestations, such as asthma. In occupational settings, direct contact with substances, and possibly inhalation may be the more common routes of exposure inducing urticaria. The pathological mechanisms may be nonimmunological, immunological, or of uncertain etiology.

EPIDEMIOLOGY

Limitations of Epidemiological Data

It can be difficult to obtain accurate epidemiological data for occupational and non-occupational urticaria, and all sources have their limitations. First of all, though a case definition is a prerequisite for the gathering of epidemiological data, there is no standard case definition in the literature to define occupational urticaria, and there is no standard approach to prove the presumed occupational-relatedness of the urticaria. Cases may be defined using a variety of criteria. These include the following: the self-reporting of current or past episodes of urticaria in the workplace; histories of urticaria associated with a specific occupational exposure or work activity; objective signs of urticaria on clinical examination in the workplace, sometimes associated with the use of the alleged etiologic substance; evidence of specific IgE to suspect occupational antigens (e.g., radioallergosorbent test (RAST) assays or skin prick testing). A case definition used in a study or a data source may be based upon one or more of these criteria. Therefore, because the epidemiological case definition for occupational urticaria varies from one data source to another, it is difficult to compare different sources of information and different findings.

The accuracy of the diagnosis of occupational urticaria is related to the skill level, experience, and knowledge of the medical professional. The diagnosis is based on the medical and exposure history, physical findings, and in vitro or in vivo testing. The lack of a standard case definition and the difficulty of diagnosis lead to potential misclassification of occupational urticaria, which can result in either over- or underestimation of disease frequency. In allergic contact urticarial syndromes, the lack of standardized occupational test allergens also contributes to the problem of vague case definitions.

Much of the literature of urticaria in the workplace is filled with anecdotal case reports and limited observations. This usually results in information about a single worker or a relatively small number of workers. Many of the cases in the literature are based upon clinical presentations, a determination that the urticaria is based upon a "probable" occupational exposure, and a "probable" allergic or nonallergic mechanism. Further attempts to prove etiology or mechanisms may be lacking or inadequate. Although the literature is filled with cases of occupational urticaria, tabulating these cases cannot be considered a basis for epidemiological assessment (2).

Because of the problems with case definition and diagnosis, the limited number of subjects, and the difficulty in proving etiologies and mechanisms, the epidemiology of occupational urticaria remains obscure. There are other problems in assessing the epidemiology of occupational urticaria and other occupational skin diseases (3):

1. Occupational urticaria is not a reportable disease (except in states that require reporting of all occupational diseases). This makes health department data sources useless for monitoring occupational urticaria.
2. Occupational urticaria is not a disease that commonly leads to mortality or hospitalization; thus, death certificates or hospital records are not potential data sources.
3. Occupational urticaria is a disease seen and treated (though not always specifically diagnosed) by medical professionals in multiple specialties, especially primary care practitioners, making review of physician-based data sources inefficient.
4. Occupational urticaria may be a disease that often goes untreated and undiagnosed; thus, many cases may never be documented in any data source.
5. Once a diagnosis of occupational urticaria is made, a case does not necessarily elicit a public health response.
6. Individuals with occupational urticaria who seek medical care may be a unique subset of those with the condition. Through this self-selection bias, the information obtained may not reflect the epidemiology of the disease in the general population.
7. Unique exposures may occur in different populations and different industries, making the epidemiology of occupational urticaria in one population or workforce not necessarily generalizable to other populations.
8. The evaluation of past exposures causing occupational urticaria may be exceedingly difficult, often relying on historical information and patient recollection, which are subject to recall and information bias.
9. Cross-sectional studies of working populations, a common epidemiological study design, are subject to survivor bias. Those with severe occupational urticaria may leave the workforce, leaving only those who are not affected or less affected to be included in the studies.
10. An occupational urticaria case, especially if treated by a company's own occupational health personnel, may not involve lost wages or any costs to the worker. Thus, there would be no workers' compensation claim, reducing the utility of this already limited data source.

Descriptive Epidemiology of Occupational Urticaria

Accurate data on the general prevalence of urticaria are not available, although it is estimated that in a lifetime 5%–23% of the U.S. population may have had an episode of acute urticaria (4). Of 1011 consecutive patients seen in a dermatology practice, 26% gave a history of at least one urticarial episode (5). Data from the National Ambulatory Medical

Care Survey, a national probability sample survey of nonfederal office-based physicians in the United States, showed that from January 1989 to December 1990 over 25 million visits (4% of the total 698 million visits) were made to dermatologists. Urticaria was listed as the seventeenth most common principal diagnosis, accounting for 240,000 visits (1% of the total visits to dermatologists) (6). Unfortunately, similar data are not available for patient visits to allergists and immunologists.

International data are also limited. Of 4600 patients seen in a Spanish dermatology clinic and referred for patch testing from 1973 to 1977, 3.5% were given a final diagnosis of urticaria (7). A questionnaire study of 4492 respondents from a population of randomly selected Norwegians showed that 9% reported at least one episode of urticaria (8).

National occupational disease and illness data are available from the U.S. Bureau of Labor Statistics (BLS), but once again data specific for occupational urticaria are limited. The BLS conducts annual surveys of approximately 250,000 employers, selected to represent most private industries in the United States (9). The survey results are then projected to estimate the number and incidence rates of occupational injuries and illnesses in the American working population. BLS data are limited because they exclude several groups, including self-employed individuals, small farms, and government agencies; they depend on misinterpretable definitions of reportable occupational injuries and illnesses; they rely to a large extent on employees reporting conditions to the employer; and they do not provide information on the etiology of the disease.

In 1993, BLS estimated 60,200 cases of occupational skin diseases or disorders in the U.S. workforce (9). Further information is available on the 12,613 cases which involved days away from work. Of this subgroup, 142 (1.1%) were diagnosed with urticaria/hives. The median time away from work for workers with urticaria was 5 days. These 142 workers included 81 from the services industry, 39 from manufacturing, 9 from transportation and public utilities, and 13 not classified. It must be emphasized that because of BLS survey limitations, it has been estimated that the number of actual occupational skin diseases may be on the order of 10 to 50 times higher than reported by the BLS (10). Only limited clinically-based epidemiological information on occupational urticaria is available in the United States. Of 250 consecutive dermatology patients who had filed workers' disability compensation benefits, 8 (3.2%) were found to have urticaria and/or dematographism (11). However, in this study none were deemed to be work-related dermatoses.

In contrast, more specific occupational data are available in Finland. Between 1990 and 1994, occupational contact urticaria was responsible for 29.5% of all reported occupational dermatoses (12). Of the 815 cases of occupational contact urticaria, 70% were in women. Table 1 lists the most common causes which include cow dander (44%); natural rubber latex (24%); flour, grains, and feed (11%); foodstuffs (3%); industrial enzymes (2%); and decorative plants (2%). Interestingly, cow protein allergens also represented the most common cause of occupational asthma in Finland (13). Other, less common causes included roots, spices, pork, vegetables, storage mites, ethylhexyl acrylate, onions, egg, fish, fish meal, poultry, chicken, and other birds. Table 2 lists the occupations with the highest number of cases per 100,000 workers, which included bakers (140 cases per 100,000 employed persons), processed-food preparers, dental assistants, veterinarians, animal attendants, farmers, chefs and cooks, dairy workers, horticultural supervisors, laboratory technicians, physicians, butchers, laboratory assistants, dentists, and nurses.

In general, risk factors for contact urticaria and contact anaphylaxis (e.g., natural rubber latex glove proteins) include a history of atopy, a compromise to the barrier function of intact skin (such as eczema, abrasions, ulcers), and in some cases, occupation (14).

Table 1 Ranking List of the Causes of Occupational Contact Urticaria and Protein Contact Dermatitis During 1990–1994 (815 cases) According to the Finnish Register of Occupational Diseases

Ranking/cause	No. of cases	%	Men/women
1. Cow dander	362	44.4	132/230
2. Natural rubber latex	193	23.7	22/171
3. Flour, grains and feed	92	11.3	ng
4. Handling of foodstuffs	25	3.1	9/16
5. Enzymes	14	1.7	ng
Cellulase	8		
Alfa-amylase	2		
Other enzymes	4		
6. Decorative plants	13	1.6	1/12
7. Roots	10	1.2	2/8
8. Spices	9	1.1	1/8
9. Pork	8	1.0	4/4
10. Vegetables	8	1.0	ng
11. Storage mites	6	0.7	5/1
12. Ethylhexyl acrylate	5	0.6	0/5
13. Onions	4	0.5	1/3
14. Egg	4	0.5	1/3
15. Fish, fish meal	3	0.4	0/3
16. Poultry, chicken, other birds	3	0.4	1/3
Total	815	100	148/567

ng: not given.
Source: Ref. 12.

Epidemiology of Natural Rubber Latex Allergy

Urticaria is an important manifestation of natural rubber latex allergy. Although many studies have been published on natural rubber latex allergy, the prevalence and incidence are still unknown. Still, some occupational epidemiological details are available. Health care workers are the occupational group with the highest risk for developing immediate hypersensitivity reactions to natural rubber latex. A survey of hospital workers showed that 2.9% of 512 employees had positive latex skin prick tests (15,16). Positive reactions were seen in 7.4% of the surgeons and 5.6% of the surgical nurses. Questionnaire data showed that 2% of operating and dental personnel reported localized contact urticaria (17) and 4% of U.S. Army dentists reported symptoms of probable latex allergy (18). Recent studies in dental students and staff revealed that 14% of 203 students and staff reported pruritus and 3% reported urticaria within minutes of exposure to latex gloves; 10% of 131 who underwent skin prick tests had a positive response to natural rubber latex (19).

A cross-sectional study of 741 registered nurses in a large U.S. metropolitan hospital showed that 8.9% were positive for antilatex IgE antibodies (20). The prevalence ranged from 6.4% for operating room nurses to 13.6% for labor and delivery nurses. In this study, the factors that were most closely associated with the presence of antilatex IgE included nonwhite race, self-reported allergy to penicillin, pruritus, conjunctivitis, localized urticaria on latex exposure, history consistent with atopy, and allergies to avocado or ragweed.

Table 2 Ranking List of Occupations with Occupational Contact Urticaria in Finland During 1990–1994 ($n = 815$) per 100,000 Employed Workers[a]

Ranking/occupation	No. per 100,000 workers (total no.)
1. Bakers	140.5
2. Preparers of processed food	101.8
3. Dental assistants	95.5
4. Veterinary surgeons	72.5
5. Domestic animal attendants	69.1
6. Farmers, silviculturalists	57.7
7. Chefs, cooks, cold buffet managers	38.5
8. Dairy workers	37.9
9. Horticultural supervisors	37.8
10. Laboratory technicians, radiographers	35.6
11. Physicians	33.0
12. Butchers and sausage makers	28.9
13. Laboratory assistants	24.6
14. Dentists	23.4
15. Nurses	21.2
16. Waiters in cafes and snack bars, etc.	15.1
17. Kitchen assistants, restaurant workers, etc.	13.6
18. Hairdressers, beauticians, bath attendants, etc.	11.8
19. Housekeeping managers, snack bar managers, etc.	11.5
20. Packers	11.2
21. Horticultural workers	10.7
22. Assistant nurses, hospital attendants	10.2
23. Industrial sewers, etc.	9.1
24. Cleaners, etc.	6.7
25. Electrical and teletechnical equipment assemblers	6.6
26. Homemakers, home helps (municipal)	6.2
27. Technical nursing assistants	4.2
28. Machine and engine mechanics, etc.	3.9
29. Shop assistants, shop cashiers	2.1
Total	3.7

[a]Occupations with at least three cases of occupational urticaria were included.
Source: Ref. 12.

Another cross-sectional study of 1351 Canadian hospital workers showed a prevalence of positive latex skin prick tests of 12.1% (21). The highest prevalence was found in laboratory workers (16.9%) and nurses and physicians (13.3%). The latex skin prick–positive workers reported work-related symptoms, including urticaria, more often than latex skin test–negative workers; 11.3% of latex skin test–positive workers reported urticaria, compared to 2.5% of latex skin test–negative workers (adjusted odds ratio 6.3; confidence interval 3.2–12.5).

Natural rubber latex allergy may be seen in other occupations as well. In a Finnish clinic, 144 adult patients (66 health care workers and 78 from other occupations) were diagnosed with natural rubber latex allergy over a 10-year period. In 88% of the 66 health care workers, but in only 24% of the other workers, was the sensitization determined to be work-related (22). The other affected occupations included kitchen workers, cleaners, workers in a rubber band plant, textile workers, farmers' wives, a papermill worker, a gardener, a food worker, a dairy worker, a secretary, and a private caretaker. In a survey of latex allergy in a surgical glove manufacturing plant, seven of 68 workers (10%) stated that they had hives at work, and seven of 64 workers who had skin testing had positive reactions to latex (23). In a study of 418 greenhouse workers who used latex gloves, 18% reported immediate symptoms associated with wearing gloves, and 5% had positive skin prick tests (24).

Epidemiology of Occupational Urticaria in Specific Occupations

The prevalence of occupational skin diseases within specific occupations is based upon the exposures inherent within those occupations. Cross-sectional studies of workers in a specific occupation or workplace may allow for an estimation of skin disease within that occupation or workplace. However, there are few studies of specific occupations where occupational urticaria is a measured endpoint. In a study of 801 car mechanics, 120 (15%) reported hand eczema and five (0.6%) had a history of contact urticaria; scratch tests were all negative (25). In 5,641 laboratory animal handlers, 1304 (23.1%) reported one or more allergic symptoms related to the animals (26). Of this symptomatic group 45.6% had skin symptoms and 16% reported contact urticaria. Various combinations of symptoms were noted—19.3% had nasal or eye and skin symptoms, and 11.6% had nasal or eye, respiratory, and skin symptoms. A study of laboratory workers handling rats showed that of 323 workers surveyed, 31% reported at least one work-related symptom with 22% reporting eye and nose symptoms, followed by skin (15%), and chest symptoms (10%) (27). In another study of biology laboratory workers, 27 (11.3%) of those who had frequent exposure to animals had reactions, of whom 15 had various skin reactions, including urticaria; 21 had positive prick tests to animal dander (28). A study of 101 laboratory technicians showed that 14 cases of contact urticaria were caused by rat, seven by mouse, four by guinea pig, and two by cat exposure (29).

Case studies alone do not allow an estimation of occupational prevalence but may describe potential high-risk occupations based upon exposures to specific allergens or urticants. In one study of nine veterinary surgeons, all nine exhibited specific IgE against cow hair and dander; seven were symptomatic (30). A study of 50 food handlers/caterers with possible immediate protein contact dermatitis showed that nine (18%) had positive prick tests, most commonly to fish (31). Another study of 33 food handlers with a similar skin condition showed that 10 had positive scratch tests to explain their dermatitis, with the major allergens being fish and shellfish (32).

CONTACT URTICARIA

Contact urticaria is defined as urticaria that occurs after direct skin contact with a substance. Table 3 lists some of the many substances that can cause contact urticaria in occupational settings. Extensive lists are available in several sources, and new etiological agents are continually being described (33,38).

There are four types of contact urticaria: (1) *nonallergic* (nonimmunological; primary urticariogenic agents); (2) *allergic* (immunological); (3) *combined allergic and nonallergic*; and (4) *combined allergic eczematous and urticarial* (35). Some contactants affect normal

Table 3   Selected Causes of Occupational Contact Urticaria

Agent	Nonimmunological	Immunological
Animals	Caterpillars Jellyfish Moths	Animal products, e.g., placenta, saliva
Foods	Cayene pepper Fish Mustard Thyme	Cheese, egg, milk Kiwi, mango Maize Peanut butter, sesame food, sunflower seed Beef, chicken, lamb, liver, turkey Seafood (e.g., fish, prowns, shrimp) Bean
Fragrances and flavorings	Balsam of Peru Cassia (cinnamon oil) Cinnamic acid Cinnamic aldehyde	Balsam of Peru Menthol Vanillin

Medications	Alcohols
	Benzocaine
	Camphor
	Capsaicin
	Dimethyl sulfoxide
	Friar's balsam
	Tincture of benzoin
		Antibiotics
		   Ampicillin
		   Bacitracin
		   Cephalosporins
		   Gentamycin
		   Idochlorhydroxyquine
		   Neomycin
		   Penicillin
		   Rifamycin
		   Streptomycin
		   Virginiamycin
		   Benzocaine
		   Phenothiazines
		      Chlorpromazine
		      Levomepromazine
		      Promethazine

Plants	Nettles
	Seaweed
		Plant products
		   Cornstarch (?)
		   Henna
		   Latex rubber
		   Teak
		   Tulip

Preservatives and disinfectants	Benzoic acid Chlorocresol Formaldehyde Sodium benzoate Sorbic acid	Benzoic acid Chlorhexidine Chlorocresol Benzyl alcohol Formaldehyde Gentian violet Sodium hypochlorite
Miscellaneous	Histamine Sulfur Turpentine	Carbonless copy paper Formaldehyde resin Paraphenylenedimine Seminal fluid

Source: Ref. 38.

skin while others require eczematized or fissured skin to produce urticaria (37,39). Small molecules may penetrate intact skin while large proteinaceous molecules may require disruption of the epidermal barrier.

There may be a variety of skin manifestations associated with contact urticaria. Because of the potential of this varied morphology, terms such as "immediate contact reactions" are also used to describe what may be different skin manifestations of urticaria (36). Contact urticaria may comprise a spectrum of manifestations "that flows continuously from wheals to erythema to pruritus" (40). Pruritus, tingling, or burning accompanied by erythema is the weakest type of immediate contact reaction. A local wheal and flare is the prototypical reaction of contact urticaria, while generalized urticaria after a local contact is considered a rare phenomenon. Symptoms in other organ systems, such as asthma, rhinitis, conjunctivitis, orolaryngeal effects, and gastrointestinal and cardiovascular symptoms, can occur (36). The term "contact urticaria syndrome" is used to describe both local and systemic immediate reactions caused by contact uticarial agents (41,42). The contact urticaria syndrome was initially divided into the following four stages:

1. Stage 1—localized urticaria at the point of contact
2. Stage 2—contact urticaria and angioedema
3. Stage 3—contact urticaria and asthma
4. Stage 4—contact urticaria and anaphylaxis (42)

Another variety of immediate reaction is termed "protein contact dermatitis." This condition had been initially described in food handlers exposed to certain food proteins (especially fish and shellfish), who developed immediate (10–30 min after exposure) pruritus and erythema, and sometimes vesicle formation (32). Other causes of protein contact dermatitis include animal proteins, enzymes, fruits, grains, plants, spices, and vegetables (43). In most cases a delayed skin reaction with patch tests is negative but scratch tests are positive.

Concomitant type I (urticarial) and type IV (allergic contact dermatitis) skin reactions have been increasingly reported. Some of the contactants that can produce both an immediate and delayed reaction include acrylic acid, benzocaine, carrot, chlorhexidine, chlorocresol, chrysanthemum, cinnamic aldehyde, epoxy resin, garlic, latex, lettuce, nickel sulfate, potato, soybean, and textile dyes (37).

In terms of pathomechanisms, contact urticaria may be caused by nonimmunological, immunological, or undetermined mechanisms. In instances where the mechanism of urticaria is undefined, both unknown nonimmunological and immunological mechanisms could be operative. Examples include urticaria due to ammonium persulfate (used as an oxidizing hair bleach) (44,45), formaldehyde, and some physical agents (2).

Nonimmunological Contact Urticaria

Nonimmunological (nonallergic) contact urticaria occurs without previous sensitization. The mechanisms of nonimmunological urticaria remain unclear. It can result from a direct influence on dermal blood vessel walls or a non-antibody–mediated release of vasoactive substances such as histamine, prostaglandins, leukotrienes, platelet-activating factor, and cytokines (35,46,47). Indirect provocation of mast-cell degranulation by complement activation or neutral reflex vasodilation can occur. Multiple stimuli can cause the nonimmunological degranulation of mast cells within the subcutaneous tissues and dermis. This causes the release of preformed mediators (e.g., histamine), which cause vasodilation and increase capillary permeability. Also, cellular regulatory factors secreted by lymphocytes, neutrophils, eosinophils, platelets, and macrophages, such as C-C chemokines (e.g., MCP-1, MCP-3), possess histamine-releasing factor (HRF) that can activate exocytosis of histamine from mast cells or basophils (48).

Nonimmunological contact urticaria needs to be distinguished from irritant reactions, although this may be difficult at times. Strong irritants, such as hydrochloric acid, formaldehyde, and phenol, can cause immediate urticaria formation. However, this reaction does not disappear within 24 hr but is followed by erythema, scaling, or crusting (49). Some substances may be both primary irritants and contact urticants.

Nonimmunological contact urticaria may be the most common form of occupational contact urticaria and is usually not associated with systemic symptoms (37). However, in one case, severe systemic immediate allergic reactions have been reported after occupational exposure to benzoic-acid–containing materials (35). A variety of agents have been shown to cause a nonimmunological contact urticaria. These include: acetic acid, ethyl and butyl alcohol, balsam of Peru, benzoic acid, butyric acid, caterpillar hair, cinnamic acid, cinnamic aldehyde, cobalt chloride, diethyl fumarate, dimethyl sulfoxide (DMSO), formaldehyde, insect stings, methyl nicotinate, moths, sodium benzoate, and sorbic acid (35,37). Exposures to these substances may occur in occupational settings, one example being contact urticaria due to airborne sodium benzoate in a pharmaceutical manufacturing plant (50). Some of the physical urticarias may also be classified as nonimmunological urticarias.

Atopic and nonatopic individuals are at equal risk for nonimmunological contact urticaria. Even with well-documented chemical urticants, such as benzoic acid, cinnamic acid, and methyl nicotinate, there is wide interindividual variation in response (51). In addition, there is regional body site variation in the response to chemical urticants (52).

Immunological Contact Urticaria

Immunological (allergic) contact urticaria occurs in individuals previously sensitized to the offending substance. The sensitization route may be through the skin or through extracutaneous organs such as the respiratory and gastrointestinal tracts (2). Confirmation of an allergic basis for contact urticaria is achieved by demonstration of specific IgE to a causative antigen either by demonstrating serum specific IgE (e.g., via a RAST assay) or by skin prick testing. In the past, immediate hypersensitivity was demonstrated by the passive transfer of allergic serum to naive skin where wheal and flare responses could be elicited by injection of allergen (Prausnitz-Küstner reaction); at that time, the transferrable allergic factor was referred to as "reagin" which is now known to be IgE.

A variety of stimuli can cause mast cell activation and release of mediators. These include specific IgE molecules which are bound to mast cell membrane via high affinity receptors for IgE. The cross linking of these IgE receptors by the interaction of the IgE antibody and its antigen initiates cell activation and subsequent degranulation. Other mechanisms that can effect histamine release in occupational urticaria are unproven. They include the activation of the complement cascade and generation of anaphylotoxins (C3a, C4a, C5a) which activate mast cells via specific complement receptors. A variety of peptides may activate mast cells including bradykinin and substance P. As mentioned, C-C chemokines secreted by mononuclear cells and neutrophils can induce histamine release.

As a rule, usually a low proportion of exposed individuals are affected by allergic contact urticaria, and it is likely that it is more common among atopic individuals. It is also likely that most cases are mediated by IgE since non-specific elevation of IgE is frequently reported. In many cases, specific IgE has also been documented (37). In other cases, specific IgG and perhaps IgM may be responsible by activating the classical complement system (37).

Based upon reviews of epidemiological studies, exposures, and patterns seen in case reported, several occupations may be at higher-risk for the development of allergic contact urticaria. These include the following:

1. food handlers, cooks, caterers, and bakers;
2. general health care workers (53), dental professionals (54), and pharmaceutical industry workers (55);
3. animal handlers such as laboratory workers or veterinarians; and
4. gardeners, florists, woodworkers, and agricultural workers.

For food handlers, cooks, caterers, and bakers the following foods have been reported to produce allergic contact urticaria: apples, bean, beer, caraway seed, carrot, egg, endive, fish, garlic, kiwi fruit, lettuce, meat (beef, chicken, lamb, liver, pork, and turkey), milk, peach, potato, rice, shellfish, spices, and strawberries (35,37). Bakers can develop contact urticaria and other systemic symptoms after exposure to cereal flours, buckwheat flour, and additive flour enzymes such as alpha-amylase (from *Aspergillus oryzae* or *Bacillus subtilis*) (37,56,57). A unique food-related contact urticaria in nontraditional "food handlers" has been described in hairdressers using egg shampoos (58).

In health care, dental, and pharmaceutical environments, handling or producing a variety of medications or chemical disinfectants can put workers at risk. Exposures that can cause allergic contact urticaria include aminothiazole, bacitracin, benzocaine gel, cephalosporins, chloramine (a sterilizer, disinfectant, and chemical reagent), chloramphenical, chlorhexidine (an antiseptic), chlorocresol (a disinfectant), ethylene oxide, gentamicin, neomycin, nitrogen mustard, penicillin, pentamidine isethionate, phenothiazines, rifamycin, and streptomycin (35,37,59). In most circumstances skin patch or prick tests were used to confirm the diagnoses. Specific IgE has not been demonstrated for most of these exposures.

The initial 1979 case report of natural rubber latex allergy occurred in a woman using gloves for hand protection during housework (60). The next reported case occurred in a nurse using surgical gloves (61). Since then, natural rubber latex has been found to be an important cause of allergic contact urticaria, asthma, and anaphylaxis in health care professionals. The most frequently reported manifestation is contact urticaria, followed by rhinoconjunctivitis (62). Atopic individuals and individuals with hand eczema seem to be at higher risk for natural rubber latex allergy.

Allergic contact urticaria has been found to be caused by animal hair (rat and guinea pig exposure in laboratory workers), dander, insects (such as cockroaches and locusts), animal placenta, saliva, seminal fluid, and serum (35). Slaughterhouse workers can develop contact urticaria to animal blood (63). Contact urticaria can be seen in veterinarians after exposure to cow's hairs and placenta, horse dander, and pig's bristles (37).

Certain woods and plants can cause allergic contact urticaria. These include the larch, limba, obeche (African maple), and teak woods (35,64) and plants such as chrysanthemum, *Ficus benjamina* (weeping fig), lilies, *Limonium tataricum, Phoenix canariensis* (canary palm), *Spathiphyllum walisii* (spathe flower), tulips and fungi (shiitake mushrooms) (65–71). High-risk occupations include agricultural workers, carpenters, florists, gardeners, and woodworkers. Caterpillar hair, insect stings, and moths can also cause an allergic contact urticaria in outdoor workers (35). In one investigation, of 46 farm workers with allergic symptoms, 17 had an allergic contact urticaria and respiratory complains and 29 had respiratory complaints resulting from contact with *Tetranychus urticae* (red spider mite) (72). Agricultural workers may also be exposed to fertilizers and pesticides, some of which can cause allergic contact urticaria.

A variety of industrial chemicals can cause allergic contact urticaria, including: acrylic monomers (plastics), aliphatic polyamines (epoxy resins), alkyl-phenol novolac resin (found in carbonless copy paper), ammonia, castor bean pomace (fertilizers), diethyltoluamide (DEET), formaldehyde (used in clothing, leather, fumigation, and resins), lindane (a parasiticide), paraphenylenediamine, phenylmercuric priopionate (an antibacterial fabric softener), plastic additives (such as butylhydroxytoluene and oleylamide), reactive dyes, sodium sulfide (used in photographs, dyes, and tanning), sulfur dioxide, vinyl pyrilidine, xylene and other solvents (35,37). Allergic contact urticaria can occur with exposure to a variety of metal salts, including iridium, nickel, platinum, and rhodium (35,73). Also, silk, wool, and nylon, which may be found in work clothing, are rare causes of allergic contact urticaria (74).

Some causes of allergic contact urticaria are well documented with in vivo and in vitro testing. An example of one of the more completely documented causes of occupational contact urticaria and asthma are the acid anhydrides, which include phthalic anhydride (PA), tetrahydrochlorophthalic anhydride (TCPA), and trimellitic anhydride (TMA). The anhydrides are used as crosslinking agents or hardeners in epoxy resins, which are used in paints, plastics, and for encapsulation of electronic components. Immediate allergy has been verified by an open test with undiluted PA, a scratch chamber test using 1% PA, prick tests, specific IgE determinations, RAST inhibition studies, and chamber provocation tests (75). Exposure to airborne acid anhydrides has been documented as causing sensitization in some workers (76).

AIRBORNE EXPOSURE URTICARIA

Contact urticaria caused by airborne exposures is an unusual condition as most agents that can cause contact urticaria are not volatile and do not easily vaporize. But in some cases airborne aerosols, dusts, fumes, mists, or vapors have been shown to cause contact urticaria (77). Examples of agents that can cause airborne contact urticaria include acrylic acid, ammonia, formaldehyde, garlic, naphtha, natural rubber latex (protein alone or protein-cornstarch powder combination), phthalic anhydrides, sodium benzoate, soybean, 1,1,1-trichloroethane, and xylene (15,50,76,78–81).

Airborne dermatoses are usually caused by direct skin contact with a substance. In some instances skin diseases may appear after inhalation of a substance (82). Inhaled agents, however, are considered rare causes of urticaria. Case reports have described generalized urticaria and metal fume fever-like symptoms in welders exposed to zinc oxide and polyurethane (83–84). Other occupational exposures that have been reported to induce inhalant urticaria include aminothiazide, ammonia, animal danders, castor bean dust and pomace, coffee bean dust, formaldehyde, lindane, mold spores, complex platinum salts, pollens, and sulfur dioxide (85–88). In many circumstances the exact etiology, route of exposure, and mechanism remain unproven (84). A precise distinction between an inhalational exposure and an epidermal exposure to airborne aerosols, dusts, fumes, mists, or vapors is seldom made in these reports.

PHYSICAL URTICARIAS

Urticarias that result from non-chemical exposures are commonly classified as "physical urticarias." Up to 17% of chronic urticarias may be attributable to physical causes (89). These include mechanical urticarias (caused by trauma, pressure, friction, and fibration) and urticaria resulting from local exposure to physical agents (such as cold, heat, and solar radiation) and water (90,91). The physical urticarias can also be classified mechanistically as immunological, nonimmunological, and uncertain. An allergic mechanism is supported for certain forms of the physical urticarias (e.g., dermatographism) by demonstration that the urticarial response can be passively transferred to a naïve donor (i.e., the Prausnitz-Küstner reaction) (92).

Causes of trauma-induced urticaria include mechanical irritants, for example fiberglass fragments that puncture the skin (93). Pressure urticaria, compromising less than 1% of all urticarias, occurs as deep, indurated, tender hives, usually on the buttocks, feet, or palms, that occur 3–12 hr after application of pressure. These lesions, which may occur after manual labor, walking, climbing stairs, and using hand tools, may persist for up to 48 hr and can be accompanied by fever, chills, and arthralgias (90). A nonimmunological mechanism seems most likely (94). Although rare, pressure urticaria can be very disabling. This condition may be associated with chronic idiopathic urticaria and dermatographism. Dermatographism, the most common form of physical urticaria (seen in 2–5% of the population), results in a linear wheal and flare at the site of firm stroking or friction. The very rare vibratory urticaria may be acquired or familial (autosomal dominant inheritance) and can occur after occupational exposure to vibration, as in metal grinding or jackhammer operation (95,96).

Cold urticaria occurs as an acquired form, an inherited form, and a secondary form associated with serum abnormalities (cryoglobulinemia, cold agglutinins, cryofibrinogens, and cold hemolysins) (97). Urticarial lesions develop during rewarming after direct cold contact or immersion and may be associated with bronchospasm, flushing, hypotension, and syncope. A positive Prausnitz-Küstner reaction shows that acquired cold urticaria, which compromises 1–3% of all urticarias, may be IgE mediated (91,97). Examples of occupational exposures causing cold urticaria include contact sprays, cold lithography solutions, and cold environments (98–100).

Localized heat urticaria is a very rare entity in which pruritic lesions occur quickly after localized heat contact. These lesions can be associated with nausea, diarrhea, abdominal pain, headache, and dizziness. Urticaria caused by heat is likely to be nonimmunological (97). Cholinergic urticaria, which may comprise 5–7% of all urticarias, is marked by a sensation of warmth followed by the appearance of small (1–3 mm) pruritic wheals (91). This condition, which can be accompanied by systemic symptoms, develops after increases in core body temperature and is induced by heat, exercise, or emotion (97). One report documented occupational exposures causing cholinergic uticaria in U.S. Air Force personnel (101). Cholinergic urticaria is mediated by cholinergic substances liberated from stimulated peripheral nerves (102). The rare exercise-induced anaphylactic syndrome needs to be distinguished from cholinergic urticaria. Some individuals develop symptoms only during exercise (or strenuous work) following the eating of certain foods, and the condition is not related to core body temperature (91).

Solar urticaria, seen in less than 1% of persons with urticaria, occurs after exposure to a variety of wavelengths of light and occurs only on exposed skin surfaces. Solar urticaria may be associated with other photosensitive disorders such as systemic lupus erythematosus and porphyria cutanea tarda (103). Solar urticaria can be associated with systemic symptoms as well; the mechanism is uncertain.

Aquagenic urticaria is a very rare disorder associated with water contact at any temperature and is not associated with any systemic symptoms. It is typically marked by punctate, perifollicular hives. There is some evidence that a water-soluble epidermal antigen permeates the skin after contact with water and activates mast cells, although the mechanism remains uncertain (91).

DIAGNOSIS OF WORK-RELATED URTICARIA

Although a reliable clinical diagnosis of urticaria may usually be established on the basis of clinical examination alone, reliable attribution of causation to an occupational exposure is generally difficult. In part, this difficulty is inherent to the investigation of urticaria in general. No cause can be identified in at least 70% of cases of chronic urticaria (94). As urticaria is common, cases will inevitably occur within the working population. In the absence of an obvious explanation, some workers and physicians will ultimately attribute the cause of the urticaria to an exposure in the workplace. While patient observation and insight may offer valuable clues to any medical investigation, the etiology of a case of urticaria may remain in question unless objective criteria can be established to support an occupational relationship.

Although no general consensus yet exists, a review of the best-documented cases of occupational urticaria cited in this review and elsewhere (104) suggests that the following seven criteria are most useful:

1. The clinical diagnosis of urticaria has been documented by medical examination. The pathognomonic lesion of urticaria is the wheal—a circumscribed, pruritic, raised, pink to erythematous, effervescent swelling of the superficial dermis, without any changes (such as scaling) in the overlying epidermis. The wheal usually lasts only a few hours, rarely more than 24 hr. The appearance of new wheals, coupled with the relatively rapid disappearance of older wheals, may give rise to the patient's perception that the rash is "moving around the body." There are no particular characteristics of wheals caused by occupational exposures that allow them to be distinguished from urticaria due to other causes (including idiopathic).

Urticaria may sometimes be confused with other acute erythematous cutaneous eruptions, such as morbilliform rashes caused by drugs or viruses, erythema multiforme, or even acute contact dermatitis. These latter conditions are more persistent and individual lesions last longer than 24 hr. A skin biopsy is not usually helpful or necessary to confirm a diagnosis of urticaria, but may sometimes be useful to exclude these other dermatological conditions (including urticarial vasculitis) when uncertainty exists. Objective medical documentation is essential since patients' self-reported histories of hives can be unreliable. Similarly, pruritus alone is not objective proof of urticaria unless wheals can be observed.

2. Exposure has occurred in the workplace to an agent that has already been documented as a potential cause of urticaria, based on published medical or toxicological studies. Published studies must be critically evaluated. Upon careful scrutiny, rigorous or convincing proof is often lacking; skin tests allegedly supporting a causal relationship may not have adequate standardization or controls, and the etiological relationship to many purported causes of occupational urticaria, such as formaldehyde, seems to be based upon subjective historical data, such as "hives occur only when working; do not occur when not working."

3. The temporal relationship between exposure and onset of symptoms should be consistent with the diagnosis of urticaria, an immediate hypersensitivity reaction. Under ordinary circumstances, hives should develop at least within 30–60 min of exposure to the putative causal agent in the workplace. However, no general consensus yet exists concerning the time lag between initial exposure and first occurrence of urticaria; symptoms may not develop for weeks, months, or even years after first exposure or date of hire.

4. Associated medical symptoms and the anatomical localization of urticaria must be consistent with the clinical route of exposure to the alleged causal agent. If the skin is the primary route of exposure, the skin should urticate first and foremost on anatomical areas (e.g., the hands and arms) where the causal substance has directly contacted the skin. Although hives may remain localized to the primary areas of direct contact (contact urticaria), generalized urticaria may develop if sufficient percutaneous absorption occurs. In the latter case, the appearance of hives elsewhere on the body surface should follow, not precede, the appearance of hives at the site of primary skin contact. If the primary route of exposure is airborne, urticaria is often associated with additional medical symptoms consistent with rhinitis, conjunctivitis, or asthma. These symptoms should precede, rather than follow, the onset of hives. Medical documentation of these associated symptoms is valuable, since self-reported symptoms are unreliable and difficult to distinguish from minor irritation caused by noxious vapors. In rare instances of alleged contamination of food from workplace exposures, the gastrointestinal tract will be the primary route of exposure. In this case, hives should be associated with nausea and abdominal cramping. Lip and oropharyngeal swelling may also occur as a result of direct contact with the mucous membranes of the mouth.

5. Urticaria should occur only in the workplace and should completely resolve on weekends, vacations, layoffs, or termination of employment. As urticaria is a common disorder in general, care should be taken to distinguish urticaria that may be aggravated by nonspecific workplace conditions that elevate skin temperature (such as hot environments and heavy physical exercise) from hives caused by an exposure that occurs only at work.

6. Nonoccupational causes of urticaria should be excluded. Unfortunately, since no specific cause is objectively documented in the majority of cases of chronic urticaria, a natural temptation exists to blame idiopathic cases on any temporal association, e.g. workplace exposures, although the scientific proof is seldom more than "guilt by association."

7. Medical testing should support a causal relationship between urticaria and a workplace exposure. The following tests may be employed in the investigation of contact or systemic urticaria suspected to be caused by an occupational exposure. In all cases where skin tests are performed, the patient should be off conventional antihistamine therapy for at least 72 hr and long-acting antihistamine therapy for at least 2 weeks. If asthma or anaphylactic symptoms have been associated with urticaria, cardiopulmonary resuscitation equipment should be readily available.

Open or closed patch test this is the primary test utilized for the diagnosis of contact urticaria and is the preferred test for the evaluation of systemic urticaria thought to be caused by skin exposure, as it most closely approximates the conditions under which exposure is actually occurring in the workplace. In the open patch test, the suspected etiological agent is placed directly on the skin "as is" and the test site observed up to 60 mins for erythema or a wheal-and-flare reaction. In the closed patch test, the suspected causal agent is placed on a standard commercial patch test device (e.g., Finn Chamber on Scanpor Tape) and occluded against the skin for 15–30 min. The device is then removed and the test site observed for a reaction for an additional 30 min (total of 60 min). The preferred test site is the ventral forearm, upper outer arm, or upper back. In cases where occupational cutaneous exposure has been occurring on eczematous skin exclusively (e.g., natural rubber latex gloves over eczemematous hand dermatitis), these tests may be cautiously repeated over the eczematous skin (e.g., cutting a finger off a latex glove and placing it over an affected finger). No standardization of test concentrations exists, and ideally the interpretation of a test as "positive" should be supported by at least 20 negative controls. In some instances, published case reports supported by negative controls may serve as "literature" controls.

With *prick or scratch tests* the skin is either pricked with a 26-gauge needle or blood lancet, or scratched (approximate 7–8-mm-length scratch) with a 20-gauge needle. If the suspected causal agent is a liquid, a drop should be placed on the skin first and the skin pricked or scratched through the liquid. If the suspected causal agent is a solid, the skin should be pricked or scratched first, and then the solid placed over it after first moistening it with water. A variation called the scratch-chamber test has been developed and is particularly useful for solids such as food substances. With this procedure, the test substance is placed into a standard patch test device (e.g., Finn Chamber on Scanpor Tape) and then taped to the skin over a 7–8-mm-length scratch and observed for response. These invasive tests may be necessary if the primary route of exposure is airborne, as mucous membranes are generally more permeable to absorption than the general skin surface and false-negative patch tests (open or closed) may occur as the result of inadequate percutaneous penetration of the test substance. Unfortunately, many industrial chemicals may be nonspecifically irritating to the skin when tested in this fashion. No prick or scratch test standardization exists for most industrial test substances in terms of vehicle or concentration, and the onus is on the investigator to test a sufficient number of control subjects, using positive histamine and negative saline controls as well as the test substance(s), which may turn a clinical evaluation into a time-consuming research project. Ideally, controls should include other subjects with chronic urticaria unrelated to workplace chemical exposure. The mean wheal diameter (i.e., longest diameter + perpendicular diameter divided by 2) should be measured for any positive reaction. Kanerva et al. (105) have recommended a test reaction grading system as follows: 1+ = reaction diameter less than 1/2 diameter of a histamine control, but at least 2 mm greater than the diameter of a saline control; 2+ = reaction diameter greater than 1/2 diameter but less than the full diameter of a histamine control; 3+ = reaction diameter greater than or equal to, but less than twice, a histamine control; 4+ = reaction diameter equal to or greater than twice a histamine control. A weak test reaction of 1+ intensity can be considered significant if other aspects of the evaluation overwhelmingly support this conclusion.

Intradermal tests should not ordinarily be performed unless standardized materials already exist (e.g., wheat antigen for evaluation of baker's asthma associated with hives). The lack of standardization for the majority of workplace allergens makes this test almost impossible to interpret reliably. Furthermore, the majority of workplace chemicals are likely to be highly irritating to tissue when injected intradermally, even in diluted aqueous vehicles, and some may be corrosive.

RAST materials are not commercially available for most workplace chemicals, with few exceptions (natural rubber latex protein, diisocyanates, acid anhydrides). Where available, the RAST can be an extremely helpful diagnostic aid, especially if generalized urticaria exists. However, the test may be negative unless there is a sufficient amount of circulating specific IgE antibody to the suspected allergen. The RAST is generally considered quite specific but not as sensitive as a properly performed and standardized skin test for the diagnosis of immediate hypersensitivity.

Miscellaneous blood tests such as increased total serum IgE levels and peripheral blood eosinophilia are sometimes suggestive of a true allergic reaction, but none are specific for any causal agent.

Skin biopsies are seldom helpful in establishing a diagnosis of urticaria, which is usually made on clinical grounds alone, unless a diagnosis of urticarial vasculitis is suspected. A biopsy is never helpful for establishing a specific etiological cause.

TREATMENT

In all cases of occupational urticaria where a specific causal agent can be identified, the treatment of obvious choice is avoidance of the offending agent. In some cases, a nonallergenic substance may simply be substituted, and the affected worker kept in the same job (e.g., substitution of nitrile gloves for natural rubber latex gloves for workers allergic to latex protein). In other cases, the affected worker will have to be removed from that part of the work environment where exposure has been occurring, even if it ultimately means changing jobs. However, medical recommendations to leave employment should not be made lightly and should be supported by adequate objective medical findings, including tests that specifically identify the causal agent.

Since the overwhelming majority of cases of urticaria occurring among workers will not be due to any occupational exposures, treatment may be instituted according to the same therapeutic principles to manage any other case of chronic urticaria. First-generation antihistamines that block H_1 receptors (e.g., diphenhydramine, hydroxyzine) should be employed initially, but they frequently cause sedation; this may present a safety issue for certain occupations (e.g., heavy-equipment operators). When sedation occurs or presents a safety concern, nonsedating, second-generation antihistamines (cetirizine, astemizole, loratadine, fexofenadine) may be employed. When H_1 histamine blockers alone are not sufficient, they may be combined with H_2 blockers (e.g., cimetidine, ranitidine, famotidine) or doxepin, a tricyclic antidepressant with potent H_1 and H_2 blocking activity. Doxepin is extremely sedating and should be used cautiously, if at all, when safety concerns arise on the job. Oral corticosteroid therapy may be employed for severe cases of chronic urticaria, especially those associated with angioedema, which are unresponsive to the above measures.

REFERENCES

1. Lever WF, Schaumburg-Lever G. Histopathology of the Skin, 7th ed. Philadelphia: Lippincott, 1990:152–153.
2. Harvell J, Bason M, Maibach H. Contact urticaria and its mechanisms. Food Chem Toxicol 1994; 32:103–112.
3. Lushniak BD. The epidemiology of occupational contact dermatitis. Dermatol Clin 1995; 13: 671–680.
4. Greaves MW. Chronic urticaria. N Engl J Med 1995; 332:1767–1771.
5. Elpern DJ. The syndrome of immediate reactivities (contact urticaria syndrome)—an historical study from a dermatology practice. Hawaii Med J 1985; 44:426–440.
6. Nelson C. Office visits to dermatologists: National Ambulatory Medical Care Survey, United States 1989–90. Vital and Health Statistics of the Centers for Disease Control and Prevention/ National Center for Health Statistics 1994; no. 240:1–12.

7. Romaguera C, Grimalt F. Statistical and comparative study of 4600 patients tested in Barcelona (1973–1977). Contact Dermatitis 1980; 6:309–315.
8. Bakke P. Gulsvik A, Eide GE. Hay fever, eczema and urticaria in southwest Norway. Allergy 1990; 45:515–522.
9. Bureau of Labor Statistics (BLS). Occupational Injuries and Illnesses in the United States. US Department of Labor, BLS, published annually since 1972; data for 1993 published August 1996 in Bulletin 2478.
10. National Institute for Occupational Safety and Health (NIOSH). National Occupational Survey—Pilot study for development of an occupational disease surveillance method. Rockville, MD: US Department of Health, Education, and Welfare, 1975; HEW Publication (NIOSH) 75–162.
11. Plotnick H. Analysis of 250 consecutively evaluated cases of workers' disability claims for dermatitis. Arch Dermatol 1990; 160:782–786.
12. Kanerva L, Toikkanen J, Jolanki R, Estlander T. Statistical data on occupational contact urticaria. Contact Dermatitis 1996; 35:229–233.
13. Kanerva L, Vaheri E. Occupational rhinitis in Finland. Int Arch Occup Environ Health 1993; 32:150–155.
14. Skinner SL, Fowler JF. Contact anaphylaxis: a review. Am J Contact Dermatitis 1995; 6:133–142.
15. Hamann CP. Natural rubber latex sensitivity in review. Am J Contact Dermatitis 1993; 4:4–21.
16. Turjanmaa K. Incidence of immediate allergy to latex gloves in hospital personnel. Contact Dermatitis 1987; 17:270–275.
17. Wrangsjo K, Osterman K, van Hage-Hamsten M. Glove-related skin symptoms among operating theatre and dental care unit personnel. Contact Dermatitis 1994; 30:102–107.
18. Berky ZT, Luciano WJ, James WD. Latex glove allergy, a survey of the US Army Dental Corps. JAMA 1992; 268:2695–2696.
19. Tarlo SM, Sussman GL, Holness DL. Latex sensitivity in dental students and staff—a cross-sectional study. J Allergy Clin Immunol 1997; 99:396–401.
20. Grzybowski M, Ownby DR, Peyser PA, Johnson CC, Schork MA. The prevalence of anti-latex IgE antibodies among registered nurses. J Allergy Clin Immunol 1996; 98:535–544.
21. Liss GM, Sussman GL, Deal K, Brown S, Cividino M, Siu S, Beezhold DH, Smith G, Swanson MC, Yunginger J, Douglas A, Holness DK. Lebert P, Keith P, Wasserman S, Turjanmaa K. Latex allergy: epidemiological study of 1351 hospital workers. Occup Environ Med 1997; 54:335–342.
22. Turjanmaa K. Update on occupational natural rubber latex allergy. Dermatol Clin 1994; 12:561–567.
23. Tarlo SM, Wong L, Roos J, Booth N. Occupational asthma caused by latex in a surgical glove manufacturing plant. J Allergy Clin Immunol 1990; 85:626–631.
24. Carillo T, Blanco C, Quiralte J, Castillo R, Cuevas M, Rodriguez de Castro F. Prevalence of latex allergy among greenhouse workers. J Allergy Clin Immunol 1995; 96:699–701.
25. Meding B, Barregard L, Marcus K. Hand eczema in car mechanics. Contact Dermatitis 1994; 30:129–134.
26. Aoyama K, Ueda A, Manda F, Matsushita T, Ueda T, Yamauchi C. Allergy to laboratory animals: an epidemiological study. Br J Ind Med 1992; 49:41–47.
27. Cullinan P, Lowson D, Nieuwenhuijsen MJ, Gordon S, Tee RD, Venables KM, McDonald JC, Newman-Raylow AJ. Work-related symptoms, sensitization and estimated exposure in workers not previously exposed to laboratory rats. Occup Environ Med 1994; 51:589–592.
28. Lincoln TA, Bolton NE, Garret AS. Occupational allergy to animal dander and sera. J Occup Med 1974; 16:465–469.
29. Agrup G, Sjostedt L. Contact urticaria in laboratory technicians. Acta Derm Venereol (Stockh) 1985; 65:114–115.
30. Prahl P, Roed-Petersen J. Type I allergy from cows in veterinary surgeons. Contact Dermatitis 1979; 5:33–38.

31. Cronin E. Dermatitis of the hands in caterers. Contact Dermatitis 1987; 17:265–269.

32. Hjorth N, Roed-Petersen J. Occupational protein contact dermatitis in food handlers. Contact Dermatitis 1976; 2:28–42.

33. Lahti A, Maibach HI. Immediate contact reactions: Immunol Allergy Clin North Am 1989; 9:463–478.

34. Lahti A, Maibach HI. Immediate contact reactions: contact urticaria and the contact urticaria syndrome. In: Marzulli FN, Maibach HI, eds. Dermatotoxicology. New York: Hemisphere, 1991:473–495.

35. Fisher AA. Contact urticaria due to occupational exposures. In: Adams RM, ed. Occupational Skin Disease. Philadelphia: W.B. Saunders, 1990:113–126.

36. Lahti A. Immediate contact reactions. In: Rycroft RJG, Menne T, Frosch PJ, eds. Textbook of Contact Dermatitis. Berlin: Springer-Verlag; 1992:62–74.

37. Reitschel RL, Fowler JF. Contact urticaria. In: Reitschel RL, Fowler JF. Fisher's Contact Dermatitis. 4th ed. Baltimore: Williams & Wilkins, 1995:778–807.

38. Hogan DJ, Tanglertsampan C. The less common occupational dermatosis. Occup Med: State of the Art Reviews 1992; 7:385–401.

39. Andersen KE, Maibach HI. Multiple application delayed onset contact urticaria: possible relation to certain unusual formalin and textile reactions. Contact Dermatitis 1984; 10:227–234.

40. Kligman AM. The spectrum of contact urticaria—wheals, erythema, and pruritus. Dermatol Clin 1990; 8:57–60.

41. Tanglertsampan C, Maibach HI. Contact urticaria. In: Hogan DJ, ed. Occupational Skin Disorders. New York: Igaku-Shoin, 1994:81–88.

42. Maibach HI, Johnson HL. Contact urticaria syndrome. Arch Dermatol 1975; 111:726–730.

43. Janssens V, Morren M, Dooms-Goosens A, Degreef H. Protein contact dermatitis: myth or reality? Br J Dermatol 1995; 132:1–6.

44. Calnan CD, Shuster S. Reactions to ammonium persulfate. Arch Dermatol 1963; 88:812–815.

45. Fisher AA, Dooms-Goosen A. Persulfate hair bleach reactions. Arch Dermatol 1976; 112:1407–1409.

46. Marks JG, DeLeo VA. Contact urticaria. In: Marks JG, DeLeo VA, eds. Contact and Occupational Dermatology. St Louis: Mosby–Year Book, 1992:309–318.

47. Beltrani VS. Urticaria and angioedema. Dermatol Clin 1996; 14:171–198.

48. Kaplan AP, Kuna P, Reddigari SR. Chemokines and the allergic response. Exp Dermatol 1995; 4:260–265.

49. Lahti A, Maibach HI. Immediate contact reactions. Immunol Allergy Clin North Am 1989; 9:463–478.

50. Nethercott JR, Lawrence MJ, Roy AM, Gibson BL. Airborne contact urticaria due to sodium benzoate in a pharmaceutical manufacturing plant. J Occup Med 1984; 26:734–736.

51. Basketter DA, Wihelm KP. Studies on non-immune immediate contact reactions in an unselected population. Contact Dermatitis 1996; 35:237–240.

52. Shriner DL, Maibach HI. Regional variation of nonimmunologic contact urticaria—functional map of the human face. Skin Pharmacol 1996; 9:312–321.

53. Cohen SR. Skin disease in health care workers. Occup Med: State of the Art Reviews 1987; 2:565–580.

54. Kanerva L, Estlander T, Jolanki R. Occupational skin allergy in the dental profession. Dermatol Clin 1994; 12:517–531.

55. Sherertz EF. Occupational skin diseases in the pharmaceutical industry. Dermatol Clin 1994; 12:533–536.

56. Valdivieso R, Moneo I, Pola J, Munoz T, Zapata C, Hinojosa M. Losada E. Occupational asthma and contact urticaria caused by buckwheat flour. Ann of Allergy 1989; 63:149–152.

57. Morren MA, Janssens V, Dooms-Goosens A, Van Hoeyveld E, Cornelis A, De Wolf-Peeters C, Heremans A. Alpha-amylase, a flour additive: an important cause of protein contact dermatitis in bakers. J Amer Acad Dermatol 1993; 29:723–728.

58. Temesvari E, Varkonyi V. Contact urticaria provoked by egg. Contact Dermatitis 1980; 6: 143–144.
59. Belsito DV. Contact urticaria from pentamidine isethionate. Contact Dermatitis 1993; 29:158.
60. Nutter AF. Contact urticaria to ruber. Br J Dermatol 1979; 101:597–598.
61. Forstrom L. Contact urticaria from latex surgical gloves. Contact Dermatitis 1980; 6:33–34.
62. Turjanmaa K. Alenius H. Makinen-Kiljunen S, Reunala T, Palusuo T. Natural ruber latex allergy. Allergy 1996; 51:593–602.
63. Goransson K. Occupational contact urticaria to fresh cow and pig blood in slaughtermen. Contact Dermatitis 1981; 7:281–282.
64. Hinojosa M, Subiza J, Moneo I, Puyana J, Diez ML, Fernandez-Rivas M. Contact urticaria caused by Obeche wood (*Triplochiton scleroxylon*). Report of eight patients. Ann of Allergy 1990; 64:476–479.
65. Blanco C, Carillo T, Quiralte J, Pascual C, Martin Estaban M, Castillo R. Occupational rhinoconjunctivitis and bronchial asthma due to *Phoenix canariensis* pollen allergy. Allergy 1995; 50:277–280.
66. Quirce S, Garcia-Figueroa B, Alaguibel JM, Muro MD, Tabar AI. Occupational asthma and contact urticaria from dried flowers of *Limonium tartaricum*. Allergy 1993; 48:285–290.
67. Kanera L. Makinen-Kiljunen S, Kiistala R, Granlund H. Occupational allergy caused by the spathe flower (*Spathiphyllum walisii*), Allergy 1995; 50:174–178.
68. Tanaka T, Moriwaki SI, Horio T. Occupational dermatitis with simultaneous immediate and delayed allergy to chrysanthemum. Contact Dermatitis 1987; 16:152–154.
69. Tarvainen K, Salonen JP, Kanerva L, Estlander T, Keskinen H, Rantenen T. Allergy and toxicodermia from shiitake mushrooms. J Am Acad Dermatol 1991; 24:64–66.
70. Lahti A. Contact urticaria and respiratory symptoms from tulips and lilies. Contact Dermatitis 1986; 14:317–319.
71. Axelsson IGK, Johansson SGO, Zetterstrom O. Occupational allergy to weeping fig in plant keepers. Allergy 1987; 42:161–167.
72. Astarita C, Di Martino P, Scala G, Franzese A, Sproviero S. Contact allergy: another occupational risk to *Tetranychus urticae*. J Allergy Clin Immunol 1996; 98:732–738.
73. Bergman A, Svedberg U, Nilsson E. Contact urticaria with anaphylactic reactions caused by occupational exposure to irridium salt. Contact Dermatitis 1995; 32:14–17.
74. Dooms-Goosens A, Duron C, Loncke J, Degreef H. Contact urticaria due to nylon. Contact Dermatitis 1986; 14:63.
75. Kanerva L, Hyry R, Jolanki R, Hytonen M. Estlander T. Delayed and immediate allergy caused by methylhexahydrophthalic anhydride. Contact Dermatitis 1997; 36:34–38.
76. Tarvainen K, Jolanki R, Estlander T, Tupasela O, Pfaffli P, Kanerva L. Immunologic contact urticaria due to airborne methylhexahydrophthalic and methyltetrahydrophthalic anhydrides. Contact Dermatitis 1995; 32:204–209.
77. Dooms-Goosens A, Deleu H. Airborne contact dermatitis: an update. Contact Dermatitis 1991; 25:211–217.
78. Lindskov R. Contact urticaria to formaldehyde. Contact Dermatitis 1982; 8:333–334.
79. Fowler JF. Contact urticaria to 1,1,1-Trichoroethane. Amer J. Contact Dermatitis 1991; 2: 239.
80. Goncalo M, Chiera L. Goncalo S. Immediate and delayed hypersensitivity to garlic and soybean. Amer J Contact Dermatitis 1992; 3:102–104.
81. Palmer KT, Rycroft RJG. Occupational airborne contact urticaria due to xylene. Contact Dermatitis 1993; 28:44.
82. Bjorkner BE. Industrial airborne dermatoses. Dermatol Clin 1994; 12:501–509.
83. Farrell FJ. Angioedema and urticaria as acute and late phase reactions to zinc fume exposure, with associated metal fume fever-like symptoms. Am J Ind Med 1987; 12:331–337.
84. Kanerva L, Estlander T, Jolanki R, Lahteenmaki MT, Keskinen H. Occupational urticaria from welding polyurethane. J Am Acad Dermatol 1991; 24:825–826.
85. Kanerva L, Estlander T, Jolanki R. Long-lasting contact urticaria from castor bean. J Amer Acad Dermatol 1990; 23:351–355.

86. Mathias CGT. Occupational dermatoses. J Am Acad Dermatol 1988; 19:1107–1114.
87. Key MM. Some unusual allergic reactions in industry. Arch Dermatol 1961; 83:3–6.
88. Morris GE. Urticaria following exposure to ammonia fumes. Arch Ind Health 1956; 13:480.
89. Champion RH, Roberts SOB, Carpenter RG, Roger JH. Urticaria and angioedema: a review of 554 patients. Br J Dermatol 1969; 81:588–595.
90. Black AK. Mechanical trauma and urticaria. Am J Ind Med 1985; 8:297–303.
91. Caslae TB, Sampson HA, Hanifin J, Kaplan AP, Kulczycki A, Lawrence ID, Lemanske RF, Levine MI, Lillie MA. Guide to physical urticarias. J Allergy Clin Immunol 1988; 5:758–763.
92. Soter NA. Physical urticaria/angioedema. Semin Dermatol 1987; 6:302–312.
93. Farkas J. Fiberglass dermatitis in employees of a project-office in a new building. Contact Dermatitis 1983; 9:79.
94. Soter NA. Urticaria and angioedema. In: Fitzpatrick TB, Eisen AZ, Wolff K, Freedberg IM, Austen KF, eds. Dermatology in General Medicine. New York: McGraw-Hill, 1993:1483–1493.
95. Wener MH, Metzger WJ, Simon RA. Occupationally acquired vibratory angioedema with secondary carpal tunnel syndrome. Ann Intern Med 1983; 98:44–46.
96. Cohen SR, Bilinski DL, McNutt NS. Vibration syndrome: cutaneous and systemic manifestations in a jackhammer operator. Arch Dermatol 1985; 12:1544–1547.
97. Page EH, Shear NH. Temperature-dependent skin disorders. J Amer Acad Dermatol 1988; 18:1003–1119.
98. Bjorkner B. Occupational cold urticaria from contact spray. Contact Dermatitis 1981; 7:338–339.
99. Fitzgerald DA, Heagerty AHM, English JSC. Cold urticaria as an occupational dermatosis. Contact Dermatitis 1995; 32:238.
100. Miller SD, Pritchard D, Crowley JP. Blood histamine levels following graded cold challenge in atypical acquired cold urticaria. Ann of Allergy 1992; 68:27–29.
101. Whinnery JE, Anderson GK. Environmentally induced cholinergic urticaria and anaphylaxis. Avia Space Environ Med 1983; 54:551–553.
102. Hirschmann JV, Lawlor F, English JSC, Louback JB, Winkelmann RK, Greaves MW. Cholinergic urticaria. Arch Dermatol 1987; 123:462–467.
103. Jorizzo JL, Smith EB. The physical urticarias. Arch Dermatol 1982; 118:194–201.
104. Amin A, Lahti A, Maibach HI, eds. Contact Urticaria Syndrome. Boca Raton, FL: CRC Press, 1997.
105. Kanerva L, Estlander E, Jolanki R. Skin testing for immediate hypersensitivity in occupational allergology. In: Menna T, Maibach HI, eds. Exogenous Dermatoses: Environmental Dermatitis. Boca Raton, FL: CRC Press, 1990.

20

Enzymes

Jonathan A. Bernstein
University of Cincinnati College of Medicine, Cincinnati, Ohio

William Gerald Gaines, Jr.
Scott and White Clinic, Texas A&M Health Sciences Center and School of Rural Public Health, and Texas A&M/National Science Foundation Industry—University Cooperative Ergonomics Research Center, College Station, Texas

INTRODUCTION

Enzymes are proteins that are commonly used in biological systems to enhance catalytic reaction rates (1). Enzymes have been used in a variety of industrial processes and consumer products in this capacity. Proteolytic enzymes were first introduced commercially in Holland as part of an application for soaking soiled linen before washing (2). In 1967, the first enzyme to be introduced commercially in the United States and England was alcalase. This enzyme, synthesized from *Bacillus subtilis* through a submerged fermentation process, was used in soap detergents. Within 3 years, 80% of all soap detergents sold in the United States contained enzymes (3,4). Shortly thereafter, Flindt and Pepys reported the first cases of respiratory symptoms in detergent workers after inhalational exposure to *B. subtilis*–derived powdered enzymes, alcalase and maxatase (5,6). Twenty of 25 workers manifesting respiratory symptoms elicited positive wheal-and-flare skin test responses to skin test reagents prepared from the enzymatic material and *B. subtilis* spore extracts (5). Inhalational challenge tests to low concentrations of these enzyme extracts resulted in dual airway responses in three of these symptomatic workers (6). Further immunological evaluation of these workers revealed that IgE-mediated mechanisms were primarily involved in the immunopathogenesis of their respiratory symptoms (6). These early index cases were strong indicators that enzymes are highly allergenic materials and that susceptible workers exposed to these agents are at increased risk for becoming sensitized and developing asthma.

The development of enzyme technology gave rise to many novel applications for use of these agents in consumer products. For example, novel uses were discovered for enzymes in food preparation, soap detergents, pharmaceutical products as well as the leather and dry-cleaning industries (7). These new applications also placed the consumer at increased risk for enzyme exposure and sensitization. Subsequent studies conducted in Europe and the United States revealed that cutaneous enzyme sensitization and clinical symptoms occurred among some consumers repeatedly using these new enzyme-containing soap detergents (3,8). Initially, reports of enzyme sensitization and development of clinical symptoms in and out of the workplace were not recognized by the manufacturers of enzyme-containing products (9). Gradually, workplace structural and procedural changes were implemented to achieve better dust control and reduce potential worker exposures. These included manufacturing equipment enclosures and improved work area exhaust ventilation systems, operational methods for safe handling of enzymes, and novel enzyme-coating methods to reduce enzyme friability and dust generation. However, plant physicians continued to report cutaneous enzyme sensitization in exposed workers at levels well below the industry's recommended threshold limit value of 3.9 Tg/m^3 even after structural modifications in the workplace and enzyme encapsulation were introduced (4). These findings led to the understanding that all workers exposed to enzymes should be medically monitored at regular intervals for enzyme sensitization in conjunction with strict control of airborne enzyme dust in the workplace (10). In fact, manufacturers of enzyme-containing products represent the first industry that voluntarily implemented immunosurveillance programs designed to identify and monitor sensitized enzyme workers. These programs enabled the immediate removal of clinically symptomatic enzyme-sensitized workers from further enzyme exposure in the workplace. Immunosurveillance programs have also been successful in establishing safer operating guidelines in the enzyme industry, which has further reduced the risk for enzyme sensitization of exposed workers (10).

PREVALENCE AND RISK FACTORS

Epidemiological surveys conducted in England, the United States, and Canada in the early 1970s demonstrated that workers exposed to *B. subtilis*–derived enzymes become sensitized at a frequency of 20–60% depending on the degree of exposure (11). Although the frequency of enzyme sensitization and enzyme-induced asthma has been substantially reduced as a result of enzyme dust control measures, this problem has not been totally eliminated.

Identification of risk factors among enzyme-exposed workers for enzyme sensitization and clinical symptoms are not entirely clear. The amount of enzyme exposure and atopy are considered the most important risk factors. The importance of enzyme exposure is based on studies that have demonstrated a reduction in skin sensitization and clinical symptoms after reduced enzyme exposure in the workplace. The importance of atopy as a risk factor is based on studies that have demonstrated a strong correlation between enzyme-specific, IgE-mediated immune responses and clinical disease (12–15). A majority of studies reported that atopic enzyme-exposed workers are more likely to exhibit specific IgE antibodies to enzymes compared to nonatopic enzyme-exposed workers. Juniper and Roberts reported a higher incidence of enzyme-induced asthma in atopic subjects but this relationship has not been consistently found by other investigators (18,19). Although most studies indicate that atopic workers are more susceptible to becoming skin-sensitized to enzymes, it is still not clear whether atopy is predictive of progression to clinical disease (12–16,18,19). Flood et al. and Johnsen et al. have reported a higher incidence of enzyme sensitization among smoking versus nonsmoking workers (16,17). Other demographic characteristics such as gender, age, and race have not been identified as risk factors for enzyme sensitization (12–16).

IMMUNOPATHOGENESIS

Three of the initial symptomatic enzyme-sensitized workers reported by Flindt were studied more extensively by Pepys et al. to define the underlying immunological mechanism(s) for these reactions (5,6). They concluded that the pulmonary symptoms exhibited by these enzyme-sensitized workers involved IgE-mediated immune responses as all three subjects demonstrated strong, immediate percutaneous reactions to the specific proteolytic enzymes in addition to dual-phase asthmatic responses after specific inhalational challenges (6). Subsequent studies have confirmed the central role of IgE-mediated immune responses in enzyme-induced allergic reactions and asthma (2,3,10). These findings are based on strong correlations between respiratory symptoms, enzyme exposure, positive percutaneous reactions to enzymes, and specific bronchial inhalational challenges (2,3,10,12–16,18).

Animal models have revealed the effects of enzymes on the respiratory tract. Kilburn et al. developed a hamster model for studying morphological changes in the lung induced by the enzyme papain (20). Papain had previously been reported to produce a lung lesion that resembled centrilobular emphysema in hamster, rabbit, and dog animal models. Hamsters injected with 1 mg of purified papain in saline developed pulmonary edema and hemorrhage. After 4 days, there was loss of collagen from the alveolar walls but total lung protein, collagen, and elastin did not change (20). Although there was evidence of digestion of alveolar basement membrane connective tissue, normal cellular mechanisms to repair this damage were also observed (20).

Other animal models have been used to study the toxicological effects of enzymes. Guinea pigs exposed to aerosolized solutions and dry powder enzyme at a concentration of 80,000 Gu/m^3 (Gu = glycine units, which is a measure of enzyme activity) for 1 hr experienced hypothermia and respiratory distress, which was histologically characterized by intra-alveolar hemorrhage and infiltration of neutrophils and eosinophils (10). When one-fourth the concentration was administered for half the time, only the inflammatory cell infiltrates were observed. Repeated 3- to 4-weekly exposures to enzyme aerosols at concentrations that induced only the inflammatory cell infiltrates resulted in systemic sensitization, which was demonstrated by immediate percutaneous reactions and passive cutaneous anaphylaxis (10). Sensitized guinea pigs later challenged with enzyme preparations manifested bronchospasm induced by the release of histamine and other bioactive mediators. This observation was confirmed by studies using specific mediator antagonists that blocked this physiological response (10). In this study, induction of guinea pig sensitization was observed at very high concentrations of enzymes (10). However, other guinea pig studies demonstrated that enzyme sensitization and production of specific IgG_{1a} antibodies can also occur after repeated low doses of enzyme exposure (10). Interestingly, tolerance, which was observed after repeated low-dose enzyme exposures, was thought to be due to the production of enzyme-specific blocking antibodies (10). Development of tolerance to enzymes after chronic low-dose enzyme exposure in the workplace might partially explain why enzyme-skin-sensitized workers have been able to safely continue working with enzymes without progression to clinical asthma (10).

The toxicological and immunological effects of enzymes have also been investigated in cynomolgus monkeys (10). Monkeys have been subjected to inhalational exposure of pure enzymes and/or detergents at varying concentrations and combinations for 6 months. There were no observed histological, pulmonary function, or biochemical effects at levels of 1 mg/m^3 detergent dust containing 200 Tg/m^3 enzyme (10). At higher concentrations there was evidence of bronchiolar constriction and histology revealed alveolar fibrosis and bronchiolar epithelial hyperplasia. Bronchiolar contriction was reversible over time after exposure was terminated. The monkeys produced precipitating antibodies at all levels of enzyme exposure (10). Emphysematous histological changes reported in the hamster model exposed to papain were not observed in animal models exposed to other enzymes (10).

Ritz et al. developed a guinea pig intratracheal test to study relative allergenic potencies of enzymes on the respiratory tract of guinea pigs (21). They found that the initial appearance of respiratory symptoms in guinea pigs after repeated intratracheal enzyme exposure coincided with the initial appearance of enzyme-specific allergic antibodies in the serum. The allergic antibody response increased with duration and concentration of exposure regardless of whether the enzyme was administered by inhalation or intratracheally (21). They concluded that the guinea pig intratracheal test was a reliable method for studying enzyme-induced respiratory disease (21). Sarlo et al. used the guinea pig intratracheal test to study allergic antibody responses to enzymes at different concentrations and exposure levels (22). This model has provided useful information for establishing operating guidelines for newer enzyme proteins being developed for the detergent industry (22). This model has been used to determine the sensitization threshold dose for new enzymes that produced comparable allergic antibody responses previously observed with alcalase and for which effective plant-operating guidelines already exist. When the new enzyme concentrations were adjusted to the known sensitization concentration established for alcalase, similar rates of percutaneous enzyme sensitization were observed among workers newly exposed to the enzymes (22).

Although animal models provide a valuable tool for studying the toxicological, histological, and immunological effects of specific enzymes, the direct extrapolation of findings in animals to humans is not possible because of marked interspecies differences and variable exposure conditions that occur in the workplace.

SPECIFIC CAUSES OF ENZYME-INDUCED OCCUPATIONAL ASTHMA

Plant-Derived Enzymes

Papain is the most widely used plant-derived enzyme in industry and research. Papain is a protease enzyme with a molecular weight of 23,000 daltons that is produced from the latex of the papaya fruit (*Carica papaya*) (23). Papain is used in hundreds of cosmetic, food, and pharmaceutical consumer products. For example, papain is found in meat tenderizers, fruit juices, beer (as a clarifying agent), digestive aids, medications, and contact-lens-cleaning agents (23–25). Papain is an important immunological reagent used to cleave immunoglobulin molecules into two Fab (antigen-binding) fragments and an Fc (crystallizable) fragment (26). Allergic reactions to papain were reported as early as 1928. However, only a handful of papain-induced asthma cases have been reported (23). Papain is known to induce pulmonary lesions resembling emphysema in rat, hamster, rabbit, and dog animal models (23,24). Because of papain's potent elastolytic activity, there were serious concerns that a similar phenomenon could occur in papain-exposed workers. Tarlo et al. studied 330 papain-exposed workers and found only seven who elicited positive percutaneous reactions to papain. Sensitization was subsequently confirmed by an in vitro RAST assay (23). Baur et al. evaluated the clinical effects of papain in a total of 33 exposed workers in two studies (24,27). In one study they observed that seven of 11 papain-exposed workers developed upper and lower respiratory symptoms after variable lengths of exposure. Papain sensitization was confirmed in all seven of these workers by percutaneous testing and papain-specific RAST. Bronchial provocation testing was performed on five of these workers, all of whom demonstrated an immediate asthmatic response (24). One worker also experienced a late asthmatic response 4 hr after challenge (24). A subsequent study revealed that the prevalence of papain sensitization was 34.5%. In this study, eight of nine symptomatic workers who underwent specific bronchial provocation testing showed immediate or dual airway responses (27). Novey et al. also reported respiratory symptoms in papain-exposed workers. These correlated with changes in pulmonary function, positive percutaneous reactions, and positive RAST tests to papain (25). All of these studies confirmed that papain acted as an inhaled allergen that could sensitize exposed workers and cause occupational asthma. Evidence of pulmonary emphysema was not observed by any of the later investigators.

The potential for enzyme-exposure subsequent health effects in the general community has been increasingly recognized. Chymopapain is a proteolytic enzyme, structurally related to papain, that has been used for intradiscal dissolution of herniated lumbar discs (28). This procedure offered a noninvasive alternative approach to surgical laminectomy. Since anaphylaxis and death were reported in 1% of patients undergoing chemonucleolysis, serious concerns were raised about the safety of this procedure (28). Bernstein et al. evaluated 84 patients prior to undergoing chemonucleolysis by chymopapain percutaneous testing and specific RAST. Three subjects elicited a positive percutaneous reaction, which was confirmed by chymopapain IgE-specific RAST in only one of these individuals (28). Thirty-seven percent of subjects who returned for repeat skin testing to chymopapain developed a positive reaction. Atopy was associated with an increased risk for chymopapain sensitization (28). They concluded that skin testing was a more sensitive screening method for detecting IgE-specific chymopapain antibodies prior to chemonucleolysis compared to RAST. It has been recommended that all subjects being considered for chemonucleolysis should be routinely screened for chymopapain sensitization by percutaneous testing (28). Because chymopapain and papain obviously cross-react, prior occupational exposure to either papain or chymopapain would constitute an additional risk factor for such patients.

Pepsin is a vegetable-derived enzyme used as an additive in the production of liquors, cheeses, and cereals. Cartier et al. reported an index case of pepsin-induced occupational asthma in an atopic pharmaceutical worker (29). Pepsin sensitization was confirmed by skin prick testing and IgE RAST. A specific inhalational challenge confirmed the diagnosis of pepsin-induced occupational asthma (29).

Bromelain is a purified protease of pineapple (*Ananas comosus*) used in the pharmaceutical industry. A case of occupational asthma in a pharmaceutical worker developed after 10 years of exposure (30). Bromelain sensitization was confirmed by percutaneous reactivity to bromelain extracts and by bromelain-specific RAST. Specific bronchial and oral challenges to bromelain in this subject elicited respiratory and gastrointestinal symptoms, respectively (30).

Galson et al. performed a cross-sectional survey of a large group of workers in a meat-tenderizing plant where exposure to airborne aerosolized papain, bromelain, and ficin was documented (7). Good correlation was reported between work-related respiratory symptoms, peak flow variability, and percutaneous reactivity to two or more meat-tenderizer-enzyme reagents. They concluded that percutaneous testing was a sensitive method for detecting workers at risk for development of occupational asthma and/or rhinitis (7).

Animal-Derived Enzymes

The majority of animal-derived enzymes are commonly produced by microorganisms such as *B. subtilis, Bacillus licheniformis*, and *Aspergillus niger* while a few animal enzymes are still extracted from mammalian solid organs (7). Similar technological advances that enabled the early manufacture of penicillin ultimately led to large-scale production of microorganisms and their by-products. Proteases derived from these microorganisms, called subtilisins or subtilopeptidases, were found to be useful in household cleaning agents because of their potent enzymatic activity, which was stable over wide ranges of pH and temperature (13). Proteolytic enzymes derived from cultures of *B. subtilis* were first introduced in laundry detergents in the 1960s. As the enzyme-manufacturing industry rapidly expanded, greater numbers of workers were being continuously exposed to high concentrations of enzyme dusts. The adverse health effects of enzymes first became apparent in 1967 when employees of an English enzyme-producing plant were reported to develop upper and lower respiratory symptoms (5). In 1969, Pepys et al. reported their findings on three symptomatic workers exposed to the *B. subtilis*–derived enzymes alcalase and maxatase (6). They confirmed enzyme sensitization of these workers by percutaneous reactivity to specific enzymes and dual airway responses following specific enzyme inhalational challenges (6). They also found that both enzyme-exposed workers and nonexposed control subjects produced serum-precipitating antibodies to these enzymes. They interpreted this to mean that type III immune-complex-mediated mechanisms were involved in these reactions (6). However, the presence of precipitating antibodies in enzyme-exposed and nonexposed subjects in these early studies could have been artifactual and were not found to have clinical significance.

Newhouse et al. surveyed 271 of 278 workers in a detergent-manufacturing plant in England and found that 21% (57 workers) exhibited percutaneous reactions to alcalase (12). Forty-two of these workers experienced lower respiratory symptoms. Atopy was twice as prevalent among enzyme-sensitized workers as in nonsensitized workers (12). Airway obstruction was demonstrated in 11 of these workers. These workers were reassessed 6 months later after modifications to reduce exposure to enzyme dusts were implemented in the workplace. No evidence of deterioration of lung function was observed in either the enzyme-sensitized or nonsensitized workers (12). In the United States, Franz et al. studied 38 detergent-manufacturing employees in the United States who developed upper and lower respiratory symptoms after exposure to high enzyme dust concentrations (13). Symptoms ranged from nasal congestion, rhinorrhea, and throat irritation to chest tightness, cough, and shortness of breath. Enzyme sensitization was confirmed by intracutaneous testing to enzymes in 22 of 25 exposed workers manifesting lower respiratory symptoms (13). The prevalence of atopy among these workers was no greater than that found for the normal population. Passive transfer studies were positive using sera from five of the symptomatic workers. Pulmonary function abnormalities were found in 70% of the enzyme-sensitized (skin test positive) workers (13). Subsequent enzyme-specific bronchial challenges revealed a dual airway response in nine of 10 sensitized workers manifesting lower respiratory symptoms (13). Serum precipitins to enzymes were observed in both enzyme-exposed and nonexposed workers confirming the previous report of Pepys et al. (6,13). Once enzyme dust control measures were implemented, the frequency of respiratory complaints dramatically decreased (13).

The pervasive use of enzymes in the manufacture of laundry detergents led investigators to query about sensitization associated with repeated use by consumers. Bernstein first reported allergic symptoms in some individuals with chronic low-level exposure to enzyme containing-laundry detergents (3). These individuals had developed enzyme sensitization and respiratory symptoms, confirmed by specific skin test reactivity and provocative challenges, similar to those that had been observed in workers with enzyme-induced occupational asthma (3). Symptoms were either significantly improved or completely abated when these individuals stopped using detergents containing enzymes (3). Belin et al. reported a similar finding among three Swedish housewives who had repeated exposure using a powdered laundry detergent containing enzymes (8). These women experienced ocular pruritus, rhinorrhea, and sneezing and one also experienced wheezing, cough, and dyspnea. Enzyme sensitization was confirmed by percutaneous testing and serum-specific

IgE antibodies to alcalase (8). Symptoms abated when the powdered laundry detergent was changed to a "granular" detergent (8).

Modification of enzymes from a powdered form to a granulated form was one method of reducing enzyme sensitization and clinical symptoms among workers and consumers. Zetterström reported 12 atopic patients with positive IgE RAST and percutaneous reactions to the detergent enzyme subtilisin (2). Eight of these subjects experienced atopic symptoms after challenge with this enzyme in the powdered form while subsequent challenge with a granulated form of this enzyme resulted in only minimal upper respiratory symptoms in three subjects (3). Furthermore, thorough rinsing of bedding after washing with powdered detergents containing enzymes was effective in reducing clinical responses after facial contact. This study indicated that granulated forms of enzyme detergents and/or thorough rinsing of fabrics laundered with powdered forms of enzyme detergents was less likely to induce clinical symptoms (3).

Enzyme-induced sensitization and clinical disease continued to occur in the workplace even though improvements in enzyme dust control were implemented. To further reduce the allergenic potential of enzymes, an encapsulation process called "marumerization" was developed to embed the enzyme into a matrix of inorganic salt, resulting in the formation of uniform solid spheres approximately 600 Tm in diameter (4). This reduced the amount of respirable airborne enzyme dust generated in the detergent-manufacturing process. Additionally, enzyme detergent manufacturers created explicit industrywide recommendations for manufacturing equipment, its enclosure and exhaust ventilation, worker education, medical monitoring, and work practices for handling enzymes and enzyme-containing detergents (31). These interventions have resulted in significant declines in prevalences of positive enzyme skin test reactions and respiratory illnesses such as asthma (4,22).

In 1985, Pepys et al. investigated the prevalence of enzyme sensitization in the general atopic population by skin-testing 136 subjects with preexisting asthma and/or seasonal allergic rhinitis to alcalase and maxitase enzymes derived from *B. licheniformis* (19). They failed to demonstrate cutaneous sensitization in these subjects. It was concluded that consumers who used the newer modified enzyme detergents on a regular basis were at minimal risk for developing enzyme sensitization and clinical symptoms (19). However, Liss et al. reported that 25% of workers exposed to encapsulated enzymes at levels well below the threshold limit value of 3.9 Tg/m^3 developed enzyme sensitization confirmed by specific percutaneous testing and RAST (4).

Mitchell and Gandevia originally addressed the significance of positive skin test responses to enzymes among enzyme-exposed workers by surveying 98 workers who were intermittently exposed to high concentrations of proteolytic enzymes. Fifty percent of these subjects experienced immediate or delayed asthma-like symptoms after enzyme exposure (15). However, there was no significant difference between symptomatic workers and asymptomatic workers in prevalences of enzyme skin test reactivity to enzymes (15). Subjects with skin test reactivity to three common aeroallergens (*Aspergillus*, dust, and grass pollen) were at significantly greater risk for sensitization to alcalase. No other risk factors for enzyme sensitization and clinical symptoms were identified (15). They found that workers could continue to work safely in an enzyme-dust-free environment even after they developed skin sensitization to enzymes, a finding subsequently confirmed in other studies (10,15,17,22). Some studies have reported that removal of asymptomatic atopic individuals from enzyme exposure was of limited value since enzyme-induced allergic reactions did not differ between atopics and nonatopics (10,17).

Allergic reactions to flour dust were reported as early as 1700 (32). Baker's asthma is one of the most common causes of occupational asthma in certain parts of the world (32). Alpha-amylase enzymes derived from *Aspergillus oryzae* is commonly added to baking flour to compensate for the low natural content of amylases and carbohydrates fermentable by yeast (32). Alpha-amylase acts to stimulate the growth of *Saccharomyces*, which improves the rising of dough and the quality of the bread (32). Of 118 bakery workers surveyed for symptoms, 35 had asthma and/or rhinitis symptoms after contact with flour (32). In all 35 subjects, IgE-mediated sensitization to wheat flour was confirmed by skin testing and RAST and in 33 of 35 subjects to rye flour (32). Twelve of 35 subjects had positive IgE antibodies by RAST to *Aspergillus*-derived amylase. Specific inhalational challenges to this enzyme reproduced either rhinitis or asthma symptoms in four of these subjects (32). All of the subjects with I-amylase-specific IgE antibodies were atopic (32). A subsequent study evaluating 140 bakery workers with either upper or lower respiratory symptoms failed to elicit signs of sensitization to wheat or rye flour allergens (33). However, testing of these individuals to the *Aspergillus*-derived enzymes I-amylase and glucoamylase revealed sensitization rates ranging between 5 and 24% (33). Other investigators have also demonstrated the importance of enzymes as major allergens in baker's asthma (34). Barber et al. reported that a 14.5-kDa, barley, salt-soluble protein related to a single protein family of I-amylase/trypsin inhibitors was a major IgE-binding allergen in patients with baker's asthma (35).

Documentation of occupational asthma has been demonstrated in pharmaceutical workers exposed to enzymes. Losada et al. reported two cases of occupational asthma induced by cellulase derived from *A. niger* (36). IgE-mediated sensitization to cellulase was confirmed by skin testing and specific IgE immunoassays. Immediate airway responses were induced by bronchial provocation with cellulase dust (36). A cross-sectional survey performed on 94 pharmaceutical workers exposed to *A. oryzae*–derived J-d-galactoside galactohydrolase revealed that 29% of exposed workers had percutaneous reactivity to this lactase (37). Sensitized lactase workers were nine times more likely to experience upper or lower respiratory symptoms compared to skin-test-negative subjects; atopic workers were four times more likely to develop lactase sensitization compared to nonatopic workers (37). Reduction of lactase exposure and restricting atopic workers from working with lactase successfully prevented lactase-induced occupational symptoms (37). Another group of investigators has recently reported lactase sensitization in the workplace (38).

Egg-processing workers are known to be at increased risk for developing occupational asthma induced by egg proteins such as ovalbumin, ovomucoid, conalbumin, and egg lysozyme (39,40). Bernstein et al. recently reported the first case of occupational asthma induced by inhaled egg lysozyme in a worker employed at a plant that manufactured hen egg-white-derived lysozyme (41). IgE sensitization was confirmed by skin test reactivity and serum-specific IgE antibodies to egg lysozyme (41). Antigen specificity of egg-lysozyme-specific IgE was demonstrated by ELISA inhibition and bronchoprovocation testing to egg lysozyme (41).

Although symptoms among workers exposed to pancreatic enzymes have not yet been documented, asthma and allergic rhinitis symptoms have occurred in five parents of cystic fibrosis children who became sensitized by inhaling pancreatic extracts sprinkled on their children's food (42). Avoidance of further exposure to these pancreatic extracts prevented asthma (42). Colten et al. studied 14 workers exposed to airborne hog trypsin in a plant that manufactured plastic polymer resins (43). Four of these workers were identified by history to have symptoms consistent with trypsin-induced occupational asthma. Hog trypsin sensitization was confirmed by skin test reactivity to trypsin antigens.

Three of the workers had immediate asthma responses after specific inhalational challenge (43). A pharmaceutical worker was reported to develop occupational asthma and rhinitis to the enzymes serratial peptidase and lysozyme. Sensitization was confirmed by percutaneous reactivity and elevated serum-specific IgE to both enzymes (44). The worker experienced a dual asthmatic response after specific bronchoprovocation (44).

CLINICAL EVALUATION AND TREATMENT

Assessment of enzyme-exposed workers who develop respiratory symptoms should be approached in an algorithmic manner. The initial evaluation should begin with a comprehensive history, which should include information pertaining to the job description, duration of exposure prior to onset of symptoms, temporal relationship between symptoms and the workplace, description of the workplace, length of daily exposure, and use of protective clothing and masks. Material safety data sheets and industrial hygiene air-sampling data identifying specific exposure(s) should always be reviewed. To assure correct workplace interventions the evaluating physician should communicate directly with health and safety personnel from the manufacturing site to determine the symptomatic worker's potential source of enzyme exposure.

As discussed in other chapters, an occupational history and skin prick testing are not sufficient to confirm a diagnosis of occupational asthma (OA). Decrements in lung functions in association with exposure to the causative agent must be demonstrated. A methacholine challenge should be performed to confirm or exclude bronchial hyperresponsiveness when airway obstruction and reversibility cannot be demonstrated. If the diagnosis of enzyme-induced OA remains in question, peak flow monitoring combined with a workplace challenge or enzyme-specific bronchial provocation test may be necessary (45). Methods for performing peak flow monitoring and bronchial challenges are described in detail in other chapters.

IMMUNOLOGICAL TESTING

Confirmatory testing should include assessment of atopic status by percutaneous testing to common seasonal and perennial aeroallergens and to the specific enzymes encountered in the workplace (45). In preparing enzyme extracts for skin testing, proper preliminary testing of nonexposed control subjects should be performed using serial dilutions of the enzymatic extract to determine the least irritating concentration (11).

Merget et al. compared the sensitivity and specificity of enzyme skin testing and in an in vitro serological test of enzyme-specific IgE using the specific bronchial challenge as the gold standard for confirming OA among 42 enzyme-exposed plant workers (46). They found that enzyme skin testing using nondialyzed aqueous enzyme extracts was 100% sensitive and 93% specific compared to enzyme allergosorbent testing, which yielded a sensitivity of only 62% and specificity of 96% (46). In addition, the predictive value of a negative test was 100%. Although the specificity of the skin test in this study far surpassed that reported in studies evaluating OA due to other natural protein allergens, these data suggest that skin prick testing is essential in diagnosing and screening for enzyme-associated respiratory disorders (46).

A significant problem in correlating enzyme exposure with sensitization has been the lack of reliable enzyme skin test reagents and a standardized approach for skin testing and interpretation of reactions. Studies that reported contradictory findings cited inconsistencies in skin test reagents or in vitro immunoassay sensitivity as reasons for these differences. Early investigations evaluating enzyme-exposed workers were performed using crude enzymatic extracts and may have elicited false-positive results (or irritant reactions) in some instances (11). The standard in vitro immunoassay used to detect specific IgE antibodies in enzyme-exposed workers was the radioallergosorbent test (RAST) (47). In one study, the RAST identified 68% of enzyme skin test positive workers whereas the enzyme-linked immunosorbent assay (ELISA) identified 86% of enzyme skin-test-positive workers (48). Therefore, neither of these immunoassays possesses adequate sensitivity for screening worker populations for enzyme sensitization (49).

Dor et al. reported potential problems in performing IgE-specific RAST to various *Bacillus*-derived proteases (47). For example, they reported that esperase derived from *B. licheniformis* undergoes autolysis, which can result in the loss of its enzyme reactivity through degradation (47). They found that pretreatment of esperase with phenylmethyl-sulfonyl fluoride (PMSF) is required to stabilize the antigen so it can function as a stable allergen (47). These investigators also found that serum IgE antibodies of sensitized subjects are cross-reactive for esperase, alcalase, and savinase which can limit the specificity of in vitro assays (47).

Sarlo et al. partially addressed the problem with in vitro assays by developing an IgE-enzyme-specific ELISA with greater sensitivity and specificity than RAST (48). Complete agreement between enzyme skin test reactivity and ELISA was demonstrated in 87% of subjects tested whereas total agreement between skin test reactivity and RAST was found only 77% of the time (48). They concluded that the ELISA was more sensitive for detecting alcalase-specific IgE antibody in detergent-enzyme-exposed workers (48).

Bernstein et al. recently confirmed that skin testing was more sensitive than in vitro methods for detecting enzyme sensitization in exposed workers (49). They found that the range of percutaneous threshold response to enzymes was able to detect "lightly" sensitized subjects whereas the IgE RAST could detect only "highly" sensitized subjects (49). It was concluded that skin prick testing was a more sensitive method for longitudinal monitoring of occupational groups at risk for enzyme sensitization (49).

Immunosurveillance

Currently enzyme skin testing is used to screen for sensitization among enzyme-exposed workers. However, workers who demonstrate percutaneous sensitivity to enzymes are not automatically removed from further enzyme exposure as clinical symptoms do not always immediately follow (10,22,49). Strict control of enzyme dust exposure in the workplace to ambient concentrations less than 60 ng/m^3 has resulted in dramatic reductions in enzyme-induced OA and in incidences of cutaneous sensitization (50). Once a sensitized worker clinically manifests upper airway symptoms, such as watering eyes or rhinitis, prompt removal from additional exposure is mandatory to prevent or retard the development of lower airway complications, such as asthma.

CONCLUSIONS

Enzymes are widely used in industry to manufacture a number of widely used consumer products. The rapid widespread use of enzymes by a spectrum of industries coupled with the lack of regulatory guidelines for safe enzyme dust exposure levels were two major reasons why enzymes readily surfaced as potent allergens. Many studies have indicated that atopic status and enzyme exposure levels are important factors for enzyme sensitization. However, risk factors that determine progression to clinical disease such as asthma remain to be determined. Modifications in synthesis of enzymes and improvements in control of airborne enzyme dust in the workplace have been successful in the reduction, but not the complete elimination, of enzyme-induced occupational asthma. Therefore, it is essential that immunosurveillance programs be implemented in the workplace for the early detection and removal of symptomatic enzyme-sensitized workers. Such programs will also provide greater insight into environmental and/or genetic risk factors that contribute to enzyme sensitization and the progression to clinical disease.

REFERENCES

1. Stryer L. Introduction to enzymes. In: Stryer L, ed. Biochemistry, 2nd ed. San Francisco: WH Freeman, 1981:109–131.
2. Zetterström O. Challenge and exposure test reactions to enzyme detergents in subjects sensitized to subtilisin. Clin Allergy 1977; 355–363.
3. Bernstein IL. Enzyme allergy in populations exposed to long-term, low-level concentrations of household laundry products. J Allergy Clin Immunol 1972; 49:219–237.
4. Liss GM, Kominsky JR, Gallagher JS, Melius J, Brooks SM, Bernstein IL. Failure of enzyme encapsulation to prevent sensitization of workers in the dry bleach industry. J Allergy Clin Immunol 1984; 348–355.
5. Flindt MLH. Pulmonary disease due to inhalation of derivatives of *Bacillus subtilis* containing proteolytic enzyme. Lancet 1969; 1177–1181.
6. Pepys J, Longbottom JL, Hargreave FE, Faux J. Allergic reactions of the lungs to enzymes of *Bacillus subtilis*. Lancet 1969; 1181–1184.
7. Bernstein DI, Malo J-L. High molecular weight agents. In: Bernstein IL, Chan-Yeung M, Malo J-L, Bernstein DI, eds. Asthma in the Workplace. New York: Marcel Dekker, 1993:373–398.
8. Belin L, Hoborn J, Falsen E, André J. Enzyme sensitization in consumers of enzyme-containing washing powder. Lancet 1970; 2:1153–1157.
9. Flindt ML. Biological miracles and misadventures: identification of sensitization and asthma in enzyme detergent workers. Am J Ind Med 1996; 29:99–110.
10. Gibson JC, Juniper CP, Martin RB, Weill H. Biological effects of proteolytic enzyme detergents. Thorax 1976; 31:621–634.
11. Belin LG, Norman PS. Diagnostic tests in the skin and serum of workers sensitized to *Bacillus subtilis* enzymes. Clin Allergy 1977; 7:55–68.
12. Newhouse ML, Tagg B, Pocock SJ. An epidemiological study of workers producing enzyme washing powders. Lancet 1970; 689–693.
13. Franz T, McMurrain KD, Brooks S, Bernstein IL. Clinical, immunologic, and physiologic observations in factory workers exposed to *Bacillus subtilis* enzyme dust. J Allergy 1971; 47:170–180.
14. Gandevia B, Mitchell C. The dangers of proteolytic enzymes to workers. Med J Aust 1971; 1032–1033.
15. Mitchell CA, Gandevia B. Respiratory symptoms and skin reactivity in workers exposed to proteolytic enzymes in the detergent industry. Am Rev Respir Dis 1971; 104:1–12.
16. Flood DGS, Blofeld RE, Bruce CF, Hewitt JI, Juniper CP, Roberts DM. Lung function, atopy, specific hypersensitivity, and smoking of workers in the enzyme detergent industry over 11 years. Br J Ind Med 1985; 42:43–50.
17. Johnsen CR, Sorensen TB, Larsen IA, Secher AB, Andreasen E, Kofoed GS, Fredslund, Gyntelberg F. Allergy risk in an enzyme producing plant: a retrospective follow up study. Occup Environ Med 1997; 9:671–675.

18. Juniper CP, Roberts DM. Enzyme asthma: Fourteen years' clinical experience of a recently prescribed disease. J Soc Occup Med 1984; 34:127–132.

19. Pepys J, Mitchell J, Hawkins R, Malo J-L. A longitudinal study of possible allergy to enzyme detergents. Clin Allergy 1985; 15:101–115.

20. Kilburn KH, Dowell AB, Pratt PC. Morphological and biochemical assessment of papain-induced emphysema. Arch Intern Med 1971; 127:884–890.

21. Ritz HL, Evans BLB, Bruce RD, Fletcher ER, Fisher GL, Sarlo K. Respiratory and immunological responses of guinea pigs to enzyme-containing detergents: a comparison of intratracheal and inhalation modes of exposure. Fund Appl Toxicol 1993; 21:31–37.

22. Sarlo K, Fletcher ER, Gaines WG, Rita HL. Respiratory allergenicity of detergent enzymes in the guinea pig intratracheal test: association with sensitization of occupationally exposed individuals. Fund Appl Toxicol 1997; 39:44–52.

23. Tarlo SM, Shaikh W, Bell B, Cuff M, Davies GM, Dolovich J, Hargreave FE. Papain-induced allergic reactions. Clin Allergy 1978; 8:207–215.

24. Baur X, Fruhmann G. Papain induced asthma: diagnosis by skin test, RAST and bronchial provocation test. Clin Allergy 1979; 9:75–81.

25. Novey HS, Keenan WJ, Fairshter RD, Wells ID, Wilson AF, Culver BD. Pulmonary disease in workers exposed to papain: clinico-physiological and immunological studies. Clin Allergy 1980; 10:721–731.

26. Goodman JW, Parslow TG. Immunoglobulin proteins. In: Stites DP, Terr AI, Parslow TG, eds. Basic and Clinical Immunology. Norwalk, CT: Appleton & Lange, 1994:66–79.

27. Baur X, Konig G, Bencze K, Fruhmann G. Clinical symptoms and results of skin test, RAST and bronchial provocation test in thirty-three papain workers: evidence for strong immunogenic potency and clinically relevant proteolytic effects of airborne papain. Clin Allergy 1982; 12: 9–17.

28. Bernstein DI, Gallagher JS, Ulmer A, Bernstein IL. Prospective evaluation of chymopapain sensitivity in patients undergoing chemonucleolysis. J Allergy Clin Immunol 1985; 76:458–465.

29. Cartier A, Malo J-L, Pineau L, Dolovich J. Occupational asthma due to pepsin. J Allergy Clin Immunol 1984; 73:574–577.

30. Baur X, Fruhmann G. Allergic reactions, including asthma, to the pineapple protease bromelain following occupational exposure. Clin Allergy 1979; 9:443–450.

31. Work Practices for Handling Enzymes in the Detergent Industry. New York: Soap and Detergent Association, 1995.

32. Bauer X, Fruhmann G, Haug B, Rasche B, Reiher W, Weiss W. Role of *Aspergillus* amylase in baker's asthma. Lancet 1986; 43.

33. Baur X, Sauer W, Weiss W. Baking additives as new allergens in baker's asthma. Respiration 1988; 54:70–72.

34. Quirce S, Cuevas M, Diez-Gomez M, Fernandez-Rivas M, Hinojosa M, Gonzalez R, Losada E. Respiratory allergy to *Aspergillus*-derived enzymes in baker's asthma. J Allergy Clin Immunol 1992; 90:970–978.

35. Barber D, Sanchez-Monge R, Gomez L, Carpizo J, Armentia A, Lopez-Otin C, Juan F, Salcedo G. A barley flour inhibitor of insectI-amylase is a major allergen associated with baker's asthma disease. FEBS Lett 1989; 248:119–122.

36. Losada E, Hinojosa M, Moneo I, Dominguez J, Gomez MLD, Ibanez MD. Occupational asthma caused by cellulase. J Allergy Clin Immunol 1986; 77:635–639.

37. Bernstein JA, Bernstein DI, Stauder T, Herd Z, Bernstein IL. Allergic sensitization to *Aspergillus oryzae* derived lactase in pharmaceutical workers. J Allergy Clin Immunol 1993; 93: 265.

38. Julian JA, Millman JM, Beaudin MA, Dolovich J. Occupational sensitization to lactase. Am J Ind Med 1997; 31:570–571.

39. Bernstein DI, Smith AB, Moller DR, Gallagher JS, Aw T-C, London M, Kopp S, Carson G. Clinical and immunologic studies among egg-processing workers with occupational asthma. J Allergy Clin Immunol 1987; 80:791–797.

40. Smith AB, Bernstein DI, Aw T-C, Gallagher JS, London M, Kopp S, Carson GA. Occupational asthma from inhaled egg protein. Am J Ind Med 1987; 12:205–218.

41. Bernstein JA, Kraut A, Bernstein DI, Warrington R, Bolin T, Warren CPW, Bernstein IL. Occupational asthma induced by inhaled egg lysozyme. Chest 1993; 103:532–535.

42. Dolan TF Jr, Meyers A. Bronchial asthma and allergic rhinitis associated with inhalation of pancreatic extracts. Am Rev Respir Dis 1974; 110:812–813.

43. Colten HR, Polakoff PL, Weinstein SF, Strieder DJ. Immediate hypersensitivity to hog trypsin resulting from industrial exposure. N Engl J Med 1973; 292:1050–1053.

44. Nahm DH. New occupational allergen in a pharmaceutical industry: serratial peptidase and lysozyme chloride. Ann Allergy Asthma Immunol 1997; 78:225–229.

45. Bernstein JA, Bernstein DI, Bernstein IL. Occupational Asthma. In: Bierman CW, Pearlman DS, Shapiro GG, Busse WW, eds. Allergy, Asthma and Immunology from Infancy to Adulthood. Philadelphia: WB Saunders, 1996:529–548.

46. Merget R, Stollfuss J, Wiewrodt R, Frühauf H, Koch U, Bolm-Audorff U, Bienfait H-G, Hiltl G, Schultze-Werninghaus G. Diagnostic tests in enzyme allergy. J Allergy Clin Immunol 1993; 92:264–277.

47. Dor PJ, Agarwal MK, Gleich MC, Welsh PW, Dunnette SL, Adolphson CR, Gleich GJ. Detection of antibodies to proteases used in laundry detergents by the radioallergosorbent test. J Allergy Clin Immunol 1986; 78:877–886.

48. Sarlo K, Clark ED, Ryan CA, Bernstein DI. ELISA for human IgE antibody to Subtilisin A (alcalase): correlation with RAST and skin test results with occupationally exposed individuals. J Allergy Clin Immunol 1990; 86:393–399.

49. Bernstein DI, Bernstein IL, Gaines WG Jr, Stauder T, Wilson ER. Characterization of skin prick testing responses for detecting sensitization to detergent enzymes at extreme dilutions: inability of the RAST to detect lightly sensitized individuals. J Allergy Clin Immunol 1994; 94:498–507.

50. Kelling CK et al. Safety assessment of enzyme-containing personal cleansing products: exposure characterization and development of IgE antibody to enzymes after a 6 month use test. J Allergy Clin Immunol 1998; 101:179–181.

21
Occupational Asthma in the Baking Industry

Dick Heederik
Wageningen University and Research Center, Wageningen, The Netherlands

Anthony J. Newman Taylor
Imperial College School of Medicine at the National Heart and Lung Institute, London, England

INTRODUCTION

One of the first descriptions of asthma in bakers was given by Ramazzinni in 1700 in *De Morbis artificum diatriba*. However, until the beginning of this century the etiology was unknown. De Besche (1) suggested for the first time that asthma in bakery workers is an allergic disease. The first systematic investigation in the baking industry was made by Baagöe in 1933 (2). Since then, numerous surveys have been undertaken with the aim of unraveling the etiology of allergic rhinitis and asthma in bakery workers and estimating the risk of developing these diseases. Asthma in bakers and bakery workers is often referred to as bakers' asthma. This terminology is better avoided because asthma caused by the same agents occurs in other occupations such as in flour millers, workers in other food-producing and -processing industries, and related industries such as the enzyme-producing and baking-ingredient industries.

Asthma in bakery workers is one of the most frequently occurring forms of occupational asthma. The annual incidence of asthma in bakery workers has been estimated to be 290–409 cases per million using data from the UK SWORD surveillance scheme (3–5). This roughly corroborates estimates from a similar surveillance scheme in the area around Birmingham, England (6), and puts bakery workers among the high-risk occupations. The Swedish Occupational Disease Register reported an incidence figure of 800 per million among bakers during 1984–1988 based on sickness leave compensation applications (7). Some indications from occupational disease registries suggest that the number of asthma cases in bakery workers is rising (8–12). Studies in bakery workers suggest incidence rates of sensitization and allergy (sensitization and symptoms) ranging from 1 to 10 per 1000 workers (13–15). In Germany more than 1200 bakers claim insurance compensation each year (9,11). A small U.S. death certificate study in 184 individuals who died between 1980 and 1990 with asthma listed as cause or contributing cause of death revealed an increased age-and-race-adjusted mortality rate in bakery workers compared to local and national mortality rates (16).

Asthma is the most important manifestation of occupational allergy in bakery workers. Work-related asthmatic symptoms are in most cases preceded by rhinitis and conjunctivitis. Allergens from cereal flours have long been regarded as the major cause of bakers' asthma. But other ingredients of the dough, such as enzymes used as dough improvers, or contaminants, such as mite allergens and possibly microorganisms, are known to cause allergies in bakers as well. Many cases of bakers' allergy, especially those with asthma, have specific IgE to the responsible proteins. Specific inhalation challenges with flour extracts in sensitized workers provoke predominantly immediate asthmatic reactions. Late and dual reactions are also reported (17,18). However, several studies suggest that a considerable number of bakery workers without positive SPTs or specific IgE to flour extracts and other allergens from the bakery environment (enzymes) have work-related asthma symptoms (19–24). This might be explained to some extent by other allergens. Nevertheless, it seems plausible that nonspecific irritation or aggravation of preexisting asthma plays at least some role in explaining the occurrence of respiratory symptoms. Some studies show that workers without positive skin prick tests (SPTs) or specific IgE to the most important allergens from the work environment are atopic (23,25).

Little is known about the epidemiology of asthma in bakery workers. The development and use of immunoassays, which use the specificity of the immunoglobulin response, to measure allergens in dust samples has led to a recent breakthrough in the study of the epidemiology of asthma in bakery workers. Wheat and α-amylase allergen levels have been measured across the baking industry. Exposure-response relationships have been established for some allergens used in the baking industry facilitating risk assessment approaches, and in the near future, possibly standard setting and the development of better preventive strategies. There is still a need for prospective studies, and preventive strategies based on recent evidence should be validated and optimized in intervention studies.

ALLERGENS: NATURE AND SOURCES

Cereal Flours

Most reports implicate cereal flours such as wheat flour (*Triticum* sp.) and other cereal flours such as rye flour (*Secale cereale*) and barley flour (*Hordeum vulgare*) as responsible agents causing allergic diseases in bakery workers. Specific IgE antibodies against extracts from these cereal flours have been demonstrated in affected workers by in vivo and in vitro tests (26–28). Although cereal flours are the most common flours bakers work with, flours from other sources may be involved as well. Buckwheat (*Fagopyrum schulentum*), a Polygonaceae belonging to the weed group and taxonomically not related to cereal grains, has been mentioned as a cause of IgE-mediated asthma in bakers involved in crepe and health food production (29). Changes in consumer demands over the last decade required production of a greater variety of products and this in its turn led to the introduction of other flours that contain allergens such as soy flour.

Strong cross-antigenicity exists between allergens from different cereals. This reflects the taxonomic relationships between at least some of the grain species (26,30,31). Some of the cereal allergens are closely related enzymes or enzyme inhibitors (31–34). The strongest in vitro reactivity had been observed with water-soluble proteins, particularly albumins (35,36). IgE against water-insoluble proteins contained in gliadin, globulin, and glutenin fractions has also been reported (37). The number of potentially relevant allergens is large (Fig. 1, p. 382). A total of 40 different antigens in wheat flour have been identified, of which 20 cross-reacted with rye flour (38). Sera of a majority of sensitized bakers show IgE reactions with many of these proteins, but reaction profiles often differ markedly between individual sera (39) (Figs. 2–4, pp. 383–385). Reactions to some components in the

12–17-kDa range are found most commonly (39–42). One of the major components of the 12–15-kDa bands belongs to the α-amylase/trypsin inhibitor family (32,43–45). The allergenicity of purified members of this enzyme inhibitor family has been shown in vitro (32, 46) and in vivo (47), and is found in other cereal species as well (48–51). A 14.5-kDa protein from barley belonging to this family has been associated with bakers' asthma (52). Allergens in the 26–28- and 35-kDa range are homologous to cereal enzymes such as acyl-CoA oxidase and fructose-bisphosphate adolase and acyl-CoA oxidase, respectively (44,45). Addition of cereal malt flours as dough improvers decreased since the introduction of fungal amylases. However, malt flours are still being used and contain potent allergens that are probably related to the cereal amylases mentioned earlier (53–55).

Enzymes

A relatively new source of occupational allergies and asthma in the baking industry are enzymes such as fungal α-amylase, proteases, and cellulases. Use of enzymes provides better control of the rising and baking processes. They modify the viscosity of the dough, volume and coloring of the baked product, and lengthen shelf life. The baking industry started using enzymes in the 1970s with rapid increases in the 1980s and 1990s. First reports of enzyme-related respiratory morbidity in bakers come in the early 1980s. Since then, several case reports have been reported of bakers' asthma caused by this enzyme, often in the absence of specific IgE to cereal allergens (53,55–62). The baking industry, along with the detergent industry, is one of the major industries where a large-scale use of enzymes occurs and causes an occupational hazard.

The most commonly used dough improver, fungal α-amylase (1,4-α-D-glucan glucanohydrolase), usually derived from *Aspergillus oryzae*, is a glycoprotein that catalyzes the hydrolysis of internal α(1,4)-glycosidic linkages in polysaccharides. Fungal α-amylase is routinely added in small amounts (mg/kg flour) to baking flour in the flour mill before shipment or by adding commercially available mixtures of dough improvers containing enzymes, fats, and sugar in the bakery. Several IgE-binding proteins have been detected in crude amylase preparations with a dominating IgE-binding band for a protein with a molecular weight between 51 and 54 kDa (56,61,63–67) (Fig. 4). This band represents the active fungal α-amylase enzyme (64). Commercially available extracts of fungal α-amylase contain several other allergenic proteins with molecular weights of 25–27 and 40 kDa (63,64,67,68). Case studies suggest that oral provocation with fungal α-amylase enzyme (69) and bread (70,71), may cause allergic respiratory symptoms in individuals sensitized through airborne amylase. Others were unable to provoke reactions by eating bread in individuals with skin test reactions to *Aspergillus fumigatus*, *A oryzae*, and fungal α-amylase (72). Some studies have shown a loss of allergenicity of heated α-amylase, suggesting that α-amylase in baked food products would indeed not be an important cause of allergic sensitization (73,74). Three other studies suggest, however, that fungal α-amylase partially retains its allergenicity and is still capable of binding IgE antibodies after being heated (71,75,76). Amylases are also present in cereal flour in its native form. IgE antibodies that bind cereal α-amylases or β-amylases from barley flour have been demonstrated. Molecular weights of these cereal amylases appeared to be 54, 59, and 64 kDa (65,74). However, cereal and fungal amylases show only minimal immunological cross-reactivity (65,74) and different allergenic behavior exists between homologous allergens such as α-amylase inhibitor allergens from rye, barley, and wheat (51).

Other allergens are being used in the baking industry and could form a respiratory hazard but seem of less importance compared to fungal α-amylase. Bauer et al. (63,77) studied asthmatic bakers and showed that 5–10% were sensitized to fungal glucoamylase and (hemi)cellulase, while sensitization to proteolytic enzymes (protease and papain) was rare. A Finnish study of 365 workers from bakeries, a flour mill, and a crisp bread factory showed that most workers sensitized to enzymes had a positive SPT to fungal α-amylase and very few workers had a positive SPT to fungal proteases, cellulase, or glucose oxidase (78).

Storage Mites

Wheat flour in bakeries can be contaminated with storage mites (79), and allergens from storage mites have been suggested as a cause of allergic symptoms in bakery workers (79,80). Epidemiological studies showed high prevalence rates of sensitization to storage mites (*Acarus siro*, *Glycophagus domesticus*, *Lepidoglyphus destructor*, *Tyrophagus longior*, *Tyrophagus putrescentiae*) in bakery workers varying from 11 to 33% (20,21,24,25). However, no difference in sensitization to storage mites could be found in two studies comparing bakery workers and controls (24,81,82). Others have also reported high prevalence rates of storage mite sensitization in non–occupationally exposed subjects (81,83,84). This suggests that storage mites are widespread in the environment and that a positive skin response to storage mites among bakers is more an indicator of atopy rather than a response to an occupational allergen specific to bakers. Moreover, part of the apparent anti-storage-mite IgE reactions may be due to cross-reactivity with house dust mites (81,84,85), although, according to some studies, storage mites also possess storage-mite-specific allergenic epitopes (81,84).

Other Allergens

Molds have also been suggested as causing asthma in some bakers but their role remains controversial (86,87). The prevalence of sensitization in symptomatic bakers significantly differed from groups of symptomatic controls (88,89). However, the study of Musk et al. (25) showed that sensitization rates were low in randomly selected bakery workers. The prevalence of positive skin prick test to bakers' yeast seems low as well (22,25). For most other allergens mentioned in the literature such as egg yolk and egg white, sesame seeds, nuts (hazelnuts and almonds), and so forth, only sporadic case reports have been presented and these allergens have only a marginal contribution to the high prevalence of respiratory allergy in bakers.

MEASUREMENT OF DUST EXPOSURE AND AIRBORNE ALLERGENS

Most studies involve large bakeries with distinctly different job categories. Some data are available for small bakeries, often family enterprises. Job rotation is common in small bakeries and family members are often involved in part of the process. Small bakeries form an important segment of the bread- and pastry-producing industry, especially in some European countries.

Until recently, dust sampling has been the only tool for exposure assessment in the baking industry. A known volume of air is drawn through a sampling head with a filter and the dust particles are retained on the filter and weighed. The design of the sampling head determines the size of the particulates sampled. For studies in occupational asthma it is now common to sample the inhalable dust fraction. This is the fraction that is able to penetrate and deposit into the airways. However, despite the widespread availability of dust measurement techniques, reliable exposure data results from large dust measurement series across the bakery industry have only become available in the 1990s (91–95).

Results of the available exposure studies show that workers at the front end of the process of larger industries (dough makers, bread formers, average inhalable dust exposures of 3–9 mg/m^3) had the highest 8-hr average dust exposures. Oven workers had intermediate dust exposures (8-hr average inhalable dust exposures of 1–3 mg/m^3), and workers involved in packing and slicing had the lowest exposures (below 1 mg/m^3). Some of these studies suggest small differences in dust exposure between bakeries that produce different products (93,95). High average dust exposure levels were found in Canadian bakeries for workers involved in the production of puff pastry ($n = 14$, arithmetic mean (AM) 23 mg/m^3), bread and buns ($n = 17$, AM 18 mg/m^3), croissants ($n = 8$, AM 5.3 mg/m^3), and cinnamon buns ($n = 6$, AM 3.6 mg/m^3) (95). Data from small bakeries show geometric mean inhalable dust levels of 3.3 mg/m^3 in bread bakers ($n = 36$, 2.0 mg/m^3) and in mixed (bread and confectionery) bakers, and 0.7 mg/m^3 in confectioners with considerable variability between bakeries (93).

Recently several assays have become available that allow measurement of allergen levels in personal dust samples (Fig. 5, p. 386). The development of these immunoassays forms an important step forward in quantifying allergen exposure in the bakery industry. These methods are valid, specific, and produce reasonably reproducible results. The sensitivity is sufficient to detect allergens quantitatively in personal samples in the μg/m^3 or even pg/m^3 range. Assays have been described for the whole specter of airborne wheat allergens (93,96) by using, respectively, polyclonal rabbit IgG antibodies and IgG$_4$ antibodies from a pool of IgG$_4$-positive bakery workers in RAST and ELISA assays. Similar assays, using affinity-purified polyclonal rabbit IgG or monoclonal antibodies, are available to measure airborne α-amylase allergens (66,67). Some semiquantitative assays have been developed to measure cellulase and xylanase in the air (78).

In two studies, personal dust exposure levels were compared with wheat allergen exposure levels. The wheat content of the inhalable dust varied strongly depending on the use of products other than wheat flour (91,93). In the second study the relationship between dust level and wheat allergen levels depended on the type of bakery (93). The correlation was strongest in bread bakeries, weakest in pastry bakeries, and intermediate for mixed bakeries. Allergen content of the dust (expressed as the ratio of wheat antigen/dust) varied from 2850 ng/mg for dough makers, to 1150 ng/mg for oven staff, to 350 ng/mg for slicers, packers, and transport workers in large bakeries. In small, family-based bakeries ratios between 1950 ng/mg (bread bakeries) and 1550 ng/mg (confectioneries) were observed. There were also considerable differences in the ratios of wheat allergen and dust between industries, dependent on the end-product. For instance, within the group of dough makers the ratio varied from 4750 ng/mg (wheat bread production), to 1900 ng/mg (crisp bake production), to 550 ng/mg (rye bread production).

For fungal α-amylase the correlation with dust exposure was only 0.19 in a sample of 357 dust measurements taken in one industry (22,67). This study illustrated that dust concentration is a poor approximation of the allergen exposure level in bakeries, and that misclassification of exposure may occur in epidemiological surveys when bakery workers are classified based on dust exposure levels only. A major drawback of the use of immunoassays is that assay characteristics differ between laboratories. The use of different standard allergen preparations and antibody sources hampers the comparison of allergen levels reported by different research groups. This requires rigid standardization and harmonization in the near future.

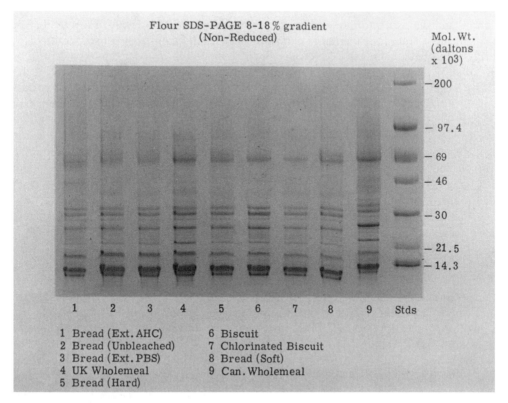

Figure 1 SDS-PAGE gel of different flours + standards. Note common proteins: (1) bread; (2) bread (unbleached) (extracted in ammonium carbonate); (3) bread; (4) U.K. wholemeal (extracted in phosphate-buffered saline); (5) bread (hard); (6) biscuit; (7) chlorinated biscuit; (8) bread (soft); (9) Canadian wholemeal.

Occasionally, particle size distribution of flour dust has been determined, showing that particles larger than 10 μm predominate (90,97). Only a small fraction of the dust (approximately 20%) belongs to the respirable fraction (roughly <5 μm). Both wheat and α-amylase allergens are predominantly present in particulates larger than 5 μm (93,97). Exposure to mainly larger particulates has a few important implications. The dust that is generated is airborne for only a short period because sedimentation occurs soon after emission of the dust, and sedimentation of particulates larger than 10 μm takes only a matter of minutes. Bystander exposures will rarely occur and background exposure levels will be extremely low. As a result, bakery workers will mainly be exposed to a series of short peaks that occur during dusty tasks. A small field study in which the dust exposure was monitored continuously showed that the 8-hr dust exposure could almost entirely be explained by the number of dust peaks that occurred during the day (98).

Little is known about exposure to airborne fungi in bakeries. A large variety of fungal species has been found in bakeries (87,99–102). The dominating mold species varied from study to study, suggesting that local circumstances in each bakery may be very important. Reliable quantitative exposure data for airborne fungi in bakeries have not been published.

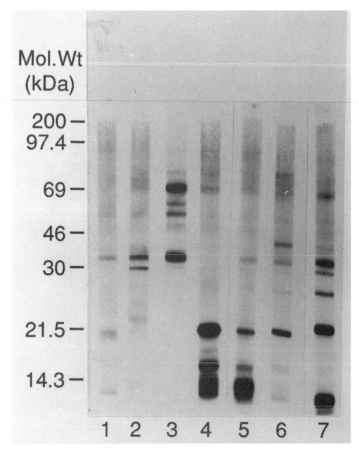

Figure 2 Western blot of Canadian western red spring flour probed with sera of seven patients allergic to flour (1–7). IgE in different sera bind to different flour proteins.

EPIDEMIOLOGY

Prevalence and Incidence Data

Sensitization to wheat flour or fungal amylase has been evaluated in a large number of cross-sectional studies, either by skin testing or by measurement of specific IgE antibodies in sera. Sensitization rates vary from 5–25% for wheat flour and from 2 to 15% for α-amylase (14,15,20–25,82,105,107). Sensitization rates for other allergens from bakeries such as and bakers' yeast (*Sacchromyces sereviciae*) and enzymes such as xylanase are considerably lower and in most cases below 1–2% (22,25,60,103,104). Sensitization to other allergens has been reported in case studies, but has not been studied routinely in epidemiological studies. A detailed comparison of the studies is not possible as these tests have been performed with different methods, extracts, and cutoff points. Moreover, little data are available about background levels of sensitization while some occupationally unexposed individuals have specific IgE to allergens possibly due to an increased propensity to develop IgE-mediated sensitization in atopic individuals, or as a result of cosensitization or cross-reactivity to other allergens, for instance pollens (105,108).

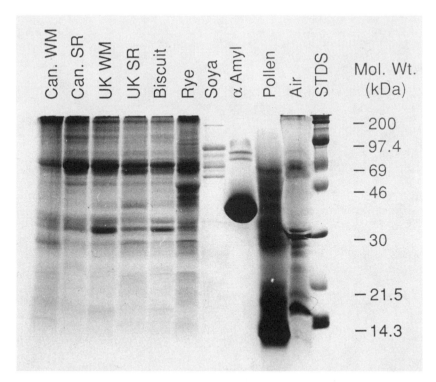

Figure 3 SDS-Page of 10 samples + standards. (1) Canadian wholemeal flour; (2) Canadian self-rising flour; (3) U.K. wholemeal flour; (4) U.K. self-rising flour; (5) biscuit flour; (6) rye flour; (7) soya flour; (8) fungal α-amylase; (9) rye grass pollen; (10) air sample eluate.

A large number of cross-sectional studies have shown that prevalence rates of respiratory symptoms are high. Rhinitis and asthma-like symptoms can be found in 5–25% of the workers (14,15,20–25,82,105–107,109). However, several of these studies have important methodological shortcomings. The participation rate is not known, methods have not been described, and information on exposure or risk modifiers (atopy, gender, smoking) is not given.

Apart from information from registry-based studies, little information is available on the incidence of asthma in bakers' asthma from studies in the industry. Gadborg (13) studied 1555 Danish bakers in Copenhagen. Of a random sample of 500, 487 could be traced and were reexamined after 5–6 years. Nineteen had developed wheat flour sensitization and seven had developed a wheat-flour-induced respiratory allergy, defined as the presence of symptoms and sensitization. The incidence rate for wheat flour sensitization was in the order of magnitude of 10 per 1000 workers per year, and for respiratory wheat allergy 3–4 per 1000 per year. A German cohort study in 880 bakers' apprentices with a 5-year follow-up and annual skin prick testing showed cumulative incidence figures for the number of positive tests of 12% in the second year, 19% in the third, 27% in the fourth, and 30% in the fifth (14,110). Symptom rates compatible with allergic rhinitis or asthma rose as well from 0.2% to 7% in year 3 and dropped to 4.8% after 5 years. A major problem of the study was the enormous loss to follow-up particularly in the later years of the study. The follow-up rates after the second year were below 33% (baseline 100%; 1st year 74%; 2nd 48%; 3rd 33%; 4th 11%; and 5th 4.2%), which could have

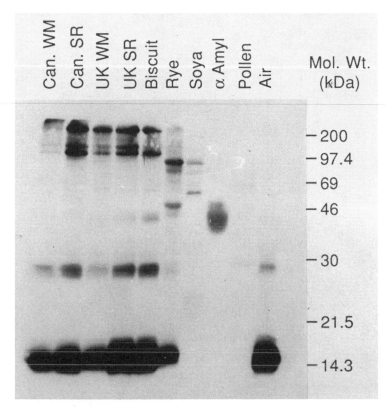

Figure 4　Western blot of the 10 samples in Figure 3 probed with pooled patients' sera allergic to flour.

biased the prevalence and cumulative incidence rates considerably. In a Swedish study the asthma incidence rates were estimated in a retrospective cohort study comprising 2226 workers trained as bakers between 1959 and 1989 and two reference categories (111). Men employed as bakers had an incidence rate of 3.0 cases per 1000 person-years, versus 0.9–1.9 for the referents. For female bakers, no increased risk was observed. In a British study incidence rates for specific sensitization and respiratory symptoms were reported for 103 newly exposed bakers (15). For chest and eye/nose symptoms incidence rates of approximately 2 and 19 per 1000 person-months, respectively, were found. The incidence of positive skin prick tests to α-amylase were more common (6 per 1000 person-months) than to flour (0.6 per 1000 person-months).

Determinants and Exposure-Response Studies

Two early studies were able to show exposure-sensitization relationships using dust exposure data. A cross-sectional study among 314 bakery workers (112,113) showed that dust exposure, measured by 2–4-hr personal dust samples, was positively associated with wheat flour sensitization in symptom-free workers. Sensitization to allergens in the work environment was more common among highly-exposed workers compared with low-exposed workers (OR = 3.0) in a U.K. study, when workers were ranked by dust exposure using information on perceived dustiness (25).

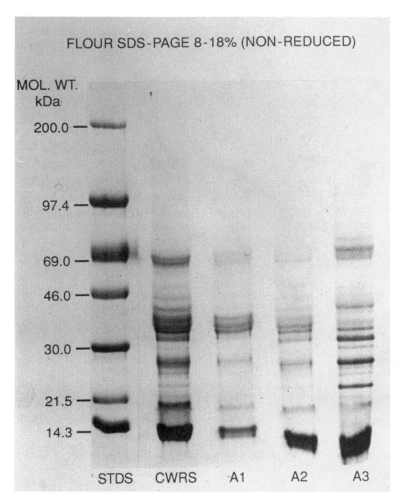

Figure 5 SDS-PAGE of four samples + standards. Canadian western red spring (CWRS); three air sample eluates (A1, A2, A3) from bakeries.

More recent studies have included quantitative exposure data on both inhalable dust and airborne allergens. Cullinan et al. (21) divided 264 workers from bakeries and flour mills without a previous flour exposure into three dust (<1 mg/m^3, 1–5 mg/m^3, >5 mg/ m^3) and wheat (<101 μg/m^3, 101–225 μg/m^3, >225 μg/m^3) exposure categories. The sensitization rate to wheat flour and α-amylase tended to increase with intensity of dust exposure and wheat allergen exposure. Work-related sensitization was more often observed in atopics than in nonatopics. Interestingly, flour and amylase sensitization in nonatopics occurred only in those with a high exposure. Work-related sensitization occurred in low-exposed atopics, but more frequently in high-exposed atopics. The authors did not test for statistical significance, but a multiple regression analysis (correcting for age, gender, smoking, and atopic status) did not reveal an independent effect of aeroallergen exposure probably because of lack of sufficient power. Respiratory symptoms were related to wheat allergen levels in atopics, but not in nonatopics.

In a Dutch study 393 bakery workers were divided into three exposure groups with mean wheat flour allergen exposure levels of 0.2, 3.5, and 11.0 μg/m^3 (mean dust exposure

Table 1 Prevalence of Wheat Flour Sensitization (Specific IgE) by Wheat Allergen Exposure Category and Atopy Defined as Total Serum IgE $\geq$100 kU/L (n = 346)

	Positive IgE for wheat flour	
Whole population (n = 346)		
Low wheat allergen exposure	4/90	4.4%
Intermediate wheat allergen exposure	5/64	7.8%
High wheat allergen exposure	27/192	14.1%
Atopic workers (n = 87)		
Low wheat allergen exposure	1/22	4.6%
Intermediate wheat allergen exposure	2/17	11.8%
High wheat allergen exposure	11/48	22.9%
Nonatopic workers (n = 259)		
Low wheat allergen exposure	3/68	4.4%
Intermediate wheat allergen exposure	3/47	6.4%
High wheat allergen exposure	16/144	11.1%

Source: From Ref. 23.

levels in these groups were 0.5, 0.8, and 2.4 mg/m^3, respectively) (23). A strong, statistically significant, and positive association was found between wheat flour allergen exposure and wheat-flour-specific sensitization (Table 1). These associations were found in both atopic and nonatopic workers, but the relationship was much steeper in atopics. This study showed that exposure levels have to be reduced at least until the exposure levels of the lowest exposure category (0.2 μg/m^3 wheat allergen exposure or 0.5 mg/m^3 dust exposure during a work shift), to achieve a considerable reduction in risk sensitization to wheat flour. The same group reported exposure-sensitization relationships for α-amylase allergens in a population of 169 workers from a rusk-producing industry (22). A strong and positive relationship was shown between α-amylase allergen exposure levels and α-amylase specific sensitization. As for wheat allergens, this relationship differed between atopic and nonatopic bakery workers.

Atopy is the most important risk modifier of work-related sensitization. In most studies atopy was defined as a positive skin prick test to one or more common allergens (grasses, trees, house dust mites). The risk of work-related sensitization was 5–20 times higher in atopics compared to nonatopics. Only one study (24) identified smoking of cigarettes as a risk factor of work-related sensitization.

DIAGNOSIS

The diagnosis of allergy in bakery and flour mill workers is based on an appropriate history of respiratory symptoms—particularly of the nose and airways—in an individual with relevant exposure at work. Symptoms develop only after an initial symptom-free period of exposure, which can range from months to several years. Rhinitis often accompanies asthma and may have developed before the onset of asthma, but asthma in the absence of rhinitis is not uncommon. The majority of subjects identify a clear relationship between periods at work and the development or worsening of their symptoms. Nasal and asthmatic symptoms can develop within minutes of exposure but asthmatic symptoms may develop after several hours. Asthmatic symptoms may resolve within a few hours of leaving work but can persist for 24 hr or more, causing nocturnal waking with asthma. In these circumstances symptomatic improvement may not be sufficient to be appreciated during a weekend away from work and only recognized during a 1- or 2-week vacation. Objective evidence in support of the diagnosis of occupational asthma can be obtained from specific IgE response, series peak flow measurements, or inhalation tests. *Specific IgE* can be identified either by an immediate wheal-and-flare response to a skin prick test with the relevant allergen or in serum by methods such as RAST. In general, specific IgE is a sensitive, but not specific, test for occupational asthma caused by protein allergens. However, in asthma in bakery and flour mill workers the large number of potentially relevant allergens—grain, flour, additives (particularly enzymes), and possibly mites and molds—limits the diagnostic value of specific IgE if absent in a patient with an appropriate history. In the majority of cases, in bakery and flour mill workers, allergy is to grain or flour proteins or to fungal α-amylase. Because the frequency of specific IgE to these allergens is greater than asthma caused by them, when present, they only have diagnostic value in those occupationally exposed with a history of work-related nasal or asthmatic symptoms. *Serial peak flow measurements*, ideally made at 2–3-hourly intervals from waking to sleep during a 4-week period, which includes periods at and away from work, can identify work-related asthma (with deterioration during periods at work and improvement during absence from work), but do not identify its cause (Fig. 6).

The diagnosis of occupational asthma in bakery and flour mill workers can usually be made on the basis of (1) relevant occupation and exposure, (2) history of work-related respiratory symptoms that have developed since initial occupational exposure, (3) serial peak flow measurements that show work-related asthma, and (4) specific IgE to extracts of relevant allergens, usually flour or grain proteins or the enzyme α-amylase. In a few patients the diagnosis remains unclear after these investigations. Medical decision-making procedures that facilitate combination on information from different diagnostic tests in decision trees may be helpful when surveillance data have to be interpreted (114). Because of the important social and financial implications of a diagnosis of occupational asthma—in particular the need to avoid further exposure and change work if asthma is caused by allergy to an agent encountered at work—inhalation testing with relevant allergens may be indicated, although this is now uncommon. Inhalation testing with the responsible allergen can provoke an immediate asthmatic response, which develops within minutes and can last 1–2 hr, a late asthmatic response, which develops after 1–2 hr, is maximal at 6–8 hr, and has usually resolved by 24 hr, or both—a dual asthmatic response. The late asthmatic reaction is often accompanied by an increase in nonspecific airway responsiveness (Fig. 7).

MANAGEMENT

The management of cases of occupational asthma in bakery and flour mill workers is based on the avoidance of further exposure to the cause of their asthma. This can in theory be achieved by (1) reduction in dust exposure at work, (2) use of respiratory protection, or (3) change of work. In practice, because, once sensitized, individuals react to very low concentrations of inhaled allergen, in the usual circumstances of work in bakeries and flour mills reduction in dust exposure is impractical. The use of respiratory protection is also usually impractical as a long-term solution in the majority of cases, but can allow an individual to continue in employment and provide time to consider and obtain alternative

PEAK FLOW RATES IN BAKER SENSITIVE TO FLOUR

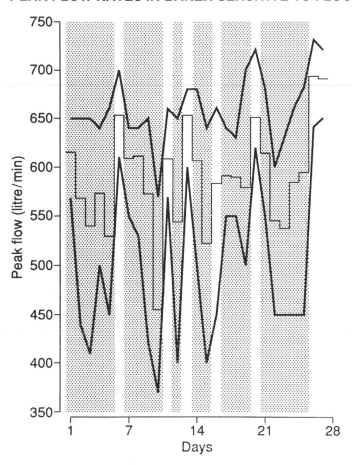

Figure 6   Serial peak flow measurements in a flour mill worker showing work-related asthma with improvement with use of respiratory protection.

employment. Avoidance of exposure usually requires a change of work. In many cases, particularly small family bakeries, an alternative site of work in the bakery, where exposure to flour can be avoided, cannot be found and exposure is only adequately avoided by leaving work. In large bakeries relocation at work is a more feasible solution, but even here, because of the dustiness of bakeries and flour mills, avoidance of exposure, sufficient not to provoke asthmatic symptoms, can be difficult to ensure. The important social and financial implications of a diagnosis of occupational asthma make it essential that the diagnosis be made only on the basis of sufficient evidence. In the United Kingdom one-third of individuals with occupational asthma were without employment 3–5 years after the diagnosis had been made (115). Loss of employment consequent upon an incorrect diagnosis can be disastrous. The consequences of misdiagnosis can be as serious as missing the diagnosis. Because of the adverse financial consequences of leaving work in economies with relatively high levels of unemployment, some bakery and flour mill workers with occupational asthma choose to remain in employment, despite being made aware that their asthma is likely to become increasingly severe and may become irreversible. In these

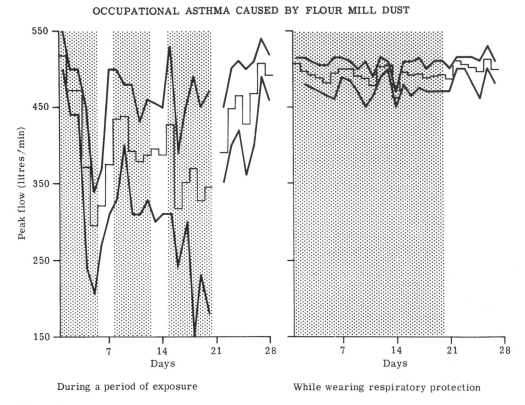

OCCUPATIONAL ASTHMA CAUSED BY FLOUR MILL DUST

Figure 7 Asthmatic reaction in a baker associated with increased airway responsiveness provoked by α-amylase.

circumstances steps should, where possible in conjunction with their employers, be taken to minimize their exposure to flour dust at work and to wear respiratory protection when in contact with dust. It is unlikely these measures alone will be sufficient to control their asthma, which should be treated in the same way as asthma not caused by work with anti-inflammatory and symptomatic treatment taken primarily by inhalation.

PREVENTION

Reduction of Dust and Allergen Exposure

Little quantitative information is available on the contribution of different determinants of exposure in the baking industry (equipment, technology, production layout). However, it is clear that several dusty tasks contribute to the high exposures of dough makers and other workers in this industry. Studies using real-time aerosol monitors showed that tasks like emptying bags, compressing empty (paper) bags containing flour or dough improvers, and dusting dough during forming to prevent dough adhesion to surfaces are among the dustiest tasks. Cleaning with brooms or the use of pressurized air leads to high exposures as well. Silo- and bin-cleaning tasks resulted in the highest dust exposure, according to one study (116). Some dough makers are involved in weighing of ingredients on simple scales and this activity can lead to high peak exposures. A recent Canadian study examined several potential determinants of dust exposure. The study shows that use of horizontal mixers is associated with higher dust exposures than use of vertical mixers (geometric mean exposure 13.0 mg/m^3 vs. 3.8 mg/m^3; $p < 0.001$) (95). Use of divider oil to prevent dough adhesion was associated with considerably lower exposures (geometric mean) than dusting with flour (geometric mean 0.43 mg/m^3 vs. 12.0 mg/m^3; $p < 0.001$) (95). Dough brakes led to exposures that were orders of magnitudes higher than use of other forming methods such as automated forming (95,116). The use of reversible sheeters lead to increased exposures as well, probably because rapid changes in direction of the machine's belt-like surface can result in emissions of dust particles.

The high exposures that occur during the performance of these tasks can be eliminated by fundamental modifications to the baking process and effective use of ventilation technology. The use of flour silos in combination with compressed air to transport flour instead of bags is potentially an effective, but fundamental change to the process. Use of exhaust ventilation in a ring around the dough mixer can reduce exposure levels considerably. General room ventilation is seldom effective. Covering dough mixers can further reduce exposure of dough makers when the flour is mixed. Automation of parts of the process is a long-term option that can lead to considerably lower exposure levels (117); however, maintenance of automated equipment seems crucial (95). A major source of wheat exposure occurs when the dough is covered with some flour, often by hand, to prevent sticking. For certain products the use of divider oil seems possible to reduce exposures. When the use of flour to dust dough is inevitable, these tasks could be performed using flow tables. This requires considerable investments. An unnecessary exposure to amylase occurs if enriched flour is used for this purpose. Exposure to enzymes could be reduced by the use of encapsulated or micropalletized or dissolved enzyme formulations. However, there seems to exist some reluctance to use these alternative enzyme formulations probably because this might also involve changes in mixing and rising times.

SUMMARY

Occupational asthma and rhinitis caused by allergens encountered in bakeries and flour mills is an important occupational health problem that may be increasing in prevalence. The nature of the responsible allergens and in particular the importance of fungal α-amylase as a cause of asthma in bakers has become clear in recent years. The identification of the responsible allergens and the development of methods to measure their concentration in air have allowed the study of exposure–response relationships. These studies, although to date few in number, have shown that the frequency of sensitization and respiratory symptoms, both nasal and asthmatic, increases with increasing exposure and implies that the disease incidence can be reduced by improved control of allergen exposure in the workplace. The physiological as well as financial and social consequences for those bakery and flour mill workers who develop occupational asthma make application of the scientific findings now available an important priority.

ACKNOWLEDGMENTS

We would like to thank Gert Doekes and Remko Houba for their useful comments and suggestions.

REFERENCES

1. Besche A de. Serologische Untersuchungen über "Allergische Krankheiten" beim Menchen. Acta Pathol Microbiol Scand 1929; 6:115–144.

2. Baagöe KH. Mehlidiosynkrasie als Ursache vasomotorischer Rhinitis und Asthma. Acta Med Scand 1933; 80:310–322.

3. Meredith SK, Taylor VM, McDonald JC. Occupational respiratory disease in the United Kingdom 1989: a report to the British Thoracic Society and the Society of Occupational Medicine by the SWORD project group. Br J Ind Med 1991; 48:292–298.

4. Meredith S. Reported incidence of occupational asthma in the United Kingdom, 1989–1990. J Epidemiol Commun Health 1993; 47:459–463.

5. Meredith SK, McDonald JC. Work-related respiratory disease in the United Kingdom, 1989–1992: report on the SWORD project. Occup Med 1994; 44:183–189.

6. Sallie BA, Ross DJ, Meredith SK, McDonald JC. SWORD '93. Surveillance of work-related and occupational disease in the UK. Occup Med 1994; 44:177–182.

7. Malmberg P. Yrken/arbetsmiljöer med hög sjuklighet i respirationsorganen. Arbete Och Hälsa 1990:6. [As quoted by Brisman J, Järvholm BG. Occurrence of self-reported asthma among Swedish bakers. Scand J Work Environ Health 1995; 21:487–493.]

8. Thiel H. Inhalationsallergien bei Bäckern—Aktuelle probleme des Mehlberufsasthmas. Lebensversicherungsmedizin 1984; 4:82–87.

9. Baur X. Allergien inm Backgewerbe. Allergologie 1993; 16:245.

10. Nordman H. Occupational asthma—time for prevention. Scand J Work Environ Health 1994; 20(special issue):108–115.

11. Grieshaber R, Rothe R. Obstruktive Atemwegserkrankungen in Bäckereien. Staub 1995; 55:403–407.

12. Mastrangelo G, Bombana S, Priante E, Gallo A, Saia B. Repeated case-control studies as a method of surveillance for asthma in occupations. J Occup Environ Med 1997; 39:51–57.

13. Gadborg E. Allergy to flour. Thesis, Copenhagen, 1956. [As quoted by Bonnevie P. Occupational allergy in bakery, 1958, and Thiel H, Kallweit C. Das Bäckerasthma—eine klassische allergische Berufskrankheit, Allergologie 1984; 7:407–414.]

14. Herxheimer H. Skin sensitivity to flour in bakers' apprentices. Lancet 1967; 1:83–84.

15. Cullinan P, Lowson D, Nieuwenhuijsen M, Sandiford C, Tee RD, Venables KM, McDonald JC, Newman Taylor AJ. Work-related symptoms, specific sensitization and exposure in a cohort of flour workers. Eur Respir J 1995; 8(Suppl 19):272s.

16. DeMers MP, Orris P. Occupational exposure and asthma mortality. JAMA 1994; 272:1575.

17. Hendrick DJ, Davies RJ, Pepys J. Bakers' asthma. Clin Allergy 1976; 6:241–250.

18. Nakamura S. On occupational allergic asthma of different kinds newly found in our allergy clinic. J Asthma Res 1972; 10:37–47.

19. Zuskin E, Mustajbegovic J, Schachter EN, Kern J. Respiratory symptoms and ventilatory function in confectionery workers. Occup Environ Med 1994; 51:435–439.

20. Zuskin E, Kanceljak B, Mustajbegovic J, Schachter EN. Immunologic findings in confectionary workers. Ann Allergy 1994; 73:521–526.

21. Cullinan P, Lowson D, Nieuwenhuijsen MJ, Sandiford C, Tee RD, Venables KM, McDonald JC, Newman Taylor AJ. Work related symptoms, sensitisation, and estimated exposure in workers not previously exposed to flour. Occup Environ Med 1994; 51:579–583.

22. Houba R, Heederik DJJ, Doekes G, van Run PEM. Exposure-sensitization relationship for α-amylase allergens in the baking industry. Am J Respir Crit Care Med 1996; 154:130–136.

23. Houba R, Heederik D, Doekes G. Wheat sensitization and work related respiratory symptoms are preventable: an epidemiological study. Am J Respir Crit Care Med 1998; 158:1499–1503.

24. De Zotti R, Larese F, Bovenzi M, Negro C, Molinari S. Allergic airway disease in Italian bakers and pastry makers. Occup Environ Med 1994; 51:548–552.

25. Musk AW, Venables KM, Crook B, Nunn AJ, Hawkins R, Crook GD, Graneek BJ, Tee RD, Farrer N, Johnson DA, Gordon DJ, Darbyshire JH, Newman Taylor AJ. Respiratory symptoms, lung function, and sensitisation to flour in a British bakery. Br J Ind Med 1989; 46: 636–642.
26. Block G, Tse KS, Kijek K, Chan H, Chan-Yeung M. Baker's asthma—studies of the cross-antigenicity between different cereal grains. Clin Allergy 1984; 14:177–185.
27. Prichard MG, Ryan G, Musk AW. Wheat flour sensitisation and airways disease in urban bakers. Br J Ind Med 1984; 41:450–454.
28. Sutton R, Skerritt JH, Baldo BA, Wrigley CW. The diversity of allergens involved in bakers' asthma. Clin Allergy 1984; 14:93–107.
29. Valdivieso R, Moneo I, Pola J, Muñoz T, Zapata C, Hinojosa M, Losada E. Occupational asthma and contact urticaria caused by buckwheat flour. Ann Allergy 1989; 63:149–152.
30. Baldo BA, Krilis S, Wrigley CW. Hypersensitivity to inhaled flour allergens—comparison between cereals. Allergy 1980; 35:45–56.
31. Sandiford CP, Tee RD, Newman Taylor AJ. Identification of crossreacting wheat, rye, barley and soya flour allergens using sera from individuals with wheat-induced asthma. Clin Exp Allergy 1995; 25:340–349.
32. Fränken J, Stephan U, Meyer HE, König W. Identification of alpha-amylase inhibitor as a major allergen of wheat flour. Int Arch Allergy Immunol 1994; 104:171–174.
33. Nakamura R, Matsuda T. Rice allergenic protein and molecular-genetic approach for hypoallergenic rice. Biosci Biotechnol Biochem 1996; 60:1215–1221.
34. García-Casado G, Armentia A, Sánchez-Monge R, Sánchez LM, Lopez-Otín C, Salcedo G. A major bakers' asthma allergen from rye flour is considerably more active than its barley counterpart. FEBS Lett 1995; 364:36–40.
35. Baldo BA, Wrigley CW. IgE antibodies to wheat flour components. Clin Allergy 1978; 8: 109–124.
36. Prichard MG, Ryan G, Walsh BJ, Musk AW. Skin test and RAST responses to wheat and common allergens and respiratory disease in bakers. Clin Allergy 1985; 15:203–210.
37. Walsh BJ, Wrigley CW, Musk AW, Baldo BA. A comparison of the binding of IgE in the sera of patients with bakers' asthma to soluble and insoluble wheat-grain proteins. J Allergy Clin Immunol 1985; 76:23–28.
38. Blands J, Diamant B, Kallós P, Kallós-Deffner L, Løwenstein H. Flour allergy in bakers—identification of allergenic fractions in flour and comparison of diagnostic methods. Int Arch Allergy Appl Immunol 1976; 52:392–406.
39. Gómez L, Martin E, Hernández D, Sánchez-Monge R, Barber D, del Pozo V, de Andrés B, Armentia A, Lahoz C, Salcedo G, Palomino P. Members of the α-amylase inhibitors family from wheat endosperm are major allergens associated with bakers' asthma. FEBS Lett 1990; 261:85–88.
40. Pfeil T, Schwabl U, Ulmer WT, König W. Western blot analysis of water-soluble wheat flour (*Triticum vulgaris*) allergens. Int Arch Allergy Appl Immunol 1990; 91:224–231.
41. Sandiford CP, Tee RD, Newman Taylor AJ. Identification of major allergenic flour proteins in order to develop assays to measure flour aeroallergen. Clin Exp Allergy 1990; 20(Suppl 1):3.
42. Sandiford CP, Tee RD, Newman Taylor AJ. Comparison of allergens detected by rabbit and human sera by western blotting of wheat flour. 1991; 132.
43. Boisen S. Comparative physico-chemical studies on purified trypsin inhibitors from the endosperm of barley, rye, and wheat. Z Lebensm Unters Forsch 1983; 176:434–439.
44. Posch A, Weiss W, Wheeler C, Dunn MJ, Görg A. Sequence analysis of wheat grain allergens separated by two-dimensional electrophoresis with immobilized pH gradients. Electrophoresis 1995; 16:1115–1119.
45. Weiss W, Huber G, Engel KH, Pethran A, Dunn MJ, Gooley AA, Görg A. Identification and characterization of wheat grain albumine/globulin allergens. Electrophoresis 1997; 18: 826–833.

46. Sanchez-Monge R, Gomez L, Barber D, Lopez-Otin C, Armentia A, Salcedo G. Wheat and barley allergens associated with bakers' asthma—glycosylated subunits of the α-amylase-inhibitor family have enhanced IgE-binding capacity. Biochem J 1992; 281:401–405.

47. Armentia A, Sanchez-Monge R, Gomez L, Barber D, Salcedo G. In vivo allergenic activities of eleven purified members of a major allergen family from wheat and barley flour. Clin Exp Allergy 1993; 23:410–415.

48. Garcia-Olmedo F, Salcedo G, Sanchez-Monge R, Gomez L, Royo J, Carbonero P. Plant proteinaceous inhibitors of proteinases and α-amylases. Oxford Surveys Plant Mol Cell Biol 1987; 4:275–334.

49. Mena M, Sanchez-Monge R, Gomez L, Salcedo G, Carbonero P. A major barley allergen associated with bakers' asthma disease is a glycosylated monomeric inhibitor of insect α-amylase: cDNA cloning and chromosomal location of the gene. Plant Mol Biol 1992; 20: 451–458.

50. Adachi T, Alvarez AM, Aoki N, Nakamura R, Garcia VV, Matsuda T. Screening of rice strains deficient in 16-kDa allergenic protein. Biosci Biotechnol Biochem 1995; 59:1377–1378.

51. García-Casado G, Armentia A, Sánchez-Monge R, Malpica JM, Salcedo G. Rye flour allergens associated with bakers' asthma. Correlation between in vivo and in vitro activities and comparison with their wheat and barley homologues. Clin Exp Allergy 1996; 26:428–435.

52. Barber D, Sánchez-Monge R, Gómez L, Carpizo J, Armentia A, López-Otín C, Juan F, Salcedo G. A barley flour inhibitor of insect α-amylase is a major allergen associated with bakers' asthma disease. FEBS Lett 1989; 248:119–122.

53. Heyer N. Backmittel als berufsbedingte Inhalationsallergene bei mehlverarbeitenden Berufen. Allergologie 1983; 6:389–392.

54. Jorde W, Heyer N, Schata M. Bäckereirohstoffe als berufsspezifische Allergene. Allergologie 1986; s552–s524.

55. Wüthrich B, Baur X. Backmittel, insbesondere α-Amylase, als berufliche Inhalationsallergene in der Backwarenindustrie. Schweiz Med Wochenschr 1990; 120:446–450.

56. Baur X, Fruhmann G, Haug B, Rasche B, Reiher W, Weiss W. Role of aspergillus amylase in bakers' asthma. Lancet 1986; 1:43.

56a. Baur X. Allergien im Backgewerbe. Allergologie 1993; 16:245.

57. Birnbaum J, Latil F, Vervloet D, Senft M, Charpin J. Rôle de l'alpha-amylase dans l'asthme du boulanger. Rev Mal Respir 1988; 5:519–521.

58. Bermejo N, Maria Y, Gueant JL, Moneret-Vautrin DA. Allergie professionnelle du boulanger à l'alpha-amylase fongique. Rev Fr Allergol 1991; 31:56–58.

59. Blanco Carmona JG, Juste Picón S, Garcés Sotillos M. Occupational asthma in bakeries caused by sensitivity to α-amylase. Allergy 1991; 46:274–276.

60. Tarvainen K, Kanerva L, Tupasela O, Grenquist-Nordén B, Jolanki R, Estlander T, Keskinen H. Allergy from cellulase and xylanase enzymes. Clin Exp Allergy 1991; 21:609–615.

61. Quirce S, Cuevas M, Díez-Gómez ML, Fernández-Rivas M, Hinojosa M, González R, Losada E. Respiratory allergy to *Aspergillus*-derived enzymes in bakers' asthma. J Allergy Clin Immunol 1992; 90:970–978.

62. Valdivieso R, Subiza J, Subiza JL, Hinojosa M, Carlos E de, Subiza E. Bakers' asthma caused by alpha amylase. Ann Allergy 1994; 73:337–342.

63. Baur X, Sauer W, Weiss W. Baking additives as new allergens in bakers' asthma. Respiration 1988; 54:70–72.

64. Baur X, Chen Z, Sander I. Isolation and denomination of an important allergen in baking additives: α-amylase from *Aspergillus oryzae* (*Asp o* II). Clin Exp Allergy 1994; 24:465–470.

65. Sandiford CP, Tee RD, Newman Taylor AJ. The role of cereal and fungal amylases in cereal flour hypersensitivity. Clin Exp Allergy 1994; 24:549–557.

66. Sander I, Baur X. Evidence for continuous B-cell epitopes on α-amylase of *Aspergillus oryzae* (*Aspo* II). Allergy Clin Immunol 1994; 93:265.

67. Houba R, van Run P, Doekes G, Heederik D, Spithoven J. Airborne levels of α-amylase allergens in bakeries. J Allergy Clin Immunol 1997; 99:286–292.

68. Moneo I, Alday E, Sanchez-Agudo L, Curiel G, Lucena R, Calatrava JM. Skin-prick tests for hypersensitivity to α-amylase preparations. Occup Med 1995; 45:151–155.

69. Losada E, Hinojosa M, Quirce S, Sánchez-Cano M, Moneo I. Occupational asthma caused by α-amylase inhalation: clinical and immunological findings and bronchial response patterns. J Allergy Clin Immunol 1992; 89:118–125.

70. Baur X, Czuppon AB. Allergic reaction after eating α-amylase (*Asp o* 2)-containing bread. Allergy 1995; 50:85–87.

71. Kanny G, Moneret-Vautrin DA. α-Amylase contained in bread can induce food allergy. J Allergy Clin Immunol 1995 95:132–133.

72. Cullinan P, Lowson D, Nieuwenhuijsen M, Sandiford C, Tee RD, Venables KM, McDonald JC, Newman Taylor AJ. Work-related symptoms, specific sensitization and exposure in a cohort of flour workers. Eur Resp J 1995; 8:272 supplement.

73. Alday E, Moneo I, Lucena R, Curiel G. Alpha-amylase hypersensitivity: diagnostic methods. Allergy 1995; 50(Suppl 26):88.

74. Baur X, Sander I, Jansen A, Czuppon AB. Sind Amylasen von Backmitteln und Backmehl relevante Nahrungsmittelallergene? Schweiz Med Wochenschr 1994; 124:846–851.

75. Baur X, Czuppon AB, Sander I. Heating inactivates the enzymatic activity and partially inactivates the allergenic activity of *Asp o* 2. Clin Exp Allergy 1996; 26:232–234.

76. Sander I, Baur X. Evidence for continuous B-cell epitopes on α-amylase of *Aspergillus oryzae* (*Asp o* II). J Allergy Clin Immunol 1994; 93(nr.1 part 2):265.

77. Baur X, Sauer W, Weiss W, Fruhmann G. Inhalant allergens in modern baking industry. Immunol Allergy Pract 1989; 11:13–15.

78. Vanhanen M, Tuomi T, Hokkanen H, Tupasela O, Tuomainen A, Holmberg PC, Leisola M, Nordman H. Enzyme exposure and enzyme sensitisation in the baking industry. Occup Environ Med 1996; 53:670–676.

79. Armentia A, Tapias J, Barber D, Martin J, de la Fuente R, Sanchez P, Salcedo G, Carreira J. Sensitization to the storage mite *Lepidoglyphus destructor* in wheat flour respiratory allergy. Ann Allergy 1992; 68:398–403.

80. Revsbech P, Dueholm M. Storage mite allergy among bakers. Allergy 1990; 45:204–208.

81. Tee RD. Allergy to storage mites—review. Clin Exp Allergy 1994; 24:636–640.

82. De Zotti R, Molinari S, Larese F, Bovenzi M. Pre-employment screening among trainee bakers. Occup Environ Med 1995; 52:279–283.

83. Korsgaard J, Dahl R, Iversen M, Hallas T. Storage mites as a cause of bronchial asthma in Denmark. Allergol Immunopathol 1985; 13:143–149.

84. Müsken H, Bergmann Kch. Vorratsmilben: Biologie, Sensibilisierung, klinische Bedeutung. Allergologie 1992; 15:s189–s196.

85. Johansson E, Johansson SGO, Hage-Hamsten M van. Allergenic characterization of *Acarus siro* and *Tyrophagus putrescentiae* and their crossreactivity with *Lepidoglyphus destructor* and *Dermatophagoides pteronyssinus*. Clin Exp Allergy 1994; 24:743–751.

86. Weiner A. Occupational bronchial asthma in a baker due to *Aspergillus*—a case report. Ann Allergy 1960; 18:1004–1007.

87. Klaustermeyer WB, Bardana EJ, Hale FC. Pulmonary hypersensitivity to *Alternaria* and *Aspergillus* in bakers' asthma. Clin Allergy 1977; 7:227–233.

88. Bergmann I, Rebohle E, Wallenstein G, Gemeinhardt H, Thürmer H. Häufigkeit und Bedeutung von Schimmelpilzsensibilisierungen bei Werktätigen in der Backwarenindustrie. Allergie Immunol 1976; 22:297–301.

89. Wallenstein G, Bergmann I, Rebohle E, Gemeinhardt H, Thürmer H. Berufliche Atemtrakterkrankungen durch Schimmelpilze bei Getreidemüllern und Bäckern. Z Erkrank Atm Org 1980; 154:229–233.

90. Burdorf A, Lillienberg L, Brisman J. Characterization of exposure to inhalable flour dust in Swedish bakeries. Ann Occup Hyg 1994; 38:67–78.

91. Nieuwenhuijsen MJ, Sandiford CP, Lowson D, Tee RD, Venables KM, McDonald JC, Newman Taylor AJ. Dust and flour aeroallergen exposure in flour mills and bakeries. Occup Environ Med 1994; 51:584–588.

92. Nieuwenhuijsen MJ, Lowson D, Venables KM, Newman Taylor AJ. Flour dust exposure variability in flour mills and bakeries. Ann Occup Hyg 1995; 39:299–305.

93. Houba R, van Run P, Heederik D, Doekes G. Wheat antigen exposure assessment for epidemiologic studies in bakeries using personal dust sampling and inhibition ELISA. Clin Exp Allergy 1996; 26:154–163.

94. Houba R, Heederik D, Kromhout K. Grouping strategies for exposure to inhalable dust, wheat allergens and α-amylase allergens in bakeries. Ann Occup Hyg 1997; 41:287–296.

95. Burstyn I, Teschke K, Kennedy SM. Exposure levels and determinants of inhalable dust exposure in bakeries. Ann Occup Hyg 1997; 41:609–624.

96. Sandiford CP, Nieuwenhuijsen MJ, Tee RD, Newman Taylor AJ. Measurement of airborne proteins involved in bakers' asthma. Clin Exp Allergy 1994; 24:450–456.

97. Sandiford CP, Nieuwenhuijsen MJ, Tee RD, Newman Taylor AJ. Determination of the size of airborne flour particles. Allergy 1994; 49:891–893.

98. Jongedijk T, Meijler M, Houba R, Heederik D. Tijdstudies en vergelijkende piekblootstellingsmetingen in ambachtelijke bakkerijen. Tijdschr Toegepaste Arbowetenschap 1995; 8:1–8.

99. Charpin J, Lauriol-Mallea M, Renard M, Charpin H. Étude de la pollution fungique dans les boulangeries. Acad Natl Méd 1971; 19:52–55.

100. Singh A, Singh AB. Airborne fungi in a bakery and the prevalence of respiratory dysfunction among workers. Grana 1994; 33:349–358.

101. Gemeinhardt H, Bergmann I. Zum Vorkommen von Schimmelpilzen in Bäckereistäuben. Zentralbl Bakt Abt II 1977; 132:44–54.

102. Wüthrich B. Enzyme: potente inhalative und ingestive Allergene—fehlende Deklarationspflicht von Backmitteln und Backmehl. Schweiz Med Wochenschr 1994; 124:1361–1363.

103. Baldo BA, Baker RS. Inhalant allergies to fungi: reactions to bakers' yeast (*Saccharomyces cerevisiae*) and identification of bakers' yeast enolase as an important allergen. Int Arch Allergy Appl Immunol 1988; 86:201–208.

104. Belchi-Hernandez J, Mora-Gonzalez A, Iniesta-Perez J. Bakers' asthma caused by *Saccharomyces cerevisiae* in dry powder form. J Allergy Clin Immunol 1996; 97:131–134.

105. Gautrin D, Infante-Rivard C, Dao TV, Magnan-Larose M, Desjardins D, Malo JM. Specific IgE-dependent sensitization, atopy, and bronchial hyperresponsiveness in apprentices starting exposure to protein-derived agents. Am J Respir Crit Care Med 1997; 155:1841–1847.

106. Smith TA, Lumley KPS. Work-related asthma in a population exposed to grain, flour and other ingredient dusts. Occup Med 1996; 46:37–40.

107. Smith TA, Lumley KPS, Hui EHK. Allergy to flour and fungal amylase in bakery workers. Occup Med 1997; 47:21–24.

108. Sander I, Raulfheimsoth M, Duser M, Flagge A, Czuppon AB, Baur X. Differentiation between cosensitization and cross reactivity in wheat flour and grass pollen sensitized subjects. Int Arch Allergy Immunol 1997; 112:378–385.

109. Bohadana AB, Massin N, Wild P, Kolopp MN, Toamain JP. Respiratory symptoms and airway responsiveness in apparently healthy workers exposed to flour dust. Eur Respir J 1994; 7:1070–1076.

110. Herxheimer H. The skin sensitivity fo flour of bakers' apprentices. Acta Allergol 1973; 28:42–49.

111. Brisman J, Järvholm BG. Occurrence of self-reported asthma among Swedish bakers. Scand J Work Environ Health 1995; 21:487–493.

112. Hartmann AL, Wüthrich B, Deflorin-Stolz R, Helfenstein U, Hewitt B, Guérin B. Atopie-Screening: Prick-Multitest, Gesamt-IgE oder RAST? Schweiz Med Wochenschr 1985; 115:466–475.

113. Hartmann AL. Berufsallergien bei Bäckern—Epidemiologie; Diagnose, Therapie und Prophylaxe; Versicherungsrecht. München-Deisenhofen, Germany: Dustri-Verlag Dr Karl Feistle,1986.

114. Post WK, KM Venables, D Ross, P Cullinan, D Heederik, A Burdorf. Stepwise health surveillance for bronchial irritability syndrome in workers atrisk of occupational respiratory disease. Occup Environ Med 1998; 55:119–125.

115. Cannon J, Cullinan P, Newman Taylor A. Consequences of occupational asthma. Br Med J 1995; 311:602–603.

116. Nieuwenhuijsen MJ, Sandiford CP, Lowson D, Tee RD, Venables KM, Newman Taylor AJ. Peak exposure concentrations of dust and flour aeroallergen in flour mills and bakeries. Ann Occup Hyg 1995; 39:193–201.

117. Jauhiainen A, Louhelainen K, Linnainmaa M. Exposure to dust and α-amylase in bakeries. Appl Occup Environ Hyg 1993; 8:721–725.

22

Animal, Insect, and Shellfish Allergy

Susan Gordon and Anthony J. Newman Taylor
Imperial College School of Medicine at the National Heart and Lung Institute, London, England

INTRODUCTION

Occupational allergy is an important health problem for those exposed to animals, insects, and shellfish in their place of work. Exposure to laboratory animals such as rats, mice, guinea pigs, rabbits, and other species occurs in the pharmaceutical industry, in universities, and in research institutes among those undertaking scientific research or those involved in animal breeding and husbandry. The majority of the cases of allergic disease among laboratory animal workers are caused by rats and mice, probably because these are the animals most commonly used in experimental studies. Within the farming industry, the important animal species causing respiratory and other allergic symptoms are cows, pigs, horses, and deer. Occupational allergy to insects and shellfish occurs in those in entomological research and the food industry.

Since January 1989, British chest physicians and occupational physicians have reported new cases of lung disease to the Surveillance of Work Related and Occupational Respiratory Disease (SWORD) project (1). Laboratory animals are consistently among the three most commonly reported agents causing occupational asthma, comprising some 5% of the cases reported (2). Occupational lung disease caused by farm animals, insects, and shellfish is relatively rare in the United Kingdom (approximately 2% of reported cases), but they are more important causes of work-related disease in other countries.

The major source of allergens is the excreta and secreta of the animals and insects, which may become airborne and are inhaled by those working with them. The most usual manifestations of allergy are rhinitis, conjunctivitis, contact urticaria, and asthma; asthma is the least common but most important, as those with severe symptoms may be unable to continue their work. Many with allergy to animal and insect species, particularly those with asthma, have specific IgE antibody to the responsible proteins. The presence of specific IgE, identified by skin or serological testing, is helpful in diagnosis. The specificity of the immunoglobulin response has been exploited both to identify allergenic proteins in different potential sources (such as urine, serum, and pelt) and to measure the concentration of airborne allergens in the workplace.

Laboratory animal allergy is the best understood of the causes of occupational asthma considered here and although its recognition as an important occupational health problem has increased considerably in the past 15 years, knowledge of the factors determining the incidence of the disease remains limited. More needs to be learned about the influence of exposure in determining the immunological and tissue responses. Such knowledge is essential to provide the scientific basis for control measures to reduce disease incidence.

ANIMAL ALLERGENS: NATURE AND SOURCES

Rat (*Rattus norvegicus*) and Mouse (*Mus musculus*)

Urine is the major source of allergenic proteins for rats and mice (3) and the low-molecular-weight constituents have been identified as major allergens (Table 1). Alpha$_{2u}$-globulin (Rat n1.02) and MUP (Mus m1) may be glycosylated (4) and are synthesized in the liver in an analogous manner in both species, under complex hormonal control (5). These proteins have recently been identified as lipocalins (6), which have pheromonal properties (7) and share 66% of their amino acid sequence in common (8,9). The cross-reactivity has been confirmed by the ability of purified alpha$_{2u}$-globulin to cause proliferation of MUP-reactive clones (10) and in RAST inhibition experiments (11,12). Both alpha$_{2u}$-globulin and MUP appear in the urine, particularly of male animals after puberty, and disappear after castration or with senility.

All male rats develop chronic renal disease spontaneously (13) due to the production of alpha$_{2u}$-globulin and its ability to bind toxic chemicals (14). Male rats therefore secrete increasing levels of serum proteins in their urine as they mature. The serum proteins albumin and transferrin found in rat urine are allergenic for nearly 30% of rat-sensitive subjects (15,16) (Fig. 1). Conversely, most strains of mice do not develop chronic renal disease and secrete serum proteins in only trace amounts.

The secretory products of salivary, sebaceous, and other glands may be sources of allergen in both rats and mice. In both species sequence homology of these products with the urinary proteins alpha$_{2u}$-globulin and MUP have been shown (17–19). The antigenic similarity between the mouse proteins from salivary and urinary sources is, however, debated (20,21). A preliminary report of the allergens in male rat hair using sera from 77

Table 1 Occupational Allergens for Which the DNA and/or Amino Acid Sequence is Known (see also Ref. 162)

Allergen	Name	Molecular weight (kDa)	Function	Ref.
Rat	Rat n1.01, prealbumin	21	Lipocalin	6, 163
(*Rattus norvegicus*)	Rat n1.02, α_{2u}-globulin	17	Lipocalin	6, 163
Cow	Bos d2	20	Lipocalin	42, 164
(*Bos domesticus*)				
Horse	Equ c1	19	Lipocalin	165
(*Equus caballus*)				
Chrionomid midges	Chi t1	16	Haemoglobin	166
(*Chironomus thummi thummi*)				
Cockroach	Bla g2	36	Aspartic	167
(*Blatella germanica*)			protease	
Shrimp				
(*Metapenaeus ensis*)	Met e1	34	Tropomyosin	84
(*Penaeus aztecus*)	Pen a1	36	Tropomyosin	168

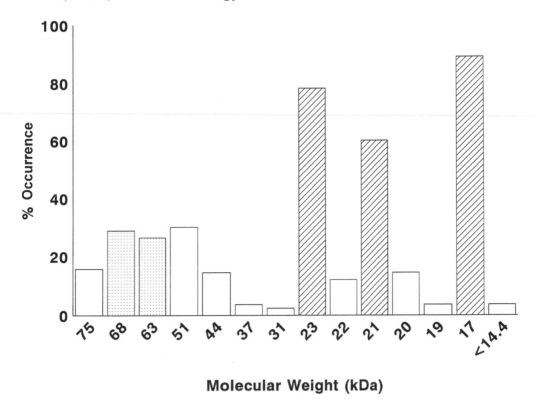

Molecular Weight (kDa)

Figure 1 Distribution of the male rat urine allergens recognized by 83 positive sera. Hatched bars, "major" allergens; dotted bars, "intermediate" allergens; open bars, "minor" allergens. The 75-kDa and 68-kDa allergens have been identified as transferrin and albumin respectively (see Ref. 16). (Data from Ref. 15.)

subjects and immunoblotting techniques identified 20 allergens with five "major" allergens at 55, 51, 19, 17 kDa, and a very-high-molecular-weight material (22). A major fur-derived allergen (Ag 3, Mus m2) (21) with a similar molecular weight to the urinary prealbumin (16 kDa), but which contains polysaccharide residues, is secreted from the hair follicle and coats the stratum corneum and the hair shafts. The allergenic composition of rat and mouse room dust has been infrequently studied. One recent study described 18 allergens in rat room dust. Three major allergens with molecular weights of 44, 21, and 17 kDa were identified, the 17-kDa protein having immunological cross-reactivity with Rat n1.02 (23). The hair (and possible salivary contaminants) was thought to be the most likely source of the high MW allergens found in airborne rat dust.

Minor differences in urinary proteins from different strains of mouse have been noted (24), but these do not affect allergenicity (25). Similarly, there are no important differences in the urinary allergens from different strains of rat (26). Whether there are differences in allergenic composition of fur and saliva from different strains of rats and mice is not known.

Other Laboratory Animals

Skin prick testing and RAST inhibition studies have confirmed that, in order of importance, fur, saliva, and urine are allergenic for most guinea pig (*Cavia porcellus*)-sensitized subjects. The major allergens in pelt have a MW of 10–22 kDa while those in urine are of a higher MW, 75–50 kDa (27). Approximately half of subjects have IgE specific for guinea pig serum and albumin. Crossed-radioimmunoelectrophoretic studies have identified 14 allergens in guinea pig–associated dust, four of which were major allergens and all of which were present in extracts of guinea pig dander, fur, saliva, and urine (28,29).

The nature and sources of rabbit *(Oryctolagus cuniculus)* allergens have been less extensively studied than those of rats, mice, and guinea pigs. The urine, fur, saliva, and dander/pelt have all been found to contain allergens (30–33). The major rabbit allergen (Ag R1) is a glycoprotein with a MW of 17 kDa and saliva and fur are the most potent sources. Albumin and immunoglobulin light-chain dimers are minor allergens that may originate from the pelt, serum, and urine. Ag R1 is a major allergenic constituent of dust collected from rabbit housing areas. Rabbit room dust exhibits some immunological cross-reactivity with rabbit saliva and urine extracts (32).

Although allergy to cats *(Felis domesticus)* and dogs *(Canis familiaris)* is generally perceived to be a domestic rather than an occupational problem, these species can be encountered in the workplace. In both species the most important allergenic sources of allergen are the pelt, dander, saliva, and urine. The biochemistry of the allergens and their relevance to laboratory animal allergy have recently been reviewed (34,35).

There have been few descriptions of allergy to gerbils (36), monkeys (37), and marmosets (Newman Taylor, unpublished data), and occupational allergy to these species is, presumably, rare. No detailed studies of the allergens involved have been undertaken, although skin prick testing with urine and dander of the animals shows these sources may contain potent allergens. Skin test (by scratch test) responses to monkey albumin have been reported among those sensitive to other mammalian albumins (38).

Farm Animals

In allergy induced by cows *(Bos domesticus)*, hair and dander are considered the most important allergenic sources. Two major allergens have been detected in cow dander extracts with MW of 20 (Bos d2) and 22 kDa (39). A major allergen with a MW of 20 kDa has also been identified in urine although urine is thought to be less potent than dander in inducing allergy (40). The 20-kDa epithelial allergen (BDA20, Bos d2) has been purified using specific monoclonal antibodies (41) and identified as a member of the lipocalin family (42). Several less important allergens have been described by immunoblotting with molecular weights of 16–24 kDa. Albumin (43) and an 11-kDa allergen, identified as an oligomycin-sensitivity-conferring protein of the mitochondrial adenosine triphosphate synthase complex (44), are thought to be minor allergens.

The allergens derived from deer (Cervidae) have been examined by immunoblotting and five allergens identified between 110 and 21 kDa (45). A study employing serum from eight deer-allergic subjects (46) showed that while urine and serum contained apparently no IgE-binding proteins, seven of the eight had IgE to proteins with a MW of 22 and 25 kDa in deer pelt and four had IgE to a 60 kDa-pelt allergen. The 22- and 25-kDa allergens had some degree of cross-reactivity with cow allergens. Cross-reactivity has also been reported with horse (47).

Although the physicochemical properties of the allergens involved in immediate hypersensitivity to pigs have not been elucidated, the urine, skin, hair, and dust of swine confinement buildings have all been shown to bind specific IgE in the serum of allergic workers (48–51).

Since the early work in the 1970s by Lowenstein and co-workers using crossed radioimmunoelectrophoresis [reviewed by Schou (34)], the importance of horse dander, hair, and skin scrapings as sources of horse allergens has been confirmed (52–54). Up to four major allergens have been described (Table 1). Albumin is thought to be a minor allergen. More detailed biochemical analysis has demonstrated the involvement of carbohydrate moieties in the binding of IgE to the 31-, 27- (possibly Equ c 1), and 14.4-kDa allergens (53).

Occupational sensitization to increasingly "exotic" species is being reported; raccoon (55), mink (56,57), and other species farmed for their fur have all recently been shown to be allergenic. The urine, fur, and epithelia again seem to be the principal sources of the allergens. In common with the observations made for the other animals discussed, significant cross-reactivity may exist between several apparently unrelated species and both low-molecular-weight allergens and albumin may contribute to this phenomenon. As mink may be susceptible to a viral disease resulting in marked proteinuria, this provides another example of how renal disease may affect the allergenic composition of urine (57).

Insects

The presence of specific IgE in cases of hypersensitivity to an increasing number of insect species has been demonstrated by skin prick tests and RAST. The species of insects identified as causing occupational hypersensitivity include flies (58–64), locusts (65), grasshoppers (66), bumblebees (67,68), mites (69–71), spiders (72), cockroaches (73), and chironimid midges (74,75).

There have been relatively few detailed biochemical studies of insect allergens. Epidemiological studies of workforces exposed to species of fly have generally employed extracts made from whole adult flies (58–60,62) and dust from the bottom of cages used to rear the flies (58,60). Immunoblot analyses of the allergens from the common housefly and blowflies show that most allergens have MWs of between 40 and 60 kDa (61,64). A major allergen for 70% of blowfly-allergic subjects was found at 67 kDa and a 20-kDa allergen may contribute to the extensive cross-reactivity found between different species of flies (59,61). An extract prepared from the salivary glands of the tsetse fly was shown to bind IgE from the serum of subjects who experienced anaphylactic symptoms after being bitten by these flies (63).

The feces and particularly the peritrophic membrane, a midgut secretion that encloses ingested food in its passage through the intestine and surrounds the feces when excreted, may be an important source of allergen for members of the order Orthoptera (65,66). Tee et al. identified multiple protein bands by SDS-PAGE in soluble extracts eluted from whole locust (65). The protein bands that bound most strongly to IgE, identified by immunoblot using sera from locust-allergic patients, were of MW 18, 29, 37, 43, 54, 66, and 68 kDa. The cockroach is more usually considered to be a domestic allergen and the allergens identified to date have been reviewed by Chapman (76) (Table 1). Laboratory workers using cockroaches for immunological investigations showed sensitization to whole-body as well as fecal extracts (73).

Honeybee body dust and venom are the major sources of allergen for those employed in the honey production industry or those using bees as a means of pollinating greenhouse crops (67,68). The role of the pollens originating from the plants used to feed the bees should not be overlooked as a potential sensitizing agent.

Although the source of the allergens involved in hypersensitivity to spider mites has not been identified in detail beyond originating from the body of these insects (69–71), the urticating hair shed from the back of the Brazilian spider is a potent source of allergen (72). Whole adult chironomids and their larvae may also elicit immediate skin prick test responses in sensitized subjects (74,75) but the hemoglobin of these insects (Chi t1) is known to be a major allergen (74,77).

As an important source of allergen for many insect species appears to be the feces, it is perhaps unsurprising that some investigators have noted some cross-reactivity of insects with the house dust mite (70). Baldo et al., who used 41 sera to investigate by immunoblotting the allergens present in extracts from seven insect species (including flies, moths, cockroaches, beetles, and silverfish), suggested that one-third of insect-sensitive subjects may have "pan allergy" to insects (78).

Shellfish

Several species of shellfish have been reported as causes of occupational asthma including snow-crab *(Chinoecetes opilis)* (79), lobster (80), shrimp *(Metapenaeus ensis)* (81,82), and clam (82). Sources of the crustacean and mollusk allergens include the water used in the preparation of the food (83) as well as the meat and exoskeleton of the animals; lyophilized meat may still contain allergens (82). The use of commercially available skin prick test solutions and research extracts both confirm that many individuals have multiple sensitivities to crustaceans and mollusks. Such multiple sensitivities may arise independently or be due to the presence of cross-reacting allergens or epitopes [e.g., in a study employing serum from food-allergic subjects the shrimp immunodominant allergen, Met e1 or tropomyosin, was found to be a common allergen among Crustacea and Mollusca (84)].

Other Allergens

A survey carried out in 1264 oyster handlers in 1964 showed that 20% had asthmatic symptoms (85). The oyster itself is not responsible for the reaction. A parasite, a Protochordae, seems the causal agent. Eighteen of 50 workers exposed to prawn had respiratory symptoms (86). A more recent survey carried out in 291 employees of a salmon-processing plant showed that 8.2% had occupational asthma attributed to an IgE-dependent reaction (87). Several other fish-derived allergens have been incriminated in case reports.

Summary

Excreta and secreta are the most important allergen sources for many animals and insects encountered in the occupational environment. While urine is probably the principal source of allergens in rodents, the fur and dander are probably allergenically more important for other mammalian species. Feces, saliva, venom, and the exoskeleton of various insects have all been shown to contain allergens. The meat and exoskeleton of shellfish and the water used in processing constitute significant sources of allergens.

MEASUREMENT OF EXPOSURE TO OCCUPATIONAL ALLERGENS

Methods

The quantification of airborne allergens was initially restricted to those with a distinct morphological appearance (e.g., pollen grains or mite bodies) or those that could be cultured (mold spores) or chemically assayed (e.g., isocyanates) (88). The measurement of amorphous allergen, such as animal allergens, became possible with the development of immunoassays. The most frequently used methods to measure airborne allergen concentration are discussed in more detail in another chapter.

The measurement of aeroallergen in the environment grows in importance as interest increases in studying the influence of aeroallergen exposure on the development of allergic disease and in controlling occupational allergen exposure. Comparison of absolute measurements of airborne allergen between studies, even for the same species, is difficult because of the different methods employed; reported levels for rat allergen under apparently comparable circumstances, for example, vary from 10^{-10} g/m^3 to 10^{-6} g/m^3. While factors such as the concentration of Tween-20 used in the filter elution buffer increase the elution of rat allergen by up to 10-fold (89), differences in the assay format and standards employed also contribute to these differences. It is currently popular to identify and quantify a "marker" protein, which ideally is also a major allergen (e.g., Bos d2, Rat n1). A recent comparison of the performance of a monoclonal antibody assay and a polyclonal assay (RAST inhibition) to measure rat airborne allergen has shown that for the same samples, the values obtained varied between approximately 10- and 3,000-fold (90,91). While these values were correlated, there was a systematic bias: as the measured value increased, the difference in measurements increased. This apparent discrepancy was not explained by any differences in the standard urine preparations employed and was due to the way different assays measure the allergens present in the airborne dust (92). In measuring occupational exposure to allergens a compromise may therefore have to be reached between accurate quantification of individual allergens (such as with monoclonal antibody–based assays for the purpose of establishing exposure limits) and obtaining an estimate of exposure of total allergen (such as with polyclonal antibody–based assays for clinical or epidemiological purposes). Monoclonal antibody–based assays, however, have obvious advantages where standardization and comparison of measurements are important.

Exposure Data

General observations about the airborne concentrations of laboratory animal allergens in the workplace are very consistent. Aeroallergen levels are highest in animal rooms, especially during disturbances such as cleaning out (93–95). Personal exposure when working directly with animals can be three- to 10-fold higher than that of static or background concentration of the room (96–99). The rat aeroallergen concentration in undisturbed rat rooms has been reported between 300 ng/m^3 (93) and 2.3 ng/m^3 (97) while personal samples collected during the handling of rats have measured rat aeroallergen concentrations between 3.6 μg/m^3 (99) and 15 ng/m^3 (97). The airborne allergen concentrations reported for mouse show similar variations (94,95,100–102) and probably reflect the analogous working practices adopted with these species. Limited data are available for guinea pig and rabbits (94,99).

It is also a consistent observation that rat, mouse, and guinea pig allergens are predominantly carried on large particles, typically 5–15 μm in aerodynamic diameter. The size distribution of the allergenic dust particles is of importance, as the aerodynamic diameter of the dust particles will determine the site of deposition in the airways, which in turn may influence the nature of symptoms provoked. The distribution of particle sizes measured in the air is dependent upon the conditions of the study; recent disturbance of animal litter encourages the dissemination of large particles, which would remain settled if undisturbed (103). Up to 30% of animal allergens have also been detected on respirable particles (<2.5 μm), which may remain airborne for long periods and are small enough to penetrate to alveoli (104,105).

Of the farm animals, the levels of bovine allergen have been the most widely studied. Airborne cow allergen has been quantified in Finnish cow sheds by Virtanen and co-workers. Using an epithelial antigen and an ELISA inhibition assay employing polyclonal rabbit antiserum (106), they made a number of observations in parallel with laboratory animals. Their principal findings were (1) that the aeroallergen exposure in the breathing zone of dairy farmers was greater than that for static sampling sites in the same cowshed, (2) that there was only moderate correlation between the airborne concentrations of total dust and bovine allergen, and (3) that there was considerable variation in aeroallergen levels between different cowsheds (107). Unlike the wide variation in levels of aeroallergen observed in animal houses, which is influenced by the activities within the animal holding rooms (108,109), individual cowsheds seem to have characteristic background levels of bovine aeroallergen (static samples $2-13$ μg/m^3, personal samples $3-22$ μg/m^3) (110), suggesting that single measurements to determine occupational exposure may be possible. Further refinement of the immunoassay to employ monoclonal antibodies to quantify the major cow allergen Bos d2 showed that the average concentration of Bos d2 was approximately 10-fold less than total epithelial antigen (111). In a recent study of asthmatic German dairy farmers (112), dust collected from the carpets of their homes was a significant source of Bos d2 (as measured by rocket immunoelectrophoresis), particularly if the barn and living quarters were in the same building.

With pig hypersensitivity it is unclear whether allergen levels or other factors are most important in eliciting respiratory disease. The composition of the dust found in swine confinement buildings is complex and comprised of numerous microorganisms, both bacteria and fungi, as well as pig-derived proteins. Ammonia and endotoxin are also important airborne contaminants although the levels of these are usually below recommended safety limits and can be effectively controlled with adequate ventilation (51). Although some workers have specific IgE to allergens of pig origin and animal feed (e.g., barley), these aeroallergens have not been adequately measured in the occupational setting. The use of disinfectants may also contribute to chronic respiratory disease (113).

Several species of insect have been linked to occupational allergy, and in some cases investigation of the aeroallergens has been undertaken primarily to demonstrate the relevant allergen in the air. Tee and co-workers, in their study of the housefly (*Musca domesticus*), demonstrated that the airborne fly allergen(s) originated in part from the dust collecting in the fly-rearing cage and were probably of fecal origin (58). Dust from filters collected in a fly-rearing room had a steeper slope than self-inhibition (fly extract), suggesting the presence of additional, but unidentified, allergens in the air. Similarly, feces and the peritrophic membrane are the most likely source of airborne locust allergens in the species *Schistocerca gregaria* and *Locusta migratoria* (65).

RAST inhibition has also been used to detect aerosolized shrimp and clam proteins in the workplace (82). The concentration of snow-crab aeroallergen has been found to be highest (1.7 μg allergen on filter equivalent to an airborne concentration of ~10 μg/m^3) in an area adjacent to the sorting and boiling of crabs, but is virtually undetectable in other areas of the factory where cooked meat is handled (114).

Exposure-Response Studies

The effect of animal and insect allergen exposure on occupational disease has only been studied in detail for allergy to laboratory animals (LAA). Initial cross-sectional studies employed qualitative estimates of exposure such as the frequency of animal contact (days per week) or job description and provided discrepant findings; more recent studies have found an association between symptoms and exposure (115,116) although earlier ones did not (117–119). A series of studies have quantified exposure to rat aeroallergen and examined the relationship with the prevalence and incidence rates of LAA (120–122). The workforce was grouped or zoned according to the similarity of the job they performed after Corn and Esmen (123). By measuring the exposure of representative workers within each zone, the exposure of the entire workforce was estimated (Fig. 2). Grouping of the aeroallergen exposure categories into low (0.04 $\mu g/m^3$), medium (1.07 $\mu g/m^3$), and high (31.80 $\mu g/m^3$) demonstrated an increasing prevalence of sensitization and symptoms with increasing exposure intensity: the odds of having skin symptoms were increased 10-fold in animal technicians and individuals handling soiled litter, and fivefold in those less frequently or indirectly exposed such as scientists. The prevalence of respiratory symptoms was greater in medium- than low-exposure groups, but did not increase further in the high-exposure group.

A recent cross-sectional study of 540 workers employed at eight separate sites in The Netherlands has reported a clear exposure-response relationship when analysis was restricted to those employed for less than 4 years (121). Case-referent analysis of 342 new

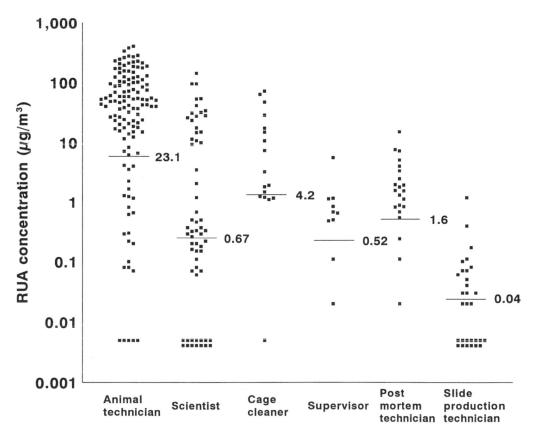

Figure 2 Rat urinary aeroallergen (RUA) exposure of a pharmaceutical workforce by exposure group. Each point represents an air sample collected at 2 L/min for the duration of each worker's shift. The RUA content of each filter eluate was determined by RAST inhibition (see Ref. 98).

employees followed at 6-monthly intervals also showed a relationship between exposure and the development of symptoms (respiratory, eye or nose, and skin). The odds ratio for those employed in the highest exposure category (animal technicians and cage cleaners) were less than those for the intermediate categories (an effect that may possibly be explained by the different perceived risk and hence use of safety equipment in the different exposure categories). However, when the analysis was confined to outcomes developing within the first 2 years of exposure, a dose-response relationship across all the exposure categories was demonstrated (122). Although the precise relationship of different exposures with the risk of disease is unknown, it is clear that sensitization can occur at any level of exposure, with increasing risk at increasing concentrations of airborne allergen.

Eggleston et al. have challenged rat-allergic individuals within rat rooms under controlled conditions and have found evidence for an apparent threshold for the provocation of both respiratory and nasal symptoms (97). Repeated challenges with the same individuals suggested a dose-response effect between intensity of exposure and the severity of nasal and bronchial symptoms (124).

Summary

Increasingly sophisticated methods of measuring animal, insect, and shellfish allergens are becoming available, although in some instances, a choice between methods to quantify individual allergens or "total allergen exposure" may have to be made. Nonstandardization of assays means that while general observations between individual studies may be consistent, absolute values obtained for allergen exposure may not be readily comparable.

Several studies have now demonstrated a convincing relationship between the intensity of exposure to animal allergens and the development of respiratory disease.

EPIDEMIOLOGY

It is difficult to estimate the incidence of occupational asthma caused by animals, insects, and shellfish in many countries owing to inadequate information about the number of people exposed and lack of a suitable reporting scheme to monitor cases of occupational respiratory disease.

In the United Kingdom, chest and occupational physicians report new cases of occupational lung disease to SWORD. During the first year of the SWORD study, 26% (554) of the 2101 cases reported were of occupational asthma, an estimated incidence of 22 cases per 10^6 U.K. workforce per year. Of these 554 cases, 21 (4%) were attributed to sensitivity to laboratory animals and insects, giving an estimated incidence of 204 cases of occupational asthma per 10^6 laboratory technicians and assistants per year. This compares with annual incidences for bakers of $409/10^6$, for chemical processors of $424/10^6$, and for coach and spray painters of $639/10^6$ (1). Allergy to laboratory animals has since remained in the top three most frequently reported causes of occupational asthma in the United Kingdom since (2). A pilot scheme in Canada attributed only four cases (3.2%) of occupational asthma to animals (125) although this may be a reflection of local patterns of occupations (e.g., the forest industry is the main employer in the province of British Columbia). Bovine allergens are, however, the most frequently reported cause of occupational asthma in Finland, accounting for 92% of the animal-related causes of occupational asthma (98/920 of the total cases) reported in 1996 (126). A recent population-based study from New Zealand showed that the highest-risk occupations for developing asthma and bronchial hyperresponsiveness associated with exposure to high-molecular-weight allergens were farm workers, laboratory workers, and food-processing workers (127). Data are not available for the other species being considered here except for published cross-sectional studies describing the prevalence of disease in individual workforces.

Laboratory Animals

Many cross-sectional studies have been reported of workforces exposed to laboratory animals, with consistent results (115–121,128–133). The prevalence rate of LAA is usually between 20 and 40%, with some 5–10% of exposed personnel developing asthma. Because those with disease, particularly asthma, may leave employment, such studies may underestimate the size of the problem by examining a "survivor" population. Recent reports have shown that this high prevalence continues (132,133). Symptoms typically occur between 1 month and several years after first exposure to animals with a mean interval of 2–3 years. The most common symptoms reported are rhinitis and conjunctivitis, which occur in most subjects. Contact urticaria appears in 5–15% of allergic subjects and can be the only manifestation of LAA. Asthma usually develops with or after the onset of other allergic symptoms and is uncommon in the absence of other symptoms. Asthma is usually associated with the presence of specific IgE. This antibody response is not necessarily found with other manifestations of LAA where up to 50% of subjects have no detectable IgE.

Atopy has consistently been identified as a risk factor for the development of allergy to laboratory animals and in particular for asthma. There is some evidence that atopy may shorten the latent period of the disease from initial exposure (134). Hollander et al. have shown in a cross-sectional study that a positive skin prick test or symptoms associated with exposure to cats and dogs and an elevated level of total IgE are risk factors for the presence of rat and mouse allergy (135). When two or more of these factors were present, an individual was 25 times more likely to have rat allergy and 40 times more likely to report mouse allergy. Evidence to suggest that smoking might be a risk factor for LAA has only been found when data were pooled from three separate studies (136).

Although atopy and intensity of exposure both contribute to the development of LAA, other factors may be involved as two-thirds of atopics who have remained in high-intensity-exposure jobs may remain healthy (Table 2). It is possible individuals may also need a specific genetic predisposition to mount an IgE response to these animal proteins.

Table 2 Data from a Cross-Sectional Survey of 323 Workers (88% of Workforce) Exposed to Rats

Exposure category	Number	Atopic status	SPT to rat +	SPT to rat −
High	77	Y $n = 28$	10 (13%)	18 (23%)
		N $n = 49$	3 (4%)	46 (60%)
Low	75	Y $n = 20$	1 (1%)	19 (25%)
		N $n = 55$	0 (0%)	55 (73%)

The rat skin-prick-test-positive subjects had had a similar duration of employment and atopic status (i.e., cat allergy) as healthy workers.
Source: Ref. 120.

Farm Animals

Asthma induced by cows is an important cause of occupational respiratory disease among Finnish farmers. While dairy farming is common in other countries, two factors are thought to be important in contributing to the high prevalence of the disease in Finland. Because of its northern location, cows are kept in cowsheds (which may form part of the farmhouse) for much of the year, grazing only during the summer months (May–September). It is also common practice for dairy farmers to brush their animals, which can result in intense exposure to cow dander allergens. Hinze and Bergmann have examined the development of asthma in 67 subjects diagnosed with asthma due to cows (137). In common with the progression of hypersensitivity to other animal species, the subjects usually experience rhinoconjunctivitis and urticaria prior to developing lower respiratory symptoms. Also, those with preexisting atopy tended to develop more severe symptoms. Skin diseases are important causes of morbidity in those with contact to cows; 44% of the cases of occupational contact urticaria reported to the Finnish Register of Occupational Diseases in 1990–1993 were attributed to cow dander (138).

Reindeer herding is another common occupation in Scandinavia where its meat is widely used as food. High exposure to reindeer epithelia only occurs in the autumn when the animals are collected from the forest, marked, and kept in fenced areas over the winter. In a random study of 211 reindeer herders from northern Finland, only one person had a positive skin prick test to reindeer epithelium. The respiratory symptoms experienced by 10–30% of the herders were attributed to the effects of working in extreme outdoor weather conditions and/or the effects of smoking (139). A case report of occupational asthma due to deer has, however, been reported in a farmer from Korea where large numbers of the animals are raised on small holdings for deerhorn, which is an important component of traditional herbal medication in Asia (45). Allergic reactions to wild animals such as deer and elk can also be an occupational disease of professional hunting guides (140). Sensitized individuals may experience asthmatic symptoms when skinning and dressing skins, or washing contaminated clothing. In a study of 15 subjects with exposure to deer and elk (140), all those studied were highly atopic. It therefore seems that subjects with preexisting allergy to domestic animals may be at increased risk of developing IgE-mediated reactions to deer when coming into professional or recreational contact with these animals.

The prevalence of asthma caused by occupational exposure to horses has not been reported. The prevalence of chronic respiratory symptoms among pig farmers is high although the etiology of the disease remains unknown. Modern methods of pig farming now mean that the animals are kept indoors at high stock densities. Studies from Yugoslavia (50), the United Kingdom (51), France (141), The Netherlands (142,143), and Denmark (144) describe symptoms of chronic cough and wheeze as well as headache and eye and nose symptoms among pig farmers. Estimates for the prevalence of wheeze and/or asthma vary between 8 and 45% of the pig-farming population. Only two proven cases of occupational asthma related to pig exposure have been reported [a butcher (49) and an agricultural student (48)] both of whom were highly atopic.

Insects

The epidemiology of occupational insect allergy has been less well studied, primarily because the size of the problem is less than that of LAA.

Individual case reports of occupational allergy to fly species include those of an atopic scientific worker who developed rhinitis when exposed to *Musca domestica* (58), a sewage plant worker who developed rhinoconjunctivitis and then asthma to sewer flies, *Psychoda alternata* (59), and a doctoral student who experienced anaphylactic symptoms after being bitten by tsetse flies, *Glossina morsitans* (63). A cross-sectional study of 22 research workers who worked with the fruitfly, *Drosophila melanogaster*, demonstrates the potency of insect allergens (60). Seven of the subjects (32%) experienced nasal symptoms, four of whom also had lower respiratory tract symptoms and three also had eye symptoms. Similarly 28% of Australian research workers involved in the breeding of the sheep blowfly (*Lucilia cuprina*) used in genetic studies and biological control programs were found to be symptomatic: 24% had upper respiratory tract symptoms, 20% had eye symptoms, 17% had skin symptoms, and 11% had asthma or experienced tightness of the chest (145). Workers exposed to large numbers of insects in outdoor locations may also be at risk of occupational allergy. At least 25% of the 57 workers employed at a hydroelectric power plant in Canada described work-related symptoms associated with exposure to caddis flies (*Hydropsyche recurvata*) (62). Seventeen of the 28 subjects tested had a positive skin prick test to caddis fly allergen. Workers were 3.7 times more likely to be sensitized if they worked in areas of high exposure to the caddis fly. Subjects with specific IgE to caddis fly were more likely to report an increased number of work-related symptoms and 10 reported "wheeze" (compared to three who were skin prick test negative).

Occupational allergy to cockroaches (73), locusts (65), and grasshoppers (*Melanoplus sanguinipes*) (66) has been described in laboratory workers. Owing to the similarity in observations and the small number of subjects studied [6 (73), 15 (65), and 17 (66), respectively], the findings will be summarized. The prevalence of a positive skin prick test in these exposed subjects is high (67%, 67%, 41%) with over half of the exposed subjects experiencing work-related allergic symptoms. Asthma was seen in 33% of the locust workforce and 24% of the grasshopper workers. All of those experiencing occupational asthma had specific IgE to the relevant antigen and had other related symptoms (typically rhinoconjunctivitis in the locust workers and skin sensitivity in the grasshopper workers). Atopy was not necessarily associated with symptomatic or immunological allergy in occupational sensitivity to Orthopterans; 2/4 skin prick test positive to cockroach, 4/10 skin prick test positive to locust, and 5/7 skin prick test positive to grasshopper were considered nonatopic.

Case reports of occupational insect allergy include a nonatopic subject who developed severe asthma coincident with the seasonal honey-packing process (67), seven subjects (five nonatopic) who experienced anaphylactic symptoms when stung by bees (68), three female subjects sensitized to spider mites (69,71), nine female subjects with occupational skin and upper respiratory tract symptoms attributed to the urticating hair from the Brazilian spider (72), and a male researcher who developed severe rhinoconjunctivitis after 10 years of collecting live adult chironomid midges (75).

Chironomids are an important environmental inhalant allergen in Japan and have been identified as a source of allergy in those occupationally or recreationally involved in the running of aquariums and fish-food factory workers (146). As subjects were recruited by advertisement, the prevalence of reported symptoms for the whole group was high (63% prevalence of rhinoconjunctivitis, 45% asthma). Of the 32 subjects employed in the fish-food factory, 15 had very high exposure to Chi t1 and of these 15, five had symptoms and specific IgE to Chi t1.

Shellfish

The first cross-sectional study to examine the prevalence of work-related respiratory symptoms in snow-crab (*Chinoecetes opilis*)-processing workers was published in 1984 by

Cartier and co-workers (79). A total of 313 subjects were employed at two industrial sites in Canada. The freshly caught crabs were boiled, cooled, and the cooked meat separated from the legs and claws before being canned. The prevalence of work-related symptoms was high in both plants with work-related asthma being confirmed in approximately 46 of the 303 workers studied [15% of the total workforce, which corresponds to nearly all (97%) of the exposed workers]. Approximately two-thirds of the workers with asthma had rhinoconjunctivitis and one-third had urticaria. No relationship was found between occupational asthma and the presence of atopy. Skin prick testing with crab antigens found specific IgE in just over half of the asthmatics suggesting that other immunological mechanisms might also be important. Smoking was a risk factor for the development of occupational asthma. Further immunological studies reported in 1986 (83) showed that specific IgE to crab antigens could be detected in the serum of the workers by RAST. An improved extract of snow-crab cooking water demonstrated that 84% of the 37 asthmatics tested had specific IgE to the extract.

The same group have also reported on clam and shrimp as causes of occupational asthma (82). In this study population, the food-processing workers handled lyophilized clam and shrimp and packed the powder into bags. Of the 61 workers employed, 25 worked on the bag production line. Less than 10% of workers reported symptoms associated with exposure to clam and shrimp. Asthma was present in two atopic subjects (4%) who had specific IgE to both clam and shrimp. The prevalence of sensitization to clam was approximately 6% and 15% to shrimp. Subjects with specific IgE to clam and/or shrimp often had specific IgE to other seafood species. Additional case reports of occupational asthma attributed to lobster and shrimp have been reported in an atopic, non-smoking women working in a fishmongers (81) and in an atopic chef (80). Both had been employed for at least 2 years before the onset of increasingly severe skin and respiratory symptoms, and both experienced gastrointestinal symptoms after the ingestion of shellfish.

Summary

Despite the diverse nature of the species causing occupational allergy, the pattern of hypersensitivity to them is remarkably consistent. The majority of subjects, particularly atopics, develop symptoms within the first 2 years of exposure to a novel allergen. Rhinoconjunctivitis and/or skin symptoms are the most common manifestations of disease and often precede, but rarely succeed, the onset of asthma. Atopy and the development of specific IgE are important risk factors for asthma. Animals are probably the most common "high molecular weight" cause of occupational asthma worldwide, although insect and seafood allergens are highly potent sensitizers for the small numbers exposed to them.

DIAGNOSIS

The diagnosis of laboratory animal, seafood, and insect allergy is based on an appropriate history of symptoms—nasal, eye, skin, or chest—in a person who encounters these allergens in his or her work. Symptoms develop after an initial asymptomatic period of exposure, commonly within the first 2 or 3 years of occupational exposure. Asthma without rhinitis is unusual and usually develops with or after the onset of rhinitis. The majority of patients identify a clear relationship between working with animals and the provocation of their symptoms. In sensitized individuals nasal and eye symptoms are commonly provoked within minutes. Asthma, at least initially, may be only manifest as increased airways responsiveness (147) (e.g., provoked by exercise or cold air) or develop only several hours after allergen contact, making identification of the provoking agent more difficult. Nasal and eye symptoms may resolve in hours, whereas asthma may resolve only after several days and cause nocturnal respiratory symptoms with sleep disturbance. Urticaria usually develops at the site of direct skin contact with the allergens. Acute anaphylaxis may rarely follow an animal bite or injury with contaminated sharps (148). Objective evidence to support a diagnosis can be obtained from a specific immunological (usually IgE) response, work-related changes in peak flow rate, and inhalation tests. In the case of small-mammal allergy, urine is the major source of allergenic protein and extracts of animal urine are the most relevant for diagnostic skin testing. Specific IgE in serum or identified by a skin prick test to a specific allergen is, in general, more sensitive (few false negatives) than a specific test (few false positives) in allergic asthma. The absence of specific IgE is therefore more helpful in excluding a specific allergen as the cause of asthma than is its presence in attributing to it.

Several studies of laboratory animal allergy have shown that an immediate skin test response and specific IgE in serum to an extract of animal urine is a sensitive indicator of asthma, but not of other manifestations (rhinitis and conjunctivitis) caused by laboratory animal allergy. The reasons for this discrepancy remain unclear. Other allergens have been less well studied than laboratory animal allergy and it is not possible to be as confident about the diagnostic value of specific IgE. Asthma caused by snow-crab has been studied by Cartier and colleagues. They found that an immediate skin prick test response was provoked by an extract of snow crab meat and of cooking-pot water in 37 of 48 cases of asthma (sensitivity 37/48 = 77%). The skin test to meat extract was negative in 33 and to water extract in 35 of the 52 without asthma (specificities: 33/52 = 63% and 35/52 = 67%) (83). The likelihood ratio for having asthma if the skin test was positive in this study population (true positive rate/false positive rate) was 2.35.

Work-related asthma can be identified by serial measurements of peak flow rates with deterioration in peak flow during periods at work and improvements during absences from work. In laboratory animal workers with work-related asthma, one or both of specific IgE or serial peak flow measurements is usually sufficient to allow a confident diagnosis to be made. Inhalation testing is now rarely necessary.

OUTCOME

Few studies have investigated the prognosis of patients who have developed occupational asthma caused by allergy to high-molecular-weight proteins. The major exceptions are the outcome studies of patients with asthma caused by allergy to snow-crab (149,150). Hudson et al. followed up 31 cases of occupational asthma caused by allergy to snow-crab. The diagnosis had been made in 24 by inhalation testing with an extract of snow-crab boiling water, and in seven by serial peak flow measurements or changes in airway responsiveness to inhaled histamine at and away from work (149). They found that after avoidance of exposure of an average of 2 years to snow-crab most cases showed improvement in symptom severity, treatment requirements, and airway responsiveness to inhaled histamine. Twelve of the 31 were asymptomatic at the time of follow-up and 19 remained symptomatic. On average, duration of exposure after the onset of symptoms was longer in the symptomatic (8 months) than in the asymptomatic (4 months) group.

In a second, more detailed study 31 cases of snow-crab asthma were followed up on three occasions at, on average, 1 year, 2.5 years, and 5 years from last exposure (150).

FEV_1 showed maximal improvement by the first year of follow-up; histamine PC_{20} showed maximal improvement at the second point of follow-up; specific IgE to snow-crab boiling water continued to fall to the third point of follow-up, on average 5 years from last exposure. By the time of the third follow-up point only 10 of the 31 cases were still receiving treatment, of whom eight were taking inhaled beta-2 agonists, supplemented in two with oral theophylline. None were taking oral or inhaled corticosteroids at the time of the second or third follow-up points.

These observations suggest that occupational asthma caused by allergy to inhaled snow-crab, in common with asthma caused by low-molecular-weight sensitizing agents, can persist in a significant proportion of cases, although this was not of sufficient severity in these cases by the second point of follow-up, 2.5 years after avoidance of exposure, to require treatment with oral or inhaled steroids. Also in common with asthma caused by low-molecular-weight agents, those who had continuing symptoms after avoidance of exposure to snow-crab were more likely to have experienced longer duration, suggesting the risk of chronic asthma is minimized by early identification of cases and their avoidance of subsequent exposure.

MANAGEMENT

It is important to distinguish cases of allergy with asthma from those without. The prognosis for cases with asthma is worse for snow-crab allergy, and possibly others (although not formally studied). Cases of asthma who continue to be exposed may develop increasingly severe asthma, which can be provoked by an increasing number of the small animal or insect species with which they work. Cases with asthma should be advised to avoid further exposure to the animals or processes that cause their symptoms. For some, immediate avoidance of animal contact is impractical; Ph.D. students, research scientists, technicians, and animal handlers may all require time to allow a change in job description to be made. In these circumstances, provided the possible consequences to their health are fully explained, support and symptomatic treatment for a short period is appropriate, so long as animal contact has not provoked a life-threatening reaction (acute-severe asthma or anaphylaxis), that there is a firm intention to make a job change within an agreed time frame, and exposure to animal products can be kept to a minimum in the interim. This usually requires, when working with animals, the use of adequate respiratory protection such as laminar flow equipment, the effectiveness of which should be monitored by several measurements of lung function. Drug treatment may also be needed primarily to prevent or reverse reactions to indirect contact, such as from animal excreta on the clothes or hair of others in direct contact with animals.

Laboratory animal allergy without asthma is generally easier to manage with respiratory and skin protection and adequate washing and changing facilities on site. The majority of such cases are able to continue to work with animals.

PREVENTION

The major occupational health goal for those responsible for the health of persons working with animals and insects must be the progressive reduction in disease incidence. The prevention of disease is most appropriately based on controlling environmental exposure to allergen rather than on the identification and exclusion of "susceptible" individuals;

the latter is poorly discriminating and identifies the individual rather than the environment as responsible for the problem.

Cross-sectional studies that have examined the relationship between atopy and LAA have consistently found the prevalence of asthma, but not its other manifestations, to be increased some fivefold in atopic individuals. Although limited by its cross-sectional design, the results from the study of Venables et al. demonstrate the poor discrimination of the use of atopy as a selection criterion for employment (131). Forty-two percent (58 of 138) of the workforce were atopic (Table 3) and chest symptoms were four times more common in atopics than nonatopics (a risk of 1 in 5 in atopics compared to 1 in 20 in nonatopics). However, LAA without chest symptoms was no more common in the atopics than in the nonatopics. Therefore, if 58 atopics were excluded (and nonatopics employed instead) and the same prevalence rates applied, only four cases of asthma would have been prevented and the prevalence of LAA without chest symptoms would have remained the same. To prevent four cases of asthma, atopics who would not have developed any manifestations of LAA and 47 who would not have developed asthma would have been excluded from employment. Total IgE and preexisting allergy to animals have been shown to be important risk factors, but again their discriminatory power is too low to be used for preemployment screening tools (135, 151).

The prevention of allergy to animals and insects and shellfish should therefore be achieved primarily by preventing animal allergens becoming airborne and being inhaled by those working with them. The observations from the exposure-response studies involving laboratory animal allergens (120,121) imply that a reduction in exposure to allergens would be associated with a reduction in the risk of developing the disease. This hypothesis is supported by Botham et al., who observed a decrease in the incidence of LAA symptoms when more stringent procedures, including changed work practices and the mandatory use of respiratory protection (e.g., disposable mask or ventilated helmet), were adopted (152, 153). The prevalence of sensitization was, however, unaffected suggesting that the threshold of exposure for sensitization may be lower than that to provoke symptoms.

It is clear from the continuing high prevalence of LAA worldwide (132,133) that individuals with animal contact remain exposed to sufficient allergen to become sensitized and develop symptoms. Highly effective and practicable methods are needed to reduce animal allergen exposure sufficiently to prevent sensitization. The development of methods to quantify aeroallergen exposure has allowed the objective assessment of interventions designed to reduce exposure to rat and mouse allergens. Litter has been shown to be an important vehicle for allergen dissemination (154,155) and the use of noncontact absorbent litters is a very effective way of reducing animal aeroallergen. The number of animals (stock density) and cage design may also directly influence aeroallergen concentrations

Table 3 Frequency of Laboratory Animal Allergy According to Atopic Status

	With chest symptoms	Without chest symptoms	No symptoms	Total
Atopics	11	17	30	58
Nonatopics	4	28	48	80
Total	15	45	78	138

Source: Data taken from Ref. 131.

(154,155); the use of well designed, individually ventilated cage systems is, although expensive, an excellent way of housing large numbers of animals while maintaining background levels of allergen at almost undetectable levels (156). Exposure associated with the handling of animals may be reduced approximately 20-fold when the procedure is undertaken in a ventilated safety cabinet as compared with on an open bench. The same study was, however, unable to show the efficacy of vacuum systems to reduce aeroallergen exposure when removing soiled litter from cages. Increasing the relative humidity of the rooms housing the animals has also been shown to be an effective way of reducing airborne rat and mouse allergens (93,157). Any steps taken to increase the local ventilation and/or the introduction of simple engineering methods to contain allergen, such as the introduction of Perspex curtains to surround animal cages (158), may be associated with a decrease in levels of airborne allergen. Several studies now suggest that such improved procedures may be sufficient to reduce aeroallergens to such a level that sensitized subjects may tolerate their symptoms (156,159). Should all other measures fail, personal protective equipment such as ventilated helmets is effective in reducing exposure to animal allergens (160,161).

Summary

The prevention of occupational allergy must be based on physical approaches to reduce the concentration of airborne allergen inhaled by those working with animals and insects or cooking or handling shellfish. Any method of containing the allergens or increasing the ventilation, or both, will be effective in reducing airborne levels of allergen.

REFERENCES

1. Meredith SK, Taylor V, McDonald JC. Occupational respiratory disease in the United Kingdom: a report to the British Thoracic Society and the Society of Occupational Medicine by the SWORD project group. Br J Ind Med 1991; 48:292–298.
2. Ross DJ, Keynes HL, McDonald JC. SWORD 96: surveillance of work-related and occupational respiratory disease in the UK. Occup Med 1997; 47:377–381.
3. Newman Taylor AJ, Longbottom JL, Pepys J. Respiratory allergy to urine proteins of rats and mice. Lancet 1977; 2:847–849.
4. Haars LJ, Pitot HC. Hormonal and developmental regulation of glycosylated $alpha_{2u}$-globulin synthesis. Arch Biochem Biophys 1980; 201:556–563.
5. Roy AK, Chatterjee B, Demyan WF, Milin BS, Motwani NM, Nath S, Schiop MJ. Hormone and age-dependent regulation of $alpha_{2u}$-globulin gene expression. Recent Prog Horm Res 1983; 39:425–461.
6. Bayard C, Holmquist L, Vesterberg O. Purification and identification of allergenic $_{2u}$-globulin species of rat urine. Biochim Biophys Acta 1996; 1290:129–134.
7. Bacchini A, Gaetani E, Cavaggioni A. Pheromone binding properties of the mouse, *Mus musculus*. Experientia 1992; 48:419–421.
8. Hastie ND, Held WA, Toole JJ. Multiple genes coding for the androgen regulated major urinary proteins of the mouse. Cell 1979; 17:449–457.
9. Clark AJ, Clissold PM, Shawi RA, Beattie P, Bishop J. Structure of mouse urinary protein genes: different splicing configurations in the 3′ non-coding region. EMBO J. 1984; 3:1045–1052.
10. Gurka G, Ohman J, Rosenwasser LR. Allergen-specific human T cell clones: derivation, specificity, and activation requirements. J Allergy Clin Immunol 1989; 83:945–954.

11. Longbottom JL. Characterisation of allergens from the urines of experimental animals. Proceedings of XIth International Congress of Allergology and Clinical Immunology. London: Macmillan 1983:525–529.

12. Gordon S, Welch JA, Tee RD, Newman Taylor AJ. Allergenic cross-reactivity between rat and mouse urine. Clin Exp Allergy 1994; 24:176.

13. Burek JD, Duprat P, Owen R, Peter CP, Van Zwieten MJ. Spontaneous renal disease in laboratory animals. Int Rev Exp Pathol 1988; 30:231–319.

14. Borghoff SJ, Short BG, Swenberg JA. Biochemical mechanisms and pathobiology of alpha$_{2u}$-globulin nephropathy. Ann Rev Pharm Toxicol 1990; 30:349–367.

15. Gordon S, Tee RD, Newman Taylor AJ. Analysis of rat urine proteins and allergens by sodium dodecyl sulfate-polyacrylamide gel electrophoresis and immunoblotting. J Allergy Clin Immunol 1993; 92:298–305.

16. Gordon S, Tee RD, Newman Taylor AJ. Analysis of rat serum allergens. J Allergy Clin Immunol 1997; 99:716–717.

17. Laperche Y, Lynch KR, Dolan KP, Feigelson P. Tissue-specific control of alpha$_{2u}$-globulin gene expression: constitutive synthesis in the submaxillary gland. Cell 1983; 32:453–460.

18. Mancini MA, Majumdar D, Chatterjee B, Roy AK. Alpha$_{2u}$-globulin in modified sebaceous glands with pheromonal functions: localisation of the protein and its mRNA in preputial, meibomian and perianal glands. J Histochem Cytochem 1989; 37:149–157.

19. Shaw PH, Held WA, Hastie ND. The gene family for major urinary proteins: expression in several secretory tissues of the mouse. Cell 1983; 32:755–761.

20. Finlayson JS, Asofsky R, Potter M, Runner CC. Major urinary protein complex of normal mice: origin. Science 1965; 149:981–982.

21. Price JA, Longbottom JL. Allergy to mice I. Identification of two major mouse allergens (Ag 1 and Ag 3) and investigation of their possible origin. Clin Allergy 1987; 17:43–53.

22. Gordon S, Tee RD, Newman Taylor AJ. Comparison of proteins and allergens in rat hair and urine. Clin Exp Allergy 1993; 23:56.

23. Gordon S, Tee RD, Newman Taylor AJ. Analysis of the allergenic composition of rat dust. Clin Exp Allergy 1996; 26:533–541.

24. Finlayson JS, Potter M, Shinnick CS, Smithies O. Components of the major urinary protein complex of inbred mice; determination of NH$_2$-terminal sequences and comparison with homologous components from wild mice. Biochem Gene 1974; 11:325–335.

25. Schumacher MJ, Tait BD, Holmes MC. Allergy to murine antigens in a biological research institute. J Allergy Clin Immunol 1981; 68:310–318.

26. Lutsky II, Fink JN, Kidd J, Dahlberg MJE, Yuninger JW. Allergenic properties of rat urine and pelt extracts. J Allergy Clin Immunol 1985; 75:279–284.

27. Swanson MC, Agarwal MK, Yuninger JW, Reed CE. Guinea pig derived allergens. Clinicoimmunologic studies, characterisation, airborne quantitation and size distribution. Am Rev Respir Dis 1984; 129:844–849.

28. Walls AF, Newman Taylor AJ, Longbottom JL. Allergy to guinea pigs. I. Allergenic activities of extracts derived from the pelt, saliva, urine and other sources. Clin Allergy 1985; 15:241–251.

29. Walls AF, Newman Taylor AJ, Longbottom JL. Allergy to guinea pigs. II. Identification of specific allergens in guinea pig dust by crossed radio-immunoelectrophoresis and the investigation of the possible origin. Clin Allergy 1985; 15:535–546.

30. Ohman JL, Lowell FC, Bloch KJ. Allergens of mammalian origin. II. Characterisation of allergens extracted from rat, mouse, guinea pig and rabbit pelts. J Allergy Clin Immunol 1975; 55:16–24.

31. Price JA, Longbottom JL. Allergy to rabbits. I. Specificity and non-specificity of RAST and crossed-radioimmunoelectrophoresis due to the presence of light chains in rabbit allergenic extracts. Allergy 1986; 41:603–612.

32. Price JA, Longbottom JL. Allergy to rabbits. II. Identification and characterization of a major rabbit allergen. Allergy 1988; 43:39–48.

33. Warner JA, Longbottom JL. Allergy to rabbits. III. Further identification and characterization of rabbit allergens. Allergy 1991; 46:481–491.

34. Schou C. Defining allergens of mammalian origin. Clin Exp Allergy 1993; 23:7–14.

35. Gordon S. Allergy to furred animals. Clin Exp Allergy 1997; 27:479–481.

36. McGivern D, Longbottom JL, Davies D. Allergy to gerbils. Clin Allergy 1985; 15:163–165.

37. Petry RW, Voss MJ, Kroutil BS, et al. Monkey dander asthma. J Allergy Clin Immunol 1985; 75:268–271.

38. Simon FA. Device for rapid performance of skin test by scratch methods. J Allergy 1941; 12:191–192.

39. Ylönen J, Mäntyjärvi R, Taivainen A, Virtanen T. Comparison of the antigenic and allergenic properties of three types of bovine epithelial material. Int Arch Allergy Immunol 1992; 99: 112–117.

40. Ylönen J, Mäntyjärvi R, Taivainen A, Virtanen T. IgG and IgE antibody responses to cow dander and urine in farmers with cow-induced asthma. Clin Exp Allergy 1992; 22:83–90.

41. Ylönen J, Virtanen T, Horsmanheimo L, Parkkinen S, Pelkonen J, Mäntyjärvi R. Affinity purification of the major bovine allergen by a novel monoclonal antibody. J Allergy Clin Immunol 1994; 93:851–858.

42. Mäntyjärvi R, Parkkinen S, Rytkönen, Pentikäinen J, Pelkonen J, Rautiainen J, Zeiler T, Virtanen T. Complementary DNA cloning of the predominant allergen of bovine dander: a new member of the lipocalin family. J Allergy Clin Immunol 1996; 97:1297–1303.

43. Wahn U, Peters T Jr, Siraganian RP. Allergenic and antigenic properties of bovine serum albumin. Mol Immunol 1981; 18:19–28.

44. Parkkinen S, Rytkönen M, Pentikäinen J, Virtanen T, Mäntyjärvi R. Homology of a bovine allergen and the oligomycin sensitivity-conferring protein of the mitochondrial adenosine triphosphate synthase complex. J Allergy Clin Immunol 1995; 95:1255–1260.

45. Nahm D-H, Park J-W, Hong C-S. Occupational asthma due to deer dander. Ann Allergy Asthma Immunol 1996; 76:423–426.

46. Spitzauer S, Valenta R, Mühl, Rumpold H, Ebner H, Ebner C. Characterization of allergens from deer: cross-reactivity with allergens from cow dander. Clin Exp Allergy 1997; 27: 196–200.

47. Huwyler T, Wuthrich B. A case of fallow deer allergy. Cross-reactivity between fallow deer and horse allergy. Allergy 1992; 47:574–575.

48. Harries MG, Cromwell O. Occupational asthma caused by allergy to pig's urine. Br Med J 1982; 284:867.

49. Brennan NJ. Pig butcher's asthma—case report and review of the literature. Irish Med J 1985; 78:321–322.

50. Zuskin E, Kanceljak B, Schachter EN, Mustajbegovic J, Goswami S, Maayani S, Marom Z, Rienzi N. Immunological and respiratory findings in swine farmers. Environ Res 1991; 56: 120–130.

51. Crook B, Robertson JF, Travers Glass SA, Botheroyd EM, Lacey J, Topping MD. Airborne dust, ammonia, microorganisms, and antigens in pig confinement houses and the respiratory health of exposed farm workers. Am Ind Hyg Assoc J 1991; 52:271–279.

52. Fjeldsgaard BE, Smestad Paulsen B. Comparison of IgE-binding antigens in horse dander and a mixture of horse hair and skin scrapings. Allergy 1993; 48:535–541.

53. Johnsen TK, Thanh DB, Ly Q, Smestad Paulsen B, Wold JK. Further characterisation of Ig-E binding antigens in horse dander, with particular emphasis on glycoprotein allergens. Allergy 1996; 49:673–674.

54. Felix K, Ferrandiz R, Einarsson R, Dreborg S. Allergens of horse dander: comparison among breeds and individual animals by immunoblotting. J Allergy Clin Immunol 1996; 98:169–171.

55. Stoger P, Schmid-Grendelmeier P, Johansson SGO, Wuthrich B. Raccoon epithelium—a new allergen source. Allergy 1994; 49:673–674.

56. Jimenez Gomez I, Anton E, Picans I, Jerez J, Obispo T. Occupational asthma caused by mink urine. Allergy 1996; 51:364–365.

57. Savolainen J, Uitti J, Halmepuro L, Nordman H. IgE response to fur animal allergens and domestic allergens in fur farmers and fur garment workers. Clin Exp Allergy 1997; 27: 501–509.

58. Tee RD, Gordon DJ, Lacey J, Nunn AJ, Brown M, Newman Taylor AJ. Occupational allergy to the common house fly (*Musca domestica*): use of imunologic responses to identify atmospheric allergen. J Allergy Clin Immunol 1985; 76:826–831.

59. Gold BL, Mathews KP, Burge HA. Occupational asthma caused by sewer flies. Am Rev Respir Dis 1985; 131:949–952.

60. Spieksma FThM, Vooren PH, Kramps JA, Dijkman JH. Respiratory allergy to laboratory fruit flies (*Drosophila melanogaster*). J Allergy Clin Immunol 1986; 77:108–113.

61. Baldo BA, Bellas TE, Tovey ER, Kaufman GL. Occupational allergy in an entomological research centre. II. Identification of IgE-binding proteins from developmental stages of the blowfly *Lucilia cuprina* and other species of adult flies. Clin Exp Allergy 1989; 19: 411–417.

62. Kraut A, Sloan J, Silviu-Dan F, Peng Z, Gagnon D, Warrington R. Occupational allergy after exposure to caddis flies at a hydroelectric power plant. Occup Environ Med 1994; 51:408–413.

63. Stevens WJ, Van den Abbeele J, Bridts CH. Anaphylactic reaction after bites by *Glossina morsitans* (tsetse fly) in a laboratory worker. J Allergy Clin Immunol 1996; 98:700–701.

64. Frigerio C, Aubry M, Gomez F, Graf I, Dayer E, de Kalbermatten N, Gaillard RC, Spertini F. Occupational allergy to the housefly (*Musca domestica*). Allergy 1997; 52:238–239.

65. Tee RD, Gordon DJ, Hawkins ER, Nunn AJ, Lacey J, Venables KM, Cooter RJ, McCaffery AR, Newman Taylor AJ. Occupational allergy to locusts: an investigation of the sources of the allergen. J Allergy Clin Immunol 1988; 81:517–525.

66. Soparkar GR, Patel PC, Cockcroft DW. Inhalant atopic sensitivity to grasshoppers in research laboratories. J Allergy Clin Immunol 1993; 92:61–65.

67. Ostrom NK, Swanson MC, Agarwal MK, Yuninger JW. Occupational allergy to honeybee-body dust in a honey processing plant. J Allergy Clin Immunol 1986; 77:736–740.

68. Kochuyt AM, Van Hoeyveld E, Stevens EAM. Occupational allergy to bumble bee venom. Clin Exp Allergy 1993; 23:190–195.

69. Reunala T, Bjorksyen F, Forstrom L, Kanerva L. IgE-mediated occupational allergy to a spider mite. Clin Allergy 1983; 13:383–388.

70. Kroidl R, Maasch HJ, Wahl R. Respiratory allergies (bronchial asthma and rhinitis) due to sensitization of type I allergy to red spider mite (*Panonychus ulmi KOCH*). Clin Exp Allergy 1992; 22:958–962.

71. Erlam AR, Johnson AJ, Wiley KN. Occupational asthma in greenhouse tomato growing. Occup Med 1996; 46:163–164.

72. Castro FFM, Antila MA, Croce J. Occupational allergy caused by urticating hair of Brazilian spider. J Allergy Clin Immunol 1995; 95:1282–1285.

73. Steinberg DR, Bernstein DI, Gallagher JS, Arlian L, Bernstein IL. Cockroach sensitisation in laboratory workers. J Allergy Clin Immunol 1987; 80:586–590.

74. Baur X. Chironomid midge allergy. Jpn J Allergol 1992; 41:81–85.

75. Teranishi H, Kawai K, Murakami G, Miyao M, Kasuya M. Occupational allergy to adult chironomid midges among environmental research workers. Int Arch Allergy Immunol 1995; 106:271–277.

76. Chapman MD. Dissecting cockroach allergens. Clin Exp Allergy 1993; 23:459–461.

77. Tee RD, Cranston PS, Kay AB. Further characterisation of allergens associated with hypersensitivity to the "green nimitti" midge (*Cladotanytarsus lewisi*, Diptera: Chironomidae). Allergy 1986; 42:12–19.

78. Baldo BA, Panzani RC. Detection of IgE antibodies to a wide range of insect species in subjects suspected of inhalant allergies to insects. Int Arch Allergy Appl Immunol 1988; 85: 278–287.

79. Cartier A, Malo J-L, Forest F, Lafrance M, Pineau L, St-Aubin J-J, Dubois J-Y. Occupational asthma in snow-crab processing workers. J Allergy Clin Immunol 1984; 74:261–269.

80. Patel PC, Cockcroft DW. Occupational asthma caused by exposure to cooking lobster in the work environment: a case report. Ann Allergy 1992; 68:360–361.

81. Lemiere C, Desjardins A, Lehrer S, Malo J-L. Occupational asthma to lobster and shrimp. Allergy 1996; 51:272–273.

82. Desjardins A, Malo J-L, L'Archeveque J, Cartier A, McCants M, Lehrer SB. Occupational IgE-mediated sensitization and asthma caused by clam and shrimp. J Allergy Clin Immunol 1995; 96:608–617.

83. Cartier A, Malo J-L, Ghezzo H, McCants M, Lehrer SB. IgE sensitization snow crab processing workers. J Allergy Clin Immunol 1986; 78:344–348.

84. Leung PS, Chow WK, Duffey S, Kwan HS, Gershwin ME, Chu KH. IgE reactivity against a cross-reactive allergen in crustacea and mollusca: evidence for tropomyosin as the common allergen. J Allergy Clin Immunol 1996; 98:954–961.

85. Jyo T, Kohmoto K, Katsutani T, Otsuka T, Oka SD, Mitsui S. Occupational asthma. In: Occupational Asthma. Frazier CA, ed. London: Von Nostrand Reinhold, 1980:209–228.

86. Gaddie J, Legge JS, Friend JAR, Reid TMS. Pulmonary hypersensitivity in prawn workers. Lancet 1980; 2:1350–1353.

87. Douglas JDM, McSharry C, Blaikie L, Morrow T, Miles S, Franklin D. Occupational asthma caused by automated salmon processing. Lancet 1995; 346:737–740.

88. Newman Taylor AJ ,Tee RD. Occupational lung disease. Curr Opin Immun 1989; 1:684–689.

89. Gordon S, Tee RD, Lowson D, Newman Taylor AJ. Comparison and optimization of filter elution methods for the measurement of airborne allergen. Ann Occup Hyg 1992; 36:575–587.

90. Renström A, Gordon S, Larsson PH, Tee RD, Newman Taylor AJ, Malmberg PL. Comparison of a radioallergosorbent (RAST) inhibition method and a monoclonal enzyme linked immunosorbent assay (ELISA) for aeroallergen measurement. Clin Exp Allergy 1997; 27:1314–1322.

91. Hollander A, Gordon S, Renström A, Thissen J, Doekes G, Larsson PH, Malmberg P, Venables KM, Heederik D. Comparison of methods to assess airborne rat or mouse allergen levels. I. Analysis of air samples. Allergy 1999; 54:in press.

92. Renström A, Gordon S, Hollander A, Spitoven J, Larsson PH, Venables KM, Heederik D, Malmberg P. Comparison of methods to assess airborne rat or mouse allergen levels. II. Factors influencing antigen detection. Allergy 1999; 54:in press.

93. Edwards RG, Beeson MF, Dewdney JM. Laboratory animal allergy: the measurement of airborne urinary allergens and the effects of different environmental conditions. Lab Animals 1983; 17:235–239.

94. Swanson MC, Agarwal MK, Reed CE. An immunochemical approach to indoor aeroallergen quantitation with a new volumetric air sampler: studies with mite, roach, cat, mouse and guinea pig antigens. J Allergy Clin Immunol 1985; 76:724–729.

95. Twiggs JT, Agarwal MK, Dahlberg MJE, Yuninger JW. Immunochemical measurement of airborne mouse allergens in a laboratory animal facility. J Allergy Clin Immunol 1982; 69:522–526.

96. Davies GE, Thompson AV, Rackham M. Estimation of airborne rat-derived antigens by ELISA. J Immunoassay 1983; 4:113–126.

97. Eggleston PA, Newill CA, Ansari AA, Pustelnik A, Lou S-R, Evans R III, et al. Task-related variation in airborne concentrations of laboratory animal allergens: studies with Rat nI. J Allergy Clin Immunol 1989; 84:347–352.

98. Gordon S, Tee RD, Nieuwenhuijsen M, Lowson D, Newman Taylor AJ. Measurement of airborne rat urinary allergen in an epidemiological study. Clin Exp Allergy 1994; 24:1070–1077.

99. Price JA, Longbottom JL. ELISA method for measurement of airborne levels of major laboratory animal allergens. Clin Allergy 1988; 18:95–107.

100. Ohman JL, Hagberg K, MacDonald MR, Jones RR, Paigen BJ, Karcergis JB. Distribution of airborne mouse allergen in a major breeding facility. J Allergy Clin Immunol 1994; 94: 810–817.

101. Gordon S, Kiernan LA, Nieuwenhuijsen MJ, Cook AD, Tee RD, Newman Taylor AJ. Measurement of exposure to mouse urinary proteins in an epidemiological study. Occup Environ Med 1997; 54:135–140.

102. Hollander A, van Run P, Spithoven J, Heederik D, Doekes G. Exposure of laboratory animal workers to airborne rat and mouse urinary allergens. Clin Exp Allergy 1997; 27:617–626.

103. Platts-Mills TAE, Heymann PW, Longbottom JL, Wilkins SR. Airborne allergens associated with asthma: particle sizes carrying dust mite and rat allergens measured with a cascade impactor. J Allergy Clin Immunol 1986; 77:850–857.

104. Corn M, Koegel A, Hall T, Scott A, Newill C, Evans R. Characteristics of airborne particles associated with animal allergy in laboratory workers. Ann Occup Hyg 1988; 32(Suppl 1): 435–446.

105. Swanson MC, Campbell AR, O'Hollaren MT, Reed CE. Role of ventilation, air filtration, and allergen production rate in determining concentrations of rat allergens in the air of animal quarters. Am Rev Respir Dis 1990; 141:1578–1581.

106. Virtanen T, Louhelainen K, Mäntyjärvi R. Enzyme-linked immunosorbent assay (ELISA) inhibition method to estimate the level of airborne bovine epidermal antigen in cow sheds. Int Arch Allergy Appl Immunol 1986; 81:253–257.

107. Virtanen T, Vilhunen P, Husman K, Happonen P, Mäntyjärvi R. Level of airborne bovine epithelial antigen in Finnish cowsheds. Int Arch Occup Environ Health 1988; 60:355–360.

108. Nieuwenhuijsen MJ, Gordon S, Harris JM, Tee RD, Venables KM, Newman Taylor AJ. Variation in rat urinary aeroallergen levels explained by differences in site, task and exposure groups. Ann Occup Hyg 1995; 39:819–825.

109. Nieuwenhuijsen MJ, Gordon S, Harris JM, Tee RD, Venables KM, Newman Taylor AJ. Determinants of airborne allergen exposure in an animal house. Occup Hyg 1995; 1:317–324.

110. Virtanen T, Eskelinen T, Husman K, Mäntyjärvi R. Long- and short-term variability of airborne bovine epithelial antigen concentrations in cowsheds. Int Arch Allergy Immunol 1992; 98:252–255.

111. Ylonen J, Virtanen T, Rytkönen M, Mäntyjärvi R. Quantification of a major bovine allergen by a two-site immunometric assay based on monoclonal antibodies. Allergy 1994; 49:707–712.

112. Hinze S, Bergmann KCh, Lowenstein H, Nordskov Hansen G. Cow hair allergen (Bos d2) content in house dust: correlation with sensitisation in farmers with cow hair asthma. Int Arch Allergy Immunol 1997; 112:231–237.

113. Preller L, Heederik D, Boleij JS, Vogelzang PF, Tielen MJ. Lung function and chronic respiratory symptoms of pig farmers: focus on exposure to endotoxins and ammonia and use of disinfectants. Occup Environ Med 1995; 52:654–660.

114. Malo J-L, Chretien P, McCants M, Lehrer S. Detection of snow-crab antigens by air sampling of a snow-crab production plant. Clin Exp Allergy 1997; 27:75–78.

115. Aoyama K, Ueda A, Manda F, Matsushita T, Ueda T, Yamauchi C. Allergy to laboratory animals: an epidemiological study. Br J Ind Med 1992; 49:41–47.

116. Kibby T, Powell G, Cromer J. Allergy to laboratory animals: a prospective and cross-sectional study. J Occup Med 1989; 31:842–846.

117. Agrup G, Belin L, Sjöstedt L, Skerfving S. Allergy to laboratory animals in laboratory technicians and animal keepers. Br J Ind Med 1986; 43:192–198.

118. Beeson MF, Dewdney JM, Edwards RG, Lee D, Orr RG. Prevalence and diagnosis of laboratory animal allergy. Clin Allergy 1983; 13:433–442.

119. Cockcroft A, Edwards J, McCarthy P, Andersson N. Allergy in laboratory animal workers. Lancet 1981 1:827–830.

120. Cullinan P, Lowson D, Nieuwenhuijsen MJ, Gordon S, Tee RD, Venables KM, et al. Work-related symptoms, sensitisation and estimated exposure in workers not previously exposed to laboratory rats. Occup Environ Med 1994; 51:589–592.

121. Hollander A, Heederik D, Doekes G. Respiratory allergy to rats: exposure-response relationships in laboratory animal workers. Am J Respir Crit Care Med 1997; 155:562–567.

122. Cullinan P, Cook A, Gordon S, Nieuwenhuijsen MJ, Tee RD, Venables KM, McDonald JC, Newman Taylor AJ. Allergen exposure, atopy and smoking as determinants of allergy to rats in a cohort of laboratory employees: a case-referent analysis. Eur Respir J 1998 (manuscript submitted).

123. Corn M, Esmen NA. Workplace exposure zones for classification of employee exposures to physical and chemical agents. Am Ind Hyg Assoc J 1979; 40:47–57.

124. Eggleston PA, Ansari AA, Adkinson NF, Wood RA. Environmental challenge studies in laboratory animal allergy. Effect of different airborne allergen concentrations. J Allergy Clin Immunol 1995; 151:640–646.

125. Contreras GR, Rousseau R, Chan-Yeung M. Occupational respiratory diseases in British Columbia, Canada in 1991. Occup Environ Med 1994; 51:710–712.

126. Karjalainen A, Aalto L, Jolanki R, Keskinen H, Savela A. Occupational diseases in Finland in 1996. Helsinki: Finnish Institute of Occupational Health, 1998.

127. Fishwick D, Pearce N, D'Souza W, Lewis S, Town I, Armstrong R, Kogevinas M, Crane J. Occupational asthma in New Zealanders: a population based study. Occup Environ Med 1997; 54:301–306.

128. Slovak AJM, Hill RN. Laboratory animal allergy: a clinical survey of an exposed population. Br J Ind Med 1981; 38:38–41.

129. Davies GE, Thompson AV, Niewola Z, Burrows GE, Teasdale EL, Bird DJ, et al. Allergy to laboratory animals: a retrospective and a prospective study. Br J Ind Med 1983; 40:442–449.

130. Bland SM, Evans RE, Rivera JC. Allergy to laboratory animals in health care personnel. Occup Med 1987; 2:525–546.

131. Venables KM, Tee RD, Hawkins ER, Gordon DJ, Wale CJ, Farrer NM, et al. Laboratory animal allergy in a pharmaceutical company. Br J Ind Med 1988; 45:660–666.

132. Fuortes LJ, Weih L, Jones ML, Burmeister LF, Thorne PS, Pollen S, Merchant JA. Epidemiologic assessment of laboratory animal allergy among university employees. Am J Ind Med 1996; 29:67–74.

133. Bryant DH, Boscato LM, Mboloi PN, Stuart MC. Allergy to laboratory animals among animal handlers. Med J Aust 1995; 163:415–418.

134. Botham PA, Davies GE, Teasdale EL. Allergy to laboratory animals: a prospective study of the incidence and of the influence of atopy on its development. Br J Ind Med 1987; 44:627–632.

135. Hollander A, Doekes G Heederik D. Cat and dog allergy and total IgE as risk factors of laboratory animal allergy. J Allergy Clin Immunol 1996; 98:545–554.

136. Venables KM, Upton JL, Hawkins ER, Tee RD, Longbottom JL, Newman Taylor AJ. Smoking, atopy and laboratory animal allergy. Br J Ind Med 1988; 45:667–671.

137. Hinze S, Bergmann K-Chr. Cow hair asthma: symptoms and clinical course. Allergol J 1995; 4:97–101.

138. Kanerva L, Susitaival P. Cow dander: the most common cause of occupational contact urticaria in Finland. Contact Dermatitis 1996; 35:309–310.

139. Reijula K, Halmepuro L, Hannuksela M, Larmi E, Hassi J. Specific IgE to reindeer epithelium in Finnish reindeer herders. Allergy 1991; 46:577–581.

140. Gillespie DN, Dahlberg MJE, Yuninger JW. Inhalant allergy to wild animals (deer and elk). Ann Allergy 1985; 55:122–125.

141. Choudat D, Goehen M, Korobaeff M, Boulet A, Dewitte JD, Martin MH. Respiratory symptoms and bronchial reactivity among pig and dairy farmers. Scand J Work Environ Health 1994; 20:48–54.

142. Bongers P, Houthuijs D, Remijn B, Brouwer R, Biersteker K. Lung function and respiratory symptoms in pig farmers. Br J Ind Med 1987; 44:819–823.

143. Preller L, Heederik D, Boleij JSM, Vogelzang PFJ, Tielen MJM. Lung function and chronic respiratory symptoms of pig farmers: focus on exposure to endotoxins and ammonia and use of disinfectants. Occup Environ Med 1995; 52:654–660.

144. Iversen M, Dahl R, Korsgaard J, Hallas T, Jensen EJ. Respiratory symptoms in Danish farmers: an epidemiological study of risk factors. Thorax 1988; 43:872–877.

145. Kaufman GL, Gandevia BH, Bellas TE, Tovey ER, Baldo BA. Occupational allergy in an entomological research centre. I. Clinical aspects of reactions to the sheep blowfly *Lucilia cuprina*. Br J Ind Med 1989; 46:473–478.

146. Liebers V, Hoernstein M, Baur X. Humoral immune response to the insect allergen Chi tI in aquarists and fish-food factory workers. Allergy 1993; 48:236–239.

147. Renström A, Malmberg P, Larsson K, Larsson PH, Sundblad B-M. Allergic sensitisation is associated with increased bronchial responsiveness. A prospective study of laboratory animal allergy. Eur Respir J 1995; 8:1514–1519.

148. Watt AD, McSharry CP. Laboratory animal allergy: anaphylaxis from a needle injury. Occup Environ Med 1996; 53:573–574.

149. Hudson P, Cartier A, Pineau L, Lafrance M, St-Aubin JJ, Dubois JY, Malo J-L. Follow-up of occupational asthma caused by crab and various agents. J Allergy Clin Immunol 1985; 76:682–687.

150. Malo J-L, Cartier A, Ghezzo H, Lafrance M, McCants M, Lehrer SB. Patterns of improvement in spirometry, bronchial hyperresponsiveness, and specific IgE antibody levels after cessation of exposure in occupational asthma caused by snow crab processing. Am Rev Respir Dis 1988; 138:807–812.

151. Renström A, Malmberg P, Karlsson A-S, Sundblad B-M, Larsson P H. Prospective study of laboratory-animal allergy: factors pre-disposing to sensitisation and development of allergic symptoms. Allergy 1994; 49:548–552.

152. Botham PA and Teasdale EL. Allergy to laboratory animals. Biologist 1987; 34:162–163.

153. Botham PA, Lamb CT, Teasdale EL, Bonner SM, Tomenson J.A. Allergy to laboratory animals: a follow up study of its incidence and of the influence of atopy and pre-existing sensitisation on its development. Occup Environ Med 1995; 52:129–133.

154. Gordon S, Tee RD, Lowson D, Wallace J, Newman Taylor AJ. Reduction of airborne allergenic urinary proteins from laboratory rats. Br J Ind Med 1992; 49:416–422.

155. Sakaguchi M, Inouye S, Miyazawa H, Kamimura M, Yamazaki S. Evaluation of countermeasures for reduction of mouse airborne allergens. Lab Animal Sci 1990; 40:613–614.

156. Gordon S, Wallace J, Cook A, Tee RD, Newman Taylor AJ. Reduction of exposure to laboratory animal allergens in the workplace. Clin Exp Allergy 1997; 27:744–751.

157. Jones RB, Kacergis JB, MacDonald MR, McKnight FT, Turner WA, Ohman JL, Paigen B. The effect of relative humidity on mouse allergen levels in an environmentally controlled mouse room. Am Ind Hyg Assoc J 1995; 56:398–401.

158. Renström A, Larsson PH, Malmberg P, Bayard C. A new amplified monoclonal rat allergen assay used for evaluation of ventilation improvements in animal rooms. J Allergy Clin Immunol 1997; 100:649–655.

159. Renström A, Karlsson A-S, Malmberg P, Larsson PH, van Hage-Hamsten M. Allergy to laboratory rodents in environments with low exposure. In: Allergy to laboratory animals. Risk factors for development of allergy and methods for measuring airborne rodent allergens. Arbete och Hälsa 1997; 26. Thesis.

160. Slovak AJM, Orr RG, Teasdale EL. Efficacy of the helmet respirator in occupational asthma due to laboratory animal allergy (LAA). Am Ind Hyg Assoc J 1985; 46:411–415.

161. Sakaguchi M, Inouye S, Miyazawa H, Kamimura H, Kimura M, Yamazaki S. Evaluation of dust respirators for elimination of mouse aeroallergens. Lab Animal Sci 1989; 39:63–66.

162. WHO/IUS Allergen Nomenclature Subcommittee World Health Organisation, Chairman T P King. Allergen nomenclature. Clin Exp Allergy 1995; 25:27–37.

163. Stewart GA, Thompson PJ. Letter to the Editors. Re: nomenclature of rat allergens. Reply to Gordon S, Jones MG, Tee RD, Newman Taylor AJ. Clin Exp Allergy 1997; 27:714–715.

164. Rautiainen J, Rytkönen M, Virtanen T, Pentikäinen J, Zeiler T, Mäntyjärvi R. BDA20, a major bovine dander allergen characterized at sequence level is Bos d2. J Allergy Clin Immunol 1997; 100:251–252.

165. Gregoire C, Rosinski Chupin I, Rabillon J, Alzari PM, David B, Dandeu JP. cDNA cloning and sequencing reveal the major horse allergen Equ c1 to be a glycoprotein member of the lipocalin superfamily. J Biol Chem 1996; 271:32951–32959.

166. Liebers V, Baur X. Chironomidae haemoglobin Chi t1—characterization of an important inhalant allergen. Clin Exp Allergy 1994; 24:100–108.

167. Arruda LK, Vailes LD, Mann BJ, Shannon J, Fox JW, Vedvick TS, Hayden ML, Chapman MD. Molecular cloning of a major cockroach (*Blatella germanica*) allergen, Bla g2. J Biol Chem 1995; 270:19563–19568.

168. Reese G, Jeong BJ, Daul CB, Lehrer SB. Characterisation of recombinant shrimp allergen Pen a1 (tropomyosin). Int Arch Allergy Immunol 1997; 113:240–242.

23
Latex Allergy

Olivier Vandenplas
University Hospital of Mont-Godinne, Yvoir, Belgium

B. Lauren Charous
Milwaukee Medical Clinic and Medical College of Wisconsin, Milwaukee, Wisconsin

Susan M. Tarlo
University of Toronto, Toronto, Ontario, Canada

INTRODUCTION

Natural rubber latex (NRL) allergy has been clearly identified in 1979 in Europe (1) and in 1989 in North America (2,3), although adverse events to natural rubber materials have been rarely described earlier (4). Over the last decade, NRL has been increasingly acknowledged as a major cause of IgE-mediated allergy in occupational and nonoccupational environments (5–9). NRL materials can cause a wide spectrum of immediate hypersensitivity reactions ranging from mild urticaria to extensive angioedema and life-threatening anaphylaxis after cutaneous, mucosal, or visceral exposure. In addition, it has been shown that NRL proteins can bind to glove powder and be dispersed as airborne allergens causing rhinitis and asthma (10).

NATURAL RUBBER LATEX

Composition

In the chemical industry nomenclature, the term "latex" applies to any emulsion of polymers, including synthetic rubbers and plastics. "Natural rubber latex" refers specifically to products derived from the milky fluid, or latex, produced by the laticifers of the tropical rubber tree *Hevea braziliensis* (botanical family of Euphorbiaceae) (11). The laticifers are specialized structures that consist of anastamosed latex-producing cells. Upon wounding, the cytoplasmic content of these cells is expelled and coagulates to seal the wounded sites.

Using high-speed centrifugation, NRL can be separated into three components: the "rubber cream" containing the rubber particles, the latex serum (C-serum), and the "bottom fraction," which consists mainly of vacuolar structures called lutoids. Rubber particles are spherical droplets containing polymers of *cis*-1,4-polyisoprene coated with a layer of hydrophylic colloid (proteins, lipids, and phospholipids). Lutoids are vacuoles with an acidic content that are involved in the coagulation of latex through the release of proteins interacting with rubber particles. Fresh NRL consists of about 30–40% rubber hydrocarbon

425

and 2–3% protein. Several of the proteins in NRL have been purified and sequenced. Prenyltransferase (38 kDa) is found in the cytosol as well as in association with rubber particles. Rubber elongation factor (14.6 kDa) is bound to the surface of rubber particles. These two enzymes play a role in the elongation of polyisoprene chains (12). The lutoid bodies contain defense-related proteins. Hevein (4.7 kDa), a major protein of the lutoid bodies, is synthesized as a preproprotein (or prohevein, 20 kDa) that is posttranslationally processed into an amino-terminal fragment, hevein (4.7 kDa), and a carboxy-terminal domain (14 kDa). Hevein is a lectin-like protein that may be involved in the coagulation of latex by bridging rubber particles (13). Hevein may also inhibit the growth of chitin-containing fungi through chitin-binding properties (14). Hevein shows structural homology to wheat germ agglutinin and other chitin-binding proteins, while the carboxyl-terminal domain demonstrates homology to wound-inducible proteins in various plants, such as WIN 1 and WIN 2 (15). Hevamine (29 kDa), an enzyme with lysozyme and chitinase properties, has been isolated from the lutoids (16). The lutoid bodies contain glycoproteins that can form complex microfibrils and microhelices.

Processing

Ammonia is added to the fresh latex obtained by tapping the rubber tree to prevent premature coagulation and bacterial growth. The resulting substance is concentrated to obtain a 60% rubber content by centrifuging. Further processing of concentrated NRL varies considerably according to the desired properties of the finished product, but usually includes the following three steps: compounding, coagulation, and vulcanization. Compounding involves the addition of a variety of chemicals including antioxidants (e.g., paraphenylenediamine), accelerators (e.g., zinc oxide, thiurams, dithiocarbamates, mercaptobenzothiazole), fillers, pigments, emulsifiers, and other ingredients. Some of these compounding agents can cause delayed type IV hypersensitivity (17). The concentrated liquid NRL is converted to a solid form during the coagulation, or curing, process by dehydration and/or addition of acids, metal ions, or surface-active agents. Vulcanization consists of a heat-catalyzed crosslinking of the *cis*-1,4-polyisoprene chains by sulfur bridges. NRL articles are produced by either dipping or extrusion compression molding. Typically, gloves are manufactured by dipping porcelain formers, pretreated with a coagulant (e.g., calcium nitrate) and a releasing agent (cornstarch powder), into the compounded liquid NRL. The gloves are then passed through ovens to complete coagulation of NRL, and through water baths to extract water-soluble proteins and processing chemicals. Finally they undergo the vulcanization process. The powder can be subsequently removed from gloves through a chlorination wash process.

PATHOGENESIS

There is convincing evidence from both in vitro and in vivo experiments that immediate hypersensitivity reactions caused by NRL materials are mediated through specific IgE antibodies directed against NRL proteins that persist in manufactured products (5–7,9). Maize allergens in cornstarch powder (18,19) and ethylene oxide used for sterilization of medical devices (20,21) have been reported as possible causes of immediate allergic reactions to gloves, but their role has never been convincingly substantiated. A recent report suggests that significant amounts of rapidly elutable endotoxin contaminate NRL gloves and are also present in glove-generated aerosols (22). However, the preliminary nature of these findings mandates further research to investigate the effects of endotoxins on IgE responses to NRL.

NRL Allergens

Immunoblotting studies conducted by several groups of investigators have identified IgE-binding proteins with molecular weights ranging from 2 to 200 kDa in raw NRL and eluates from NRL-manufactured products (22–33). Antigenic peptides with molecular weights of 14, 20, 24, 27, 30, 36, and 46 kDa have been identified most consistently. Variations in protein antigen profile may be due to differences in source materials, including fresh latex, ammoniated latex, and finished products. Ammonia treatment and other manufacturing procedures can cause denaturation or precipitation of NRL peptides (25,29,33–36). Antigenic variability may also result from the methods used for extracting and identifying antigens from NRL products as these methods can lead to conformational alteration and degradation of NRL proteins (35). Furthermore, significant differences can be detected in the pattern of IgE reactivity between subjects with NRL allergy (32,33, 37–40), possibly as a result of differences in the patients' mode of sensitization. Although most studies failed to demonstrate a correlation between the pattern of IgE reactivity to NRL proteins and clinical manifestations of NRL allergy, some investigations suggest that spina bifida is more specifically associated with the development of IgE antibodies against 24-kDa and 27-kDa proteins (30,36,41).

In recent years, substantial progress has been made in the purification and molecular characterization of NRL allergens (Table 1). Several potential allergens have been identified in *Hevea* latex and finished products, including rubber elongation factor (Hev b 1) (35,36,42), β-1,3-glucosidase (Hev b 2) (43,44), a protein associated with small rubber particles (Hev b 3) (36), a component of the microhelix glycoprotein complex in lutoids (Hev b 4) (44), an acidic protein (Hev b 5) (35,45), prohevein (Hev b 6.01) and its C-terminal fragment (Hev b 6.03) (32,43,46), hevein (Hev b 6.02) (43), a patatin homolog (Hev b 7) (32), and hevamine (32,43). The clinical relevance of these various allergens warrants further investigation.

Table 1 Allergenic Proteins of Natural Rubber Latex

Allergen[a] *Hevea braziliensis* protein			Molecular weight (kDa)	Prevalence of IgE reactivity (%)	Ref.
Hev b 1		Rubber elongation factor (REF)	14.6,58	20–100	35,36,42
Hev b 2		β-1,3-glucosidase	34–36	~30	43,44
Hev b 3		Rubber particle protein	24–27	?	36
Hev b 4		Microhelix component	100,110,115	~30	44
Hev b 5		Acidic protein	16–24	~60	35,45
Hev b 6	6.01	Prohevein	20	50–90	32,43,46
	6.02	Hevein	5	~60	46
	6.03	Prohevein C domain	14	~20	46
Hev b 7		Patatin homologue	43–46	~20	32

[a]Allergen designation by the International Union of Immunological Societies (IUIS)

Exposure to NRL Allergens

NRL is widely used in the manufacturing of medical devices (gloves, catheters, drainage tubes, anesthetic masks, tourniquets, dental dams), as well as in the production of a variety of everyday articles (household gloves, toys, balloons, condoms, baby pacifiers, sports equipment, elastic straps, mattresses, tires, adhesives) (Table 2). Various in vitro methods have been used to estimate the allergenic content of NRL materials, including total protein measurements and immunochemical methods (47). Standard protein assays are reproducible but lack sensitivity and specificity. The results of these assays are affected by the presence of various chemicals in NRL products that can interfere in these tests (48), although precipitation techniques can remove interfering substances (49). The majority of studies have found at most only a modest association between the total amount of protein eluting from NRL devices and their allergenic potential, as assessed by skin-prick testing (50–53). ELISA and RAST inhibition methods have been used to estimate the antigen content in NRL products (48,52,54). Immunochemical assays provide a more sensitive and biologically relevant method for determining allergen levels in NRL products (48). These methods have shown considerable variations in the allergen content between different brands of gloves or even between different batches of the same brand of gloves (48,52,54,55). At present, there is no standardized method for quantifying the allergenic potential of latex materials. Inhibition assays are affected by the sources of specific IgE and the type of allergen reference standard. Furthermore, it remains uncertain whether the results of in vitro methods for quantitative assessment of NRL allergens correlate with the in vivo effects of NRL materials. In vivo and in vitro methods have shown that the content of total protein and allergen in NRL gloves can be significantly reduced by washing the gloves during the manufacturing process (51,54,56). Exposure to NRL allergens can occur from direct contact of NRL materials with the skin, and mucosal and serosal membranes (Table 2). It has been also demonstrated that NRL protein allergens can bind to powder particles of gloves (or to any dusted rubber product, such as toy balloons) and become potent airborne allergens (27,57–59). Using an inhibition assay, Swanson and co-workers quantified airborne NRL allergens collected with personal and area samplers at various

Table 2   Exposure to NRL Allergens

Route of exposure	Sources of exposure (examples)
Skin	Any direct contact with NRL materials
	Medical devices: gloves, catheters, drainage tubes, anesthetic mask, tourniquets, dental dams
	Consumer products: household gloves, toys, balloons, condoms, baby pacifiers, sports equipment (diving mask, handle cover of squash racket), elastic straps, tyres, adhesives
Mucous membranes	
Oral	Dental care (gloves, dental dams), blowing of toy balloon
Gynecological	Pelvic examination, sexual intercourse (condom), delivery
Rectal	Barium enema (balloon-tipped catheter), rectal manometry
Inhalation	Glove powder particles, grinding of NRL devices
Visceral	Surgical procedure, cesarean section
Parenteral	Injection ports in intravenous lines, plungers on syringes, stoppers on medication vials

work sites in a hospital (60). The amount of airborne NRL allergens correlated with the frequency of glove use, although considerable variation was found among subjects with the same type of job. Substantial amounts of allergens were recovered from coats and surgical scrub suits suggesting that resuspension from clothing and settled dust may lead to secondary or even remote inhalation exposure. Twenty percent of airborne powder particles were in a respirable size and therefore capable of causing asthma. The authors found that airborne allergens were predominantly of high molecular weight (70–100 kDa) although it has not yet been shown that subjects with asthma are more specifically sensitized to these allergens as compared with subjects with other symptoms of NRL allergy. Exposure to airborne NRL has also been documented to result from inhalation of dust generated by grinding NRL articles (61). A recent study suggests that NRL allergens could be present in respirable particulate air pollution resulting from the abrasion of rubber tires on road surfaces (62). At this time, their role in the development of respiratory hypersensitivity to NRL appears speculative, and the fact that the vast majority of NRL-allergic individuals have prior occupational or patient exposure suggests that this is not a major source of sensitization.

EPIDEMIOLOGY

Prevalence

A number of studies have documented a high incidence of NRL allergy in individuals with occupational exposure to NRL, particularly glove wearers and manufacturers, as well as patients undergoing multiple surgical procedures, particularly in early infancy, such as children with spina bifida and urogenital abnormalities (Table 3) (61,63–82). Epidemiological studies have documented NRL allergy in about 10% of workers manufacturing medical gloves and NRL toys (61,63). Prevalence figures for NRL allergy have ranged from 2.8 to 17% among health-care workers, including physicians, nurses, laboratory technicians, hospital housekeepers, and dental-care providers (64–73). The highest prevalence rates, ranging from 29 to 65%, have been found in children with spina bifida (75–79). In addition, NRL allergy due to gloves is increasingly described in nonmedical environments, including workers exposed to chemicals (24,83,84), hairdressers (85), and greenhouse workers (74). The prevalence of sensitization to NRL in the general population varied from 0 to 9% (64,65,77,80–82), with the highest figures being found in atopic individuals (65,77,80,81).

The advent of "universal precautions" in the last half of the 1980s resulted in increased use of NRL devices as a protective barrier against viral infections. While this rise in exposure to NRL certainly played a role in the consequent dramatic rise in incidence of NRL allergy, it fails to explain cases of anaphylactic reactions induced by retention balloons used in barium enema procedures or by rubber gloves, which occurred in patients without significant histories of prior exposure to NRL. Even among patients and health-care workers with continuing exposure to NRL, recognizable allergic reactions appeared rather abruptly in about 1987 in the United States (86), suggesting that some intrinsic alteration in the NRL may play a role in the origin of this new disease. Changes in manufacturing processes (87,88) and *Hevea* growing methods may play a role in altering the antigenicity of the final products. For example, treatment of *Hevea* trees with phytohormones to stimulate the production of latex can enhance the biosynthesis of some proteins by laticifers, especially defense-related proteins (13). An increased recognition of

Table 3 Prevalence of Allergy and Occupational Asthma Due to NRL

Populations	No. of subjects studied	NRL allergy[a] (%)	NRL-induced occupational asthma (%)	Country/ Ref.
NRL industry workers				
Glove manufacture	64	10.9	6.0	Canada (63)
Doll manufacture	22	9.0	9.0	USA (61)
Health-care workers				
Hospital employees	512	2.8		Finland (64)
Operating room nurses	71	5.6		Finland (64)
Surgeons	54	7.4		Finland (64)
Physicians	101	9.9		Canada (65)
Operating room nurses	197	10.7		France (66)
Laboratory tecnologists	230	1.3[a]		Canada (67)
Hospital employees	224	16.9		USA (68)
Hospital employees	273	4.7	2.5	Belgium (69)
Dental care providers	176	2.1		Sweden (70)
Dental care providers	34	11.7		USA (71)
Dental students and staff	131	10.0		Canada (72)
Hospital housekeepers	50	8.0		Canada (73)
Other glove-wearing workers				
Greenhouse workers	418	5.0		Spain (74)
Multiple surgical procedures				
Spina bifida children	32	34.3[a]		USA (75)
Spina bifida children	76	64.5		USA (76)
Spina bifida children	25	32.0		France (77)
Spina bifida children	86	48.8		USA (78)
Spina bifida children	100	29.0		Spain (79)
General population				
Dermatology clinic	30	0.8		Finland (64)
Nonatopics (allergy clinic)	272	0.4		France (77)
Nonatopics (allergy and asthma clinic)	78	0		Canada (80)
Nonatopics (children, allergy clinic)	127	0		Italy (81)
Atopics (allergy clinic)	100	3.0		Canada (65)
Atopics (allergy clinic)	180	9.4		France (77)
Atopics (allergy and asthma clinics)	146	7.0		Canada (80)
Atopics (children, allergy clinic)	326	3.0		Italy (81)
Blood donors	1000	3.9[a]		USA (82)

[a]Prevalence of NRL allergy based on skin-prick tests, except in Refs. 67, 75, and 82, where in vitro assessment of specific IgE was used to confirm NRL sensitization.

NRL allergy by exposed workers and physicians might also have contributed to the apparent increase in the prevalence of the disease.

Risk Factors

The highest prevalence rates of NRL allergy have been found in operating-room workers, who presumably have the highest level of exposure (64,66). It has recently been shown that dental students with increasing exposure to NRL have an increasing incidence of NRL allergy (72), although a clear dose-response relationship between exposure to NRL and IgE-mediated sensitization has not been consistently demonstrated in prevalence surveys (69). Thus, assessment of exposure based on self-reported use of NRL gloves may not reflect the actual level of exposure (69), since colleagues working in the same environment represent a significant source of airborne allergen. Furthermore, it has been shown that sensitization to NRL can result purely from indirect airborne exposure in subjects who have no direct contact with NRL materials (89). Immunological techniques for quantitative assessment of environmental NRL allergens (60) should help to further clarify exposure-response relationships.

In addition to repeated exposure to NRL products, atopy seems to be the principal determinant for the development of NRL sensitization. Atopy (defined either by immunological tests to common inhalant allergens or by the history) is two- to fivefold more frequent in health-care personnel with NRL allergy than in their co-workers without NRL allergy (64–66,68,69,72). However, the predictive value of atopy with regard to the presence of immunological sensitization and occupational asthma due to NRL is low as only about 10% of atopic hospital workers had NRL allergy (69). Preexisting dermatitis of the hands is thought to enhance the risk of NRL allergy by facilitating the transcutaneous passage of NRL proteins (90). Hand eczema has been found two- to fourfold more frequently in subjects with NRL allergy than in their nonallergic co-workers (64,68,69,72). In spina bifida children, the development of NRL allergy is associated with atopy, the number of surgical procedures, and daily exposure to NRL materials used for bladder catheterization and rectal disimpaction (76,79,86). Exposure to NRL in infancy is likely to be the crucial factor leading to the high prevalence of NRL sensitization in spina bifida children as compared with adults affected by similar neurological disorders and NRL exposure (91). Multiple anecdotal reports strongly suggest that allergy to foods known to cross-react with NRL is likely an independent risk factor for the development of NRL allergy (92–95). In recent years, clinical NRL allergy has been reported in subjects, usually atopic children, with no recognizable exposure risk (94,96,97). The presence of NRL-specific IgE antibodies has been documented in normal blood donors and others with no identifiable history of NRL allergy (82,98) although the clinical relevance of this finding requires further clarification.

CLINICAL MANIFESTATIONS

Skin Symptoms

Contact urticaria or one of its clinical variants is the most frequent, and usually the initial, manifestation of IgE-mediated allergy to NRL. In glove wearers, skin symptoms usually take the form of contact hives almost always beginning within 30 min after donning gloves, which characteristically do not extend beyond the level of the glove cuff. This reaction may also be expressed as extensive pruritic erythema or angioedema. Some individuals develop an acute dyshidrotic reaction consistent with a protein contact dermatosis (90).

A high proportion (13–53%) of health-care workers experience glove-related skin symptoms consistent with contact dermatitis, including localized itching and/or redness (64,66–69) in the absence of any demonstrable allergic sensitization to NRL. For this reason, symptoms of glove-induced itching and redness of the hands, particularly if indolent in character and nonimmediate in onset, have a low predictive value with regard to the presence of NRL allergy. In addition to immediate skin reactions, NRL-exposed workers can also present with persistent dermatitis related to irritant contact dermatitis or delayed hypersensitivity reaction to NRL additives or disinfectants (17).

Anaphylactic Reactions

The severity of clinical manifestations of NRL allergy varies according to the route of exposure (99), although the number of reports of anaphylaxis suggest an unusual propensity of this antigen to evoke potentially catastrophic reactions. Cutaneous exposure to NRL causes local urticaria, although systemic reactions have occasionally been reported (3,100,101). Mucosal, visceral, and parenteral exposures are associated with the greatest risk for developing severe systemic reactions. Anaphylactic reactions have been documented during surgical procedures (2,86,99,102–104), delivery (105,106), gynecological examination (100,107), dental treatment (100), barium enema using balloon-tipped catheters (108,109), condom-protected sexual intercourse (110), exposure to toy balloons and baby pacifiers (111). Identification of the agent responsible for anaphylactic reaction during surgery can be difficult, since such reactions can be caused by various agents, including anesthetic agents, muscle relaxants, antibiotics, and ethylene oxide. NRL-induced reactions are characterized by a delayed onset after induction of anaesthesia (2,103,104), although reactions occurring before surgical incision have been reported (86). Intravenous exposure to NRL allergens can result from injection ports in intravenous lines, plungers on syringes, and stoppers on medication vials (112,113). Systemic reactions have been described after ingestion of foods contaminated by NRL allergens when handled by personnel wearing gloves in restaurants (114). Finally, it should be kept in mind that urticaria and anaphylaxis can occur after remote exposure to NRL allergens transferred from the workplace on hands and clothes (115).

Respiratory Symptoms

Rhinoconjunctivitis and asthma have been described primarily among workers manufacturing or using gloves (Table 3). Occupational asthma has been diagnosed in 6% of workers in a glove-manufacturing plant on the basis of positive skin-prick tests associated with changes in spirometry and nonspecific bronchial responsiveness related to workplace exposure (63). In a survey of hospital employees, including nurses, members of the cleaning staff, and laboratory technologists, the presence of occupational asthma due to NRL was demonstrated in 2.5% of the participants using specific inhalation challenges (69). These findings illustrate that NRL-induced asthma represents a significant respiratory health hazard in health-care providers. Although powdered NRL gloves are the most frequent source of exposure to airborne NRL, the possibility of respiratory reactions to NRL in other industrial environments should be considered. In a recent survey, NRL-induced asthma was documented in 2/22 workers exposed to NRL dust in a latex-doll-manufacturing plant (61). In nonoccupational environments, respiratory symptoms can result from exposure to deflating or bursting balloons.

Subjects with NRL-induced asthma may experience the classic patterns of asthmatic reactions. Among 20 subjects who showed a positive inhalation challenge with NRL gloves, the pattern of bronchial response included immediate ($n = 14$), dual ($n = 5$), and isolated late ($n = 1$) reactions (10). The natural history of NRL-induced asthma remains largely uncertain. There is some suggestion that health-care workers have a progression of symptoms from cutaneous reactions to rhinoconjunctivitis and asthma, although rhinitis and asthma can be the inaugural symptomatology in workers who have only indirect exposure to airborne NRL allergens. Among subjects with confirmed NRL-induced asthma, rhinitis preceded the onset of asthma by an average of 6 months (range: 2–20 months) (10). Studies using quantitative assessment of airborne NRL allergens at work or during inhalation challenges are required to determine the minimum dose of allergen that can provoke respiratory reactions.

Food Allergy

Serious allergic reactions to banana, kiwi, avocado, and chestnut were noted to occur with unusual frequency among NRL-allergic individuals (83,92,93,95,116–121). In recent years, the list of cross-reacting agents is the most extensive of any known allergens and now includes potato, tomato, passion fruit, hazelnut, peanut, celery, melons, figs, peaches, plums, and other stone fruits (95,116,120,122). Several reports have described an association between NRL allergy and sensitization to latex from the weeping fig (*Ficus benjamina*) (123,124) and to enzymes extracted from the latex of papaya (*Carica papaya*) (95,125–127). Investigation into this phenomenon has revealed that the unexpectedly high prevalence of food allergies in NRL-allergic subjects is due to immunological cross-reactivity between NRL allergens and food allergens, particularly in tropical fruits and vegetables (119,121,128), even though these diverse plants are botanically unrelated. The potential for serious allergic reactions to foods should be strongly considered in patients sensitized to NRL. The degree of sensitivity to NRL appears, however, to be a poor predictor of developing cross-reacting food allergy. Allergy to cross-reacting foods may also precede the onset of identifiable NRL allergy (92–95). For this reason, progressive oral allergy syndrome or anaphylactic reactions provoked by foods known to cross-react with NRL should be viewed as indicating a heightened likelihood of allergic reactions to NRL materials and appropriate safeguards should be instituted.

DIAGNOSIS

Immunological Tests

Most studies have shown that in vitro measurement of NRL-specific IgE using RAST or ELISA methods is less reliable than skin testing. The sensitivity of in vitro tests ranged from 14 to 84% as compared with skin-prick tests (27,66,77,78,90,97,129,130). Although anaphylactic events have been reported after skin tests with NRL extracts (78), most investigators agree that skin testing can be performed safely and should be, for the time being, the recommended procedure for demonstrating IgE sensitization to NRL. The severity of symptoms on exposure to NRL materials can help in determining a safe starting dilution of NRL extract for prick testing to prevent occasional cases of anaphylaxis (131). The use of home-made extracts of NRL materials is not recommended for routine testing, because these extracts are of variable allergenic activity (132). Laboratory manipulation of raw latex solution can reduce the skin test bioequivalence (133). Standardized and validated extracts of NRL are becoming commercially available (134). Further characterization of relevant NRL allergens will make it possible to achieve proper allergen standardization for in vivo and in vitro investigation of NRL allergy. A cross-sectional study of health-care workers skin-tested with an unstandardized NRL glove extract and a commercial NRL extract demonstrated that the test had excellent sensitivity (100%) but inadequate specificity for identifying NRL-induced asthma (69). The negative predictive value of the NRL skin test for occupational asthma has not yet been determined although multicenter studies are being performed to define test characteristics of various NRL extracts.

Inhalation Challenges

The clinical history has proved to be a sensitive but not a specific diagnostic tool in the individual assessment of occupational asthma (135). In the case of NRL-induced asthma among health-care workers, it is our experience that the clinical history is frequently misleading. The work-relatedness of asthmatic symptoms can be confused by the fact that exposure to airborne NRL allergens is intermittent. On the other hand, NRL often remains unidentified as the responsible agent, because exposure may be indirect, resulting from inhalation of NRL allergens disseminated in the air by co-workers handling NRL gloves (89). Subjects with skin allergy to NRL often ascribe their asthma to substances other than NRL (136), because they still experience asthma at work despite using NRL-free gloves. Respiratory symptoms can be the initial manifestation of NRL allergy without ever having experienced contact urticaria (87,89). On the other hand, the presence of NRL-specific IgE does not necessarily indicate that NRL is involved in the development of asthmatic reactions, even when the subject has nonspecific bronchial hyperresponsiveness.

Diagnosing asthma due to occupational agents, including NRL, has considerable medical, professional, and financial consequences. The causal relationship between exposure to airborne NRL allergens and asthmatic reactions can be ascertained using either monitoring peak expiratory flow rate combined with serial assessment of nonspecific bronchial hyperresponsiveness during periods at work and off work or specific inhalational challenges (SIC) in the laboratory (10). SIC should be performed only in specialized centers with facilities to treat severe asthmatic reactions and anaphylactic responses (137,l38). SIC with NRL proved to be a simple and safe technique, provided safety requirements and stringent protocols of exposure and monitoring are carefully observed (10). SIC can be performed either by handling NRL gloves (10,27,53,69,139,140) or by inhaling aqueous extracts of gloves (141,142). The ''handling'' method is more likely to reproduce the mode of exposure encountered in the workplace (i.e., airborne particles) than is the inhalation of nebulized glove extracts. At present, however, no standardized methodology exists for performing SIC with NRL, as standardization would require quantifing the amount of NRL allergen delivered to the tested subjects.

MANAGEMENT

Complete and definitive avoidance of exposure to NRL allergens is the most effective treatment, but it is difficult to implement because NRL is ubiquitous in medical and nonmedical environments. Since continued exposure may result in increasing sensitivity over time, treatment with antiallergic medications, such as antihistamines, is not a safe alternative to a program of allergen avoidance (143). Their use may also mask early expression of allergic reactions due to inadvertent exposures. Once NRL allergy has been firmly established, NRL-allergic patients should receive complete information about the sources of exposure to NRL (Table 2) and the possibility of cross-reactivity with certain foods. All surgical procedures, diagnostic investigations, and dental treatments should be performed in latex-free environments even if the reactions induced by skin exposure have been mild (144). NRL-allergic individuals should wear a Medic Alert bracelet or another "allergy identification card" and should be prescribed an autoinjectable epinephrine kit with careful instructions on how to use it.

Affected workers should be instructed to use only nonlatex gloves. However, personal avoidance of NRL gloves should not be considered sufficient to prevent exposure to airborne NRL allergens. As the major source of NRL aeroallergen in the medical setting is powdered NRL gloves (60,145), their continued use by co-workers may disseminate significant amounts of NRL-contaminated powder particles, which are capable of triggering respiratory reactions in allergic workers. For this reason, workers suffering from NRL-induced occupational asthma should not return to work until all workers in their geographic area or work unit are using nonlatex or low-allergen NRL gloves as well. Thus, strict avoidance of exposure to airborne NRL implies both personal professional and institutional policy changes. Every effort should be made to avoid direct exposure to NRL and to reduce indirect exposure to airborne NRL. Nonpowdered NRL gloves with lower protein content should be used by all staff members working in the environment of affected subjects. It has been shown that nonpowdered, low-protein gloves are effective in reducing the concentration of airborne NRL allergens (60,145,146) and in preventing the development of asthmatic reactions in health-care workers with NRL-induced asthma (5,146) (Fig. 1). Powdered, low-protein gloves should be used with more caution and evaluated on an individual basis, as highly sensitive subjects may still develop asthmatic reactions after prolonged exposure (53). Transfer of highly allergic individuals to smaller worksites, such as outpatients clinics, where control of NRL aeroallergen can be more easily accomplished, should be viewed as a reasonable accommodation that permits retention of highly trained individuals without sacrificing safety. Further investigation is required to determine whether reduction of exposure to airborne NRL allergens allows for preventing long-term deterioration of asthma. The natural history of NRL allergy remains largely unknown. In general, symptoms progress from urticaria through rhinoconjunctivitis to asthma and anaphylaxis (90) but either anaphylaxis and asthma can represent the inaugural symptomatology. Prospective studies are needed to determine whether subjects with urticaria and/or rhinitis will develop asthma if they remain exposed to low levels of airborne NRL.

PREVENTION

The use of NRL-free materials is undoubtedly the most effective means of preventing sensitization to NRL. Most NRL devices for medical or consumer purposes can be easily replaced by latex-free materials with similar properties, with the notable exception of medical gloves. At present, the widespread use of NRL-free gloves does not appear to be feasible, because synthetic elastomer gloves with satisfactory mechanical and tactile properties are much more expensive than NRL gloves. Vinyl gloves are not as strong as latex gloves, nor do they provide a satisfactory tactile feel. Nevertheless, vinyl or other synthetic gloves should be used where possible for nonsterile procedures, as examination gloves are a significant source of exposure to airborne NRL outside operating rooms. Unless mandated by accepted universal precautions standards, the routine use of NRL gloves by workers and other individuals, such as food handlers and housekeeping personnel, should be discouraged. The American College of Allergy, Asthma, and Immunology and the American Academy of Allergy, Asthma, and Immunology strongly recommend the exclusive use of nonpowdered, low-allergen gloves or non-NRL gloves.

Widespread switching to NRL gloves with a low allergen content in all exposed health-care workers would appear to be a logical intervention to reduce exposure to NRL

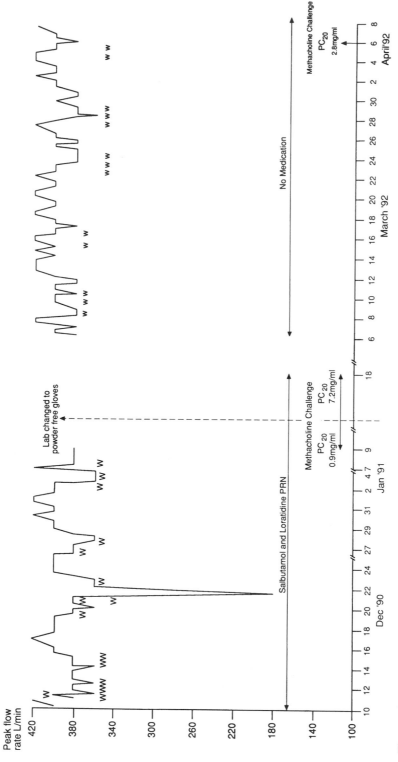

Figure 1 Peak flow responses, symptoms, and medication use in a patient with NRL-induced anaphylaxis. She was working in a medical laboratory, initially with powdered NRL glove used by co-workers, and then, after her vacation, with powder-free gloves used by co-workers. PC_{20} = provocative concentration of methacholine causing a 20% fall in forced expiratory volume in 1 sec.

allergens. However, it has not been determined if this will completely prevent sensitization of naïve workers to NRL. On a practical level, selecting gloves with low allergen content remains a challenge, as clinically relevant allergens have not been precisely identified and characterized. Immunological methods for quantitative in vitro assessment of allergen content in NRL devices have not yet been validated and demonstration that their results correlate with in vivo allergenic potential remains to be confirmed. Further complicating this problem is the fact that the content of total protein may not accurately reflect their allergen content (50–53). At present, however, measurement of total protein content in NRL materials remains the most practical and simple option until more specific methods are validated. Regulatory agencies should establish international standards for the labeling of NRL-containing devices and for measurement of their protein and allergen content. Published data regarding allergen and protein levels in gloves may also prove to be a valuable tool to guide procurement decisions (47,54,55).

Although cost considerations are frequently cited as an objection to converting to nonlatex or low-allergen NRL gloves, one recent report from a major United States medical center documented substantial savings attendant to institution of policies designed to reduce aeroallergen levels (147). Furthermore, indirect costs such as workers' compensation, disability, loss of work, and medical treatment resulting from NRL exposure must be added into any strict accounting of costs incurred to reduce NRL exposure.

The high prevalence of NRL allergy among exposed workers justifies regular medical surveillance by questionnaire and immunological assessment. Children requiring early frequent surgical and medical procedures due to spina bifida and other congenital abnormalities are at such high risk for developing NRL allergy that complete avoidance of exposure to NRL products should be implemented from birth. Further research is needed to clarify the relationship of food allergies, particularly if manifested in childhood, and the subsequent development of NRL allergy.

CONCLUSION AND PERSPECTIVES

There is accumulating evidence that NRL represents a significant cause of immediate hypersensitivity reactions among individuals who are repeatedly exposed to NRL-containing materials in medical and nonmedical environments. Considering the number of exposed individuals throughout the world, especially health-care providers, NRL allergy should be considered a cause of major medical concern. Furthermore, the condition may lead to considerable socioeconomic consequences. Preventive strategies are therefore urgently required to reduce exposure to NRL allergens below the level that elicits reactions in already sensitized subjects and, preferably, below the level that initiates sensitization.

Further characterization of relevant NRL allergens should be considered a priority, as greater knowledge of the relevant allergens will make it possible to: (1) develop methods for quantitative assessment of allergen content in NRL devices and workplace environments, (2) help manufacturers reduce the NRL-allergen content of their products, and (3) establish international quality standards and precise labeling regulations. Alternatively, the development of synthetic rubber devices with satisfactory mechanical properties at lower expense should be strongly encouraged.

REFERENCES

1. Nutter AF. Contact urticairia to rubber. Br J Dermatol 1979; 101:597–598.
2. Slater JE. Rubber anaphylaxis. N Engl J Med 1989; 320:1126–1130.

3. Spaner D, Dolovich J, Tarlo S, Sussman G, Buttoo K. Hypersensitivity to natural latex. J Allergy Clin Immunol 1989; 83:1135–1137.

4. Fuchs T. Latex allergy. J Allergy Clin Immunol 1994; 93:951–952 (letter).

5. Levy DA, Charpin D, Pecquet C, Levnadier F, Vervloet D. Allergy to latex. Allergy 1992; 47:579–587.

6. Hamann CP. Natural rubber latex proteins sensitivity in review. Am J Contact Dermatitis 1993; 4:4–21.

7. Slater JE. Latex allergy. J Allergy Clin Immunol 1994; 94:139–149.

8. Charous BL, Banov C, Bardana EJ, Blaiss M, Hamilton R, Kim K, Kwittken P, Melton A, Randolph C, Selner JC, Steinberg P, Sullivan T, Williams B, Yassin M. Latex allergy—an emerging healthcare problem. Ann Allergy Asthma Immunol 1995; 75:19–21.

9. Turjanmaa K, Alenius H. Makinen-Kiljunen S, Reunala S, Palosuo T. Natural rubber allergy. Allergy 1996; 51:593–602.

10. Vandenplas 0. Occupational asthma due to natural rubber latex. Eur Respir J 1995; 8:1957–1965.

11. St Cyr DR. Rubber, natural. In: Kirk-Othmer, ed. Encyclopedia of Chemical Technology. New York: Wiley, 1982:468–491.

12. Dennis MS, Light DR. Rubber elongation factor from *Hevea braziliensis*. Identification, characterization, and role in rubber biosynthesis. J Biol Chem 1989; 264:18608–18617.

13. Gidrol X, Chrestin H, Tan HL, Kush A. Hevein, a lectin-like protein from *Hevea braziliensis* (rubber tree) is involved in the coagulation of latex. J Biol Chem 1994; 269:9278–9280.

14. Lee H, Broekaert WF. Raikhel NV. Co- and post-translational processing of the hevein pre-proprotein latex of the rubber tree (*Hevea braziliensis*). J Biol Chem 1991; 24:15944–15948.

15. Beezhold DH, Kostyal DA, Sussman GL. IgE epitope analysis of the hevein preprotein, a major latex allergen. Clin Exp Immunol 1997; 108:114–121.

16. Jekel PA, Hartmann JBH, Beintma JJ. The primary structure of hevamine, an enzyme with lysozyme/chitinase activity from *Hevea braziliensis* latex. Eur J Biochem 1991; 200:123–130.

17. Fisher AA. Allergic contact reactions in health personnel. J Allergy Clin Immunol 1992; 90:729–738.

18. Van der Meeren HLM, Van Erp PEL. Life-threatening contact urticaria from glove powder. Contact Dermatitis 1986; 14:323–324.

19. Fisher AA. Contact urticaria due to cornstarch surgical glove powder. Cutis 1986; 38:307–308.

20. Moneret-Vautrin DA, Laxenaire MC, Bavoux F. Allergic shock to latex and ethylene dioxide during surgery for spina bifida. Anesthesiology 1990; 73:556–558.

21. Dugue P, Faraut C, Figueredo M, Bettendorf A, Salvadori JM. Asthme professionnel a l'oxyde d'ethylene chez une infirmiere. Presse Med 1991; 20:1455.

22. Williams P, Halsey, J. Endotoxin as a factor in adverse reactions to latex gloves. Ann Allergy Asthma Immunol 1997; 79:303–310.

23. Carrillo T, Cuevas M, Munoz T, Hinojosa M, Moneo I. Contact urticaria and rhinitis from latex surgical gloves. Contact Dermatitis 1986; 14:69–72.

24. Morales C, Basomba A, Carreira J, Sastre A. Anaphylaxis produced by rubber glove contact: case reports and identification of the antigen involved. Clin Exp Allergy 1989; 19:425–430.

25. Alenius H, Turjanmaa K, Palosuo T, Makinen-Kiljunen S, Reunala T. Surgical latex glove allergy: characterization of rubber protein allergens by immunoblotting. Int Arch Allergy Appl Immunol 1991; 96:376–380.

26. Chambeyron C, Dry J, Leynadier F, Pecquet C, Thao TX. Study of the allergenic fractions of latex. Allergy 1992; 47:92–97.

27. Jaeger D, Czuppon AB, Baur X. Latex-specific proteins causing immediate-type cutaneous, nasal, bronchial, and systemic reactions. J Allergy Clin Immunol 1992; 89:759–767.

28. Makinen-Kiljunen S, Turjanmaa K, Palosuo T, Reunala T. Characterization of latex antigens and allergens in surgical gloves and natural rubber by immuoelectrophoretic methods. J Allergy Clin Immunol 1992; 90:230–235.

29. Slater JE, Chhabra SK. Latex antigens. J Allergy Clin Immunol 1992; 89:673–678.

30. Alenius H, Palosuo T, Kelly K, Kurup V, Reunala T, Makinen-Kiljunen S, Turjanmaa K, Fink J. IgE reactivity to 14-kD and 27-kD natural rubber proteins in latex-allergic children with spina bifida and other congenital anomalies. Int Arch Allergy Immunol 1993; 102:61–66.

31. Alenius H, Turjanmaa K, Makinen-Kiljunen S, Reunala T, Paluoso T. IgE immune response to rubber proteins in adult patients with latex allergy. J Allergy Clin Imniunol 1994; 93:859–863.

32. Beezhold DH, Sussman GL, Kostyal DA, Chang NS. Identification of a 46-kD latex protein allergen in healthcare workers. Clin Exp Immunol 1994; 98:408–413.

33. Tomazic VJ, Withrow TJ, Hamilton RG. Characterization of the allergen(s) in latex protein extracts. J Allergy Clin Immunol 1995; 96:635–642.

34. Lu L, Kurup VP, Fink JN, Kelly KJ. Comparison of latex antigens from surgical gloves, ammoniated and nonammoniated latex: effect of ammonia treatment on natural rubber latex proteins. J Lab Clin Med 1995; 126:161–168.

35. Akasawa A, Hsieh LS, Lin Y. Serum reactivities to latex proteins. J Allergy Clin Immunol 1995; 95:1196–1205.

36. Yeang HY, Cheong KF, Sunderasan E, Hamzah S, Chew NP, Hamid S, Hamilton RG, Cardosa MJ. The 14.6-kd rubber elongation factor (Hev b 1) and 24 kd (Hev b 3) rubber particle proteins are recognized by IgE from patients with spina bifida and latex allergy. J Allergy Clin Immunol 1996; 98:628–639.

37. Kurup VP, Kelly KJ, Turjanmaa K, Alenius H, Reunala T, Paluoso T, Fink JN. Immunoglobulin E reactivity to latex antigens in the sera of patients from Finland and the United States. J Allergy Clin Immunol 1993; 91:1128–1134.

38. Charous BL, Steven GC, Beezhold DH. Anti-latex IgE specificity does not correlate with clinical history. J Allergy Clin Immunol 1995; 95:156 (abstract).

39. Akasawa A, Hsieh LS, Lin Y. Comparison of latex-specific IgE binding among nonammoniated latex, ammoniated latex, and latex glove allergenic extracts by ELISA and immunoblot inhibition. J Allergy Clin Immunol 1996; 97:1116–1120.

40. Kurup V, Alenius H, Kelly K. Castillo L, Fink J. A two-dimensional electrophoretic analysis of latex peptides reacting with IgE and IgG antibodies from patients with latex allergy. Int Arch Allergy Immunol 1996; 109:58–67.

41. Alenius H, Kalkkinen N, Lukka M, Turjanmaa K, Reunala T, Makinen-Kiljunen S, Palosuo T. Purification and partial amino acid sequencing of a 27-kD natural rubber allergen recognized by latex-allergic children with spina bifida. Int Arch Allergy Immunol 1995; 106:258–262.

42. Czuppon AB, Rennert S, Engelke T, Meier H, Heber M, Baur X. The rubber elongation factor of rubber trees (*Hevea brasiliensis*) is the major allergen in latex. J Allergy Clin Immunol 1993; 92:690–697.

43. Alenius H, Kalkkinen N, Lukka M, Reunala T, Turjanmaa K, Yip E, Makinen-Kiljunen S, Paluoso T. Prohevein from the rubber tree (*Hevea braziliensis*) is a major latex allergen. Clin Exp Allergy 1995; 25:659–665.

44. Sunderasan E, Hamzah S, Hamid S, Ward MA, Yeang HY, Cardosa MJ. Latex B-serum J-1,3-glucanase (Hev b II) and a component of the microhelix (Hev b IV) are major latex allergens. J Natl Rubber Res 1995; 10:82–89.

45. Akasawa A, Hsieh LS, Martin BM, Liu T, Lin Y. A novel acidic allergen, Hev b 5, in latex. Purification, cloning and characterization. J Biol Chem 1996; 271:25389–25393.

46. Alenius H, Kalkkinen N, Reunala T, Turjanmaa K, Palosuo T. The main IgE binding epitope of a major latex allergen, prohevein, is present in its N-terminal 43-amino acid fragment, hevein. J Immunol 1996; 156:1618–1625.

47. Patterson P. Allergy issues complicate buying decisons for gloves. OR Manager 1995; 11(6).

48. Beezhold D, Swanson M, Zehr BD, Kostyal D. Measurement of natural rubber proteins in latex glove extracts: comparison of the methods. Ann Allergy Asthma Immunol 1996; 76:520–526.

49. Yeang HY, Yussof F, Abdullah L. Precipitation of *Hevea braziliensis* latex proteins with trichloroacetic acid and phophotungstic acid in preparation for the Lowry protein assay. Ann Biochem 1995; 226:35–43.

50. Turjanmaa K, Laurila K, Makinen-Kiljunen S, Reunala T. Rubber contact urticaria: allergenic properties of 19 brands of latex gloves. Contact Dermatitis 1988; 19:362–367.

51. Leynadier F, TranXuan T, Dry J. Allergenicity suppression in natural latex surgical gloves. Allergy 1991; 46:619–625.

52. Alenius H, Makinen-Kiljunen S, Trujanmaa K, Palosuo T, Reunala T. Allergen and protein content of latex gloves. Ann Allergy 1994; 73:315–319.

53. Vandenplas O, Delwiche JP, Depelchin S, Sibille Y, Vande Weyer R, Delaunois L. Latex gloves with a lower protein content reduce bronchial reactions in subjects with occupational asthma due to latex. Am J Respir Crit Care Med 1995; 151:887–891.

54. Yunginger JW, Jones RT, Fransway AF, Kelso JM, Warner MA, Hunt LW. Extractable latex allergens and proteins in disposable medical gloves and other rubber products. J Allergy Clin Immunol 1994; 93:836–842.

55. Jones RT, Scheppmann DL, Heilman DK, Yumginger JW. Prospective study of extractable latex allergen contents of disposable medical gloves. Ann Allergy 1994; 73:321–325.

56. Bubak ME, Reed CE, Fransway AF, Yunginger JW, Jones RT, Carlson CA, Hunt LW. Allergic reactions to latex among health-care workers. Mayo Clin Proc 1992; 67:1075–1079.

57. Turjanmaa K, Reunala T, Alenius H, Brummer-Korvenkontio H, Palosuo T. Allergens in latex surgical gloves and glove powder. Lancet 1990; 336:1588.

58. Beezhold D, Beck WC. Surgical glove powder bind latex antigens. Arch Surg 1992; 127: 1354–1357.

59. Tomazic VJ, Shampaine EL, Lamanna A, Withrow TJ, Adkinson F, Hamilton RG. Cornstarch powder on latex products is an allergen carrier. J Allergy Clin Immunol 1994; 94:751–758.

60. Swanson MC, Bubak ME, Hunt LW, Yunginger JW, Warner MA, Reed CE. Quantification of occupational latex aeroallergens in a medical center. J Allergy Clin Immunol 1994; 94: 445–451.

61. Orfan NA, Reed R, Dykewlcz MS, Ganz M, Kolski GB. Occupational asthma in a latex doll manufacturing plant. J Allergy Clin Immunol 1994; 94:826–830.

62. Williams PB, Buhr MP, Weber RW, Volz MA, Koepke JW, Selner JC. Latex allergen in respirable particulate air pollution. J Allergy Clin Immunol 1995; 95:88–95.

63. Tarlo SM, Wong L, Roos J, Booth N. Occupational asthma caused by latex in a surgical glove manufacturing plant. J Allergy Clin Immunol 1990; 85:626–631.

64. Turjanmaa K. Incidence of immediate allergy to latex gloves in hospital personnel. Contact Dermatitis 1987; 17:270–275.

65. Arellano R, Bradley J, Sussman G. Prevalence of latex sensitization among hospital physicians occupationally exposed to latex gloves. Anesthesiology 1992; 77:905–908.

66. Lagier F, Vervloet D, Lhermet I, Poyen D, Charpin D. Prevalence of latex allergy in operating room nurses. J Allergy Clin Immunol 1992; 319:319–322.

67. Salkle ML. The prevalence of atopy and hypersensitivity to latex in medical laboratory technologists. Arch Pathol Lab Med 1993; 117:897–899.

68. Yassin MS, Lierl MB, Fisher TJ, O'Brien K, Cross J, Steinmetz C. Latex allergy in hospital employees. Ann Allergy 1994; 72:245–249.

69. Vandenplas O, Delwiche JP, Evrard GI, Aimont P, van der Brempt X, Jamart J, Delaunois L. Prevalence of occupational asthma due to latex among hospital personnel. Am J Respir Crit Care Med 1995; 151:54–60.

70. Wrangsjo K, Osterman K, van Hage-Hamsten M. Glove-related skin symptoms among operating theatre and dental care unit personnel. II. Clinical examination, tests and laboratory findings indicating latex allergy. Contact Dematitis 1994; 30:139–143.

71. Safadi GS, Safadi TJ, Terezhalmy GT, Taylor JS, Battisto JR, Melton AL. Latex hypersensitivity: its prevalence among dental professionals. J Am Dent Assoc 1996; 127:83–88.

72. Tarlo SM, Sussman GL, Holness DL. Latex sensitivity in dental students and staff: a crosssectional study. J Allergy Clin Immunol 1997; 99:396–401.

73. Sussman GL, Lem D, Liss G, Beezhold D. Latex allergy in housekeeping personnel. Ann Allergy Asthma Immunol 1995; 74:415–418.

74. Carrillo T, Blanco C, Quiralte J, Castillo R, Cuevas M, Rodriguez de Castro F. Prevalence of latex allergy among greenhouse workers. J Allergy Clin Immunol 1995; 96:699–701.

75. Slater JE. Mostello LA, Shaer C. Rubber-specific IgE in children with spina bifida. J Urol 1991; 146:578–579.

76. Yassin MS, Sanyurah S, Lierl MB, Fischer TJ, Oppenheimer S, Cross J, O'Brien K, Steinmetz C, Khoury J. Evaluation of latex allergy in patients with meningomyelocele. Ann Allergy 1992; 69:207–211.

77. Moneret-Vautrin D, Beaudouin E, Widmer S, Mouton C, Kanny G, Prestat F, Kohler C, Feldmann L. Prospective study of risk factors in natural rubber latex hypersensitivity. J Allergy Clin Immunol 1993; 92:668–677.

78. Kelly KJ, Kurup V, Zacharisen M, Resnick A, Fink JN. Skin and serologic testing in the diagnosis of latex allergy. J Allergy Clin Immunol 1993; 91:1140–1145.

79. Nieto A, Estornell F, Mazon A, Relo C, Nieto A, Garcia-Ibarra F. Allergy to latex in spina bifida: a multivariate study of associated factors in 100 consecutive patients. J Allergy Clin Immunol 1996; 98:501–507.

80. Hadjiliadis D, Khan K, Tarlo S. Skin test responses to latex in an allergy and asthma clinic. J Allergy Clin Immunol 1995; 96:431–432.

81. Novembre E, Bernardini R, Brizzi I, Bertini G, Mugnaini L, Azzari C, Vierucci A. The prevalence of latex allergy in children seen in a university hospital allergy clinic. Allergy 1997; 52:101–105.

82. Ownby DR, Ownby HE, McCullough J, Shafer AW. The prevalence of anti-latex IgE antibodies in 1000 volunteer blood donors. J Allergy Clin Immunol 1996; 97:1188–1192.

83. Fernandez de Corres L, Moneo I, Munoz D, Bernaola G, Fernandez E, Audicana M, Urrutia I. Sensitization from chestnuts and bananas in patients with urticaria and anaphylaxis from contact with latex. Ann Allergy 1993; 70:35–39.

84. Vandenplas 0, Delwiche JP, Dejonghe M. Occupational asthma to latex and amoxicillin. Allergy 1997; 52:1147–1149.

85. van der Walle H, Brunsveld V. Latex allergy among hairdressers. Contact Dermatitis 1995; 32:177.

86. Kelly KJ, Pearson ML, Kurup VP, Havens PL, Byrd RS, Setlock MA, Butler JC, Slater JE, Grammer LC, Resnick A, Roberts M, Jarvis WR, Davis JP, Fink JN. A cluster of anaphylactic reactions in children with spina bifida during general anesthesia: epidemiologic features, risk factors, and latex hypersensitivity. J Allergy Clin Immunol 1994; 94:53–61.

87. Hunt LW, Fransway AF, Reed CE, Miller LK, Jones RT, Swanson MC, Yunginger JW. An epidemic of occupational allergy to latex involving health-care workers. J Occupat and Environ Med 1995; 37:1204–1209.

88. Ttruscott W. The industry perspective on latex. Immunol Allergy Clin North Am 1995; 15: 89–122.

89. Vandenplas O, Delwiche JP, Sibille Y. Occupational asthma due to latex in a hospital administrative employee. Thorax 1996; 51:452–453.

90. Charous BL, Hamilton RG, Yunginger JW. Occupational latex exposure: characteristics of contact and systemic reactions in 47 workers. J Allergy Clin Immunol 1994; 94:12–18.

91. Konz KR, Chia JK, Kurup VP, Resnick A, Kelly KJ, Fink JN. Comparison of latex hypersensitivity among patients with neurologic defects. J Allergy Clin Immunol 1995; 95:950–954.

92. M'Raihi ML, Charpin D, Pons A, Bongrand P, Verloet D. Cross-reactivity between latex and banana. J Allergy Clin Immunol 1991; 87:129–130.

93. Rodriguez M, Vega F, Garcia MT, Panizo C, Laffond E, Montalvo A, Cuevas M. Hypersensitivity to latex, chestnut, and banana. Ann Allergy 1993; 70:31–34.

94. Charous BL. Latex sensitivity in low-risk individuals. Ann Allergy 1994; 74:50 (abstract).

95. Blanco C, Carillo T, Castillo R, Quiralte J, Cuervas M. Latex allergy: clinical features and cross-reactivity with fruits. Ann Allergv 1994; 73:309–311.

96. Sorva R, Makinen-Kiljunen S, Suvilehto K, Juntunen-Backman K, Haahtela T. Latex allergy in children with no known risk factors for latex sensitization. Pediatr Allergy Immunol 1995; 6:36–38.

97. Kadambi A, Field S, Charous BL. Diagnostic testing in latex allergy. J Allergy Clin Immunol 1997; 99:S503 (abstract).

98. Reinheimer G, Ownby DR. Prevalence of latex-specific lgE antibodies in patients being evaluated for allergy. Ann Allergy Asthma Immunol 1995; 74:184–187.

99. Sussman GL, Tarlo S, Dolovich J. The spectrum of IgE-mediated responses to latex. JAMA 1991; 265:2844–2847.

100. Axelsson JGK, Johansson SGO, Wrangsjo K. IgE-mediated anaphylactold reactions to rubber. Allergy 1987; 42:40–50.

101. Beuers U, Baur X, Schrandolph M, Richter W. Anaphylactic shock after a game of squash in an atopic woman with latex allergy. Lancet 1990; 335:1095.

102. Leynadier F, Pecquet C, Dry J. Anaphylaxis to latex during surgery. Anaesthesia 1989; 44: 547–550.

103. Gerber AC, Jorg W, Zbinden S, Seger RA, Dangel PH. Severe intraoperative anaphylaxis to surgical gloves: latex allergy, an unfamiliar condition. Anesthesiology 1989; 71:800–802.

104. Gold M, Swartz JS, Braude BM, Dolovich J, Shandling B, Gilmour RF. Intraoperative anaphylaxis: an association with latex sensitivity. J Allergy Clin Immunol 1991; 87:662–666.

105. Turjanmaa K, Reunala T, Tuimala R, Karkkainen T. Allergy to latex gloves: unusual complication during delivery. Br Med J 1988; 297:1029.

106. Laurent J, Malet R, Smiejan JM, Madelenat P, Herman D. Latex hypersensitivity after natural delivery. J Allergy Clin Immunol 1992; 89:779–780.

107. Mansell PI, Reckless JPD, Lovell CR. Severe anaphylactic reaction to latex rubber surgical gloves. Br Med J 1994; 308:246–247.

108. Lozynski OA, Dupuis L, Shandling B, Gilmour RF, Zimmerman B. Anaphylactold and systemic reaction following saline enema administration: six case reports. Ann Allergy 1986; 56:62–66.

109. Ownby DR, Tomlanovich M, Sammons N, McCullough J. Anaphylaxis associated with latex allergy during barium enema examinations. Am J Roentgenol 1991; 156:903–908.

110. Turjanmaa K, Reunala T. Condoms as a source of latex allergens and cause of contact urticaria. Contact Dermatitis 1989; 20:360–364.

111. Sullivan TJ, Magera BE. Recurrent allergic reactions to latex in a hospitalized pediatric patient. J Allergy Clin Immunol 1995; 96:423–425.

112. Schwartz HA, Zurowski D. Anaphylaxis to latex in intravenous fluids. J Allergy Clin Immunol 1993; 92:358–359.

113. Vassallo SA, Thurston TA, Kim SH, Todres ID. Allergic reaction to latex from stopper of a medication vial. Anesth Analg 1995; 80:1057–1058.

114. Schwartz HJ. Latex: a potential hidden "food" allergen in fast food restaurants. J Allergy Clin Immunol 1995; 95:139–140.

115. Karathanasis P, Cooper A, Zhou K, Mayer L, Kang BC. Indirect latex contact causes urticaria/anaphylaxis. Ann Allergy 1993; 71:526–528.

116. Ceuppens JL, Van Durme P, Dooms-Goossens A. Latex allergy in patients with allergy to fruit. Lancet 1992; 339:493 (letter).

117. Lavaud F, Cossart C, Reiter V, Bernard J, Deltour G, Holmquist I. Latex allergy in patients with allergy to fruit. Lancet 1992; 339:492–493 (letter).

118. Anibarro B, Garcia-Ara MC, Pascual C. Associated sensitization to latex and chestnut. Allergy 1993; 48:130–131.

119. Makinen-Kiljunen S. Banana allergy in patients with immediate-type hypersensitivity to natural rubber latex: characterization of cross-reacting antibodies and allergens. J Allergy Clin Immunol 1994; 93:990–996.

120. Beezhold DH, Sussman GL, Liss GM, Chang NS. Latex allergy can induce clinical reactions to specific foods. Clin Exp Allergy 1996; 26:416–422.

121. Ahlroth M, Alenius H, Turjanmaa K, Makinen-Kiljunen S, Reunala T, Palosuo T. Cross-reacting allergens in natural rubber latex and avocado. J Allergy Clin Immunol 1995; 96: 167–173.

122. Weiss SJ, Halsey JF. A nurse with anaphylaxis to stone fruits and latex sensitivity: potential diagnostic difficulties to consider. Ann Allergy Asthma Immunol 1996; 77:504–508.

123. Axelsson IGK, Johanson SGO, Larsson PH, Zetterstrom O. Characterization of allergenic components in sap extract from the weeping fig (*Ficus benjamina*). Int Arch Allergy Appl Immunol 1990; 91:130–135.

124. Delbourg MF, Moneret-Vautrin DA, Guilloux L, Ville G. Hypersensitivity to latex and *Ficus benjamina* allergens. Ann Allergy Asthma Immunol 1995; 75:496–500.

125. Baur X, Chen Z, Rozynek P, Duser M, Raulf-Heimsoth M. Cross-reacting IgE antibodies recognizing latex allergens, including Hev b 1, as well as papain. Allergy 1995; 50:604–609.

126. Quarre JP, Lecomte J, Lauwers D, Gilbert P, Thiraux J. Allergy to latex and papain. J Allergy Clin Immunol 1995; 95:922 (letter).

127. Vandenplas O, Vandezande LM, Halloy JL, Delwiche JP, Jamart J, Looze Y. Association between sensitization to natural rubber latex and papain. J Allergy Clin Immunol 1996; 97: 1421–1424.

128. Lavaud F, Prevost A, Cossart C, Guerin L, Bernard J, Kochman S. Allergy to latex, avocado pear, and banana: evidence for a 30 kd antigen in immunoblotting. J Allergy Clin Immunol 1995; 95:557–564.

129. Turjanmaa K, Reunala T, Rasanen L. Comparison of diagnostic methods in latex surgical glove contact urticaria. Contact Dermatitis 1988; 19:241–247

130. Hamilton RG, Adkinson NF. Natural rubber latex skin testing reagents: safety and diagnostic accuracy of nonammoniated latex, ammonlated latex, and latex rubber glove extracts. J Allergy Clin Immunol 1996; 98:872–883.

131. Hadjiliadis D, Banks DE, Tarlo SM. The relationship between latex skin prick test responses and clinical allergic responses. J Allergy Clin Immunol 1996; 97:1202–1206.

132. Fink JN, Kelly KJ, Elms N, Kurup VP. Comparative studies of latex extracts used in skin testing. Ann Allergy Asthma Immunol 1996; 76:149–152.

133. Wai YC, Tarlo SM. A comparison of the skin test bioequivalence of ammoniated raw latex and a filtered, glycerinated extract. Can J Allergy Clin Immunol 1997; 2:110–113.

134. Turjanmaa K, Palosuo T, Alenius H, Leynadier F, Autegarden JE, Andre C, Sicard H, Hrabliia M, Tran TX. Latex allergy diagnosis: in vivo and in vitro standardization of a natural rubber latex extract. Allergy 1997; 52:41–50.

135. Malo J-L, Ghezzo H, L'Archeveque J, Lagier F, Perrin B, Cartier A. Is the clinical history a satisfactory means of diagnosing occupational asthma? Am Rev Respir Dis 1991; 143:528–532.

136. Hayes JP, Fitzgerald MX. Occupational asthma among hospital health-care personnel: a cause for concern? Thorax 1994; 49:198–200.

137. Cartier A, Bernstein IL, Burge PS, Cohn JR, Fabbri LM, Hargreave FE, Malo J-L, McKay RT, Salvaggio JE. Guidelines for bronchoprovocation in the investigation of occupational asthma. Report of the subcommittee on bronchoprovocation for occupational asthma. J Allergy Clin Immunol 1989; 84:823–829.

138. Sterk PJ, Fabbri LM, Quanjer PH, Cockcroft DW, O'Byrne PM, Anderson SD I, Juniper EF, Malo J-L. Airway responsiveness. Standardized challenge testing with pharmacological, physical and sensitizing stimuli in adults. Official statement of the European Respiratory Society. Eur Respir J 1993; 6(Suppl 16):53–83.

139. Lagier F, Badier M, Charpin D, Martigny J, Vervloet D. Latex as acroallergen. Lancet 1990; 2:516–517.

140. Brugnami G, Marabini A, Siracusa A, Abbritti G. Work-related late asthmatic response induced by latex allergy. J Allergy Clin Immunol 1995; 96:457–464.

141. Marcos C, Lazaro M, Fraj J, Quirce S, de la Hoz B, Fernandez-Rivas M, Losada E. Occupational asthma due to latex surgical gloves. Ann Allergy 1991; 67:319–323.

142. Pisati G, Baruffini A, Bernabeo F, Stanizzi R. Bronchial provocation testing in the diagnosis of occupational asthma due to latex surgical gloves. Eur Respir J 1994; 7:332–336.

143. Setlock MA, Cotter TP, Rosner D. Latex allergy: failure of prophylaxis to prevent severe reaction. Anesth Analg 1993; 76:650–652.

144. Task Force on Allergic Reactions to Latex. American Academy of Allergy and immunology. J Allergy Clin Immunol 1993; 92:16–18.

145. Heilman DK, Jones RT, Swanson MC, Yunginger JW. A prospective, controlled study showing that rubber gloves are the major contributor to latex aeroallergens in the operating room. J Allergy Clin Immunol 1996; 98:325–330.

146. Tarlo SM, Sussman G, Contala A, Swanson MC. Control of airborne latex by use of powder-free latex gloves. J Allergy Clin Immunol 1994; 93:985–989.

147. Hunt LW, Boone-Orke JL, Fransway AF, Fremstad CE, Jones RT, Swanson MC, McEvoy MT, Miller LK, Majerus ET, Luker PA, Scheppmann DL, Webb MJ, Yunginger JW. A medical-center-wide, multidisciplinary approach to the problem of natural rubber latex allergy. J Occupat Environ Med 1996; 38:765–770.

24

High-Molecular-Weight Protein Agents

David I. Bernstein
University of Cincinnati College of Medicine, Cincinnati, Ohio

Jean-Luc Malo
Université de Montréal and Sacré-Coeur Hospital, Montréal, Quebec, Canada

INTRODUCTION

High-molecular-weight (HMW) agents are protein-derived agents that cause sensitization through an IgE-mediated mechanism. This represents an interesting and useful model of allergic asthma. Discussions of some HMW agents are excluded here and are addressed in specific chapters on: enzymes, flour, and baking additives; laboratory animal allergens; and insect and shellfish emanations. All other proteinaceous agents causing occupational asthma (OA) will be discussed in this chapter.

ANIMAL-DERIVED ANTIGENS

Mammalian Proteins

These are important sources of occupational allergens that can cause OA. The most important of these is laboratory animal allergens, reviewed extensively in another chapter. Allergens in cow dust are important causes of occupational asthma in farmers in Finland and estimated to account for 40% of all new cases of OA in that country; the major purified allergen is designated BDA20 or Bos d2. Specific IgE to the purified cow allergen, BDA20, is a sensitive and specific diagnostic marker of OA (1). Asthmatic dairy farmers have been demonstrated to be sensitized to the major allergen of cow and to other cow-derived proteins. The use of purified BDA20 marginally increases the performance of diagnostic tests that measure specific IgE in respiratory cow allergy (1). Specific IgG, on the other hand, is unable to distinguish healthy farm workers from those with OA. Farmers who develop cow-hair-specific IgE improve following complete avoidance of cow exposure (2).

Severe asthma during milking of sheep has been described in a worker sensitized to sheep milk proteins, lactoglobulin and casein (3). OA and rhinoconjunctivitis have been reported in a candy worker exposed to dried cow's milk proteins and was confirmed by percutaneous sensitivity to lactalbumin and a positive bronchial challenge test to the same antigen (4). A farmer raising deer was reported to be sensitized to a deer dander extract and to have OA confirmed by bronchoprovocation testing with deer dander extract. Multiple allergens were identified (size range: 21–110 kDa) (5).

Avian Proteins

Exposure to raw poultry has recently been reported as a cause of occupational dermatitis, rhinitis, and asthma (6). Eggs were first reported to cause OA in eight of 13 bakers spraying egg protein, although sensitization to egg protein was not confirmed (7). In 1987, a survey of 25 egg-processing workers was described in an egg-processing plant where high exposures to egg white and egg yolk aerosols were generated (8). Five workers had definite OA confirmed by symptoms and work-related decrements in peak expiratory flow rates (9). Four of the workers exhibited skin prick test reactions to purified egg proteins including ovalbumin, conalbumin, lysozyme, and ovomucoid. In this study, cutaneous reactivity to purified proteins was a sensitive immunological marker of OA. Specific IgG responses to the aforementioned purified egg white proteins were detected in the sera of egg-processing workers, but their presence did not discriminate between symptomatic and asymptomatic workers. In a cross-industry survey of egg-processing workers, Smith and co-workers reported a 34% prevalence of cutaneous sensitization to egg white proteins (10). Fourteen of the combined workforce of 188 subjects (7%) employed at two plants showed evidence of OA as assessed by questionnaire, a physician diagnosis of OA, and IgE-mediated sensitization to at least one egg protein. A higher prevalence of egg asthma was found in the "transfer" and "breaking" areas where liquid protein aerosols were generated (12% and 10%, respectively) compared to drying areas where there was exposure principally to egg powder (5%).

Lummus and co-workers reported extremely high exposure to ambient egg protein (47–774 μg/mm^3 of ovalbumin) to particulates of respirable size, which were increased in areas of a plant where egg protein aerosols were generated (egg breaking and transfer rooms) (11). In this study, atopic egg-processing-factory workers were at significantly increased risk for cutaneous sensitization to egg protein allergens (12), a finding that was not identified in similar surveys of egg workers. It is possible that the lack of an association in previous cross-sectional surveys of egg sensitivity with atopic status could reflect survivor effects; atopic may have been more likely than nonatopic workers to become clinically sensitized and quit their jobs. Purified hen egg white lysozyme used in the pharmaceutical industry has been reported as a cause of allergic OA in a worker exposed to lysozyme powder (13).

Crustaceans, Seafood, and Fish-Derived Allergens

OA is a frequent occurrence in snowcrab (14), prawn (15), oyster (16), trout (17), salmon (18), red soft coral (19), and cuttlefish (20) processors. Trout processors can be affected by occupational rhinitis and asthma. The mechanism remains unexplained, but inhalation of an endotoxin from gram-negative bacteria may be the cause (17).

OA has been described in salmon processing-workers. In a plant with 291 workers, 24 (8.2%) were suspected of having OA. The respirable aerosols of salmon proteins were generated during processing. Specific IgE responses to salmon protein are associated with asthma symptoms and cigarette smoking status. Nearly all workers improved after cessation and removal to low-exposure work areas (18). Allergic reactions to cuttlefish, including asthma, have been reported in 61 Polish crew members harvesting the fish in the South Atlantic. An increasing incidence was noticed between 1983 and 1987; the estimated incidence was 1% in the last year of survey. Five fishermen had to be evacuated from the boats because of severe asthma (20). Cuttlefish bone dust was linked to asthma in a goldsmith who was exposed to it while polishing gold jewelry. Immediate skin reactivity was documented (21).

In 1950, oyster handlers in Hiroshima who developed work-related asthma were described (16). This is a seasonal industry (November–April). The oysters are contaminated by a parasite (protochordae). When the workers open the oysters, particles of protochordae ("hoya" or "sea-squirt") are aerosolized. A survey carried out in 1964 showed that 20% of 1416 workers had asthmatic symptoms. Subjects often had rhinoconjunctivitis as well. Extracts of protochordae were prepared. A strong association was seen between the results of skin testing and increased specific IgE antibodies, on the one hand, and the presence of work-related asthmatic symptoms, on the other. Oyster itself does not seem to be the causal agent. Desensitization was felt to be useful.

A survey carried out among 50 subjects exposed to prawn ("Norway lobster," *Nephrops norwegicus*) showed that 18 of them had respiratory symptoms (15). Seven of the 18 had skin reactions to a prawn extract, as compared to six of 32 asymptomatic subjects and none of 30 nonexposed control subjects. The two subjects who underwent specific inhalation challenges had either dual or isolated late reactions. In a survey of 61 workers exposed to clam and shrimp in a food-production company preparing soups, Desjardins and co-workers found that three subjects (5%) had immediate skin reactivity to clam and nine (16%) to shrimp (22). Two subjects had OA due to clam and one to shrimp as confirmed by specific inhalation challenges in the laboratory. Shrimpmeal used as foodstuff in intensive aquaculture was the etiological agent of OA in a technician as confirmed by specific inhalation challenges and the presence of specific IgE antibodies (23).

Dried daphnia, which is used as a fish food, can also cause OA (24). Onizuka et al. described two cases of OA due to red soft coral among spiny lobster fishermen. Of 72 subjects who underwent a questionnaire, 9% had symptoms compatible with OA (19). Baldo and co-workers describe a subject with OA due to a powdered marine sponge with evidence of IgE-mediated sensitization (25).

Respiratory symptoms were first described in several employees handling Alaska king crab in 1976 by R. R. Orford and J. J. Wilson, Jr., in a thesis; a first account in the medical literature appeared in 1982 (26). There are several crab species. Snow-crab (*Chinoecetes opilis*) is found on the East Coast of North America, more precisely in the Gulf of St. Lawrence. Snow-crab has been harvested commercially since 1980. Once it is harvested, it is sent to the processing plants where it is brushed and boiled. It is then cooled and the flesh is either canned or frozen. Boiling the snow-crab releases a vapor. The first two cases of OA caused by snow crab were identified after the 1981 harvesting season. Two plants on the Magdalen Islands in the Gulf of St. Lawrence were subsequently contacted and the employees investigated. The first survey was carried out before the season using a questionnaire and skin tests with commercial crab preparations (14). The majority (303/313) of the workers agreed to participate. Table 1 summarizes the questionnaire responses. A diagnosis of OA was considered for all subjects who had a history suggesting work-related asthma. Forty-six (16%) were found to have OA, the diagnosis being confirmed by specific inhalation challenges in 33 and by monitoring peak expiratory flow rates in the rest. In a subsequent study (27), we showed a strong association between the presence of asthma due to snow-crab and cutaneous reactivity to specific snow-crab extracts prepared by Sam Lehrer in New Orleans. Findings are tabulated in Table 2. The same association was also demonstrated by assessing specific IgE levels.

Table 1 Summary of Clinical Findings in Snow-Crab Processors

Symptom group	Number of subjects	Number of subjects with confirmed OA
Asymptomatic	119	5
Chronic bronchitis	57	2
Asthma not related to work	24	2
Asthma possibly related to the workplace	39	4
Asthma likely to be related to the workplace	64	33
Total	303	46

Two follow-up studies of snow-crab workers no longer exposed to the offending agent showed that symptomatology, the need for medication, and bronchial hyperresponsiveness persisted in the vast majority of them, the plateau of improvement being reached approximately 2 years after exposure ended (28,29).

MOLD-DERIVED ALLERGENS

There are rare reports of mold or yeasts as causes of OA. A case of baker's yeast asthma was proven to be caused by respiratory sensitization to powdered baker's yeast, *Saccharomyces cerevisiae*. Immediate-onset asthma was reported during mixing of yeast with additives and flour (30). Occupational rhinoconjunctivitis and asthma occurred in a research microbiologist working with a slime mold that produced allergenic lysosomal enzymes (31). *Aspergillus* and *Alternaria* mold spores have been isolated from the room air of bakeries. Klaustermeyer and co-workers reported two bakers with work-related asthma in whom inhalation challenges with wheat or rye antigens were negative but in whom intracutaneous and bronchial sensitivity were demonstrable to *Aspergillus* and *Alternaria* antigens (32). In another case report of baker's asthma attributed to respiratory sensitization to *Aspergillus*, a favorable response was observed to allergen immunotherapy with *Aspergillus* antigens (33).

Table 2 Summary of Immunological Findings as Shown by Immediate Skin Reactivity in Asthma Caused by Snow-Crab

Characteristic	Snow-crab boiling water		Snow-crab meat	
	Positive	Negative	Positive	Negative
Presence of OA	37	11	37	11
Absence of OA	17	35	19	33
Odds of OA in a skin-test-positive subject	69%		66%	
Odds of no OA in a skin-test-negative subject	76%		75%	

PLANT-DERIVED ALLERGENS

Grain dust as well as various cereals (wheat, rye, soya, buckwheat) can cause OA in bakers. Gluten (34) can also be responsible for OA in bakers. *Chlorella* algae has caused OA in a pharmacist (35).

Coffee beans have been reported repeatedly to cause OA, as was thoroughly reviewed by Zuskin and co-workers (36). These authors found a 9% prevalence of asthma and a 25% prevalence of skin reactivity among 45 coffee workers. In the largest epidemiological survey to date, 10% of a group of workers had skin reactions to green coffee bean extract and 14%, to the dust that was collected (37). Those subjects who had been employed for a longer period and therefore exposed to the dust of green (unroasted) coffee for a longer time and with increased specific serum IgE values, had lower FEV_1 results. The extraction of allergens from coffee beans used for bronchoprovocation tests has been described (38,39). Water soluble extracts from the dust of coffee beans have been used in proving the causal relationship of symptoms in 22 coffee roastery workers, eight of whom had positive bronchial provocation tests and 18 of whom had positive prick tests (40). Zuskin and co-workers studied nine coffee workers who complained of job-related respiratory symptoms. Four had immediate bronchospastic reactions on exposure to green coffee allergens and six showed skin reactivity to green coffee allergens (41). Roasted coffee can cause OA (42). The latter report illustrated that the allergens of green coffee can also be found in roasted coffee, although at a lesser concentration.

Other beans and seeds from oleaginous plants are also incriminated in the genesis of OA. Several such cases have been reported in the harbor of Marseille (43,44). The prevalence of asthma caused by handling the fruit from which castor oil is extracted by agricultural workers harvesting it has been estimated at 15% of 3000 Rumanian workers. The prevalence of skin reactivity was much higher among symptomatic than asymptomatic workers and reached 80% in those with asthma (45). Castor oil is derived from castor beans (*Ricinus communis*) and principally used in the production of cosmetics, nylon, explosives, paints, and inks. It was recognized to cause allergic symptoms early in the twentieth century, as reviewed by Davison and co-workers (46).

Five cases of asthma caused by castor oil were described by these authors in seamen and laboratory workers (46). IgE antibodies specific to castor bean extracts have been identified (47,48).

Although hypersensitivity pneumonitis has been described in cheese workers, OA and bronchitis also seems to represent a significant respiratory ailment (49). Tea dust can cause respiratory symptoms among workers involved in the primary processing of tea in countries where it is grown (50). The prevalence of OA has been estimated at 6% of 125 workers (51). The secondary process, tea packing, can be responsible for OA as demonstrated by objective means in four case reports (52,53). Herbal teas made of sage, camomile, dog rose, and mint can also cause OA as documented in a subject who underwent specific inhalation challenges (54). Various molds that grow on tobacco leaves can be responsible for asthmatic symptoms. These symptoms were reported by a subject who had a positive inhalation challenge to a fungal extract of *S. brevicaulis* (55).

Florists can be exposed to various flowers that can cause sensitization. This includes *Lathyrus* (56,57), baby's breath (*Gypsophila paniculata*) (58), freesia and paprika (59), amaryllis (60), *Limonium tataricum* (61), spathe flowers (62), and various decorative flowers (63). Weeping fig is a green plant from the genus *Ficus* belonging to the mulberry family. It is used as a decorative house plant. After reporting two cases of OA (64), Axelsson and co-workers found that 18 of 84 subjects (21%) had immunological sensitization to the latex of the plant (65). Lander and Gravesen described 16 tobacco workers, including 11 who reported asthma symptoms; sensitization was felt to be due to microfungi and/or mites (66).

Newmark reported an interesting case of OA due to hops, presumed to be caused by terpene (67). Seeds of onion (68), sesame (69), and cacoon (70) can act as sensitizers. Pectin powder used in fruit jam causes OA (71).

Garlic dust has been reported to cause OA (72,73). Specific IgE antibodies have been found. Aniseed powder used as a spice caused OA confirmed by inhalation challenge (74). Concurrent sensitization and development of IgE-mediated asthma due to multiple spices (paprika, coriander, and mace) have been documented in a single worker (75). Spices and aromatic herbs have also been reported to cause IgE-mediated sensitization and asthma (76). Mushroom powder caused occupational rhinoconjunctivitis and asthma (77) among eight food-manufacturing workers who had an immediate skin reaction to a dried mushroom extract. This was also found by others (78). Various vegetable products can cause OA: onion (79), potato (80), chicory (81), sarsaparilla root (82), rose hips (83), ginseng (84), sunflower (85), fenugreek (86), and kapok (87).

Lycopodium powder derived from the herbaceous plant *Lycopodium clavatum* L. has been reported to cause OA in two workers employed by a firm making contraceptive sheaths for men (88). "Maiko" is a dust derived from a tuberous root, devil's tongue (*Amorphophalus konjac*), which is used in the production of a Japanese food product. It has been demonstrated that this agent causes OA through an IgE-mediated mechanism (89). Sensitization to the herbal medicines sanyak and banha resulted in OA in herbal pharmacists (90).

Various pharmaceutical products cause OA. Some of these are proteins. Ipecacuanha, a protein product derived from the roots of *Cephaelis ipecacuanha*, is used as an expectorant or emetic. A survey of 42 employees at a pharmaceutical company was carried out by Luczynska et al. (91). Nineteen subjects (45%) had work-related symptoms (rhinitis, conjunctivitis, and/or chest tightness), 10 of whom had skin reactions to ipecacuanha. Three subjects without symptoms also had skin reactions. Specific IgE assessments revealed a similar significant relationship between the presence of symptoms and increased immunological sensitization. Maiko has been reported to cause OA in Japanese workers (92).

VEGETABLE GUMS

Several gums have been incriminated as causes of OA. Gums are derived from plants and contain carbohydrates that produce mucilages when they react with water. The various types of gums can be distinguished in the following way: (1) gums obtained from an exudate: (a) acacia or arabic gum derived from *Acacia senegal*, a vegetable grown in Africa, and used in food, pharmaceuticals, and printing; (b) tragacanth, derived from *Astragalus gummifer*, a vegetable grown in Asia and widely used in the printing industry; (c) karaya, derived from *Sterculea urens* (Sterculiacae family), which grows in India and can be used instead of tragacanth; and (2) gums obtained from seeds: (a) carob gum, derived from the carob that grows in the Mediterranean region; (b) guar gum, derived from *Cyamopsis tetragonolobus*, a vegetable grown in India and used in numerous pharmaceutical and food products as well as by carpet manufacturers.

Natural gums are high polymer carbohydrates, which are used as protective colloids and emulsifying agents in food products and pharmaceuticals. In 1933, Spielman and

Baldwin described a case of asthma caused by acacia gum (93). Later, cases of OA among printers exposed to acacia gum were documented. Bohner and co-workers described 10 such cases, all of whom had positive skin tests (94). Similar cases were later found (95,96). In 1934, Bullen described a case of asthma in a hairdresser exposed to karaya (97). In 1943, Gelfand described one case of asthma caused by tragacanth in a subject working for an import firm (98).

In 1952, Fowler described 32 subjects, all of them printers, who had OA caused by acacia gum (99). More recently, guar gum, which is widely used, has been incriminated as causing occupational rhinitis (100) and asthma (101). The prevalence of sensitization to guar gum among 162 carpet manufacturers has been estimated to vary between 5% (skin testing) and 8% (specific IgE assessments) (102). In the same survey, it was found that the prevalence of OA as confirmed by specific inhalation challenges was 2%.

Psyllium is a high-molecular-weight gum widely used as a laxative, which has been associated with OA, rhinitis, and urticaria associated with sensitization to allergens in the psyllium seed embryo and seed endospore (99). Allergens are not found in the husk of psyllium seeds. Work-related exposure to psyllium products occurs in several ways: in processing plants that produce psyllium; and in nurses chronically handling psyllium when distributing it to patients. The prevalence in pharmaceutical workers has been estimated to vary between 28 and 44% (103) whereas the prevalence of OA confirmed by specific inhalation challenges is 4% (104).

Nasal, ocular, and chest symptoms in subjects handling this product have been documented in several case reports (105–112). IgE immunological sensitization can usually be demonstrated. A self-administered questionnaire showed that 18% of 743 nurses had allergic episodes while handling psyllium, 5% of whom reporting respiratory symptoms or hives (113). A recent survey of 193 nurses employed by four chronic care hospitals showed that the prevalence of immunological sensitization to psyllium varied between 5% (skin testing) and 12% (increased specific IgE levels), whereas 4% had OA as confirmed by specific inhalation challenges (100).

REFERENCES

1. Virtanen T, Zeiler T, Rautiainen J, Taivainen A, Pentikajnen J, Rytkonen M, Parkkinen S, Pelkonen J, Mantyjarvi R. Immune reactivity of cow-asthmatic dairy farmers to the major allergen of cow (BDA20) and to other cow-derived proteins. The use of purified BDA increases the performance of diagnostic tests in respiratory cow allergy. Clin Exp Allergy 1996; 26:188–196.
2. Hinze S, Bergmann KC, Lowenstein H, Hansen GN. Cow hair allergen (Bos d2) content in house dust: correlation with sensitization in farmers with cow hair asthma. Int Arch Allergy Immunol 1997; 112:231–237.
3. Vargiu A, Vargiu G, Locci F, Giacco S, Giacco GS Del. Hypersensitivity reactions from inhalation of milk proteins. Allergy 1994; 49:386–387.
4. Bernaola G, Echechipia S, Urrutia I, Fernandez E, Audicana M, Corres L Fernandez de. Occupational asthma and rhinoconjunctivitis from inhalation of dried cow's milk caused by sensitization to alpha-lactalbumin. Allergy 1994; 49:189–191.
5. Nahm DH, Park JW, Hong CS. Occupational asthma due to deer dander. Ann Allergy Asthma Immunol 1996; 76:423–426.
6. Schwartz HJ. Raw poultry as a cause of occupational dermatitis, rhinitis and asthma. J Asthma 1994; 31:485–486.
7. Edwards JH, McConnochie K, Trotman DM, Collins G, Saunders MJ, Latham SM. Allergy to inhaled egg material. Clin Allergy 1983; 13:427–432.

8. Bernstein DI, Smith AB, Moller DR, Gallagher JS, Tar-Ching AW, London M, Kopp S, Carson G. Clinical and immunologic studies among egg-processing workers with occupational asthma. J Allergy Clin Immunol 1987; 80:791–797.
9. Smith AB, Bernstein DI, Aw Tar-Ching, Gallagher JS, London M, Kopp S, Carson GA. Occupational asthma from inhaled egg protein. Am J Ind Med 1987; 12:205–218.
10. Smith A Blair, Bernstein DI, London MA, Gallagher J, Ornella GA, Gelletly SK, Wallingford D, Newman MA. Evaluation of occupational asthma from airborne egg protein exposure in multiple settings. Chest 1990; 98:398404.
11. Lummus ZL, Boeniger M, Biagini R, Massoudi M, Berntein DI. Environmental survey of occupational exposure to aerosolized egg allergens in the egg processing industry. J Allergy Clin Immunology 1997; 99(1):S502.
12. Pinkerton LE, Massoudi M, Bernstein D, Biagini R, Hull RD, Ruder A, Brown M, Boeniger M, Ward E. Occupational ashtma and rhinitis amoung egg-processing workers. J Allergy Clin Immunol 1997; 99:S501.
13. Bernstein JA, Kraut A, Bernstein DI, Warrington R, Bolin T, Warren CPW, Bernstein IL. Occupational asthma induced by inhaled egg lysozyme. Chest 1993; 103:532–535.
14. Cartier A, Malo J-L, Forest F, Lafrance M, Pineau L, St-Aubin JJ, Dubois J-Y. Occupational asthma in snow crab-processing workers. J Allergy Clin Immunol 1984; 74:261–269.
15. Gaddie J, Legge JS, Friend JAR, Reid TMS. Pulmonary hypersensitivity in prawn workers. Lancet 1980; 2:1350–1353.
16. Jyo T, Kohmoto K, Katsutani T, Otsuka T, Oka SD, Mitsui S. Hoya (sea-squirt) asthma. In: Occupational Asthma. London: Von Nostrand Reinhold, 1980:209–228.
17. Sherson D, Hansen I, Sigsgaard T. Occupationally related respiratory symptoms in trout-processing workers. Allergy 1989; 44:336–341.
18. Douglas JDM, McSharry C, Blaikie L, Morrow T, Miles S, Franklin D. Occupational asthma caused by automated salmon processing. Lancet 1995; 346:737–740.
19. Onizuka R, Inoue K, Kamiya H. Red soft coral-induced allergic symptoms observed in spiny lobster fishermen. Aerugi 1990; 39:339–347.
20. Tomaszunas S, Weclawik Z, Lewinski M. Allergic reactions to cuttlefish in deep-sea fishermen. Lancet 1988; 1:1116–1117.
21. Beltrami V, Innocenti A, Pieroni MG, Civai R, Nesi D, Bianco S. Occupational asthma due to cuttle-fish bone dust. Med Lav 1989; 80:425–428.
22. Desjardins A, Malo JL, L'Archevêque J, Cartier A, McCants M, Lehrer SB. Occupational IgE-mediated sensitization and asthma due to clam and shrimp. J Allergy Clin Immunol 1995; 96:608–617.
23. Carino M, Elia G, Molinini R, Nuzzaco A, Ambrosi L. Shrimpmeal asthma in the aquaculture industry. Med Lav 1985; 76:471–475.
24. Meister W. Professional asthma owing to Daphnia-allergy. Allerg Immunol (Leipz) 1978; 24:191–193.
25. Baldo BA, Krilis S, Taylor KM. IgE-mediated acute asthma following inhalation of a powdered marine sponge. Clin Allergy 1982; 12:179–186.
26. Anonymous. Asthma-like illness among crab-processing workers—Alaska. Morbid Mortal Wkly Rep 1982; 31:95–96.
27. Cartier A, Malo JL, Ghezzo H, McCants M, Lehrer SB. IgE sensitization in snow crab-processing workers. J Allergy Clin Immunol 1986; 78:344–348.
28. Hudson P, Cartier A, Pineau L, Lafrance M, St-Aubin JJ, Dubois JY, Malo JL. Follow-up of occupational asthma caused by crab and various agents. J Allergy Clin Immunol 1985; 76:682–687.
29. Malo JL, Cartier A, Ghezzo H, Lafrance M, Mccants M, Lehrer SB. Patterns of improvement on spirometry, bronchial hyperresponsiveness, and specific IgE antibody levels after cessation of exposure in occupational asthma caused by snow-crab processing. Am Rev Respir Dis 1988; 138:807–812.
30. Belchi-Hernandez J, Mora-Gonzalez A, Iniesta-Perez J. Baker's asthma caused by Saccharomyces cerevisiae in dry powder form. J Allergy Clin Immul 1996; 97:131–134.

31. Gottlieb SJ, Garibaldi E, Hutcheson PS, Slavin RG. Occupational asthma to the slime mold dictyostelium discoideum. J Occup Med 1993; 35:1231–1235.

32. Klaustermeyer WB, Bardana EJ, Hale FC. Pulmonary hypersensitivity to alternaria and aspergillus in baker's asthma. Clin Allergy 1977; 7:227–233.

33. Weiner A. Occupational bronchial asthma in a baker due to *Aspergillus*. Ann Allergy 1960; 18:1004–1007.

34. Lachance P, Cartier A, Dolovich J, Malo J-L. Occupational asthma from reactivity to an alkaline hydrolysis derivative of gluten. J Allergy Clin Immunol 1988; 81:385–390.

35. Ng TP, Tan WC, Lee YK. Occupational asthma in a pharmacist induced by *Chlorella*, a unicellular algae preparation. Respir Med 1994; 88:555–557.

36. Zuskin E, Valic F, Kanceljak B. Immunological and respiratory changes in coffee workers. Thorax 1981; 36:9–13.

37. Jones RN, Hughes JM, Lehrer SB, Butcher BT, Glindmeyer HW, Diem JE, Hammad YY, Salvaggio J, Weill H. Lung function consequences of exposure and hypersensitivity in workers who process green coffee beans. Am Rev Respir Dis 1982; 125:199–202.

38. Karr RM. Bronchoprovocation studies in coffee worker's asthma. J Allergy Clin Immunol 1979; 64:650–654.

39. Lehrer SB, Karr RM, Salvaggio JE. Extraction and analysis of coffee bean allergens. Clin Allergy 1978; 8:217–226.

40. Osterman K, Johansson SGO, Zetterstrom O. Diagnostic tests in allergy to green coffee. Allergy 1985; 40:336–343.

41. Zuskin E, Kanceljak B, Mataija M, Tonkovic-Lojovic M. Specific bronchial reactivity in coffee workers. Arh Hig Rada Toksikol 1989; 40:3–8.

42. Lemière C, Malo JL, McCants M, Lehrer S. Occupational asthma caused by roasted coffee: immunologic evidence that roasted coffee contains the same antigens as green coffee, but at a lower concentration. J Allergy Clin Immunol 1996; 98:464–466.

43. Charpin J, Zafiropoulo A, Simon L. Asthmes professionnels dus aux oléagineux. J Franç Méd Chir Thor 1961; 15:47–50.

44. Charpin J, Zafiropoulo A, Luccioni R. Asthmes professionnels dans l'industrie des corps gras. Poumon Coeur 1966; 22:513–521.

45. Lupu NG, Dinischiotu GT, Paun R, Popescu IG, Fotescu L, Zamfirescu-Gherghiu M, Olaru C, Iota CG, Moscovici B, Molner C, Ursea N. L'asthme professionnel des cultivateurs de ricin. Concours Méd 1962; 84:5843–5846.

46. Davison AG, Britton MG, Forrester JA, Davies RJ, Hughes DTD. Asthma in merchant seamen and laboratory workers caused by allergy to castor beans: analysis of allergens. Clin Allergy 1983; 13:553–561.

47. Lehrer SB, Karr RM, Muller DJG, Salvaggio JE. Detection of castor allergens in castor wax. Clin Allergy 1980; 10:33–41.

48. Panzani R, Johansson SGO. Results of skin test and RAST in allergy to a clinically potent allergen (castor bean). Clin Allergy 1986; 16:259–266.

49. Dalphin JC, Illig S, Pernet D, Dubiez A, Debieuvre D, Teyssier-Cotte C, Depierre A. Symptômes et fonction respiratoires dans un groupe d'affineurs de gruyère de Comté. Rev Mal Respir 1990; 7:31–37.

50. Uragoda CG. Tea maker's asthma. Br J Ind Med 1970; 27:181–182.

51. Uragoda CG. Respiratory disease in tea workers in Sri Lanka. Thorax 1980; 35:114–117.

52. Roberts JA, Thomson NC. Tea-dust induced asthma. Eur Respir J 1988; 1:769–770.

53. Cartier A, Malo JL. Occupational asthma due to tea dust. Thorax 1990; 45:203–206.

54. Blanc PD, Trainor WD, Lim DT. Herbal tea asthma. Br J Ind Med 1986; 43:137–138.

55. Lander F, Jepsen JR, Gravesen S. Allergic alveolitis and late asthmatic reaction due to molds in the tobacco industry. Allergy 1988; 43:74–76.

56. Valdivieso R, Quirce S, Sainz T. Bronchial asthma caused by *Lathyrus sativus* flower. Allergy 1988; 43:536–539.

57. Jansen A, Vermeulen A, vanToorenenbergen AW, Dieges PH. Occupational asthma in horticulture caused by *Lathyrus odoratus*. Allergy Proc 1995; 16:135–139.

58. Twiggs JT, Yunginger JW, Agarwal MK, Reed CE. Occupational asthma in a florist caused by the dried plant, baby's breath. J Allergy Clin Immunol 1982; 69:474–477.

59. Toorenenbergen AW van, Dieges PH. Occupational allergy in horticulture: demonstration of immediate-type allergic reactivity to freesia and praprika plants. Int Arch Allergy Appl Immunol 1984; 75:44–47.

60. Jansen APH, Visser FJ, Nierop G, Jong NW De, Raadt J Waanders-De Lijster De, Vermeulen A, Toorenenbergen AW van. Occupational asthma to amaryllis. Allergy 1996; 51:847–849.

61. Quirce S, Garcia-Figueroa B, Olaguibel JM, Muro MD, Tabar AI. Occupational asthma and contact urticaria from dried flowers of *Limonium tataricum*. Allergy 1993; 48(4):285–290.

62. Kanerva L, Makinen-Kijunen S, Kiistala R, Granlund H. Occupational allergy caused by spathe flower (*Spathiphyllum wallisii*). Allergy 1995; 50:174–178.

63. Piirila P, Keskinen H, Leino T, Tupasela O, Tuppurainen M. Occupational asthma caused by decorative flowers: review and case reports. Int Arch Occup Environ Health 1994; 66:131–136.

64. Axelsson G, Skedinger M, Zetterström O. Allergy to weeping fig—a new occupational disease. Allergy 1985; 40:461–464.

65. Axelsson IGK, Johansson SGO, Zetterström O. Occupational allergy to weeping fig in plant keepers. Allergy 1987; 42:161–167.

66. Lander F, Gravesen S. Respiratory disorders among tobacco workers. Br J Ind Med 1988; 45:500–502.

67. Newmark FM. Hops allergy and terpene sensitivity: an occupational disease. Ann Allergy 1978; 41:311–312.

68. Navarro JA, Pozo MD del, Gastaminza G, Moneo I, Audicana MT, Corres LD de. Allium cepa seeds: a new occupational allergen. J Allergy Clin Immunol 1995; 96:690–693.

69. Alday E, Curiel G, Lopez-Gil MJ, Carreno D. Occupational Hypersensitivity to sesame seeds. Allergy 1996; 51:69–70.

70. Rubin JM, Duke MB. Unusual cause of bronchial asthma. Cacoon seed used for decorative purposes. NY State J Med 1974; 538–539.

71. Cohen AJ, Forse MS, Tarlo SM. Occupational asthma caused by pectin inhalation during the manufacture of jam. Chest 1993; 103:309–311.

72. Falleroni AE, Zeiss CR, Levitz D. Occupational asthma secondary to inhalation of garlic dust. J Allergy Clin Immunol 1981; 68:156–160.

73. Lybarger JA, Gallagher JS, Pulver DW, Litwin A, Brooks S, Bernstein IL. Occupational asthma induced by inhalation and ingestion of garlic. J Allergy Clin Immunol 1982; 69:448–454.

74. Fraj J, Lezaun A, Colas C, Duce F, Dominguez MA, Alonso MD. Occupational asthma induced by aniseed. Allergy 1996; 51:337–339.

75. Sastre J, Olmo M, Novalvos A, Ibanez D, Lahoz C. Occupational asthma due to different spices. Allergy 1996; 51:117–120.

76. Lemière C, Cartier A, Lehrer SB, Malo JL. Occupational asthma caused by aromatic herbs. Allergy 1996; 51:647–649.

77. Symington IS, Kerr JW, McLean DA. Type I allergy in mushroom soup processors. Clin Allergy 1981; 11:43–47.

78. MIchils A, Vuyst P De, Nolard N, Servais G, Duchateau J, Yernault JC. Occupational asthma to spores of *Pleurotus cornucopiae*. Eur Respir J 1991; 4:1143–1147.

79. Valdivieso R, Subiza J, Varela-Losada S, Subiza JL, Narganes MJ, Martinez-Cocera C, Cabrera M. Bronchial asthma, rhinoconjunctivitis, and contact dermatitis caused by onion. J Allergy Clin Immunol 1994; 94:928–930.

80. Quirce S, Gomez ML Diez, Hinojosa M, Cuevas M, Urena V, Rivas MF, Puyana J, Cuesta J, Losada E. Housewives with raw potato-induced bronchial asthma. Allergy 1989; 44:532–536.

81. Cadot P, Kochuyt AM, Deman R, Stevens EAM. Inhalative occupational and ingestive immediate-type allergy caused by chicory (*Cichorium intybus*). Clin Exp Allergy 1996; 26:940–944.

82. Vandenplas O, Depelchin S, Toussaint G, Delwiche JP, Weyer R Vande, Saint-Remy JM. Occupational asthma caused by sarsaparilla root dust. J Allergy Clin Immunol 1996; 97: 1416–1418.

83. Kwaselow A, Rowe M, Sears-Ewald D, Ownby D. Rose hips: a new occupational allergen. J Allergy Clin Immunol 1990; 85:704–708.

84. Subiza J, Subiza JL, Escribano PM, Hinojosa M, Garcia R, Jerez M, Subiza E. Occupational asthma caused by Brazil ginseng dust. J Allergy Clin Immunol 1991; 88:731–736.

85. Bousquet OJ, Dhivert H, Clauzel AM, Hewitt B, Michel FB. Occupational allergy to sunflower pollen. J Allergy Clin Immunol 1985; 75:70–75.

86. Dugue J, Bel J, Figueredo M. Le fenugrec responsable d'un nouvel asthme professionnel. Presse Méd 1993; 22:922.

87. Kern DG, Kohn R. Occupational asthma following kapok exposure. J Asthma 1994; 31:243–250.

88. Catilina P, Chamoux A, Gabrillargues D, Catilina MJ, Royfe MH, Wahl D. Contribution à l'étude des asthmes d'origine professionnelle: l'asthme à la poudre de lycopode. Arch Mal Prof 1988; 49:143–148.

89. Kobayashi S. Different aspects of occupational asthma in Japan. In: CA Frazier, ed. Occupational Asthma. New York: Van Nostrand Reinhold, 1980:229–244.

90. Park HS, Kim MJ, Moons HB. Occupational asthma caused by two herb materials, *Dioscorea batatas* and *Pinellia ternata*. Clin Exp Allergy 1994; 24:575–581.

91. Luczynska CM, Marshall PE, Scarisbrick DA, Topping MD. Occupational allergy due to inhalation of ipecacuanha dust. Clin Allergy 1984; 14:169–175.

92. Kobayashi S, Y Yamamura, OL Frick, Y Horiuchi, S Kishimoto, T Miyamoto, ed, Naranjo P, ed, De Weck A. Occupational asthma due to inhalation of pharmacological dusts and other chemical agents with some reference to other occupational asthmas in Japan. Allergology. Proceedings of the VIII International Congress of Allergology, Tokyo, October 1973, 1974. Amsterdam: Excerpta Medica, 1974:124–132.

93. Spielman AD, Baldwin HS. Atopy to acacia (gum arabic). JAMA 1933; 101:444–445.

94. Bohner CB, Sheldon JM, Trenis JW. Sensitivity to gum acacia, with a report of ten cases of asthma in printers. J Allergy 1941; 12:290–294.

95. Hinault G, Blacque-Bélair A, Buffe D. L'asthme à la gomme arabique dans un grand atelier de typographie. J Franç Méd Chir Thor 1961; 15:51–61.

96. Gaultier M, Fournier E, Gervais P, Vignolet. Un cas d'asthme à la gomme arabique. Histoire clinique, tests cutanés, épreuves fonctionnelles respiratoires. Arch Mal Prof 1960; 21:55–56.

97. Bullen SS. Perennial hay fever from indian gum (Karaya gum). J Allergy 1934; 5:484–487.

98. Gelfand HH. The allergenic properties of vegetable gums: a case of asthma due to tragacanth. J Allergy 1943; 14:203–219.

99. Fowler PBS. Printers'asthma. Lancet 1952; 2:755–757.

100. Kanerva L, Tupasela O, Jolanki R, Vaheri E, Estlander T, Keskinen H. Occupational allergic rhinitis from guar gum. Clin Allergy 1988; 18:245–252.

101. Lagier F, Cartier A, Somer J, Dolovich J, Malo JL. Occupational asthma caused by guar gum. J Allergy Clin Immunol 1990; 85:785–790.

102. Malo JL, Cartier A, L'Archevêque J, Ghezzo H, Soucy F, Somers J, Dolovich J. Prevalence of occupational asthma and immunologic sensitization to guar gum among employees at a carpet-manufacturing plant. J Allergy Clin Immunol 1990; 86:562–569.

103. Morgan MS, Arlian LG, Vyszenski-Moher DL, Deyo J, Kawabata T, Fernandez-Caldas E. English plantain and psyllium: lack of cross-allergenicity by crossed immunoelectrophoresis. Ann Allergy Asthma Immunol 1995; 75:351–359.

104. Bardy JD, Malo JL, Séguin P, Ghezzo H, Desjardins J, Dolovich J, Cartier A. Occupational asthma and IgE sensitization in a pharmaceutical company processing psyllium. Am Rev Respir Dis 1987; 135:1033–1038.

105. Malo JL, Cartier A, L'Archevêque J, Ghezzo H, Lagier F, Trudeau C, Dolovich J. Prevalence of occupational asthma and immunologic sensitization to psyllium among health personnel in chronic care hospitals. Am Rev Respir Dis 1990; 142:1359–1366.

106. Gauss WF, Alarie JP, Karol MH. Workplace allergenicity of a psyllium-containing bulk laxative. Allergy 1985; 40:73–76.
107. Scott D. Psyllium-induced asthma. Postgrad Med 1987; 82:160–167.
108. Terho EO, Torkko M. Occupational asthma from psyllium laxatives. Duodecim 1980; 96: 1213–1216.
109. Schwartz HJ, Arnold JL, Strohl KP. Occupational allergic rhinitis reaction to psyllium. J Occup Med 1989; 31:624–626.
110. Bernton HS. The allergenicity of psyllium seed. Med Ann DC 1970; 39:313–317.
111. Nelson WL. Allergic events among health care workers exposed to psyllium laxatives in the workplace. J Occup Med 1987; 29:497–499.
112. Breton JL, Leneutre F, Esculpavit G, Abourjaili M. Une nouvelle cause d'asthme professionnel chez un préparateur en pharmacie. Presse Méd 1989; 18:433.
113. Busse WW, Schoenwetter WF. Asthma from psyllium in laxative manufacture. Ann Intern Med 1975; 83:361–362.

25
Polyisocyanates and Their Prepolymers

Cristina Elisabetta Mapp
University of Padova, Padova, Italy

Brian T. Butcher
Arthritis Foundation, Atlanta, Georgia

Leonardo M. Fabbri
University of Ferrara, Ferrara, Italy

INTRODUCTION

The most important low-molecular-mass agents that induce occupational asthma are polyisocyanates and their oligomers (1,2). They are a group of low-molecular-weight aromatic or aliphatic organic chemical compounds, synthesized by reaction of amines or their hydrochlorides with phosgene, which readily form esters of substituted carbamic acid or urethanes. A common feature of these chemicals is the presence of an $-N{=}C{=}O$ group. The importance of polyisocyanates lies in the property of readily forming plastics, adhesives, elastomers, and flexible or rigid foams via this chemical group.

Diisocyanates, the forerunners of all polyisocyanates, were first discovered in 1849 by Wurtz. Use of the prototype of these compounds, toluene diisocyanate (TDI), for manufacturing polyurethane foam was first developed by I. G. Farben in Germany during World War II. A number of related compounds have subsequently been developed and utilized commercially, the most important of which are 2,4- and 2,6-toluene diisocyanate (TDI), hexamethylene diisocyanate (HDI), methylene diphenyldiisocyanate (MDI), naphthalene diisocyanate (NDI), isophorone diisocyanate (IPDI), and prepolymers derived from HDI and MDI (Fig. 1).

Diisocyanates are used worldwide in a number of important industries. They are used extensively in the automobile industry for production of foam rubber cushions, dashboards, body parts, and for finish coatings. Almost all mold and core processes in modern steel foundries require MDI. They also have growing application as insulating materials in the building industry. Prepolymers of HDI, MDI, and their respective polyisocyanate oligomers (see Fig. 1) now rank among the most important sources of exposure in spray paint. Prepolymerized TDI and vapors of TDI are also used in spray lacquering. Additionally, diisocyanates are present in a number of products used by hobbyists. Worldwide production of diisocyanates is unknown, but, in the United States alone, it is estimated that use will exceed 2 million tons by the year 2000, and that as many as 200,000 workers will be exposed (3). It can be anticipated that other isocyanates will be developed and that new applications will be found for these chemicals.

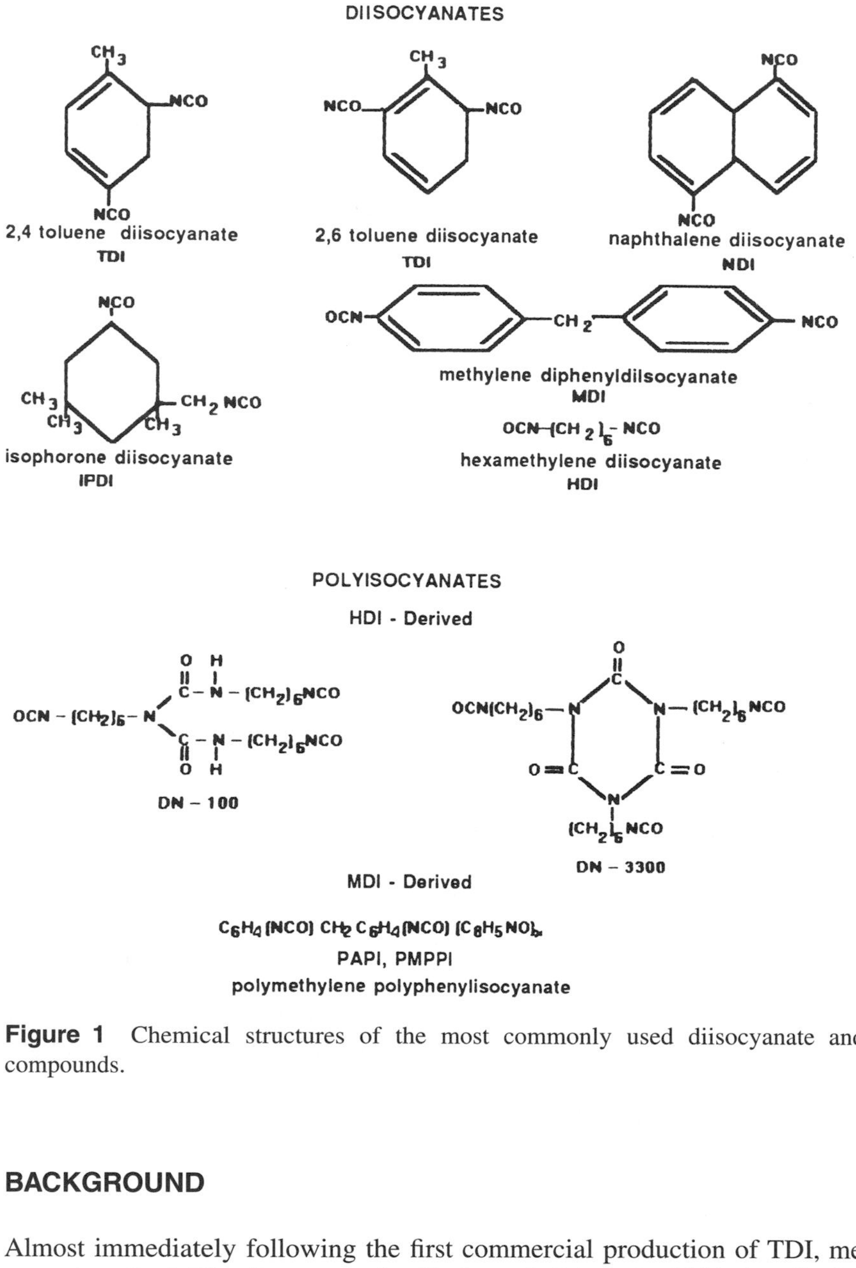

DIISOCYANATES

2,4 toluene diisocyanate
TDI

2,6 toluene diisocyanate
TDI

naphthalene diisocyanate
NDI

isophorone diisocyanate
IPDI

methylene diphenyldiisocyanate
MDI

OCN—(CH$_2$)$_6$—NCO

hexamethylene diisocyanate
HDI

POLYISOCYANATES

HDI - Derived

DN – 100

DN – 3300

MDI - Derived

C$_6$H$_4$(NCO) CH$_2$ C$_6$H$_4$(NCO) (C$_8$H$_5$NO)$_x$

PAPI, PMPPI

polymethylene polyphenylisocyanate

Figure 1 Chemical structures of the most commonly used diisocyanate and polyisocyanate compounds.

BACKGROUND

Almost immediately following the first commercial production of TDI, medical problems were described. The first report by Fuchs and Valade in 1951 described development of asthma in seven of nine workers exposed to TDI (4). Later citations documented respiratory symptoms to the other major diisocyanates. Continuation of exposure of sensitized subjects, even in areas of lower exposure, is associated with persistence of asthma (5–9) and may be fatal (10).

Today, exposure to diisocyanates is recognized as a leading cause of occupational asthma (3,11,12). Diisocyanates have diverse function profiles as sensitizers, irritants, or both. They are widely produced and used in industrialized nations. In some countries, diisocyanates are the most frequent recognized cause of occupational asthma (12). Although incidence varies widely depending on the form of diisocyanate and type of manufacture or use, it is generally accepted that approximately 5% of exposed workers develop occupational asthma after exposure to TDI, the most widely studied of the diisocyanates (13,14). Estimates as high as 15% have been proposed (15). For other polyisocyanates, prevalence is usually considered to be lower and is thought to be related to whether the compound is in monomeric or polymeric form and to the vapor pressure of the chemical (16). For example, TDI and HDI are volatile at room temperature, whereas MDI must be heated above 60°C before vapors are given off. In all cases, estimates may be low due to self-selection by sensitized workers leaving the industry and the difficulty of diagnosing the disease.

Because adverse respiratory effects were known to be associated with exposure to isomeric isocyanate compounds having high vapor pressure properties, new high-molecular-weight isocyanates with low vapor pressure were synthesized to be used in spray polyurethane paint formulations, which are currently in widespread use. These included polyisocyanate oligomers of HDI and MDI (see Fig. 1) having multiple isocyanate reactive sites. Several recent cross-sectional surveys of spray painters in the automobile and aeronautical industries revealed a significant prevalence of asthma despite the fact that most of the workers were using recommended respiratory hazard protection equipment (16). In one of these investigations, occupational asthma was documented by positive broncho-provocation responses after controlled laboratory exposures to HDI- and MDI-derived polyisocyanates in six asthmatic patients (16). These investigations demonstrated that car painters are exposed to high concentrations of airborne prepolymers and that these compounds induce asthma at the same or greater frequency in exposed workers as inhaled isocyanate monomers.

There are numerous anecdotal reports from symptomatic workers suggesting that a high exposure, such as might be experienced in an industrial accident or spill, may induce asthma. Single exposure to high levels has been documented to induce asthma similar to other agents that cause reactive airways dysfunction syndrome (RADS), or irritant-induced asthma (17). It has been suggested that such levels may alter integrity of the tight junctions in the epithelium allowing free passage of the diisocyanate (18). Interestingly, in animals exposed for 4 hr to levels of 2 ppm, sloughing of the superficial epithelium occurred and higher exposures induced foreign body inflammatory responses (19). When humans are exposed to such levels, symptoms include lacrimation, acute inflammation, rhinitis, coughing, and burning in the throat and upper chest. The most widely known accidental high concentration exposure was the 1984 disaster in Bhopal, India where a massive quantity of a monofunctional isocyanate, methyl isocyanate, was discharged from a pesticide plant (20). The consequences ranged from irritant symptoms of the upper respiratory tract to lethal lung injury manifested by pulmonary edema and widespread inflammation.

CLINICAL MANIFESTATIONS OF POLYISOCYANATE HYPERSENSITIVITY

The spectrum of lung diseases that can be induced by diisocyanates is broad, including asthma, RADS or irritant-induced asthma, hypersensitivity pneumonitis, chemical bronchitis, a dose-dependent excess annual decline in FEV_1, and pulmonary edema (13,20–25). Asthma is the most common syndrome linked to exposure to diisocyanates. The symptoms include rhinorrhea, cough, chest tightness, wheeze, and dyspnea. The clinical picture of these asthmatics is compatible with that of an allergic disease: (1) only a small proportion of exposed subjects develop asthma; (2) there is a latency period between the onset of exposure and the onset of asthma; and (3) exposure to low levels of the sensitizing agent can induce an attack of asthma. Once an individual has developed asthma, small amounts of diisocyanate, as low as 1 ppb for short periods, may initiate a response (26). Thus, even exposures below those mandated by regulatory agencies or those attainable by industrial hygiene methods are often sufficient to stimulate a reaction in a sensitized worker. The majority of affected subjects are nonatopic and nonsmokers (27).

The pulmonary responses fall into three categories: (1) an immediate response, usually occurring within minutes following the exposure; (2) a delayed or isolated late response occurring at least one and often a number of hours after the exposure; or (3) a dual response with characteristics of both immediate and delayed reactions. There have been reports of diurnal association of responses and instances of recurrent late responses over a period of days. An increase in nonspecific airway hyperresponsiveness (NSBH) is usually seen in conjunction with diisocyanate asthma, but this is not a consistent finding, since NSBH may return to the normal range after removal from the isocyanate environment and there have been reports of diisocyanate asthma without NSBH (28,29). TDI responders are more responsive to methacholine than TDI nonresponders (30,31), and those responding with immediate asthmatic reactions had the greatest methacholine sensitivity (30). From 40% to 67% of workers respond to a TDI challenge (30). The interval between the last occupational exposure to diisocyanates and response to specific inhalation challenge was shorter in responders (31) in contrast with the findings of Banks and co-workers (32). Another explanation for a negative response in a subject with symptoms of asthma could be related to factors such as level and duration of exposure. Also, the type of isomer used could be inadequate to induce an asthmatic reaction in some subjects. TDI-specific IgE and IgG isotypic antibodies, assessed by well-characterized haptenated serum albumin conjugates, were found in only a few individuals and were not associated with response to TDI challenge. However, a more recent study has shown that, providing the blood sample is obtained within a month from last exposure, TDI specific IgE may provide very specific and sensitive results in detecting TDI-induced asthma (33).

Also, TDI is different from other diisocyanates such as MDI and HDI, which elicit specific antibody responses to both IgE and IgG isotypes in 36% and 80% of occupational asthma patients, respectively. In multiple studies, the presence of elevated HDI-HSA- and MDI-HSA-specific IgE antibodies in sera of diisocyanate workers is a specific diagnostic marker of occupational asthma induced by HDI or MDI (33,34).

Once asthma is symptomatic, its persistence is variable. In some workers, there is evidence that the asthma resolves following removal from the isocyanate environment (35), but in others asthma persists (5–8). If exposure continues after diagnosis, isocyanate-induced asthma usually persists or often worsens (6,18). The majority of patients with occupational asthma do not recover even after several years of cessation of diisocyanate exposure (Table 1). The prognosis of occupational asthma is better in subjects who, at the time of diagnosis, have better lung function, milder degree of NSBH, shorter duration of exposure and symptoms, and who develop an early (as compared to a late or dual) asthmatic reaction after inhalation challenge with the specific agent. Prognosis is not influenced by race, sex, or atopy, and it is not improved by relocation to working areas with lower exposure (18,27). Interestingly, persistence of asthma is associated with an eosinophilic inflammation of the airways even after cessation of exposure (18).

EPIDEMIOLOGY

Shortly after the widespread industrial application of diisocyanates, it was determined that about 5–10% of exposed workers developed asthma. In the decade of the 1960s, long-

Table 1 Persistence of Symptoms and Airway Hyperresponsiveness in Subjects with Isocyanate-Induced Asthma, After Cessation of Exposure

Agent	Number of subjects	Duration of follow-up (yrs)	Persistence of symptoms (%)	Persistence of hyperresponsiveness
Isocyanates	50	>4	82	12/19 (63%)
Isocyanates	20	0.5–4	50	9/12 (75%)
Isocyanates	22	1	77	17/22 (77%)
Isocyanates	12	1.3	66	7/12 (58%)
Various	32	0.5–4	93	31/32 (97%)

Source: Modified from Ref. 8.

term epidemiological studies were undertaken to establish safe occupational threshold limits, which were then set at 20 ppb by the Occupational Safety and Health Administration. A recent study suggested that isocyanate workers are still at risk under work conditions defined as safe by these limit values (35). Most of the recent cross-sectional studies and several longitudinal epidemiological studies have not uncovered special risk factors for occupational asthma such as preexisting atopy, NSBH, and smoking history.

UPTAKE AND DISTRIBUTION OF DIISOCYANATES

Recent studies have shown that most of the diisocyanates (e.g., MDI and TDI) are absorbed in the upper airways, particularly in noses of guinea pigs and rats, and that the uptake, as reflected by the concentration of ^{14}C in the blood, correlates linearly with time and concentration in inhaled air (36). Tissue distribution suggests that primary targets of inhaled diisocyanates are airway tissues and blood, even though traces of ^{14}C may be found in other viscera. In the airways, labeled diisocyanates can be found in the epithelium and the subepithelial level from the nose down to the terminal bronchioles, but not in the alveolar space. Labeled compounds may persist up to 2 weeks after a single exposure. After TDI inhalation, most of the ^{14}C is found in the plasma, but a small proportion of it links to cells, particularly red blood cell hemoglobin. A stable conjugate found in plasma after exposure is a 70,000-kDa protein. In airway tissue, most of the diisocyanate remains at the subepithelial level where it apparently conjugates with a 70,000-kDa protein subsequently identified as laminin (37). Exposure of laminin to TDI vapor modifies both the structure and the cell-binding capacity of this protein (38), suggesting that alteration of laminin could be an intermediate mechanism of epithelial desquamation induced by exposure to TDI in animals and humans (39,40).

Although these studies were performed in animals, they provide the first information regarding uptake and distribution of inhaled diisocyanates. Biological monitoring of urinary polyisocyanate metabolites has recently been described in exposed workers and will be discussed in the next section.

PATHOGENESIS AND AIRWAY INFLAMMATION

Dual and late asthmatic reactions are more frequent than early asthmatic reactions after challenge with diisocyanates and, like allergen-induced dual and late asthmatic reactions, are more relevant to natural asthma than immediate asthmatic reactions (28). In fact, compared with early asthmatic reactions, dual and late asthmatic reactions induced by diisocyanates are usually more severe, longer, are associated with a transient increase of airway responsiveness to nonspecific stimuli such as methacholine, and are more resistant to therapy. In addition, TDI-reactive subjects who develop dual or late asthmatic reactions upon specific inhalation challenge are more likely to have persistent asthma upon cessation of exposure (6,27,41). Although the precise mechanisms of diisocyanate asthma and the late component of the asthmatic response are not clear, airway inflammation has been found in affected subjects (42). Indeed, airway inflammation is a pathophysiological feature common to both occupational and nonoccupational asthma. Bronchoalveolar lavage (BAL) fluid obtained during late asthmatic reactions induced by diisocyanates has shown a significant increase of neutrophils, eosinophils, and albumin concentration (40–43). Bronchial biopsies have also demonstrated a cellular influx in the airways of TDI asthmatics. In fact, in bronchial biopsies obtained in subjects with occupational asthma induced by TDI, eosinophils are increased in the epithelium, in the most superficial layer of the submucosa and in the total submucosa, whereas CD45+ cells (mainly mononuclear cells) are increased in the epithelium and in the most superficial layer of the submucosa, and mast cells are increased only in the epithelium (44).

Immunohistochemical analysis of bronchial biopsy specimens from TDI asthmatics revealed an increase in CD25+ve cells (i.e., activated lymphocytes expressing the IL-2 receptor) as well as in total and activated eosinophils (45). Eosinophil activation has also been demonstrated by increased levels of eosinophil cationic protein (ECP) in the serum of subjects who developed a late asthmatic reaction after exposure to TDI in the laboratory (46). In sensitized subjects, sputum eosinophilia is present in early and late reactors, and declines to near baseline values 48 hr after challenge (47). The degree of airway eosinophilia is similar in asthma and exacerbations of chronic bronchitis, but only in asthma is increased bronchial mucosal expression of IL-5 protein observed (48).

Mast cell activation has been suggested by an increased neutrophil chemotactic activity (NCA) in the serum of subjects exposed to TDI in the laboratory (49). Proinflammatory cytokines such as TNF-α and IL-1β were increased in the submucosa of TDI asthmatics (50). Moreover, the majority of T-cell clones, derived from the bronchial mucosa of two TDI asthmatics, were CD8+ve producing INF-γ and IL-5 in response to nonspecific stimulation (51). An increase in circulating CD8+ve T Lymphocytes has also been observed after the development of a late asthmatic reaction, at a time when airflow obstruction has resolved (52). The presence of activated lymphocytes and eosinophils in bronchial biopsies of TDI asthmatic suggests that a T-lymphocyte–eosinophil interaction may be important in occupational asthma induced by low-molecular-weight agents.

Diisocyanate asthma may be fatal. Postmortem examination of the lungs of one sensitized subject who died after exposure to TDI in the workplace showed denudation of airway epithelium and thickening of the basement membrane, with infiltration of the lamina propria by eosinophils, and diffuse mucous plugging of the bronchioles. Bronchial smooth muscle was hyperplastic and disarrayed, and lung parenchyma showed focal areas of alveolar destruction adjacent to areas of intact alveolar walls (10). Recently, a case of fatal asthma induced by exposure to MDI has also been reported (53). Similarly to nonoccupational asthma death, epithelial desquamation, infiltration of the mucosa of eosinophils and neutrophils, dilation of bronchial vessels, edema, hypertrophy, and disarray of smooth muscle were observed (10,54).

Bronchial biopsies obtained from one subject with HDI-induced asthma 24 hr after challenge revealed airway inflammation and the presence of HDI adducts in human lung tissue, suggesting that the identification and the characterization of the macromolecules to which diisocyanates bind could be helpful for a better understanding of the mechanism of diisocyanate-induced asthma (55). The frequent occurrence of late asthmatic responses in subjects sensitized to diisocyanates suggests a role for cellular immune mechanisms (56). Histamine-releasing activity attributable to monocyte chemoattractant peptide 1 (MCP-1) has been demonstrated in peripheral blood mononuclear cells (PBMC) of workers with occupational asthma as has IL-8 and TNF-α following in vitro stimulation by hapten-specific antigens (57,58).

An underlying genetic susceptibility is suggested by the fact that diisocyanate-induced asthma develops in approximately 5–20% of the exposed workers. Two related studies have provided evidence for a role of HLA class II molecules in TDI-induced asthma (59,60). Evaluation of HLA class II gene products showed a positive association with HLA DQB1*0503 and a negative association with HLADQB1*0501 alleles, which differed at residue 57 for a single amino acid, i.e., aspartic acid in DQB1*0503 and valine in DQB1*0501, suggesting that HLADQB1*0503 has a role in conferring susceptibility in TDI-induced asthma and that residue 57 is a potentially critical location. The results of these studies suggest that the basic molecular and cellular mechanisms of diisocyanate-induced asthma are immunological, as is IgE-mediated asthma, in which the association with HLA class II genes has been well documented (56,61).

Isocyanates themselves may be involved in antibody binding or in the induction of structural changes in an unidentified protein. TDI could behave as a hapten and alter the structure or the specificity of the T-cell receptor (TcR) directly or indirectly at the gene level, or it could react with membrane proteins such as adhesion molecules, amplifying T-cell–B-cell interactions. As residue 57 is a negatively charged residue, it may directly interact with TDI itself. Other explanations include the possibility that TDI could modify the structure of HLA class II molecules or self-peptides at the surface of the antigen-presenting cells (APC) in such a way that the modified epitopes are recognized as foreign by T cells, or it could cause dysfunction in the suppressor-induced network, since DQ molecules act as dominant immunosuppressor genes (Is). Whatever the exact mechanisms of the association of HLA-DQ and TDI asthma may be, the data is consistent with the hypothesis that both exposure to the chemical and inheritance of the genetic marker are necessary to cause the expression of the disease. Most of the TDI asthmatics (59,60) have the marker in both haplotypes (i.e., a homozygous phenotype). The fact that healthy subjects may carry the predisposing marker and some affected individuals lack the same marker may be partially explained by the complex, multifactorial/polygenic nature of asthma.

Recently, the role of HLA class II molecules and of TcR V-beta-gene-segment usage has been examined in workers with diisocyanate-induced asthma (62). The conclusions of this study were that antigen-specific T-cell subpopulations could be sequestered in the lungs of the affected subjects and clonally expand after further exposure to diisocyanates.

The dose and duration of diisocyanate exposure that induce occupational asthma are unknown. More workers exposed to western red cedar and diisocyanates develop work-related symptoms in the first 2 years of exposure than do those exposed to high-molecular-weight agents (i.e., allergenic proteins). However, after 5 years of exposure, the rate of developing symptoms is similar for high-molecular-weight agents and diisocyanates (63). Moreover, there is a lack of good estimates of human exposure to diisocyanates. Since monitoring of aerial TDI concentration itself does not exclude various adverse health effects on exposed workers, biological monitoring may be a useful preventive measure. It has recently been reported that biological monitoring of urinary hexane diamine (HDA), a metabolite of HDI, is sensitive enough to detect HDI at and below the current allowable exposure limits (64). In another study, isocyanate metabolites were measured in biological samples of workers exposed to MDI, TDI, and HDI in a factory using isocyanate-based polyurethane glue. The results showed that metabolites of 4,4'-methylene diphenyl diisocyanate in plasma were useful as biomarkers for isocyanate exposure (65). Specific IgG to MDI-HSA has also been correlated with ambient exposure to MDI among asymptomatic urethane foam workers. These results suggest that specific IgG levels are indirect markers of exposure (66). It has been suggested that the increase in NSBH after a specific inhalation challenge can be an early and sensitive marker of bronchial response to occupational agents, including diisocyanates, especially in subjects removed from workplace exposure for a long time. Thus nonspecific airway responsiveness should be systematically assessed after specific inhalation challenge in the absence of changes in airway caliber (67).

ANIMAL MODELS

To study the mechanism of action of diisocyanates, animal models have been developed in several species. It has been shown that, in the guinea pig, TDI is capable of inducing airway changes obtained by intraperitoneal (68) inhalation (69–71), dermal contact (72,73), and intradermal (74) or intranasal administration (75). In the guinea pig, sensitization and multiple challenge with TDI produced immediate and late respiratory responses and the eosinophil was the key cell of the late response (75). In one inhalation model NSBH and an eosinophil response were observed without concurrent evidence of IgE or IgG_1 antibodies (69). Airway inflammation has been characterized in detail in the guinea pig immunized with intradermal injections of TDI (74). Specific IgG and IgG_1 antibodies against TDI were present only in immunized animals. In these animals, TDI challenge caused an increase in the number of metachromatic cells (at 24 hr) and a late increase of eosinophils (at 48 hr) in the peripheral blood. Mast cells and eosinophils were increased in the submucosa of immunized TDI-challenged animals. A similar pattern was observed in the animals' peripheral airways. At 6 hr after TDI challenge, an increase of T lymphocytes (CD4+ve T cells) and of eosinophils was found in the lamina propria, indicating that these cells are the key cells in the immunopathological alterations induced by TDI in the guinea pig lung. After administration of anti-IL-5, EPO+ eosinophilic cells were significantly different from controls treated with an irrelevant control antibody, suggesting a role for IL-5 in the accumulation of eosinophils in the lungs of TDI-immunized animals. In this model, sensory neuropeptides play an important role. The immunization and TDI challenge decreased the density of substance P- and calcitonin gene-related peptide (CGRP)-immunostained nerves. The number of eosinophils correlated inversely with neuropeptide changes in the central airways of immunized TDI-challenged guinea pigs (76).

An animal model of HDI-induced asthma has also been developed in the guinea pig (77). In this model, HDI-induced airway hyperresponsiveness to acetylcholine was reversible within 8 weeks of HDI avoidance. the effect of HDI has also been evaluated in the isolated, perfused, and ventilated guinea pig lung (78). In this experimental model, HDI-induced bronchoconstriction was mediated via arachidonic acid release and thromboxane formation.

Airway changes induced by TDI inhalation have also been reported in rats and rabbits (79,80). Recently a murine model of TDI-induced asthma has been described (81). Interestingly, TDI was capable of inducing lymphocyte-dependent and IgE-independent tracheal hyperreactivity that was not associated with cellular infiltration in the airways. No influx of lymphocytes could be detected in the trachea, lung tissue, or airway lumen at 2, 24, or 48 hr after the challenge. Tracheal hyperreactivity was associated with a marked increase in myeloperoxidase activity in the lung tissue and in the cells of bronchoalveolar lavage fluid at 24 hr after the challenge. In this model, tachykinins are essential for the development of TDI-induced tracheal hyperreactivity during the effector phase. However, the airways and the skin behaved differently with respect to the sensory neuropeptides (82).

Systemic immunization of mice with TDI induced both haptenic and neoantigenic specific IgG_1 antibodies (83). The sensitizing potential of phenyisocyanate (PI) has also been investigated in mice (84). In this species, PI was found to be the most potent isocyanate tested yielding an SD_{50} (dose predicted to sensitize 50% of the mice) of 0.04 μmol/kg. In mice, the repeated topical administration of different chemicals, including TDI, elicited divergent cytokine secretion patterns consistent with the selective stimulation of distinct Th subsets (85). The skin sensitizer dinitrofluorobenzene (DNFB) provoked substantial amounts of IFN-γ (a TH1-type product), but only low levels of IL-10 and mitogen inducible IL-4 (TH2-type cytokines), whereas exposure to TDI resulted in the converse profile of cytokine section.

In the rat, the increased production of the free radical nitric oxide (NO) was evaluated after a single, sublethal isocyanate inhalation. The animals were exposed to 2 ppm of TDI for 4 hr. At 20 hr after exposure, bronchoalveolar lavage was performed. Exposure to TDI was associated with an increase in the number of alveolar macrophages, lymphocytes, and polymorphonuclear leukocytes. NO levels in the lavage fluid and NO synthase (NOS)-dependent production of reactive species by alveolar macrophages were increased following TDI exposure. In addition, inducible NO production by BAL cells, assessed by both mRNA in cells and nitrite levels in BAL fluid, was elevated following TDI treatment (86). These interesting findings indicate that the airway inflammatory response induced by TDI exposure is associated with increases in inducible NO production.

In vitro experiments have proven useful in investigating pharmacological effects of diisocyanates, especially TDI. This chemical enhanced the muscarinic response to methacholine in the rat trachea whereas the isoprenaline-induced relaxation was decreased (87). The authors suggested an imbalance between bronchoconstrictor and bronchodilator mechanisms. In different preparations, such as rat isolated urinary bladder and guinea pig and human bronchi, it has been found that TDI activated the efferent function of capsaicin-sensitive primary afferents (CSPA) (88–90), confirming the reports of Sheppard and coworkers, who demonstrated a role for tachykinins and for neutral endopeptidase (NEP) in airway responses to TDI (91,92). In isolated guinea pig bronchial smooth muscle, pretreatment with capsaicin or a substance P inhibitor inhibited the TDI-induced contractions (93), whereas they were enhanced by a NEP inhibitor (94). The authors suggested that the action of TDI on sensory nerves is indirect through the release of prostanoids (95). A role for tachykinins has also been demonstrated in the rabbit (96).

In the guinea pig, incubation of bronchi with serum obtained from both nonimmunized and TDI-immunized guinea pigs, followed by washing, modified the in vitro bronchial smooth muscle response to TDI from contraction to relaxation (97). By contrast, after incubation with both normal and immune serum, followed by indomethacin, TDI produced contraction of the bronchial smooth muscle. It is likely that the action of TDI on bronchial smooth muscle is indirect through the release of prostanoids, and that serum or its components (i.e., albumin) are able to change the profile of released prostanoids.

Recently, the effect of immunization and challenge with TDI in guinea pigs on serum proteins has been investigated. Immunized TDI-challenged animals had a significant increase of total serum proteins. Albumin and alpha$_1$ and alpha$_2$ globulins were increased whereas $beta_1$ and $beta_2$ globulins were decreased in these animals. Moreover, in immunized TDI-challenged guinea pigs, albumin was modified by TDI and migrated faster on gel electrophoresis than albumin from nonimmunized animals. Western blotting of TDI-specific antibodies (IgG and IgG_1) induced in these animals revealed reactivity against TDI and TDI-BSA conjugates without reactivity against native or denatured protein of immunized guinea pig serum or bovine serum albumin alone (BSA) (98). If these results are confirmed in humans, routine electrophoresis on agarose gel may be a simple and useful tool to detect the presence of acute inflammation, characterized by an increase in serum proteins, suggesting that these findings may be used in the biological monitoring of subjects sensitized to isocyanates. Of five adducted proteins identified in the BAL of guinea pigs following inhalation exposure to TDI, the most prevalent was TDI adducted to serum albumin (99). The mechanism underlying sensitization to isocyanates remains controversial. Recently, it has been reported that exposure to TDI in the guinea pig results in detectable adducts, and that the tissue localization of adducts is dependent upon both the concentration of TDI inhaled and the number or exposures (100). Isolation and characterization of the cellular adducts should assist in elucidation of the role of adducts in the sensitization process, and provide identification of the protein carriers involved in the sensitizing process.

DIAGNOSIS

Diagnosis of diisocyanate asthma is often difficult, especially when the asthma is of the delayed type occurring hours after exposure. Occasionally, a clear diagnosis can be made in the office if the patient is observed soon after an acute episode of asthma at work. Sometimes a confirmatory diagnosis with identification of the diisocyanate as the offending agent requires special testing, such as a provocative inhalation challenge test, which can only be undertaken by a limited number of specialized centers (101). Under certain conditions, workplace challenges may facilitate diagnosis.

During the diagnostic medical evaluation, the dictum of Ramazzini—"ask the patient about his occupation"—is still valid (102). Much essential information can be derived from the history to determine possible contributory host factors, types of agents in the work environment, and the potential for and level of exposure. History should include length and type of present and past employment, including military service and duration of exposure to diisocyanate agents. Past and current hobbies are worth evaluating, as asthma has been reported in individuals exposed to diisocyanates used in these pursuits (103). Development of diisocyanate-induced asthma has even been documented in office workers in a building whose atmosphere was contaminated by diisocyanate discharges from a nearby factory (104).

Often, the worker can provide a comprehensive list of agents, some of which may also be asthma inducers or aggravants used in the job, a precise description of the job duties, details of the manufacturing process, environmental controls employed in the factory, whether there are detectable fumes or odors, and the frequency of spills. Thus, a worker with diisocyanate asthma can usually associate his or her asthma with a particular process and can sometimes relate onset of symptoms after exposure to high levels of diisocyanates during an accident or spill (13,14).

Personal or family history of atopy, allergic disease, and other possible risk factors such as smoking do not appear to be related to development of diisocyanate asthma and are not useful in diagnosis. A detailed history of respiratory symptoms and their temporal relationship to occupational exposure, however, often provides important clues by indicating whether symptoms occur during or after the work shift, are worse on some workdays than others, or abate during time off (i.e., weekends and vacations). Sometimes, the patient will relate that co-workers in the factory, especially those working at a similar process or location, are experiencing similar respiratory problems.

On physical examination, chest auscultation reveals wheezing only if the worker has continuous symptoms. Chest X-rays are usually negative. If interstitial or patchy infiltrates are observed, hypersensitivity pneumonitis should be suspected. This complication is not necessarily associated with preexistent or current asthma. Rhinitis and conjunctivitis are not infrequent and may be exposure related. The prevalence of upper airway symptoms or signs induced by diisocyanates has not been systematically investigated, but a surprisingly high prevalence was found in one longitudinal study (35). Urticaria, anaphylaxis, eczema, and contact dermatitis have occasionally been reported, but the presence of such findings is not useful in diagnosis of diisocyanate asthma (35).

Pulmonary function testing should always be performed to confirm airway obstruction, but airway dysfunction alone is not sufficient to establish a definitive diagnosis of diisocyanate asthma. Demonstration of pre/post-bronchodilator pulmonary function improvement has been used to confirm reversibility of the airway obstruction, although it is not necessarily an indication of diisocyanate asthma. Determination of NSBH, while not usually diagnostic, has also been used as an indicator of asthma, but it cannot confirm the occupational nature of the disease. Nevertheless, increase of NSBH within 24 hr after a controlled laboratory challenge or a known workplace challenge may have diagnostic significance, especially if the increase in NSBH subsides in the ensuing weeks (67).

As previously discussed, skin testing with diisocyanates has not proved useful. Although there have been occasional reports of positive patch testing, interpretation of this finding could only be applied to patients with contact dermatitis.

LABORATORY TESTING

Hemolysis-free serum is required for specific antibody assays measuring IgG and IgE isotypes. Measurements of total serum IgE are of modest clinical value. However, a total serum IgE should be performed in all samples tested for specific IgE by the radioallergosorbent test because high levels of total IgE can result in nonspecific binding in this assay.

Commercially available assays for allergen-specific IgE are based on the principle of immunoabsorption (e.g., RAST, EAST, CAP, ELISA). In detecting polyisocyanate immunological reactions, the role of the polyisocyanate protein conjugate is extremely important. Precise methods are available to avoid under- or oversubstitution of protein carrier moieties (105). At the very least, all assays for polyisocyanate-specific IgE should have known positive and negative sera run with each new lot of reagents. Preferably, positive or negative sera should be included in each individual assay for each polyisocyanate allergen.

Clinical interpretation of polyisocyanate-specific IgE results varies depending on the specific agent. Very few TDI-sensitive workers develop specific IgE antibodies. In contrast, specific polyisocyanate IgE antibodies to diisocyanate-HSA antigens are found in approximately 20% and 50% of workers with proven occupational asthma induced by MDI and HDI, respectively (34). If workers are exposed primarily to polyisocyanate prepolymers, specific IgE antibodies may be detectable to antigens prepared with mono- or bifunctional isocyanates. Recently, direct comparison of specific IgE in challenge positive or negative workers revealed a high positive predictive value but a low to moderate negative predictive value for the immunoassay (33). In the case of TDI asthma false positive tests have been reported in a few workers (106).

Polyisocyanate-specific IgG can be measured and interpreted using immunoassays similar to those used to measure specific IgE. Significant amounts of specific IgG indicate that the worker has been exposed to enough polyisocyanate antigen to induce a measurable IgG antibody response. In the case of polyisocyanate-induced hypersensitivity pneumonitis, very large amounts of polyisocyanate-specific IgG or precipitins are produced.

Both specific IgE and IgG antibodies may appear in diisocyanate-exposed workers, particularly in those with a positive inhalation challenge (34). Because specific IgE antibodies are present in 24% of workers with a negative inhalation challenge, specific IgG antibodies are poor predictors of diisocyanate asthma. In addition, the prevalence of different isotypic classes of specific antibodies was different among subjects reacting to different diisocyanates. In one study, diisocyanate antigen–specific IgE was present mainly in subjects sensitized to HDI (Table 2). Very few subjects with TDI occupational asthma had specific antibodies of any isotypic class. Recent investigations of occupational asthma induced by MDI disclosed a wider spectrum of specific isotypic antibodies including IgG and IgM (66,107). The high prevalence of MDI-specific IgG antibodies in exposed asymptomatic workers suggests the possibility that assays for such antibodies could be used as a biological markers of exposure (66).

Car painters exposed to combined mixtures of HDI oligomers and HDI develop high titers of IgG antibodies against a human serum albumin (HSA) conjugate of an HDI prepolymer, DN (see Fig. 1), but not to HDI-HSA (108). These antibody results correlated with exposure studies, which determined that exposure to DN was 2–3 orders of magnitude higher than to HDI. Similar to diisocyanate-induced asthma, polyisocyanate-specific IgE antibodies appeared in only a relatively few symptomatic workers.

In vitro tests that correlate with cellular or delayed hypersensitivity reactions are used chiefly for research purposes in workers with polyisocyanate sensitivity reactions (51,56). The currently available tests that quantify cell-mediated lymphocyte function are: (1) proliferation; (2) production of proinflammatory mediators, cytokines, and chemokines; (3) cytotoxic reactions; and (4) those that regulate specific IgE or IgG responses. Some of these tests are currently being evaluated as possible clinical markers of polyisocyanate sensitivity but these techniques require systematic standardization before they can be applied to the clinical situation of sensitized workers.

Table 2 Relationship Between Specific IgE Antibodies Against the Low-Molecular-Weight Sensitizers Hexamethylene Diisocyanate (HDI) and Occupational Asthma Induced by HDI

	Specific IgE	
	Increased	Normal
HDI exposed	7 (47%)	8 (53%)
HDI exposed, no asthma	1 (4%)	23 (96%)

Source: Modified from Ref. 33.

BRONCHOPROVOCATION TESTING

Inhalation challenges may cause early (10–20%), dual (30–50%), or late (30–50%) asthmatic reactions in about 40% of individuals with history of asthma induced by TDI (27). The challenge is highly specific because no reaction is induced in normal subjects or in asthmatics not sensitized to TDI. Similarly to non-occupational asthma, dual and late, but not early, TDI-induced asthmatic reactions are associated with transient increase of NSBH to methacholine, which lasts for at least 24 hr (109–111), and such increase of NSBH is specific because it does not occur in normal subjects or in non-TDI-exposed asthmatics (41).

While inhalation challenge remains the "gold standard" for confirming a diagnosis of diisocyanate asthma in an individual workers, it is also an important research tool for confirming the diagnosis and monitoring the disease (109–112). Such testing is not without risk to the patient and should not be lightly undertaken because transient increases in NSBH may persist as long as 30 days after diisocyanate challenge (11). It is advisable to obtain informed consent from the subject before the test is undertaken. Testing should be performed in specialized centers with all safety measures recommended by international guidelines (101,113). Although challenges with diisocyanates are highly specific if the test is positive, they may not be sufficiently sensitive especially if they are performed with subthreshold concentrations. Thus, a negative inhalation challenge does not necessarily exclude the presence of occupational asthma.

The patient should be observed at least 12 hr in an outpatient setting or hospitalized throughout the procedure to permit monitoring and treatment of asthmatic reactions. Thus, the cost of this test is high. Testing often requires the patient's cooperation for a week and withdrawal of medication for sufficient time prior to testing to ensure that there is no artifactual interference with results. If severe respiratory impairment is present, challenge should not be performed. These caveats preclude routine utilization of this test. As there is currently no standardized method of provocation testing, it is difficult to interpret and compare results from different centers. Generation and monitoring of the challenge atmosphere must be undertaken only by environmental experts in facilities designed especially for challenge procedures and depend on the type of diisocyanate being tested. For some isocyanates such as MDI, it is difficult to deliver the agent in an aerosol or vapor phase (113) and special delivery systems have been devised. Sometimes, such as with paint spraying, it has been possible to reproduce the conditions of occupational exposure in the laboratory but, as with all bronchoprovocation tests, it is vital that diisocyanate levels be measured. In all environmental challenges, the importance of appropriate control exposures must be emphasized.

Extreme caution must be exercised in performing the challenge. Initially, diisocyanate exposures are those that reasonably could be expected not to induce a severe asthmatic reaction, usually 5 ppb; subsequent challenges are stepwise increases of dose and/or exposure time. Except in special circumstances, the combination of dosage exposure and time should not exceed the established permissible workplace exposure level of 20 ppb (101). Severe reactions can occur even at low exposure levels; patients should be immediately removed from the test environment when symptoms occur. Most importantly, a placebo exposure should always be performed and the patient should be unaware of the nature of the exposure throughout the challenge protocol.

Bronchoprovocation testing demonstrates the type of asthma and the degree of sensitivity. As a research tool, it has proved useful in monitoring the progress of workers removed from diisocyanate-containing environments and possible treatments, but it is not practical as a method of routine monitoring of individuals.

It may be possible to do a less expensive (but also less precise) occupational exposure at the worksite with the patient performing serial peak flow rates and/or spirometry during the work shift and at periods away from work. Burge et al. have shown that occupational exposure studies, where worksite pulmonary function testing has been performed, can be of value (114). It should be emphasized, however, that it is not usually possible to monitor these tests and that workers may have a personal interest in the type of result obtained. Results should be evaluated with care, since testing is effort dependent and results may be less than ideal in a patient seeking to prove disability. Because the worksite usually contains other potential asthma-inducing agents, this technique is not sufficient for identification of diisocyanate as the asthma-inducing agent, but, if performed in conjunction with environmental measurements, it can give an indication of the level of reactivity. The advantages of this type of challenge are that it is relatively inexpensive and the worker is exposed to environmental levels of agent normally encountered during work.

INDUSTRIAL HYGIENE

There continues to be discussion on the appropriate threshold limit value (TLV) of diisocyanates. The current TLV of 20 ppb aims to prevent chronic respiratory symptoms in workers, but there is evidence to suggest that this level should be reduced to 5 ppb. Whether these levels are appropriate to stop induction of asthma is not known, although, as described above, many workers can relate onset of their asthma to an industrial accident or spill where levels far exceed the TLV. While levels below the TLV may be appropriate to arrest development of chronic lung effects, there is strong evidence that once a worker has developed diisocyanate asthma, exposure to levels far below the TLV can initiate the asthmatic response (101,109–111). Nevertheless, improvement in industrial hygiene technology and surveillance promises to be a means of reducing diisocyanate-induced lung disease. Better-controlled methods of avoiding exposure, such as more efficient extractor hoods, masks, and use of positive-pressure hoods, may decrease incidence of both chronic and acute disease. Nevertheless, prepolymerized HDI-specific antibody responses were detected in car painters "effectively" protected by respirators (108).

TREATMENT

Because it is often difficult for a sensitized subject to avoid partial exposure to the inciting agent in the workplace, it may be helpful to know the most effective pharmacological treatment that prevents late asthmatic reactions induced by specific exposure (43,115–120). Oral and topical steroids prevent both TDI-induced late asthmatic reactions and the associated increase in airway responsiveness, whereas slow-release theophylline only partially inhibits the early and late asthmatic reactions and has no effect on the increased airway responsiveness (115,116,118–120). Salbutamol alone, cromolyn, verapamil, and ketotifen do not prevent TDI-induced asthmatic reactions and the associated increase of NSBH (119–121).

Although late asthmatic reactions, increased NSBH, and airway inflammation are all inhibited by steroids, airway hyperresponsiveness already present in subjects before exposure to TDI is not associated with leukocytosis in bronchoalveolar lavage and is not modified by steroids (40,43). Thus, it is speculated that this long-lasting component of airway hyperresponsiveness is probably caused by mechanisms different from airway inflammation. Interestingly, in some subjects with late asthmatic reactions NSBH becomes normal away from exposure to TDI and increases only after exposure to TDI at the time when airways are inflamed (29). In these subjects, the NSBH may be caused entirely by airway inflammation.

Beta$_2$ agonists may be used to prevent or reverse intermediate asthmatic reactions, but more severe asthma induced by diisocyanates should be treated as any asthma occurrence, i.e., with high-dose inhaled beta$_2$ agonists and high-dose steroids. Drug treatment of chronic occupational asthma is identical to drug treatment of nonoccupational asthma (122,123).

In conclusion, the management of occupational asthma is identical to the management of nonoccupational asthma, i.e., avoidance is preferable to medical treatment, and medical treatment is similar in occupational and nonoccupational asthma.

LEGAL CONSIDERATIONS

The physician is frequently asked for advice on disposition of workers who have developed diisocyanate asthma. Ideally, a worker who develops diisocyanate asthma should be removed from the work environment. There may be occasions, however, when the worker, for personal or financial reasons, does not wish to change employment. In such cases, where the worker chooses not to heed the advice of avoiding the diisocyanate-containing environment, a number of strategies have been tried, usually with little success.

In cases where there is workmen's compensation or other legal dispute, a physician may be called to confirm a diagnosis of diisocyanate asthma. Since it is difficult to make a diagnosis at a time far removed from the event, it is apparent that there is overdiagnosis by those not having experience with this disease. Where the evidence of the occupational asthma is good, the patient should be encouraged to avoid reexposure and to seek employment elsewhere. Often companies will undertake to train the worker for employment in a nondiisocyanate environment. However, it should be borne in mind that in workers who have developed concurrent and persistent NSBH, the factory environment often contains other agents that will trigger the asthmatic response.

SUMMARY

Polyisocyanate-induced asthma is the leading cause of occupational asthma. The prevalence of asthma depends upon the chemical structure of the polyisocyanate and its vapor pressure. Approximately 5–10% of workers exposed to toluene diisocyanate develop asthma. The dose and length of exposure to polyisocyanates necessary to induce asthma are not known. Radioactivity labeled TDI is found in the plasma and in specific airway tissues after inhalation. Among the possible pathogenetic mechanisms of polyisocyanate-induced asthma are immunological reactions, airway inflammation, and possible augmentation of nonimmunological neurogenic inflammation. The diagnosis of polyisocyanate asthma is based on careful history, pulmonary function testing, and both specific and nonspecific bronchoprovocation. Early recognition of the problem is essential because persistent asthma may occur in patients whose workplace exposure is prolonged.

REFERENCES

1. Bernstein IL. Isocyanate-induced pulmonary disease: a current perspective. J. Allergy Clin Immunol 1982; 70:24–32.
2. Bernstein JA. Overview of diisocyanate occupational asthma. Toxicology 1996; 111:181–189.
3. Seta JA, Young RO. The United States National Exposure Survey (NOES) data base. In: Bernstein IL, Chan-Yeung M, Malo J-L, Bernstein DI, eds., 1st ed. Asthma in the Workplace. New York: Marcel Dekker, 1993:627–634.
4. Fuchs S, Valade P. Etude clinique et experimentale sur quelque cas d'intoxication par le desmodur T (diisocyanate de toluylene 1-12-4 et 1-2-6). Arch Mal Profess 1951; 12:191–196.
5. Moller DR, McKay RT, Bernstein IL, Brooks SM. Persistent airways disease caused by toluene diisocyanate. Am Rev Respir Dis 1986; 134:175–176.
6. Mapp CE, Chiesura Corona P, De Marzo N, Fabbri LM. Persistent asthma due to isocyanates. A follow-up study of subjects with occupational asthma due to toluene diisocyanate (TDI). Am Rev Respir Dis 1988; 137:1326–1329.
7. Banks DE, Rando RJ, Barkman HW. Persistence of toluene diisocyanate-induced asthma despite negligible workplace exposure. Chest 1990; 97:121–125.
8. Allard C, Cartier A, Ghezzo H, Malo J-L. Occupational asthma due to various agents. Absence of clinical and functional improvement at an interval of four or more years after cessation of exposure. Chest 1989; 96:1046–1049.
9. Paggiaro PL, Loi AM, Rosso O, et al. Follow-up study of patients with respiratory disease due to toluene diisocyanate (TDI). Clin Allergy 1984; 14:463–469.
10. Fabbri LM, Danieli D, Crescioli S, Bevilacqua P, Meli S, Saetta M, Mapp CE. Fatal asthma in a toluene diisocyanate sensitized subject. Am Rev Respir Dis 1988; 137:1494–1498.
11. Fabbri LM, Mapp CE, Saetta M, Allegra L. Occupational asthma. In: O'Byrne PM, ed. Asthma as an Inflammatory Disease. New York: Marcel Dekker, 1990.
12. Sallie B, Ross D, Meredith S, et al. SWORD '93, Surveillance of work-related and occupational respiratory disease in the UK. Occup Med 1994; 44:177–182.
13. Diem JE, Jones RN, Hendrick DJ, Glindmeyer HW, Dharmarajan V, Butcher BT, Salvaggio JE, Weill H. Five year longitudinal study of workers employed in a new toluene diisocyanate manufacturing plant. Am Rev Respir Dis 1982; 126:420–428.
14. Butcher BT, Jones RN, O'Neil CE, Glindmeyer HW, Diem JE, Dharmarajan V, Weill H, Salvaggio JE. Longitudinal study of workers employed in the manufacture of toluene diisocyanate. Am Rev Respir Dis 1977:116:411–421.
15. Peters JM, Wegman DH. Epidemiology and toluene diisocyanate (TDI) induced respiratory disease. Environ Health Perspect 1975; 11:97–100.
16. Seguin P, Allard A, Cartier A, Malo J-L. Prevalence of occupational asthma in spray painters exposed to several types of isocyanates, including polymethylene polyphenylisocyanate. J Occup Med 1987; 29:340–344.
17. Luo JC, Nelsen KG, Fischbein A. Persistent reactive airway dysfunction syndrome after exposure to toluene diisocyanate. Br J Ind Med 1990; 47:239–241.
18. Paggiaro PL, Bacci E, Paoletti P, et al. Bronchoalveolar lavage and morphology of the airways after cessation of exposure in asthmatic subjects sensitized to toluene diisocyanates. Chest 1990; 98:536–542.
19. Duncan G, Scheel LD, Fairchild EJ, et al. Toluene diisocyanate inhalation toxicity: pathology and mortality. Am Ind Hyg Assoc J 1962; 23:447–456.
20. Weill H. Disaster at Bhopal: the accident, early findings and respiratory health outlook in those injured. Bull Eur Physiopathol Respir 1987; 23:587–590.
21. Vandenplas O, Malo, J-L, Saetta M, Mapp CE, Fabbri LM. Occupational asthma and extrinsic alveolitis due to isocyanates: current status and perspectives. Br J Ind Med 1993; 50:213–228.

22. Luo JCJ, Nelson KG, Fischbein A. Persistent reactive airways dysfunction syndrome after exposure to toluene diisocyanate. Br J Ind Med 1990; 47:239–241.
23. Mapp CE, Saetta M, Maestrelli P, Ciaccia A, Fabbri LM. Low molecular weight pollutants and asthma: pathogenetic mechanisms and genetic factors. Eur Respir J. 1994; 7:1559–1563.
24. Henschler D, Assman W, Meyer KO. The toxicology of toluene diisocyanate. Arch Toxicol 1962; 19:364–387.
25. Vandenplas O, Malo J-L, Saetta M, Mapp CE, Fabbri LM. Occupational asthma and extrinsic alveolitis due to isocyanates: current status and perspectives. Br J Industr Med 1993; 50:213–228.
26. Butcher BT, Karr RM, O'Neill CE, Wilson MR, Dharmarajan V, Salvaggio JE, Weill H. Inhalation challenge and pharmacologic studies of TDI sensitive workers. J Allergy Clin Immunol 1979; 64:146.
27. Mapp CE, Boschetto P, Dal Vecchio L, Maestrelli P, Fabbri LM. Occupational asthma due to isocyanate. Eur Respir J 1988; 1:273–279.
28. Smith AB, Brooks SM, Blanchard J, Bernstein IL, Gallagher JS. Absence of airway hyper-reactivity to methacholine in a worker sensitized to toluene diisocyanate (TDI). J Occup Med 1980; 22:237–241.
29. Mapp CE, Dal Vecchio L, Boschetto P, De Marzo N, Fabbri LM. Toluene diisocyanate-induced asthma without airway hyperresponsiveness. Eur J Respir Dis 1986; 68:89–95.
30. Karol MH, Tollerud DJ, Campbell TP, Fabbri LM, Maestrelli P, Saetta M, Mapp CE. Predictive value of airways hyperresponsiveness and circulating IgE for identifying types of responses to toluene diisocyanate inhalation challenge. Am J Respir Crit Care Med 1994; 149:611–615.
31. Moscato G, Dellabianca A, Vinci G, Candura SM, Bossis MC. Toluene diisocyanate-induced asthma: clinical findings and bronchial responsiveness studies in 113 exposed subjects with work-related respiratory symptoms. J Occup Med 1991; 33(6):720–725.
32. Banks DE, Sastre J, Butcher BT, Ellis E, Rando RJ, Barkman HW, Hammad YY, Glindmeyer HW, Weill H. Role of inhalation challenge testing in the diagnosis of isocyanate-induced asthma. Chest 1989; 95:414–423.
33. Tee RD, Cullinan P, Welch J, Burge PS, Newman-Taylor AJ. Specific IgE to isocyanates: a useful diagnostic role in occupational asthma. J Allergy Clin Immunol 1998; 101:709–715.
34. Cartier A, Grammar L, Malo J-L, et al. Specific serum antibodies against isocyanates: association with occupational asthma. J Allergy Clin Immunol 1989; 84:507–514.
35. Bernstein DI, Korbee L, Stauder T, Bernstein JA, Scinto J, Herd ZL, Bernstein IL. The low prevalence of occupational asthma and antibody-dependent sensitization to diphenylmethane diisocyanate in a plant engineered for minimal exposure to diisocyanate. J Allergy Clin Immunol 1993; 92:387–396.
36. Kennedy AL, Stock MF, Alarie Y, Brown WE. Update and distribution of ^{14}C during and following inhalation exposure to radioactive toluene diisocyanate. Toxicol Appl Pharmacol 1989; 100:280–292.
37. Kennedy AL, Brown WE. Modification of airway proteins and induction of secondary responses by inhalation exposure to isocyanates. Am Rev Respir Dis 1989; 139:387A.
38. Kennedy AL, Wilson TR, Brown WE. Analysis of functional alterations of laminin modified by isocyanates in vitro and in vivo. Am Rev Respir Dis 1990; 141:706A.
39. Gordon T, Sheppard D, MacDonald DM, Distefano S, Scypinski L. Airway hyperresponsiveness and inflammation induced by toluene diisocyanate in guinea pigs. Am Rev Respir Dis 1985; 132:106–112.
40. Fabbri LM, Boschetto P, Zocca E, Milani GF, Pivirotto F, Burlina A. Plebani M, Licata B, Mapp CE. Bronchoalveolar neutrophilia during late asthmatic reactions induced by toluene diisocyanate (TDI). Am Rev Respir Dis 1987; 136:36–42.
41. Mapp CE, Di Giacomo R, Borseghini, et al. Late, but not early, asthmatic reactions induced by toluene diisocyanate (TDI) are associated with increased airway responsiveness. Eur J Respir Dis 1986; 68:276–284.

42. Mapp CE, Saetta M, Maestrelli P, Di Stefano A, Chitano P, Boschetto P, Ciaccia A, Fabbri LM. Mechanisms and pathology of occupational asthma. Eur Respir J 1994; 7:544–554.

43. Boschetto P, Fabbri LM, Zocca E, Milani GF, Pivirotto F, Dal Vecchio A. Plebani M, Mapp CE. Prednisone inhibits late asthmatic reactions and airway inflammation induced by toluene diisocyanate in sensitized subjects. J Allergy Clin Immunol 1987; 80:261–267.

44. Saetta M, Stefano A, Maestrelli, De Marzo N, Milani GF, Pivirotto F, Mapp CE, Fabbri LM. Airway mucosal inflammation in occupational asthma induced by toluene diisocyanate. Am Rev Respir Dis 1992; 145:160–168.

45. Bentley, AM, Maestrelli P, Saetta M, Fabbri LM, Robinson DS, Bradely BL, Jeffery PK, Durham SR, Kay AB. Activated lymphocytes-T and eosinophils in the bronchial mucosa in isocyanate-induced asthma. J Allergy Clin Immunol 1992; 89:821–828.

46. Mapp CE, Plebani M, Faggian D, Maestrelli P, Saetta M, Calcagni PG, Borghesan F, Fabbri LM. Eosinophil cationic protein (ECP), histamine and tryptase in peripheral blood before and during inhalation challenge with toluene diisocyanate (TDI) in sensitized subjects. Clin Exp Allergy 1994; 24:730–736.

47. Maestrelli P, Calcagni PG, Saetta M, Stefano AD, Hosselet J-J, Santonastaso, A, Fabbri LM, Mapp CE. Sputum eosinophilia after asthmatic responses induced by isocyanates in sensitized subjects. Clin Exp Allergy 1994; 24:29–34.

48. Saetta M, Di Stefano A, Maestrelli P, Turato G, Mapp CE, Pieno M, Zanguochi G, Del Prete G, Fabbri LM. Airway eosinophilia and expression of interleukin 5 protein in asthma and in exacerbations of chronic bronchitis. Clin Exp Allergy 1996; 26:774–776.

49. Sastre J, Banks DE, Lopez M. Barkman HW, Salvaggio JE. Neutrophil chemotactic activity in toluene diisocyanate (TDI)-induced asthma. J Allergy Clin Immunol 1990; 85:567–572.

50. Maestelli P, Di Stefano A, Occari P, Turato G, Milani GF, Pivirotto F, Mapp CE, Fabbri LM, Saetta M. Cytokines in the airway mucosa of subjects with asthma induced by toluene diisocyanate. Am J Respir Crit Care Med 1995; 151:607–612.

51. Del Prete GF, De Carli M, D'Elios MM, Maestrelli P, Ricci M, Fabbri LM, Romagnani S. Allergen exposure induces the activation of allergen-specific Th2 cells in the airway mucosa of patients with allergic respiratory disorders. Eur J Immunol 1993; 23:1445–1449.

52. Finotto S, Fabbri LM, Rado V, Mapp CE, Maestrelli P. Increase in numbers of CD8 positive lymphocytes and eosinophils in peripheral blood of subject with late asthmatic reactions induced by toluene diisocyanate. Br J Ind Med 1991; 48:116–121.

53. Carino M, Aliani M, Licitra C, Sarno N, Ioli F. Death due to asthma at work place in a diphenylmethane diisocyanate sensitized subject, Respiration 1997; 64:111–113.

54. Saetta M, Rosina C, DiStefano A, Thiene G, Fabbri LM. Quantitative structural analysis of peripheral airway and arteries in sudden fatal asthma. Am Rev Respir Dis 1991; 143:138–143.

55. Redlich CA, Karol MH, Graham C, Homer RJ, Holm CT, Wirth JA, Cullen MR. Airway isocyanate adducts in asthma induced by exposure to hexamethylene diisocyanate. Scand J Work Environ Health 1997; 23:227–231.

56. Mapp CE, Balboni A, Baricordi R, Fabbri LM. Human leukocyte antigen associations in occupational asthma induced by isocyanates. Am J Respir Crit Care Med 1997; 156:s139–s143.

57. Lummus ZL, Alam R, Bernstein JA, Bernstein DI. Characterization of histamine releasing factors in diisocyanate induced occupational asthma. Toxicology 1996; 111:191–206.

58. Lummus ZL, Alam R, Bernstein JA, Bernstein DI. Diisocyanate antigen–enhanced production of monocyte chemoattractant protein-1, IL-8, and tumor necrosis factor-α by peripheral mononuclear cells of workers with occupational asthma. J Allergy Clin Immunol 1998; 102: 265–274.

59. Bignon JS, Aron Y, Ju LY, Kopferschmitt MC, Graneir RGR, Mapp CE, Fabbri LM, Pauli G, Lockart A, Charron D, Swierczewski E. HLA class II alleles in isocyanate-induced asthma. Am J Respir Crit Care Med 1994; 49:71–75.

60. Balboni A, Baricordi OR, Fabbri LM, Gandini E, Ciaccia, A, Mapp CE. Association between toluene diisocyanate-induced asthma and DQB1 markers: a possible role for aspartic acid at position 57. Eur Respir J 1996; 9:207–210.

61. Marsh DG. Immunogenetic and immunochemical factors determining immune responsiveness to allergens: studies in unrelated subjects. In: Marsh DG, Blumenthal MN, eds. Genetic and Environmental Factors in Clinical Allergy. Minneapolis: University of Minnesota Press, 1990: 97–123.

62. Bernstein JA, Munson J, Lummus ZL, Balakrishnan K, Leikauf G. T cell receptor V beta gene segment expression in diisocyanate induced occupational asthma. J Allergy Clin Immunol 1997; 99:245–250.

63. Malo J-L, Ghezzo H, D'Aquino C, et al. Natural history of occupational asthma: relevance of type of agent and other factors in the rate of development of symptoms in affected subjects. J Allergy Clin Immunol 1992; 90:937–943.

64. Maitre A, Berode M, Perdrix A, Stoklow M, Mallion JM, Savolainen H. Urinary hexane diamine as an indicator of occupational exposure to hexamethylene diisocyanate. Int Arch Occup Environ Health 1996; 69:65–68.

65. Skarping G, Dalene M, Svensson GB, Littorin M, Akesson B, Welinder H, Skerfvin S. Biomarkers of exposure, antibodies, and respiratory symptoms in workers heating polyurethane glue. Occup Environ Med 1996; 53:180–187.

66. Lushniak BD, Reh CM, Bernstein DI, Gallagher JS. Indirect assessment of 4,4'-diphenylmethane diisocyanate (MDI) exposure by evaluation of specific humoral immune responses to MDI conjugated to human serum albumin. Am J Ind Med 1998; 33:471–477.

67. Vandenplas O, Delwiche JP, Jamart J, Vandeweyer R. Increase in nonspecific bronchial hyperresponsiveness as an early marker of bronchial response to occupational agents during specific inhalation challenges. Thorax 1996; 51:472–478.

68. Chen SE, Bernstein IL. The guinea pig model of diisocyanate sensitization. I. Immunologic studies. J Allergy Clin Immunol 1982; 69:123.

69. Cibulas W, Murlas CG, Miller ML, et al. Toluene diisocyanate-induced airway hyperreactivity and pathology in the guinea pig. J Allergy Clin Immunol. 1986; 77:828–834.

70. McKay RT, Brooks SM. Hyperreactive airway smooth muscle responsiveness after inhalation of toluene diisocyanate vapours. Am Rev Respir Dis 1984; 129:296–300.

71. Raulf M, Tennie L, Marczynski B, Potthast J, Marek W, Baur X. Cellular and mediator profile in bronchoalveolar lavage of guinea pigs after toluene diisocyanate (TDI) exposure. Lung 1995; 173:57–68.

72. Karol MH, Hauth BA, Riley EJ, Magreni CM. Dermal contact with toluene diisocyanate (TDI) produces respiratory tract hypersensitivity in guinea pigs. Toxicol Appl Pharmacol 1981; 58:221–230.

73. Sugaware Y, Okamoto Y, Sawahata T, Kanaka K. Skin reactivity in guinea pigs sensitized with 2,4-toluene diisocyanate. Int Arch Allergy Immunol 1993; 100:190–196.

74. Mapp CE, Lapa e Silva JR, Lucchini RE, Chitano P, Rado V, Saetta M, Pretolani M, Karol MH, Maestrelli P, Fabbri LM. Inflammatory events in the blood and airways of guinea pigs immunized to toluene diisocyanate. Am J Respir Crit Care Med 1996; 154:201–208.

75. Nimi A, Amitani R, Yamada K, Tanaka K, Kuze F. Late respiratory response and associated eosinophilic inflammation induced by repeated exposure to toluene diisocyanate in guinea pigs. J Allergy Clin Immunol 1996; 97:1308–1319.

76. Mapp CE, Lucchini RE, Miotto D, Chitano P, Jovine L, Saetta M, Maestrelli P, Springall DR, Polak J, Fabbri LM. Immunization and challenge with toluene diisocyanate decrease tachykinins and calcitonin gene-related peptide immunoreactivity in guinea pig central airways. Am J Respir Crit Care Med 1998; 158:263–269.

77. Marek W, Mensing T, Riedel F, Viso N, Barczynski B, Baur X. Hexamethylene diisocyanate induction of transient airway hyperresponsiveness in guinea pigs. Respiration 1997; 64:35–44.

78. Lastbom L, Skarping G, Moldeus P, Ryrfeldt A. Hexamethylene diisocyanate (HDI) induced lung impairment: studies in isolated perfused and ventilated guinea pig lungs. Pharmacol Toxicol 1997; 81:85–89.

79. Brondeau MT, Bana M, Simon P, Bonnet P, Ceaurriz J. Decrease in the rat bronchial acetylcholinesterase activity after toluene diisocyanate inhalation. J Appl Toxicol 1990; 10: 423–427.

80. Marek W, Potthast J, Marczynski B, Baur X. Toluene diisocyanate induction if airway hyperresponsiveness at the threshold limit value (19 ppb) in rabbits. Lung 1995; 173:333–346.

81. Scheerens H, Bucklet TL, Davidse EM, Garseen J, Nijkamp FP. The involvement of sensory neuropeptides in toluene diisocyanate induced tracheal hyperreactivity in the mouse. Am J Respir Crit Care Med 1996; 154:858–865.

82. Scheerens H, Buckley TL, Muis T, Vanlovern H, Nijkamp FP. The involvement of sensory neuropeptides in toluene diisocyanate induced tracheal hyperreactivity in the mouse airways. Br J Pharmacol 1996; 119:1665–1671.

83. Dearman RJ, Basketter DA, Kimber I. Characterization of chemical allergens as a function of divergent cytokine secretion profiles induced in mice. Toxicol Appl Pharmacol 1996; 138: 308–316.

84. Karol MH, Kramark JA. Phenyl isocyanate is a potent chemical sensitizer. Toxicol Lett 1996; 89:139–146.

85. Dearman RJ, Basketter DA, Kimber I. Characterization of chemical allergens as a function of divergent cytokine secretion profiles induced in mice. Toxicol Appl Pharmacol 1996; 138: 308–316.

86. Huffman LJ, Judy DJ, Frazer D, Shapiro RE, Castranova V, Billie M, Dedhia HV. Inhalation of toluene diisocyanate is associated with increased production of nitric oxide by rat bronchoalveolar lavage cells. Toxicol Appl Pharmacol 1997; 145:61–67.

87. Borm PJ, Bast A, Zuiderveld OP. In vitro effect of toluene diisocyanate on beta adrenergic and muscarinic receptor function in lung tissue of the rat. Br J Ind Med 1989; 46:56–59.

88. Mapp CE, Chitano P, Fabbri LM, Patacchini R, Santicioli P, Geppetti P, Maggi CA. Evidence that toluene diisocyanate activates the efferent function of capsaicin-sensitive primary afferents. Eur J Pharmacol 1990; 180:113–118.

89. Mapp CE, Graf PD, Boniotti A, Nadel JA. Toluene diisocyanate contracts guinea pig bronchial smooth muscle by activation of capsaicin-sensitive sensory nerves. J Pharmacol Exp Ther 1991; 256:1082–1085.

90. Chitano P, Di Blasi P, Lucchini RE, Calabro F, Saetta M, Maestrelli P, Fabbri LM, Mapp CE, The effects of toluene diisocyanate and of capsaicin on human bronchial smooth muscle in vitro. Eur J Pharmacol Environ Toxicol Pharmacol Section 1994; 270:167–173.

91. Sheppard D, Scypinski L. A tachykinin receptor antagonist inhibits and an inhibitor of tachykinin metabolism potentiates toluene diisocyanate-induced airway hyperresponsiveness in guinea pigs. Am Rev Respir Dis 1988; 138:547–551.

92. Sheppard D, Thompson JE, Scypinski L, Dusser D, Nadel JA, Borson DB. Toluene diisocyanate increases airway responsiveness to substance P and decreases airway neutral endopeptidase. J Clin Invest 1988; 81:1111–1115.

93. Mapp CE, Chitano P, Fabbri LM, Patacchini R, Maggi CA. Pharmacological modulation of the contractile response to toluene diisocyanate in the rat urinary bladder. Br J Pharmacol 1990; 100:886–888.

94. Mapp CE, Boniotti A, Papi A, Chitano P, Saetta M, Di Stefano A, Ciaccia A, Fabbri LM. The effect of phosphoramidon and epithelium removal on toluene diisocyanate-induced contractions in guinea pig bronchi. Eur Respir J 1992; 5:331–333.

95. Mapp CE, Boniotti A, Masiero M, Plebani M, Burlina A, Papi A, Maestrelli P, Saetta M, Ciaccia A, Fabbri LM. Toluene diisocyanate-stimulated release of arachidonic acid metabolites in the organ bath of isolated guinea-pig airways. Eur J Pharmacol Environ Toxicol Pharmacol Section 1993; 248:277–280.

96. Marek W, Potthast JJW, Marczynski B, Baur X. Role of substance P and neurokinin A in toluene diisocyanate-induced increased airway responsiveness in rabbits. Lung 1996; 174: 83–97.

97. Mapp CE, Jovine L, Lucchini RE, De Marzo N, Miotto D, Saetta M, Maestrelli P, Fabbri LM. Pre-incubation with serum changes the effect of toluene diisocyanate (TDI) in guinea pig bronchi: relaxation instead of contraction. Am J Respir Crit Care Med 1997; 155:A483.

98. Mapp CE. Personal observations (unpublished data).

99. Jin R, Day BW, Karol MH. Toluene diisocyanate protein adducts in the bronchoalveolar lavage of guinea pigs exposed to vapors of the chemical. Chem Res Toxicol 1993; 6:906–912.

100. Karol MH, Jin RZ, Lantz RC. Immunohistochemical detection of toluene diisocyanate (TDI) adducts in pulmonary tissue of guinea pigs following inhalation exposure. Inhal Toxicol 1997; 9:63–83.

101. Tarlo SM, Boulet LP, Cartier A, Cockcroft D, Cote J, Hargreave FE, Holness L, Liss G, Malo JL, Chan-Yeung M. Canadian Thoracic Society Guidelines for occupational asthma. Can Respir J 1998; 5:397–410.

102. Ramazzini B. De Morbis Artificum, translated from the Latin text by Wilmer Cave Wright. New York: Hafner, 1964.

103. Pepys J, Pickering CAC, Terry DJ. Asthma due to inhaled chemical agents—tolylene diisocyanate. Clin Allergy 1972; 2:225–236.

104. Carroll KB, Secombe CJP, Pepys J. Asthma due to non-occupational exposure to toluene (tolylene) diisocyanate. Clin Allergy 1976; 2:99–104.

105. Tse CST, Pesce AJ. Chemical characterization of isocyanate-protein conjugates. Toxicol Appl Pharmacol 1979; 51:39–46.

106. Butcher BT, O'Neil CE, Reed MA, Salvaggio JE. Radioallergosorbent testing with p-tolyl monoisocyanate in toluene diisocyanate workers. Clin Allergy 1983; 13:31–34.

107. Liss GM, Bernstein DI, Moller DR, Gallagher JS, Stephenson RL, Bernstein IL. Pulmonary and immunologic evaluation of foundry workers exposed to methylene diphenyldiisocyanate (MDI). J Allergy Clin Immunol 1988; 82:55–61.

108. Welinder H, Nielsen J, Bensryd I, Skerfving S. IgG antibodies against polyisocyanates in car painters. Clin Allergy 1988; 18:85–93.

109. Sterk PJ, Fabbri LM, Quanjer PH, Cockcroft DW, O'Byrne PM, Anderson SD, Juniper EF, Malo JL. Airway Responsiveness. Standardized challenge testing with pharmacological, physical, and sensitizing stimuli in adults. Eur Respir J 1993; 6(Supplement 16):53–83.

110. Vandenplas O, Malo JL. Inhalation challenges with agents causing occupational asthma. Eur Respir J 1997; 10:2612–2629.

111. Mapp CE, Polato R, Maestrelli P, Hendrick DJ, Fabbri LM. Time course of the increase in airway responsiveness associated with late asthmatic reactions to toluene diisocyanate in sensitized subjects. J Allergy Clin Immunol 1985; 75:568–572.

112. Butcher BT, Hammad YY, Hendrick DJ. Occupational asthma: identification of the agent. In: Gee JBL, ed. Occupational Lung Disease. New York: Churchill Livingston, 1984:111.

113. Hammad YY, Rando RJ, Abdel-Kader H. Considerations in the design and use of human inhalation challenge delivery systems. Folia Allergol Immunol Clin 1985; 32:37–44.

114. Burge PS, O'Brien IM, Harries MG. Peak flow rate records in the diagnosis of occupational asthma due to isocyanates. Thorax 1979; 34:317–323.

115. Fabbri LM, Chiesura-Corona P, Dal Vecchio L, Di Giacomo GR, Zocca E, De Marzo N, Maestrelli P, Mapp CE. Prednisone inhibits the late asthmatic reaction and the associated increase in bronchial responsiveness induced by toluene-diisocyanate in sensitized subjects. Am Rev Respir Dis 1985; 132:1010–1014.

116. Fabbri LM, Giacomo R, Dal Vecchio L, Zocca E, De Marzo N, Maestrelli P, Mapp CE. Prednisone, indomethacin and airway responsiveness in toluene diisocyanate sensitized subjects. Bull Eur Physiopathol Respir 1985; 21:421–426.

117. De Marzo N, Fabbri LM, Crescioli S, Plebani M, Testi R, Mapp CE. Dose response inhibitor effect of inhaled beclomethasone on late asthmatic reactions and increased airway responsiveness to methacholine induced by toluene diisocyanate in sensitized subjects. Pulm Pharmacol 1988; 1:15–20.

118. Tossin L, Leproux GB, DeMarzo N, Crescioli S, Mapp CE, Fabbri LM. Dexamethasone isonicotinate inhibits late asthmatic reactions induced by toluene diisocyanate in sensitized subjects. Ann Allergy 1989; 63:292–296.

119. Mapp CE, Boschetto P, Dal Vecchio L, Crescioli S, De Marzo N, Paleari D, Fabbri LM. Protective effect of antiasthmatic drugs on late asthmatic reaction and increase responsiveness to methacholine induced by toluene diisocyanate in sensitized subjects. Am Rev Respir Dis 1987; 136:1403–1407.

120. Moscato G, Gherson G, Dellabiaca, et al. Salbutanol plus beclomethasone inhibits early and late asthmatic reactions to toluene diisocyanate (TDI) whereas salbutamol alone inhibits neither. Eur Respir J 1989; 2(Suppl 5):398 (abstract).

121. Tossin L, DeMarzo N, Crescioli S, Mapp CE, Fabbri LM. Ketotifen does not inhibit asthmatic reactions induced by toluene diisocyanate in sensitized subjects. Clin Experim Allergy 1989; 19:177–182.

122. Sheffer AL (ed.). Global strategy for asthma management and prevention. NIHLBI/WHO Workshop Report. National Institute of Health, 1995, Pub. 95-3659.

123. National Heart, Lung and Blood Institute, National Asthma Education and Prevention Program. Expert Panel Report 2: Guidelines for the Diagnosis and Management of Asthma, National Institutes of Health, pub. No. 97-4051 Bethesda, MD, 1997.

26
Acid Anhydrides

C. Raymond Zeiss
*Northwestern University Medical School and VA Chicago Health Care System/
Lakeside Division, Chicago, Illinois*

Roy Patterson
Northwestern University Medical School, Chicago, Illinois

Katherine M. Venables
*Imperial College School of Medicine at the National Heart and Lung Institute,
London, England*

OVERVIEW

The acid anhydrides form a family of low-molecular-weight reactive chemicals. The chemical structures of the major anhydrides are shown in Figure 1. They are capable of both irritating and sensitizing the respiratory tract; the health effects reported are summarized in Table 1. They are of major interest because a spectrum of immunologically mediated lung disease caused by acid anhydrides, together with associated well-defined immunological changes, has been extensively studied. Research has been carried out on affected patients, on exposed populations, and in animal models by centers in several countries worldwide; reviews have been published previously (1–6).

USES

These reactive organic chemicals have had industrial uses for over 50 years. Production and trade are international (6). For example, world production of trimellitic anhydride (TMA) is currently confined to one site in the United States with an annual production capacity of about 22,500 tons, used in the United States and also exported. U.K. industry manufactures phthalic anhydride (PA) in two sites with an annual capacity of about 85,000 tons, around half exported; maleic anhydride (MA) is imported to the United Kingdom from countries including France, Germany, and Italy. This pattern of trade in PA and MA is probably repeated in other industrialized countries.

Acid anhydrides are versatile chemicals with major uses as intermediates in the manufacture of plasticizers, of alkyd, epoxy, and polyester resins, and in a variety of processes making, for example, dyes, insecticides, pharmaceuticals, lubricating oil additives, and paper size (6). Resins, in turn, are used in paints, varnishes, reinforced plastics, surface coatings, adhesives, casting, encapsulation, sealants, and powder coatings. Differ-

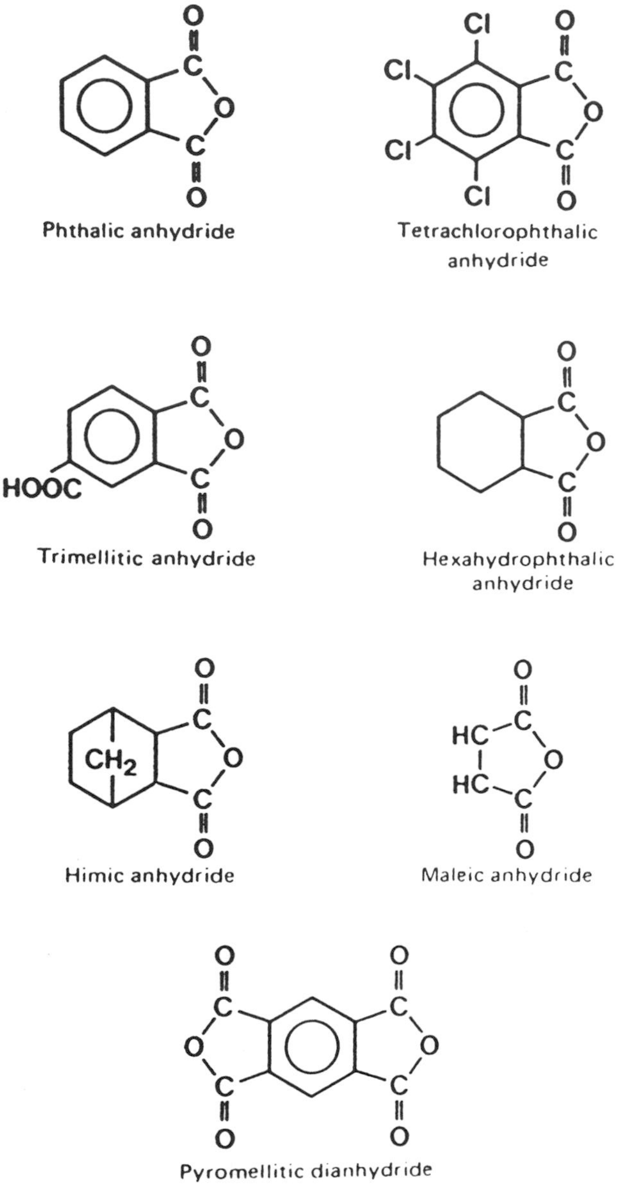

Figure 1 Chemical structures of some industrially important acid anhydrides. (From Ref. 2.)

ent acid anhydrides confer different properties. For example, trimellitates withstand high temperatures, are flexible at low temperature, and poorly soluble in water, so they have advantages as plasticizers in wire coatings compared to the corresponding phthalate esters. It has been estimated that 170,000 workers are exposed to acid anhydrides in the United States alone (7,8). A more recent review from the United Kingdom (6) provides evidence that it can be difficult to assess the size of an exposed workforce; for example, of several thousand employed at sites that handle PA, about 750 are likely to be exposed on a regular basis and about 1000 on an occasional basis. In large sites, PA may be handled in molten

Table 1 Health Effects of Acid Anhydrides

Attributed to direct toxicity:
   Skin irritation, burns, vesicles
   Conjunctivitis, keratitis, corneal burns and ulcers
   Rhinitis, pharyngitis
   Epistaxis
   Cough
   Dyspnea, wheezing
   Pulmonary congestion
   Hemoptysis
   Bronchitis, emphysema
   Transient increase in airway resistance
   Dyspepsia, nausea, vomiting, anorexia, weight loss
   Anemia, reticulocytosis
   Fever, chills, malaise, weakness, headache, dizziness
Attributed to hypersensitivity:
   Asthma, rhinitis, conjunctivitis
   Urticaria
   Possible contact dermatitis
   Fever, chills, malaise, anorexia, weight loss, myalgia
   Hemoptysis/hemolysis

Source: From Ref. 2.

form, limiting the numbers exposed, and TMA may be handled with semiautomatic bag-handling and disposal equipment by workers wearing either air-fed hoods or high-efficiency, full-face respirators.

EXPOSURE, UPTAKE, AND TOXICOKINETICS

Exposure

Levels of exposure to acid anhydrides have rarely been studied systematically and most data are from large firms with the resources to control and measure exposure. Air concentrations of acid anhydrides in small firms are likely to be much higher. van Tongeren et al. (9) reviewed the literature for PA, TMA, and MA. Arithmetic mean values ranging from less than 0.001 mg/m^3 for TMA (10) to 13 mg/m^3 for PA (11) had been reported. However, much of the exposure data were difficult to interpret because too little information was provided on air-sampling methodology. They also reported an exposure survey in the United Kingdom showing that, in the large factories studied, exposure to PA, TMA, and MA was low on average, though this concealed high short-term exposures during specific tasks. For example, full-shift personal exposures for TMA in four factories were in the range 0.0004–0.21 mg/m^3 but charging the reactors to make alkyd resin led to 15-min levels in the range 0.15–20 mg/m^3. Air-fed hoods were worn during this activity, however, so actual personal exposure should have been negligible. Several different sampling devices have been used in exposure studies, and several methods for determining acid anhydrides in air. Jonsson et al. have summarized the methodology and comment that there is no obvious choice of one method for all purposes (12).

Occupational Exposure Limits

Several countries have included one or more acid anhydrides on their lists of occupational exposure standards. The long-term exposure limit (8-hr time-weighted average reference period) recommendation for PA in the United Kingdom, for example, is 4 mg/m^3 and the short-term exposure limit (15-min reference period) is 12 mg/m^3 (6). Equivalent recommendations for TMA are 0.04 and 0.12, and for MA, 1 and 3 mg/m^3. These figures vary somewhat between countries and over time as knowledge of current exposure levels and health effects develops and changes in technology alter cost-benefit assessments.

Urinary Excretion and Biological Monitoring

Very little is known about the absorption, distribution, metabolism, and elimination of acid anhydrides. Workers exposed to PA absorb it, presumably mainly by inhalation, and some is excreted in the urine as phthalic acid (13). The concentration of phthalic acid in the urine increased preshift to postshift and the half-life was about 14 hr. The urine of unexposed control subjects had a low concentration of phthalic acid, presumably from phthalate plasticizers in food, cosmetics, and plastics. Similarly, a tool for biological monitoring for hexahydrophthalic anhydride (HHPA) exposure was reported by quantifying HHP acid in urine, which increased rapidly with exposure and fell rapidly at the end of exposure (14). There was a close correlation between time-weighted average levels of HHPA in air and HHP acid in urine samples adjusted for creatinine.

Conjugation with Proteins

Acid anhydrides have repeatedly been shown to form conjugates in vitro with a range of human proteins. This property has long been exploited by protein chemists, for example, Habeeb et al. in 1958 (15) and Palacian et al. in 1990 (16). Acid anhydrides bind mainly to lysine and the binding can be made reversible by manipulating experimental conditions. Methyltetrahydrophthalic anhydride (MTHPA) has been shown to form adducts with lysine in collagen in guinea pig lung tissue (17). Workers exposed to HHPA and/or to methylhexahydrophthalic anhydride (MHHPA) were shown to form hemoglobin adducts whose concentration correlated well with urinary HHP acid (18).

ADVERSE EFFECTS

The toxic effects of acid anhydride exposure, both direct toxicity and hypersensitivity, were noted in classical descriptions in the 1930s. The Chief Inspector of Factories and Workshops in the United Kingdom in his report for 1937 (19) described direct toxicity in eight men with mucosal irritation and a blistering skin rash after working with MA, three requiring sick leave for up to 40 days. The first description of a hypersensitivity response was Kern's (20) case report in 1939 of an American paint chemist exposed to PA dust from the factory next to his laboratory.

Kern's report (20) was noted in the laboratory of the pioneer of hapten immunology, Karl Landsteiner, by then working in the United States. Landsteiner and Jacobs (21) had developed a method in 1935 for sensitizing guinea pigs by repeated intracutaneous injection. PA, MA, citraconic anhydride, and other acid anhydrides were used successfully, sensitized animals showing immediate wheal-and-flare responses on skin testing and also late skin responses at 6–8 hr (22). Some guinea pigs developed generalized urticaria after scratch tests, occasionally with cough and shivering (23). Further experiments showed that sensitivity could be transferred to naïve animals by a heat-labile factor in serum, that there was cross-reactivity between acid anhydrides but not with other chemicals, and that the use of protein conjugates made these animal models more sensitive (24–26).

Direct Toxicity

Between the 1930s and 1970s, most reports of toxicity by acid anhydrides appear to be of direct mucosal or skin irritation. A recent review comments that PA, TMA, and MA are severe eye irritants in animal studies (6). In a toxicological study in 1946 of damage to the rabbit eye, only two of 180 chemicals scored 10 out of 10 in the authors' scale, MA and sodium hydroxide (27). Ten years later, Tanaka (28) reported that almost three-quarters of 265 printers exposed to MA reported eye pain, lacrimation, and blurring of vision. Almost half of a group of Swedish workers exposed to PA dust at about 6 mg/m^3 had symptoms suggestive of conjunctivitis (29). One case of reactive airways dysfunction syndrome (RADS) has been reported in a tanker driver accidentally exposed to a high concentration of gaseous PA (30). After acute mucosal symptoms she then developed symptoms of asthma and measurable bronchial hyperresponsiveness to histamine, which slowly resolved over 3.5 years.

Potentially even more serious symptoms of epistaxis, hemoptysis, and "pulmonary congestion" in PA-exposed workers were frequently reported in the 1940s and 1950s (2), a time when occupational exposures must have been high in the emerging postwar organic chemical and plastics industries. The reports are not sufficiently detailed to derive exposure-response relationships or to distinguish between acid anhydrides. More recently, TMA at 1.7–2.6 mg/m^3 (31,32) has caused irritant and allergic symptoms in exposed workers.

The acute inhalation toxicity of acid anhydrides in animals has not been extensively studied. A TMA-acetone aerosol showed some features of a pulmonary irritant in a study of mice exposed once for 30 min to concentrations ranging from 2 to 150 mg/m^3 (33) but there were no acute histopathological lesions or features of sensory irritation. This is in marked contrast to animal studies with multiple exposures that result in pulmonary lesions in association with immunological evidence of sensitization (see below).

Hypersensitivity

Patterson and co-workers have outlined the immunological considerations related to the reaction of antibody classes with these reactive chemicals that combine with self-proteins (4,5). The immunological considerations can be considered within the conceptual framework of the Gell and Coombs classification of four types of possible immunological injury, as illustrated for TMA in Table 2 (34).

Type I, or immediate hypersensitivity, is mediated by IgE antibody, which is fixed to tissue mast cells and basophils with the combining sites of the IgE antibody directed against specific determinants generated by the reactive anhydride and a self-protein. Classically, the crosslinking of IgE molecules by the antigen results in release of mediators and clinical symptoms. A second pathway that could lead to mast cell mediator release received experimental support in a study in 1984 (35). Here the anhydride, TMA, reacts with IgE on the mast cell surface, and a second antibody (IgG) is directed against the TMA-modified IgE, which bridges adjacent IgE molecules with subsequent mediator release. This is similar to the histamine release induced by anti-IgE (36). In addition, the

Table 2 Diseases Caused by TMA Based Upon Gell and Coombs Classification

| Type | Terminology | Mechanism | TMA reactions | |
			In vitro or in vivo tests	Diseases
I	Anaphylactic, immediate-type, IgE antibody-mediated	IgE antibody-sensitized mast cells react with TM-protein and bioactive mediators are released	Immediate-type skin test; in vitro histamine release	Asthma, rhinitis, conjunctivitis
II	Cytotoxic	Antibody against hapten cell results in cell damage or destruction	Antibodies against TM-E lyse cells in the presence of complement	Anemia or pulmonary disease anemia syndrome? Other?
III	Toxic antigen-antibody complex reaction	Immune complexes fix complement, attract poly-morphonuclear leukocytes, which results in tissue damage	Experimental skin reaction	Probable cause of LRSS associated with increase in total antibody and IgG and IgA antibodies against TM proteins
IV	Lymphocyte-mediated, delayed, tuberculin-type	Sensitized T lymphocytes stimulated by antigen, resulting in tissue damage	In vitro lymphocyte transformation	Uncertain; possible component of LRSS and pulmonary disease anemia syndrome

Source: From Ref. 4.

reactive anhydride could combine in a third pathway with the mast cell or basophil Fc receptor proteins for IgE. An antibody directed against the IgE receptor, modified by the anhydride, could result in the apposition of IgE receptors and mediator release (36). A fourth hypothetical pathway having some experimental support involves bifunctional, reactive anhydrides, such as pyromellitic dianhydride (PMDA), that would crosslink two or three IgE molecules in the fluid adjacent to a mast cell, creating dimers and trimers of IgE. This configuration of IgE has been shown to be a potent stimulus for histamine release from human basophils (37).

In this model, the type II, or cytotoxic, reaction is assumed to occur when the reactive anhydride combines with proteins on a tissue cell surface, and antibody, directed against that modified cell surface, results in cytotoxic injury, mediated by complement activation and influx of inflammatory cells.

In producing type III, or immune complex injury, the reactive chemical could combine with respiratory tract immunoglobulin such as IgA, and IgG antibody could be directed against the chemically modified IgA resulting in immune complex formation. TMA has been shown to react with IgA and IgG proteins, with the demonstration of IgG and IgA antibody to these modified human immunoglobulins (38).

Type IV immunological injury could hypothetically result when reactive chemicals combine with a variety of self-proteins to induce a TH1 lymphocyte response with the expansion of T-cell clones that could participate in a delayed hypersensitivity reaction.

Fundamental to these immunological considerations is the way in which the reactive chemical can modify self-proteins. Two pathways have been demonstrated experimentally. First, the anhydride can act as a hapten, with antibody recognizing the hapten as foreign (39,40). Second, the reactive anhydride can combine with self-proteins to generate new, carrier-dependent antigenic determinants with antibody-combining sites being directed against a conformational change in the self-proteins (41). It is characteristic of a new antigenic determinant (NAD) that the simple chemical is necessary, but not sufficient, to form the complete determinant.

ANIMAL MODELS

Several animal models have been used to study the effects of the acid anhydrides. Guinea pigs have some advantages because their airway responses to irritant and allergen challenge have been well documented. On the other hand, their anaphylactic antibodies are mainly IgG1, not IgE as in the human. The rat, however, has IgE and IgG anaphylactic antibodies. Nonhuman primates are the closest species to humans but are studied only rarely because of the expense of maintaining them and because of their conservation importance. Some of the significant studies are discussed below.

Guinea Pig

The early work on guinea pigs by Landsteiner's group (21–26) showed that a range of acid anhydrides can induce sensitization experimentally. This has been examined in detail by large studies in Sweden of structure-activity relationships in the experimental sensitization of guinea pigs (42,43) and rats (44). The studies used up to 14 different acid anhydrides and measured serum antibodies in guinea pigs and rats, together with measures of response to airway provocation in the guinea pigs. They concluded that there is considerable variation in the sensitizing potential of different acid anhydrides and that the ring structure and the positions of double bonds and of methyl groups are important. This work has important implications not only for understanding the response to acid anhydrides, but also for making recommendations for primary prevention of disease by substituting one chemical by another in industrial processes.

The guinea pig model has been used to explore the pathogenesis of immediate hypersensitivity to anhydrides induced by the intradermal injection of the anhydride in an oil vehicle. Studies (45,46) with PA and TMA indicated that the dose and route of anhydride used for sensitization might be critical for inducing an immediate airway response in this species. Studies of TMA-induced airway responses demonstrated that IgG1 antibody levels were significantly correlated with the extravasation of Evans blue dye in the airway of animals challenged via the airway with TMA linked to guinea pig serum albumin (GPSA) and blockage of the airway response by antihistamine and Evans blue dye extravasation by a leukotriene receptor antagonist (47–49). An increase in inducible nitric oxide synthase in the lung and bronchial tissues was demonstrated at 15–17 hr post challenge to TMA-GPSA (50). Zhao et al. (51) demonstrated that guinea pigs sensitized to MTHPA or HHPA developed marked immediate airway responses and hypoxemia on inhalation or intravenous challenge with the respective GPSA-conjugated anhydride, similarly to TMA. As with TMA, these airway responses correlated with serum levels of IgG1, suggesting that the antibody may mediate the airway response (44).

Rat

In the rat, inhalation of repeated doses of TMA (see below) leads to lung pathology characterized by intense interstitial inflammation and pulmonary hemorrhage. The development of pulmonary hemorrhagic foci in this model was directly related to the TMA inhalation exposure concentration. There was healing of lung lesions 2 weeks after exposure and a marked return of lung lesions only 18 hr after a subsequent inhalation reexposure. The underlying lung pathology was interstitial pneumonitis with pulmonary hemorrhage as the end result of marked interstitial inflammation (52). Neither lung lesions nor antibody responses were seen with trimellitic acid inhalation at identical doses. A major technical breakthrough in these studies was the ability to deliver accurately, inhalation doses of TMA powder from 10 to 500 $\mu g/m^3$ to rats in large inhalation chambers without disturbing the animals (53).

The time course of lung injury and immune response in this model has been explored (54). Sprague-Dawley rats inhaled micronized TMA powder, 100 $\mu g/m^3$, 6 hr a day, for 2, 6, or 10 days and were sacrificed. At each time period, total IgG, IgA, and IgM antibody to TMA-rat serum albumin (TMA-RSA) were measured by radiolabeled antigen binding and enzyme-linked immunosorbent assay (ELISA) in serum and bronchoalveolar lavage fluid (BAL). Hemorrhagic lung foci, weight, and displacement volume were determined and lungs were examined by light and electron microscopy. There was no apparent lung injury or antibody response at 2 days. There was minimal lung injury at 6 days with low levels of antibody in BAL and serum. At 10 days, there was a marked increase in hemorrhagic foci, lung weight, and volume, and in BAL and serum antibody levels, suggesting that sensitization had taken place. BAL antibody levels at 6 and 10 days had higher correlations with measures of lung injury than serum levels. Antibody levels in BAL were always higher than the corresponding serum level (55). There was minimal ultrastructural change at 6 days but by day 10, there was marked intra-alveolar hemorrhage, macrophage infiltration, and evidence of endothelial and epithelial cell injury.

The Sprague-Dawley rat can be sensitized with short-term (high-dose) TMA inhalation on day 1, 5, and 10. This may mimic short-term high-exposure peaks experienced by workers in some industries. These sensitized animals developed significant lung pathology on TMA rechallenge, which was highly correlated with all classes of antibody to TMA-RSA (Fig. 2) (56). Using this model, investigators have been able to passively transfer (using high-titer serum) to naïve rats the ability to develop lung lesions after one acute, nontoxic TMA inhalation exposure (100 $\mu g/m^3$ for 6 hr) and completely suppress lung lesions and the antibody response by pretreatment of the animals with cyclophosphamide (57), thus confirming the immunological basis for the lung injury.

Swedish workers have established a model of IgE-mediated disease in the Brown Norway (BN) rat sensitized by intradermal injections of TMA in oil resulting in an IgE and IgG response that could be attenuated with glucocorticoid and cyclosporin A (58). Sensitization with TMA resulted in the accumulation of eosinophils in the bronchial wall of animals challenged with aerosolized TMA-RSA and in the skin of animals challenged intradermally with TMA (59). The BN rat has been used in the United Kingdom to explore

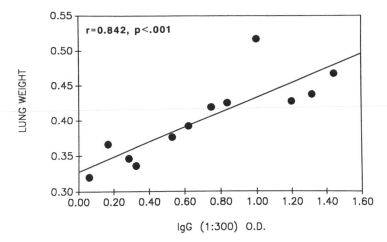

Figure 2 Correlation of IgG serum antibody to TMA-RSA as measured by ELISA and lung injury expressed as fractional lung weight in sensitized rats re-exposed to TMA by inhalation. (From Ref. 56.)

the differential response of these animals to a contact sensitizer oxazolone and TMA (60). Only TMA elicited an IgE response with mast cell sensitization and an IL-4/IL-5 mRNA increase in lymph node lymphocytes.

Rhesus Monkey

In 1980, Patterson et al. (61) demonstrated that intrabronchial TMA administration led to both a systemic and pulmonary immune response. They used TMA-haptenized erythrocytes to demonstrate a systemic IgG, IgA, and IgM response. The local pulmonary immune response was that of IgM and IgA. In addition, a lymphocyte response to TMA-HSA was demonstrated but no IgE response. This group (62) later showed that passive transfer of human IgE to TMA to the rhesus monkey airway led to the development of airway reactivity to inhaled TMA-HSA 24 hr after passive transfer. This demonstrated the importance of IgE antibody for the pathogenesis of airway responses to TMA challenge. In addition, passive transfer to rhesus monkey skin of human sera containing IgE antibodies to TMA has been used to study cross-reactivity to other anhydrides. Using this in vivo assay cross-reactivity was detected that was not apparent with immunoassay (63).

Other Animals

Liu et al. (64) sensitized mice to TMA by intraperitoneal injection and demonstrated both IgE and IgG antibodies. They also showed that giving TMA coupled to an amino acid copolymer suppressed the secondary IgE and IgG responses and proposed that this approach might be useful therapy for sensitized workers. Their work was later confirmed by Wei et al. (65). Dogs have been sensitized by intrabronchial TMA, developing a systemic IgG, IgA, and IgM response to TMA and hemorrhagic pneumonitis; rabbits were less responsive (66).

CLINICAL MANIFESTATIONS OF ACID ANHYDRIDE HYPERSENSITIVITY

The responses in animals described above have parallels in the clinical syndromes reported in patients exposed to acid anhydrides. A spectrum of lung disease has been described in TMA workers that fitted the conceptual framework described by Gell and Coombs (Table 2). Case descriptions from the 1930s to 1970s suggested that other acid anhydrides were capable of causing this spectrum of reactions and the approach of synthesizing clinical and toxicological research, so productive for TMA, is increasingly being applied to other acid anhydrides.

Asthma and Related Conditions

All acid anhydrides appear capable of causing classic asthma, with or without rhinitis, conjunctivitis, and/or urticaria. There is a latent period of exposure of weeks to years before the onset of symptoms; once the subject is sensitized, symptoms occur with exposure, sometimes immediately or after the work shift, often waking the patient at night or in the early morning. Symptoms improve at weekends or on vacation but it may take several days before a significant improvement is noted.

The first case report, Kern's in 1939 (20), demonstrated what we now know as specific IgE; the patient had a positive prick test and Prausnitz-Kustner test. In 1976, specific IgE antibody to PA-HSA was shown by modern methods for the first time by Maccia and colleagues (67). Since then IgE and IgG antibodies have been detected against a number of acid anhydrides. Bernstein and colleagues showed that IgE antibody can be directed against the phthalyl group acting as a hapten or against new antigenic determinants (NADs) that arise when PA combines with human serum albumin (68). In 1993, Drexler et al. demonstrated that PA in acetonic solution elicited positive prick skin tests in workers with serum IgE by RAST to PA-HSA (69). Studies in workers exposed to other acid anhydrides using a variety of hapten-modified human protein conjugates have also shown that IgE antibody is directed not only against hapten, but also against NADs.

Inhalation Challenge Tests

The first inhalation tests with acid anhydrides carried out by modern standards in a chamber and with lung function monitored for 24 hr were performed by Pepys's group in the United Kingdom in 1977 (70). They reported three cases of PA asthma and the first case of TMA asthma and demonstrated the late asthmatic response, which had previously been suggested in case histories, for example by Kern (20) and by Maccia et al. (67). They also noted a lack of in vivo cross-reactivity between PA and TMA in a patient with PA asthma who showed no response to TMA.

Inhalation challenge tests in patients with acid-anhydride-induced asthma usually result in dual asthmatic responses with an immediate asthmatic response within minutes and a late response peaking at approximately 4–12 hr after exposure (2). There have been reports of isolated late asthmatic responses in TCPA asthma (71,72) and one of an isolated immediate response to TMA (73). However, the precise response pattern seen in exposure chamber studies is unlikely to be a fixed pattern and may depend on exposure and patient characteristics. Sensitized patients may respond to very low exposures, for example one breath of PA or TMA vapor (70). Few studies have had a sufficiently large number of dose steps to study dose-response relationships for the provoked airway response, but one that did showed that the size of immediate and late asthmatic responses to TCPA dust increased with increasing challenge exposure (74). In common with other causes of asthma, late asthmatic responses provoked by acid anhydrides, but not isolated immediate responses, have been shown to increase nonspecific bronchial responsiveness (73). Illustrations of inhalation challenge responses are shown in Figure 3.

Related Conditions

Few studies have focused on rhinitis but nasal challenge with HHPA was reported by Nielsen et al. to correlate with serum IgE antibody to HHPA-HSA and challenged sensitized subjects had nasal symptoms, increased nasal lavage levels of tryptase, albumin, eosinophils, and neutrophils (75). The same group has reported similar findings for MTHPA (76). Contact urticaria was mentioned in older anecdotal case reports and two cases recently described in detail (77). The patients worked with MTHPA and MHHPA and after 2 months noted urticarial lesions and itching on exposed skin. Later, they developed eye, nose, and chest symptoms. Both had positive skin prick tests and a positive RAST to MTHPA-HSA and MHHPA-HSA.

Genetic Background

Some authors have reported an association between acid-anhydride-induced asthma and atopy and others have not. The developing research field of the genetics of asthma and

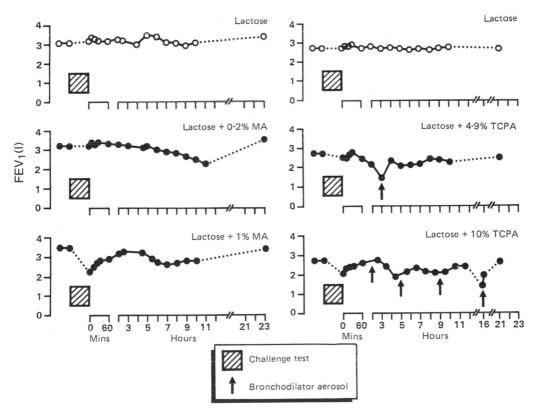

Figure 3 Inhalation challenge test responses in occupational asthma caused by acid anhydrides. Dust challenge tests were carried out with the relevant acid anhydride diluted in lactose powder. (From Refs. 2, 72, and 73.)

allergy may give interesting findings. An association between the HLA antigen DR3 and IgE-mediated sensitization by acid anhydrides has been reported by Young et al. (78). The association was driven by those sensitized to TMA with eight of 11 workers with IgE to TMA-HSA positive for HLA DR3 and only two of 14 referents positive, giving an odds ratio of 16. This suggests the possibility of important structure-activity differences in humans, as in animals (42–44).

Prognosis

The acid anhydrides are the only group of asthmagenic chemicals where it has been possible to follow both antibody decay and changes in symptoms over time after cessation of exposure. In a group of patients with TCPA asthma, symptoms improved but did not completely remit, similarly to findings in follow-up studies in other causes of occupational asthma (79). IgE to TCPA-HSA also fell, with a half-life of 1 year at 5 years (79) and longer at 12 years (80). This study also showed that skin prick test responses fell over time (81). Figure 4 shows antibody decay over time.

The predictable decay of specific antibody with cessation of exposure and rise after reexposure, for example in challenge tests, suggests that specific antibodies are a good biomarker of prevailing exposure in industry. Grammer et al. have reported the outcome of TMA workers in a large industrial setting, with TMA-induced immunological lung

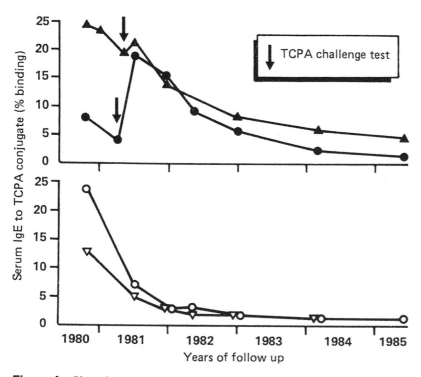

Figure 4 Slow decay over time in IgE antibody levels to TCPA-HSA in patients with occupational asthma after complete cessation of exposure. Two patients in the top panel had low exposures during inhalation challenge tests with TCPA and IgE levels rose afterward, then fell again, suggesting that IgE antibody has a role in biological monitoring. (From Refs. 2 and 79.)

disease, removed from the direct manufacture or packaging of TMA to other areas of the complex. Most workers did well, with an abatement of symptoms and a fall in IgG and IgE serum antibody level to TMA-HSA, but only five of 12 with the asthma/rhinitis syndrome improved. Elevated IgE antibody level against TMA-HSA was a marker for those with asthma/rhinitis that did not improve (82). Elsewhere, environmental control procedures have been shown to decrease the number of workers sensitized to TMA in a plant mixing TMA with resins to make coating material (83).

Late Respiratory Systemic Syndrome

A second immunological syndrome has been reported in TMA workers, the late respiratory systemic syndrome (LRSS), or "TMA flu" as named by the workers (31). Possibly, it may be similar to the febrile symptoms noted in the early literature in asthma induced by acid anhydrides (2). It is characterized by cough, occasional wheezing dyspnea, mucus production, and systemic symptoms of malaise, chills, myalgias, and arthralgias occurring 4–12 hr after TMA inhalation exposure. The authors reporting the syndrome noted that it symptomatically resembled hypersensitivity pneumonitis and requires a latent period following exposure before the onset of symptoms. But, in contrast to hypersensitivity pneumonitis, clinical examinations and chest radiographs were normal (31). The syndrome is accompanied by elevated levels of IgG, IgA, and IgM antibody directed against TMA-HSA.

Pulmonary Hemorrhage and Anemia

The early literature, before the development of immunological tests, contained repeated references to hemoptysis or epistaxis in PA workers but without sufficient detail for diagnosis (2). In the 1970s, 12 TMA workers in several plants in Canada and the United States were reported with a potentially fatal pulmonary presentation characterized by hemoptysis, dyspnea, pulmonary infiltrates, restrictive lung disease, and anemia; it has been termed the pulmonary disease–anemia (PDA) syndrome (84–87). Understanding of this syndrome has been greatly aided by animal toxicology, as described above. In particular, work with rats demonstrated that pulmonary hemorrhage occurs on rechallenge and that this can be transferred passively to naive rats and suppressed by cyclophosphamide (57). Without this work, it was possible to suggest that PDA could be a result of direct chemical toxicity rather than immunologically mediated (2).

This illness develops with high-dose TMA fume exposure, which occurs when heated metal surfaces are sprayed with TMA-containing materials. The syndrome requires a latent period of exposure, with a range of clinical severity from mild to severe. High levels of IgG, IgA, and IgM antibody to TMA protein and TMA erythrocytes have been identified in these individuals (88).

In Germany, PDA has been described in a worker exposed to epoxy resin vapor containing PMDA. The worker's serum contained high levels of IgG that on immunoblotting had specificity for a number of PMDA-modified serum proteins (89,90). A syndrome of hemorrhagic rhinitis in workers exposed to heated epoxy resin containing HHPA (91) with high levels of serum IgG and IgE to HHPA-HAS has been reported, which may be an upper airway equivalent to PDA.

Clinical Immunology

Cross-reactivity between acid anhydrides has been noted in animal (43) and human (41,68,92) studies indicating a relationship between antibody binding and the chemical structure of the acid anhydride. The type of protein conjugated to the anhydride also influences the specificity of the antibody response in humans (38,92). The practical implication of this observation is that workers sensitized to one acid anhydride may experience a clinical response if reexposed to a similar acid anhydride. A challenge study in 1977 suggested no cross-reactivity between PA and TMA in one of the patients studied who was allergic to PA and responded only to PA and not TMA (70). In a recent cross-reactivity study (63), serum was transferred from a patient sensitized to TMA to rhesus monkeys and cross-reactivity with PA was detected by passive cutaneous transfer, although it had not in in vitro cross-inhibition studies. Passive transfer to animals may offer a way of doing in vivo experimental work that would be unacceptable in humans. In the meantime, it would be wise to recommend that patients sensitized by one acid anhydride may well respond to others so that patients can either avoid exposure in the future or experience exposure only under medical surveillance.

EPIDEMIOLOGICAL STUDIES

Epidemiology can describe the frequency with which occupational asthma or another health outcome occurs, exposure-response relationships, the role of other risk factors, and the effect of measures to control the problem in industry. The well-described tests for specific antibody against acid anhydrides can be used in population studies, adding a dimension that has not been available in research on other low-molecular-weight causes of asthma, for example diisocyanates or solder fume.

Several cross-sectional studies were reported in the early literature. The first appears to be one of eye symptoms in Japanese printers (28). Of 265, 73% reported eye pain, lacrimation, and blurring of vision. The first to include a test for specific antibody appears to be one of TCPA workers, where the prevalence of detectable specific IgE antibody was 8% in 300 exposed workers making capacitors using a powder epoxy resin (93). The prevalence is influenced both by hiring and firing practices and also by decisions about what is a "significant" level of antibody. This plant had recently retired seven workers with occupational asthma on medical grounds (72) whose inclusion would have increased the prevalence, but on the other hand, a higher laboratory cutoff for detectable specific IgE would have reduced the prevalence. In this and other epidemiological studies, specific IgE presents with a continuous, unimodal, approximately log-normal distribution and decisions on cutoff values are inevitably somewhat arbitrary. However, study of more populations with a high prevalence of specific IgE may show whether two populations can be defined: sensitized and unaffected.

The study of electronics workers exposed to TCPA (93) showed an increasing prevalence of anti-TCPA IgE by plant area with increasing exposure. It also showed a strong association between smoking and specific IgE. Smokers had a significant fivefold increased risk of having specific IgE and there was some, nonsignificant, evidence that also being atopic further increased the risk. This finding of an increased risk in smokers has not been confirmed for other acid anhydrides but has been observed for sensitization by complex platinum salts (94), snow-crabs (95), green coffee beans (96), and ispaghula (96), and the reasons for these differing associations between IgE-mediated sensitization and smoking may be a fruitful field for research.

Surveillance over several years is also informative. Zeiss and co-workers have followed workers involved in the manufacture of TMA at a single site since 1976 (31,32,82,97,98). These studies have been based on a voluntary surveillance program evaluating workers presenting with TMA-related respiratory symptoms. Table 3 illustrates some of the complexities related to the study of anhydride occupational immunological lung disease. This table summarises a 12-year experience in evaluation and classification of workers involved in the manufacture of TMA (97). It is apparent that the development of immunological lung disease to TMA is sporadic and uncommon and many years are needed to obtain a comprehensive picture at any given facility. The latent period prior to the development of symptoms had a wide range from one-half month to 14 years (32). The asthma/rhinitis syndrome was the most common followed by LRSS. Three workers developed isolated late asthma. It is clear that a survey done at this facility in 1981 and 1983 would have given a widely different picture of the incidence of TMA-induced immunological lung disease.

In a cross-sectional study (98) of the entire work force at this facility, 474 employees were surveyed in 1 year related to the presence of TMA immunological lung disease. This study included 153 employees who had joined the previous voluntary surveillance program and 321 who had not. The prevalence of TMA immunological lung disease was 7% in the total population. In the 321 employees who had not previously been surveyed only 1% had a TMA-related immunological syndrome. In addition, the level of total and IgE antibody to TMA-HSA was compared to occupational exposure. There was a marked trend in mean total and IgE antibody levels across five exposure classes. This result allowed the targeting of further environmental control measures to job classifications in the groups with the highest potential TMA exposure.

Follow-up also gives information helpful in evaluating control measures in industry and factors influencing prognosis in individual patients. In a recent survey, of a solenoid

Table 3 Voluntary Clinical Surveillance in One Industrial Site Manufacturing TMA with a Workforce of Almost 500, 1976–1987

Year	Asthma/Rhinitis	LRSS	Both	LA	PD-A	LAMS	Irritant	No Symptoms	Other	Enrolled
1976	2	1	2				5	1	3	14
1977	2	3	1				10	5		21
1978		1					1			2
1979		1					2	2		5
1980	2	1	1				24	3	1	32
1981	6			2	1		15	13		37
1982	1						9	5		15
1983						1	23	11		35
1984							6	4		10
1985							5			5
1986	4						4	2		10
1987				1			9			10
Totals	17	7	4	3	1	1	113	46	4	196

Source: From Ref. 97.

coil manufacturing plant utilizing a TCPA hardener, Liss et al. (99) reported that 15 of 49 workers (31%) had IgE and 19 (39%) had IgG antibodies to TCPA-HSA, with no new cases and a decrease in symptoms with improved ventilation and a reduction in exposure levels to less than 0.1 mg/m^3. In a study of 59 workers exposed to HHPA during a molding operation, only exposure and specific antibody level were associated with an immunological syndrome while atopy, smoking status, age, and race were not predictive (100). In these workers there were no permanent physiological or anatomical sequelae after removal from exposure (101). In a survey of 92 workers exposed to PMDA, PA, MA, and TMA (102,103), 56 reported work-related symptoms but specific IgE in only 15. A follow-up of 23 symptomatic workers showed improvement in symptoms and lung function in a subset whose exposure ceased but no change in those whose exposure continued.

It is clear that irritant and immunologically mediated symptoms coexist in the same workforces and that workers may be sensitized but without symptoms. Wernfors et al. (104), for example, surveyed 118 Swedish workers exposed to PA and found that 18% had symptoms suggestive of occupational asthma. Scratch tests on a sample suggested that only about a quarter had immunologically mediated disease. The authors suggested that short-term high exposure might have caused asthma in some workers. In another example, Drexler et al. reported a survey of 110 workers exposed to both HHPA and MTHPA where 15% were found to have IgE against these anhydrides, but only six (5%) were positive on a workplace inhalation challenge (105). This study also included nasal lavage and challenge; MTHPA-sensitized workers had high levels of tryptase in nasal lavage fluid on initial evaluation compared to nonsensitized controls and were positive on nasal challenge with MTHPA-HSA with airflow obstruction and increased symptoms.

Longitudinal studies of disease incidence can give a clearer picture of exposure-response relationships, the role of other risk factors, and the time course of development of disease but they require major resources for repeated surveys and follow-up of workers who leave employment. Barker and colleagues have carried out a survey in four sites in the United Kingdom, one with exposure only to TMA in cushioned flooring manufacture (106,107). This showed a clear increase in risk of sensitization by TMA and of work-related respiratory symptoms as air concentration of TMA increased.

SUMMARY

Acid anhydrides are a valuable model of occupational lung disease because they provoke a variety of symptomatic and physiological responses as well as a variety of immunological responses. The interrelationships between responses, the risk factors for response, and the outcome after developing a response have been studied in detail in clinical and epidemiological studies and in animal models.

REFERENCES

1. Bernstein IL, Bernstein DI. Respiratory allergy to synthetic resins. Clin Immunol Allergy 1984; 4:83–101.
2. Venables KM. Low molecular weight chemicals, hypersensitivity, and direct toxicity: the acid anhydrides. Br J Ind Med 1989; 46:222–232.
3. Gillner M. Trimellitic anhydride (TMA) a hazard analysis. In: Freig L, ed. The KEMI Report. Stockholm: The Swedish National Chemicals Inspectorate, 1989:1–48.

4. Patterson R, Zeiss CR, Pruzansky JJ. Immunology and immunopathology of trimellitic anhydride pulmonary reactions. J Allergy Clin Immunol 1982; 70:19–23.

5. Zeiss CR. Reactive chemicals in industrial asthma. J Allergy Clin Immunol 1991; 87:775–761.

6. Ridgway P, Morris L, Ogunbiyi AO, Brown RH, Cocker J. Acid Anhydrides: Criteria Document for an Occupational Exposure Limit. London: Health and Safety Executive, HMSO, 1996.

7. OSHA. Occupational Public Health Guideline for Phthalic Anhydride. US Department of Health and Human Services, Public Health Service, Centers for Disease Control and US Department of Labor, 1978:1–5.

8. Documentation of the Threshold Limit Values and Biological Exposure Indices, 5th ed. Cincinnati: American Conference of Governmental Industrial Hygienists, 1986:353, 487, 606.

9. van Tongeren MJA, Barker RD, Gardiner K, Harris JM, Venables KM, Newman Taylor AJ, Harrington JM. Exposure to acid anhydrides in three resin and one cushioned flooring manufacturing plants. Ann Occup Hyg 1995; 39:559–571.

10. Boxer MB, Grammer LC, Karris KE, Roach DE, Patterson R. Six-year clinical and immunologic follow-up of workers exposed to trimellitic anhydride. J Allergy Clin Immunol 1987; 80:147–152.

11. Nielsen J. Airways effects in workers exposed to organic acid anhydrides. Doctoral dissertation, Lund University, Sweden, 1992.

12. Jonsson BAG, Welinder H, Pfaffli P. Determination of cyclic organic acid anhydrides in air using gas chromatography. Part 1. A review. Analyst 1996; 121:1279–1284.

13. Pfaffli P. Phthalic acid excretion as an indicator of exposure to phthalic anhydride in the work atmosphere. Int Arch Occup Environ Health 1986; 58:209–216.

14. Jonsson BA, Welinder H, Hansson C, Stahlbom B. Occupational exposure to hexahydrophthaic anhydride: air analysis, percutaneous absorption, and biological monitoring. Int Arch Occup Environ Health 1993; 65:43–47.

15. Habeeb AFSA, Cassidy HG, Singer SJ. Molecular structural effects produced in proteins by reaction with succinic anhydride. Biochim Biophys Acta 1958; 29:587–593.

16. Palacian E, Gonzalez MP, Pineiro M, Hernandes F. Dicarboxylic acid anhydrides as dissociating agents of protein-containing structures. Mol Cell Biochem 1990; 97:101–111.

17. Jonsson BAG, Wishnok JS, Skipper PL, Stillwell WG, Tannenbaum SR. Lysine adducts between methyltetrahydrophthalic anhydride and collagen in guinea pig lung. Toxicol Appl Pharmacol 1995; 135:156–162.

18. Jonsson BAG, Lindh CH, Welinder H. Haemoglobin adducts and specific immunoglobulin G in humans as biomarkers of exposure to hexahydrophthalic anhydride. Biomarkers 1997; 1–6.

19. Chief Inspector of Factories and Workshops. Annual Report for 1937. London: HMSO, 1938: 62.

20. Kern RA. Asthma and allergic rhinitis due to sensitization to phthalic anhydride: report of a case. J Allergy 1939; 10:164–165.

21. Landsteiner K, Jacobs J. Studies on the sensitization of animals with simple chemical compounds. J Exp Med 1935; 61:337–351.

22. Jacobs JL, Golden TS, Kelley JJ. Immediate reactions, to anhydrides, of wheal-and-erythema type. Proc Soc Exp Biol Med 1940; 43:74–77.

23. Jacobs JL. Immediate generalised skin reactions in hypersensitive guinea pigs. Proc Soc Exp Biol Med 1940; 43:641–643.

24. Landsteiner K, Chase MW. Experiments on transfer of cutaneous sensitivity to simple compounds. Proc Soc Exp Biol Med 1942; 49:688–690.

25. Chase MW. Studies on the sensitization of animals with simple chemical compounds. X. Antibodies inducing immediate-type skin reactions. J Exp Med 1947; 86:489–514.

26. Chase MW. Models for hypersensitivity studies. In: Lawrence HS ed. Cellular and Humoral Aspects of the Hypersensitive States. London: Cassell, 1959:251–278.

27. Carpenter CP, Smyth HF Jr. Chemical burns of the rabbit cornea. Am J Ophthalmol 1946; 29:1363–1372.

28. Tanaka S. Lesion of the eye caused by maleic anhydride vapour. J Sci Labor 1956; 32: 117–126.

29. Neilsen J, Welinder H, Schitz A, Skerfving S. Specific serum antibodies against phthalic anhydride in occupationally exposed subjects. J Allergy Clin Immunol 1988; 82:126–133.

30. Frans A, Pahulycz C. Apparition transitoire d'un syndrome d'irritation aigue des bronches induit par une inhalation unique et massive d'anhydride phtalique. Rev Pneum Clin 1993; 49:247–251.

31. Zeiss CR, Patterson R, Pruzansky JJ, Miller MM, Rosenberg M, Levitz D. Trimellitic anhydride-induced airway syndromes: clinical and immunologic studies. J Allergy Clin Immunol 1977; 60:96–103.

32. Zeiss CR, Wolkonsky P, Chacon R, Tuntland PA, Levitz D, Pruzansky JJ, Patterson R. Syndromes in workers exposed to trimellitic anhydride: a longitudinal clinical and immunologic study. Ann Intern Med 1983; 98:8–12.

33. Schaper M, Brost MA. Respiratory effects of trimellitic anhydride aerosols in mice. Arch Toxicol 1991; 65:671–677.

34. Gell PGH, Coombs RRA. The classification of allergic reactions underlying disease. In: Gell PGH, Coombs RRA eds. Clinical Aspects of Immunology. Oxford: Blackwell, 1963:317–337.

35. Akiyama K, Pruzansky JJ, Patterson R. Hapten-modified basophils: a model of human immediate hypersensitivity that can be elicited by IgG antibody. J Immunol 1984; 133:3286–3290.

36. Ishizaka T. The Robert A Cooke memorial lecture. Analysis of triggering events in mast cells for immunoglobulin E–mediated histamine release. J Allergy Clin Immunol 1981:67:90–96.

37. Kagey-Sobotka A, Dembo M, Goldstein B, Metzger H, Lichtenstein LM. Qualitative characteristics of histamine release from basophils by covalently cross-linked IgE. J Immunol 1981; 127:2285–2291.

38. Zeiss CR. Occupational lung disease induced by reactive chemicals. Clin Rev Allergy 1985; 3:217–226.

39. Naor D, Galili N. Immune response to chemically modified antigens. Prog Allergy 1977; 22: 107–146.

40. Patterson R, Zeiss CR, Roberts M, Pruzansky JJ, Wolkonsky P, Chacon R. Human antihapten antibodies in trimellitic anhydride inhalation reactions: immunoglobulin classes of anti-trimellitic anhydride antibodies and hapten inhibition studies. J Clin Invest 1978; 62:971–978.

41. Zeiss CR, Levitz D, Chacon R, Wolkonksky P, Patterson R, Pruzansky JJ. Quantitation and new antigenic determinant specificity of antibodies induced by inhalation of trimellitic anhydride in man. Int Arch Allergy Appl Immunol 1980; 61:380–388.

42. Welinder H, Zhang X-D, Gustavsson C, Bjork B, Skerfving S. Structure-activity relationships of organic acid anhydrides as antigens in an animal model. Toxicology 1995; 103:127–136.

43. Zhang X-D, Lotvall J, Skerfving S, Welinder H. Antibody specificity to the chemical structures of organic acid anhydrides studied by in-vitro and in-vivo methods. Toxicology 1997; 118:223–232.

44. Zhang X-D. Relationship between chemical structure and airway sensitizing potential for organic acid anhydrides: an animal model. Doctoral dissertation, Lund University, Sweden, 1997.

45. Sarlo K, Clark ED. Guinea pig inhalation and injection models for the detection of low molecular weight chemical sensitizers. J Allergy Clin Immunol 1990; 85:257 (abstract).

46. Botham PA, Hext PM, Rattray NJ, Walsh ST, Woodcock DR. Sensitisation of guinea pigs by inhalation exposure to low molecular weight chemicals. Toxicol Lett 1988; 41:159–173.

47. Arakawa H, Lotvall J, Kawikova I, Morikawa A, Lofdahl CG, Skoogh BE. Airway responses following intradermal sensitization to different types of allergens: ovalbumin, trimellitic anhydride and *Dermatophagoides farinae*. Int Arch Allergy Immunol 1995; 108:274–280.

48. Arakawa H, Lotvall J, Kawikova I, Tee R, Hayes J, Lofdahl CG, Newman Taylor AJ, Skoogh BE. Airway allergy to trimellitic anhydride in guinea pigs: different time courses of IgG1 titer and airway responses to allergen challenge. J Allergy Clin Immunol 1993; 92:425–434.

49. Arakawa H, Lotvall J, Linden A, Kawikova I, Lofdahl CG, Skoogh BE. Role of eicosanoids in airflow obstruction and airway plasma exudation induced by trimellitic anhydride-conjugate in guinea-pigs 3 and 8 weeks after sensitization. Clin Exp Allergy 1994; 24:582–589.

50. Yan ZQ, Hansson GK, Skoogh BE, Lotvall JO. Induction of nitric oxide synthase in a model of allergic occupational asthma. Allergy 1995; 50:760–764.

51. Zhao H, Zhang XD, Welinder H, Jonsson B. Anaphylactic bronchoconstriction in immunized guinea pigs provoked by inhalation and intravenous administration of hexahydrophthalic anhydride and methyltetrahydrophthalic anhydride. Allergy 1997; 52:18–26.

52. Leach CL, Hatoum NS, Ratajczak HV, Zeiss CR, Roger JC, Garvin PJ. The pathologic and immunologic response to inhaled trimellitic anhydride in rats. Toxicol Appl Pharmacol 1987; 87:67–80.

53. Ledbetter AD, Leach CL, Hatoum NS, Roger JC. The generation and detection of particulate aerosol of trimellitic anhydride and trimellic acid for inhalation exposures. Am Ind Hyg Assoc J 1987; 48:35–38.

54. Zeiss CR, Leach CL, Smith LJ, Levitz D, Hatoum NS, Garvin PJ, Patterson R. A serial immunologic and histopathologic study of lung injury induced by trimellitic anhydride. Am Rev Respir Dis 1988; 137:191–196.

55. Chandler MJ, Zeiss CR, Leach CL, Hatoum NS, Levitz D, Garvin PJ, Patterson R. Levels and specificity of antibody in bronchoalveolar lavage (BAL) and serum in an animal model of trimellitic anhydride-induced lung injury. J Allergy Clin Immunol 1987; 80:223–229.

56. Zeiss CR, Leach CL, Levitz D, Hatoum NS, Garvin PJ, Patterson R. Lung injury induced by short-term intermittent trimellitic anhydride (TMA) inhalation. J Allergy Clin Immunol 1989; 84:219–223.

57. Leach CL, Hatoum NS, Ratajczak HV, Zeiss CR, Garvin PJ. Evidence of immunologic control of lung injury induced by trimellitic anhydride. Am Rev Respir Dis 1988; 137:186–190.

58. Pullerits T, Dahlgren U, Skoogh BE, Lotvall J. Development of antigen-specific IgE after sensitisation with trimellitic anhydride in rats is attenuated by glucocorticoids and cyclosporin A. Int Arch Allergy Immunol 1997; 112:279–286.

59. Andius P, Arakawa H, Molne J, Pullerits T, Skoogh BE, Lotvall J. Inflammatory responses in skin and airways after allergen challenge in Brown Norway rats sensitized to trimellitic anhydride. Allergy 1996; 51:556–562.

60. Vento KL, Dearman RJ, Kimber I, Basketter DA, Coleman JW. Selectivity of IgE responses, mast cell sensitization, and cytokine expression in the immune response of Brown Norway rats to chemical allergens. Cell Immunol 1996; 172:246–253.

61. Patterson R, Roberts M, Harris KE, Levitz D, Zeiss CR. Pulmonary and systemic immune responses of rhesus monkeys to intrabronchial administration of trimellitic anhydride. Clin Immunol Immunopathol 1980; 15:357–366.

62. Dykewicz MS, Patterson R, Harris KE. Induction of antigen-specific bronchial reactivity to trimellityl-human serum albumin by passive transfer of serum from humans to rhesus monkeys. J Lab Clin Med 1988; 111:459–465.

63. Lowenthal M, Shaughnessy MA, Harris KE, Grammer LC. Immunologic cross-reactivity of acid anhydrides with immunoglobulin E against trimellityl-human serum albumin. J Lab Clin Med 1994; 123:869–873.

64. Liu F-T, Bargatze RF, Katz DH. Induction of immunologic tolerance to the trimellitate haptenic group in mice: model for a therapeutic approach to trimellitic anhydride–induced hypersensitivity syndromes in humans? J Allergy Clin Immunol 1980; 66:322–326.

65. Wei B-Y. Holford-Strevens V, Carter BG, Sehon AH. Suppression of the anti-trimellityl (TM) IgE response in mice by conjugates of TM with polyvinyl alcohol. Immunology 1984; 51:687–696.

66. Sale SR, Patterson R, Zeiss CR, Fiore M, Harris KE, Yawn D. Immune response of dogs and rabbits to intrabronchial trimellitic anhydride. Int Arch Allergy Appl Immunol 1982; 67: 329–334.
67. Maccia CA, Bernstein IL, Emmett EA, Brooks SM. In vitro demonstration of specific IgE in phthalic anhydride hypersensitivity. Am Rev Respir Dis 1976; 113:701–704.
68. Bernstein DI, Gallagher JS, D'Souza L, Bernstein IL. Heterogeneity of specific-IgE responses in workers sensitized to acid anhydride compounds. J Allergy Clin Immunol 1984; 74:794–801.
69. Drexler H, Schaller KH, Weber A, Letzel S, Lehnert G. Skin prick tests with solutions of acid anhydrides in acetone. Int Arch Allergy Immunol 1993; 100:251–255.
70. Fawcett IW, Newman Taylor AJ, Pepys J. Asthma due to inhaled chemical agents—epoxy resin systems containing phthalic acid anhydride, trimellitic acid anhydride and triethylene tetramine. Clin Allergy 1977; 7:1–14.
71. Schlueter DP, Banaszak EF, Fink JN, Barboriak J. Occupational asthma due to tetrachlorophthalic anhydride. J Occup Med 1978; 20:183–188.
72. Howe W, Venables KM, Topping MD, Dally MB, Hawkins R, Law JS, Newman Taylor AJ. Tetrachlorophthalic anhydride asthma: evidence for specific IgE antibody. J Allergy Clin Immunol 1983; 71:5–11.
73. Durham SR, Graneek BJ, Hawkins R, Newman Taylor AJ. The temporal relationship between increases in airway responsiveness to histamine and late asthmatic responses to occupational agents. J Allergy Clin Immunol 1987; 79:398–406.
74. Venables KM, Newman Taylor AJ. Exposure-response relationships in asthma caused by tetrachlorophthalic anhydride. J Allergy Clin Immunol 1990; 85:55–58.
75. Nielsen J, Welinder H, Ottosson H, Bensryd I, Venge P, Skerfving S. Nasal challenge shows pathogenetic relevance of specific IgE serum antibodies for nasal symptoms caused by hexahydrophthalic anhydride. Clin Exp Allergy 1994; 24:440–449.
76. Neilsen J, Welinder H, Bensryd I, Andersson P, Skerfving S. Symptoms and immunologic markers induced by exposure to methyltetrahydrophthalic anhydride. Allergy 1994; 49:281–286.
77. Tarvainen K, Jolanki R, Estlander T, Tupasela O, Pfaffli P, Kanerva L. Immunologic contact urticaria due to airborne methylhexahydrophthalic and methyltetrahydrophthalic anhydrides. Contact Dermatitis 1995; 32:204–209.
78. Young RP, Barker RD, Pile KD, Cookson WOCM, Newman Taylor AJ. The association of HLA-DR3 with specific IgE to inhaled acid anhydrides. Am J Respir Crit Care Med 1995; 151:219–221.
79. Venables KM, Topping MD, Nunn AJ, Howe W, Newman Taylor AJ. Immunologic and functional consequences of chemical (tetrachlorophthalic anhydride)-induced asthma after four years of avoidance of exposure. J Allergy Clin Immunol 1987; 80:212–218.
80. Barker RD, Harris JM, Welch JA, Venables KM, Newman Taylor AJ. Occupational asthma caused by tetrachlorophthalic anhydride—a twelve year follow-up. J Allergy Clin Immunol 1998; 101.
81. Venables KM. Occupational asthma caused by tetrachlorophthalic anhydride. Doctoral dissertation, London University, London, 1987.
82. Grammer LC, Shaughnessy MA, Henderson J, Zeiss CR, Kavich DE, Collins MJ, Pecis KM, Kenamore BD. A clinical and immunologic study of workers with trimellitic-anhydride-induced immunologic lung disease after transfer to low exposure jobs. Am Rev Respir Dis 1993; 148:54–57.
83. McGrath KG, Roach D, Zeiss CR, Patterson R. Four-year evaluation of workers exposed to trimellitic anhydride: a brief report. J Occup Med 1984; 26:671–675.
84. Rice DL, Jenkins DE, Gray JM, Greenberg SD. Chemical pneumonitis secondary to inhalation of epoxy pipe coating. Arch Environ Health 1977; 32:173–178.

85. Herbert FA, Orford R. Pulmonary hemorrhage and edema due to inhalation of resins containing trimellitic anhydride. Chest 1979; 76:546–551.

86. Rivera M, Nicotra MB, Byron GE, Patterson R, Yawn DH, Franco M, Zeiss CR, Greenberg SD. Trimellitic anhydride toxicity: a cause of acute multisystem failure. Arch Intern Med 1981; 141:1071–1074.

87. Ahmad D, Morgan WKC, Patterson R, Williams T, Zeiss CR. Pulmonary haemorrhage and haemolytic anaemia due to trimellitic anhydride. Lancet 1979; 2:328–330.

88. Patterson R, Addington W, Banner AS, Byron GE, Franco M, Herbert FA, Nicotra MB, Pruzansky JJ, Rivera M, Roberts M, Yawn D, Zeiss CR. Antihapten antibodies in workers exposed to trimellitic anhydride fumes: a potential immunopathogenetic mechanism for the trimellitic anhydride pulmonary disease-anemia syndrome. Am Rev Respir Dis 1979; 120: 1259–1267.

89. Kaplan V, Baur X, Czuppon A, Ruegger M, Russi E, Speich R. Pulmonary hemorrhage due to inhalation of vapor containing pyromellitic dianhydride. Chest 1993; 104:644–645.

90. Czuppon AB, Kaplan V, Speich R, Baur X. Acute autoimmune response in a case of pyromellitic acid dianhydride-induced hemorrhagic alveolitis. Allergy 1994; 49:337–341.

91. Grammer LC, Shaughnessy MA, Lowenthal M. Hemorrhagic rhinitis. An immunologic disease due to hexahydrophthalic anhydride. Chest 1993; 104:1792–1794.

92. Topping MD, Venables KM, Luczynska CM, Howe W, Newman Taylor AJ. Specificity of the human IgE response to inhaled acid anhydrides. J Allergy Clin Immunol 1986; 77:834–842.

93. Venables KM, Topping MD, Howe W, Luczynska CM, Hawkins R, Newman Taylor AJ. Interaction of smoking and atopy in producing specific IgE antibody against a hapten protein conjugate. Br Med J 1985; 290:201–204.

94. Venables KM, Dally MB, Nunn AJ, Stevens JF, Stephens R, Farrer N, Hunter JV, Stewart M, Hughes EG, Newman Taylor AJ. Smoking and occupational allergy in workers in a platinum refinery. Br Med J 1989; 299:939–942.

95. Cartier A, Malo J-L, Forest F, Lafrance M, Pineau L, St-Aubin J-J, Dubois J-Y. Occupational asthma in snow crab processing workers. J Allergy Clin Immunol 1984; 74:261–269.

96. Zetterstrom O, Nordvall SL, Bjorksten B, Ahlstedt S, Stelander S. Another smoking hazard: raised serum IgE concentration and increased risk of occupational allergy. Br Med J 1981; 283:1215–1217.

97. Zeiss CR, Mitchell JH, Van Peenen PFD, Harris J, Levitz D. A twelve-year clinical and immunologic evaluation of workers involved in the manufacture of trimellitic anhydride (TMA). Allergy Proc 1990; 11:71–77.

98. Zeiss CR, Mitchell JH, Van Peenen PFD, Kavich D, Collins MJ, Grammer L, Shaughnessy M, Levitz D, Henderson J, Patterson R. A clinical and immunologic study of employees in a facility manufacturing trimellitic anhydride. Allergy Proc 1992; 13:193–198.

99. Liss GM, Bernstein D, Genesove L, Roos JO, Lim J. Assessment of risk factors for IgE-mediated sensitization to tetrachlorophthalic anhydride. J Allergy Clin Immunol 1993; 92: 237–247.

100. Grammer LC, Shaughnessy MA, Yarnold PR. Risk factors for immunologically mediated disease in workers with respiratory symptoms when exposed to hexahydrophthalic anhydride. J Lab Clin Med 1996; 127:443–447.

101. Grammer LC, Shaughnessy MA. Study of employees with anhydride-induced respiratory disease after removal from exposure. J Occup Environ Med 1996; 38:771–774.

102. Baur X, Czuppon AB, Rauluk I, Zimmermann FB, Schmitt B, Egen-Korthaus M, Tenkhoff N, Degens PO. A clinical and immunological study on 92 workers occupationally exposed to anhydrides. Int Arch Occup Environ Health 1995; 67:395–403.

103. Baur X, Czuppon A. Diagnostic validation of specific IgE antibody concentrations, skin prick testing, and challenge tests in chemical workers with symptoms of sensitivity to different anhydrides. J Allergy Clin Immunol 1995; 96:489–494.

104. Wernfors M, Nielsen J, Schutz A, Skerfving S. Phthalic anhydride-induced occupational asthma. Int Arch Allergy Appl Immunol 1986; 79:77–82.

105. Drexler H, Weber A, Letzel S, Kraus G, Schaller KH, Lenhert G. Detection and clinical relevance of a type I allergy with occupational exposure to hexahydrophthalic anhydride and methyltetrahydrophthalic anhydride. Int Arch Occup Environ Health 1994; 65:279–283.

106. Barker RD, van Tongeren MJA, Harris JM, Gardiner K, Venables KM, Newman Taylor AJ. Risk factors for sensitisation and respiratory symptoms among workers exposed to acid anhydrides: a cohort study. Occup Environ Med 1998; 55:684–691.

107. van Tongeren M, Barker RD, Gardiner K, Venables KM, Harrington JM, Newman Taylor AJ. Retrospective exposure assessment of acid anhydride exposure. Occup Environ Med 1998; 55:692–696.

27
Metals

I. Leonard Bernstein
University of Cincinnati College of Medicine, Cincinnati, Ohio

Benoit Nemery
Katholieke Universtiteit Leuven, Leuven, Belgium

Stuart Brooks
University of South Florida, Tampa, Florida

INTRODUCTION

Occupational asthma induced by inhalation exposure to metals may have been first described by Georgius Agricola, who published "De Re Metallica" in 1556 (1). He described the possible harmful effects of metallic dust as follows: "On the other hand, some mines are so dry that they are entirely devoid of water and this dryness causeth the workmen even greater harm, for the dust, which is stirred and beaten up by digging, penetrates into the windpipe and lungs and produces difficulty in breathing and the disease the Greeks call 'asthma.'" Admittedly, this excerpt is more likely to pertain to mineworkers' pneumoconiosis than to what would now be called asthma. Nevertheless, although many forms of pulmonary toxicity have been noted after exposure to metals, metalloids, and their respective oxides, salts, and coordination complexes, the occurrence of occupational asthma induced by these substances has only been recognized as a medical entity in the early part of the twentieth century. While the numerical contribution of metal-induced asthma to the overall prevalence of occupational asthma appears to be relatively small, the number of literature citations of these problems continues to increase each year. In addition, significant numbers of workers are exposed to these agents according to the NIOSH 1981–1983 National Exposure Survey (Table 1).

GENERAL PROPERTIES OF METALS

Workers are rarely exposed to pure metals or metalloids, but usually to oxides, sulfides, halides, hydrides, carbides, or other salts of these elements (2). Transition metals also form coordination complexes with ligands such as ammonia, carbon monoxide, cyanogen, organic nitrogen, or sulfur molecules. Bioavailability is also an important determinant of the possible effects resulting from exposure to these substances. Thus, deposits of insoluble metallic compounds in the airways are more likely to be cleared by the mucociliary apparatus, while soluble metallic salts may readily dissociate and be transported as metal

Table 1 Estimated Number of Workers Exposed to Metals and Metallic Salts in the United States, 1981–1983

Agent	All durations		Full-time	
	Total	Female	Total	Female
Nickel: welding, soldering, brazing	139,771	30,830	31,829	8,960
Chromium				
Metal (Cr III)	395,612	11,800	42,181	639
Welding, soldering brazing	6,876	162	3,774	153
Cobalt: metal, dust fume	79,659	2,718	9,976	44
Vanadium	54,160	2,657	14,867	717
Zinc oxide	1,305,837	248,087	41,410	2,610
Platinum				
Metal	24,836	4,135	1,964	108
Compounds	37,402	18,286	539	
Aluminum				
Metal	1,104,885	102,130	217,084	27,165
Total dust	20,321	1,643	3,374	1,179

ions into lung tissues. Some metals such as cobalt (Co), zinc (Zn), and chromium (Cr) may act as essential trace elements or coenzymes for important metabolic enzyme pathways (3). Indeed, specific metal-binding sites in enzymatic proteins could possibly play a role in the pathogenesis of some metal-related allergic reactions (e.g., platinum interaction with endogenous malic dehydrogenase enzymes) (4). Interaction of metallic ions with other body transport proteins and macromolecules may also lead to the development of antigenicity similar to other organic low-molecular-weight compounds, which may function as haptens (e.g., platinum, chromium, nickel, and cobalt). The biological activity and impact of some metals are also predicated on their abilities to change oxidation states by oxidation (loss of electrons) and reduction (gain of electrons) (2). Inasmuch as transition metals are electronically stable in more than one oxidation state, these metals play important roles in the catalysis of biological oxidation reactions. Moreover, their ability to enhance the production of toxic species of oxygen could also be involved in the pathogenesis of nonimmunological asthma.

DIFFERENTIAL DIAGNOSIS OF METAL-INDUCED ASTHMA

The spectrum of pulmonary toxicity due to inhalation of metallic compounds encompasses a wide range of acute and chronic obstructive syndromes, which in some instances may mimic asthma (2). Inhalation of fumes or dusts from many metallic salts and hydrides may cause chemical tracheobronchitis or chemical pneumonitis with a picture resembling the adult respiratory distress syndrome (5). Similarly, chronic exposure to cobalt (hard metal), aluminum, manganese, titanium dioxide, beryllium, and cadmium is associated with chronic obstructive lung diseases such as chronic bronchitis and pulmonary emphysema (6). Small airway involvement in these diseases may at times be confused with asthma. In the case of occupational exposure to cobalt, alveolitis and asthma may coexist (7). Although the pathogenesis of metal fume fever is not entirely understood, there have been recent reports of associated or superimposed bronchial asthma with this condition.

Specific examples of these concurrent entities will be discussed in separate sections under respective individual metals. Finally, small airway disease may at times be a prominent feature of pneumoconiosis with features of diffuse interstitial pneumonitis such as hard metal lung disease or pneumoconiosis with sarcoid-like granuloma formations such as berylliosis (8).

OCCUPATIONAL EXPOSURE VARIABLES

Asthma in workers occupationally exposed to metals may not necessarily be due to the metallic exposure. Prior or current cigarette smoking may obfuscate the diagnosis of occupational asthma in some workers. There are other examples of mixed exposures to metals and nonmetals. For example, workers in foundries are far more likely to develop asthma due to methylenediphenyl diisocyanate (MDI), used in some molding resins, than they are to metal oxides. In certain industries, concurrent exposure to sulfur oxide, ozone, chlorine, or nitrogen dioxide may constitute as much or greater risk than specific metallic compounds. In the platinum-refining industry, for example, workers are exposed not only to the platinum halide salts but also to significant concentrations of chlorine and sulfur dioxide gases (9).

On the other hand, exposure to metals is not necessarily confined to workers involved in metal mining or metallurgical industries. Thus, cobalt-induced bronchial asthma has been described in diamond polishers who use cobalt-containing polishing discs (10). Metallic compounds are used as pigments in the paint and ceramic industry, as catalysts in the chemical industry, or as additives in the plastic industry (11). Finally, significant exposure to metals is not confined to the work environment. Hobbies and domestic activities may lead to clinical sensitivity in susceptible individuals. It has also been suspected that persistence of platinum-induced asthma could be due to continued contact with former platinum workers who continue to have small amounts of platinum on their clothing (12).

CLASSIFICATION

Because recognition of occupational asthma induced by a variety of metals and their derivatives is relatively recent, a generally acceptable system of classification has not yet evolved. Thus far, this category of occupational asthma has been identified according to specific etiological agents and such terms as "transitional" metals, "precious" metals (platinum, palladium), and hard metals (tungsten carbide, cobalt) have been used to define specific asthmatic problems. However, because the vast majority of workplace asthma induced by metallic compounds is caused by metallic elements (and their derivatives) in specific sections of the periodic table of elements, a new classification based on a specific metallic element's position in the periodic table is proposed as a frame of reference for the following discussion of occupational asthma induced by specific agents (Table 2). Thus far, all metallic elements that cause asthma can be classified as follows:

1. First long period of transitional elements (also referred to as the "iron group transition metals" between scandium and zinc). This group includes metals such as vanadium, chromium, cobalt, nickel, copper, and zinc.
2. Second long period of transitional elements (also referred to as the "palladium group transition metals" between yttrium and cadmium). This group includes ruthenium, rhodium, palladium, silver, and cadmium.

Table 2   Periodic Table of Elements

	Ia	IIa	IIIb	IVb	Vb	VIb	VIIb	VIII			Ib	IIb	IIIa	IVa	Va	VIa	VIIa	0
1	1 H																	2 He
2	3 Li	4 Be											5 B	6 C	7 N	8 O	9 F	10 Ne
3	11 Na	12 Mg											*13* *Al*	14 Si	15 P	16 S	17 Cl	18 Ar
4	19 K	20 Ca	21 Sc	22 Ti	**23** **V**	**24** **Cr**	25 Mn	26 Fe	**27** **Co**	**28** **Ni**	29 Cu	**30** **Zn**	31 Ga	32 Ge	33 As	34 Se	35 Br	36 Kr
5	37 Rb	38 Sr	39 Y	40 Zr	41 Nb	42 Mo	43 Tc	44 Ru	45 Rh	**46** **Pd**	47 Ag	48 Cd	49 In	50 Sn	51 Sb	52 Te	53 I	54 Xe
6	55 Cs	56 Ba	57 La	72 Hf	73 Ta	74 W	75 Re	76 Os	77 Ir	**78** **Pt**	79 Au	80 Hg	81 Tl	82 Pb	83 Bi	84 Po	85 At	86 Rn
7	87 Fr	88 Ra	89 Ac															

Lanthanides	58 Ce	59 Pr	60 Nd	61 Pm	62 Sm	63 Eu	64 Gd	65 Tb	66 Dy	67 Ho	68 Er	69 Tm	70 Yb	71 Lu
Actinides	90 Th	91 Pa	92 U	93 Np	94 Pu	95 Am	96 Cm	97 Bk	98 Cf	99 Es	100 Fm	101 Md	102 No	103 Lr

Occupational asthma may be caused after exposure to some of the metal species indicated in boldface; for the elements presented in italics, there is no evidence that asthma is based on immunological sensitization to the metal itself.

3. Third long period of transitional elements (also referred to as the "platinum group transition metals" between hafnium and thallium). This group includes osmium, iridium, platinum, gold, mercury, and lead.
4. Second short period of elements (aluminum is the sole agent in this series).
5. Indeterminate (due to mixtures of alloys or contaminants in manufactured metallic products).

Table 3 is a compilation of metals according to their respective orbital structures in the periodic table and the various obstructive airways diseases that can occur after occupational exposure to these agents. According to this classification, it is apparent that the majority of metal-induced asthmatic problems are associated with metals in the group of the first long transitional series of metallic elements. However, it should be emphasized

Table 3 Metals Known to Induce Occupational Asthma

Classification	Periodic system		Chemical form exposed to:	TLV/TWA (mg/m^3)	IgE-mediated
	Atomic number	Classifi-cation			
Nickel	28	1	Elemental/metal (inhalable)	*1.5*	No
			Soluble compounds, as Ni (inhalable)	*0.1*	Yes
			Insoluble compounds, as Ni (inhalable)	*0.2*[a]	No
			Nickel subsulfide, as Ni (inhalable)	*0.1*[a]	No
			Nickel carbonyl (inhalable)	*0.12* (0.05 ppm)	Equivocal
Chromium	24	1	Metal and CrIII compounds, as Cr	0.5	No
			Water-soluble CrVI compounds, as Cr	0.05[a]	Yes
			Insoluble CrVI compounds, as Cr	0.01[a]	No
Cobalt	27	1	Metal and inorganic compounds	0.02	Yes
Vanadium	23	1	As V_2O_5 (respirable dust or fumes)	0.05	No
Zinc oxide	30	1	Fume	5	No
			Dust	10	No
Platinum	78	3	Metal	1	No
			Soluble salts, as Pt	0.002	Yes
Aluminum	13	4	Metal dust	10	No
			Pyro powders, as Al	5	No
			Welding fumes, as Al	5	No
			Alkyl	2	No
			Soluble salts, as Al	2	No

TLV/TWA = threshold limit value/time-weighted average: the time-weighted average concentration for a conventional 8-hr workday and a 40-hr workweek, to which it is belived that nearly all workers may be repeatedly exposed, day after day, without adverse effect. Data in italics concern substances for which a change has been proposed ("notice of intended change").
[a]Human carcinogen.
Source: 1998 updated TLV/TWA data were supplied by the ACGIH Cincinnati, Ohio.

that the absolute number of medical reports of asthma caused by platinum and asthma associated with aluminum far outnumbers other metals (13–16).

FIRST LONG PERIOD OF TRANSITIONAL ELEMENTS

Nickel

Primary nickel industries include mining, milling, smelting, and refinishing processes whereby nickel ores are removed from the ground and transformed into marketable, unfabricated materials such as nickel metal, nickel oxide, and nickel alloy (17). Workers in electroplating industries are commonly exposed to nickel sulfate. Workers involved in the production of nickel catalysts (used in the food industry for hardening of edible oils by hydrogenation) are exposed to both nickel sulfate and nickel hydroxide-carbonate complex. Nickel workers may also be exposed to vapors of nickel carbonyl. The latter compound is extremely toxic to the central nervous system and lung, and the permitted exposure limit is a time-weighted concentration of 0.12 mg/m³. For nickel-soluble salts, the exposure limit is 0.1 mg/m³ as the time-weighted average concentration for up to an 8-hr workday, 40-hr workweek (18).

Although it is estimated that 140,000 workers in the United States are potentially exposed to nickel, the occurrence of asthma induced by exposure to these salts is uncommon. Moreover, relatively few cases of nickel-induced asthma have been associated with or preceded by contact dermatitis, a frequent outcome of nickel sensitization (19). However, no conclusions can be drawn about the association of nickel dermatitis and asthma because the number of documented asthma reports is too sparse.

Apart from one case of nickel-related Löffler's syndrome and asthma due to exposure to nickel carbonyl, there have been about a dozen recorded cases of asthma occurring after exposure to nickel sulfate (19–28). Eight of these were documented by controlled bronchial challenge tests (19,21–24,27,28). Four workers demonstrated immediate broncho-provocation response, and four workers experienced an isolated late asthmatic reaction. Several of these patients also manifested an increase in bronchial hyperresponsiveness for varying periods after the nickel sulfate challenge.

Four of the reported cases demonstrated evidence of immediate skin reactivity. Nickel-reactive hemagglutinating antibodies were first demonstrated by McConnell et al. (20). Modest levels (twice the negative control) of nickel-specific-IgE-associated antibodies were demonstrated by Dolovich et al., who showed specific reactivity to a nickel-human serum albumin conjugate (29), while Novey et al. obtained significantly higher IgE antibody using an ionic-exchange resin as a nonspecific binding agent for the nickel antigen (23). Specific IgE antibodies were also demonstrated in two other instances (19,27). Detailed investigations of possible cell-mediated immune mechanisms were not undertaken in any of these cases.

Chromium

Chromium is a transition metal that is widely used for electroplating processes, metal alloys, pigments, tanning of leather, and production of chromate salts (30). Moreover, many varieties of cement contain traces of chromium, which are responsible for allergic sensitization and contact dermatitis in construction workers. Chromium metal is nonallergic, but chromium salts have been investigated extensively as causative agents in occupational contact dermatitis. Chromium salts exist naturally in three valency forms: 2, 3, and 6. Bivalent compounds are unstable and have little commercial value. Hexavalent chromium compounds (e.g., chromium trioxide and mono- and bichromates) may have an increased potential for allergenicity because they are more soluble and presumably have easier access into body tissues. It is estimated that 400,000 workers are potentially exposed to hexavalent chromium (18). Work place standards distinguish between carcinogenic and noncarcinogenic species of hexavalent chromate. Monochromates and bichromates (dichromates of hydrogen, lithium, sodium, potassium, rubidium, cesium, and ammonium as well as chromium oxide) are considered noncarcinogenic. The workplace environmental limit for hexavalent chromium is a time-weighted average of 0.05 mg of hexavalent chromium/m^3 for up to an 8-hr workday, 40-hr workweek (18).

Although hexavalent chromium is generally acknowledged to be the most frequent skin sensitizer of male industrial workers, it is an uncommon cause of occupational asthma. Documentation of chromium-induced asthma by controlled laboratory bronchial challenge testing has been published in 19 cases (23,28,31–33,36). Five workers demonstrated immediate-type bronchoconstrictive responses after inhaling chromium sulfate fumes. A transient, reversible asthmatic response after bronchial challenge was observed in a metal-plating worker (34). Nine workers experienced dual asthmatic responses and four had isolated late reactions. Methacholine-induced hyperresponsiveness was demonstrated in four of these cases (31). Another worker experienced a unique late wheezing reaction 6 hr after the challenge (32). This was accompanied by a generalized urticarial eruption, facial edema, and periorbital swelling. Cement asthma has been described in building workers (35). Occupational asthma was also reported in a floorer who had both occupational dermatitis and occupational asthma. In this case, it was proposed that the inhalation exposure to chromates occurred by means of smoking rolled cigarettes contaminated with cement (36).

Chromium-specific IgE antibodies were demonstrated in the worker showing immediate bronchoconstrictive response (23). In these studies, the chromium salt was absorbed to a cationic exchange resin. Prick tests with 10 mg/ml solutions of chromate salts were positive in two cases (31). In contrast to nickel-induced asthma, a prior history of contact dermatitis and positive patch tests (using 0.5% solution of potassium dichromate) were noted in five cases (33). Evidence of cell-mediated mechanisms was also suggested in a patient who exhibited an isolated delayed response after chromate challenge (32). In this instance, significant leukocyte inhibitory factor activity to hexavalent chromate was obtained in a dose-response fashion.

Cobalt

Cobalt is used in the manufacture of alloys for the electrical, automobile, and aircraft industries (2,6,8). Steel-containing cobalt is used for safety razor blades and surgical instruments. Cobalt is also used in the manufacture of pigment, coloring glass, and enamel. One of the chief uses of cobalt is as a binder for tungsten carbide in sintered hard metals (also called cemented carbides or cemets) and more recently, also in diamond tools. Thus, cobalt incorporated into high-speed polishing discs represents a significant source of exposure for diamond polishers (10). The largest work population exposed to cobalt dust is in the hard metal industry, because hard metals are used for tools and engine parts that need to sustain high temperatures.

Significant exposure to cobalt-containing dust occurs not only during the various stages of the manufacturing of hard metal tools, but also during their maintenance and resharpening. During the latter operations the use of coolants and their continuous recycling has been shown to lead to an enrichment in dissolved cobalt and hence a higher potential for exposure to ionic cobalt in the aerosolized fluids (37).

NIOSH estimates that approximately 80,000 workers are exposed to cobalt materials and reports of occupational asthma are not infrequent (6,38). In a large industrial survey, Kusaka et al. observed that 5% of hard metal workers had work-related asthma (39). This should be distinguished from hard metal disease, which is also caused by cobalt. Hard metal disease is an interstitial pneumonia with clinical presentations resembling hypersensitivity pneumonitis and the potential to evolve to irreversible fibrosis (40). A characteristic pathological feature of hard metal lung disease is the presence of "bizarre" multinucleated giant cells in the interstitium and alveoli, and hence in the bronchoalveolar lavage. Hard metal lung disease has never been reported to occur in subjects exposed to cobalt alone and it is, therefore, likely that the simultaneous presence of cobalt and other particles (such as tungsten carbide or diamond) is required for the interstitial pneumonia. However, it is well established by several investigators that cobalt alone can induce asthma in susceptible workers.

Cobalt-induced asthma has been documented in workers involved in the production of cobalt, the manufacture and use of cobalt pigments, the production and maintenance of hard metal and diamond tools, and the polishing of diamonds (10,38,41–44). Provocation tests performed separately with both cobalt and tungsten carbide powder revealed that only cobalt provoked the asthmatic response (45). In addition, investigators have shown that controlled positive challenge to cobalt temporarily increased nonspecific bronchial hyper-responsiveness. It has also been demonstrated that affected workers will react not only to inhaled powder but also water-soluble cobalt. Late bronchial challenge reactions appear to be common (37).

Shirakawa et al. investigated possible immunopathogenesis in 12 cobalt broncho-provocation-positive patients (46). None of the patients had positive immediate-type skin tests to cobalt reagents. Six patients demonstrated evidence of cobalt-specific IgE to a cobalt human serum albumin conjugate. One patient showed a borderline significant reaction to cobalt adsorbed to a resin reagent. Of interest also was that five of these workers were considered to be atopic by virtue of high total IgE titers and positive RAST scores when tested to a battery of common aeroallergens. In a recent cross-sectional survey of 706 workers exposed to hard metal dust, there was no correlation between cobalt specific IgE antibodies and cigarette smoking (47). Kusaka et al. observed that two of the patients who had specific IgE antibodies to cobalt also exhibited lymphocyte proliferation responses when their peripheral blood lymphocytes were incubated with either free cobalt or a cobalt human serum albumin conjugate (48). In a few cases, bronchoalveolar lavage revealed an increase in T lymphocytes with an inverted CD4+/CD8+ ratio (49). These results suggested that cobalt-sensitized lymphocytes may play a role in the immunopathogenesis of some hard metal asthmatics. However, in the combined studies of Shirakawa et al. and Kusaka et al., it should be noted that five hard metal asthmatic patients demonstrated neither cobalt-specific IgE nor sensitized lymphocytes. The recent in vitro finding that cobalt and metallic carbides interact with oxygen to produce activated toxic oxygen species suggests that some workers with lower antioxidant defensive mechanisms may be more susceptible to hard metal disease (50). However, it is not clear whether cobalt-induced asthma is related to the interstitial lung disease associated with cobalt. Since occasional workers exhibit both asthmatic reactions and parenchymal involvement, it is possible that cobalt asthma may be an "airway variant" of hard metal disease (7,51,52).

Shirakawa et al. demonstrated that some workers with cobalt-induced asthma also manifested specific IgE sensitization and positive bronchial responses to nickel sulfate

(53). It is known that nickel is sometimes added to hard metal as a matrix in addition to cobalt. Further evaluation of these workers revealed that four showed evidence of specific IgE antibodies to both cobalt and nickel. Although the authors postulated that cross-reactivity between these two metals was a possibility, it is more likely that these workers developed concurrent hypersensitivity reactions after exposure to both metals.

Vanadium

Vandium pentoxide is the most important chemical derivative of vanadium in commercial use. It is used as a catalyst for a variety of reactions in the chemical and petroleum refinery industries (54). It is particularly prominent in the production of high-strength steel alloys. Occupational exposure to vanadium pentoxide is primarily an inhalation hazard causing irritation of the upper respiratory tract. The recommended threshold limit of vanadium pentoxide dust is 0.5 mg/m^3 of air (18). Acute tracheitis and bronchitis with persistent bronchial hyperresponsiveness can be caused by exposure to vanadium pentoxide. Vanadium-induced asthma is associated with the cleaning of oil tanks ("boilermaker's bronchitis") (55).

Information about vanadium-induced asthma is available only from case reports (56). It has been established that asthma develops in workers without prior history of asthma. The majority of affected workers thus far have been nonatopic. Increased bronchial hyperresponsiveness has been demonstrated in at least two cases. Evidence of positive skin tests or any other immunopathogenetic mechanism has not been described. In addition, there are no reports of controlled laboratory challenges to vanadium pentoxide. However, subhuman primates exposed to vanadium pentoxide over a period of weeks develop a pattern of increased hyperresponsiveness to the agent (57).

Zinc

A major use for zinc is for galvanizing, which consists of depositing a fine layer of zinc onto a metal surface (steel sheet, structural sections, nails) to protect it from corrosion. Other important uses of zinc include various alloys (die castings used in automotive parts) and in brass. Further uses of zinc are as pigments and salts in paints, and for wood preservation. Zinc chloride is a component of smoke bombs. The most significant exposure to zinc occurs as a result of welding or burning (galvanizing) metals, the fumes of which contain various metal oxides including zinc oxide.

Exposure to fumes of zinc oxide is most often associated with metal fume fever, which typically begins 4–12 hr after exposure. The manifestations of metal fume fever resemble a flu-like illness, but coughing and shortness of breath may also be present. Episodes may persist anywhere from 24 to 48 hr.

Several cases of occupational asthma have been described, but considering the extensive usage of zinc-containing metals, the overall prevalence of this problem is negligible (58–60). The threshold limit value of zinc is 5 mg/m^3.

In the available cases of suspected wheezing due to zinc oxide fumes, two patients were subjected to controlled bronchial challenge under laboratory conditions (59). Both workers demonstrated objective evidence of bronchial constriction 4–9 hr after the exposure. Fever and leukocytosis occurred in one of the patients, so this individual may have had a combination of occupational asthma and metal fume fever. Increased bronchial hyperresponsiveness was also observed in one patient 24 hr after the exposure. Environmental measurements at the workplace of these two individuals revealed significantly elevated concentrations of zinc after a work-simulated episode of soldering on galvanized iron (22 mg/m^3). Another recent case report fulfilled the criteria of occupational asthma, as indexed by a postshift fall of FEV$_1$, bronchial hyperresponsiveness to methacholine, and an immediate asthmatic response after bronchial challenge (61). Although positive immediate skin tests were demonstrated in this case, it is not certain that IgE-mediated mechanisms were involved (61).

SECOND LONG PERIOD OF TRANSITIONAL ELEMENTS

The occurrence of either skin or clinical sensitization after exposure to precious metals in this category (ruthenium, rhodium, palladium, and silver) is rare (62). Several groups of Russian investigators have reported that some salts of these metals—chiefly palladium—may induce both immediate and delayed hypersensitivity skin reactions and may also elicit direct histamine release from human leukocytes (63–66). The immunogenic potential of palladium was partially corroborated by Biagini et al., who demonstrated that sera from some platinum-sensitive, palladium-exposed workers also elicited a positive PCA response to palladium in subhuman primates (12). However, these investigators did not have direct evidence that workers exposed to a variety of precious metal salts other than platinum developed allergic symptoms or asthma to these salts. One of us (BN) recently investigated a case of occupational asthma that was clearly related to fumes of an electrolysis bath containing palladium chloride. This worker exhibited an isolated positive skin test to tetrammminepalladium (II) chloride (1 µg/ml) as well as a positive bronchial provocation test to this salt administered as an aerosol (10 µg/ml) for 3.5 min (67).

Asthma has not been reported after exposure to salts or fumes of cadmium, one of the metallic elements in the second long series. Acute exposure to cadmium fumes may cause life-threatening chemical pneumonitis. Recent studies suggest that there is excess of impaired respiratory function and diffusing capacity as well as radiological signs of emphysema in workers with chronic inhalation exposure to cadmium, compared to appropriate controls (2).

THIRD LONG PERIOD OF TRANSITIONAL ELEMENTS

Platinum

Exposure to platinum occurs in the mining and metallurgical industries (68). Since platinum is also used extensively as a catalyst in the chemical industry, chemists and chemical workers may be exposed. Although platinum oxide is an essential component of catalytic converters used for control of automobile exhaust fumes, automobile workers are at no additional risk from this particular platinum salt. The chief occupational exposure to platinum salts occurs in the primary and secondary refining of platinum. In the secondary refining process, precious metals such as platinum, palladium, rhodium, and ruthenium are reclaimed from scrap metal and expended automobile exhaust catalysts for use in the electrical and chemical industries (9). The scrap is burned to remove carbon and other combustible components. The resultant fine powder is dissolved in hydrochloric acid and chlorine followed by separation, sequential solubilization, and precipitation to yield halide platinum salts. This manufacturing process also involves exposure to chlorine gas, formaldehyde, sulfur dioxide, hydrazine, hydrogen chloride, and nitric acid. Presumably, the halide moiety in these salts confers strong allergic properties to platinum salts. Because of the specialized supply-and-demand nature of platinum products, it is estimated that only several thousand workers have significant exposure to the specific salts that have been incriminated as causes of occupational asthma. The threshold limit value for platinum salts is 2 $\mu g/m^3$.

Since platinum salts have such a high propensity for inducing IgE-mediated sensitivity, the prevalence of platinum salt skin sensitization alone does not necessarily correlate with occupational asthma (9,12,69). However, workers with positive platinum salt skin tests had significantly higher prevalences of rhinitis, asthma, and positive cold air challenges compared to negative skin test workers (9,12,70). In a cross-sectional survey of a secondary refinery, it was determined that 15 of 107 (14%) current employees and eight of 29 (28%) medically terminated workers exhibited positive skin test reactivity to platinum salts (12). Moreover, it was also found that 10% of workers in the production areas were medically terminated each year due to upper and large airways symptoms. A similar study revealed that 41% of newly hired workers had developed clinical respiratory symptoms after 24 months of exposure and had to be medically separated (13). Thus, the platinum salts industry is a primary example of how the "healthy worker" effect can interact with cross-sectional industrial surveys (9). Another factor that may confound the evaluation of respiratory symptoms in workers exposed to platinum salts is the fact that the halide platinum salts may cause bronchial hyperresponsiveness by direct effects on human and subhuman primate mucosal permeability and bronchial smooth muscle. Moreover, Biagini et al. demonstrated that concurrent exposure of subhuman primates to irritants such as those commonly used in the secondary platinum-refining industry could potentiate the effects of platinum salt exposure by increasing pulmonary mucosal permeability (71).

Among all metal salts that have been reported to induce occupational asthma, platinum salts have received the greatest attention and documentation in the medical literature. Platinum-induced occupational asthma has been recognized since 1911 (72–82). Soon after the initial reports appeared, it was also recognized that sensitization to platinum was frequently associated with airways symptoms in exposed workers. In these early reports, it was clearly demonstrated that direct skin tests (scratch and prick) with the appropriate platinum salts were positive in many of these workers. Indeed, this appeared to be one of the few instances in which simple, unconjugated chemicals (haptens) could be used as reliable reagents for detection of immediate, IgE-mediated hypersensitivity responses in the skin. Prick test reactivity has been observed at concentrations as low as 10^{-9} g/ml (12). The general consensus among investigators in this field is that prick testing is a useful technique for surveillance and early detection of sensitized workers. A direct comparison between skin prick and bronchial challenge tests revealed that the skin prick test has excellent specificity (69).

The majority of past industrial surveys focused on the role of respiratory allergy in exposed workers. A combined physiological, immunological, and industrial sampling cross-sectional survey contributed significant information about risk factors, prevalence odds ratios of developing asthma, and persistence of symptoms in medically terminated workers (9). In this investigation, each worker received a work exposure medical questionnaire (administered by a physician), physical examination, spirometry before and after a work shift, cold air bronchial inhalation challenge test, and skin prick testing to platinum salts and common aeroallergens (ragweed, timothy, and house dust mite). Serum total IgE, platinum-specific IgE, and specific IgE to several aeroallergens were determined. These examinations were conducted in 107 of 123 available current employees and 29 of 59 employees terminated for medical reasons. Five years previous to the study, the number of medical terminations due to allergic problems represented 9.8% of the employees in the production areas per year. Environmental air sampling for 3 years before the study revealed elevated platinum salt measurements in various production areas of the plant. These often exceeded the OSHA standard of 2 $\mu g/m^3$.

Positive skin tests were observed in 15 of 107 current employees and eight of the 29 terminated workers. Platinum salt skin sensitivity generally varied directly with the environmental air concentration of platinum salts in the current employees' production work areas, and the risk of demonstrating platinum salt skin test reactivity increased 1.13 times per 1 $\mu g/m^3$ increment in work area concentration of platinum salts ($p = 0.01$). Prevalence of symptoms and medical test results were compared between platinum skin test-positive and -negative workers. Skin test reactivity to platinum was associated with increased symptoms of rhinitis, asthma, and dermatitis, abnormal FEV_1, positive cold air challenge, and elevated total serum IgE. The medically terminated workers reported more symptoms and demonstrated more adverse test results than nonsensitized current employees. A significant change in FEV_1 across work shifts was specific for overall atopic status but not for platinum salt sensitization. The prevalence of aeroallergen skin test reactivity (atopy) was similar among positive and negative platinum skin test groups and the general population. This finding did not corroborate previous reported recommendations for excluding prospective employees having a positive medical history of atopy (80). On the other hand, cigarette smoking status was strongly associated with platinum skin sensitization. Furthermore, cigarette smoking prevalence was markedly increased among the medically terminated workers. This risk factor was confirmed in other prospective studies (13,80).

Prevalence odds ratios for health outcomes adjusted for aeroallergen skin test reactivity and cigarette smoking status were compared between platinum skin test-positive and -negative employees. The prevalence odds ratio for asthma (11.3) was significantly increased in platinum skin test-positive workers when the case definition of asthma was restricted to asthma symptoms with onset occurring after date of hire (17.9; $p = 0001$). The prevalence odds ratio for a positive cold air challenge in skin test-positive workers was 7.77, and the average decrease in FEV_1 following cold air challenge was more than twice as much in skin test-positive as in skin test-negative workers.

A striking observation of this investigation was the persistence of positive platinum skin tests among medically terminated workers (9,12). This risk factor was confirmed in a recent prospective study (13). This occurred despite the apparent lack of further exposure to platinum during an average of 5 years since respective termination dates. These medically terminated subjects also demonstrated a high prevalence of airway symptoms, abnormal FEV_1/FVC ratios, and positive cold air challenges. These observations suggested that allergic sensitization to platinum salts leading to termination may have prolonged consequences. This long-term adverse health effect had not been observed previously by investigators concerned with surveillance of platinum refinery workers (78,79,81). The most likely reasons for these differences are that exposures of platinum salts may be higher in certain plants and that medical screening may vary in terms of detecting early sensitization and prompt removal from further exposure. It was therefore concluded that persistence of symptoms in the terminated workers of this study occurred presumably because of a delay in removal from further exposure after they had been sensitized to platinum salts. To understand the dynamics of sensitization to platinum salts, a proportion (63%) of this study population underwent repeat platinum skin testing 1 year later. In this group, there was conversion of platinum skin tests from negative to positive in five employees, with three conversions occurring in workers who showed a positive cold air challenge test the year before.

Cold air challenge was performed as an index of bronchial hyperresponsiveness in these workers (67). The test was positive in one-third of the patients with positive platinum skin tests and in one-fifth of the patients reporting asthma symptoms at the time of the survey. The test was positive in only six of 107 patients with negative skin tests to platinum. Thus, the prevalence odds ratio of a positive cold air challenge in positive versus negative platinum skin test-positive workers was 7.7 ($p = 0.003$). There was a strong association between a positive cold air challenge test at baseline measurement and subsequent conversion to a positive platinum skin test 1 year later. Of the four workers in the follow-up study with a positive cold air challenge and a negative skin test at the initial visit, three skin test conversions occurred. In comparison, only two of 63 workers with negative cold air and negative skin tests converted. It was noteworthy that the sensitivity of cold air challenge for selecting workers reporting asthma symptoms was 68% compared to platinum skin test alone, which was 35%. If one analyzed both tests together, the sensitivity increased to 78%. Nevertheless, the cold air challenge test itself cannot be used as a predictor of platinum sensitization and respiratory symptoms, especially in view of the strong effect of cigarette smoking in these studies. The latter variable confounded the cold challenge results because it is known that cigarette smoking alone can cause increase in cold challenge response. The conclusion of this detailed cross-sectional analysis was that the platinum skin test used in conjunction with the cold air challenge and a validated respiratory questionnaire seemed to offer a good screening protocol for identifying workers with occupational asthma caused by platinum salts. It also appeared to constitute a useful paradigm for cross-sectional studies of occupational asthma induced by metals and other substances. The other interesting finding that emerged from this study was that the possible direct bronchial irritative effect of platinum did not appear to predict the subsequent development of skin test reactivity because positive cold challenge tests occurred in 10 of 114 skin test-negative workers.

Several recent investigations also addressed the relationship of bronchial hyperresponsiveness, as indexed by methacholine challenge, with both positive platinum prick and specific challenge tests (14,15). There was no correlation between nonspecific bronchial hyperresponsiveness and skin reactivity or specific platinum bronchial challenge. Moreover, a subset of the same workers who were reevaluated 19 months after removal from platinum exposure revealed that both nonspecific and specific bronchial hyperresponsiveness did not decrease after removal (16).

The allergenicity of platinum salts is well documented. The immunological pathogenesis of the allergic reaction is considered to be a type 1 IgE-mediated hypersensitivity reaction with a possible reaginic IgG_4 component (5). The role of IgE in this disease has been corroborated by both positive passive transfer tests in humans and monkeys with sera from affected workers and IgE radioimmunoassay. Several RAST procedures have been used for the detection of platinum sensitivity. These include two studies using hapten protein conjugates and one investigation in which platinum was adsorbed nonspecifically to an ion exchange resin (12,78,79). The sensitivity and specificity of these various RAST procedures varied somewhat between investigators. In all studies, some overlapping between the amount of serum binding to various reagents occurred in platinum-exposed, skin test-negative patients and normal, nonexposed subjects. Nevertheless, RAST inhibition experiments clearly showed that these tests were specific for the respective platinum conjugates. In one investigation, the sensitivity of the specific IgE radioimmunoassay was improved by preabsorption of free platinum in serum specimens by polyacrylamide gel (12). It was postulated that small amounts of freely circulating serum platinum competitively competed with the platinum salt conjugate for binding to test substrate. All studies agreed that the specific radioimmunoassay is less sensitive than skin testing in the clinical diagnosis of platinum hypersensitivity. One of the cross-sectional investigations revealed that total IgE levels were elevated in all groups of previous metal refinery workers (82). Mean levels of serum IgE were highest in former skin test positive workers who left the plant because of platinum-associated symptoms (12). Unusually high values (1840 ng/ml or more) were observed in 50% of these medically terminated workers. It was suggested that chronic exposure to platinum group salts may result in nonspecific immunopotentiation of the isotypic IgE response. This phenomenon had been noted in a rodent experimental model of platinum sensitization (83). The presence of heat-stable, short-term sensitizing antibodies to platinum was also demonstrated by two independent groups of investigators (12,78). Further research is required to determine whether these antibodies are analogous to human IgG_4.

SECOND SHORT PERIOD OF ELEMENTS

Aluminum

Asthma was first recognized as an occupational health hazard for workers in potrooms of Norwegian aluminum smelters in 1936 (84). Subsequently, the existence of asthma has also been reported in Australian, Dutch, French, Italian, North American, and New Zealand smelters (85–89). The major components of the potroom environment include fluorides in particulate and gaseous forms, dust containing cryolite (Na_3AIF_6), alumina, sulfur dioxide, oxides of carbon, and particulate organic matter (85). Initially, it was thought that an allergic reaction to fluoride in the work environment of the smelter was the cause of potroom asthma, but this widely held belief has yet to be confirmed (84). Whatever the ultimate cause may prove to be, asthma occurring in aluminum smelter workers is now known as "potroom asthma." Since the exact etiological agent is unknown, it is customary to use representative time-weighted averages of known pulmonary hazards such as gaseous and particulate fluorides, respirable dust, sulfur dioxide, and cold tar pitch volatiles as an estimate of permissible exposure (85).

There is a large variation in the prevalence and incidence of occupational asthma in the aluminum industry. The estimated incidence of potroom asthma ranged from 0.06 to 4% of exposed workers per year. There is a lower prevalence of potroom asthma reported in North American studies compared to European studies (85). This could be related to different preemployment medical criteria, prevailing climatic conditions, or the degree of potroom environmental controls. The population at risk also poses problems. This is confounded by high labor turnover in this industry. Forty-four percent of potroom workers in New Zealand left within 12 months, and 71% of Australian smelter workers within 3 years (85). The results of some cross-sectional analyses are also difficult to interpret because of the healthy survivor effect. Thus, Chan-Yeung et al. were not able to demonstrate any potroom asthma in their study, but this is possibly explained by the fact that five workers left the plant just prior to the study (87). The relative paucity of documented potroom asthma cases in other Canadian aluminum smelter plants has also been observed by an editor (JLM) of this book. However, his investigative team recently demonstrated a pattern of dual hyperresponsiveness after workplace challenge in a symptomatic, nonsmoking potroom worker 6 months after he had been removed from further exposure (88).

Symptoms of potroom asthma consist of shortness of breath, wheezing, chest tightness, and cough. While these may occur immediately after exposure, generally the symptoms are of delayed onset. The symptoms become more frequent and severe with repeated exposure. The duration of potroom exposure before the first attack ranges from 1 week to 10 years (89,90). When asthma becomes fully established, it is easy to confirm by objective pulmonary function tests as well as tests measuring bronchial hyperresponsiveness. Risk factors have not been satisfactorily defined. Although early workers suggested allergy as a possible cause, this association is not convincing because skin tests with house and potroom dust are negative, and only a minority of workers demonstrate eosinophilia and/ or elevated total IgE (91–93). Although in most series the majority of asthmatic cases appeared in smokers, the potential effects of cigarette smoking are not yet proven because the effect of smoking has not been studied simultaneously in matched, unexposed controls. The prognosis of potroom asthma is variable. In some cases, as many as 40% of workers may continue to have asthma after terminating further exposure (69). Bronchial hyperresponsiveness also may persist in many workers (94,95). Some authors have postulated that differences in individual patterns of exposure may account for persistence of asthma. An analogy between this type of persistent asthma and the reactive airways dysfunction syndrome described by Brooks et al. has also been suggested (94,95). A recent report showing that high plasma fluoride levels in potroom workers are associated with a steeper bronchial hyperresponsiveness dose-response curve may reflect the fact that high airborne fluoride levels are associated with persistent asthma (96). Persistence of asthma after work stoppage has also been reported from industries where smokers have been exposed to other aluminum fluoride compounds ($K_3ALF_6ALF_3$). Apparently, most of these cases occurred when there were high airborne concentrations of total dust up to 53 mg/m^3. Such high peak exposures would certainly be consistent with the onset of reactive airways dysfunction syndrome (RADS).

Complete immunological surveys have been conducted in aluminum smelter workers. Mean levels of IgG, IgA, IgE, recall-delayed hypersensitivity, immune complexes, and antinuclear and/or other autoantibodies were identical in asthmatic and nonasthmatic workers (92). Thus, immune function was normal in both symptomatic and asymptomatic workers in an aluminum smelter. Immediate skin tests to aluminum and fluoride salts were uniformly negative. In one study, six workers showed positive patch tests to 2% NaF (91). The significance of this finding is unknown.

In summary, both cross-sectional and longitudinal studies now indicate that working in aluminum smelters causes occupational asthma. The actual causative agent(s) are unidentified, but it is recognized that dust and fume controls may lessen the overall prevalence of this problem.

INDETERMINATE EXPOSURE TO STEEL PRODUCTS

Workers exposed to several processes unique to the steel-manufacturing industry may develop occupational asthma after varying periods of exposure ranging from less than 1 year to 8 years. A significant outbreak of industrial asthma occurred in 21 workers exposed to coating materials of rolled steel sheets (97). The coverings were known to contain epoxy resins, acrylics, phenol, formaldehyde chromates, and polyvinyl chloride. Of great interest, however, was the fact that 8 years after the onset of asthmatic symptoms in this plant, it was discovered that toluene diisocyanate (TDI) was liberated during the curing process. Subsequently, two workers in this group demonstrated delayed-onset asthma after a bronchial challenge with TDI. Follow-up survey in this plant after the TDI exposure was eliminated demonstrated that about 40% of the workers still had some work-related asthma, but in the vast majority of cases this was much improved. Although TDI appeared to be the responsible agent for many of these workers, it is possible that employees with residual symptoms of asthma at work could still have increased reactive airways after exposure to some of the other substances in the coating process.

Occupational asthma has been reported in welders after exposure to solid particles emanating from stainless steel welding fumes (98,99). Six workers using the manual metal arc-welding technique developed symptoms only after welding operations of stainless steel and not "mild" steel. Challenge tests in three of these workers revealed immediate-type and dual reactions in two and one worker(s), respectively. Two of these workers had positive history and patch tests to chromates in the past. Inasmuch as stainless steel welding fumes contain significantly higher amounts of chromium and nickel than "mild" steel, the investigators of this industrial problem postulated that either the chromium or nickel in stainless welding fumes might be the actual etiological factor. However, challenge tests to these metallic elements were not performed, so the actual etiological agent in this group of workers was unknown.

WELDING IN GENERAL

In addition to the occurrence of occupational asthma in steel manufacturing processes, welding is often mentioned as a cause of occupational asthma or as a risk factor for asthma (100–103). It is not clear whether these asthma reports are due to specific metallic sensitization or work-related RADS.

SUMMARY

Occupational asthma occurs after exposure to a variety of metallic compounds. Apart from aluminum, the majority of these agents are salts of elements found in the first, second, and third long series of transitional elements. The prevalence of occupational asthma to various metallic agents varies from rare to as high as 35% in the platinum industry. Both immunological and nonimmunological factors contribute to the pathogenesis of metal-induced occupational asthma. IgE-mediated mechanism have been demonstrated in nickel-, chromium-, cobalt-, and platinum-induced asthma. The possible contributory role of delayed hypersensitivity is less well understood. Asthma in several metal-fabricating industries has been shown to be due to nonmetallic components. Persistence of asthma in several forms of metal-induced asthma may occur if recognition and removal from further exposure are not accomplished as promptly as possible.

REFERENCES

1. Agricola G. De re metallica. The Mining Magazine, (translated by HC Hoover and LH Hoover). London: Mining Journal Ltd, 1912:1556.
2. Nemery B. Metal toxicity and the respiratory tract. Eur Respir J 1990; 3:202–219.
3. Spivey-Fox MR. Nutritional aspects of metals. In: Lee DHK, ed. Metallic Contaminants and Human Health. New York: Academic Press, 1972:191–208.
4. Friedman ME, Musgrove G, Lee K, Teggins JE. Inhibition of malate dehydrogenase by platinum (II) complexes. Biochem Biophys Acta 1971; 250:286–296.
5. Editorial. Metals and the lung. Lancet 1984; 903:904.
6. Brooks SM. Lung disorders resulting from the inhalation of metals. Clin Chest Med 1981; 2:235–254.

7. Van Cutsem EJ, Ceuppens JL, Lacquet LM, Demedts M. Combined asthma and alveolitis induced by cobalt in a diamond polisher. Eur J Respir Dis 1987; 70:54–61.

8. Morgan WKC. Other pneumoconioses. In: Morgan WKC, Seaton A, eds. Occupational Lung Diseases. Philadelphia: WB Saunders, 1975:217–250.

9. Baker DB, Gann PH, Brooks SM, Gallagher J, Bernstein IL. Cross-sectional study of platinum salts sensitization among precious metals refinery workers. Am J Ind Med 1990; 18: 653–664.

10. Gheysens B, Auwerx J, Van den Eeckhout A, Demedts M. Cobalt-induced bronchial asthma in diamond polishers. Chest 1985; 88:740–744.

11. Smith RG. Five metals of potential significance. In: Lee DHK, ed. Metallic Contaminants and Human Health. New York: Academic Press, 1982:139–162.

12. Biagini RE, Bernstein IL, Gallagher JS, Moorman WJ, Brooks S, Gann PH. The diversity of reaginic immune responses to platinum and palladium metallic salts. J Allergy Clin Immunol 1985; 76:794–802.

13. Calverley AE, Rees D, Dowdeswell RJ, Linnett PJ, Kielkowski D. Platinum salt sensitivity in refinery workers: incidence and effects of smoking and exposure. Occup Environ Med 1995; 52:661–666.

14. Merget R, Caspari C, Kulzer R, Breitstadt R, Rueckmann, A, Schultze-Werninghaus G. The sequence of symptoms, sensitization and bronchial hyperresponsiveness in early occupational asthma due to platinum salts. Int Arch Allergy Immunol 1995; 107:407–407.

15. Merget R, Dierkes A, Rueckmann A, Bergmann EM, Schultze-Werninghaus G. Absence of relationship between degree of nonspecific and specific bronchial responsiveness in occupational asthma due to platinum salts. Eur Respir J 1996; 92:211–216.

16. Merget R, Reineke M, Rueckmann A, Bergmann EM, Schultze-Werninghaus G. Nonspecific and specific bronchial responsiveness in occupational asthma caused by platinum salts after allergen avoidance. Am J Respir Crit Care Med 1994; 150:1146–1149.

17. Nriagu JO. Nickel in the Environment. New York: Wiley, 1980: 1–833.

18. American Conference of Government Industrial Hygienists, 1997 TLVs and BEIs, Threshold Limit Values for Chemical Substances and Physical Agents. Biological Exposure Indices, ACHIG, Cincinnati, OH, 1998.

19. Estlander T, Kanerva L, Tupasela O, Keskinen H, Jolanki R. Immediate and delayed allergy to nickel with contact urticaria, rhinitis, asthma and contact dermatitis. Clin Exp Allergy 1993; 23:306–310.

20. McConnell LH, Fink JN, Schlueter DP, Schmidt MG Jr. Asthma caused by nickel sensitivity. Ann Intern Med 1973; 78:888–890.

21. Malo J-L, Cartier A, Doepner M, Nieboer E, Evans S, Dolovich J. Occupational asthma caused by nickel sulfate. J Allergy Clin Immunol 1982; 69:55–59.

22. Block GT, Yeung M. Asthma induced by nickel. JAMA 1982; 247:1600–1602.

23. Novey HS, Habib M, Wells ID. Asthma and IgE antibodies induced by chromium and nickel salts. J Allergy Clin Immunol 1983; 72:407–412.

24. Malo J-L, Cartier A, Gagnon G, Evans S, Dolovich J. Isolated late asthmatic reaction due to nickel sulphate without antibodies to nickel. Clin Allergy 1985; 15:95–99.

25. Davies JE. Occupational asthma caused by nickel salts. J Occup Med 1986; 36:29–30.

26. Sunderman FW, Sunderman FW Jr. Loffler's syndrome associated with nickel sensitivity. Arch Intern Med 1961; 107:405–408.

27. Shirakawa T, Morimoto K. Brief reversible bronchospasm resulting from bichromate exposure. Arch Environ Health 1996; 51:221–226.

28. Bright P, Burge PS, O'Hickey SP, Gannon PF, Robertson AS, Boran A. Occupational asthma due to chrome and nickel electroplating. Thorax 1997; 52:28–32.

29. Dolovich J, Evans SL, Nieboer E. Occupational asthma from nickel sensitivity. I. Human serum albumin in the antigenic determinant. Br J Ind Med 1984; 41:51–55.

30. Burrows D. The dichromate problem. Int J Dermatol 1984; 23:215–220.

31. Park HS, Yu HJ, Jung KS. Occupational asthma caused by chromium. Clin Exp Allergy 1994; 24:676–681.

32. Moller DR, Brooks SM, Bernstein DI, Cassedy K, Enrione M, Bernstein IL. Delayed anaphylactoid reaction in a worker exposed to chromium. J Allergy Clin Immunol 1986; 77: 451–456.

33. Olaguibel JM, Basomba A. Occupational asthma induced by chromium salts. Allergol Immunopathol 1989; 17:133–136.

34. Shirakawa T, Morimoto K. Brief reversible bronchospasm resulting from bichromate exposure. Arch Environ Health 1996; 51:221–226.

35. Lob M. Allergie respiratoire au ciment. Z Unfallchir Vers Med Berufskr 1985; 78:47–50.

36. Nemery B, De Raeve H, Demedts M. Dermal and respiratory sensitization to chromate in a floorer. Eur Respir J 1995; 8(Suppl 19):222s.

37. Sjogren I, Hillerdal G, Andersson A, Zetterstrom O. Hard metal lung disease: importance of cobalt in coolants. Thorax 1980; 35:653–659.

38. Cirla AM. Cobalt-related asthma: clinical and immunological aspects. Sci Tot Environ 1994; 150:85–94.

39. Kusaka Y, Yokayama K, Sera Y, Yamamoto S, Sone S, Kyono H, Shirakawa T, Goto S. Respiratory diseases in hard metal workers: An occupational hygiene study in a factory. Br J Ind Med 1986; 43:474–485.

40. Newman LS, Maier LA, Nemery B. Interstitial lung disorders due to beryllium and cobalt. In: Schwartz MI, King TE Jr, eds. Interstitial Lung Disease, 3rd ed. St Louis: CV Mosby, 1998:367–392.

41. Cullen MR. Respiratory diseases from hard metal exposure. A continuing enigma. Chest 1984; 86:513–514.

42. Roto P. Asthma, symptoms of chronic bronchitis and ventilatory capacity among cobalt and zinc production workers. Scand J Work Environ Health 1980; 6(Suppl):11–36.

43. Pillière F, Garnier R, Rousselin X, Dimerman S, Rosenberg N, Efthymiou ML. Asthme aux sels de cobalt. A propos d'un cas dû au résinate de cobalt. Arch Mal Prof 1990; 51:413–417.

44. Bruckner HC. Extrinsic asthma in a tungsten carbide worker. J Occup Med 1967; 9:518–519.

45. Shirakawa T, Kusaka Y, Fujimura N, Goto S, Kato M, Heki S, Morimoto K. Occupational asthma from cobalt sensitivity in workers exposed to hard metal dust. Chest 1989; 95:29–37.

46. Shirakawa T, Kusaka Y, Fugimura N, Goto S, Morimoto K. The existence of specific antibodies to cobalt in hard metal asthma. Clin Allergy 1988; 18:451–460.

47. Shirakawa T, Morimoto K. Interplay of cigarette smoking and occupational exposure on specific immunoglobulin E antibodies to cobalt. Arch Environ Health 1997; 52:124–128.

48. Kusaka Y, Nakano Y, Shirakawa T, Morimoto K. Lymphocyte transformation with cobalt in hard metal asthma. Ind Health 1989; 27:155–163.

49. Forni A. Bronchoalveolar lavage in the diagnosis of hard metal disease. Sci Tot Environ 1994; 150:69–76.

50. Lison D, Lauwerys R, Demedts M, Nemery B. Experimental research into the pathogenesis of cobalat/hard metal lung disease. Eur Respir J 1996; 9:1024–1028.

51. Davison AG, Haslam PL, Corrin B, Coutts H, Dewar A, Riding WD, Studdy PR, Newman-Taylor AJ. Interstitial lung disease and asthma in hard-metal workers: bronchoalveolar lavage, ultrastructural, and analytical findings and results of bronchial provocation tests. Thorax 1983; 38:119–128.

52. Rivolta G, Nicoli E, Ferretti G, Tomasini M. Hard metal lung disorders: analysis of a group of exposed workers. Sci Tot Environ 1994; 150:161–165.

53. Shirakawa T, Kusaka Y, Fujimura N, Kato M, Heki S, Morimoto K. Hard metal asthma: cross immunological and respiratory reactivity between cobalat and nickel? Thorax 1990; 45: 267–271.

54. Hudson TFG. Vanadium: Toxicology and Biological Significance. New York: Elsevier, 1964.

55. Kiviluoto M, Rasanen O, Rinne A, Rissanen M. Effects of vanadium on the upper respiratory tract of workers in a vanadium factory. Scand J Work Environ Health 1982; 5:50–58.

56. Musk AW, Tees JG. Asthma caused by occupational exposure to vanadium compounds. Med J Aust 1982; 1:183–184.

57. Knecht EA, Moorman WJ, Clark JC, Lynch DW, Lewis TR. Pulmonary effects of acute vanadium pentoxide inhalation in monkeys. Am Rev Respir Dis 1985; 132:1181–1185.

58. Weir DC, Robertson AS, Jones S, Burge PS. Occupational asthma due to soft corrosive soldering fluxes containing zinc chloride and ammonium chloride. Thorax 1989; 44:220–223.

59. Malo J-L, Cartier A. Occupational asthma due to fumes of galvanized metal. Chest 1987; 92:375–377.

60. Kawane H, Soejima R, Umeki S, Niki Y. Metal fume and asthma. Chest 1988; 93:1116–1117.

61. Malo J-L, Cartier A, Dolovich J. Occupational asthma due to zinc. Eur Respir J 1993; 6:447–450.

62. Murdoch RD, Pepys J. Platinum group metal sensitivity: reactivity to platinum group metal salts in platinum halide salt-sensitive workers. Ann Allergy 1987; 59:464–469.

63. Bruevich TS, Bogomolets NN, Berezovski B. Sensitizing influence of compounds of noble metals (gold, platinum, ruthenium, rhodium, and silver). Gig Tr Prof Zabol 1980; 5:42–44.

64. Tomilets VA, Dontsov VI, Zakharova IA. Immediate and delayed allergic reactions to group VIII metals in an experiment. Fiziol Zh 1979; 25:653–657 (translation).

65. Tomilets VA, Dontsov VI, Zakharova IA, Klevtsov AV. Histamine releasing and histamine binding action of platinum and palladium compounds. Arch Immunol Ther Exp 1980; 28:953–957.

66. Tomilets VA, Zakharova IA. Anaphylactic and anaphylactoid properties of palladium complexes. Farmakol Toksikol 1979; 42:170–173.

67. Daenen M, Rogiers P, Van De Walle C, Rochette F, Demedts M, Nemery B. Occupational asthma caused by palladium. Eur Respir J 1999; 13:213–216.

68. Gafaefer WM. Occupational Diseases. A Guide to Their Recognition. Washington, DC: U.S. Department of Health, Education and Welfare, 1964:1–375.

69. Merget R, Schultze-Werninghaus G, Bode F, Bergmann EM, Zachgo W, Meier-Sydow J. Quantitative skin prick and bronchial provoation tests with platinum slat. Br J Ind Med 1991; 48:830–837.

70. Brooks SM, Baker DB, Gann PH, Jarabek AM, Hertzberg V, Gallagher J, Biagini RE, Bernstein IL. Cold air challenge and platinum skin reactivity in platinum refinery workers. Chest 1990; 97:1401–1407.

71. Biagini RE, Moorman WJ, Lewis TR, Bernstein IL. Ozone enhancement of platinum asthma in primate model. Am Rev Respir Dis 1986; 135:719–725.

72. Karasek SR, Karasek M. The use of platinum paper. Report of Illinois State commission of Occupational Diseases, Springfield, IL, 1911:97.

73. Hunter D, Milton R, Perry KMA. Asthma caused by complex salats of platinum. Br J Ind Med 1945; 2:92–98.

74. Roberts, AE. Platinosis. Arch Ind Hyg 1951; 4:549–559.

75. Freedman SO, Kropey J. Respiratory allergy caused by platinum salts. J Allergy 1968; 42:233–237.

76. Parrott JL, Hebert R, Saindelle A, Ruff F. Platinum and platinosis. Allergy and histamine release due to some platinum salts. Arch Environ Health 1969; 19:685–691.

77. Pepys J, Pickering CAC, Hughes EG. Asthma due to inhaled chemical agents—complex salts of platinum. Clin Allergy 1972; 2:391–396.

78. Cromwell O, Pepys J, Parish W, Hughes EG. Specific IgE antibodies to platinum salts in sensitized workers. Clin Allergy 1979; 9:109–117.

79. Hughes EG. Medical surveillance of platinum refinery workers. J Soc Occup Med 1980; 30:27–30.

80. Venables KM, Dally MB, Nunn AJ, Stevens JF, Stephens R, Farrer N, Hunter JV, Stewart M, Hughes EG, Newman Taylor, AJ. Smoking and occupational allergy in workers in a platinum refinery. Br Med J 1989; 299:939–942.

81. Murdoch RD, Pepys J, Hughes EG. IgE antibody responses to platinum group metals: a large scale refinery survey. Br J Ind Med 1986; 143:37–43.

82. Merget R, Schultze-Werninghaus G, Muthorst T, Friedrich W, Meier-Syndow J. Asthma due to the complex salts of platinum—a cross-sectional survey of workers in a platinum refinery. Clin Allergy 1988; 18:569–580.

83. Murdoch RD, Pepys J. Enhancement of antibody production by mercury and platinum group metal halide salts. Kinetics of total and ovalbumin-specific IgE synthesis. Int Arch Allergy Appl Immunol 1986; 80:405–411.

84. Frostad EW. Fluorine intoxication in Norwegian aluminum plant workers. Tidsskr Nor Laegefor 1936; 56:179–182.

85. Abramson MJ, Wlodarczyk JH, Saunders NA, Hensley MJ. Does aluminum smelting cause lung disease? Am Rev Respir Dis 1989; 139:1042–1057.

86. Gispen JGW. Respiratory problems at Pechiney Nederland. In: Coulon J-P, ed. Seminar on Aluminum Respiratory Disorders. St. Nicholas Aluminum, Greece. Aluminum Penchiney, Paris, 1980:49–57.

87. Chan-Yeung M, Wong R, MacLean L, Tan F, Schulzer M, Enarson D, Martin A, Dennis R, Grzybowski S. Epidemiologic health study of workers in an aluminum smelter in British Columbia—effects on the respiratory system. Am Rev Respir Dis 1989; 127:465–469.

88. Desjardins A, Bergeron JP, Ghezzo H, Cartier A, Malo J-L. Aluminum potroom asthma confirmed by monitoring of forced expiratory volume in one second. Am J Respir Crit Care Med 1994; 150:1714–1717.

89. O'Donnell TV, Welford B, Coleman ED. Potroom asthma: New Zealand experience and follow-up. Am J Ind Med 1989; 15:43–49.

90. Kongerud J, Boe J, Soyseth V, Naalsund A, Magnus P. Aluminum potroom asthma: the Norwegian experience. Eur Respir J 1994; 7:165–172.

91. Saric M, Godnic-Cvar J, Gomzi M, Stilinovic L. The role of atopy in potroom workers' asthma. Am J Ind Med 1986; 9:239–242.

92. Mackay IR, Ollihant RC, Laby B, Smith MM, Fisher JN, Mitchell RJ, Propert DN, Tait BD. An immunologic and genetic study of asthma in workers in an aluminium smelter. J Occup Med 1990; 32:1022–1026.

93. Sorgdrager B, Pal TM, de Looff AJ, Dubois AE, de Monchy JG. Occupational asthma in aluminium potroom workers related to pre-employment eosinophil count. Eur Respir J 1995; 8:1520–1524.

94. Wergeland E, Lund E, Waage JE. Respiratory dysfunction after potroom asthma. Am J Ind Med 1987; 11:627–636.

95. Simonsson BG, Sjöberg A, Rolf C, Haeger-Aronson B. Acute and long-term airway hyperreactivity in aluminum-salt exposed workers with nocturnal asthma. Eur J Respir Dis 1985; 66:105–118.

96. Hydro Aluminium, Health Department, Ardal Aluminium Planat, Norway. Relation between exposure to fluoride and bronchiala responsiveness in aluminium potroom workers with work-related asthma-like symptoms. Thorax 1994; 49:984–989.

97. Venables KM, Dally MB, Burge PS, Pickering CA, Newman Taylor AJ. Occupational asthma in a steel coating plant. Br J Ind Med 1985; 42:517–524.

98. Keskinen H, Kalliomaki P-L, Alanko K. Occupational asthma due to stainless steel welding fumes. Clin Allergy 1980; 10:151–159.

99. Vandenplas O, Dargent F, Auverdin JJ, Boulanger J, Bossiroy JM, Roosels D, Vande Weyer R. Occupational asthma due to gas metal arc welding on mild steel. Thorax 1995; 50:587–588.

100. Beach JR, Dennis JH, Avery AJ, Bromly CL, Ward RJ, Walters EH, Stenton SC, Hendrick DJ. An epidemiologic investigation of asthma in welders. Am J Respir Crit Care Med 1996; 154:1394–1400.

101. Meredith S. Reported incidence of occupational asthma in the United Kingdom, 1989–1990. J Epidemiol Commun Health 1993; 47:459–463.

102. Meredith SK, Taylor VM, McDonald JC. Occupational respiratory disease in the United Kingdom 1989: a report to the British Thoracic Society and the Society of Occupational Medicine by the SWORD project group. Br J Ind Med 1991; 48:292–298.

103. Wang ZP, Larsson K, Malmberg P, Sjögren B, Hallberg BO, Wrangskog K. Asthma, lung function and bronchial responsiveness in welders. Am J Ind Med 1994; 26:741–754.

28

Other Chemical Substances Causing Occupational Asthma

Jean-Luc Malo
Université de Montréal and Sacré-Coeur Hospital, Montréal, Quebec, Canada

I. Leonard Bernstein
University of Cincinnati College of Medicine, Cincinnati, Ohio

INTRODUCTION

Various chemical substances can cause occupational asthma. Chemicals most often found include polyisocyanates and acid anhydrides. These agents are discussed in other chapters. Most of the other agents have been documented as individual case reports. The frequency of occupational asthma caused by these agents has generally not been determined either because they are not used extensively or because no sufficient interest was found in carrying out the studies. The mechanism of sensitization has only been determined for some of the agents. Some substances have been found to mediate sensitization through an IgE-dependent mechanism. Low-molecular-weight agents, which represent the majority of these miscellaneous chemical substances, may cause sensitization by acting as haptens. However, the mechanism of asthma induction remains inconclusive for many other low-molecular-weight agents.

Agents that have been the subject of a larger number of publications are dealt with under specific headings of this chapter, including the chemical agents that have been reported to cause occupational asthma together with the evidence.

AZOBISFORMAMIDE OR AZODICARBONAMIDE

The chemical formula of this compound is $H_2N-CH-O-N=N-O-CH-NH_2$. The product is used in the plastic industry to introduce gas into the plastic to make a product that foams when heated. In 1977, Ferris and co-workers first described that all but one of 11 workers exposed to azodicarbonamide had symptoms characterized by a productive cough (1). In three subjects, FEV_1 recordings on the first day back at work after a period of 4 days off work showed a fall of 21%. In 1981, a survey of 151 workers exposed to this product showed that 19% had symptoms of late-onset asthma (2). No significant changes in spirometry were recorded. Atopy was not a predisposing factor and skin prick tests with the product were negative. Malo and co-workers described two subjects who underwent specific inhalation challenges and developed either an isolated late or a dual asthmatic reaction

(3). Another case report, also published in 1985, documented a late asthmatic response in a worker who was challenged with the product (4). Although blockade of the reaction by cromolyn sodium might suggest that mast cells are involved, sensitization has not been proven (4). More recently, four other cases were described, one of whom had a late asthmatic reaction after exposure to the product (5).

Azobisformamide or azodicarbonamide can cause occupational asthma as confirmed by specific inhalation challenges in a total of four subjects reported in the literature. The prevalence of occupational asthma to this product has been estimated based on questionnaires only and not by objective means. As it is not water soluble and is insoluble in virtually every diluent, skin prick tests and in vitro testing to search for antibodies are not possible (3).

AMINES

As reviewed by Hagmar and co-workers (6) (Table 1), various (approximately 40) secondary, tertiary, and quarternary amines, either aliphatic, heterocyclic, or aromatic, have been reported to cause occupational asthma. These products are handled in the primary manufacturing as well as in secondary industries (rubber industry, beauty culture industry, shellac handling, developing of color photographs, aluminium soldering, use of acrylate paints, manufacturing of antihelminthic drugs, fur industry and hair dyes, rubber additive). Dermatitis caused by ethylenediamine was diagnosed as early as in 1951 in 14 subjects with exposure to this product (7). In the same article, Dernehl describes three cases of asthma. In 1963, the same author documented asthma in workers exposed to epoxy resins.

Table 1 Occupational Asthma Caused by Amines

Amine	Occupational setting	Ref.
Aliphatic amines		
Ethylenediamines		
Ethylenediamine (EDA)	Manufacturing, rubber industry, cosmetics industry, shellac handling, color photograph development	7, 8, 9, 12
Diethylenetriamine and Triethylenetriamine	Manufacturing	8, 14
Hexamethylenetetramine	Cosmetics	9
Ethanolamines		
Monoethanolamine	Cosmetics	9
Aminoethylethanolamine	Aluminum soldering	10, 11
Dimethylethanolamine	Acrylate paints	13
Other		
3-Dimethylamino-propylamine	Manufacturing	15, 16
Heterocyclic amines		
Piperazine	Antihelminthic-drug manufacturing	17, 18, 19, 20, 21
Aromatic amines		
p-Phenylenediamine	Fur industry and hair dyes, oil and rubber additives	22

Source: Slightly modified from Ref. 6.

Production of epoxy resin is initiated by amines or other materials that act as crosslinking agents, binding the resin molecules together and becoming an intimate part of the polymer molecule (8). In the same year, Gelfand showed that exposure to ethylenediamine, a solvent for shellac, can cause occupational asthma, confirmed by specific inhalation challenges (9). Seven other subjects underwent specific inhalation challenges and experienced dual and late asthmatic reactions (10–13). Sargent and co-workers described lower respiratory tract symptoms and significant changes in bronchial caliber in 25 workers exposed to a mixture of propylamine and triethylenediamine (14). Environmental controls at the workplace later resulted in the disappearance of significant symptoms and changes in airway caliber in the same workforce (15). Ng et al. found that 3/12 (25%) plus an index case had occupational asthma on exposure to various aliphatic polyamines (ethylenediamine, diethylenetriamine, and thiethylenetetramine) (16). Savonius and co-workers described three cases of asthma caused by ethanolamines, which are amino alcohols (17).

McCullagh described a case of cutaneous and respiratory sensitivity to piperazine, a heterocyclic amine used as an antihelminthic drug (18). In another report, two subjects who underwent specific inhalation challenges in the laboratory developed late asthmatic reactions (19). Benzalkonium chloride, a quaternary amine, also caused a combined cutaneous and respiratory hypersensitivity syndrome (20).

A survey carried out in 131 subjects exposed to piperazine and ethylenediamine revealed that 8% were asthmatic or had experienced asthma associated with exposure to chemicals during their employment (21). Specific IgE antibodies to a piperazine-human serum albumin conjugate were detected in five of 72 exposed workers (7%) (22). In a cohort sample of 602 workers employed in a piperazine-producing plant between 1942 and 1979, Hagmar and co-workers showed a strong exposure-response association between the presence of respiratory symptoms and the degree of exposure (23). Furthermore, long-term exposure seemed to result in symptoms of chronic bronchitis. Using logistic regressions, the authors showed that age, length of employment, smoking habits, and previous work-related symptoms all increased the likelihood of developing symptoms. Paraphenylene diamine can also cause asthma in fur workers (24); 37 of 80 workers (46%) described by Silberman and Sorrell had symptoms of asthma; 74% of the tested subjects experienced nasal or chest symptoms during specific inhalation challenges.

It is still controversial as to whether amines can cause work-related asthma in employees exposed to isocyanates. In a group of 48 workers exposed to toluene diisocyanate and amines, 13 (27%) had respiratory symptoms and eight (17%) showed increased methacholine reactivity (25). Airborne concentrations of isocyanates were below 0.005 ppm whereas concentrations of amines were 10,000 times greater. Belin and co-workers therefore concluded that exposure to amines was more likely to have been the cause of the respiratory syndrome than exposure to isocyanates (25). These results were later contested by Candura and Moscato (26), who documented 12 instances of occupational asthma to toluene diisocyanate and no occurrence of occupational asthma to toluenediamine in workers who underwent inhalation challenges to both products.

The mechanism by which amines cause asthma remains controversial, although evidence of immediate skin reactivity has been seen in some studies.

COLOPHONY AND FLUXES

Colophony is the resin obtained from pine trees and which mainly contains abietic acid and pumaric acid. This product is widely used as a "flux" in the electronics industry to

Table 2 Colophony Fluxes and Occupational Asthma[a]

Evidence	Ref.
First report: 4 workers with immediate reactions	27
First larger survey in 21 subjects	28
Epidemiological surveys:	
Prevalence of symptoms = 22% vs. 4% in controls	29
Prevalence of symptoms in those who left = 4% vs. 1% of other shop workers	30
Lower Monday morning FEV_1 and more pronounced changes in FEV_1 during a work shift; atopy is a weak predisposing factor, smoking is not	31
Evidence that PEFR monitoring is a useful means of assessment	32
Abietic acid as a possible causal agent	33
Association between the degree of exposure and work-related symptoms	34
Evidence for the persistence of asthma after removal from exposure	35

[a]Summary of the original studies, including those of P. S. Burge.

prevent corrosion. The first report that it caused occupational asthma came from Fawcett and co-workers; they performed specific challenges on four workers who experienced isolated immediate bronchospastic reactions (27). Burg and colleagues later described in detail 21 subjects who had undergone specific inhalation challenges and developed either isolated immediate (in five subjects), isolated late (in two subjects), or dual (in 12 subjects) asthmatic reactions or an alveolitis type of reaction (28). The same group of investigators has since thoroughly investigated several aspects of this form of occupational asthma (Table 2). Work-related symptoms were found in 22% of 446 exposed workers as compared to 6% of a control group of 86 office workers (29) (Fig. 1). In a study of 1339 workers who had left the factory during the 3 previous years, 4% of solderers had left because of respiratory symptoms as compared to 1% of other shop floor workers and none of the office workers (30). A case-control study comparing 58 affected workers and 48 controls showed that affected workers had a significantly lower preexposure FEV_1 on Monday morning and a more pronounced fall in FEV_1 during shift at work. Atopy was a weak predisposing factor and smoking was not a statistically significant factor (31). In a

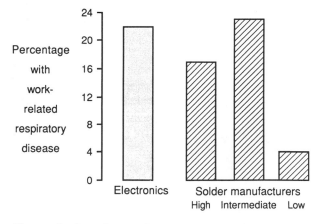

Figure 1 Prevalence of work-related wheeze and breathlessness in electronic workers and manufacturers of colophony fluxes. Significantly lower prevalence seen in the low-exposure group.

subsequent article, Burge et al. validated the use of serial peak expiratory flow rates in the diagnosis of the condition (32). Specific bronchial provocation tests were also used by the authors (33). They found that exposure to colophony for 15 min or less was sufficient to elicit a reaction in all 34 workers tested. Reactions were encountered in six workers tested with abietic acid, the principal resin acid in colophony. There was a poor correlation between the level of nonspecific bronchial responsiveness and the response to colophony but there was an association between the degree of exposure as assessed by the level of resin acid and the likelihood of having work-related symptoms. Work-related symptoms were present in 21% of the two higher-exposure groups and in only 4% of the lowest-exposure group (34). Moreover, exposed workers had a significantly lower FEV_1 than unexposed workers (Fig. 2). Follow-up of 39 workers showed that symptoms persisted in half of the affected workers up to 4 years after exposure ended. Bronchial responsiveness to histamine returned to normal in half of the workers who were no longer exposed ($n = 20$) but it returned to normal in only one of the eight workers who were still indirectly exposed to colophony, thus suggesting that a nonspecific bronchial hyperresponsiveness was the result rather than the cause of the occupational asthma (35). Results of these original works were latter summarized by Burge (36). Others have also described cases of occupational asthma caused by colophony (37,38). Colophony-induced asthma was also confirmed in a poultry vender (39). The mechanism of reaction to colophony remains unknown as no specific antibodies have been found.

More recently, it was found that unheated colophony can also cause occupational asthma (40). The variability of peak expiratory flow rates was assessed by cosinor analysis in workers who were asked to assess their breathing every 1–2 hr for periods of up to 1 year (41). Several parameters calculated from peak expiratory flow data including mesor (24-hr mean), amplitude (24-hr variation), and acrophase (peak time) were different at work and off work.

Burge and co-workers described two cases of occupational asthma caused by another soldering flux containing zinc chloride and ammonium chloride (42). The diagnosis was confirmed by serial monitoring of peak expiratory flows and specific inhalation challenges. Another soldering flux containing polyether alcohol–polypropylene glycol has also been reported to cause occupational asthma (43).

FORMALDEHYDE

Formaldehyde is a chemical used in a wide variety of occupational settings (hospitals, furniture manufacturing, textiles). Formaldehyde can have irritant effects at higher concentrations as described by Harris in 1953 (44) and reviewed more recently (45). A level of 3.0 ppm for the onset of toxic effects has been proposed as a standard. Formaldehyde has been used as insulation in many buildings. Acute (46–50) and chronic (51,52) exposure to formaldehyde in normal and asthmatic subjects at concentrations <3.0 ppm can cause irritation of the nasal and conjunctival mucosa but does not generally result in bronchoconstriction. Some normal subjects may develop acute bronchial obstruction after being exposed to 3.0 ppm of formaldehyde during exercise (53). Challenging workers routinely exposed to formaldehyde at concentrations of 2.0 ppm for 40 min did not cause significant airway constriction (54) although others have found some effect on airway caliber in workers at a carpentry shop after a day at work as compared with a control group (55). Gamble and co-workers found an increase in respiratory symptoms and a decrease in expiratory flow rates at low lung volumes in rubber workers exposed to a

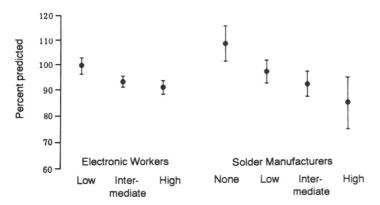

Figure 2 FEV$_1$ values for electronic workers and solder manufacturers, related to exposure to colophony fumes. Significantly higher FEV$_1$ values demonstrated in the no-exposure (none) group.

phenol-formaldehyde resin (56). Schoenberg and Mitchell also found evidence of lower expiratory flow rates in a sample of 63 workers exposed to a phenol-formaldehyde resin (57). Wallenstein and Rebohle nevertheless concluded that the low percentage of work-related symptoms was evidence of formaldehyde's low risk in causing occupational diseases (58).

Formaldehyde can cause occupational asthma as suspected initially by Sakula (59) and Kerfoot and Mooney (60) and reviewed elsewhere (61,62). Hendrick and Lane (63,64) have reported cases where subjects underwent specific inhalation challenges and developed late asthmatic reactions. These were later confirmed by exposing subjects to low concentrations of formaldehyde, which had not been done in the initial reports (65). Subsequent to these early reports, the documentation of formaldehyde asthma was a rare occurrence. Frigas and co-workers were unsuccessful in reproducing bronchial obstruction in 13 subjects with work-related asthma (66). In a study of 230 subjects reporting asthma-like symptoms while being exposed to formaldehyde at work, only 12 had significant bronchoconstriction at levels of 1.0–2.0 ppm during specific inhalation challenges (67). Urea formaldehyde particles can also cause occupational asthma in subjects exposed to this product incorporated in houses (68) and in carpenters (69) as has been confirmed by specific inhalation challenges. Attempts to detect specific antibodies in the sera of subjects exposed to formaldehyde and to relate it to the symptomatology have so far been unfruitful (70–72) except in two case reports (73). However, exposure to gaseous formaldehyde can induce IgE-mediated sensitization in schoolchildren (74). The physical state of formaldehyde is relevant in causing occupational asthma. Cases of occupational asthma caused by formaldehyde resin dust with or without reaction to gaseous formaldehyde were recently described (75). Interestingly, Gannon and co-workers reported seven subjects with occupational asthma to glutaraldehyde (76); of these, three also experienced an asthmatic reaction on exposure to formaldehyde, which suggests cross-reactivity.

CHLORAMINE T AND OTHER BIOCIDES

Chloramine T is a sterilizing agent in the food and beverage industries. It was reported as a cause of occupational asthma in 12 workers of a pharmaceutical company be Feinberg and Watrous in 1945 (77). Other cases of occupational asthma have been observed by different authors (78,79). Late and dual asthmatic reactions to inhalation testing have been documented (80). The mechanism of the reaction is IgE mediated as demonstrated by skin testing (77) and specific IgE assessments. The antigenic determinant is felt to be the *p*-toluenesulfonyl group (81), and no evidence of new antigenic determinants related to the carrier could be demonstrated by Wass and co-workers (82).

Glutaraldehyde and chlorhexidine are disinfectants commonly used by hospital staff in endoscopy units and radiology departments (83–86). Hexachlorophene, a topical disinfectant, can cause occupational asthma as reported and confirmed through specific inhalation challenges, which cause an immediate reaction that was blocked by the use of sodium cromoglycate (87). Lauryl dimethyl benzyl ammonium chloride, a cleaning agent, caused occupational asthma in a pharmacist who was indirectly exposed (88).

Case reports of occupational asthma due to three fungicides, tetrachloroisophthalonitrile (89), tributyl tin oxide (90), and captafol (Difolatan) (91), and organic phosphate insecticides (92) have been described.

PERSULFATE

Individual case reports of occupational asthma due to ammonium persulfate were published as early as in 1957 (93–97) (Pepys, 1976 #7097). Hairdressers are also exposed to henna, a powder derived from the leaves and roots of a shrub that can cause occupational asthma as has been confirmed by specific inhalation challenges in two subjects (98). Paraphenylenediamine is another product handled by hairdressers and has been reported to cause occupational asthma (9). Blainey and co-workers found that four of 23 workers (17%) at a hairdressing salon had occupational asthma, confirmed by specific inhalation challenges carried out in 22 employees with ammonium persulfate (99). However, Merget et al. did not document any case of occupational asthma in 32 employees of a chemical industry in which persulfates were used (100). Some, but not all, workers with occupational asthma to persulfate have evidence of immediate skin reactivity to this product.

DIAZONIUM SALTS AND REACTIVE DYES

Diazonium salts are used in the photocopying process; an azo dye results from their coupling with light. Armeli originally described four cases of workers with lower respiratory tract symptoms on exposure to diazonium salts (101). Graham and co-workers (102) described occupational asthma in one subject who underwent specific inhalation challenges and developed a late asthmatic reaction with recurrent symptoms over the next 2 days. The prevalence of work-related respiratory symptoms and increased specific IgE antibodies to diazonium tetrafluoroborate–HSA conjugates was found to be 57% and 20%, respectively, among 45 workers in the polymer industry (103). All workers with increased specific IgE antibodies ($n = 9$) had work-related respiratory symptoms, whereas none of the asymptomatic workers ($n = 10$) and none of those with irritant symptoms only ($n = 10$) had increased specific IgE levels.

Alanko and co-workers first described and confirmed occupational asthma in four workers exposed to reactive dyes, which are used to create brilliant colors in the textile industry (104). They and others have shown that it is IgE mediated as demonstrated by immediate skin reactivity and increased specific IgE antibodies in the majority of affected workers (105). Recent surveys were carried out in a dye-producing plant (106) and in textile plants (107) where dyes are used. In a survey of a producing plant employing 309 workers, Park and colleagues found that 8% had skin reactivity to Black GR and 7% to Brilliant orange 3R. Slightly more had increased specific IgE levels to Black GR (17%) and to Brilliant orange 3R (13%) (106). Specific inhalation challenges were positive in 13 workers. In a survey of 162 textile plant workers exposed to reactive dyes, Nilsson and co-workers found that 10 had work-related symptoms (107). Of these, five had evidence of immediate allergic reactivity. Park and Hong found increased levels of specific IgG and of specific IgG4 in 23% and 14%, respectively, of the 309 workers who were assessed (108). The presence of increased specific IgG antibodies was associated with increased specific IgE levels and work-related symptoms, although not perfectly so (108).

PHARMACEUTICAL PRODUCTS

The capacity of various pharmaceutical products to induce respiratory sensization has been touched on by several authors (109–111). Chida also found through prospective assessment that the risk of sensitization increases with the degree of exposure (112). Pharmaceutical products derived from proteins or gums (psyllium, ipecacuanha, pancreatic and glandular extracts) are covered in another chapter.

Several antibiotics can cause occupational asthma. In 1946, Rosberg described two nurses with occupational asthma due to sulfathiazoles (113). In 1957, Tara described four subjects who had clinical evidence of asthma after being exposed to penicillin dust (114). Two other cases with evidence of skin and bronchial reactivity to penicillin were described in 1960 (115). Synthetic penicillins can also be the cause of work-related asthma. Carlesi and co-workers described six subjects with asthma caused by amoxicillin (116). Davies and co-workers confirmed the diagnosis of occupational asthma due to ampicillin in three subjects who underwent specific inhalation challenges and experienced isolated late asthmatic reactions (117). Cross-reactivity of ampicillin with penicillin was also demonstrated by the subjects. Penicillamine, which is a synthetic derivative of penicillin, has also been reported as a cause of occupational asthma as demonstrated by a late asthmatic reaction after exposure (118). Piperacillin, a semisynthetic penicillin, can also cause occupational asthma (119). Cephalosphorins induced immediate asthmatic reactions in two pharmaceutical workers (120). The prevalence of occupational asthma due to cephalosporins was found to be 8% (7/91) in 91 workers examined by Briatico-Vangosa and co-workers (121). A third-generation cephalosphorin, ceftazidine, was also incriminated (122). Phenylglycine acid chloride makes up the side chains of ampicillin and other antibiotics. An investigation of 24 workers producing it was performed by Kammermeyer and Mathews (123). Seven subjects had respiratory symptoms and two underwent specific inhalation challenges, which were both positive. Nine subjects had definite immediate skin reactions to phenylglycine acid chloride. In another study, an immediate skin and bronchospastic reaction was documented in a worker exposed to tetracycline (124). Davies and Pepys described one pharmaceutical worker in whom the diagnosis of occupational asthma caused by the macrolide antibiotic spiramycin was confirmed by specific inhalation challenge (125). Evidence of dermatitis and asthma due to spiramycin was also observed in a chick breeder (126). Two other cases were described by Moscato and co-workers, and in one of them, specific inhalation challenges with adipic acid, an additive used to bind spiramycin, elicited an immediate reaction (127). Investigation of all 51 employees at a pharmaceutical company processing spiramycin revealed that four (8%) had occupational asthma as confirmed by specific inhalation tests (128). The mechanism of the reaction has not been determined. Tylosin tartrate is used in animal food as an antibiotic to prevent dysentery. It has been described as causing asthma in a laboratory technician in whom specific inhalation challenges induced a late asthmatic reaction (129).

Alpha-methyldopa can induce late asthmatic reactions, as was shown by Harries and co-workers (130). A glycyl compound used in the preparation of salbutamol has also been incriminated in causing asthma, confirmed by specific challenges that induced a late reaction (131). Amprolium hydrochloride is used as a food additive in poultries to prevent coccidiodomycosis. It has been reported to cause an immediate bronchoconstriction on bronchial challenges (132).

Coutts and co-workers found that eight of 55 subjects (15%) exposed to cimetidine had lower respiratory tract symptoms. In one subject, the diagnosis of occupational asthma was confirmed by specific inhalation challenges that caused a late asthmatic reaction (133). Agius described a pharmaceutical worker exposed to morphine dust who developed symptoms and spirometric changes compatible with occupational asthma (134). Specific IgG and IgG4 antibodies were also demonstrated in workers exposed to morphine with lowering of this level after exposure diminished (135). Two cross-sectional surveys by Moneo and co-workers (136) and Biagini and colleagues (137) found a significant association between the presence of immediate skin wheal and flare and symptoms of lung function abnormalities in 28 and 33 opiate workers, respectively. Isonicotinic acid hydrazide (INH) used for the treatment of tuberculosis can cause occupational asthma as was demonstrated by immediate bronchospasm in a pharmacist for whom evidence of type I sensitization was also confirmed by in vivo and in vitro tests (138,139). Rosenberg and co-workers described two subjects who developed asthma after handling powdered aminophylline (140). Delayed reactions to bronchial challenges were observed. Hydralazine, an antihypertensive drug, has been shown to cause asthma, eliciting a late reaction after a challenge (141). The mechanism of the reaction is unknown. Finally, as discussed in the section on amines, piperazine hydrochloride is used as an antihelminthic drug and can cause occupational asthma.

POLYVINYLCHLORIDE

Polyvinylchloride (PVC) has been reported to cause occupational asthma due to thermal degradation products. Several studies of occupational asthma due to PVC were published between 1973 and 1977. Sokol and co-workers published the first evidence of so-called "meat-wrapper's asthma" in 1973. They described three female subjects who developed symptoms after heating PVC with hot wires (142). Johnston and Anderson described symptoms reported among 15 women employees at a meat-packing plant (143). Similar symptoms were described in another group of meat wrappers and cutters (144). Identification of the thermal degradation products was later made. Although trace amounts of phthalic anydride among several other products were identified, none of the exposed workers had specific IgE antibodies to this chemical (145). Andrasch and co-workers were able to reproduce bronchoconstriction by serial monitoring of FEV_1 after exposure to PVC and to the price label adhesive fumes in some of the workers (146). Unheated PVC dust can cause occupational asthma (147).

ACRYLATES

Kopp and co-workers first described asthma in a subject who used ethylcyanoacrylate instant glue while building model airplanes as a hobby. He developed an isolated late asthmatic reaction after bronchial challenges (148). Pickering and co-workers (149) and Nakazawa (150) described similar individual cases. The largest series was published by Lozewicz and co-workers, who described six subjects as experiencing either isolated late or dual reactions after exposure to methyl methachrylate and cyanoacrylates (151). Artificial nail makers and health professionals are exposed to acrylates. The mechanism of sensitization is unknown. A report of six cases of physician-diagnosed occupational asthma in cosmetologists working with ethyl methacrylate prompted ventilation modifications that would significantly control nail salon technician exposure (152). Ninhydrin used as a laboratory reagent in detection of proteins and peptides caused rhinitis in a laboratory technician (153).

OTHER CHEMICALS

Various chemicals have been incriminated as causes of occupational asthma, primarily in individual case reports or surveys. The list includes:

> Freon contained in propellants (154) and hair-sprays (155)(156) as causing irritation of the airways. Only one case of occupational asthma due to heated freon has been described and confirmed by specific inhalation challenges (157).
>
> Furan used in the production of molds in foundries (158); the diagnosis was confirmed by specific inhalation challenges and serial monitoring or peak expiratory flows.
>
> Paraphenylenediamine in fur workers (24); 37 of 80 workers (46%) had symptoms of asthma; 74% of subjects tested experienced nasal or chest symptoms on specific inhalation challenges performed by inhalation.
>
> Styrene in two plastics manufacturers who had isolated immediate bronchospastic reaction (159).
>
> Enflurane in an anesthesiologist who experienced an asthmatic reaction 11 hr after a specific challenge (160).
>
> Methyl blue contained in ECG ink (161,162) and terpene contained in rubber gloves (163) in hospital employees.
>
> Workers exposed in a fiberglass plant in whom the causative agent could not be identified (164) as well as one worker exposed to plexiglas in whom specific inhalation challenges elicited a dual asthmatic reaction (165); plexiglas is a polyacrylic resin that contains methylmetacrylate, which can cause occupational asthma.
>
> Tetrazene, a powder produced by detonator manufacturers, as demonstrated by suggestive peak flows changes and specific inhalation challenges that induced a late asthmatic reaction (166).
>
> Sodium iso-nonanoyl oxybenzene sulphonate (SINOS) in detergent workers, as confirmed by specific inhalation challenges in three workers; the mechanism of the late reaction remains unexplained (167,168).
>
> Polyethylene (169), polypropylene (170), and polyester contained in electrostatic paints (171).
>
> Various machining fluids reported to cause acute pulmonary responses in some (172), but not others (173); oil mists have also been incriminated in occupational asthma (174,175); for at least one subject, the causal agent may be a pine odorant additive (176,177).

Various acids (hydrochloric, hydrofluoric, nitric, perchloric, and sulfuric) although it is not clear whether these reactions are "irritant" or reflect true sensitization (178).

STRUCTURE-ACTIVITY RELATIONSHIPS OF RESPIRATORY SENSITIZATION POTENTIAL

Agius and co-workers have set various hypothetical mechanisms, based on structure-activity relationship, for the interactions of low-molecular-weight agents, mainly chemical agents, with human machomolecules (179). Karol and co-workers have introduced a model for predicting respiratory sensitization by comparing structure-activity relationships of chemicals as potential sensitizers in a computer-based expert system, Multi Case (180). This system enables prediction of sensitizing activity based on structural fragments and physicochemical properties of chemicals in the database. Approaches to the identification of chemical respiratory sensitizers in a mouse model have been proposed by Kimber et al. (181). Contact allergens, which do not generally cause sensitization of the respiratory tract, provoke a TH1-type immune response with high levels of interferon-gamma. Exposure of mice to chemical respiratory sensitizers results in the generation of selective TH2 immune responses with the production of cytokines (IL-4 and IL-10). This differential response, referred to as "cytokine fingerprinting," may provide a clue on the likelihood that a chemical product will cause predominant skin or respiratory sensitization.

MULTIPLE CHEMICAL SENSITIVITY (MCS) SYNDROME

There are claims that an unusual assortment of symptoms such as headaches, rashes, food intolerance, confusion, chronical vaginal yeast infections, depression, confusion, fatigue, and mental disorientation occur after single or chronic exposures such as factory workers commonly experience in contact with low levels of organic solvents used in various manufacturing processes (182). A rash of MCS claims may also occur after exposure to unknown agent(s) associated with the sick building syndrome. Multiple synonyms have been used for MCS. These include total environmental allergy, ecological illness, environmental illness, twentieth-century disease, and the immune dysregulation syndrome. No clear-cut pattern of symptoms has emerged to distinguish a homogeneous group of patients that would be suitable for epidemiological investigation. Claims of altered immune responses after exposure to certain chemicals have not been substantiated. One hypothesis that has been proposed is that MCS symptoms represent a chemically triggered syndrome that could alter brain levels of neurotransmitters such as serotonin or acetylcholine. This speculation has not been tested. Several series of typical patients with this syndrome have been evaluated. The common denominator of these clinical reports is a patient presenting with somatoform symptoms as a physical explanation for either unrecognized or self-denied psychiatric disorder. Despite these inconsistencies, patients with this problem claimed to be relieved when they avoid many common environmental agents. Sometimes patients with this disorder have gone to extremes of building "safe rooms" and wearing charcoal filter or full head gas masks. Patients having these symptoms also claim that prior exposures to one or several chemicals were the triggers of current responses to a broad range of unrelated chemicals or odors. None of these multiple chemical reactions have been documented by objective immune or provocative responses (183). It should be emphasized that the atypical and at times bizarre spectrum of nonpulmonary symptoms associated with the MCS syndrome bears no relationship to RADS or other chemically induced cases of occupational asthma. Therefore, disability compensation of MCS symptoms based on prior occupational exposure alone is not justified by the available facts.

CONCLUSION

With the increased use of new chemical products steadily appearing in workplace settings, it is highly probable that the list of agents categorized under the heading of miscellaneous chemical products causing occupational asthma will grow. It is also likely that the increased use of these products will result not only in more documentation of individual cases but also proper surveys of workplaces where the products are used. As for other low-molecular-weight agents, more studies exploring the mechanism of sensitization are needed.

REFERENCES

1. Ferris BG, Peters JM, Burgess WA, Cherry RB. Apparent effect of an azodicarbonamide on the lungs. A preliminary report. J Occup Med 1977; 19:424–425.
2. Slovak AJM. Occupational asthma caused by a plastics blowing agent, azodicarbonamide. Thorax 1981; 36:906–909.
3. Malo JL, Pineau L, Cartier A. Occupational asthma due to azobisformamide. Clin Allergy 1985; 15:261–264.
4. Valentino M, Comai M. Occupational asthma from azodicarbonamide: casereport. G Ital Med Lav 1985; 7:97–99.
5. Normand J-C, Grange F, Hernandez C, Ganay A, Davezies P, Bergeret A, Prost G. Occupational asthma after exposure to azodicarbonamide: report of four cases. Br J Ind Med 1989; 46:60–62.
6. Hagmar L, Nielsen J, Skerfving S. Clinical features and epidemiology of occupational obstructive respiratory disease caused by small molecular weight organic chemicals. In: Epidemiology of Allergic Diseases. Monogr Allergy, 1987:42–58.
7. Dernehl CU. Clinical experiences with exposures to ethylene diamines. Ind Med Surg 1951; 20:541–546.
8. Dernehi CU. Hazards to health associated with the use of epoxy resins. J Occup Med 1963; 5:17–21.
9. Gelfand HH. Respiratory allergy due to chemical compounds encountered in the rubber, lacquer, shellac, and beauty culture industries. J Allergy 1963; 34:374–381.
10. Sterling GM. Asthma due to aluminium soldering flux. Thorax 1967; 22:533–537.
11. Pepys J, Pickering CAC. Asthma due to inhaled chemical fumes—amino-ethil ethanolamine in aluminium soldering flux. Clin Allergy 1972; 2:197–204.
12. Lam S, Chan-Yeung M. Ethylenediamine-induced asthma. Am Rev Respir Dis 1980; 121:151–155.
13. Vallières M, Cockcroft DW, Taylor DM, Dolovich J, Hargreave FE. Dimethyl ethanolamine–induced asthma. Am Rev Respir Dis 1977; 115:867–871.
14. Sargent EV, Mitchell CA, Brubaker RE. Respiratory effects of occupational exposure to an epoxy resin system. Arch Environ Health 1976; 31:236–240.
15. Brubaker RE, Muranko HJ, Smith DB, Beck GJ, Scovel G. Evaluation and control of a respiratory exposure to 3-(dimethylamino)propylamine. J Occup Med 1979; 21:688–690.

16. Ng TP, Lee HS, Malik MA, Chee CBE, Cheong TH, Wang YT. Asthma in chemical workers exposed to aliphatic polyamines. Occup Med 1995; 45:45–48.

17. Savonius B, Keskinen H, Tuppurainen M, Kanerva L. Occupational asthma caused by ethanolamines. Allergy 1994; 49:877–881.

18. McCullagh SF. Allergenicity of piperazine: a study in environmental aetiology. Br J Ind Med 1968; 25:319–325.

19. Pepys J, Pickering CAC, Loudon HWG. Asthma due to inhaled chemical agents—piperazine dihydrochloride. Clin Allergy 1972; 2:189–196.

20. Bernstein JA, Stauder T, Bernstein DI, Bernstein IL. A combined respiratory and cutaneous hypersensitivity syndrome induced by work exposure to quaternary amines. J Allergy Clin Immunol 1994; 94:257–259.

21. Hagmar L, Bellander T, Bergöö B, Simonsson BG. Piperazine-induced occupational asthma. J Occup Med 1982; 24:193–197.

22. Hagmar L, Welinder H. Prevalence of specific IgE antibodies against piperazine in employees of a chemical plant. Int Arch Allergy Appl Immunol 1986; 81:12–16.

23. Hagmar L, Bellander T, Ranstam J, Skerfving S. Piperazine-induced airway symptoms: exposure-response relationships and selection in an occupational setting. Am J Ind Med 1984; 6:347–357.

24. Silberman DE, Sorrell AH. Allergy in fur workers with special reference to paraphenylenediamine. J Allergy 1959; 30:11–18.

25. Belin L, Wass U, Audunsson G, Mathiasson L. Amines: possible causative agents in the development of bronchial hyperreactivity in workers manufacturing polyurethanes from isocyanates. Br J Ind Med 1983; 40:251–257.

26. Candura F, Moscato G. Do amines induce occupational asthma in workers manufacturing polyurethane foams. Br J Ind Med 1984; 41:552–553.

27. Fawcett IW, Newman Taylor AJ, Pepys J. Asthma due to inhaled chemical agents—fumes from "Multicore" soldering flux and colophony resin. Clin Allergy 1976; 6:577–585.

28. Burge PS, Harries MG, O'Brien IM, Pepys J. Respiratory disease in workers exposed to solder flux fumes containing colophony (pine resin). Clin Allergy 1978; 8:1–14.

29. Burge PS, Perks W, O'Brien IM, Hawkins R, Green M. Occupational asthma in an electronics factory. Thorax 1979; 34:13–18.

30. Herks WH, Burge PS, Rehahn M, Green M. Work-related respiratory disease in employees leaving an electronics factory. Thorax 1979; 34:19–22.

31. Burge PS, Perks WH, O'Brien IM, Burge A, Hawkins R, Brown D, Green M. Occupational asthma in an electronics factory: a case control study to evaluate aetiological factors. Thorax 1979; 34:300–307.

32. Burge PS, O'Brien IM, Harries MG. Peak flow rate records in the diagnosis of occupational asthma due to colophony. Thorax 1979; 34:308–316.

33. Burge PS, Harries MG, O'Brien I, Pepys J. Bronchial provocation studies in workers exposed to the fumes of electronic soldering fluxes. Clin Allergy 1980; 10:137–149.

34. Burge PS, Edge G, Hawkins R, White V, Taylor AN. Occupational asthma in a factory making flux-cored solder containing colophony. Thorax 1981; 36:828–834.

35. Burge PS. Occupational asthma in electronics workers caused by colophony fumes: follow-up of affected workers. Thorax 1982; 37:348–353.

36. Burge PS. Occupational asthma due to soft soldering fluxes containing colophony (rosin, pine resin). Eur J Respir Dis 1982; 63(Suppl 123):65–67.

37. Innocenti A, Loi F. Occupational allergic asthma due to colophony. Med Lavoro 1978; 69: 720–722.

38. Maestrelli P, Alessandri MV, Vecchio L Dal, Bartolucci GB, Cocheo V. Occupational asthma due to colophony. Med Lavoro 1985; 76:371–378.

39. So SY, Lam WK, Yu D. Colophony-induced asthma in a poultry vender. Clin Allergy 1981; II:395–399.

40. Burge PS, Wieland A, Robertson AS, Weir D. Occupational asthma due to unheated colophony. Br J Ind Med 1986; 43:559–560.

41. Randem B, Smolensky MH, Hsi B, Albright D, Burge S. Field survey of circadian rhythm in PEF of electronics workers suffering from colophony-induced asthma. Chronobiol Int 1987; 4:263–271.

42. Weir DC, Robertson AS, Jones S, Burge PS. Occupational asthma due to soft corrosive soldering fluxes containing zinc chloride and ammonium chloride. Thorax 1989; 44:220–223.

43. Stevens JJ. Asthma due to soldering flux: a polyether alcohol-polypropylene glycol mixture. Ann Allergy 1976; 36:419–422.

44. Harris DK. Health problems in the manufacture and use of plastics. Br J Ind Med 1953; 10: 255–268.

45. Niemelä R, Vainio H. Formaldehyde exposure in work and the general environment. Scand J Work Environ Health 1981; 7:95–100.

46. Sheppard D, Eschenbacher WL, Epstein J. Lack of bronchomotor response to up to 3 ppm formaldehyde in subjects with asthma. Environ Res 1984; 35:133–139.

47. Witek TJ, Schachter EN, Tosun T, Beck GJ, Leaderer BP. An evaluation of respiratory effects following exposure to 2.0 ppm formaldehyde in asthmatics: lung function, symptoms, and airway reactivity. Arch Environ Health 1987; 42:230–237.

48. Sauder LR, Green DJ, Chatham MD, Kulle TJ. Acute pulmonary response of asthmatics to 3.0 ppm formaldehyde. Toxicol Ind Health 1987; 3:569–578.

49. Harving H, Korsgaard J, Dahl R. Low concentrations of formaldehyde in bronchial asthma: a study of exposure under controlled conditions. Br Med J 1986; 293:310.

50. Harving H, Korsgaard J, Pedersen OF, Molhave L, Dahl R. Pulmonary function and bronchial reactivity in asthmatics during low-level formaldehyde exposure. Lung 1990; 168:15–21.

51. Uba G, Pachorek D, Bernstein J, Garabrant DH, Balmes JR, Wright WE, Amar RB. Prospective study of respiratory effects of formaldehyde among healthy and asthmatic medical students. Am J Ind Med 1989; 15:91–101.

52. Tuthill RW. Woodstoves, formaldehyde, and respiratory disease. Am J Epidemiol 1984; 120: 952–955.

53. Green DJ, Sauder LR, Kulle TJ, Bascom R. Acute response to 3.0 ppm formaldehyde in exercising healthy nonsmokers and asthmatics. Am Rev Respir Dis 1987; 135:1261–1266.

54. Schachter EN, Witek Jr TJ, Brody DJ, Tosun T, Beck GJ, Leaderer BP. A study of respiratory effects from exposure to 2.0 ppm formaldehyde in occupationally exposed workers. Environ Res 1987; 44:188–205.

55. Alexandersson R, Kolmodin-Hedman B, Hedenstierna G. Exposure to formaldehyde: effects on pulmonary function. Arch Environ Health 1982; 37:279–284.

56. Gamble JF, McMichael AJ, Williams T, Battigelli M. Respiratory function and symptoms: an environmental-epidemiological study of rubber workers exposed to a phenol-formaldehyde type resin. Am Ind Hyg Assoc J 1976; 37:499–513.

57. Schoenberg JB, Mitchell CA. Airway disease caused by phenolic (phenol-formaldehyde) resin exposure. Arch Environ Health 1975; 30:574–577.

58. Wallenstein G, Rebohle E. Sensibilisierungen durch formaldehyd bei beruflicher inhalativer exposition. Allerg Immunol 1976; 22:287–295.

59. Sakula A. Formalin asthma in hospital laboratory staff. Lancet 1975; 2:816.

60. Kerfoot EJ, Mooney TF. Formaldehyde and paraformaldehyde study in funeral homes. Am Ind Hyg Assoc J 1975; 36:533–537.

61. Editorial. Formalin asthma. Lancet 1977; 1:790.

62. Editorial. Formaldehyde toxicity. Lancet 1979; 620.

63. Hendrick DJ, Lane DJ. Occupational formalin asthma. Br J Ind Med 1977; 34:11–18.

64. Hendrick DJ, Lane DJ. Formalin asthma in hospital staff. Br Med J 1975; 1:607–608.

65. Hendrick DJ, Rando RJ, Lane DJ, Morris MJ. Formaldehyde asthma: challenge exposure levels and fate after five years. J Occup Med 1982; 24:893–897.

66. Frigas E, Filley WV, Reed CE. Bronchial challenge with formaldehyde gas: lack of bronchoconstriction in 13 patients suspected of having formaldehyde-induced asthma. Mayo Clin Proc 1984; 59:295–299.

67. Nordman H, Keskinen H, Tuppurainen M. Formaldehyde asthma—rare or overlooked? J Allergy Clin Immunol 1985; 75:91–99.

68. Frigas E, Filley WV, Reed CE. Asthma induced by dust from urea-formaldehyde foam insulating material. Chest 1981; 79:706–707.

69. Cockcroft DW, Hoeppner VH, Dolovich J. Occupational asthma caused by cedar urea formaldehyde particle board. Chest 1982; 82:49–53.

70. Patterson R, Pateras V, Grammer LC, Harris KE. Human antibodies against formaldehyde–human serum albumin conjugates or human serum albumin in individuals exposed to formaldehyde. Int Arch Allergy Appl Immunol 1986; 79:53–59.

71. Kramps JA, Peltenburg LTC, Kerklaan PRM, Spieksma FTM, Valentijn RM, Dijkman JG. Measurement of specific IgE antibodies in individuals exposed to formaldehyde. Clin Allergy 1989; 19:509–514.

72. Grammer LC, Harris KE, Shaughnessy MA, Sparks P, Ayars GH, Altman LC, Patterson R. Clinical and immunologic evaluation of 37 workers exposed to gaseous formaldehyde. J Allergy Clin Immunol 1990; 86:177–181.

73. Wüthrich EIB. Formaldehyd- und phthalisches anydrid-asthma. Schweiz Med Wochenschr 1988; 118:1568–1572.

74. Wantke F, Demmer CM, Tappler P, Gotz M, Jarisch R. Exposure to gaseous formaldehyde induces IgE-mediated sensitization to formaldehyde in school-children. Clin Exp Allergy 1996; 26:276–280.

75. Lemière C, Desjardins A, Cloutier Y, Drolet D, Perrault G, Cartier A, Malo JL. Occupational asthma due to formaldehyde resin dust with and without reaction to formaldehyde gas. Eur Respir J 1995; 8:861–865.

76. Gannon PFG, Bright P, Campbell M, O'Hickey SP, Burge P Sherwood. Occupational asthma due to glutaraldehyde and formaldehyde in endoscopy and X ray departments. Thorax 1995; 50:156–159.

77. Feinberg SM, Watrous RM. Atopy to simple chemical compounds-sulfonechloramides. J Allergy 1945; 16:209–220.

78. Bourne MS, Flindt MLH, Walker JM. Asthma due to industrial use of chloramine. Br Med J 1979; 2:10–12.

79. Charles TJ. Asthma due to industrial use of chloramine. Br Med J 1979; 1:334.

80. Dijkman JG, Vooren PH, Kramps JA. Occupational asthma due to inhalation of chloramine-T. 1. Clinical observations and inhalation-provocation studies. Int Archs Allergy Appl Immunol 1981; 64:422–427.

81. Kramps JA, van Toorenenbergen AW, Vooren PH, Dijkman JH. Occupational asthma due to inhalation of chloramine-T. II. Demonstration of specific IgE antibodies. Int Arch Allergy Appl Immunol 1981; 64:428–438.

82. Wass U, Belin L, Eriksson NE. Immunological specificity of chloramine-T-induced IgE antibodies in serum from a sensitized worker. Clin Allergy 1989; 19:463–471.

83. Jachuck SJ, Bound PG, Steel J, Blain PG. Occupational hazard in hospital staff exposed to 2 per cent glutaraldehyde in an endoscopy unit. J Soc Occup Med 1989; 39:69–71.

84. Burge PS. Occupational risks of glutaraldehyde. Br Med J 1989; 299:1451.

85. Waclawski ER, McAlpine LG, Thomson NC. Occupational asthma in nurses caused by chlorhexidine and alcohol aerosols. Br Med J 1989; 298:929–930.

86. Cullinan P, Hayes J, Cannon J, Madan L, Heap D, Taylor A Newman. Occupational asthma in radiographers. Lancet 1992; 340:1477.

87. Nagy L, Orosz M. Occupational asthma due to hexachlorophene. Thorax 1984; 39:630–631.

88. Burge PS, Richardson MN. Occupational asthma due to indirect exposure to lauryl dimethyl benzyl ammonium chloride used in a floor cleaner. Thorax 1994; 49:842–843.

89. Honda I, Kohrogi H, Ando M, Araki S, Ueno T, Futatsuka M, Ueda A. Occupational asthma induced by the fungicide tetrachloroisophthalonitrile. Thorax 1992; 47:760–761.

90. Shelton D, Urch B, Tarlo SM. Occupational asthma induced by a carpet fungicide—tributyl tin oxide. J Allergy Clin Immunol 1992; 90:274–275.

91. Royce S, Wald P, Sheppard D, Balmes J. Occupational asthma in a pesticides manufacturing worker. Chest 1993; 103:295–296.

92. Weiner A. Bronchial asthma due to the organic phosphate insecticides. Ann Allergy 1961; 19:397–401.

93. Pichat R, Chatanay R. A propos d'un asthme au persulfate d'ammonium. Arch Mal Prof 1957; 18:280–282.

94. Hardel PJ, Reybet-Degat O, Jeannin L, Paqueron M-J. Asthme des coiffeurs: danger des décolorants capillaires contenant des persulfates alcalins. Nouv Presse Med 1978; 7:4151.

95. Gaultier M, Gervais P, Mellerio F. Deux causes d'asthme professionnel chez les coiffeurs: persulfate et soie. Arch Mal Prof 1966; 27:809–813.

96. Baur X, Fruhmann G, Liebe VV. Occupational asthma and dermatitis after exposure to dusts of persulfate salts in two industrial workers. Respiration 1979; 38:144–150.

97. Parra FM, Igea JM, Quirce S, Ferrando MC, Martin JA, Losada E. Occupational asthma in a hairdresser caused by persulphate salts. Allergy 1992; 47:656–660.

98. Starr JC, Yunginger J, Brahser GW. Immediate type I asthmatic response to henna following occupational exposure in hairdressers. Ann Allergy 1982; 48:98–99.

99. Blainey AD, Ollier S, Cundell D, Smith RE, Davies RJ. Occupational asthma in a hairdressing salon. Thorax 1986; 41:42–50.

100. Merget R, Buenemann A, Kulzer R, Rueckmann A, Breitstadt R, Kniffka A, Kratisch H, Vormberg R, Schultze-Werninghaus G. A cross sectional study of chemical industry workers with occupational exposure to persulphates. Occup Environ Med 1996; 53:422–426.

101. Armeli G. Bronchial asthma from diazonium salts. Med Lav 1968; 59:463–466.

102. Graham V, Coe MJS, Davies RJ. Occupational asthma after exposure to a diazonium salt. Thorax 1981; 36:950–951.

103. Luczynska CM, Hutchcroft BJ, Harrison MA, Dornan JD, Topping MD. Occupational asthma and specific IgE to diazonium salt intermediate used in the polymer industry. J Allergy Clin Immunol 1990; 85:1076–1082.

104. Alanko K, Keskinen H, Byorksten F, Ojanen S. Immediate-type hypersensitivity to reactive dyes. Clin Allergy 1978; 8:25–31.

105. Topping MD, Forster HW, Ide CW, Kennedy FM, Leach AM, Sorkin S. Respiratory allergy and specific immunoglobin E and immunoglobin G antibodies to reactive dyes used in the wool industry. J Occup Med 1989; 31:857–862.

106. Park HS, Lee MK, Kim BO, Lee KJ, Roh JH, Moon YH, Hong CS. Clinical and immunologic evaluations of reactive dye-exposed workers. J Allergy Clin Immunol 1991; 87:639–649.

107. Nilsson R, Nordlinder R, Wass U, Meding B, Belin L. Asthma, rhinitis, and dermatitis in workers exposed to reactive dyes. Br J Ind Med 1993; 50:65–70.

108. Park HS, Hong CS. The significance of specific IgG and IgG4 antibodies to a reactive dye in exposed workers. Clin Exp Allergy 1991; 21:357–362.

109. Romanski B, Zegarski W. Etiologie de l'asthme et des lésions allergiques de la peau chez les ouvriers d'une usine pharmaceutique. Toulouse Méd 1963; 64:802–804.

110. Kobayashi S, Yamamura Y, Frick OL, Horiuchi Y, Kishimoto S, Miyamoto T, (ed) Naranjo P, (ed) De Weck A. Occupational asthma due to inhalation of pharmacological dusts and other chemical agents with some reference to other occupational asthmas in Japan. Allergology. Proceedings of the VIII International Congress of Allergology, Tokyo, October 1973. Amsterdam: Excerpta Medica, 1974:124–132.

111. Fueki R. Different Aspects of Occupational Asthma in Japan. Occupational Asthma. London: Von Nostrand Reinhold, 1980:229–244.

112. Chida TA. A study on dose-response relationship of occupational allergy in pharmaceutical plant. Jpn J Ind Health 1986; 28:77–86.

113. Rosberg M. Asthma bronchiale caused by sulphathiazole. Acta Med Scand 1946; 126:185–190.

114. Tara S. Asthme à la pénicilline. Arch Mal Prof 1957; 18:274–277.

115. Gaultier M, Fournier E, Gervais P. L'asthme professionnel par allergie à la pénicilline. Arch Mal Prof 1960; 21:13–23.

116. Carlesi G, Ferrea E, Melino C, Messineo A, Pacelli E. Aspects of environmental health and of pathology caused by pollution with amoxicillin in a pharmaceutical industry. Nuovi Ann Igiene Microbiol 1979; 30:185–196.

117. Davies RJ, Hendrick DJ, Pepys J. Asthma due to inhaled chemical agents: ampicillin, bensyl penicillin, 6 amino penicillanic acid and related substances. Clin Allergy 1974; 4:227–247.

118. Lagier F, Cartier A, Dolovich J, Malo J-L. Occupational asthma in a pharmaceutical worker exposed to penicillamine. Thorax 1989; 44:157–158.

119. Moscato G, Galdi E, Scibilia J, Dellabianca A, Omodeo P, Vittadini G, Biscaldi GP. Occupational asthma, rhinitis and urticaria due to piperacillin sodium in a pharmaceutical worker. Eur Respir J 1995; 8:467–469.

120. Coutts II, Dally MB, Taylor AJ Newman, Pickering CAC, Horsfield N. Asthma in workers manufacturing cephalosporins. Br Med J 1981; 283:950.

121. Briatico-Vangosa G, Beretta F, Bianchi S, Cardani A, Marchisio M, Nava C, Talamo F. Bronchial asthma due to 7-aminocephalosporanic acid (7-ACA) in workers employed in cephalosporine production. Med Lav 1981; 72:488–493.

122. Stenton SC, Dennis JH, Hendrick DJ. Occupational asthma due to ceftazidime. Eur Respir J 1995; 8:1421–1423.

123. Kammermeyer JK, Mathews KP. Hypersensitivity to phenylglycine acid chloride. J Allergy Clin Immunol 1973; 52:73–84.

124. Menon MPS, Das AK. Tetracycline asthma—a case report. Clin Allergy 1977; 7:285–290.

125. Davies RJ, Pepys J. Asthma due to inhaled chemical agents—the macrolide antibiotic Spiramycin. Clin Allergy 1975; 1:99–107.

126. Paggiaro PL, Loi AM, Toma G. Bronchial asthma and dermatitis due to spiramycin in a chick breeder. Clin Allergy 1979; 9:571–574.

127. Moscato G, Naldi L, Candura F. Bronchial asthma due to spiramycin and adipic acid. Clin Allergy 1984; 14:355–361.

128. Malo J-L, Cartier A. Occupational asthma in workers of a pharmaceutical company processing spiramycin. Thorax 1988; 43:371–377.

129. Lee HS, Wang YT, Yeo CT, Tan KT, Ratnam KV. Occupational asthma due to tylosin tartrate. Br J Ind Med 1989; 46:498–499.

130. Harries MG, Newman Taylor A, Wooden J, MacAuslan A. Bronchial asthma due to alpha-methyldopa. Br Med J 1979; 1461.

131. Fawcett IW, Pepys J, Erooga MA. Asthma due to "glycyl compound" powder—an intermediate in production of salbutamol. Clin Allergy 1976; 6:405–409.

132. Greene SA, Freedman S. Asthma due to inhaled chemical agents—amprolium hydrochloride. Clin Allergy 1976; 6:105–108.

133. Coutts II, Lozewicz S, Dally MB, Newman Taylor AJ, Burge PS, Flind AC, Rogers DJH. Respiratory symptoms related to work in a factory manufacturing cimetidine tablets. Br Med J 1984; 288:1418.

134. Agius R. Opiate inhalation and occupational asthma. Br Med J 1989; 298–323.

135. Biagini RE, Klincewicz SL, Henningsen GM, MacKenzie BA, Gallagher JS, Bernstein DI, Bernstein IL. Antibodies to morphine in workers exposed to opiates at a narcotics manufacturing facility and evidence for similar antibodies in heroin abusers. Life Sci 1990; 47:897–908.

136. Moneo I, Alday E, Ramos C, Curiel G. Occupational asthma caused by *Papaver somniferum*. Allergol Immunopathol 1993; 21:145–148.

137. Biagini RE, Bernstein DM, Klincewicz SL, Mittman R, Bernstein IL, Henningsen GM. Evaluation of cutaneous responses and lung function from exposure to opiate compounds among ethical narcotics-manufacturing workers. J Allergy Clin Immunol 1992; 89:108–117.

138. Asai S, Shimoda T, Hara K, Fujiwara K. Occupational asthma caused by isonicotinic acid hydrazide (INH) inhalation. J Allergy Clin Immunol 1987; 80:578–582.

139. Fujiwara K, Saita T, Shimoda T, Asai S, Hara K. Isonicotinic acid hydrazide as an antigen. J Allergy Clin Immunol 1987; 80:582–585.

140. Rosenberg M, Aaronson D, Evans C. Asthmatic responses to inhaled aminophylline: a report of two cases. Ann Allergy 1984; 52:97–98.

141. Perrin B, Malo JL, Cartier A, Evans S, Dolovich J. Occupational asthma in a pharmaceutical worker exposed to hydralazine. Thorax 1990; 45:980–981.

142. Sokol WN, Aelony Y, Beall GN. Meat-wrapper's asthma. A new syndrome? JAMA 1973; 226:639–641.

143. Johnston CJ, Anderson HW. Meat-wrappers asthma: a case study. J Occup Med 1976; 18: 102–104.

144. Brooks SM, Vandervort R. Polyvinyl chloride film thermal decomposition products as an occupational illness. 2. Clinical studies. J Occup Med 1977; 19:192–196.

145. Vandervort R, Brooks SM. Polyvinyl chloride film thermal decomposition products as an occupational illness. 1. Environmental exposures and toxicology. J Occup Med 1977; 19: 188–191.

146. Andrasch RH, Bardana EJ, Koster F, Pirofsky B. Clinical and bronchial provocation studies in patients with meatwrapper's asthma. J Allergy Clin Immunol 1976; 58:291–298.

147. Lee HS, Yap J, Wang YT, Lee CS, Tan KT, Poh SC. Occupational asthma due to unheated polyvinylchloride resin dust. Br J Ind Med 1989; 46:820–822.

148. Kopp SK, McKay RT, Moller DR, Cassedy K, Brooks SM. Asthma and rhinitis due to ethylcyanoacrylate instant glue. Ann Intern Med 1985; 102:613–615.

149. Pickering CAC, Bainbridge D, Birtwistle IH, Griffiths DL. Occupational asthma due to methyl methacrylate in an orthopaedic theatre sister. Br Med J 1986; 292:1362–1363.

150. Nakazawa T. Occupational asthma due to alkyl cyanoacrylate. J Occup Med 1990; 32:709–710.

151. Lozewicz S, Davison AG, Hopkirk A, Burge PS, Boldy D, Riordan JF, McGivern DV, Platts BW, Davies D, Newman Taylor AJ. Occupational asthma due to methyl methacrylate and cyanoacrylates. Thorax 1985; 40:836–839.

152. Spencer AB, Estill CF, McCammon JB, Mickelsen RL, Johnston OE. Control of ethyl methacrylate exposures during the application of artificial fingernails. Am Ind Hyg J 1997; 58: 214–218.

153. Hytonen M, Martimo KP, Estlander T, Tupasela O. Occupational IgE-mediated rhinitis caused by ninhydrin. Allergy 1996; 51:114–116.

154. Sterling GM, Batten JC. Effect of aerosol propellants and surfactants on airway resistance. Thorax 1969; 24:228–231.

155. Zuskin E, Bouhuys A. Acute airway responses to hair-spray preparations. N Engl J Med 1974; 290:660–663.

156. Schlueter DP, Soto RJ, Baretta ED, Herrmann AA, Ostrander LE, Stewart RD. Airway response to hair spray in normal subjects and subjects with hyperreactive airways. Chest 1979; 75:544–548.

157. Malo JL, Gagnon G, Cartier A. Occupational asthma due to heated freon. Thorax 1984; 39: 628–629.

158. Cockcroft DW, Cartier A, Jones G, Tarlo SM, Dolovich J, Hargreave FE. Asthma caused by occupational exposure to a furan-based binder system. J Allergy Clin Immunol 1980; 66: 458–463.

159. Moscato G, Biscaldi G, Cottica D, Pugliese F, Candura S, Candura F. Occupational asthma due to styrene: two case reports. J Occup Med 1987; 29:957–960.

160. Schwettmann RS, Casterline CL. Delayed asthmatic response following occupational exposure to enflurane. Anesthesiology 1976; 44:166–169.

161. Keskinen H, Nordman H, Terho EO. ECG ink as a cause of asthma. Allergy 1981; 36:275–276.

162. Rodenstein D, Stanescu DC. Bronchial asthma following exposure to ECG ink. Ann Allergy 1982; 48:351–352.

163. Seaton A, Cherrie B, Turnbull J. Rubber glove asthma. Br Med J 1988; 296:531–532.

164. Finnegan MJ, Pickering CAC, Burge PS, Goffe TRP, Austwick PKC, Davies PS. Occupational asthma in a fibre glass works. J Soc Occup Med 1985; 35:121–127.

165. Kennes B, Garcia-Herreros P, Sierckx P. Asthma from plexiglas powders. Clin Allergy 1981; 11:49–54.
166. Burge P Sherwood, Hendy M, Hodgson ES. Occupational asthma, rhinitis, and dermatitis due to tetrazene in a detonator manufacturer. Thorax 1984; 39:470–471.
167. Hendrick DJ, Connolly MJ, Stenton SC, Bird AG, Winterton IS, Walters EH. Occupational asthma due to sodium iso-nonanoyl oxybenzene sulphonate, a newly developed detergent ingredient. Thorax 1988; 43:501–502.
168. Stenton SC, Dennis JH, Walters EH, Hendrick DJ. Asthmagenic properties of a newly developed detergent ingredient: sodium iso-nonanoyl oxybenzene sulphonate. Br J Ind Med 1990; 47:405–410.
169. Gannon PFG, Burge P Sherwood, Benfield CFA. Occupational asthma due to polyethylene shrink wrapping (paper wrapper's asthma). Thorax 1992; 47:759.
170. Malo JL, Cartier A, Pineault L, Dugas M, Desjardins A. Occupational asthma due to heated polypropylene. Eur Respir J 1994; 7:415–417.
171. Cartier A, Vandenplas O, Grammer LC, Shaughnessy MA, Malo JL. Respiratory and systemic reaction following exposure to heated electrostatic polyester paint. Eur Respir J 1994; 7:608–611.
172. Kennedy SM, Greaves IA, Kriebel D, Eisen EA, Smith TJ, Woskie SR. Acute pulmonary responses among automobile workers exposed to aerosols of machining fluids. Am J Ind Med 1989; 15:627–641.
173. Dumas JP, Smolik HJ, Camus P, Jeannin L, Marin A, Klepping J. Réctivité bronchique et exposition professionnelle aux fluides de coupe. Arch Mal Prof 1987; 48:213–221.
174. Massin N, Bohadana AB, Wild P, Goutet P, Kirstetter H, Toamain JP. Airway responsiveness, respiratory symptoms, and exposures to soluble oil mist in mechanical workers. Occup Environ Med 1996; 53:748–752.
175. Rosenman KD, Reilly MJ, Kalinowski D. Work-related asthma and respiratory symptoms among workers exposed to metal-working fluids. Am J Ind Med 1997; 32:325–331.
176. Hendy MS, Beattie BE, Burge PS. Occupational asthma due to an emulsified oil mist. Br J Ind Med 1985; 42:51–54.
177. Robertson AS, Weir DC, Burge PS. Occupational asthma due to oil mists. Thorax 1988; 43:200–205.
178. Musk AW, Peach S, Ryan G. Occupational asthma in a mineral analysis laboratory. Br J Ind Med 1988; 45:381–386.
179. Agius RM, Nee J, McGovern B, Robertson A. Structure activity hypothesis in occupational asthma caused by low molecular weight substances. Ann Occup Hyg 1991; 35:129–137.
180. Karol MH, Graham C, Gealy R, Macina OT, Sussman N, Rosenkranz HS. Structure-activity relationships and computer-assisted analysis of respiratory sensitization potential. Toxicol Lett 1996; 86:187–191.
181. Kimber I, Bernstein IL, Karol MH, Robinson MK, Sarlo K, Selgrade MK. Identification of respiratory allergens. Fund Appl Toxicol 1996; 33:1–10.
182. Black DW, Rathe A. Total environmental allergy: 20th century disease or deception. Res Staff Phys 1990; 34:47–54.
183. Barinaga M. Better data needed on sensitivity syndrome. Science 1991; 251:1558.

29

Western Red Cedar (*Thuja plicata*) and Other Wood Dusts

Moira Chan-Yeung
Vancouver General Hospital and University of British Columbia, Vancouver, British Columbia, Canada

INTRODUCTION

Exposure to wood dust is common in all countries because of its traditional use for fuel and for construction for human habitation. Respiratory illnesses associated with exposure to wood dust include asthma, hypersensitivity pneumonitis, organic dust toxic syndrome, chronic bronchitis, and mucous membrane irritation syndrome (1). In most instances respiratory illness is caused by exposure to chemical compounds in the wood dust; in others, the disease is caused by exposure to molds growing on the wood chips, bark, or sawdust. By far, the most common respiratory illness reported from wood dust exposure is asthma. The disease usually arises as a result of occupational exposure although in some individuals it may result from exposure as a hobby.

Many different species of wood have been identified as being associated with occupational asthma. They are often highly prized for durability and quality of appearance. The extent to which they are used in construction and in furniture industries is not known. A study of Swedish men found an increase in asthma mortality among wood-working machine operators with a smoking-adjusted mortality ratio of 226 (95% confidence interval 108–344).

Most cases of occupational asthma caused by wood dusts were published as case reports, with the exception of occupational asthma due to Western red cedar (WRC) (*Thuja plicata*), which has been studied extensively. For this reason, WRC asthma will be discussed in detail first.

OCCUPATIONAL ASTHMA DUE TO WESTERN RED CEDAR

WRC is an important wood species in the Pacific Northwest region, particularly in the coastal areas. In these areas, cedar accounts for 21% of the total volume of sound wood. It has been used extensively for poles, shakes, shingles, and lumber for exterior construction because of its well-known high durability. WRC asthma affects sawmill workers, shingle and shake mill workers, workers in remanufacturing plants, carpenters, construction workers, and cabinet makers.

543

Chemical Composition of Western Red Cedar

The structural constituents of wood substances, namely cellulose, hemicellulose, and lignan, occur in cedar in roughly the same proportion as they do in other coniferous woods. WRC is different from other species because of its unusually high content of chemical extractives. These extractives of wood are minor nonstructural components that can be extracted from the wood without impairing its structure or strength and include a variety of materials, such as tannin, dyes, pitch, resins, and gums. They are responsible for the smell, taste, and color of the wood (2,3).

Cedar wood extractives may be separated by steam distillation into volatile and nonvolatile fractions (Table 1). The volatile fractions account for only 1–1.5% of the heartwood (without bark) while the nonvolatile fractions account for 5–15%. The volatile fractions contain at least nine compounds. Some of them have interesting chemical properties. The tropolones, for example, are excellent natural fungicides and are likely to be responsible for the resistance of the wood against decay. They were found to have beta-adrenergic-receptor-blocking properties (4). Nezucone, an aromatic compound in red cedar, was found to give asthmatic reaction on inhalation challenge test in a patient (5). The significance of the tropolones and nezucone in the pathogenesis of WRC asthma has yet to be determined with careful clinical studies. On the other hand, plicatic acid (PA), a nonvolatile compound, constitutes about 90% by weight of the nonvolatile components. It has a molecular weight of 440 daltons; the structural formula is shown in Figure 1. Inhalation challenge test with PA induced similar types of asthmatic reaction as an aqueous

Table 1   Composition of Western Red Cedar Extract

Volatile components
  Methyl thujate
  Thujic acid
  Tropolones
    β-Thujaplicinol
    γ-Thujaplicin
    β-Thujaplicin
    α-Thujaplicin
    β-Dolabrin
  Nazukone
  Carvacrol methyl ether
Nonvolatile components (water-soluble)
  Phenolic fraction
    Plicatic acid
    Plicatin
    Thujaplicatin
    Thujaplicatin methyl ether
    Other lignans
  Nonphenolic fraction
    Pectic acid
    Starch
    Hemicellulose
    Arabinase
    Simple sugars

Source: Adapted from Ref. 3.

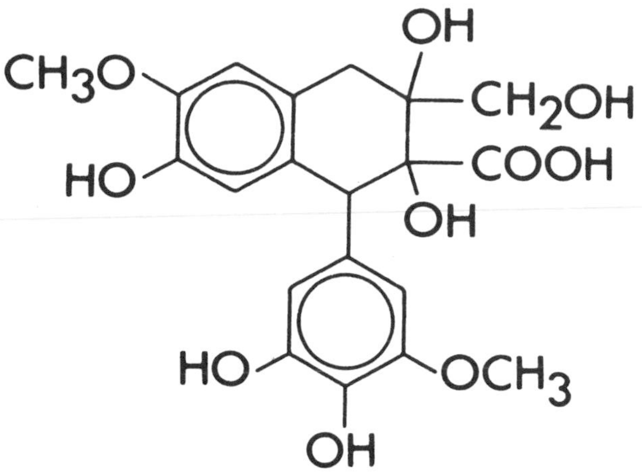

Figure 1   Structural formula of plicatic acid.

extract of the WRC dust in patients with the disease (6). The asthmatic reaction was found to be specific since patients with asthma and chronic bronchitis without history of exposure did not react on inhalation challenge test (6). PA is, therefore, the most important chemical compound present in the extract of WRC causing asthma.

Clinical Features

The clinical picture of patients with WRC asthma is characteristic. Many patients have worked with other wood dusts without respiratory symptoms. After a period of steady exposure, usually between 6 weeks and 3 years, but sometimes as long as 10 years, they develop cough, chest tightness, and wheeze. Some patients experience rhinorrhea several weeks before the onset of respiratory symptoms. In the majority of patients, respiratory symptoms occur initially after work and at night waking them with cough and wheeze. Later, cough, wheeze, and dyspnea occurr during the day and the nocturnal symptoms become more distressing. Symptoms usually improve during weekends and holidays initially; with continued exposure, they become persistent with no remission. At that stage, many patients complain of cough and wheeze immediately on exposure.

The characteristics of the 232 patients proven to be suffering from WRC asthma by inhalation provocation test are shown in Table 2 (7). The proportion of atopic subjects (those with positive skin prick test to one or more common allergens) in this group of patients was 31.4%, not different from those of the general population. This finding suggests that atopic status is not a predisposing factor in WRC asthma. The other interesting observation is the high proportion of nonsmokers and ex-smokers (94%) among this patient population—a feature that is similar to occupational asthma caused by isocyanate exposure but distinct from occupational asthma caused by high-molecular-weight compounds (8).

Inhalation challenge tests with an extract of WRC or PA induce three main types of asthmatic reaction; isolated immediate, isolated late, and biphasic or continuous asthmatic reaction (Fig. 2). Systemic or alveolar reaction has not been observed. Unlike occupational asthma due to high-molecular-weight compounds, the proportion of patients with late asthmatic reaction is high (89.2%) either as isolated late or part of biphasic or continuous reaction (Table 2). While the usual timing of onset of late asthmatic reaction is 4–6 hr after inhalation challenge, it can be as early as 2 hr or as late as 12 hr. Some patients

Table 2 Characteristics of 232 Patients with Documented
Red Cedar Asthma

Age, years	41.9 ± 11.8
Duration of exposure before onset of symptoms, years	4.1 ± 5.6
Smoking habit (%)	
Nonsmoker	66.8
Ex-smokers	28.0
Current smokers	5.2
Atopy[a] (%)	
Positive	31.4
Negative	68.6
Type of asthmatic reaction induced (%)	
Isolated immediate	10.8
Isolated late	42.3
Biphasic or continuous	46.9
Specific IgE antibodies against PA-HSA[b] (%)	20.1

[a]Defined as positive prick skin test against one or more common allergens.
[b]PA-HSA = plicatic acid-human serum albumin conjugate. RAST value greater than 2 was considered as a positive test (20).
Source: Adapted from Ref. 7.

develop an asthmatic reaction immediately after challenge and do not recover in the usual time of 1–2 hr before the development of the late asthmatic reaction. The lung function tests show airflow obstruction immediately after challenge and persist for over 24 hr. Recurrent nocturnal asthma over several nights after one single inhalation challenge test has been documented (9).

Patients with a biphasic asthmatic reaction usually have a significantly lower lung function, a greater degree of nonspecific bronchial hyperresponsiveness (NSBH), and a longer period between the onset of symptoms and diagnosis than patients with isolated immediate or late asthmatic reactions (10). These findings suggest that the occurrence of biphasic asthmatic reaction at the time of diagnosis is indicative of a greater severity of the disease.

Diagnosis

The diagnosis of WRC asthma is based on the presence of a compatible history and objective evidence that exposure to WRC dust causes acute respiratory symptoms and lung function changes. In general, any individual who is exposed to WRC dust in the workplace or as a hobby and develops asthma should be suspected of suffering from WRC asthma.

Skin tests and immunological tests are not helpful in the confirmation of diagnosis. Both crude WRC extract and PA or PA conjugated to human serum albumin (PA-HSA) failed to give reactions on skin testing. Specific IgE antibodies to PA-HSA conjugate were detected in only 30% of the red cedar asthma patients proven by inhalation challenge test (11) and they were also detected in 6% of exposed workers without respiratory symptoms (12).

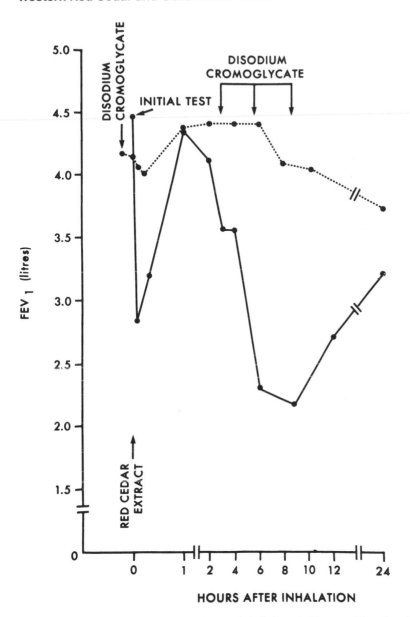

Figure 2   "Dual" asthmatic reaction to inhalation challenge with red cedar extract in one patient. Disodium cromoglycate 20 mg administered by inhalation before and at 3-hourly intervals after challenge inhibited the immediate asthmatic reaction and partially inhibited the late reaction in the same patient.

Prolonged recording of peak expiratory flow (PEF) every 2 hr during waking hours for 2 weeks at work and 1 week away from work has been proven by Côté et al. (13) to be both sensitive and specific in the diagnosis of WRC asthma when compared with the results of specific challenge test with PA. Although serial measurements of NSBH have been used together with prolonged monitoring of PEF effectively in the diagnosis of other types of occupational asthma, Côté et al. (13) did not find that the addition of this measurement improves the sensitivity and specificity of PEF monitoring in this group of patients. This is possibly due to the fact that NSBH persists for a long time in patients with WRC asthma compared to those with asthma due to other agents (14,15). Côté and co-workers (13) concluded that if both history and PEF monitoring are negative there is no need to perform specific challenge test to disprove the diagnosis. However, if only the history or the PEF monitoring is positive, it would be necessary to do a specific challenge test.

Specific challenge tests can be performed either using fine red cedar dust or using a crude extract of WRC dust or PA. The exposure test with fine WRC dust can be performed using a simple method described by Pepys and Hutchcroft (16) by pouring the dust from one container to another, or by a more sophisticated method as described by De Luca et al. (17) in another chapter. Specific challenge test can also be performed by aerosolization of the crude WRC extract or with PA (18). At present PA is not available commercially (18). All specific challenge tests should be carried out in a standardized manner to ensure the safety of the patients and the reproducibility of the results.

Outcome

The majority of the patients with WRC asthma failed to recover several years after they left exposure. A follow-up study of 232 patients about 4 years after the diagnosis showed that of the 136 patients who left the industry, only 55 (40.4%) recovered completely while the remaining 81 (59.6%) continued to have asthma (7). Table 3 shows the lung function and PC_{20} of patients who became asymptomatic and patients who remained symptomatic after they left industry at the time of diagnosis and at the time of the follow-up examination. The mean lung function results at the time of diagnosis and the mean PC_{20} were significantly higher among the asymptomatic group compared to the symptomatic group. These findings suggest that the patients in the asymptomatic group were diagnosed at an earlier stage of the disease. Race, smoking status, immediate skin reactivity, and the presence of specific IgE antibodies did not influence the outcome of the disease.

Table 3 Pulmonary Function Tests (adjusted for smoking and race) and Methacholine Challenge Test at Diagnosis and at Follow-Up

	No exposure		Exposed	
	Asymptomatic	Symptomatic	Daily	Intermittent
FEV_1[a] N	55	81	54	42
Initial	99.3 ± 2.7*	90.5 ± 2.2	90.2 ± 2.8*	100.5 ± 3.0
Follow-up	102.4 ± 2.7**	87.7 ± 2.2	86.4 ± 3.1	97.8 ± 3.3
PC_{20}[b] N	20	32	19	15
Initial	1.46 ± 3.96	0.77 ± 4.52	0.86 ± 8.94	1.14 ± 4.45
Follow-up	4.35 ± 4.58**	0.45 ± 10.8	0.61 ± 9.75	0.64 ± 3.99

[a]% predicted.
[b]mg/ml methacholine.
*Difference between asymptomatic and symptomatic or daily and intermittent statistically significant at $p < 0.05$ by analysis of covariance.
**Differences between initial and follow-up visits statistically significant at $p < 0.05$ by analysis of covariance.
Source: Adapted from Ref. 7.

Patients who failed to recover after they left exposure continued to require medications for their asthma. Bronchoalveolar studies of these patients showed a higher total cell count, eosinophil and neutrophil count, and an increase in protein and albumin in the lavage fluid compared to those who recovered (19) suggesting persistent airway inflammation in these patients.

All patients who continued to work with WRC had respiratory symptoms and required medications even though most patients used personal protection. They showed a reduction in FEV_1 and FVC and an increase in NSBH on follow-up examinations. Côté et al. (20) found that use of the twin-cartridge respirator offered better protection than the airstream helmet. This may be due to the poor compliance to the need for continuous use of the airstream helmet.

A recent follow-up study of 280 patients with WRC asthma has shown that the longitudinal decline in FEV_1 was significantly greater in those who were still exposed to red cedar compared to those who were exposed but did not have asthma (21). The diagnosis of occupational asthma has considerable socioeconomic implications for the worker and his/her family (22).

The results of the follow-up study emphasize the importance of early diagnosis and early removal from exposure in the management of patients with WRC asthma. Removal from exposure should be complete since partial removal did not prevent the deterioration of symptoms and lung function.

Pathogenesis

WRC asthma is a prototype of asthma caused by exposure to a low-molecular-weight compound. As in isocyanate-induced asthma, the pathogenetic mechanism is not entirely clear. Both nonimmunological and immunological mechanisms are likely involved.

Immunological Mechanisms

The clinical feature of WRC asthma is one of allergic disease. It affects only a small proportion of exposed workers (prevalence rate <2% in sawmill with low dust exposure) (23); reexposure to a small amount of dust may trigger a severe attack of asthma in sensitive subjects. There is a latent period between the onset of exposure and the onset of symptoms. Animals can be sensitized to parenteral administration of PA-HSA conjugate with the production of specific IgG_1 antibodies in guinea pigs and IgE antibodies in rabbits (24). So far, investigations failed to clarify which specific immunological mechanism(s) is responsible.

The changes in the airway in patients with WRC asthma are similar to those found in patients with allergic asthma. During late asthmatic reactions induced by PA, increase in eosinophils and albumin and increase in the sloughing of bronchial epithelial cells were found in the bronchoalveolar lavage fluid (25). Although there was a slight increase in neutrophils 48 hr after challenge, neutrophil infiltration was not a prominent feature earlier. Multiple bronchial biopsies were carried out in three of the patients 24 hr after inhalation challenge. The major findings were denudation of the bronchial epithelium, a thickened basement membrane, and infiltration of eosinophils in the bronchial epithelium and submucosa (Fig. 3). The occurrence of these inflammatory changes was associated with the development of NSBH. Mediators, predominantly histamine, and LTE_4 were found in the bronchoalveolar lavage fluid during the immediate asthmatic reaction induced by PA (26).

Despite these findings, skin tests with extract of WRC or PA did not produce im-

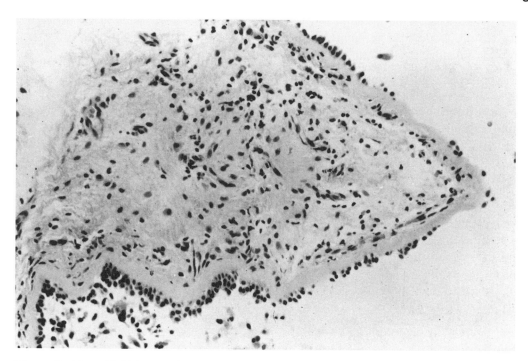

Figure 3 Bronchial biopsy of a patient with WRC asthma taken during the late asthmatic reaction showing thickened epithelium, increased thickness of basement membrane and cellular infiltration with mostly eosinophils.

mediate wheal-and-flare reaction in patients and controls (6). Using the RAST method, specific IgE antibodies to PA-HSA were found in only 30% of WRC asthma patients proven by specific challenge tests (11). Specific IgG antibodies to PA-HSA conjugate were not detected. Skin tests using PA-HSA as antigen also failed to induce positive immediate reaction in these patients. There was no difference in the frequency of specific IgE antibodies between patients with isolated late reaction and those with biphasic asthmatic reaction (11). The immediate component of the biphasic reaction can be induced on a second challenge in patients who had isolated late reaction alone during the first challenge test in the absence of specific IgE antibodies (Fig. 4). These findings cast some doubt as to the role of specific IgE antibodies in the pathogenesis of red cedar asthma.

Although PA was found to release histamine from basophils of most patients with WRC asthma and not from those of patients with allergic asthma, inactivation of basophilic IgE receptors by prior incubation with anti-IgE failed to inhibit histamine release induced by PA (27). Moreover, passive sensitization of human lung fragments with sera from patients with WRC asthma followed by challenge with PA failed to release histamine. These findings suggest that specific IgE antibodies to PA-HSA conjugate are unlikely to be responsible for the pathogenesis of the disease. Recent studies have shown that T lymphocytes play an important role in the pathogenesis of allergic asthma not only in the production of specific IgE antibodies, but also in participating in the airway inflammatory response. IL-5 produced by CD4+ cells is necessary for the maturation of eosinophils that cause airway damage. The role of T lymphocytes in the pathogenesis of WRC asthma has been studied (28). Increased numbers of T lymphocytes and acti-

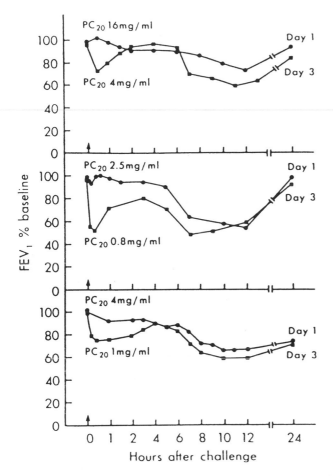

Figure 4 Effect of repeated challenge with plicatic acid on three separate patients with red cedar asthma showing the occurrence of isolated late reaction after the first challenge and biphasic reaction after the second challenge. PC_{20} decreased after the late asthmatic reaction of the first challenge.

vated T lymphocytes were found in the bronchial mucosa of patients with recently diagnosed WRC disease (28) similar to patients with isocyanate-induced asthma (29). Proliferation of T lymphocytes was found when stimulated with PA-HSA conjugate in less than 30% of patients (30).

Nonimmunological Mechanisms

In high concentrations PA has several biological activities. It activates the complement system via the classic pathway (31), leading to the generation of biologically active fragments such as C3a and C5a, both of which can induce histamine release from peripheral human basophils and mast cells, an increase in vascular permeability, and vasodilation. PA has been found to be toxic to the bronchial epithelium in high concentrations (32). WRC dust has been shown to release histamine from human and pig lung fragments in vitro (33). These properties of PA or WRC dust are unlikely to be solely responsible for the pathogenesis of asthma as only a small proportion of exposed subjects develop the disease. They may, however, account for the chronic airway inflammation and airflow obstruction in some of the exposed workers.

It is likely that both immunological and nonimmunological mechanisms are involved in the pathogenesis of WRC asthma. In a small proportion of patients, probably those with isolated immediate asthmatic reaction to inhalation challenge, specific IgE antibodies and T cells may be involved. In patients with isolated late asthmatic reaction and biphasic reaction, nonimmunological mechanisms are likely to be responsible. Inhalation of PA and possibly other chemicals present in the WRC dust may be toxic to the epithelium of the airways. Cytokines released by the epithelial cells such as IL-8 and GM-CSF may recruit cells, including eosinophils, to the airways leading to an inflammatory response. With time, these inflammatory changes may lead to structural changes in the airways resulting in the development of NSBH. This hypothesis can explain the clinical features of the majority of patients with WRC asthma. At the early stage of the disease, these patients complain of symptoms of asthma after work and at night and develop an isolated late asthmatic reaction on inhalation challenge test. They also have a mild degree of NSBH. As the disease progresses, these patients complain of symptoms earlier during the day and their symptoms persist into the evening. At this stage, they develop a biphasic or a continuous asthmatic reaction on inhalation challenge test. The immediate component of the biphasic or continuous reaction is likely to be due to heightened NSBH.

Prevalence and Determinants

The prevalence of occupational asthma in workers exposed to WRC dust has been the subject of several studies (23,34–37). The results of these studies are presented in Table 4. In these studies, a close relationship was found between the prevalence of work-related asthma and the level of dust exposure; the higher the dust concentration, the higher the prevalence of work-related asthma.

Chan-Yeung and colleagues (23) examined workers in a cedar sawmill yearly for 3 years and again at 6 years. After the initial survey in 1982, 26 workers with NSBH and work-related asthma as defined by Brooks et al. (35), were invited to have further tests. Eleven workers developed a specific reaction to PA challenge. The prevalence rate of WRC asthma, defined as specific responsiveness to PA, was 1.68%. During the subsequent 6 years, six workers developed WRC asthma at the rate of one per year giving an incidence of 0.3% per year even though the level of exposure in the sawmill was low with very few personal samples above 2.5 mg/m^3.

Given the same degree of exposure, only a small percentage of workers develop asthma. Host susceptibility factors play an important part. As discussed earlier, atopy is not a predisposing host factor in WRC asthma since the prevalence of atopy in these patients is not different from that of the general population (14). Smoking is not a predisposing host factor in WRC asthma as in occupational asthma due to large-molecular-weight compounds. On the contrary, the majority of patients with WRC asthma are lifelong nonsmokers. NSBH is unlikely to be a predisposing host factor as workers who developed WRC asthma did not have NSBH at the onset of a prospective study (14).

A recent study showed that individuals with HLA class II antigen DQB 0302 and DQB 0603 are more susceptible to WRC asthma while those with DQB 0501 are protected from the disease (38). Similar results were found in patients with isocyanate-induced asthma; the HLA class II antigen that confers susceptibility to the disease was DQB 0503

Table 4 Epidemiological Studies of Workers Exposed to Western Red Cedar

Year	Site	Type of industry	No. of subjects	Age (mean or range)	Smoker (%)	Chronic cough (%)	Chronic phlegm (%)	Wheeze (%)	Work-related asthma (%)	Lung Function FEV$_1$	Lung Function FVC	Dust concentration (mg/m³ or range)	Ref.
1973	Japan	Furniture	1797	17-60	NA	NA	NA	N	3.4	NA	NA	NA	34
1978	Vancouver, B.C.	Cedar sawmill	405	36.8	53.8	27.4	30.4	13.1	1.1	101%[a]	98.5%[a]	NA	21
		Former cedar mill	65	36.8	57.0	23.1	29.7	6.2	4.9			NA	
		Other wood dust	187	42.1	48.7	18.2	17.1	8.6	0	104%[a]	103.4%[a]		
1981	Washington State	Shake and shingle, cedar	74	NA	NA	20.2[b]			13.5	Cross-shift decrease in FEV$_1$ greater in WRC workers		4.7 ± 7.45	35
		Planer mill, noncedar	58	NA	NA	26.4		5.2				1.3 ± 3.10	
		No wood dust	22	NA	NA	9.0		0				NA	
1984	Vancouver, B.C.	Cedar sawmill	511[c]	44 ± 14	38.2	16.9	16.4	14.7	4.1	−206 ml[d]	−163 ml[d]	0–6	36
		Office	394[c]	43 ± 12	30.7	8.9[e]	12.0[e]	12.7	1.6[e]			NA	

[a]Nonsmokers only.
[b]Chronic bronchitis, %.
[c]White men only.
[d]Effect of cedar dust exposure versus no exposure adjusted for age, height, and smoking differences.
[e]Differences between cedar sawmill and office workers statistically significant, $p < 0.05$.

FEV$_1$, forced expiratory volume in 1 sec; FVC, forced vital capacity; NA, not available; WRC, western red cedar.

Source: Reproduced with permission from Chan-Yeung M, Malo JL. Occupational respiratory diseases associated with forest products industries. In: Harber P, Schenker M, Balmes J, eds. Occupational and Environmental Respiratory Disease. St. Louis: Mosby, 1996:637–653.

Table 5　Wood Dusts Causing Occupational Asthma

Species name	Common name	No. of subjects	Diagnostic test				Ref
			Inhalation	Skin test	Serology	Other features	
Aningeria robusta	Mukali	1	Immediate	Negative	Positive RAST	—	40
Bal fourodendron riedelianum	Pau marfim	1	Immediate	Negative	Negative RAST	—	41
Caesalpinia echinata	Fernam bouc	12	Immediate in 1	Negative	NA	—	42
Cedra libani	Cedar of Lebanon	6	NA	Negative in 5 Positive in 1	Negative ppt	—	43
Chlorophora excelsa	Iroko	1	Late	Positive immediate	Negative ppt	—	44,45
Cinnamomum zeylanicum	Cinnamon bark	9/40	NA	NA	NA	—	46
Dalbergia nigra	Palisander	1	Late	Positive immediate	NA	—	47
Dalbergia retusa	Cocobolla	3	NA	Positive immediate Positive patch test	NA	Responded to hypo-sensitization	48
Diospyros crassiflora	Ebony	1	Late	Negative	NA	—	49
Fraxinus americana	Ashwood	1	Immediate	Negative	Negative	—	50
Gonystyllus bacanus	Ramin	1	Late	Negative	Negative ppt	Decrease diffusing capacity on challenge	51
Juglans olanchana	Central American walnut	1	Biphasic	Negative	Negative ppt Negative RAST	—	52
Microberlinia	African zebrawood	1	Biphasic	Positive immediate	Negative ppt	—	53

Species	Common name						Ref.
Myrocarpus fastigiatus	Cabreuva	1	Late and systemic	NA	NA	↑ Leukocytes, ↑ neutrophils on challenge	54
Nesorgordonia papaverifera	Kotibe	1	Late	NA	NA	—	55
Pouteria	Abirucana	2	NA	Positive immediate	Negative ppt	—	56
Pterocarpus angolensis	Kejaat	1	NA	Positive immediate	NA	Responded to hyposensitization	57
Sequoia sempervirens	California redwood	2	Biphasic	Negative	Negative ppt	—	58
Tanganyike aningre	—	3	Immediate	Positive immediate	Negative ppt	—	59
Thuja occidentalis	Eastern white cedar	1	Late	NA	Negative specific IgE	Plicatic acid present in extract of wood	60
Thuja plicata	Western red cedar	See text	Biphasic immediate	Negative	Positive RAST in 30%	—	61–64
Triplochiton scleroxylon	Obeche or African maple	2	Immediate	Positive immediate	Positive specific IgE	—	65
NA	Mahogany	1	Late	Negative	Positive ppt	—	66
NA	Oak	1	Immediate	Negative	Positive ppt	—	66
NA	Quillaja bark	1	Immediate	NA	Positive	—	67

NA, not available; ppt, precipitins; RAST, radioallergosorbent test.

Source: Reproduced with permission from Chan-Yeung M, Malo J-L. Occupational respiratory diseases associated with forest products industries. In: Harber P, Schenker M, Balmes J, eds. Occupational and Experimental Respiratory Disease. St. Louis: Mosby, 1996:637–653.

(39). These findings further support the importance of T cells in the pathogenesis of occupational asthma due to low-molecular-weight compounds.

Permissible Concentration of Red Cedar Dust

Is there a level of WRC dust that is safe, below which no sensitization can occur? Very few epidemiological studies address this important issue. The Workers' Compensation Board of British Columbia has arbitrarily lowered the threshold limit value of cedar dust from 5 mg/m^3 to 2.5 mg/m^3. Despite a low dust concentration in a red cedar sawmill with very few samples greater than 2.5 mg/m^3, the incidence of asthma remained at 0.3% per year (24) in a longitudinal study carried out for 6 years. More study is required to confirm this finding in a relatively small number of exposed workers.

OCCUPATIONAL ASTHMA DUE TO OTHER WOOD DUSTS

Many other types of wood dust have been shown to cause occupational asthma (Table 5). The extent to which these types of wood are being used in the construction and furniture industry is not known. Most of the cases of occupational asthma due to other wood dusts were published as case reports. The diagnoses were made by inhalation challenge test or by history and positive skin test reaction to the appropriate extracts of wood dust.

Aqueous extracts of some wood dust such as abirucana (56), African maple wood (65), African zebrawood (53), kejaat wood (57), mahogany (66), and quillaja bark (67) gave immediate wheal-and-flare reaction on skin tests in sensitive subjects. In some patients specific IgE antibodies were demonstrated in the sera using the RAST method. In these patients, a type I allergic reaction is likely to be responsible for the asthma reaction. However, aqueous extracts of other wood dusts such as California redwood (58), cedar of Lebanon (43), Central American walnut (52), cocabolla (48), Eastern white cedar (60), and iroko (44,45), failed to give positive immediate skin reaction or specific IgE antibodies; precipitating antibodies were not detected in the sera of affected subjects. The pathogenetic mechanism of asthma induced by these wood dusts is likely to be similar to that of red cedar asthma. One or several of the chemical compounds present in these trees may be the causative agent(s).

Malo and associates (68) described 11 individuals with work-related asthma from 10 different sawmills of northwestern and southwestern Quebec and northern Maine where coniferous trees, spruce, firs, and pines, are cut into boards. Although the causative agent is not identified in each case, the study illustrates the point that many cases of occupational asthma due to wood dust exposure are not recognized.

The prevalence of occupational asthma due to wood dust exposure is not known. A study was conducted on furniture workers exposed to rimu, *Dacrydium cupressinum*, in Wellington, New Zealand (69). About 10% had a history compatible with work-related asthma confirmed by appropriate changes in the PEF recording. Nouaigui et al. (70) reported 5.6% of 197 woodworkers in four plants in Tunisia had asthma. The type of wood the workers were exposed to was not documented in the report.

OCCUPATIONAL ASTHMA DUE TO OTHER AGENTS PRESENT IN WOOD DUST

Woodworkers can also be sensitized to other living organisms growing on the wood, such as molds, and develop asthma. Côté et al. (71) reported a case of occupational asthma in a plywood factory worker due to a mold of *Neurospora* species growing on the wood under wet conditions. This worker had a positive skin reaction and bronchial reaction to challenge with an extract of the mold and the wood dust.

HYPERSENSITIVITY PNEUMONITIS ASSOCIATED WITH WOOD DUST EXPOSURE

Hypersensitivity pneumonitis often affects sawmill trimmers and pulp and paper mill workers in the woodroom and sometimes farmers who handle wood chips. The antigens responsible for these diseases are often not the wood dust themselves, but the molds growing in the wood dust or the bark of the wood such as *Cryptostroma corticale* in maple bark disease (72–73), *Penicillium frequentans* in suberosis (74), *Graphium* and *Pullularia* on redwood bark in sequoias (75), *Alternaria* in woodmills (76), *Aspergillus* and *Thermoactinomyces vulgaris* in moldy wood chips (77,78) and *Rhizopus* and *Paecilomyces* in wood trimmer's disease in Sweden (79–81). Of the different types of hypersensitivity pneumonitis, the maple bark disease and wood trimmer's disease were better investigated compared to the others. Maple bark disease was first described in 1932 by Towey and co-workers (72) and later by Emanuel et al. (73) in workers in the woodrooms of paper mills. The workers were involved in peeling bark from maple logs infected with fungal spores identified as *Cryptostroma corticale*. High levels of precipitating antibodies were found in the sera of patients with hypersensitivity pneumonitis against extracts of this fungus.

Wood trimmer's disease has been described among sawmill workers in Sweden in the late 1960s when conventional outdoor wood drying during the summer was changed to artificial indoor wood drying in special kilns (79). Spores of molds, *Rhizopus* and *Paecilomyces*, growing on the wood when it was wet, were found in high concentrations in the sawmills (79). A survey in 1976–1978 revealed that in 10 of 17 Swedish sawmills employing 280 workers, about 50% of the wood trimmers had precipitating antibodies mainly to the Rhizopus antigens while 10–20% had suffered symptoms compatible with hypersensitivity pneumonitis (80). In British Columbia, six cases of hypersensitivity pneumonitis have been seen from the inland sawmills where spruce, pine, fir, and hemlock are being processed. In three cases precipitating antibodies were found in the sera against *Aspergillus fumigatus* and *Thermoactinomyces vulgaris* (81).

ORGANIC DUST TOXIC SYNDROME

Organic dust toxic syndrome, which is characterized by fever, sometimes shaking chills, dry cough, and fatigue, is common among grain handlers and farmers (82). It has also been reported among sawmill workers in Sweden (79). Exposure to high concentration of fungal spores was thought to be the causative factor in the pathogenesis of this condition (83).

CHRONIC BRONCHITIS WITH AND WITHOUT AIRFLOW OBSTRUCTION

Exposure to cedar dust causes not only bronchial asthma in a proportion of workers, but increased prevalence of chronic cough and phlegm production (35). There is controversy as to whether chronic airflow limitation develops as a result of exposure to wood dust.

Little information is available on this subject except for WRC workers. The odds ratios of cough and phlegm in cedar workers compared to office workers were 2.18 and 1.44, respectively ($p > 0.001$ and 0.05, respectively, controlled for age and smoking). Cedar workers had significantly lower lung function compared to office workers after adjusting for differences in age, height, race, and smoking habits. The decrease in lung function was not due to the increased prevalence of asthma in cedar mills since exclusion of these subjects from analysis failed to influence the results. The annual decline in lung function in cedar workers was also significantly greater than in the control group in the longitudinal study (13). There is also a dose-response relationship between cumulative exposure to cedar dust and the longitudinal decline in lung function in an 11-year follow-up study of workers in a cedar sawmill (84).

There have been several epidemiological studies of respiratory health effects of exposure to wood dusts other than WRC. Whitehead et al. (85) conducted an epidemiological study on 354 workers exposed to hardwood dust (mostly maple) and on 220 workers exposed to varying levels of soft wood dust (pine). These workers did not have exposure to other industrial agents such as adhesives and finishing agents. Although an unexposed group was not studied as controls, workers in the high-exposure category to both hard wood and pine dust were associated with two to four times the prevalence of low expiratory flow rates compared to those exposed to lower levels of dust irrespective of their smoking habits. These findings indicated that both hard and soft wood exposure is associated with airflow obstruction.

Holness et al. (86) studied 50 cabinet workers exposed to different types of wood dust and 50 controls. Woodworkers reported more cough, phlegm, and wheeze but their mean lung function was not significantly different from that of the controls. Woodworkers, however, had a significant acute decline in lung function over a work shift. A positive correlation was found between baseline lung function and the degree of exposure. Paggiaro et al. (87) studied respiratory symptoms and lung function of 239 workers exposed to wood dust in a furniture plant. Significantly higher prevalence rates of cough, phlegm, and wheeze in nonsmoking workers were found compared to the control group derived from a population sample. Although mean lung function results were within normal limits, a lower $FEV_1\%$ was found in subjects with more years of employment suggestive of a dose-responsive relationship. More recently, Shamssain (88) demonstrated that exposure to pine and fiber board dust was associated with a higher prevalence of chest symptoms and lower lung function among furniture factory workers in Umtata, Republic of Transkei, compared with a group of unexposed subjects.

The results of most of the above studies have shown that exposure to different types of wood dust is associated with chronic respiratory symptoms and some impairment of lung function compared to the unexposed. A dose-response relationship was observed between the level of exposure and the level of lung function in some studies, an indication that the relationship was significant. Although asthma is the most disabling lung disease among woodworkers one should realize that inhalation of wood dusts also give rise to chronic bronchitis with and without airflow obstruction.

SUMMARY

In this chapter, the respiratory effects of wood dust exposures were reviewed. Many wood dusts can give rise to asthma by sensitization via type I allergic reaction or by an undetermined immunological mechanism. Chronic bronchitis with or without airflow obstruction unrelated to smoking is not that uncommon among exposed workers. Hypersensitivity pneumonitis and organic dust toxic syndrome are found among woodworkers but they are due to molds contaminating the wood dust.

Allergic conjunctivitis and rhinitis are also problems among woodworkers. Contact dermatitis from wood dust exposure, however, is the most common compensable disease in British Columbia among woodworkers. In many cases it is not the wood dust itself that is causing the dermatitis but contaminants, e.g., lichens growing on the bark of red cedar trees (89). Adenocarcinoma of the nasopharynx is a known disease among woodworkers (90). These conditions cannot be discussed in this chapter in depth, but have been described in detail by Hausen (91).

ACKNOWLEDGMENTS

The author wishes to thank Mrs. C. Bassett for her assistance in the preparation of this manuscript. The Workers' Compensation Board of British Columbia, National Health and Research Developement Program, Health and Welfare Canada, British Columbia Lung Association, and the Medical Research Council of Canada have contributed to the support of these studies over the years.

REFERENCES

1. Enarson DA, Chan-Yeung M. Characterization of health effects of wood dust exposures. Am J Ind Med 1990; 17:33–38.
2. Gardner JA. Chemistry and utilization of Western Red Cedar. Department of Forestry Publication no. 1023. Ottawa: Ottawa Department of Forestry, 1963.
3. Barton GM, MacDonald BF. The Chemistry of Utilization of Western Red Cedar. Department of Fisheries and Forestry, Publication no. 1023, Ottawa: Ottawa Department of Forestry, 1971.
4. Belleau B, Burba J. Occupancy of adrenergic receptors and inhibition of catechol o-methyl transferase by toropolones. J Med Chem 1963; 6:755–759.
5. Shida T, Mimaki K, Sasaki N, Nakagawa Y, Hattovi O. Western red cedar asthma: occurrence in Oume City, Tokyo and results of inhalation test using "nezucone" aromatic substance of western red cedar. Areugi Jpn J Allergol 1971; 20:915–921.
6. Chan-Yeung M, Barton G, MacLean L, Grzybowski S. Occupational asthma and rhinitis due to western red cedar (*Thuja plicata*). Am Rev Respir Dis 1973; 108:1094–1102.
7. Chan-Yeung M, MacLean L, Paggiaro PL. Follow up study of 232 patients with occupational asthma caused by western red cedar (*Thuja plicata*). J Allergy Clin Immunol 1987; 79:792–796.
8. Chan-Yeung M, Lam S. Occupational asthma—state of the art. Am Rev Respir Dis 1986; 133:686–703.
9. Cockcroft DW, Cotton DJ, Mink JT. Nonspecific bronchial hyperreactivity after exposure to western red cedar. Am Rev Respir Dis 1979; 119:505–510.
10. Paggiaro PL, Chan-Yeung M. Pattern of specific airway response in asthma due to western red cedar (*Thuja plicata*): relationship with length of exposure and lung function measurements. Clin Allergy 1987; 17:333–339.
11. Tse KS, Chan H, Chan-Yeung M. Specific IgE antibodies in patients with occupational asthma due to western red cedar (*Thuja plicata*). Clin Allergy 1982; 12:249–258.
12. Vedal S, Chan-Yeung M, Enarson D, Chan H, Dorken E, Tse K. Plicatic acid-specific IgE and nonspecific bronchial hyperresponsiveness in Western red cedar workers. J Allergy Clin Immunol 1986; 78:1103–1109.

13. Côté J, Kennedy S, Chan-Yeung M. Sensitivity and specificity of PC_{20} and peak expiratory flow rate in cedar asthma. J Allergy Clin Immunol 1990; 85:592–598.

14. Chan-Yeung M, Lam S, Koerner S. Clinical features and natural history of occupational asthma due to western red cedar (*Thuja plicata*). Am J Med 1982; 72:411–415.

15. Cartier A, L'Archevêque J, Malo JL. Exposure to a sensitizing occupational agent can cause a long-lasting increase in bronchial responsiveness to histamine in the absence of significant changes in airway caliber. J Allergy Clin Immunol 1986; 78:1185–1189.

16. Pepys J, Hutchcroft BJ. Bronchial provocation tests in etiologic diagnosis and analysis of asthma. Am Rev Respir Dis 1975; 112:829–859.

17. De Luca S, Caire N, Cloutier Y, Cartier A, Ghezzo H, Malo JL. Acute exposure to sawdust does not alter airway calibre and responsiveness to histamine in asthmatic subjects. Eur Respir J 1988; 1:540–546.

18. Chan-Yeung M, Barton GM, MacLean L, Grzybowski S. Bronchial reactions to western red cedar (*Thuja plicata*). Can Med Assoc J 1971; 105:56–61.

19. Chan-Yeung M, LeRiche J, MacLean L, Lam S. Comparison of cellular and protein changes in bronchial lavage fluid of symptomatic and asymptomatic patients with red cedar asthma on follow up examination. Clin Allergy 1988; 18:359–365.

20. Côté J, Kennedy S, Chan-Yeung M. Outcome of patients with cedar asthma with continuous exposure. Am Rev Respir Dis 1990; 141:373–376.

21. Lin FJ, Dimich-Ward H, Kennedy S, Chan-Yeung M. Longitudinal decline in lung function in patients with occupational asthma due to western red cedar. Occup Environ Med 1996; 53: 753–756.

22. Marabini A, Ward H, Kwan S, Kennedy S, Wexler-Morrison N, Chan-Yeung M. Clinical and socio-economical features of subjects with red cedar asthma: a follow up study. Chest 1993; 104:821–824.

23. Chan-Yeung M, Kennedy S, Vedal S. A longitudinal study of red cedar sawmill workers. Am Rev Respir Dis 1990; 141:A80.

24. Chan H, Tse KS, Oostdam JV, Moreno R, Pare P, Chan-Yeung M. A rabbit model of hypersensitivity to plicatic acid, the agent responsible for red cedar asthma. J Allergy Clin Immunol 1987; 79:762–767.

25. Lam S, LeRiche J, Phillips D, Chan-Yeung M. Cellular and protein changes in bronchial lavage fluid after late asthmatic reaction in patients with red cedar asthma. J Allergy Clin Immunol 1987; 80:44–50.

26. Chan-Yeung M, Chan H, Salari H, Lam S. Histamine and leukotrienes release in bronchial fluid during plicatic acid-induced bronchoconstriction. J Allergy Clin Immunol 1989; 84: 762–768.

27. Frew A, Chan H, Dryden P, Salari S, Lam S, Chan-Yeung M. Immunologic studies of the mechanisms of occupational asthma caused by western red cedar. J Allergy Clin Immunol 1993; 92:466–478.

28. Frew A, Chan H, Lam S, Chan-Yeung M. Bronchial inflammation in occupational asthma due to western red cedar. Am J Respir Crit Care Med 1994; 151:340–344.

29. Mapp CE, Saetta M, Maestrelli P, Di Stefano A, Chitano P, Boschetto P, Ciaccia A, Fabbri L. Mechanisms and pathology of occupational asthma. Eur Respir J 1994; 7:544–554.

30. Frew A, Chan H, Chan-Yeung M. Specificity of antigen-induced T-cell proliferation in western red cedar asthma. J Allergy Clin Immunol 1993; 91:A314.

31. Chan-Yeung M, Giclas P, Henson P. Activation of the complement by plicatic acid, the chemical compound responsible for asthma due to western red cedar (*Thuja plicata*). J Allergy Clin Immunol 1980; 65:333–337.

32. Ayars GH, Altman LC, Frazier CE, Chi EY. The toxicity of constituents of cedar and pine woods to pulmonary epitheliium. J Allergy Clin Immunology 1989; 83:610–618.

33. Evans E, Nicholls PJ. Histamine release by western red cedar (*Thuja plicata*) from lung tissue in vitro. J Ind Med 1974; 31:28–30.

34. Ishizaka T, Shida T, Miyamoto T, Matsumara Y, Mizuno K, Tomaru M. Occupational asthma

from western red cedar dust (*Thuja plicata*) in furniture factory workers. J Occup Med 1973; 15:580–585.

35. Brooks SM, Edwards JJ, Apol A, Edwards FH. An epidemiologic study of workers exposed to western red cedar and other wood dust. Chest 80 1981; (Suppl):30–32.

36. Chan-Yeung M, Vedal S, Kus J, MacLean L, Enarson D, Tse KS. Symptoms, pulmonary function, and bronchial hyperreactivity in western red cedar workers compared with those in office workers. Am Rev Respir Dis 1984; 130:1038–1041.

37. Vedal S, Chan-Yeung M, Enarson D, Fera T, MacLean L, Tse KS, Langille R. Symptoms and pulmonary function in western red cedar workers related to duration of employment and dust exposure. Arch Environ Health 1986; 41:179–183.

38. Horne C, Quintana J, Keown P, Dimich-Ward H, Chan-Yeung M. Distribution of HLA class II DQB1 and DRBq alleles in patients with occupational asthma due to western red cedar. Am J Respir Crit Care Med 1997; 155:A135.

39. Balboni A, Baricordi OR, Fabbri LM, Gandini E, Ciaccia C, Mapp CE. Association between toluene diisocyanate-induced asthma and DQB1 markers: a possible role for aspartic acid at position 57. Eur Respir J 1996; 9:207–210.

40. Sotillos GMM, Carmona BJG, Picon JS, Gaston RP, Gimenez PR, Gil AL. Occupational asthma and contact urticaria caused by mukali wood dust (*Aningeria robusta*). J Invest Allergol Clin Immunol 1995; 5(2):113–114.

41. Bascomba A, Burches E, Almodovar A, Rojas D, Hemandez FD. Occupational rhinitis and asthma caused by inhalation of *Balfourdendron riedelianum* (Pau marfim) wood dust. Allergy 1991; 46:316–318.

42. Hausen BM, Herrmann B. Bowmaker's disease: An occupational disease in the manufacture of bows for string instruments. Dtsch Med Wochenschr 1990; 115:169–173.

43. Greenberg M. Respiratory symptoms following brief exposure to cedar of Lebanon (*Cedra libani*) dust. Clin Allergy 1972; 2:219–224.

44. Azofra J, Olaquibel JM. Occupational asthma caused by iroko wood. Allergy 1989; 44:156–158.

45. Pickering CAC, Batten JL, Pepys J. Asthma due to inhaled wood dusts—Western red cedar and iroko. Clin Allergy 1972; 2:213–218.

46. Uragoda C. Asthma and other symptoms in cinnamon workers. Br J Ind Med 1984; 41:224–227.

47. Godnic-Cvar J, Gomzi M. Case report of occupational asthma due to palisander wood dust and bronchoprovocation challenge by inhalation of pure wood dust from a capsule. Am J Ind Med 1990; 18:541–545.

48. Eaton KK. Respiratory allergy to exotic wood dust. Clin Allergy 1973; 3:307–310.

49. Maestrelli P, Mercer G, Dal Vecchio L. Occupational asthma due to ebony wood (*Diospyros crassiflora*) dust. Ann Allergy 1987; 59:347–349.

50. Malo J-L, Cartier A. Occupational asthma caused by exposure to ashwood dust (*Fraxinus americana*). Eur Respir Dis 1989; 2:385–387.

51. Howie AD, Boyd G, Moran F. Pulmonary hypersensitivity to ramin (*Gonystylus bancanus*). Thorax 1976; 31:585–587.

52. Bush RK, Clayton D. Asthma due to Central American walnut (*Juglans olanchana*) dust. Clin Allergy 1983; 13:389–394.

53. Bush R, Yunginger JW, Reed C. Asthma due to African zebrawood (*Microberlinia*) dust. Am Rev Respir Dis 1978; 227:601–604.

54. Innocenti A, Romeo R, Mariano A. Asthma and systemic toxic reaction due to cabreuva (*Myrocarpus fastigiatus* Fr. All.) wood dust. Med Lavoro 1991; 82:446–450.

55. Reques FG, Fernandez RP. Asthma professionel a un bois exotique. Rev Mal Respir 1988; 5:71–73.

56. Booth BH, LeFoldt RH, Moffitt EM. Wood dust hypersensitivity. J Allergy Clin Immunol 1973; 57:352–357.

57. Ordman D. Wood dust as an inhalant allergen: Bronchial asthma caused by kejaat wood (*Pterocarpus angolensis*). S Afr Med J 1949; 23:973–975.

58. Chan-Yeung M, Abboud R. Occupational asthma due to California redwood (*Sequoia sempervirens*) dusts. Am Rev Respir Dis 1976; 114:1027–1031.
59. Paggiaro PL, Cantalupi R, Filieri M, Loi AM, Parlanti A, Toma G, Baschieri L. Bronchial asthma due to inhaled wood dust: *Tanganyika aningre*. Clin Allergy 1981; 11:605–610.
60. Cartier A, Chan H, Malo J-L, Pineau L, Tse KS, Chan-Yeung M. Occupational asthma caused by eastern white cedar (*Thuja occidentalis*) with demonstration that plicatic acid is present in this wood and is the causative agent. J Allergy Clin Immunol 1986; 77:639–645.
61. Milne J, Gandevia B. Occupational asthma and rhinitis due to western (Canadian) red cedar (*Thuja plicata*). Med J Aust 1969; 2:741–744.
62. Gandevia B, Milne J. Occupational asthma and rhinitis due to western cedar (*Thuja plicata*) with special reference to bronchial reactivity. Br J Ind Med 1970; 27:235–244.
63. Blainey AD, Graham VA, Phillips MJ, Davies RJ. Respiratory tract reactions to western red cedar. Hum Toxicol 1981; 1:41–51.
64. Mue S, Ise T, Ono Y, Akasaka K. A study of western red cedar induced asthma. Ann Allergy 1975; 34:296–304.
65. Hinojosa M, Moneo I, Domingues J, Delgrado E, Losada E, Alcover R. Asthma caused by African maple (*Triplochiton scleroxylon*) wood dust. J Allergy Clin Immunol 1984; 74:782–786.
66. Sosman AJ, Schlueter DP, Fink JN, Barboriak JJ. Hypersensitivity to wood dust. N Engl J Med 1969; 281:977–980.
67. Raghuprasad PD, Brooks SM, Litwin A, Edwards JJ, Bernstein IL, Gallagher J. Quillaja bark (soap bark) induced asthma. J Allergy Clin Immunol 1980; 65:285–287.
68. Malo JL, Cartier A, Boulet LP. Occupational asthma in sawmills of Eastern Canada and United States. J Allergy Clin Immunol 1986; 78:392–298.
69. Norrish AE, Beasley R, Hodgkinson EJ, Pearce N. A study of New Zealand wood workers: exposure to wood dust, respiratory symptoms, and suspected cases of occupational asthma. NZ Med J 1992; 105:185–187.
70. Nouaigui H, Gharbi R, M'Rizak N, Jaafar K, Ghachem A, Nemery B. Etude transversale de la pathologie respiratoire hez les travailleurs du bois en Tunisie. Arch Mal Prof 1998; 49:69–75.
71. Côté J, Chan H, Brochu G, Chan-Yeung M. Occupational asthma caused by exposure to neurospora in a plywood factory worker. Br J Ind Med 1991; 48:279–282.
72. Towey JW, Sweany HC, Huraon WH. Severe bronchial asthma apparently due to fungus spores found in maple bark. JAMA 1932; 99:453–459.
73. Emanuel DA, Wenzel FJ, Lawton BR. Pneumonitis due to *cryptostroma corticale* (maple-bark disease). N Engl J Med 1966; 274:1413–1418.
74. Avila R, Villar TG. Suberosis. Respiratory disease in cork workers. Lancet 1968; 1:620–621.
75. Cohen HI, Merigan TC, Kosek JC, Eldridge F. Sequoiosis. A granulomatous pneumonitis associated with redwood sawdust inhalation. Am J Med 1967; 43:785–794.
76. Schlueter DP, Fink JN, Hensley GT. Wood-pulp workers' disease: a hypersensitivity pneumonitis caused by *alternaria*. Ann Intern Med 1972; 77:907–914.
77. Thiede WH, Banaszak EF, Fink JN, Unger GF, Scanlon GT. Hypersensitivity studies in Popple (Aspen tree) peelers. Chest 1975; 67:405–407.
78. Enarson DA, Chan-Yeung M. Characterization of health effects of wood dust exposures. Am J Ind Med 1990; 17:33–38.
79. Belin L. Clinical and immunologic data on "wood-trimmer's disease": in Sweden. Eur J Respir Dis 1980; 61:169–176.
80. Belin L. Health problems caused by actinomycetes and moulds in the industrial environment. Allergy 1985; 40 (Suppl.3):24–29.
81. Belin L. Sawmill alveolitis in Sweden. Int Arch Allergy Appl Immunol 1987; 82:440–443.
82. doPico GA, Reddan W, Flaherty D, Tsiatis A, Peters NE, Roa P, Rankin J. Respiratory abnormalities among grain handlers: A clinical, physiologic and immunologic study. Am Rev Respir Dis 1977; 115:915–927.

83. Malmberg P, Palmgren U, Rask-Anderson A. Relationship between symptoms and exposure to moldy dust in Swedish farmers. Am J Ind Med 1986; 10:316–317.

84. Noertjojo K, Dimich-Ward H, Dittrick M, Peelan S, Kennedy SM, Chan-Yeung M. Western red cedar dust exposure—a dose response relationship. Am J Respir Crit Care Med 1996; 154:968–973.

85. Whitehead LW, Ashikaga T, Vacek P. Pulmonary function status of workers exposed to hardwood or pine dust. Am Ind Hyg Assoc J 1981; 42:178–186.

86. Holness DL, Sass-Kortsak AM, Pilger CW, Nethercott JR. Respiratory function and exposure effect relationships in wood dust-exposed and control workers. J Occup Med 1985; 27:501–506.

87. Paggiaro P, Vellutini M, Viegi G, Zoi D, Di Pede F, Gregori G, Diviggiano E, Di Pede C, Sbrana C, Pistelli G. Indagine epidemiologica trasversale sui sintomi e la funzione respiratoria nei lavoratori di un mobilificio. G Ital Med Lav 1986; 8:145–148.

88. Shamssain MH. Pulmonary function and symptoms in workers exposed to wood dust. Thorax 1992; 47:84–87.

89. Mitchell J, Chan-Yeung M. Contact allergy from *Frullania* and respiratory allergy from *Thuja*. Can Med Assoc J. 1974; 110:653–657.

90. Acheson ED, Cowdell RH, Hadfield E, Macbeth RG. Nasal cancer in woodworkers in the furniture industry. Br Med J 1968; 2:587–597.

91. Hausen B. Woods Injurious to Human Health—A manual. Walter de Gruyter, 1981.

30

Reactive Airways Dysfunction Syndrome, or Irritant-Induced Asthma

Denyse Gautrin
Université de Montréal, Montréal, Quebec, Canada

I. Leonard Bernstein
University of Cincinnati College of Medicine, Cincinnati, Ohio

Stuart Brooks
University of South Florida, Tampa, Florida

INTRODUCTION

Although irritant-induced nonimmunological asthma without a latency period had previously been reported, the acronym for this form of occupational asthma was first derived from the descriptive term "reactive airways dysfunction syndrome" (RADS) in 1985 (1). It was originally defined as asthma occurring after a single exposure to high levels of an irritating vapor, fume, or smoke. While the designation "irritant-induced airways disease" is actually more consistent with the definitions of occupational asthma described in Chapter 1 (2), the RADS terminology was retained by the editors because of the high recognition index that it has engendered among the occupational health community. Initial symptoms developed within minutes or hours after exposure. In the majority of cases there was continuation of obstructive symptoms and persistent airways hyperreactivity for more than 1 year. The condition is defined as nonimmunological occupational asthma in this book, and according to this definition, it should be distinguished from other nonimmunological occupational asthma entities occurring after latent periods of exposure (e.g., meat wrapper's asthma, potroom asthma) and/or fixed obstructive disorders such as bronchiolitis obliterans resulting from chemical inhalation injury. As more investigators recognize RADS as a unique form of occupational asthma, future nomenclature will most likely refer to it as irritant-induced occupational asthma (2).

CLINICAL DESCRIPTION OF THE SYNDROME

The initial report included 10 individuals who developed a persistent asthma-like illness after a single exposure to high levels of an irritant vapor, fume, gas, or smoke. Respiratory symptomatology and continued presence of nonspecific bronchial hyperresponsiveness (NSBH) was documented in all subjects for a mean follow-up of 3 years. In one person, the persistence of disease was documented to have lasted at least 12 years. Generally, the incriminated exposure was short-lived, often lasting just a few minutes but, on occasion, was as long as 12 hr. There usually was a time interval between the exposure and development of symptoms; this time period was immediate in three subjects but several hours in the other seven subjects (mean of 9 hr). In almost all instances, the exposure was due to an accident or a situation where there was very poor ventilation and limited air exchange in the work area. Although the incriminating etiological agents varied in each case, all were irritants and included uranium hexafluoride gas, floor sealant, spray paint containing significant concentrations of ammonia, heated acid, 35% hydrazine, fumigating fog, metal coating remover, and smoke inhalation. When tested, all subjects displayed a positive methacholine challenge test. There was no identifiable evidence of preexisting respiratory complaints in any patient studied. Two subjects were found to be atopic, but in all others no evidence of allergy was identified. Pulmonary function was normal in 3 of 10 and showed airflow limitation in seven.

Typical Courses of Two Cases

A previously healthy 41-year-old painter and his partner, a 45-year-old man, worked together spray-painting a poorly ventilated apartment during the late fall when the weather was cold. The room was sealed and there was poor fresh air recirculation; the windows were covered with a heavy plastic material, duct tape was placed around the edges to ensure a seal, and the main entrance to the apartment was covered to conserve heat. The painters did not wear approved respiratory protective devices but only paper masks covering their nose and mouth while they spray-painted. The paint used was a one-stage vinyl latex primer, reported to be rapid-drying, and said to contain 25% ammonia, 16.6% aluminum chlorhydrate, and other additives, many of which were documented irritants.

Both men spray-painted for a total of 12 hr: 4 hr the first day and 8 hr the second. Each individual noted the appearance of an illness beginning the end of the second day of work, with symptoms consisting of nausea, cough, shortness of breath, paint taste in the mouth, chest tightness, wheezing, and generalized weakness of the limbs. Each worker was subsequently hospitalized for about 2 weeks with provisional diagnosis of "chemical bronchitis." A chest roentgenogram of one patient showed "increased bronchovascular markings" consistent with "chemical pneumonitis." After being discharged from the hospital, both painters consulted private physicians and each was eventually treated with prednisone, oral theophylline, and aerosol beta$_2$-adrenergic bronchodilators.

When they were evaluated 4 months later, there remained persistent symptomatology of wheezing, cough, and exertional dyspnea; in one painter there was also chest discomfort. Separately, each reported newly developed bronchial irritability symptoms, i.e., respiratory manifestations after exposure to many and varied nonspecific stimuli such as cold air, dusts, aerosol sprays, smoke, and fumes. The bronchial irritability symptoms were not present before the heavy exposure. Each painter denied a past history of asthma, allergies, rhinitis, frequent colds, dyspnea, or other respiratory symptoms. One of the painters recalled a transient episode of bronchitis 11 years previously without recurrence. Each worker denied a family history of allergy, asthma, or previous respiratory problems. Each person worked only as a painter in the past, one for 20 years and the other for 25 years. Each stated he never previously spray-painted under the environmental conditions of the inciting incident. One subject was a cigarette smoker with a 21-pack/year history; the other person was essentially a nonsmoker, having smoked only 20–40 cigarettes in his life. A physical examination in one worker disclosed expiratory rhonchi. Laboratory tests of the

Table 1 Methacholine Reactivity[a]

Date	Subject 1	Subject 2
March 4, 1982	15 inhalation units	29 inhalation units
March 25, 1982	30 inhalation units	28 inhalation units
March 1, 1983	232 μg	52 μg
April 15, 1983	232 μg	—

[a]Positive tests are defined by methacholine doses of less than 200 inhalation units of 750 μg methacholine.

subjects included normal complete blood counts with 5% eosinophilia in one, normal chest roentgenograms, and negative RAST battery for common airborne allergens. Pulmonary function testing showed mild airways obstruction; FEV_1/FVC was 67.7% in one man and 70.3% in the other; FEF_{25-75} was 39.8 and 31.7% of predicted, respectively.

Over the next year, the two men were followed with serial clinical evaluations, lung function testing, and methacholine bronchial challenges. The asthmatic symptoms and airway hyperresponsiveness were noted to persist. Results of methacholine challenges shown in Table 1 demonstrate that NSBH persisted for at least 1 year in both workers. Because one of the painters reported spray-painting with a polyurethane-based paint several years before, the possibility of isocyanate-induced airway disease was entertained. Response to subsequent toluene diisocyanate (TDI) bronchial challenge testing in this person was negative. When last evaluated about 16–17 months after the accident, both continued to experience symptoms and had not returned to the painting occupation.

OTHER REPORTS OF RADS

Harkonen et al. followed seven mine workers who were involved in a pyrite dust explosion and sustained SO_2-induced lung injury (3). Four years after the accident, an asthma-like condition characterized by reversible airway obstruction was observed in three persons; four workers showed positive histamine challenges, while two subjects responded neither to histamine nor to bronchodilators. The authors concluded that NSBH was a frequent sequel of high-level SO_2 exposure and could persist for years.

Subsequent to the 1985 description of RADS, other occurrences of RADS were reported. Tarlo and Broder performed a retrospective review of the files of 154 consecutive workers assessed four "occupational asthma" (2). Of 59 subjects considered to have occupational asthma, a subset of 10 persons (and possibly an additional 15) with asthma symptoms for an average of 5 years were characterized by disease initiated by an exposure to high concentrations of an irritant. The RADS clinical criteria were modified in this study, and exposure was not limited to just a single accident or incident or work. It was concluded that "irritant-induced" occupational asthma is not uncommon in a population referred for assessment of possible occupational asthma. The prevalence was estimated to be 6% for definite irritant-induced asthma and 10% for those with a possible diagnosis. Boulet implied there was prolonged induction of increased NSBH after the inhalation of high concentrations of irritants in four "normal" subjects and aggravation of airway hyperresponsiveness in another person with "mild" preexisting asthma (4). Two of the persons were believed to have developed hyperresponsiveness after only an intense short-term exposure. Gilbert and Auchincloss reported a case of RADS occurring after a single massive silo dust exposure. In addition to objective evidence of NSBH, flow volume loops revealed a mixed obstructive/restrictive pattern in this worker, presumably on the basis of constriction of bronchioles or alveolar ducts (5). Other case examples reported as RADS included: (1) three Philadelphia police officers exposed to "toxic fumes" from a roadside truck accident (6); (2) a female computer operator exposed to a floor sealant (7); (3) workers exposed to TDI (8); and (4) possible exposures to acetic acid (9). Moisan described RADS after smoke inhalation in three subjects (10). Bernstein et al. evaluated four previously healthy, nonatopic men after acute exposure to toxic levels of anhydrous ammonia fumes (11). All of these workers exhibited obstructive symptoms, decreases in airway caliber, and persistent NSBH. Many other cases and case series have been reported. By the midnineties both the number of case reports and irritant agents have expanded. For example, inhalation accidents reported by SWORD were most commonly caused by chlorine, smoke, and oxides of nitrogen (12). A complete list of agents associated with RADS and/or irritant-induced asthma is shown in Table 2.

PATHOLOGY

The first descriptions of the pathological features of RADS were mostly those of the chronic stage of the syndrome (1). Brooks and co-workers were the first to perform bronchial biopsies in patients with RADS. Later, bronchial biopsy data reported by Bernstein et al. revealed typical histopathological features of asthma including marked denuded epithelium, submucosal chronic inflammation, and collagen proliferation below the basement membrane (11). The latter finding had developed in one anhydrous ammonia-exposed patient who had a bronchial biopsy within 2 weeks after the acute exposure (11).

Deschamps and co-workers performed biopsies on two subjects, the first case 3 years after exposure to toxic concentrations of ethylene oxide (13), the second several months after inhalation of a mixture of sodium hypochlorite and hydrochloric acid (14). They reported severe injury of the epithelial layer as well as inflammatory infiltrates containing lymphocytes. Electron microscopic examination of these biopsy specimens revealed a thickening of connective tissue with collagen fibers. There was no thickening of the basement membrane itself. Histopathological changes in the case of irritant-induced asthma secondary to multiple exposures to an irritant agent have also been described at the chronic stage of the disease. In five workers studied by Gautrin and colleagues 2 years after cessation of repeated exposure to high concentrations of chlorine, desquamation of bronchial epithelium and squamous cell metaplasia was found as well as inflammatory infiltrates consisting of lymphocytes and polynuclear cells with reticulocollagenic fibrosis in the bronchial wall and thickening of the basement membrane (15). The biopsy specimens of four subjects with irritant-induced asthma and RADS have been examined with immunohistochemial techniques to characterize structural changes further (M. Boulet, personal communication, 1995). Collagen type I, III, IV, V, and VII; fibronectin; desmin; and laminin beneath the basement membrane, between smooth muscle fibers, and around nerves were observed. These findings indicate marked airway remodeling. Three workers with irritant-induced asthma were investigated by Chan-Yeung and co-workers 5 months– 1 year after exposure to sulfur dioxide, hydrogen peroxide, and acetic acid, respectively; thickening of the basement membrane and cellular infiltration in the mucosa and submucosa were shown (16). In contrast to earlier findings, the inflammatory infiltrates consisted of eosinophils, shown by immunohistology to be activated, and a few T lymphocytes (both CD8+ and CD4+). Recently, two subjects suffering from RADS after a single exposure

Table 2 Agents Associated with RADS and/or Irritant-Induced Asthma

Agent	Type of study	Evidence	Ref.
Acetic acid	Case report	H, S, P	(9)
	Epidemiological	H, S, BHR	(54)
Acids (various)	Case report	H, S, BHR	(2)
	Case report	H, S, BHR, P	(14)
Acid (heated) (+ welding fumes)	Case report	H, S, BHR, P	(1)
Ammonia	Case report	H, S	(58)
		H, S, BHR, P	(11)
		H, S, P	(103)
Bleaching agent	Case report	H, S, BHR	(4)
Calcium oxide	Case report	H, S, BHR	(2)
Chlorine	Case report	H, S, BHR	(2)
	Case report	H, S, BHR, P	(19)
	Epidemiological	H, S, BHR	(41)
Chloropicrin	Experimental	P	(104)
Cleaning agents	Case report	H, S	(60)
Diesel exhaust	Case reports	H, S, BHR	(105)
Diethylaminoethanol	Epidemiological	H, S	(106)
Epichlorohydrin	Experimental	P	(104)
Ethylene oxide	Case report	H, S, BHR, P	(13)
Floor sealant (aromatic hydrocarbons)	Case report	H, S, BHR	(1)
Formalin	Case report	H, S	(107)
Fumigating agent	Case report	H, S, BHR	(1)
Hydrazine	Case report	H, S, BHR	(1)
Hydrochloric acid	Case reports	H, S, BHR	(2,4,6)
Isocyanates	Case report	H, S	(108)
	Case reports	H, S, BHR	(2,109)
	Case report	H, S, BHR, P	(18)
	Experimental	S	(110)
Metal coat remover	Case report	H, S, BHR	(1)
Metam sodium	Epidemiological	H, S, BHR	(111)
Spray paint	Case report	H, S, BHR, P	(1)
Paint (fumes)	Case report	H, S, BHR	(2)
Perchloroethylene	Case report	H, S, BHR	(4)
Phthalic anhydride	Case report	H, S, BHR	(112)
Sulfur dioxide	Case reports	H, S, BHR, P	(3)
	Case report	H, S, BHR	(2)
	Case reports	H, P	(113)
Sulfuric acid	Case report	H, S, BHR	(2,4)
Uranium hexafluoride	Case report	H, S, BHR	(1)
Urea fumes	Case report	H, S, BHR, P	(17)
Fire/smoke (pyrolysis products)	Case report	H, S, BHR	(1)
	Case reports	H, S	(10)
Gases (chlorine, phosgene, mustard, etc)	Case reports	H, P	(114)
	Case reports	H, S, BHR	(2)

H: clinical history; S: spirometry; BHR: bronchial hyperresponsiveness; P: pathology.
Source: From Ref. 115, with permission.

to toxic fumes were studied by Lemière and co-workers (17,18). Bronchial biopsies were performed 46 days and 2 months after the event, respectively. Immunohistochemistry stains revealed that most inflammatory cells were T lymphocytes; no degranulated eosinophils were detected.

Table 3 summarizes the time course of changes in pathophysiological features shortly after accidental inhalation in two cases of RADS caused by chlorine and isocyanates, respectively (Figs. 1 and 2) (18,19). Briefly, there was rapid denudation of the mucosa with fibrinohemorrhagic exudates in the submucosa followed by signs of regeneration of the epithelial layer with proliferation of basal and parabasal cells and subepithelial edema. Five months after the inhalation accident and 3 months after treatment with inhaled corticosteroids, regeneration of the bronchial epithelium was complete in the first case but only partial in the second case. The time course of the pathological features in these two cases suggests that histological injuries of RADS could be almost completely reversible. Yet, in the specimens described by Brooks and co-workers from biopsies performed several years after the offending exposure, injuries of the epithelial layer and inflammatory infiltrate were still present (1). An important difference in the series of cases investigated by Brooks and co-workers (1) and those by Lemière and co-workers (18,19) is the medical management. In the latter series, both subjects were prescribed inhaled corticosteroids after the first bronchoscopy, at day 3 and day 45 after exposure to chlorine and isocyanates, respectively (18,19). It can be hypothesized that early institution of inhaled corticosteroid treatment may have enhanced the regeneration of bronchial epithelium and reduced the inflammatory reaction (20).

The acute change of RADS were confirmed in a model in which rats were exposed to high concentrations of chlorine (21). Histological evaluation revealed epithelial flattening, necrosis, and evidence of epithelial regeneration. Bronchoalveolar lavage (BAL) showed an increased number of neutrophils. Maximal abnormality in the appearance of the epithelium occurred between 1 and 3 days and corresponded to the timing of maximal functional changes in lung resistance and increased bronchial hyperresponsiveness (Fig. 3) (21). Although the functional and pathological abnormalities resolved in the majority of animals after a variable period, some animals were left with persisting epithelial abnormalities. Furthermore, in the animal model of RADS, it was shown that institution of parenteral steroids for 1 week significantly reduced the increased percentage of neutrophils in BAL and had partial beneficial effects on airway wall damage, as evidenced by the decrease in the extent of epithelial changes (epithelial flattening, necrosis, and stratification), in goblet cell number, and in the amount of smooth muscle (22a).

HYPOTHESIS OF PATHOGENETIC MECHANISMS

The pathogenesis of RADS is entirely speculative primarily because the clinical descriptions of the syndrome thus far have been retrospective. Although bronchial damage in the rat model described above appears to confirm the acute changes occurring in RADS, it does not address the diversity of causative agents and the uncertainties concerning susceptibility and risk factors. Moreover, since the initial clinical cases were observed only after high-level irritant exposures, it cannot yet be claimed that the asthma-like reactions caused by low-level respiratory irritants, for which there are some good animal models, are equivalent to RADS. From the meager amount of bronchial biopsy histopathological data currently available, it appears that the micropathological outcome of RADS is similar

Table 3 Time Course of Histological Lesions After Accidental Inhalation

Interval After Accidental Inhalation

Case 1: Exposure to toxic concentrations of chlorine (19)

60 hr	15 days	60 days	150 days
Superficial fibrinohemorrhagic layer replacing bronchial epithelium that is sloughed, degeneration of connective tissue	Persistence of superficial hemorrhage, bronchial epithelial sloughing. Increased deposition of collagen	Regeneration of the epithelial cells (basal, parabasal), collagen degeneration. Spots of lymphocytes. Few polynuclear cells. Increase in collagen of basement membrane	Complete regeneration of the epithelium layer. Numerous basal cells indicating regeneration

Case 2: Exposure to toxic concentrations of solvents and isocyanates (18)

45 days	98 days
Severe damage of the epithelial layer with few remaining basal cells Subepithelial edema with inflammatory cells underneath the basement membrane	Incomplete regeneration of the epithelial layer with few ciliated cells Inflammatory cells persisting in epithelium and connective tissue

Source: Adapted from Lemière C, Malo J, Gautrin D. Nonsensitizing causes of occupational asthma. Med Clin North Am 1996; 80(4):755. From Ref. 20, with permission.

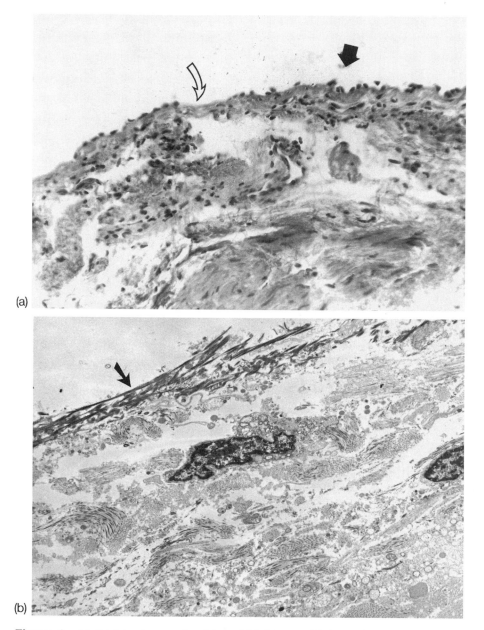

(a)

(b)

Figure 1   (a) Light micrograph of bronchial biopsy 46 days after single massive exposure to isocyanates. Severe loss of epithelial cells (open arrow) with few remaining basal cells (shaded arrow). Subepithelial edema with inflammatory cells (mainly lymphocytes) underneath basement membrane [hematoxylin-eosin (H-E) stain × 250]. (b) Electron micrograph of first biopsy. Epithelial cell loss at luminal surface with fibrin deposition and intrafibrillar edema (arrow). Epon-embedded material stained with uranyl acetate and lead citrate (×2700). (From Ref. 18, with permission.)

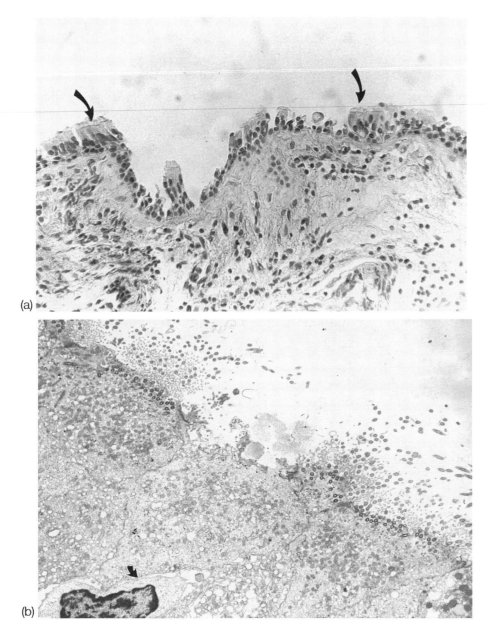

Figure 2 (a) Light micrograph of second bronchial 98 days after isocyanate exposure. Incomplete regeneration of epithelial layer with few ciliated cells (arrows). Inflammatory cells (mainly lymphocytes) persist in epithelia and connective tissue (H-E stain ×250). (b) Electron micrograph of second biopsy. Epithelial cells with incomplete cilia genesis and dilatation of smooth endoplasmine reticulum. Lymphocytes at bottom (arrow) (uranyl acetate and lead citrate staining, ×2700). (From Ref. 18, with permission.)

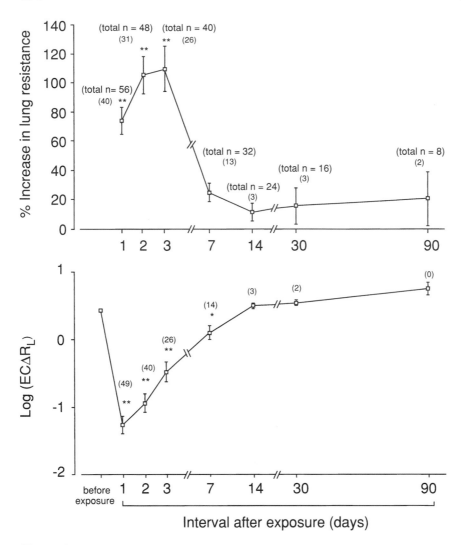

Figure 3 (Upper panel) Time course of lung resistance changes after acute chlorine exposure; (lower panel) time course of the effective concentration of methacholine required to induce an increase in R_L of 0.20 cmH$_2$O ml/sec from postsaline inhalation value (EC ΔR_L). Data are expressed as mean $\pm$ SEM. Statistically significant differences between measured value and baseline value are expressed as **$p < 0.01$, *$p < 0.05$. The total number of rats included and the number of rats with abnormal findings (in brackets) are given at each time interval. (From Ref. 21, with permission.)

to asthma. It may therefore be appropriate to propose a pathogenetic hypothesis commensurate with current knowledge about naturally occurring asthma.

Assuming that RADS is a "big bang" affair occurring after accidental single or multiple exposures to noxious agents, the high levels of irritant exposure will initiate massive airway injury (Fig. 4). The initial massive epithelial damage and destruction will be followed by direct activation of nonadrenergic, noncholinergic (NANC) pathways via axon reflexes and onset of neurogenic inflammation. Nonspecific macrophage activation and mast cell degranulation may also occur with release of proinflammatory chemotactic

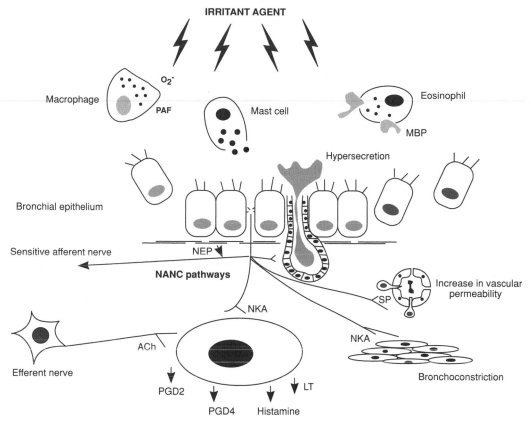

Figure 4 Pathophysiological hypothesis in RADS. See text for detailed description. Ach = acetylcholine; LT = leukotriene; MBP = major basic protein; NANC = nonadrenergic, noncholinergic; NEP = neutral endopeptidase; NKA = neurokinin A; PAF = platelet-activating factor; PGD = prostaglandin; SP = substance P. (From Ref. 20, with permission.)

and toxic mediators. Secondary recruitment of inflammatory cells will then enhance the subsequent profound inflammatory response.

The important inaugural event involves initiation of bronchial epithelial injury. What exactly transpires is not completely understood, but the injury in some way impairs intrinsic respiratory epithelial function (i.e., loss of ciliary activity, reduced neutral endopeptidase activity, decreased availability of epithelial-derived relaxing factor) and also initiates epithelial cell release of inflammatory mediators with subsequent activation of NANC nerves and transmitter release (neurokinins A and B, substance P, etc.). These combined effects not only induce changes in microvascular permeability but also cause increased mucus cell secretion.

The chronic inflammatory process observed in bronchial wall biopsies is probably the end result of secretions from the major effector cells: alveolar macrophages, mast cells, and eosinophils. Many of the inflammatory mediators released by these cells are directly toxic. Others lead to lymphocyte recruitment and subsequent release of a complex cascade of cytokines, which enhance the inflammatory response. It is therefore not surprising that a chronic state of NSBH occurs as an aftermath of RADS.

During the recovery process there may be resolution of inflammation, epithelial cell repair, neural activity inhibition, and improvement of vascular integrity. However, the greater the degree and extent of the initial injury, the more unlikely that such a complete recovery will occur. Under the latter conditions there may be deposition of type III collagen under the basement membrane, and such changes may be irreversible. In most cases of RADS due to high-level irritant exposure, the sequelae of the inflammatory response are obviously severe enough to cause chronic persistent asthma with concurrent NSBH.

DIAGNOSIS OF RADS

The clinical criteria for confirming the diagnosis of RADS are listed in Table 4. They are determined after a thorough medical and occupational history, abnormal pulmonary function tests, and objective evidence of NSBH.

Although there are no rigorous validity data about the predictive value of history, there is no question that it is crucial for the diagnosis of RADS. In contrast to other forms of occupational asthma, where the onset of the illness cannot be precisely determined, the onset of RADS usually can be specifically dated. The patient may even by able to identify the exact time of the day that the illness began. The reason for this clear-cut time discrimination is that RADS is a dramatic event, generally following an accident or unusual precipitous incident. The details remain vividly clear in the subject's mind. The exposure is irritant and generally a vapor or gas, but on occasion a high-level smoke or dust exposure may be responsible. The original criteria have been modified to encompass both single high toxic exposures and repetitive exposures to either high toxic or somewhat lower concentrations—yet still above permissible exposure levels—of the same irritant. Multiple exposures to low levels of irritants are not included in the current case definition. Moreover, the terminology of "RADS-consistent symptoms" cannot be rigorously defined and should be discouraged.

Similar to other types of occupational asthma, the symptoms of cough, dyspnea, and wheezing may occur. Characteristically, cough is a predominant symptom and may lead to an incorrect diagnosis of "acute bronchitis." Some RADS patients develop an intractable cough, which even interferes with the medical interview and precludes proper spirometric measurements.

Table 4 Cardinal Diagnostic Features of RADS

Identification of date, time(s), frequency, and extent of exposure; the latter may be a single high exposure, multiple high exposures, or multiple somewhat less high exposures (yet still higher than either TLV or PEL concentrations)
Symptoms appear within 24 hr
No latency period between exposure and symptoms
Symptoms less likely to improve away from work
Objective (pulmonary function) tests demonstrate obstruction
Presence and persistence of nonspecific bronchial hyperresponsiveness (as measured by methacholine or histamine challenge tests)

The response of symptoms to removal from work may not have the same significance for RADS patients as it does for other types of occupational asthma. Workers with RADS are less likely to improve away from work, at least for several months after the symptoms first appear. Symptoms usually do not improve over a 2-day weekend or an occasional day off but might gradually taper off within a period of months. Some workers with RADS may note improvement away from work because their newly induced hyperresponsiveness makes them more susceptible to other low-level irritants and physical stimuli in the workplace.

The most important historical feature that distinguishes RADS from immunological occupational asthma is whether there has been a latency period between the initial exposure and disease onset. Therefore, as much knowledge as possible about the suspected etiological agent, the time of exposure, and the subsequent onset of symptoms is essential for an acceptable diagnosis of RADS. Confusion may occur after a single massive exposure to an agent known to cause immunological occupational asthma in certain cases (22). For example, although workers with exposures to one or more large spills of TDI are more likely to report asthma symptoms or show changes in lung function tests, an immune mechanism may or may not be demonstrated in such cases (23,24).

Changes in airway caliber and airway reversibility are variable in RADS. Abnormalities usually can be demonstrated soon after the initial exposure event. Long-term persistence of airflow limitation depends upon the inciting agent and the initial duration of exposure, both of which determine the degree of epithelial damage and subsequent inflammatory response. Resolution of airways obstruction depends upon the quality and efficiency of the recovery process. Thus, if the recovery is complete, the spirometric tests should become normal. When a RADS patient is well enough to return to work, cross-shift changes in FEV_1 or other obstructive parameters should not be expected to vary because the industrial event that originally caused RADS is no longer an inciting risk factor for the worker. Thus, in contrast to other forms of occupational asthma (both immunological and nonimmunological), pulmonary function tests in RADS workers usually do not vary significantly at or away from work. However, during the active phases of RADS, exaggerated diurnal variation of spirometric values will be present just as in other types of asthma. Therefore, serial peak expiratory flow rate tests are particularly useful in this group of patients for prognosis of the obstructive process (25–27).

Testing for the presence of NSBH in RADS workers is vital for following the course of the disease (28,29). Since airway obstruction may resolve within a matter of months, a finding of increased NSBH may be the only objective finding in such patients. In the reported cases that have been followed up, significant NSBH, as measured by methacholine or histamine challenge tests, may be demonstrated for years after the initial inhalation episode (1,11). The waning or disappearance of NSBH is a good harbinger of recovery (30).

MANAGEMENT

Because RADS is usually precipitated by an unforeseen industrial accident, removal of the worker is automatic. Emergency treatment of the acute obstructive symptoms might require inhaled or parenteral beta$_2$-agonists, intravenous aminophylline, and/or steroids and oxygen. The specific requirements of each of these agents depends upon the severity of the worker's symptoms. Long-term medical management of RADS cases may require inhaled corticosteroids and cromolyn or tapering doses of systemic steroids to reduce the severity of NSBH (31,32). However, medical therapy is not a substitute for environmental control. This is particularly important for RADS patients who may wish to return to work, because they are particularly susceptible to other, nonspecific irritants in the workplace as a result of the original RADS-induced bronchial hyperresponsiveness (33). Workers should also be instructed to minimize exposure to environmental irritants at home and elsewhere. In some cases, good protection against the effects of nonspecific irritants may be provided by an airstream helmet (34).

PROGNOSIS

Individuals with RADS generally continue to report bronchial irritability symptoms and demonstrate evidence of NSBH for years after the inciting incident. The persistent symptoms are analogous to TDI, snow-crab processors, or western red cedar workers who have persistent asthma after their exposures have been terminated (35–38). In contrast to immunological asthma in which a more favorable prognostic outcome is associated with a shorter duration of symptoms prior to diagnosis, it is not yet possible to predict which RADS workers will have persistent symptoms and permanent hyperresponsiveness on the basis of the agent itself or the duration of exposure (39).

The functional sequelae of subjects with RADS or with a suspected syndrome of RADS are due not only to hyperresponsiveness but also to persisting airway obstruction (20). Airway obstruction has been documented after inhalation to high levels of irritant agents (14,40). This alteration can persist for several years (1,4,41). Four of the 10 subjects investigated by Brooks and co-workers had a decreased FEV_1 and FVC 4 months—11 years after the offending exposure (1). Among three subjects suffering from RADS studied by Boulet, one presented with airway obstruction 6 years after the inhalation accident (4). Bhérer and co-workers demonstrated airway obstruction in 16 of 51 bleach plant workers in a survey that took place 18–24 months after these workers had been repeatedly exposed to high concentrations of chlorine and had experienced nasal, conjunctival, and respiratory symptoms within minutes of exposure (41). In these 16 workers, no improvement was found in spirometry 30–36 months after the first survey (42).

A restrictive syndrome in association with airway obstruction after exposure to an irritant agent has been described (5,43). Gilbert and Auchincloss hypothesized that the onset of a restrictive pattern could be related to the site of bronchial obstruction (5). Large airway obstruction is more likely to result in an obstructive pattern with a restrictive component if the site of constriction also involves smaller airways. Associated decreases of FEV_1 and FVC have frequently been observed after exposure to high levels of irritant agents (9,16). The concurrent decrease of FVC suggesting a restrictive pattern could be due to hyperinflation with an increased residual volume and therefore not truly restrictive. Thus it has been demonstrated that 10% of patients with pure obstruction may have a restrictive type of spirogram (44).

Airway responsiveness can either persist for several years after the exposure (1,15) or be reversible within months to years after an inhalation accident (45,46). Bhérer and co-workers studied the time course of clinical and functional behavior of a group of 71 bleach plant workers with suspected RADS on the basis of the clinical history (exposure to toxic concentrations of an irritant material with the onset of respiratory symptoms in a subject without preceding respiratory symptoms) (41). At 18–24 months after these workers were identified and withdrawn from exposure, 22 of 51 (43%) subjects showed normal airway hyperresponsiveness. Nineteen of the 29 workers with increased airway hyperresponsiveness at the time of the first follow-up were investigated 30–36 months after removal from work: six men had a significantly improved PC_{20} including five for whom the PC_{20} value had returned to a normal range. The six men had normal FEV_1 values on both assessments (42). These subjects had not received either oral or inhaled corticosteroids.

It is still unknown whether treatment with oral or inhaled corticosteroids affects the prognosis of the condition. Randomized studies on RADS are needed to evaluate the efficacy of inhaled corticosteroids. There have been few reports of improvement in pulmonary function with corticosteroid therapy in patients suffering from RADS. Chester and co-workers reported on two subjects exposed to toxic concentrations of chlorine (47). One was treated with corticosteroids and oxygen therapy while the other received only oxygen therapy. The FEV_1 showed an initial marked improvement in both patients. The first subject continued to improve progressively until her values reached the normal range at the end of the first year while the second subject (although improved at the end of 1 year) reached a plateau and stabilized at less than 80% of predicted. There is recent evidence that parenteral and/or inhaled steroids may modify the outcome of the condition. In a subject with RADS, treatment with inhaled corticosteroids normalized the heightened bronchial hyperresponsiveness with exacerbation when the treatment was stopped (19).

COMPARISON BETWEEN RADS AND OTHER FORMS OF OCCUPATIONAL ASTHMA

Common and distinguishing features of RADS and other types of occupational asthma are listed in Table 5. From a histopathological point of view, desquamation of the epithelium is found in both conditions. In the acute stage, desquamation is much more extensive in RADS; consequently, the phenomenon or regeneration of basal cells is prominent in RADS. The inflammatory exudate, on the other hand, is less intense in RADS. Neutrophils are found in BAL, at least in the acute stage of RADS. Lymphocytes are encountered in both occupational types of asthma, although they are more numerous in nonoccupational asthma. Although eosinophils are commonly found in both natural and occupational asthma, their presence in RADS has only been reported in two series of cases (16,15). Thickening of the basement membrane is common in both conditions but is more pronounced in RADS. Subepithelial fibrosis is much more pronounced in RADS (15).

Table 5 Similarities and Differences Between Occupational Asthma with a Latency Period and RADS

	Occupational asthma with a latency period	RADS
Latency period	Present	Absent
Diagnosis	Various: PEF monitoring; SIC	History; functional
Pathology	Like asthma	Acute: more epithelial shedding hemorrhage; Chronic: more connective tissue
Functional	Better reversibility to BDT	Less reversibility to BDT
Treatment	Steroids useful	Steroids useful

PEF: peak expiratory flows; SIC: specific inhalation challenge; BDT: bronchodilator.
Source: Adapted from Ref. 115, with permission.

From a functional point of view, if airway obstruction is present, it is less responsive to bronchodilators in the case of RADS. Gautrin and co-workers compared 15 subjects with RADS and 30 subjects with occupational asthma with a latency period, all with a $FEV_1 < 80\%$ of predicted normal and with similar intervals from the end of exposure (15). The mean improvement in FEV_1 after bronchodilator was close to 20% in occupational asthma with a latency period, but only 10% in subjects with RADS. As in occupational asthma with a latency period, there may be improvement in bronchial hyperresponsiveness, up to 2–3 years after cessation of exposure (42). Finally, recent clinical evidence (19) coupled with experimental findings (22a) suggests that corticosteroids can improve airway caliber and hyperresponsiveness in RADS similar to their effects in both occupational asthma with a latency period and natural asthma.

OTHER AIRFLOW OBSTRUCTIVE SYNDROMES WITH FEATURES SIMILAR TO RADS

A clinical picture compatible with RADS has been described in several studies following accidental exposures in the community (48–50) and in the workplace (51). In a number of studies, the original diagnostic criteria of RADS have been modified to include asthma after repeated exposures to high and somewhat lower concentrations of the same irritant agent (2,41,52,53). When airway responsiveness could not be documented objectively but the other criteria were met, affected individuals were characterized as having symptoms similar to RADS (54) or at risk of developing the syndrome (41). However, the clinical criteria of RADS were not satisfied in such cases. Interestingly, in a series of cases who were repeatedly exposed to the same agent, atopy was found to be a significant risk factor (53). Since many atopic patients are known to exhibit the pathological and physiological hallmarks of asthma, it is possible that exposure to high concentrations of irritants will induce symptoms more readily in these patients than in normal, nonatopic subjects.

Incidence

It is difficult to estimate the incidence of RADS or a syndrome similar to RADS because of variability of target populations: i.e., nonoccupational exposure to an accidental spill (48,50) with populations subsequently reporting to a poison control medical center (55) or a worker population (54). In the former instance, a true incidence rate for RADS cannot be calculated because only those self-reporting to a poison or a medical center are evaluated (56). Similarly, in worker populations, airway hyperresponsiveness has not been objectively assessed in the entire exposed population but only among subjects consenting to the test (54) or among selected groups of workers at risk of developing RADS (41). However, Kern's study provided a better estimate of the incidence of RADS following a single accidental exposure to high concentrations of glacial acetic acid, as 51 of the 56 hospital employees exposed within 2.5 hr after the accident were assessed (54). Eight workers (16%), with no history of asthma, reported symptoms consistent with RADS within 24 hr after the accident and symptomatic status was related to the degree of exposure. Among the 24 workers who accepted a bronchial challenge test, RADS was confirmed in four subjects and a dose-response relationship was shown with acetic acid exposure levels.

In the United Kingdom the SWORD data offer a basis for estimating the incidence and outcome of inhalation accidents (57). Between 1990 and 1994, 1180 inhalation accidents were reported; this represented 10% of all lung diseases reported, the fifth most common category. The highest rates were among chemical processors (163.5/million/year), followed by engineers and electricians (32.1/million year). An investigation of over 700 inhalation accidents (1990–1993) indicated that symptoms lasted for 1 month or more in 26% of cases, including 9% with asthma or RADS (12).

Consequences of High-Level Irritant Exposures

Case Reports

Before RADS was defined in 1985, there were a number of reports concerning workers developing asthma after exposure to high levels of irritants. Although these workers demonstrated evidence of airflow obstruction and symptoms of airway hyperresponsiveness for varying periods after the challenge, they differed from subjects with RADS because the airway hyperresponsiveness was not documented by methacholine or histamine challenge tests. Charan and co-workers described five cases of accidental high levels of SO_2 exposure with three survivors developing severe and another showing mild airway obstruction (43). Flury et al. described a 50-year-old man who inhaled substantial quantities of concentrated ammonia vapors. Over the next 5 years serial pulmonary function testing documented the development of an obstructive lung disorder (58). While methacholine challenges were not performed, the authors indicated that hyperreactive airways were present and likely the direct result of the inhalation injury. Donham et al. described an acute toxic exposure to high levels of hydrogen sulfide after agitation of liquid manure (59). One survivor had respiratory symptoms persisting more than 2 months after the incident. Murphy et al. reported persistent obstructive disease after high-level irritant exposures (60).

Epidemiological Studies

Some epidemiological studies addressing the question of the persistence of RADS, or a syndrome with similar features, are summarized in Table 6; in selecting studies for this review, the authors gave preference to those in which nonspecific airway responsiveness was assessed. More often than not, there was a lack of information on duration of exposure and concentrations of an irritant agent after an accident (61). Levels of exposure have been assessed only indirectly through a description of location and employee's movements during the episode (61) or through an analysis of the characteristics of the site (54). In some instances, exposure has been estimated through self-reporting or first-aid reports (52,62,63). In the absence of estimates of exposure, clinical changes (i.e., dyspnea) associated with accidental inhalations have been used as predictors of lung diseases (51,61).

From the workforce-based studies, there is some evidence that accidental inhalation to high concentration of irritant leads to persistent symptoms and/or long-term lung function abnormalities (42,52,61,64,65). By contrast, in the large population-based study considered to be the most comprehensive follow-up study to date (205 subjects, 145 exposed, spirometry initially and at follow-up), no changes were seen in pulmonary function testing over the 6-year follow-up period. Airway responsiveness, however, was not assessed in this population (66). However, comparisons between population-based and occupational-based studies are limited owing to differences in exposure characteristics and prevalence of risk factors (64,65). In addition to a single and brief occupational exposure to high concentrations of an irritant, there may be chronic low-level exposure to the same or another agent in the workplace (56). Under these conditions, it has been hypothesized that

Table 6 Workforce-Based Surveys of Reactive Airways Dysfunction Syndrome: Long-Term Effects of High-Level Irritant Exposure

No. studied/ population	Type of population	Longest follow-up period	Outcome Symptoms	Outcome Functional tests	Outcome Bronchial responsiveness	Persistence of effects (%)	Type of irritant exposure; estimated level	Host facators: smoking, personal asthma	Ref.
59/150 exposed	Longshoremen	2 years	dyspnea: 35% vs. 0%	No data	No data	Dyspnea: 27%; deficits related to level of exposure	Chlorine; severe vs. minimal	46% smoking, effect not controlled	(61)
13/20	Construction workers at a pulp mill	12 years	Not reported	RV <80% in 67% (significant change over 12-year period); FEV$_1$/FVC < 80% in 62% (loss in FEV$_1$ not > the expected 25 ml/yr)	NSBH 38% (5/13) related to initial airway obstruction (p < 0.05) and airway trapping (p < 0.05)	No initial nonspecific bronchial challenge test	Chlorine	70% smoking	(65)
51/56	Hospital employees	8 months	No symptoms (70%) vs. transient symptoms (14%) vs. persistent symptoms for at least 3 months (16%)	Not reported	NSBH 37% (9/24)	RADS in 4/51 (7.8%) ~1 yr after accident; relative risk in those with high exposure: 9.8 (CI: 0.9–264.6)	Glacial acetic acid; graded by industrial hygienist	No confounding due to preexposure risk factors or smoking	(54)
90/174	Pulp mill workers	7 years	First-aid reports related to work-related chest symptoms (odds ratio: >4.4, significant)	FEV$_1$/FVC less in workers with first-aid reports (p < 0.05)	No data	Greater decline in FEV$_1$/FVC in gassed group (p < 0.05)	Chlorine/ClO$_2$, SO$_2$; welding smoke; first-aid reports/ self-reports of gassing/ nonexposed	Control for age and smoking	(52)
64/71 at risk of developing RADS	Bleach plant workers (survey II)	18–24 months	Respiratory symptoms: 91%	FEV$_1$ < 80% predicted: 31% (16/51)	NSBH 57% (29/51)	RADS: 57%, related to severity of initial outcome	Chlorine, ClO$_2$; no. of accidents, severity of initial outcome	53% smokers no effect of smoking	(41)
20/29 with RADS	Bleach plant workers (survey III)	2–3 years	Frequency of dyspnea: 80%	No change in FEV$_1$ after 1 year	Significant decrease in 6/ 19 (32%) (PC$_{20}$ ≥ 3.2-fold)	NSBH 74% (14/19)	Chlorine, ClO$_2$; no such exposure during follow-up	No previous history of asthma	(42)

VC = vital capacity; W$_{el}$ = elastic work of breathing; D$_L$CO = diffusing capacity for carbon monoxide; RV = residual volume; FEV$_1$ = forced expiratory volume in 1 sec; FVC = forced vital capacity; NSBH = nonspecific bronchial hyperresponsiveness; RADS = reactive airways dysfunction syndrome.
Adapted from Lemière C, Malo J, Gautrin D. Nonsensitizing causes of occupational asthma. Med Clin North Am 1996; 80(4):755. From Ref. 20, with permission.

the inflammatory reaction occurring in small airways after an accidental exposure to high concentrations of an irritant does not resolve completely because of continuous exposure to the offending stimulus (62).

Consequences of Low-Level Irritant Exposures With or Without High-Level Exposures

Before the entity of RADS was recognized, repetitive exposure to low concentrations of work-related irritant agents was not thought to give rise to occupational asthma. These early epidemiological studies of workers with low-level exposure and subsequent accidental high-level exposure to an irritant were conducted to compare the relative frequency of chest symptoms, increased airway obstruction, and nonspecific airway responsiveness between affected workers and those not exposed to the accidental spill. These studies did not demonstrate major differences between these groups (67,68). Nevertheless, there is an alternative hypothesis that RADS should include a "low-dose reactive airways dysfunction" syndrome, which is defined as a subtype of adult-onset asthma that develops after repeated low-dose exposure to one or more bronchial irritants (69). As discussed previously, individuals with this condition do not currently meet the criteria of RADS.

Several more recent epidemiological surveys that were conducted in workers exposed to both low and high levels of chlorine in pulp mills and papermills demonstrated adverse outcomes. The main findings are summarized in Table 7. A significantly greater prevalence of persistent wheezing was shown in workers who reported on or more episodes of accidental exposure to chlorine compared to other pulp mill workers with chronic low-level exposure to this irritant, regardless of smoking habits (62). Significantly lower values for maximal midexpiratory flows and FEV_1/FVC were found among nonsmokers and ex-smokers who reported at least one accidental gassing episode. These findings were confirmed in a longitudinal study in which first-aid reports of symptomatic inhalation accidents were used as estimates of exposure (52). Henneberger and co-workers found significant changes in FEV_1 and FEV_1/FVC to be associated with high-level irritant gas accidental exposures and cumulative pulp mill exposure and smoking. The changes in lung function appeared to have persisted beyond cessation of exposure to irritant gases (70). A further study among younger and current workers at the same plant showed that airway obstruction was related to gassing in those with high and moderate pack-year histories of cigarette smoking (71).

Gautrin and co-workers assessed 239 workers who had experienced repeated exposure to chlorine in a metal-processing plant (72). Data from first-aid records and a detailed occupational history focusing on the occurrence of chlorine puffs made it possible to identify the intensity of exposure. A mild reduction in expiratory flow rates and an increase in airway responsiveness, as assessed through the methacholine dose-response slope, were documented. The changes were significantly greater in workers who experienced mild symptoms than in those who were asymptomatic after exposure to chlorine puffs. In a 2-year follow-up study of these workers, a fall in lung function was associated with gassing incidents and the number of chlorine puffs causing mild symptoms among cigarette smokers of 20 pack-years or more. Also, a detectable increase in airway responsiveness (PC_{20} decrease ≥ 1.5-fold) was associated with gassing events (73). A surveillance program for workers experiencing gassing incidents was initiated after the first survey to describe the time course of lung function changes. After 4 years, 13 workers had reported a gassing incident at the first-aid unit among 278 workers at risk. Three of these workers whose

Table 7 Workforce-Based Surveys of Reactive Airways Dysfunction Syndrome: Chronic Low-level Irritant Exposures With or Without (Repeated) High-levels Irritant Exposure(s)

No. studied (exposed vs. nonexposed)	Type of population	Type of study	Outcome			Persistence of a syndrome consistent with RADS (%)	Type of irritant exposure and duration	Host factors: smoking, personal asthma	Ref.
			Symptoms	Functional tests	Bronchial responsiveness				
147 vs. 124	Pulp mill and papermill workers	Cross-sectional with control group	n.s. difference for chronic nonspecific respiratory disease	n.s. difference between groups for selected measures of lung function	Not assessed	No. of men with obstructive lung disease too small —no rates	Chlorine, ClO_2/SO_2; average Cl exposure duration 20 years	Current smokers (69%); control for smoking	(67)
58 with gassing vs. 81 with low exposure	Chlorine plant workers	Cross-sectional	Not related to exposure	Small decrease in MMF related to high exposure plus smoking*	Not assessed	Prevalence of ventilatory function impairment (3/139)	Chlorine- background: <1 ppm vs. background plus accidental gassing	Ever smokers (73%)	(68)
392 vs. 310	Pulp mill and railyard workers	Cross-sectional with control group	Prevalence of wheezing greater in pulp mill work*	FEV_1/FVC and MMF less in young, nonsmoking bleach plant workers*	Not assessed	Attack rate of asthma in pulp mill workers (2.7/1000) greater than in railyard workers (0.8/1000) n.s.	Chlorine, SO_2, H_2S, CH_3SH; average exposure duration 8.9 years	Current smokers (47%), atopy (17%)	(63)
316 vs. 237	Pulp mill and railyard workers	Cross-sectional with control group	Increased prevalence of wheezing in pulp mill with gassing incidents*	MMF and $FEV_1/$ FVC less in nonsmoking and ex-smoking pulp mill workers with gassing incidents	Not assessed	Not reported	Chlorine/ClO_2, H_2S, SO_2, and other; average exposure duration 13 years	Control for smoking and childhood asthma	(62)

No.	Population	Study design	Symptoms	Spirometry	Bronchial responsiveness	Other findings	Exposure	Control for confounders	Ref.
230	Pulp mill and papermill workers	Cross-sectional	Not reported	Changes in FEV_1 and FEV_1/FVC related to gassing*	Not assessed	Not reported	Chlorine or SO_2; duration: up to 54 years; cumulative exposure index, never vs. cumulative exposure and accidentally gassed (21%)	Control for smoking and assessment of interaction with cumulative exposure and gassing	(70)
273	Bleach plant workers (survey I)	Cross-sectional	Irritation of the throat (78%), eyes (77%), cough (67%), shortness of breath (54%), headache (63%)	Not performed	Not assessed	Symptoms predictive of irritant-induced chronic lung disease: dyspnea (54%)	Chlorine, ClO_2; most significant exposure episode	Current smokers (53%); asthma or chronic bronchitis (7%), dyspnea not related to smoking or personal asthma	(51)
239/255 grouped according to exposure	Metal plant workers	Cross-sectional	Low prevalence, not related to exposure	FVC less in subjects with mild vs. no symptomatic gassing; FEV_1, FVC, $FEV_1/FVC <$ in workers with frequent gassing with mild symptoms*	In 239 workers; proportion with $PC_{20} \leq 32$ mg/ml and dose-response slope related to exposure*	No new cases of RADS	Chlorine, HCl; duration ≤ 3 years; accidental gassing plus self-evaluation of exposure	Ever smokers (55%), preexistent asthma (3%); control for both	(72)

*Significant difference, $p < 0.05$.

RADS = reactive airways dysfunction syndrome; n.s. = nonsignificant; MMF = midmaximal flow; FEV_1 = forced expiratory volume in 1 sec; FVC = forced vital capacity; PC_{20} = provocative concentration of methacholine inducing a 20% fall in FEV_1.

Adapted from Lemière C, Malo J, Gautrin D. Nonsensitizing causes of occupational asthma. Med Clin North Am 1996; 80(4):755. From Ref. 20, with permission.

spirometry and bronchial responsiveness were within normal range prior to the inhalation accident showed transient but significant changes in lung function (46).

Although repetitive exposures to varying concentrations of chlorine gas exhibited irritative effects, it is noteworthy that appearance of RADS was not uniformly observed. Other chemically unrelated substances also appear to act primarily as irritants without fulfilling the case definition of RADS. In one of these instances there is borderline evidence of immune activity (i.e., formaldehyde), and in other cases, sensitization cannot yet be ruled out (e.g., meat wrapper's and pot-room asthma). These irritants may also interact with other known occupational agents. Because of the possibility that asthma by these agents may be due to mixed mechanisms, these entities do not yet fulfill the criteria of RADS.

Meat Wrapper's Asthma

This was the term coined for three meat wrappers who were treated in an emergency room because of asthma (74). Initial epidemiological investigations recounted a 10–57% prevalence of respiratory symptomatology among meat wrappers. The etiological agent was believed to be in the emissions from the polyvinylchloride (PVC) meat-wrapping film when it was cut with a hot wire, thus vaporizing a fine particulate fume containing di-2-ethylhexyladipate combined with an aerosol or vapor of hydrogen chloride (75). Subsequently, a clinical investigation concluded a component of the emitted fumes from thermally activated price labels was the principal cause of meat wrapper's asthma (76). The major ingredient of the incriminated price label adhesive is dicylohexylphthalate. When heated, it emits irritants, mainly cyclohexyl ether (dicyclohexyl ether) and cyclohexylbenzoate (cyclohexyl of ether of benzoic acid) (75). A potential sensitizer was postulated to be phthalic anhydride, a minor emission product from the heat label (77,78).

Later investigations failed to demonstrate objective evidence of any major airways disease or chronic respiratory hazard among meat wrappers (75,79–81). For instance, in one study, while lower respiratory symptoms were observed in one-third of the meat wrappers, no cross-shift change in FEV_1 was detected, even in the most symptomatic workers (79). Phthalic anhydride was not measurable in the vicinity of the heated price label emissions (75). Thus, it seems unlikely that this emission product is actually present in significant concentrations or that it is present in the air for any reasonable period or even remains stable during heating. Another independent investigation failed to find any evidence of phthalic anhydride–specific IgE and IgG antibodies in exposed workers (79).

Formaldehyde

This chemical has myriad applications including use in the chemical and plastics industries, textile processing, disinfectants, the tanning industry, the vulcanization process in the rubber industry, and as a preservative of anatomical and pathological material. A major application was in the production of urea-formaldehyde foam for mobile home insulation and phenol formaldehyde resin for particle board production. Formaldehyde monomer as well as the degassing of formaldehyde from urea-formaldehyde foam insulation has been reported to cause a variety of symptoms, including asthma (82–85). Asthma caused by low-level exposure is uncommon, but asthma has been reported in workers with high exposures such as pathologists and nurses working in a dialysis unit (85). There have been very few reported cases of formaldehyde-induced asthma proven by bronchial challenge tests. For example, among 230 exposed workers, positive challenges were obtained in only 12 workers (86). Formaldehyde-specific IgE antibodies have been reported in a case of anaphylactic shock occurring after long-term hemodialysis and in the two dialysis nurses cited above (85,87,88). However, exposure to low levels of indoor formaldehyde does not result in significant levels of specific IgE antibody (89). Low titers of specific IgG anti-bodies and autoantibodies have been reported in subjects exposed to formaldehyde in various settings (90). The clinical significance of these findings is unclear because no definite correlations can be made between symptoms or other objective findings (88,90). Thus the current evidence indicates that occupational asthma from formaldehyde is rare and that most respiratory complaints are the result of the irritative effects of formaldehyde (82,91).

Pot-Room Asthma

Although an asthmatic "irritation" syndrome was first observed over 50 years ago in the Norwegian literature, there is still disagreement about how this entity should be classified (92). Pot fume emissions contain particulate and gaseous fluorides, hydrofluoric acid, sulfur dioxide, and cold tar volatiles. Although each of these agents has been suspected as playing a role, there is no convincing evidence that a single agent induces symptoms. The duration of pot-room exposure prior to the first attack ranges from 1 week to 10 years. Thus, those workers who develop symptoms soon after exposure to high peak levels of dust (as high as 53 mg/m^3) could possibly represent a small subset of RADS (93). However, because of the variability of prevalence and prognosis of pot-room asthma, the possibility that some workers develop RADS after exposure to aluminum smelter emissions can only be addressed by future prospective epidemiological studies specifically designed to detect and characterize this entity. Pot-room asthma is discussed in more detail in another chapter.

Machining Fluids

Machine lubricants may have irritant properties because of contamination with trace quantities of metals, additives (i.e., odorants, corrosion inhibitors, antifoam agents, emulsifiers, antioxidants, detergents, viscosity index improvers, antiwear agents, extreme pressure agents), and bactericidal substances. Occupational asthma has been documented in workers exposed to several varieties of machine oil. In one plant where clean suds oil was used, there was a latent period before the workers experienced symptoms (94). Some workers also exhibited asthma after controlled exposures to 1% nebulized aerosols of the clean suds oil. One worker showed a reaction to a pine odorant component in this oil. Other contaminating constituents of the oil were suspected but not proven in some of the other cases (94).

If bactericidal substances are not present in sufficient concentrations, oil-in-water machine fluid emulsions will act as good growth media for bacteria and fungi. A study by Kennedy et al. reported significant FEV_1 cross-shift changes in 23.6% of heavily exposed machinists and 9.5% in minimally exposed assembly workers in the same plant (95). The exact etiological agent in machining fluids responsible for the FEV_1 cross-shift changes was not determined, but it was speculated that chemical irritants or endotoxin from contaminating gram-negative bacteria could be potential causes. Similar to the above discussion of pot-room asthma, it is not clear whether this entity should be considered a subtype of RADS or simply an asthma-like disorder.

Other Workplace Irritants

Many airborne irritants may have the same irritant potential as cigarette smoking. Hypothetically, multiple exposures to such irritants could presumably lead to bronchial mucosal injury and increased permeability to sensitizing agents. Industrial operations utilizing irritant agents are therefore doubly dangerous because of the risk of heavy exposures, and occurrence of accidental spills may lead to either nonimmunological or immunological asthmatic conditions, or both. Irritant gases (e.g., chlorine and ammonia) are required in the platinum-refining process. Their presence may initiate bronchial epithelial injury. Biagini et al. reported that platinum salt immunological sensitization in monkeys required concomitant exposure to ozone before sensitization to platinum salts could be induced (96). Other animal studies have documented that an antecedent exposure to an airborne irritant enhances the capacity for sensitization to an allergen. Exposure to low levels of SO_2 promotes sensitization in guinea pigs and rats and leads to increased epithelial permeability (97,98). Similar enhancement of allergic sensitization has also been reported to occur after ozone exposure (99). Recently, it has also been determined that exposure to low ozone concentrations increases bronchial hyperresponsiveness to allergen in atopic asthmatic patients (100). Other investigations employing prolonged low-level ozone exposure have documented a striking individual variability among normal subjects with a considerable range and response, suggesting that there are subpopulations that are very sensitive to low levels of ozone (101,102). These combined experimental and clinical experiences suggest that the future definition of RADS may require modification to accommodate the possible asthma inducibility effects of multiple exposures to low-level irritants in susceptible patients in the general population (i.e., atopic patients or "normal subjects" with preexisting but asymptomatic NSBH). It should be emphasized that this possible effect of multiple exposures to low-level irritants has no relationship to the multiple chemical sensitivity syndrome, which involves a variety of nonspecific and nonpulmonary symptoms.

SUMMARY

The reactive airways dysfunction syndrome is a clinical pathological entity characterized by exposure to a toxic or irritant chemical, negative history of obstructive symptoms prior to exposure, persistence of obstructive symptoms after exposure, objective evidence of obstructive airways disease, NSBH, and abnormal bronchial biopsy results. It differs from typical occupational asthma because of the absence of a preceding latent period and the onset of the illness after a single or several exposures. As the syndrome evolves, workers also react nonspecifically to other irritants presumably because of the underlying persistent bronchial hyperresponsiveness. Workers with RADS also report that symptoms are equivalent at home and at work. Similar to other types of occupational asthma, NSBH may persist for relatively long periods after cessation of exposure.

REFERENCES

1. Brooks S, Weiss MA, Bernstein IL. Reactive airways dysfunction syndrome: persistent asthma syndrome after high-level irritant exposure. Chest 1985; 88:376–384.
2. Tarlo S, Broder IB. Irritant-induced occupational asthma. Chest 1989; 96:297–300.
3. Harkonen H, Nordman H, Korhonen O, et al. Long-term effects from exposure to sulfur dioxide: lung function four years after a pyrite dust explosion. Am Rev Respir Dis 1983; 128:840–847.

4. Boulet LP. Increases in airway responsiveness following acute exposure to respiratory irritants. Reactive airway dysfunction syndrome or occupational asthma. Chest 1988; 94:476–481.

5. Gilbert R, Auchincloss J Jr. Reactive airways dysfunction syndrome presenting as a reversible restrictive defect. Lung 1989; 167:55–61.

6. Promisloff R, Phan A, Lenchner G, et al. Reactive airways dysfunction syndrome in three police officers following a roadside chemical spill. Chest 1990; 98:928–929.

7. Lerman S, Kipen H. Reactive airways dysfunction syndrome. Am Fam Phys 1988; 38:135–138.

8. Luo J-C, Nelson K, Fischbein A. Persistent reactive airways dysfunction after exposure to toluene diisocyanate. Br J Ind Med 1988; 47:239–241.

9. Rajan K, Davies B. Reversible airways obstruction and interstitial pneumonitis due to acetic acid. Br J Ind Med 1989; 46:67–68.

10. Moisan T. Prolonged asthma after smoke inhalation: a report of three cases and a review of previous reports. J Occup Med 1991; 33:458–461.

11. Bernstein IL, Bernstein DI, Weiss M, Campbell GP. Reactive airways disease syndrome (RADS) after exposure to toxic ammonia fumes. J Allergy Clin Immunol 1989; 83:173.

12. Sallie B, McDonald C. Inhalation accidents reported to the SWORD surveillance project 1990–1993. Ann Occup Hyg 1996; 40:211–221.

13. Deschamps D, Rosenberg N, Soler P, et al. Persistent asthma after accidental exposure to ethylene oxide. Br J Ind Med 1992; 49:523–525.

14. Deschamps D, Questel F, Baud F, et al. Persistent asthma after acute inhalation of organophosphate insecticide. Lancet 1994; 344:1712.

15. Gautrin D, Boulet L, Boutet M, et al. Is reactive airways dysfunction syndrome (RADS) a variant of occupational asthma? J Allergy Clin Immunol 1994; 93:12–22.

16. Chan-Yeung M, Lam S, Kennedy S, et al. Persistent asthma after repeated exposure to high concentrations of gases in pulpmills. Am J Respir Crit Care Med 1994; 149:1676–1680.

17. Lemière C, Malo J-L, Garbe-Galanti L. Syndrome d'irritation bronchique consécutif à l'inhalation d'urée. Rev Mal Respir 1996; 13:595–597.

18. Lemière C, Malo J-L, Boulet L, et al. Reactive airways dysfunction syndrome induced by exposure to a mixture containing isocyanate: functional and histopathologic behaviour. Allergy 1996; 51:262–265.

19. Lemière C, Malo J-L, Boutet M. Reactive airways dysfunction syndrome due to chlorine: sequential bronchial biopsies and functional assessment. Eur Respir J 1997; 10:241–244.

20. Lemière C, Malo J-L, Gautrin D. Nonsensitizing causes of occupational asthma. Med Clin North Am 1996; 80:749–774.

21. Demnati R, Fraser R, Ghezzo H, et al. Time-course of functional and pathological changes after a single high acute inhalation to chlorine in rats. Eur Respir J 1998; 11:1–7.

22. Moller DR, McKay RT, Bernstein IL, Brooks SM. Persistent airways disease caused by toluene diisocyanate. Am Rev Respir Dis 1986; 134:175–176.

22a. Demnati R, Fraser R, Martin JG, Plaa G, Malo J-L. Effects of dexamethasone on functional and pathological changes in rat bronchi caused by high acute exposure to chlorine. Toxicol Sci 1998; 45:242–246.

23. Brooks SM, et al. Epidemiologic study of workers exposed to isocyanates. NIOSH Health Hazard Evaluation Report, 1980.

24. Karol M. Survey of industrial workers for antibodies to toluene diisocyanate. J Occup Med 1981; 23:741–747.

25. Canadian Thoracic Society. Occupational asthma: recommendations for diagnosis, management and assessment of impairment. Can Med Assoc J 1989; 140:1029.

26. Burge P. Single and serial measurements of lung function in the diagnosis of occupational asthma. Eur J Respir Dis 1982; 63(Suppl):47–59.

27. Cartier A, Pineau L, Malo J-L. Monitoring of maximum expiratory peak flow rates and histamine inhalation tests in the investigation of occupational asthma. Clin Allergy 1984; 14:193–196.

28. Brooks SM. Bronchial asthma of occupational origin. In: Rom WN, ed. Environmental and Occupational Medicine. Boston: Little, Brown. 1992.

29. Cockcroft D. Bronchial inhalation tests. I. Measurement of nonallergic bronchial responsiveness. Ann Allergy 1985; 55:527.

30. Lam S, Wong R, Chan-Yeung M. Nonspecific bronchial reactivity in occupational asthma. J Allergy Clin Immunol 1979; 63:28–48.

31. Cockcroft D, Murdock K. Comparative effects of inhaled salbutamol, sodium cromoglycate and beclomethasone on allergen-induced early asthmatic response, late asthmatic response and increased bronchial responsiveness to histamine. J Allergy Clin Immunol 1987; 79: 734–739.

32. Mapp C, Boschetto P, dal Vecchio L, et al. Protective effects of antiasthma drugs in late asthmatic reactions and increased airway responsiveness induced by toluene diisocyanate in sensitized subjects. Am Rev Respir Dis 1987; 136:1403–1450.

33. Smith D. Medical-legal definition of occupational asthma. Chest 1990; 98:1007–1011.

34. Slovak A, Orr R, Teasdale R. Efficacy of the helmet respiratory in occupational asthma due to laboratory animal asthma. Am Ind Hyg Assoc J 1985; 46:411–451.

35. Cote J, Kennedy S, Chan-Yeung M. Outcome of patients with cedar asthma and continuous exposure. Am Rev Respir Dis 1990; 141:373–376.

36. Paggiaro P, Loi A, Rossi O, et al. Followup study of patients with respiratory disease due to toluene diisocyanate (TDI). Clin Allergy 1984; 14:463–469.

37. Malo J-L, Cartier A, Ghezzo H, et al. Patterns of improvement in spirometry, bronchial hyperresponsiveness and specific IgE antibody levels after cessation of exposure in occupational asthma caused by snowcrab processing. Am Rev Respir Dis 1988; 138:807–812.

38. Chan-Yeung M, MacLean L, Pagariaro P. A followup of 232 patients with occupational asthma due to western red cedar. J Allergy Clin Immunol 1987; 79:792.

39. Chan-Yeung M. Immunologic and nonimmunologic mechanisms in asthma due to western red cedar (Thuja plicata). J Allergy Clin Immunol 1982; 70:32–37.

40. Kaufman J, Burkons D. Clinical, roentgenologic and physiologic effects of acute chlorine exposure. Arch Environ Health 1971; 23:29–34.

41. Bhérer L, Cushman R, Courteau J, et al. Survey of construction workers repeatedly exposed to chlorine over a three to six month period in a pulpmill. II. Follow up of affected workers by questionnaire, spirometry and assessment of bronchial responsiveness 18 to 24 months after exposure. Occup Environ Med 1994; 51:225–228.

42. Malo J-L, Cartier A, Boulet L, et al. Bronchial hyperresponsiveness can improve while spirometry plateaus two to three years after repeated exposure to chlorine causing respiratory symptoms. Am J Respir Crit Care Med 1994; 150:1142–1145.

43. Charan N, Meyers C, Lakshminarayan S, et al. Pulmonary injuries associated with acute sulfur dioxide inhalation. Am Rev Respir Dis 1979; 119:555–560.

44. Gilbert A, Auchincloss J. The interpretation of the spirogram. Arch Intern Med 1985; 145: 1635–1639.

45. Blanc P, Galbo M, Hiatt P, et al. Symptoms, lung function, and airway responsiveness following irritant inhalation. Chest 1993; 103:1699–1705.

46. Leroyer C, Malo J-L, Infante-Rivard C, et al. Changes in airway function and bronchial responsiveness after acute occupational exposure to chlorine leading to treatment in a first aid unit. Occup Environ Med 1998; 55:356–359.

47. Chester E, Kaimal J, Payne C, et al. Pulmonary injury following exposure to chlorine gas. Possible beneficial effects of steroid treatment. Chest 1977; 72:247–250.

48. Hasan F, Cehshan A, Fulechan F. Resolution of pulmonary dysfunction following acute chlorine exposures. Arch Environ Health 1983; 38:76–80.

49. Chasis H, Zapp J, Bannon J, et al. Chlorine accident in Brooklyn. Occup Med 1947; 4: 152–170.

50. Charan N, Lakshminarayan S, Myers G, et al. Effects of accidental chlorine inhalation on pulmonary function. West J Med 1985; 143:333–336.

51. Courteau J, Cushman R, Bouchard F, et al. Survey of construction workers repeatedly exposed to chlorine in a pulpmill over a three to six month period. I. Exposure and symptomatology. Occup Environ Med 1994; 51:219–224.

52. Salisbury D, Enarson D, Chan-Yeung M, et al. First-aid reports of acute chlorine gassing among pulpmill workers as predictors of lung health consequences. Am J Ind Med 1991; 20:71–81.

53. Brooks S, Hammad Y, Richards I, et al. The spectrum of irritant-induced asthma, sudden and not-so-sudden onset, and the role of allergy. Chest 1998; 113:42–49.

54. Kern D. Outbreak of the reactive airways dysfunction syndrome after a spill of glacial acetic acid. Am Rev Respir Dis 1991; 144:1058–1064.

55. Blanc P, Galbo M, Hiatt P, et al. Morbidity following acute irritant inhalation in a population-based study. JAMA 1991; 266:664–669.

56. Kennedy S. Acquired airway hyperresponsiveness from nonimmunologic irritant exposure. Occup Med State of Art Rev 1992; 7:287–300.

57. Sallie B, Ross D, Meredith S, et al. SWORD '93. Surveillance of work-related and occupational respiratory disease in the UK. Occup Med 1994; 44:177–182.

58. Flury K, Ames D, Rodarte J, et al. Airway obstruction due to ammonia. Mayo Clin Proc 1983; 58:389–393.

59. Donham K, Knapp L, Monson R, et al. Acute toxic exposure to gasses from liquid manure. J Occup Med 1982; 24:142–145.

60. Murphy D, Fairman R, Lapp N, et al. Severe airways disease due to the inhalation of fumes from cleaning agents. Chest 1976; 69:372–376.

61. Kowitz T, Reba R, Parker R, et al. Effects of chlorine gas upon respiratory function. Arch Environ Health 1967; 14:545–558.

62. Kennedy S, Enarson D, Janssen R, et al. Lung health consequences of reported accidental chlorine gas exposure among pulpmill workers. Am Rev Respir Dis 1991; 143:74–79.

63. Enarson D, MacLean L, Dybuncio A, et al. Respiratory health at a pulpmill in British Columbia. Arch Environ Health 1984; 39:325–330.

64. Kaufman J, Burkons D. Clinical, roentgenologic and physiologic effects of acute chlorine exposure. Arch Environ Heath 1971; 23:29–34.

65. Schwartz D, Smith D, Lakshminarayan S. The pulmonary sequelae associated with accidental inhalation of chlorine gas. Chest 1990; 97:820–825.

66. Jones R, Hughes J, Glindmeyer H, et al. Lung function after acute chlorine exposure. Am Rev Respir Dis 1986; 134:1190–1195.

67. Ferris B, Burgess W, Worcester J. Prevalence of chronic respiratory disease in a pulp mill and a paper mill in the United States. Br J Ind Med 1967; 24:26–37.

68. Chester E, Gillespie D, Krause F. The prevalence of chronic obstructive pulmonary disease in chlorine gas workers. Am Rev Respir Dis 1969; 99:365–373.

69. Kipen H, Blume R, Hutt D. Asthma experience in an occupational environmental medicine clinic. Low-dose reactive airways dysfunction syndrome. J Occup Med 1994; 36:1133–1137.

70. Henneberger P, Ferris JBG, Sheehe P. Accidental gassing incidents and the pulmonary function of pulp mill workers. Am Rev Respir Dis 1993; 148:63–67.

71. Henneberger P, Lax M, Ferris B. Decrements in spirometry values associated with chlorine gassing events and pulp mill work. Am J Respir Crit Care Med 1996; 153:225–231.

72. Gautrin D, Leroyer C, L'Archevêque J, et al. Cross-sectional assessment of workers with repeated exposure to chlorine over a three year period. Eur Respir J 1995; 8:2046–2054.

73. Gautrin D, Leroyer C, Malo J-L. Longitudinal assessment of workers at risk of chlorine exposure. Am J Respir Crit Care Med 1996; 153:A-185.

74. Sokol WN, Aelony Y, Beall GN. A new syndrome. JAMA 1973; 226:639.

75. Vandervort R, Brooks SM. Investigation of polyvinyl chloride film thermal decomposition products as an occupational illness of meat wrappers. I. Environmental exposures and toxicology. J Occup Med 1979; 19:189.

76. Andrasch RH, Bardana EJ. Meat wrapper's asthma: an appraisal of a new occupational syndrome. J Allergy Clin Immunol 1975; 55:130.

77. Maccia CA, Bernstein IL, Emmett EA, et al. In vitro demonstration of specific IgE in phthalic anhydride hypersensitivity. Am Rev Respir Dis 1976; 113:701.

78. Pauli G, Bessot JC, Kopferschmitt MC, et al. Meat wrapper's asthma: identification of the causal agent. Clin Allergy 1980; 10:263.

79. Brooks SM, Vandervort R. Investigation of polyvinyl chloride film thermal decomposition products as an occupational illness of meat wrappers. II. Clinical studies. J Occup Med 1977; 19:192.

80. Jones RN. Respiratory health and polyvinyl chloride fumes. JAMA 1977; 238:1826.

81. Krumpe PE, Finley TN, Martinez N. The search for expiratory obstruction in meat wrappers studied on the job. Am Rev Respir Dis 1979; 199:611.

82. Committee on Adlehydes. Formaldehyde and other aldehydes. Board on Toxicology and Environmental Health Hazards. National Academy of Science, 1981.

83. Day JH, Lees REM, Clark RH. Respiratory effects of formaldehyde and UFFI off-gas following controlled exposure. J Allergy Clin Immunol 1983; 7(Suppl):159.

84. Frigas E, Filley WV, Reed CE. Asthma induced by dust from urea-formaldehyde foam insulating material. Chest 1981; 79:706.

85. Hendrick DJ, Lane DJ. Occupational formalin asthma. Br J Ind Med 1977; 34:11.

86. Nordman H, Keskinen H, Tuppurainen M. Formaldehyde asthma—rare or overlooked? J Allergy Clin Immunol 1985; 75:91.

87. Maurice F, Rivory JH, Larson PH, et al. Anaphylactic shock caused by formaldehyde in a patient undergoing long-term hemodialysis. J Allergy Clin Immunol 1986; 77:594–597.

88. Patterson R, Pateras V, Grammar LC, Harris KE. Human antibodies against formaldehyde-human serum albumin conjugates or human serum albumin in individuals exposed to formaldehyde. Natl Arch Allergy Appl Immunol 1986; 79:53–59.

89. Kramps JA, Peltenburg LT, Kerklaan PR, et al. Measurement of specific IgE antibodies in individuals exposed formaldehyde. Clin Exp Allergy 1989; 19:509–514.

90. Thrasher JD, Wojdani A, Cheung G, Hueser G. Evidence for formaldehyde antibodies and altered cellular immunity in subjects exposed to formaldehyde in mobile homes. Arch Environ Health 1987; 42:347–350.

91. Newhouse MI. UFFI dust? Nonspecific irritant only? Chest 1982; 82:511.

92. Abramson MJ, Wlodarczyk JH, Saunders NA, Hensley MJ. Does aluminum smelting cause lung cancer? Am Rev Respir Dis 1989; 139:1042–1057.

93. Wergelund E, Lung E, Waage JE. Respiratory dysfunction after potroom asthma. Am J Ind Med 1987; 11:627–636.

94. Robertson AS, Weir DC, Burge PS. Occupational asthma due to oil mist. Thorax 1988; 43:200–205.

95. Kennedy S, Greaves I, Kreibel D, et al. Acute pulmonary response among automobile workers exposed to aerosols of machining fluids. Am J Ind Med 1989; 15:627–641.

96. Biagini R, Moorman W, Lewis T, et al. Ozone enhancement of platinum asthma in a primate model. Am Rev Respir Dis 1986; 134:719–725.

97. Riedel F, Kramer M, Scheibenbogen C, et al. Effect of SO_2 exposure on allergic sensitization in the guinea pig. J Allergy Clin Immunol 1988; 82:527–534.

98. Vai F, Fournier MF, Lafuma JC, Touaty E, et al. SO_2-induced bronchopathy in rat: abnormal permeability of the bronchial epithelium in vivo and in vitro after anatomic recovery. Am Rev Respir Dis 1980; 121:851–858.

99. Osebold J, Gershwin L, Zee Y. Studies on the enhancement of allergic lung sensitization by inhalation of ozone and sulfuric acid aerosol. J Environ Pathol Toxicol Oncol 1990; 3:221–234.

100. Molfino NA, Wright SC, Katz I, Tarlo S, Silverman F, McClean PA, Szalai JP, Raizenne M, Slutsky AS, Samel N. Effect of low concentrations of ozone on inhaled allergen responses in asthmatic subjects. Lancet 1991; 338:199–203.

101. Horstman D, Folinsbee J, Ives P, et al. Ozone concentration and pulmonary response relationships for 6.6-hour exposures with five hours of moderate exercise to 0.08, 0.10, and 0.12 ppm. Am Rev Respir Dis 1990; 142:1158–1163.

102. Devlin R, McDonnell W, Mann R. et al. Exposure of humans to ambient levels of ozone for 6.6 hours causes cellular and biochemical changes in the lung. Am J Respir Mol Biol 1991; 4:72–81.

103. Leduc D, Gris P, Lheureux P, et al. Acute and long term respiratory damage following inhalation of ammonia. Thorax 1992; 47:755–756.

104. Buckley L, Jiang X, James R, et al. Respiratory tract lesions induced by sensory irritants at the RD50 concentration. Toxicol Appl Pharmacol 1984; 74:417–429.

105. Wade J, Newman L. Diesel asthma. Reactive airways disease following overexposure to locomotive exhaust. J Occup Med 1993; 35:149–154.

106. Gadon M, Melius J, McDonald G, et al. New-onset asthma after exposure to the steam system additive 2-diethylaminoethanol. J Occup Med 1994; 36:623–626.

107. Porter J. Acute respiratory distress following formalin inhalation. Lancet 1975; 2:603–604.

108. Luo JC, Nelsen K, Fischbein A. Persistent reactive airway dysfunction syndrome after exposure to toluene diisocyanate. Br J Ind Med 1990; 47:239–241.

109. Berlin L, Hjortsberg LV, Wass V. Life-threatening pulmonary reaction to car paint containing a prepolymerized isocyanate. Scand J Work Environ Health 1981; 7:310–312.

110. Ferguson J, Schaper M, Alarie Y. Pulmonary effects of a polyisocyanate aerosol: hexamethylene diisocyanate trimer (HDIt) or desmodur-N (DES-N). Toxicol Appl Pharmacol 1987; 89:332–346.

111. Cone J, Wugofski L, Balmes J, et al. Persistent respiratory health effects after a metam sodium pesticide spill. Chest 1994; 106:500–508.

112. Frans A, Pahulycz C. Apparition transitoire d'un syndrome d'irritation aiguë des bronches induit par une inhalation unique et massive d'ahydride phtalique. Rev Pneumol Clin 1993; 49:247–251.

113. Berghoff R. The more common gases; their effect on the respiratory tract. Arch Int Med 1919; 24:678–684.

114. Black J, Glenny E. Observations on 685 cases of poisoning by noxious gases used by the enemy. Br Med J 1915; 165:165–167.

115. Malo J-L, Chan-Yeung M, Lemière C, et al. Reactive airways dysfunctions syndrome. In: Rose BD, ed. Pulmonary and Critical Care Medicine, CD-ROM version. Wellesley, MA: UpToDate, 1998.

31
Cotton and Other Textile Dusts

James A. Merchant
University of Iowa, Iowa City, Iowa

I. Leonard Bernstein
University of Cincinnati College of Medicine, Cincinnati, Ohio

Anthony Pickering
Northwest Lung Centre, Wythenshawe Hospital, Manchester, England

INTRODUCTION

Byssinosis is a generic term applied to acute and chronic airway disease among those occupationally exposed to vegetable dust arising from the processing of cotton, flax, hemp, and possibly other textile fibers. Observations regarding respiratory disease attributable to these vegetable dusts date to the early eighteenth century (1).

Today the production of cotton products is commercially important to developed and developing countries alike. Processing of flax and hemp remain regionally important industries, which continue to provide traditional textile products. Thus, several million workers are occupationally exposed to these vegetable dusts worldwide. In the United States more than 300,000 workers are directly exposed to cotton dust, primarily in the textile industry, but also in cotton ginning, cotton warehousing and compressing, cotton classing offices, cottonseed oil and delinting mills, bedding and batting manufacturing, and utilization of waste cotton for a wide variety of products.

Two febrile syndromes characterized by fever, cough, and other constitutional symptoms including headache and malaise are also associated with byssinosis and textile manufacturing. These occur most frequently with exposure to low-grade, spotted cotton. Mattress-maker's fever and weaver's cough may be considered together because of their characteristically high attack rate and probable similar etiology. Mill fever, which is characterized by fever, malaise, myalgia, fatigue, and often cough, was a common complaint among workers first exposed to high levels of these vegetable dusts; with the prevailing cotton dust levels in the Western world it now rarely occurs. These febrile syndromes are similar to other febrile syndromes described among agricultural workers exposed to high levels of contaminated vegetable dusts.

It is now clear that symptoms typical of byssinosis are observed among others occupationally exposed to vegetable dusts. Many of those exposed are employed in agriculture, which typically involves daily exposure, rather than the cyclical work-week exposure of textile workers. It is also clear that exposure to organic dusts in textile and nontextile operations will often result in asthma-like symptoms. This often results in self-selection

595

or transfer of the affected worker out of dusty jobs or entirely out of the industry. There is also now evidence that exposure to textile dusts results in heightened airway reactivity and that atopy is a risk factor for the development of vegetable dust–induced broncho-constriction (2). These observations are likely to become more relevant with regulation of cotton dust to lower levels. This may allow toleration of lower exposure to cotton dust by many of those who were previously selected out of these industries because of asthma, thereby resulting in increased risk to the development of chronic airway disease.

EPIDEMIOLOGY

The term "byssinosis" was first used by Proust in 1877 to describe respiratory disease among textile workers (3). It arises from the Latin *byssus*, which means fine and valuable textile fiber known to the ancients, usually referring to flax, but also cotton, silk, and other natural textile fibers. Ramazzini was the first to describe asthma and chronic respiratory disease arising from the processing of textiles, and there are abundant important historical descriptions of respiratory disease among textile workers. These were variously described as tracheal phthisis, spinner's phthisis, cotton pneumonia, stripper's asthma, or stripper's and grinder's asthma. The first description of the symptom pattern now associated with byssinosis—that is, respiratory symptoms most severe at the start of the working week—was given in 1845 by Mareska and Heyman: "All the workers have told us that the dust bothered them much less on the last days of the week than on the Monday and Tuesday. The masters find the cause of this increased sensitivity to be in the excesses of the Sunday, but the workers never fail to attribute it to the interruption of work which, they say, makes them lose, in part, their habituation to the dust" (4).

The British Home Office established a Departmental Committee on Dust in Card-rooms in the Cotton Industry (5), which in its 1932 report described the disease as re-spiratory with three stages: (1) The stage of irritation, characterized by "a cough and tight feeling in the chest. This is usually temporary in duration; passing off in one or two days, but the susceptibility returns during a short absence from work, such as occurs at the weekend." This stage developed after approximately 5 years' exposure to cotton dust in the opening and cardroom areas and entirely disappeared on removal from a dusty at-mosphere. (2) The state of temporary disablement or incapacity, which was described as that occurring after being "exposed to the dust for some ten or more years" where the worker "suffers from early bronchitis or asthma, or both combined, associated with cough and mucous expectoration. This condition may . . . lead in time to partial incapacity" (3). The stage of total disablement or incapacity. In this advanced stage there is chronic bron-chitis, with emphysema. Cough is present with mucous or mucopurulent expectoration and shortness of breath on exertion. This condition is incurable and at this stage work in the dusty atmosphere becomes impossible, but improvement may take place and further prog-ress of the disease be arrested or retarded by removal from the dusty environment of the cardroom. In the final stage of the malady the continued strain on the right side of the heart is likely to lead ultimately to cardiac failure (5).

Mortality studies began with the collection of data on those exposed to cotton dust found in the Decennial Supplements to the Annual Report of the Registrar General of Births, Deaths, and Marriages in England and Wales between the years 1880 and 1932. Caminita et al. reviewed these data and found a "marked excess" of deaths in higher age groups, particularly from bronchitis and pneumonia (6). Later reports emphasized that excess mortality from respiratory disease occurred chiefly among cardroom and blowing room operators, strippers, and grinders, rather than among other cotton workers. These observations were reconfirmed by Schilling and Goodman, who showed that a substantial proportion of cardiovascular deaths should have been classified as respiratory deaths because cardiovascular disease was traditionally given priority in multiple certifications prior to 1939 (7,8).

Barbero and Flores studied 100 consecutive deaths among hemp workers and compared the results with 100 consecutive deaths among farm workers from the same region of Spain for the years 1938–1943 (9). The mean age of death for hemp workers was 39.6 years; that for farm workers, 67.6 years. Cardiorespiratory disease was listed as the cause of death twice as often among hemp workers.

Contemporary studies of cotton textile workers' mortality have not revealed consistent excesses in overall mortality. Assessment of respiratory mortality has been difficult to determine because of a lack of adequate work history data and lack of smoking histories. Enterline and Kendrick studied 6281 white male cotton textile workers employed in Georgia mills (10). They found an overall mortality similar to that of asbestos building product and asbestos friction material workers but less than that of asbestos textile workers. There was no evidence of excess respiratory deaths among all cotton workers when cause-specific rates were compared to U.S. white male mortality rates. There was, however, an increase in cardiovascular and all causes of death with increasing duration of exposure. Of interest was a deficit in lung cancer deaths that led Enterline et al. to suggest that there may be a cancer inhibitor, possibly endotoxin, in cotton dust (11). Recent studies of lung cancer in China have confirmed significantly less lung cancer among cotton textile workers after controlling for smoking (12). While methodological factors were considered, these authors concluded that their findings are consistent with Enterline's hypothesis that some tumor-inhibiting factor(s) may be present in dusts from cotton and other vegetable fibers.

Daum investigated a South Carolina cohort exposed primarily to cotton processing and employed between 1943 and 1949 (13). In this small cohort, moderate increases in respiratory deaths were found among male carders with 10–20 years' exposure, and from respiratory and cardiovascular disease among female spinning room workers with greater than 20 years' exposure. A study of two North Carolina mills assessing exposure between 1936 and 1970 found no increase in respiratory mortality, but did report a trend toward increased respiratory mortality with increasing duration of exposure (14). Excesses in cardiovascular mortality were also observed and accounted for a high proportion of deaths. A proportionate mortality study of Rhode Island male textile workers who died during the period 1968–1978 reported a statistically significant increase in nonmalignant respiratory mortality that appeared to be consistent with cotton dust exposure (15). Prospective evaluation of mortality among Finnish women cotton workers hired between 1950 and 1971 found no excess in respiratory disease mortality but did report a fourfold excess in disability from respiratory disease (16). Mortality from cardiovascular diseases was lower than expected, and mortality from specific cancers did not differ from that expected. All of these mortality studies suffer from the selection biases of the healthy worker effect, which becomes more pronounced with years of follow-up (14,17). In a prospective mortality study of a cohort of British textile workers, initially enrolled between 1968 and 1970, both the overall mortality and the respiratory disease mortality of the whole cohort were less than expected (18). However, there was an excess mortality from respiratory disease in those initially reporting byssinotic symptoms.

Early morbidity studies of cotton and flax workers found an unusually high prevalence of respiratory disease, particularly among those working in high-dust-exposure areas (4,19,20). In Great Britain, byssinosis was made a compensable disease in 1942 and, on the basis of the number of cases compensated, was thought to be a disappearing disease. Schilling and Goodman rediscovered byssinosis when they studied Lancashire mills to investigate an apparent increase in cardiovascular mortality (7,8). In a series of studies extending over a 10-year period, Schilling contributed significantly to our understanding of the epidemiology of respiratory diseases among textile workers. He developed, and tested for reliability and validity, a series of questions that were added to the British Medical Research Council (BMRC) respiratory questionnaire, which provided the basis for his byssinosis grading scheme (21):

Grade 0: No symptoms of chest tightness or breathlessness on Mondays
Grade 1/2: Occasional chest tightness on Mondays, or mild symptoms such as irritation (cough) of the respiratory tract on Mondays
Grade 1: Chest tightness and/or breathlessness on Mondays only
Grade 2: Chest tightness and/or breathlessness on Mondays and other workdays

Schilling's questionnaire and grading scheme has been the standard for worldwide epidemiological studies of workers exposed to textile and other vegetable dusts. To validate the grading scheme, he demonstrated that cotton workers with increasing grades of byssinosis have corresponding increases in airway obstruction. Together with Roach, he was the first to quantify a strong linear dose-response relationship between total and respirable cotton dust and the prevalence of byssinosis, which largely explained differences in prevalence in various mill work areas (22). He was also the first to report that smoking was an important risk factor in determining byssinosis prevalence (8,21).

However Schilling's clinical grading does have deficiencies, in that it does not take into account either the irritant effects of dust exposure or the lung function changes that may occur in asymptomatic workers. To address these deficiencies a new classification has been proposed (23). This classification grades byssinosis, respiratory tract irritation, and acute and chronic lung function changes separately. Grade 1/2 byssinosis has been removed from the classification. This new proposed classification is as follows:

Classification	Symptoms
Grade 0	No symptoms
Byssinosis	
Grade B1	Chest tightness and/or SOB on most of first days back at work
Grade B2	Chest tightness and/or SOB on the first and other days of the working week
Respiratory tract irritation	
Grade RTI 1	Cough associated with dust exposure
Grade RTI 2	Persistent phlegm (i.e., on most days during 3 months of the year) initiated or exacerbated by dust exposure
Grade RTI 3	Persistent phlegm initiated or made worse by dust exposure either with exacerbations of chest illness or persisting for 2 years or more
Lung function	
1. Acute changes	
No effect	A consistent[a] decline in FEV_1 of less than 5% or an increase in FEV_1 during the work shift
Mild effect	A consistent[a] decline of between 5 and 10% in FEV_1 during the work shift

Classification	Symptoms
Moderate effect	A consistent[a] decline of between 10 and 20% in FEV_1 during the work shift
Severe effect	A decline of 20% or more in FEV_1 during the work shift
2. Chronic changes	
No effect	FEV_1[b] 80% of predicted value[c]
Mild to moderate effect	FEV_1 60–79% of predicted value[c]
Severe effect	FEV_1[b] less than 60% of predicted value[c]

SOB = shortness of breath.

[a]A decline occurring in at least three consecutive tests made after an absence from dust exposure of 2 days or more.

[b]Predicted values should be based on data obtained from local populations or similar ethnic and social class groups.

[c]By a preshift test after an absence from dust exposure of 2 days or more.

Since Schilling's publications, similar findings have been reported among textile workers from many countries around the world. Recent studies confirm the presence of byssinosis, but especially nonspecific respiratory symptoms and associated lung function abnormalities among Chinese cotton textile workers (24,25). While byssinosis is now much less prevalent, it is still found among Lancashire cotton textile workers (26) and flax workers in Normandy, France (27). In addition to those exposed in primary textile mill operations, the disease has been reported among cotton ginners (28,29), cottonseed oil and delinting workers (28,30), workers in waste cotton operations (31), those in garneting (bedding and batting operations) (32), and those processing soft hemp (33,34) and flax (35–38). Byssinosis has not been typically found among those processing "hard" fibers of sisal or jute (39,40). However, one study reported typical byssinosis among Tanzanian sisal workers with very high dust exposure (41). In addition, symptoms consistent with byssinosis have been reported among workers exposed to herbal tea processing and among workers engaged in swine confinement housing operations (42,43).

Several investigations (29,37,44–47) have now confirmed Schilling's early dose-response findings with remarkable uniformity, despite differences in dose-measurement technique, study population composition, and source of raw product. More recent studies have demonstrated that reliance on total dust measurement may provide a misleading indication of risk, as much of the mass may be composed of cotton lint (48).

In the United States measurement of inhalable dust (<15 μ in aerodynamic diameter) has proven to be a reliable and valid dust measurement for assessment of vegetable dust dose-response (49). Most of these studies have concentrated on preparation and yarn-production workers, with little attention given to weavers and others exposed to cotton dust. One study examined both preparation and yarn processors, who were found to have similar dose-response relationships, and weavers, who were found to have a quantitatively different dose-response relationship (49) (see Fig. 1). Studies of changes in lung function over a Monday working shift have provided objective data on dose-related declines in FEV_1, which were consistent with the dose-response relationships based on byssinosis prevalence (49). Based on these data, a permissible exposure limit for exposure to raw cotton dust has been promulgated by the U.S. Department of Labor: for preparation and yarn operations, a time-weighted concentration of 0.2 mg/m^3 of air; and for weavers, 0.75 mg/m^3 of air (50).

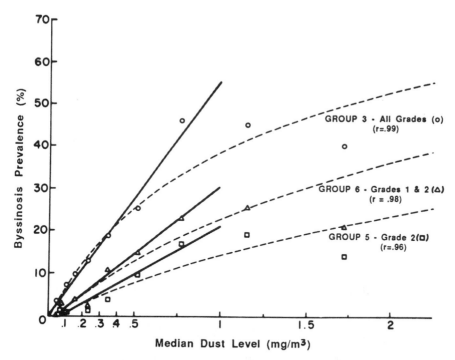

Figure 1 Byssinosis prevalence by grade and by median dust level among cotton preparation and yarn area workers: linear regressions and fitted probit dose-response curves.

In the United Kingdom a different approach was taken. In a study comparing work area and personal sampling techniques, a 7.8-fold difference in measurement between the two techniques was found in the earliest cotton spinning processes, falling to a ratio of 1.4 in ring spinning. This suggested that work area sampling may underestimate an individual's exposure in the earlier processes where byssinosis is most prevalent. This work has led to the introduction of a new cotton exposure standard in the United Kingdom, based on a personal sampling technique (51).

Dose-response data are less available for cotton dust exposures outside the cotton textile industry, but there is evidence of a dose-response relationship for other cotton operations and for processing of flax and hemp (52,53). Based on all available data, the World Health Organization has recommended limits for several of these exposures (54).

Assessment of chronic cough and phlegm, as defined from the British Medical Research Council (BMRC) respiratory questionnaire, has been an integral part of most epidemiological studies of cotton, hemp, and flax textile workers (55). While not a uniform observation, most surveys have reported increased rates of chronic cough and phlegm among those with heavy cotton dust exposure, especially among those with symptoms of byssinosis (56,57). Similarly, indices of dyspnea, as assessed by the BMRC questionnaire, have been shown to be strongly associated with dustier exposures and have been found to be increased among those with more severe grades of byssinosis (33,34,36,53). As with many other epidemiological studies of respiratory disease, smoking has been found to be a powerful risk factor for chronic cough and phlegm and for measures of dyspnea (49,58).

Two major effects of vegetable dust on lung function have been reported in epidemiological studies. The first is a chronic effect characterized by airway obstruction and manifested by reductions in FEV_1, FVC, and FEV_1/FVC with increased dust concentration and duration of exposure. The second is an acute effect characterized by measures demonstrating bronchoconstriction over a working shift of exposure to cotton dust, especially after an absence from exposure for 2 or more days (Fig. 2) (59,60). Spirometric evaluation, typically conducted prior to the Monday shift in Western countries, has confirmed Schilling's observation that those with symptoms of byssinosis, as a group, may be expected to have lower expiratory flow rates than comparable controls. Furthermore, those with chronic cough and phlegm, in addition to symptoms of chest tightness, have been found to have a further decrease in lung function (56–58,61). In large cross-sectional studies, smoking has also been found to exert a significant additive decrease in preshift lung function (48,49,62). Studies by Schacter et al. suggest that smoking may be more related to abnormalities in maximum expiratory flows at 50% and 25%, whereas cotton dust appears to be either more important than or as important as the smoking effect on FVC and FEV_1 among cotton textile workers with long exposures (63).

McKerrow et al. were the first to observe a reduction in expiratory flow rates over a work shift, a reduction that was most marked after an absence from exposure and especially among workers in areas with higher dust levels (64). From these observations they suggested that symptoms of Monday chest tightness and dyspnea might be explained by the reduction in expiratory flow rate. This hypothesis has been questioned, as many persons with symptoms of byssinosis do not exhibit work shift decrements and because the degree of reduction, although statistically significant in epidemiological studies, is typically not considered clinically significant (decrement of 10% or more) (65).

It has been further observed that subjects with bronchitis and byssinosis tend to have greater cross-shift decrements in expiratory flow than those with byssinosis alone (56,61).

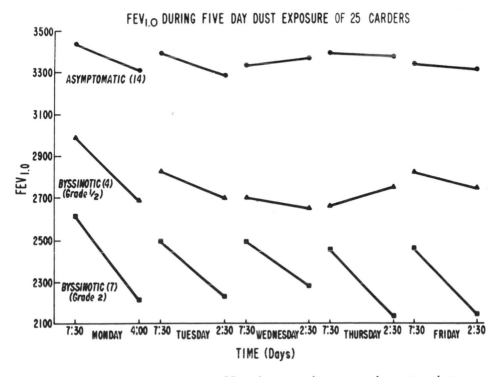

Figure 2 Pattern of response among 25 cardroom workers exposed to cotton dust.

On the basis of the epidemiological association between byssinosis grade and mean decrement in expiratory flow, Bouhuys et al. proposed a functional grading scheme (66). Subsequent reports have shown that the relationship between a Monday decline in FEV_1 of 200 cc, as proposed by Bouhuys et al., is highly variable. An appreciable proportion of those without symptoms of byssinosis have a Monday decrement of greater than 200 cc or 5%, whereas many with byssinosis symptoms do not show even a modest decline (56,67). Nevertheless, because expiratory flow can be easily measured in untrained subjects and provides an objective indicator of biological response to vegetable dusts, spirometry before and following exposure has been widely used in epidemiological studies. Those exposed to cotton, soft hemp, and flax dusts usually have greater decrements in expiratory flow than those exposed to similar dust levels from "hard fibers" (52,53). Those exposed at higher dust levels have been found to show more marked decrements, and the dose-response relationship between respirable dust and decrement in flow rates approximates that for byssinosis symptoms (29,32,49).

In a series of experimental cardroom studies utilizing volunteer subjects exposed to a wide variety of cottons at different levels of dust exposure, Castellan et al. have demonstrated a stronger dose-response relationship between vertically elutriated endotoxin than vertically elutriated dust and have concluded that these observations strongly support the hypothesis that endotoxin plays a causative role in the acute pulmonary response to cotton dust (68,69). As the volunteer subjects were not textile workers, these investigators were unable to assess the pattern of symptoms characteristic of byssinosis. Kennedy et al., in a dose-response study in Shanghai, reported a significant association with current endotoxin level and the prevalence of byssinosis and chronic bronchitis, but not with dust alone (70). While smoking clearly affects baseline spirometric levels, there is conflicting evidence regarding the influence of smoking on acute changes in lung function (56,60,70). Cross-shift decline in FEV_1 remains a useful epidemiological tool, and despite its limitations in its application to individual workers, it has been incorporated as one feature of the medical surveillance examinations required by the U.S. Cotton Dust Standard (50).

Several studies have evaluated lung function prospectively (46,71–73). In each of these studies, conclusions were necessarily based upon survivor populations and include other selection biases, which usually tend to minimize occupational effects. Prospective assessments of decline in lung function have been carried out on workers exposed to high levels of cotton dust in Yugoslavia, India, and China, all of which demonstrated accelerated mean annual declines in FEV_1, which were associated with dust exposures that were several times higher than the U.S. Cotton Dust Standard (74–76). Berry et al. reported roughly twice the annual decline in FEV_1 among cotton textile workers as among synthetic textile workers (72). The decline attributable to cotton dust was slightly greater, but similar in magnitude, to that attributable to smoking, and was somewhat greater among those working in dustier areas and among those exposed for shorter periods of time than longer periods. Merchant et al., who studied a single cotton textile mill several times over a single year, found that those exposed to high levels of cotton dust (many of whom were new employees) had 10-month declines as high as 280 cc, and that smaller dose-related, increased 10-month declines in FEV_1 occurred among workers in three other work areas with less dust exposure and longer tenure (46). A community study of active and retired older cotton textile workers found cotton textile workers to have a higher prevalence and attack rate of respiratory symptoms than controls, and that both men and women cotton textile workers had greater annual declines than did community controls. This study confirmed the cross-sectional assessment of this community and reported a significantly higher proportion of textile workers than nontextile worker controls to be severely impaired (62,71).

In the first published prospective study of lung function among cotton textile workers exposed at or below the U.S. Cotton Dust Standard, Glindmeyer et al. found no accelerated decline in FEV_1 among slashers and weavers exposed below the cotton dust standard and no accelerated decline among nonsmoking yarn-processing workers exposed at the cotton dust standard (73). However, smoking yarn-processing workers were found to have accelerated loss in annual FEV_1, even below the cotton dust standard of 0.2 mg/m^3; dose-related increases in decline in annual FEV_1 were observed among men and women smokers and nonsmokers, thereby unambiguously confirming the dose-response findings from the cross-sectional studies of byssinosis prevalence and cross-shift decline in FEV_1 on which the U.S. Cotton Dust Standard was based (44,50). While these aggregate data support the hypothesis that those with increased acute responses are at increased risk for increased declines in lung function over time, as suggested by Bouhuys (34,75,77), this question is not fully resolved.

CLINICAL EVALUATION

Signs and Symptoms

The hallmark of byssinosis is the characteristic symptom of chest tightness that typically occurs following a weekend away from exposure. Chest tightness is described by workers, often accompanied by placing a hand over their chest, as a heaviness on their chest, as chest congestion, as difficulty taking a deep breath, and sometimes as a band-like feeling around their chest. The onset of chest tightness is variable, as noted in the British Home Office report, which described the symptoms in 100 cardroom workers, 93% of whom described respiratory symptoms (5). Of these, 59% experienced their most severe symptoms during the first half of the working shift and 41% during the second half of the shift. In all workers, symptoms were most severe on the first day of the working week. This time period is important as it distinguishes byssinosis from occupational asthma, which tends to increase in severity over the working week. Affected workers often compare the feeling of chest tightness to that of a chest cold. Frequently chest tightness is accompanied by a cough, which is more prominent on Monday. Indeed, a Monday cough may be the only symptom. A history of chronic productive cough is frequently obtained. Among older workers who have been exposed to cotton dust for many years, a history of exertional dyspnea is a common finding. Among those severely affected, chest tightness and dyspnea occur on all workdays, with relief coming only on weekends and holidays, if then.

All of these symptoms become more severe if the period away from cotton dust exposure is prolonged; i.e., the affected individual appears to lose exposure tolerance. Conversely, Monday symptoms do not occur if exposure occurs 7 days a week, as often occurs with cotton ginning. Symptoms are more severe and more frequent among smokers (46,47). Occasionally, a worker with typical byssinosis will report that symptoms of Monday chest tightness disappeared when he or she stopped smoking without an apparent change in dust exposure (58).

There are no typical or characteristic signs found upon physical examination of workers with symptoms of byssinosis. While the symptomatic worker frequently exhibits a productive cough, on examination the chest is usually relatively quiet. Wheezing is not commonly found early in the course of the disease. Among those severely affected, all the physical findings of advanced chronic airflow limitation may be observed.

A number of nonspecific symptoms are observed among those exposed to cotton dust, apart from byssinosis. Work-related ocular and nasal irritation are now the most common symptoms complained of in U.K. textile mills (78). In this study of 1452 textile workers, 17.5% of cotton workers complained of eye irritation and 11% of nasal irritation. There was no relationship between these symptoms and atopy, byssinosis, or dust concentration, suggesting the presence of unidentified agents in textile dusts that are unrelated to the concentration of dust. Chronic bronchitis was first documented in cotton textile workers by Molyneux and Tombleson in 1970 (67). Even at the dust exposure levels currently prevailing in Lancashire textile mills, an excess of chronic bronchitis is still demonstrable. A study of 2991 cotton and synthetic textile workers reported a prevalence of chronic bronchitis of 6.9% in cotton workers and 4.5% in synthetic fiber workers (79). After controlling for smoking, cotton workers were significantly more likely to suffer from chronic bronchitis. This was most marked in workers over 45 years of age and was significantly associated with cumulative cotton dust exposure. In the cotton population the presence of chronic bronchitis was associated with a small, significant decrement in lung function when symptomatic workers were compared to age-, sex-, and smoking-matched asymptomatic workers.

Febrile syndromes that have been associated with cotton processing include mattress maker's fever and weaver's cough. These conditions occur among experienced workers and are characterized by a high attack rate, a clear-cut febrile episode, severe cough, and dyspnea. Most of these outbreaks have been attributed to mildewed yarn. These febrile syndromes are similar to those common among agricultural workers who are frequently exposed to high concentrations of moldy grain, hay, or silage (80–83). Because the clinical presentation is the same, and because the etiology of all of these febrile syndromes is probably from microorganism toxins, the term "organic dust toxic syndrome" (ODTS) has recently been suggested in an attempt to codify this condition (84) (see Chapter 33). It is likely that the febrile syndromes arising from high levels of cotton or grain dust are also attributable to endotoxins, which are now well-known constituents of these vegetable dusts.

Newly hired workers, and those who first go into dusty cotton-processing areas for a period of a few hours, may experience mill fever (85), which has also been called cardroom fever, dust chills, dust fever, cotton cold, cotton fever, weaver's fever, and, among flax workers, heckling fever (6). A similar syndrome has been described among those exposed to high concentrations of grain dust (84). Symptoms, which typically occur 8–12 hr following heavy dust exposure, consist of chills, headache, thirst, malaise, sweating, nausea, which may be accompanied by vomiting, and a transient fever, followed by fatigue. Without further exposure, these symptoms subside spontaneously within a day or two, but the fatigue may continue for several days. With repeated exposure, such as that experienced by a newly hired textile worker, these symptoms may occur for several days until the worker is "seasoned" or develops a tolerance (85). This "seasoning" is well recognized by workers exposed to high dust concentrations.

Another common complaint of new workers or visitors to mills with high exposures to cotton dust is tobacco intolerance (58). Also a common finding among mill visitors who have a history of asthma, and who may not have had an asthma attack for years, is immediate onset of clinical asthma, which may be severe and often requires medical intervention (80). With the improved dust control achieved through implementation of the U.S. Cotton Dust Standard, mill fever and tobacco intolerance are now infrequently observed. However, it has been suggested that better dust control may allow many more workers with airway hyperresponsiveness to remain in vegetable dust–processing operations and that these workers may constitute a high-risk group for future development of airway obstruction (86).

Lung Function

A series of studies of volunteer textile and nontextile workers in experimental cardrooms have provided a good understanding of lung function abnormalities with cotton dust exposure (59,87–90). These studies have documented a linear decline in expiratory flow over the period of exposure, which is most consistently and significantly discriminated by the FEV_1 (59). Measures of expiratory flow rates have been found to be more sensitive indicators, but the well-recognized increased variability of these measurements decreases their discrimination. Closing capacity and total lung capacity have been found to increase and oxygen tension decrease, but not significantly, with exposure. Body plethysmography before and following exposure suggests that those who exhibit decreased expiratory flow with exposure have increased resistance primarily in peripheral airways, while increased resistance among those who do not have an expiratory flow response occurs primarily in central airways (88). Helium-oxygen spirometry in these subjects found significant decrements in specific airways conductance and greater spirometric responses in smokers than nonsmokers (87).

A temporal association between a peripheral leukocytosis and recruitment of leukocytes to the nasal mucosa and decline in FEV_1 has been noted with heavy dust exposure (59). Evaluation of a selected population of nonasthmatic volunteers demonstrated that atopy, defined as positive prick tests to at least two allergens, and cross-shift decline in FEV_1 were independent. However, those with atopy had significantly greater long-term declines in FEV_1, and the degree of atopy, as measured by the number of positive skin tests, was significantly associated with cotton-induced decrements in FEV_1 (2). It was suggested that this finding may reflect airways hyperresponsiveness described in nonasthmatic, atopic individuals. Studies by Boehlecke et al. (personal communication) postulate that exposure to cotton dust heightens airways hyperresponsiveness, as has been previously reported with other organic dust exposures (91). However, since this tends to be transient rather than persistent, it is an important distinguishing feature between cotton dust–induced airways disease and other forms of occupational asthma.

Only one detailed physiological study has been done of an asthmatic with exposure to cotton dust (76). This followed an unexpected asthma attack triggered by cotton dust exposure in an investigator who had not had asthma since childhood. Highly significant declines in FEV_1 accompanied by marked declines in oxygen tension occurred within 15 min of exposure (Fig. 3). Both FEV_1 and PaO_2 remained depressed following exposure and over 3 more days of cotton dust exposure. No significant change was noted in temperature, leukocyte, or eosinophil count. FEV_1 and PaO_2 returned to baseline level, without bronchodilation, after 3 days away from dust exposure.

Assessment of lung function in those with byssinosis and cotton textile workers with long-duration exposure has usually demonstrated a pattern of mild to moderate airways obstruction, but occasionally this may be severe (92,93). A significant proportion of older cotton textile workers (50% of men and 37% of women) have been found to have some lung function abnormality (93). One study of women with byssinosis assessed transfer capacity for carbon monoxide (TLCO) and found that smokers had significantly lower TLCO, despite shorter cotton dust exposure, while nonsmoking women had normal levels of TLCO. The authors concluded these results support the hypothesis that emphysema

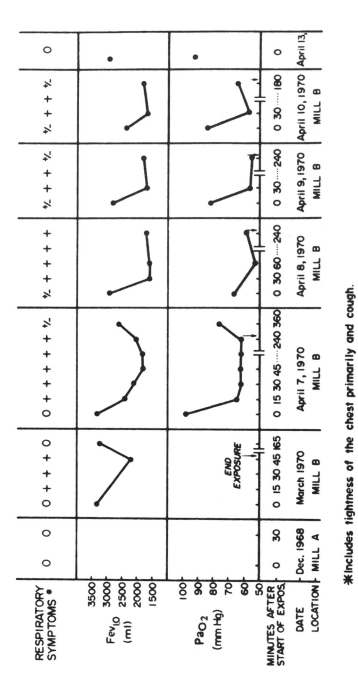

Figure 3 Pattern of response to cotton dust in a nontextile worker with a childhood history of asthma.

among cotton textile workers is probably due to concomitant cigarette smoking and is not itself a feature of byssinosis (94).

Treatment

Research on medical treatment for byssinosis has been confined to acute events. Clinical trials have relied almost exclusively on changes in flow rates among active workers as the indicators of effect. While propranolol has been shown to increase bronchoconstriction with hemp dust exposure, antihistamines and ascorbic acid have been found to protect against this effect (95,96). Similarly, inhaled bronchodilators (salbutamol, isoprenaline, and orciprenaline) will prevent or reverse flow rate changes (95–97). Finally, preexposure treatment with cromolyn sodium tends to block bronchoconstriction (95–97). Inhaled beclomethasone also appears to reduce the flow rate response to cotton dust exposure (97). It must be emphasized that these beneficial physiological effects occur without similar documentation in regard to symptoms. Thus, while the bronchoconstricting effect of these organic dusts, which is usually not severe, may be blocked or reversed, there is no evidence that use of these drugs will necessarily suppress byssinosis symptoms or retard the progression of cotton dust–induced obstructive airway disease. Therefore, these drugs cannot be considered as preventive measures. Management of severe cases of byssinosis does not differ from that for chronic bronchitis and emphysema.

Pathology

Schilling and Goodman reviewed pathological observations on lungs of workers with long cotton dust exposure, as made by several early investigators, and concluded that the pulmonary pathology was that of chronic bronchitis and emphysema (7). In one report lungs were fixed in inflation from 10 autopsies of workers with over 20 years of cotton dust exposure. Nine of these workers were found to have chronic bronchitis and/or emphysema, which was more marked among those working in high-dust-exposure areas. These five and two others had evidence of right ventricular hypertrophy, and four of these workers were judged to have died of cor pulmonale. Gough and Woodcock described lungs of cotton textile workers with histories of byssinosis as having inflammation of the bronchi with squamous metaplasia and generalized emphysema, which was somewhat more prominent in proximity to dust deposits (7).

Three more recent studies of lung pathology in cotton textile workers have been reported (98–100). Edwards et al. studied lungs from 43 patients who had long exposures to cotton dust and had been receiving industrial benefits for byssinosis (98). The lungs were distended with formalin at necropsy. Gross examination revealed 27 (63%) with no significant emphysema, 10 (23%) with varying degrees of centrilobular emphysema, and six (14%) with panacinar emphysema. Most workers showed heavy black dust pigmentation, often associated with centrilobular dilation of distal airspaces. There was, however, significantly more mucous gland hyperplasia and hypertrophy of smooth muscle in the upper and lower lobar bronchi and significantly less connective tissue and cartilage in cases than in controls. While the authors suggested that both smoking (17 cases) and air pollution from living in the Lancashire region could have contributed to these pathological lesions, this study did not assess these possible risk factors.

Pratt and colleagues studied lungs fixed in inflation from 44 textile workers and 521 nontextile workers (99). Their study had the advantage of using lungs properly prepared for evaluation of emphysema and knowledge of smoking status. It was limited, however, by lack of documentation of cotton dust exposure, the extent of that exposure, and the small numbers of nonsmoking textile workers (eight cases). Nevertheless, significantly more mucous gland hyperplasia and goblet cell metaplasia was found among textile workers. Centrilobular emphysema was slightly, but insignificantly, increased among textile workers. Moran, who conducted a study of cotton textile workers over an 18-year period, reported an odds ratio of 2.2 for emphysema among active and highly exposed cotton textile workers compared to a group of noncotton workers (100). The results of this study suggested that there may be a shift to an earlier age of onset of emphysema among certain exposed cotton textile workers, but details regarding specific cotton dust and smoking exposures were not available. Of relevance to the question of emphysema among cotton textile workers is a recent animal model of intratracheally instilled cotton dust endotoxin in hamsters. This revealed both functional and morphological evidence of mild emphysematous lesions (101).

In summary, the available pathological data consistently provide evidence of considerably more airway disease (both large and small airway lesions of chronic bronchitis), while the data regarding emphysema are incomplete. There appears to be historical evidence for the existence of emphysema and some recent clinical and animal morphological evidence for an increase in emphysema among those with heavy cotton dust exposure. An autopsy study of a larger number of cotton textile workers with well-documented occupational and smoking histories is needed to resolve this issue.

Etiology

Although there is consensus that some component(s) of the cotton plant, or an associated plant contaminant, is responsible for the acute symptoms of byssinosis, a single causal etiology has not yet been fully established. Etiological hypotheses have focused on plant-derived materials chiefly in the bract (the fine leaves below the cotton boll) or contaminating microorganisms and/or their constituents (chiefly gram-negative-derived bacterial endotoxin). Both in vivo and in vitro investigations with water-soluble extracts from cotton bracts have revealed their ability to cause both acute airways obstruction and inflammation. Early experiments with water-soluble cotton bract extracts (CBE) suggested that biological activity induced by such substances was similar to histamine itself or an intermediate substance causing histamine release (102). As research in this area progressed, a number of other pharmacological smooth muscle agonists were isolated from various types of CBE. These include agonists having properties similar to 5-hydroxytryptamine, prostaglandins, thromboxane, and acetylcholine. Of these substances, the 5-hydroxytryptamine-like agonist had the most potent effects (103). It was found primarily in presenescent cotton extracts as well as standard cotton dust extracts prepared for research purposes. Research about smooth muscle agonist substances in CBE has also raised the possibility that such substances could work as primary releaser agonists on a variety of human cells and therefore indirectly cause release of 5-hydroxytryptamine, thromboxane, histamine, and various leukotrienes. The latter hypothesis has yet to be proven. Several non-water-soluble substances have also been purported to contract smooth muscle and act as proinflammatory agents. These include tannins, terpenoid aldehydes, and the phytoalexin lacinilene C methylester (LCME) (104). These lipid-soluble materials stimulate recruitment of polymorphonuclear leukocytes to the airways in experimental animals. In addition, LCME also has been shown to have potent smooth muscle–contracting properties that are slow to develop but result in very strong contractility. β-1.3 glucan, a component of fungal cell walls, is also found in cotton dust (105) and has been reported to have biological activity on alveolar macrophages (106). However, exposure experiments in guinea pigs and mice have failed to show evidence of airway inflammation (107).

Major scientific interest in the role of endotoxin as a causative agent has emanated from a series of studies by Rylander and colleagues (108–112). Endotoxin is a lipopolysaccharide present in bacterial cell walls of gram-negative bacteria. It is assayed by the *Limulus* lysate method and can be demonstrated in dusts or aerosolized in liquids. Endotoxin is present in all parts of cotton plants, but particularly high concentrations are found in microorganisms on cotton bracts. The airborne concentration of endotoxin in cotton mill dust depends upon the degree of contamination of the cotton (usually lower-grade cotton) processed, ventilation, and the textile process. Much of the current knowledge about the effects of inhaled endotoxin derives from results of several experimental animal models (108,113,114). Inhalation exposure to endotoxin or lipopolysaccharide in guinea pigs and hamsters causes an accumulation of neutrophils in the lungs and airways with peak concentrations occurring 12–24 hr after exposure. Similarly, platelets accumulate in both of these animal species within 2 hr after exposure. Long-term inhalation of endotoxin causes both airway and alveolar changes in several animal models. Intratracheal instillation of endotoxin in the hamster has produced functional morphological evidence of mild emphysema (101). There have been a few experiments on the effects of inhaled endotoxin in humans. One of these investigations demonstrated objective evidence of airway obstruction after short-term cotton dust challenge (64). In another human study, short-term inhalation exposure to bacterial endotoxin in subjects with no previous occupational exposure history to organic dusts produced a significantly reduced methacholine provocation dose threshold response at 4 and 24 hr after the exposure in half the tested subjects (115). Most of the human studies have been performed in worker populations stratified by current and cumulative dust or endotoxin exposure. Castellan et al. reported that decline in FEV_1 correlated highly with dustborne endotoxin concentration among volunteers selected for reactivity to cotton dust (68). Similarly, Rylander and Haglind observed respiratory function decreases among cotton workers in experimental cardrooms (90). However, cotton bract extracts purified to remove endotoxin may still cause bronchoconstriction in human volunteers (116). In another study, the level of endotoxin exposure significantly correlated with the prevalence of chronic bronchitis and a decrease in FEV_1 among exposed cotton workers (108). However, this study also found that workers in the highest endotoxin exposure category had less byssinosis, a smaller cross-shift change in FEV_1, and better baseline pulmonary function than other workers. This suggested that this particularly high-exposure group had become less reactive, as a result of tolerance to repeated high exposures, or that the group represented a healthy survivor population. The latter effect appeared more likely as company officials had instituted an early retirement program for older workers, and there was also an active program of medical removal for workers with ''asthma.''

Current data suggest that while endotoxin may be an important etiological factor, it may not be the only one in cotton dust. A number of agricultural industries involve exposures to similar or higher levels of endotoxin in which the symptoms of byssinosis are not described (117).

Prevention

Given our current state of knowledge regarding the etiology of byssinosis and the lack of practical biological assays, risk assessment depends on measurement of dust concentrations, and prevention depends largely on dust control in the workplace (118). Significant improvements in exhaust ventilation and in dust control technology and application have resulted in reduced risk in most areas of textile mills in the United States. A second control technology, which appears promising in experimental studies, is cotton washing (60). Although this preprocessing has been found to reduce symptoms and functional changes among experimentally exposed subjects (largely through removal of fine dust), it is not yet clear whether cotton washing will be technically feasible prior to spinning. It is recognized to be efficacious for certain cotton products (medicinal cotton and cotton batting) that do not require spinning and is so recognized by the U.S. Cotton Dust Standard (50).

While dust control is the foundation of a respiratory disease prevention program in the cotton-processing industries, medical surveillance and employee education also play important roles. Smoking, and the interaction between smoking and cotton dust exposure, are clearly important risk factors in byssinosis and chronic lung disease arising from cotton dust exposure. Therefore, it is essential that information regarding the adverse effects of smoking, and the combined effects of smoking and cotton dust exposure, be made available to workers through employee education and smoking cessation programs. Workers who continue to smoke should be placed in low-dust-exposure areas (49,73). It is also essential to stress the use of appropriate work practices to reduce dust exposure. Periodic medical examinations designed to detect those acutely affected and those with chronic lung disease are important and can be effective (73). Through the use of a standard questionnaire, it is possible to ascertain a sound occupational and smoking history and to screen for byssinosis, bronchitis, dyspnea, and other common medical conditions. Simple, routine spirometry will identify many of those acutely affected and should detect all with significant impairment.

All of these prevention provisions—allowable dust concentrations, work practices, and medical surveillance—are detailed in the Department of Labor Cotton Dust Standard promulgated in 1978 (50). With the 4-year grace period given the industry to implement all provisions, this standard has now been in place for more than 15 years. Evaluation of the efficacy of the standard has been examined by Glindmeyer et al., who found that the standard provided protection from progressive declines in lung function for all of those working in slashing and weaving areas and for all yarn-processing workers, except for smokers, who still showed progressive losses in lung function below the 0.2 mg/m³ standard (73). This finding, which is consistent with previous cross-sectional and prospective studies of smoking cotton textile workers, points up the importance of medical surveillance and appropriate placement of smoking textile workers, but raises the possibility that dust levels may need to be further controlled to protect this sector of the workforce.

SUMMARY

Byssinosis is the term given to the acute and chronic respiratory disease arising from occupational exposure to textile vegetable dusts. It is characterized by chest tightness following an absence from regular exposure to dust. Symptoms of chest tightness have also been observed with a variety of other organic dusts, but this finding has not been referred to as byssinosis in nontextile processing settings. Also observed with exposure to textile vegetable dusts is an increased prevalence of nonspecific airway symptoms, modest cross-shift declines in spirometry, and progressive declines in lung function that may result in significant lung impairment among those with long exposure to these dusts. Linear dose-response relationships have been observed between byssinosis prevalence, cross-shift decline in FEV_1, and concentration of inhalable cotton dust. Similar findings for various dust fractions have been observed in other industries. These findings have led to regulation of cotton dust in the United States and in several other countries. While dust control is the hallmark of prevention of lung disease among textile workers, placement of smokers in low-dust areas, periodic medical surveillance, and appropriate work practices are essential components of an overall program to prevent lung disease among textile workers.

REFERENCES

1. Ramazzini B. A Treatise of the Diseases of Tradesmen. London: Bell, 1705.
2. Sepulveda M-J, Castellan RM, Hankinson JL, Cocke JB. Acute lung function response to cotton dust in atopic and non-atopic individuals. Br J Ind Med 1984; 41:487–49.
3. Proust AA. Traite d'Hygiene Publique et Privee. Paris: G. Masson, 1877.
4. Mareska J, Heyman J. Enquête sur le travail et la condition physique et morale des ouvriers employes dans les manufacturers de coton, à Gand. Ann Soc Med Gand 1845; 16: 11:5, 199.
5. Report of the Departmental Committee on Dust in Cardrooms in the Cotton Industry. London: Great Britain Home Office, 1932.
6. Caminita BH, Baum WF, Neal PA, Schneiter R. A review of the literature relating to affection of the respiratory tract in individuals exposed to cotton dust. Public Health Bulletin no. 297. Washington, DC: U.S Government Printing Office, 1949.
7. Schilling RSF, Goodman N. Cardiovascular disease in cotton workers, Part I. Br J Ind Med 1952; 9:146–153.
8. Schilling RSF. Byssinosis in cotton and other textile workers. Lancet 1956; 2:261–265, 319–324.
9. Barbero A., Flores R. Dust disease in hemp workers. Arch Environ Health 1967; 14:529–532.
10. Enterline PE, Kendrick MA. Asbestos-dust exposures at various levels and mortality. Arch Environ Health 1967; 15:181–186.
11. Enterline PE, Kykor JL, Keleti O, Lange JH. Endotoxins, cotton dust, and cancer. Lancet 1985; 265:934–935.
12. Levin LI, Gao Y-T, Blot WJ, Wei Z, Fraumeni JF. Decreased risk of lung cancer in the cotton textile industry in Shanghai. Cancer Res 1987; 47:5777–5781.
13. Daum S. Proceedings of the A.C.G.I.H. Conference on Cotton Dust, Atlanta, GA, 1975.
14. Merchant JA, Ortmeyer C. Mortality of employees of two cotton mills in North Carolina. Chest 1981; 79:65–115.
15. Dubrow R, Gute DM. Cause-specific mortality among male textile workers in Rhode Island. Am J Ind Med 1988; 13:439–454.
16. Koskela R-S, Klockars M, Jarvinen E. Mortality and disability among cotton mill workers. Br J Ind Med 1990; 47:384–391.
17. Koskela R-S, Klockars M, Jarvinen E. Response to letter to editor. Br J Ind Med 1991; 48: 143–144.
18. Hodgson JT, Jones RD. Mortality of workers in the British cotton industry in 1968–84. Scand J Environ Health 1990; 16:113–120.
19. Hill AB. Sickness amongst operatives in Lancashire cotton spinning mills (with special reference to the cardroom). Rep Ind Health Res Bd Rept no. 59. London: HMSO, 1930.
20. Malcolm AG. The influence of factory life on the health of the operative as founded upon the medical statistics of the class in Belfast. J R Statist Soc 1856; 19:170.
21. Schilling RSF, Hughes JPW, Dingwall-Fordyce I, Gilson JC. An epidemiological study of byssinosis among Lancashire cotton workers. Br J Ind Med 1955; 12:217–227.
22. Roach SA, Schilling RSF. A clinical and environmental study of byssinosis in the Lancashire cotton industry. Br J Ind Med 1960; 17:1–9.
23. Recommended health-based occupational exposure limits for selected vegetable dusts. Report of a WHO study group, WHO Technical Report Series 684. Geneva: World Health Organization, 1983.

24. Christiani DC, Eisen EA, Wegman DH, Ye T-T, Lu P-L, Gong Z-C, Dai H-L. Respiratory disease in cotton textile workers in the People's Republic of China. Scand J Work Environ Health 1986; 12:40–45.

25. Christiani DC, Eisen EA, Wegman DH, Ye T-T, Lu P-L, Gong Z-C, Dai H-L. Respiratory disease in cotton textile workers in the People's Republic of China. II. Pulmonary function results. Scand J Work Environ Health 1986; 12:46–50.

26. Fishwick D, Fletcher AM, Pickering CAC, Niven R, McL R, Faragher EB. Lung function in Lancashire cotton and man made fibre spinning mill operatives. Occup Environ Med 1996; 53:46–50.

27. Cinkotai FF, Emo P, Gibbs ACC, Caillard J-F, Jouany JM. Low prevalence of byssinotic symptoms in 12 flax scutching mills in Normandy, France. Br J Ind Med 1988; 45:325–328.

28. El Batawi MA. Byssinosis in the cotton industry in Egypt. Br J Ind Med 1962; 19:126–130.

29. El Batawi MA, Schilling RSF, Valic F, Wolfod J. Byssinosis in the Egyptian cotton industry: changes in ventilatory capacity during the day. Br J Ind Med 1964; 21:13–19.

30. Noweir MH, El-Sadek Y, El-Dakhakhry AA. Exposure to dust in the cottonseed oil extraction industry. Arch Environ Health 1969; 19:99–102.

31. Engleberg AL, Piacitelli GM, Petersen M, Zey J, Piccirillo R, Marcy PR, Carlson ML, Merchant JA. Medical and industrial hygiene characterization of the cotton waste utilization industry. Am J Ind Med 1985; 7:93–108.

32. U.S. Department of Health, Education and Welfare, Public Health Service, National Institute for Occupational Safety and Health. Health Hazard Evaluation Determination. Report no. 76-73-523. Cincinnati, OH: Stearns & Foster, 1978.

33. Bouhuys A, Lindell SD, Lundin G. Experimental studies in byssinosis. Br Med J 1960; 1:324–326.

34. Bouhuys A. Experimental studies in byssinosis. Arch Environ Health 1963; 6:56–61.

35. Carey OCR, Elwood PC, McAuley JR, Merrett JD, Pemberton J. Byssinosis in flax workers in Northern Ireland. A Report to the Minister of Labour and National Insurance, the Government of Northern Ireland. Belfast: HMSO, 1965.

36. Elwood PC. Respiratory symptoms in men who had previously worked in a flax mill in Northern Ireland. Br J Ind Med 1965; 22:38–42.

37. Elwood PC, Pemberton J, Merrett JD, Carey OCR, McAuley JR. Byssinosis and other respiratory symptoms in flax workers in Northern Ireland. Br J Ind Med 1965; 22:27–37.

38. Elwood PC, Pemberton J, Merrett JD, Carey OCR, McAuley JR. Prevalence of byssinosis and dust levels in flax preparers in Northern Ireland. Br J Ind Med 1966; 23:188–193.

39. Mair A, Smith DH, Wilson WA, Lockhart W. Dust diseases in Dundee textile workers. Br J Ind Med 1960; 17:272–276.

40. McKerrow CB, Gilson JC, Schilling RSF, Skidmore JW. Respiratory function and symptoms in rope workers. Br J Ind Med 1965; 22:204–209.

41. Khogoli M, Lakha AS, Milla MH, Dahoma A. Byssinosis, respiratory symptoms and spirometric lung function tests in Tanzanian sisal workers. Br J Ind Med 1976; 35:123–128.

42. Castellan RM, Boehlecke BA, Petersen MR, Merchant JA. Herbal tea workers pulmonary function and symptoms. Proceedings of the International Conference on Byssinosis. Chest 1981; 79:815–855.

43. Merchant JA, Donham KJ. Health risks from animal confinement units. In: Dosman JA, Cockcroft DW, eds. Principles of Health and Safety in Agriculture. Boca Raton, FL: CRC Press, 1989:56–61.

44. Merchant JA, Lumsden JC, Kilburn KH, O'Fallon WM, Ujda JR, Germino VH, Hamilton JD. Dose response studies in cotton textile workers. J Occup Med 1973; 15:222–230.

45. Fox AJ, Tombelson JBL, Watt A, Wilke AO. A survey of respiratory disease among cotton operatives. Part II. Symptoms, dust estimations, and the effect of smoking habit. Br J Ind Med 1973; 30:48–53.

46. Merchant JA, Lumsden JD, Kilburn KH, O'Fallon WM, Germino FH, McKenzie WN, Baucom D, Currin P, Stilman J. Intervention studies of cotton steaming to reduce biological effects of cotton dust. Br J Ind Med 1974; 31:261–274.

47. Molyneux MBK, Berry O. The correlation of cotton dust exposure with the prevalence of respiratory symptoms. Proceedings of the International Conference on Respiratory Disease in Textile Workers, Alicante, Spain, 1968, pp 177–183.

48. Merchant JA, Kilburn KH, O'Fallon WM, Hamilton JD, Lumsden JC. Byssinosis and chronic bronchitis among cotton textile workers. Ann Intern Med 1972; 76:423–433.

49. Merchant JA, Lumsden J, Kilburn K, O'Fallon W, Ujda J, Germino V, Hamilton J. An industrial study of the biological effects of cotton dust and cigarette smoke exposure. J Occup Med 1973; 15:212–221.

50. U.S. Department of Labor, National Institute for Occupational Safety and Health. Cotton Dust Title 29: Code of Federal Regulations. Part 1910.1043.

51. Niven R, McL, Fishwick D, Pickering CAC, Fletcher AM, Warburton CJ, Crank P. A study of the performance and comparability of the sampling response to cotton dust of work area and personal sampling techniques. Ann Occup Hyg 1992; 36(4):349–362.

52. Gilson JC, Stott H, Hopwood BEC, Roach SA, McKerrow CB, Schilling RSF. Byssinosis: the acute effect of ventilatory capacity of dusts in cotton ginneries, cotton, sisal and jute mills. Br J Ind Med 1962; 18:9–18.

53. Valic F, Zuskin E. Effect of different vegetable dust exposures. Br J Ind Med 1972; 29: 293–297.

54. WHO Study Group, Recommended Health-Based Occupational Exposure Limits for Selected Vegetable Dusts. WHO Technical Report Series 684. Geneva, Switzerland: World Health Organization, 1983.

55. Medical Research Council Committee on Aetiology of Chronic Bronchitis. Standardized questions on respiratory symptoms. Br Med J 1960; 2:1665.

56. Imbus HR, Suh MW. Byssinosis: a study of 10,133 textile workers. Arch Environ Health 1973; 26:183–191.

57. Lammers B, Schilling RSF, Wolford J. A study of byssinosis, chronic respiratory symptoms, and ventilatory capacity in English and Dutch cotton workers, with special reference to atmospheric pollution. Br J Ind Med 1964; 21:124–134.

58. Merchant JA. Epidemiological studies of respiratory diseases among cotton textile workers, 1970–1973. Dissertation, University of North Carolina, 1973.

59. Merchant JA, Halprin GM, Hanson AR, Kilburn KH, McKinzie WM, Bermanzohn P, Hurst DJ. Evaluation before and after exposure-the pattern of physiological response to cotton dust. Ann NY Acad Sci 1974; 221:38–43.

60. Merchant JA, Lumsden JC, Kilburn KH, Germino VH, Hamilton JD, Baucom D, Byrd H, Lynn W. Preprocessing cotton to prevent byssinosis. Br J Ind Med 1973; 30:237–247.

61. Valic F, Zuskin E. Pharmacological prevention of acute ventilatory capacity reduction in flax dust exposure. Br J Ind Med 1973; 30:381–384.

62. Bouhuys A, Gilson JC, Schilling RSF. Byssinosis in the textile industry. Arch Environ Health 1970; 21:475–478.

63. Schacter EN, Kapp MC, Maunder LR, Beck G, Witek TJ. Smoking and cotton dust effects on cotton textile workers: an analysis of the shape of the maximum expiratory flow volume curve. Environ Health Perspect 1986; 66:145–148.

64. McKerrow EB, McDermott M, Gilson JC, Schilling RSF. Respiratory function during the day in cotton workers: a study in byssinosis. Br J Ind Med 1958; 15:75–83.

65. Bates DV, Macklem PT, Christie RV. Respiratory Function in Disease, 2nd ed. Philadelphia: WB Saunders, 1971.

66. Bouhuys A, Gilson JC, Schilling RSF, van de Woestijne KP. Chronic respiratory disease in hemp workers. Am J Med 1969; 46:526–537.

67. Molyneux MKB, Tombleson JBL. An epidemiological study of respiratory symptoms in Lancashire mills, 1963–1966. Br J Ind Med 1970; 27:225–234.

68. Castellan RM, Olenchock AA, Hankinson JL, Millner PD, Cocke JB, Bragg CK, Perkins HH. Acute bronchoconstriction induced by cotton dust: dose-related responses to endotoxin and other dust factors. Ann Intern Med 1984; 101:157–163.

69. Castellan RM, Olenchock SA, Kinsley KB, Hankinson JL. Inhaled endotoxin and decreased spirometric values. N Engl J Med 1987; 317:605–610.

70. Kennedy SM, Christiani DC, Eisen EA, Wegman DH, Greaves IA, Olenchock SA, Ye T-T, Lu P-L. Cotton dust and endotoxin exposure-response relationships in cotton textile workers. Am Rev Respir Dis 1987; 135:194–210.

71. Beck GJ, Schachter EN, Maunder LR, Bouhuys A. The relation of lung function to subsequent employment status and mortality in cotton textile workers. Chest 1981; 79:265–305.

72. Berry G, McKerrow CB, Mollyneux MKB, Rossiter CE, Tombleson JBL. A study of the acute and chronic changes in ventilatory capacity of workers in Lancashire cotton mills. Br J Ind Med 1973; 301:25–36.

73. Glindmeyer HW, Lenfante JJ, Jones RN, Rando RJ, Kader HAA, Weill H. Exposure-related declines in the lung function of cotton textile workers. Am Rev Respir Dis 1991; 144:675–683.

74. Zuskin E, Ivankovic D, Schacter EN, Witek TJ. A ten-year follow-up study of cotton textile workers. Am Rev Respir Dis 1991; 143:301–305.

75. Kamat SR, Kamat GR, Salpekar VY, Lobo E. Distinguishing byssinosis from chronic obstructive pulmonary disease. Am Rev Respir Dis 1981; 124:31–40.

76. Christiani DC, Wegman DH, Eisen EA. Cotton dust exposure and longitudinal change in lung function. Am Rev Respir Dis 1990; 141:A589.

77. Bouhuys A, Schoenberg JB, Beck GJ, Schilling RSF. Epidemiology of chronic lung disease in a cotton mill community. Lung 1977; 154:167–186.

78. Fishwick D, Fletcher AM, Pickering CAC, Niven R, McL R, Faragher EB. Ocular and nasal irritation in operatives in Lancashire cotton and synthetic mills. Occup Environ Med 1944; 51:744–748.

79. Niven R, McL R, Fletcher AM, Pickering CAC, Fishwick D, Warburton CJ, Simpson JCG, Francis H, Oldham LA. Chronic bronchitis in textile workers. Thorax 1997; 52:22–27.

80. Hamilton JD, Germino VH, Merchant JA, Lumsden JC, Kilborn KH. Byssinosis in a non-textile worker. Am Rev Respir Dis 1973; 107:464–466.

81. Dutkiewicz J. Exposure to dust-borne bacteria in agriculture. I. Environmental studies. Arch Environ Health 1978; 33:250–259.

82. Olenchock AA, Lenhart SW, Mull JC. Occupational exposure to airborne endotoxins during poultry processing. J Toxicol Environ Health 1982; 9:339–349.

83. Pratt DS, May JJ. Feed-associated respiratory illness in farmer. Arch Environ Health 1984; 39:43–48.

84. do Pico GA. Health effects of organic dusts in the farm environment. Report on diseases. Am J Ind Med 1986; 10:261–265.

85. Arlidge JT. The Hygiene Diseases and Mortality of Occupations. London: Percival & Company, 1982.

86. Rylander R, Schilling RSF, Pickering CAC, Rooke GB, Dempsey AN, Jacobs RR. Effects after acute and chronic exposure to cotton dust: the Manchester criteria. Br J Ind Med 1987; 44:577–579.

87. Sepulveda MJ, Hankinson JL, Castellan RM, Cocke JB. Hellium oxygen spirometry in experimental cotton dust exposure. Lung 1984; 162:347–356.

88. Sepulveda MJ, Hankinson JL, Castellan RM, Cocke JB. Cotton induced bronchoconstriction detected by a forced random noise oscillator. Br J Ind Med 1984; 41:480–486.

89. Rylander R, Haglind P, Lundholm M. Endotoxin in cotton dust and respiratory function decrement among cotton workers in an experimental card-room. Am Rev Respir Dis 1985; 131:209–213.

90. Rylander R, Haglind P. Exposure of cotton workers in an experimental cardroom with reference to airborne endotoxins. Environ health Perspect 1986; 66:83–86.

91. Chan-Yeung M, Vedal S, MacLean L, Enarson DA, Tse K. Symptoms, pulmonary function and bronchial hyperreactivity in western red cedar workers compared with those in office workers. Am Rev Respir Dis 1984; 40:53–57.

92. Hamilton JD, Haiprin GM, Kilburn KH, Merchant JA, Ujda JR. Differential aerosol challenge studies in byssinosis. Arch Environ Health 1973; 26:120–124.

93. Schacter EN, Maunder LR, Beck G. The pattern of lung function abnormalities in cotton textile workers. Am Rev Respir Dis 1984; 129:523–527.

94. Honeyborne D, Pickering CAC. Physiological evidence that emphysema is not a feature of byssinosis. Thorax 1986; 41:6–11.

95. Zuskin E, Valic F, Bouhuys A. Byssinosis and airway responses to exposure to textile dust. Lung 1976; 154:17–24.

96. Zuskin E, Bouhuys A. Protective effect of disodium cromoglycate against airway constriction induced by hemp dust extract. J Allergy Clin Immunol 1976; 57(5):473–479.

97. Fawcett IW, Merchant JA, Simmonds SP, Pepys J. The effect of sodium cromoglycate, beclomethasone diproprionate and salbutamol on the ventilatory response to cotton dust in mill workers. Br J Dis Chest 1978; 29:29–38.

98. Edwards C, MacArtney J, Rooke G, Ward F. The pathology of the lung in byssinotics. Thorax 1975; 30:612–623.

99. Pratt PC, Vollmer RT, Miller JA. Epidemiology of pulmonary lesions in nontextile and cotton textile workers: a retrospective autopsy analysis. Arch Environ Health 1980; 35:133–138.

100. Moran TM. Emphysema and other chronic lung disease in textile workers: an 18-year autopsy study. Arch Environ Health 1983; 38:267–276.

101. Milton DK, Godleski JJ, Feldman HA, Greaves IA. Toxicity of intratracheally instilled cotton dust, cellulose and endotoxin. Am Rev Respir Dis 1990; 142:184–192.

102. Bouhuys A. Byssinosis. In: Breathing, Physiology, Environmental and Lung Disease. New York: Grune & Stratton, 1976:416–440.

103. Russell JH, Gilberstadt ML, Rolstad RA, Rohrbach MS. Airway smooth muscle and platelet responses to several varieties of cotton bracts. Lung 1984; 162:89–97.

104. Russell JA, McCormick JP. Lacinilene C methyl ether (LCME) constricts tracheal smooth muscle. Environ Res 1988; 45(1):118–126.

105. Rylander R, Bergstrom R, Goto H, Yuasa K, Tanaka S. Studies on endotoxin and beta-1,3 glucan in cotton dust. Proceedings of the 13th Cotton Dust Research Conference, Nashville, TN, 1989, pp 46–47.

106. Di Luzio NR. Lysozyme, glucan-activated macrophages in neoplasia. J Reticuloendothel Soc 1979; 26:67–81.

107. Castronova V, Robinson VA, Frazer DG. Pulmonary reactions to organic dust exposures: development of an animal model. Environ Health Perspect 1996; 104(1):41–53.

108. Rylander R, Snella M. Acute inhalation toxicity of cotton plant dusts. Br J Ind Med 1976; 33:175–180.

109. Rylander R, Nordstrand A, Snella M. Bacterial contamination of organic dusts. Arch Environ Health 1975; 30:137–140.

110. Rylander R. Bacterial toxins and etiology of byssinosis. Chest 1981; 79:345–385.

111. Cinkotai FF, Lockwood MG, Rylander R. Airborne microorganisms and prevalence of byssinotic symptoms in cotton mills. Am Ind Hyg Assoc J 1977; 38:554–559.

112. Rylander R. The role of endotoxin for reactions after exposure to cotton dust. Am J Ind Med 1987; 12:687–697.

113. Snella MC, Rylander R. Endotoxin inhalation induces neutrophil chemotaxis by alveolar macrophages. Agents Actions 1985; 16:521–526.

114. Lantz RC, Birch K, Hinton DE, Burrell R. Morphometric changes of the lung induced by inhaled bacterial endotoxin. Exp Mol Pathol 1985; 43:305–320.

115. Bake B, Rylander R, Fischer J. Airway hyperreactivity and bronchoconstriction after inhalation of cell-bound endotoxin. In: Jacobs RR, Wakelyn PJ, eds. Proceedings of the Eleventh Cotton Dust Research Conference. Memphis, TN: National Cotton Council, 1978:12–14.

116. Buck MG, Wall JH, Schachter EN. Airway constrictor response to cotton bract extracts in the absence of endotoxin. Br J Ind Med 1986; 43:220–226.
117. Simpson JCG, Niven R, McL, Oldham CAC, Fletcher LA, Franci HC. Animal workers respiratory symptoms, dust and endotoxin exposures. Proceedings of the 19th Cotton and Other Organic Dusts Research Conference, Memphis, TN, 1995, pp 331–333.
118. Merchant JA. Byssinosis: progress in prevention. Am J Public Health 1983; 73(2):37–138 (editorial).

32
Grain Dust–Induced Lung Diseases

Moira Chan-Yeung
Vancouver General Hospital and University of British Columbia, Vancouver, British Columbia, Canada

Susan M. Kennedy
University of British Columbia, Vancouver, British Columbia, Canada

David A. Schwartz
University of Iowa, Iowa City, Iowa

INTRODUCTION

In North America there are several million farmers, about 250,000 grain elevator workers, 50,000 people engaged in grain milling and baking, and an unknown number of workers in feedmills and dockworkers loading and unloading grain. These individuals are at risk of exposure to grain dust and flour dust. It has been known for a long time that exposure to grain dust is harmful to the lungs. Ramazzini (1) in 1713 described a disease among "sifters and measurers of grain" that led to dyspnea and early death. In this chapter, we review the current knowledge of the effects of grain dust exposure on respiratory health, describe the clinical syndromes associated with this exposure, and discuss the possible pathogenesis of these syndromes.

Emissions from agricultural operations in the United States ranked third, after fuel combustion and rock crushing. These emissions are mostly contributed by grain elevators (2). Grain is processed in three different types of elevators, country, terminal, and transfer. The process is basically the same in each type of elevator: receiving, grading, weighing, transferring, binning, drying, cleaning, and shipping. Country elevators store and clean grain trucked to them by farmers before being shipped to terminal elevators or local mills. Most country elevators are manned by one or two workers and are not ventilated. Dust levels in these elevators are high (2). Terminal elevators process grain from country elevators, clean, grade, and store grain before shipping to other parts of the country or for export. Transfer elevators do not process grain although they resemble terminal elevators in other respects.

Grain dust is generated by the abrasion of kernels when grain is being handled. It has been estimated that when passing through a typical elevator, each ton of grain handled generates 3–4 lb of dust (2). Levels of dust in elevators are influenced by the type of grain handled, the degree of activity, the extent of enclosure at transfer points when grain falls freely from one conveying system to another, the efficiency and upkeep of exhaust ventilation provided at transfer points, and work and housekeeping practices (2).

CHARACTERISTICS OF GRAIN DUST

The physical and chemical compositions of grain dust vary depending on the geographic site, the type of grain, the wetness of the season, storage temperature, and many other factors. The major components of grain dust include fractured grain kernels, fractured weed seeds, husks, storage mites, insects, bacteria, molds, chemicals such as pesticides and insecticides, and silica.

All types of grain dust contain husk or pericarp fragments in addition to respirable particles. Scanning electron microscopy has shown that each type of dust consists of a distinct assortment of particles. Small husk fragments and "trichome-like" objects are common (3). Many grain workers complain that their respiratory symptoms are worse when they handle barley and oats. These two types of grain dust contain many fine, needle-like fragments compared to other types of grain dust.

The microflora of grain dust change from harvesting, storage, and handling. During harvest, many fungi produce spores that become airborne in large quantities. *Cladosporium* and *Alternaria* are found in all samples of harvester dust (4). Once the grain is placed in storage, the microflora change depending on the water content and the degree of spontaneous heating, the aeration of the grain bulk. The predominant fungus is *Ustilago*. Others include *Cladosporium* and *Alternaria*.

Storage mites are found in grain dust. They belong to the genera *Glycyphagus*, *Tyrophagus*, *Acarus*, and *Goheiria* (5). The number of mites in grain dust is directly related to the water content of the dust. Particles from weevils, insects, rodents, birds, and their excreta are also found in grain dust. In addition, grain workers are also exposed to herbicides, aluminum phosphide, and other types of pesticides such as malathion. The pathogenic role of these various components of grain dust on respiratory health of grain workers is not known.

CLINICAL SYNDROMES CAUSED BY GRAIN DUST EXPOSURE

Acute Airway Diseases

Grain dust has been shown to induce acute airway disease by sensitization to one of its proteins, or direct airway injury and inflammation from one of the toxins present in the contaminated dust.

Allergen-Induced Airflow Obstruction (Grain Dust Asthma)

Grain dust asthma has been described by several investigators (6–10). These cases were documented by specific challenge tests with either crude grain dust or grain dust extract. Table 1 shows a summary of results of inhalation challenge studies of these studies. Immediate, late, and biphasic asthmatic responses have been described. Systemic responses (fever and leukocytosis) occurred in some grain workers (6,10). A few control subjects also had fever and leukocytosis after challege when exposure levels were high (10).

The mechanisms of these reactions were further evaluated by inhibition studies (7). The immediate asthmatic response was inhibited by pretreatment with disodium cromoglycate, while the late response was partially inhibited by treatment with beclomethasone diproprionate before and at intervals after challenge similar to those found in allergic asthma. Grain workers who had an asthmatic response on challenge had a marked degree of nonspecific bronchial hyperresponsiveness (NSBH, methacholine PC$_{20}$ 0.36 ± 0.34 mg/

Table 1 Inhalation Challenge Studies of Grain Workers

| Group | n | Testing Material | Inhalation reaction (n) 2 | | | Ref. | Author |
			Isolated immediate	Isolated late	Dual		
Grain-symptomatic	15	Crude gain dust extract	3	0	5	6	Warren
Controls	5		0	0	0		
Grain-symptomatic	1	Grain dust	0	0	1	9	Davies
Grain-symptomatic	22	Grain dust	3	3	3	7	Chan-Yeung
Grain-symptomatic	11		0	0	0		
Grain-symptomatic	11	Durum wheat	1	4	0	13	doPico
Grain-grain fever	6	Grain dust (high conc.)	4	0	2	20	doPico
Controls	6		3	0	2		

ml); those without such a response to challenge but who had respiratory symptoms and/ or lung function abnormality before challenge had some degree of NSBH (methacholine PC_{20} 1.87 ± 6.88 mg/ml). The comparison group had no NSBH (methacholine PC_{20} > 16 mg/ml). Moreover, those who had an asthmatic response to grain dust challenge tended to have a higher peripheral blood eosinophil count than those who had no such response (244 and 156/mm^3, respectively). These findings suggest that the reactions to grain dust challenge in these patients are likely to have an allergic basis. Most studies, however, were unable to demonstrate positive skin test reaction to grain dust extract or a correlation between an asthmatic response to grain dust and immediate skin reaction to grain dust extract (7–10). Specific antibodies have not been found in the sera of patients with an asthmatic response on inhalation challenge (6,7).

Studies to identify the responsible airborne allergens in grain dust have been difficult and have met with little success. Only three studies have demonstrated specific allergens in the grain dust. Davies et al. (9) reported a farmer who developed recurrent nocturnal asthma after inhalation challenge with grain dust. Examination of the grain samples together with the skin and serological tests suggested the grain mite, *Glycyphagus destructor*, to be an important allergen. Warren and co-workers (10) reported a grain handler with asthma due to the Canadian storage mite, *Lepidoglyphus destructor*. They tested 100 asthmatics for frequency of sensitization to this storage mite and found it in 12%; in addition, 4% of these asthmatics were also sensitized to another storage mite, *Acarus siro*. It is likely that sensitization to storage mites is responsible for asthma in some grain workers. Sensitization to a weevil, *Sitophilus oryzae*, which infests granaries, has been reported to cause immediate and late-phase reactions after inhalation of grain dust (11,12).

doPico and co-workers (13) studied 11 grain workers including using extracts of durum wheat, durum wheat airborne dust, and grain insects and mites for specific inhalation challenge tests. Only one subject had a positive bronchial response to durum wheat airborne dust extract and none reacted to mites or insect extracts. No parenchymal or systemic reaction was found. No other studies have successfully identified allergen(s) in grain dust that have been shown to produce asthmatic response on inhalation challenge.

There is virtually no information on the prevalence of allergic grain dust asthma. It has been suggested that asthmatics are likely to seek other employment and leave the industry shortly after starting employment. The results of the prevalence study of 669 male grain workers and 560 male office workers in Vancouver (14) support this notion. The prevalence of atopy (defined as immediate skin reactivity to one or more common allergens) was 17.3 versus 31.3%, respectively; while the prevalence of current asthma was 2.4 versus 2.7%, respectively. Eleven (1.6% of total) of 26 asthmatic grain workers claimed that their asthma started after employment. The prevalence of grain dust asthma is likely to be low even though the prevalence of wheeze, which may be also be due to asthma-like syndrome, in grain workers is high in many epidemiological studies (15–16).

Non-Allergen-Induced Airflow Obstruction (Asthma-like Syndrome)

A number of studies (17–21) show that some grain workers demonstrate an acute change in lung function over a work shift. The acute changes in lung function may or may not be associated with respiratory symptoms such as cough, sputum production, wheeze, or chest tightness and are not related to an asthmatic response on grain dust inhalation challenge (Table 2). In 1966, Gandevia and Ritchie (17) found a mean fall in forced expiratory volume in 1 sec (FEV_1) of -291 ml over a work shift following exposure to grain dust in a group of dockworkers. Their findings were subsequently confirmed by several investigators.

The acute changes in lung function in grain workers appear to be directly related to the level of dust exposure (20,21) or endotoxin (22) and are associated with an increase in peripheral blood leukocyte count but unrelated to age, smoking habit, duration of employment, atopic status, or skin test reactivity to grain dust antigens. In addition, previously unexposed individuals also developed acute decreases in lung function when exposed to high concentrations of grain dust (20,21). These characteristics suggest that, in most individuals, the acute change in lung function across a work shift is not a type I immediate hypersensitivity reaction but a nonallergic response to some constitutent(s) of grain dust. This syndrome is similar to byssinosis, described in workers with cotton dust exposure, but different from "classic" asthma since it is not associated with eosinophilia and is not clearly related to NSBH. Enarson and co-workers (23) studied the relationship between acute change in lung function over a work shift and NSBH. They found that among the

Table 2 Cross–Work Shift or Cross–Workweek Change in Lung Function

Group	n	Cross-shift change in FEV_1[a]	Cross–work week change in FEV_1[a]	Ref.
Dockworkers	24	-291.0	NA	17
Grain	248	-8.0	NA	20
Civic	192	$+36.3$	NA	
Grain	485	-22.0	-34.0	18
Sawmill	65	$+71.0$	$+100.0$	
Grain	582	NA	-87.0	75
Control	153	NA	$+82.0$	
Grain	47	Significant reduction in V_{50} and V_{75} on Monday and Wednesday within days; significant reduction in FVC within week.		19
Civic	15	No similar changes		

NA = not available
[a]FEV_1 in ml.

21 workers with a large decline in FEV$_1$ (>100 ml) over a work shift, 12 had evidence of NSBH (PC$_{20}$ ≤ 8 mg/ml) while the remaining nine did not. It is clear from this study that not all subjects with acute change in lung function over one work shift had NSBH. This syndrome is therefore clinically and pathogenetically different from allergic grain dust asthma.

In fact, these epidemiological studies are supported by recent exposure-response studies in humans. Among healthy grain handlers, Clapp and colleagues (24) found that inhalation of corn dust extract resulted in airflow obstruction within 30 min of the inhalation challenge. Clapp et al. also found that healthy volunteers had similar degrees of airflow obstruction following inhalation of corn dust extract (25). Moreover, the degree of airflow obstruction following inhalation of corn dust extract was similar to that observed following inhalation of equivalent concentrations of endotoxin (25,26). Interestingly, Deetz et al. showed that among health volunteers, a single inhalation of corn dust extract resulted in significant airflow obstruction within 10 min of the challenge that persisted for 48 hr (27). Comparing healthy, nonatopic volunteers to healthy, atopic volunteers, Blaski et al. showed that the atopic status does not appear to be an important determinant of airflow obstruction following inhalation of corn dust (28). These exposure-response studies demonstrate that the airflow obstruction following inhalation of corn dust extract can occur through nonallergic mechanisms—absent latency period and occurring in health volunteers regardless of atopy status.

The pathogenesis of grain dust–induced nonallergic airway disease is not known; several lines of evidence indicate that the physiological response to grain dust is primarily mediated by an acute inflammatory response in the lower respiratory tract. In vitro, grain dust can activate complement through the alternate and classic pathways (29–31); however, activation of complement does not appear to be important in the development of grain dust–induced airflow obstruction (32–34). Moreover, in vitro studies have demonstrated that grain dust can induce macrophages to release neutrophil chemotactic factors (31) and IL-1 (35), and animal studies have shown that inhaled grain dust causes a neutrophilic response in the lower respiratory tract (31,36). Finally, human inhalation studies have demonstrated that grain dust can induce airflow obstruction in previously unexposed individuals (24,33,37); this airway response is dependent on the inhaled dose of grain dust (24,32,33,37); and neutrophils rapidly accumulate in the upper and lower respiratory tract following inhalational challenges with aerosols of grain dust (37,38). These findings strongly suggest that a specific toxin(s), capable of inducing neutrophil chemotaxis in previously exposed and also unexposed individuals, is responsible for the development of airway inflammation and airflow obstruction in grain handlers.

Several lines of evidence indicate that endotoxin is one of the primary agents in organic dust that causes airway inflammation and airflow obstruction (Fig. 1). First, the concentration of inhaled endotoxin in the bioaerosol is strongly associated with the development of acute decrements in airflow among cotton workers (39–41), swine confinement workers (42), and poultry workers (43). The concentration of endotoxin in the bioaerosol appears to be the most important occupational exposure associated with the development (22) and progression (44) of airway disease in agricultural workers. In addition, the concentration of endotoxin in the domestic environment adversely effects asthmatics, with higher concentrations of ambient endotoxin associated with greater degrees of airflow obstruction (45,46). Second, inhaled endotoxin (45,47–50), grain dust (24,33,37), or cotton dust (40,51–53) can cause airflow obstruction in naïve or previously unexposed subjects. Furthermore, asthmatic individuals develop airflow obstruction at lower concentrations of inhaled endotoxin than normal controls (50). Finally, exposure-response studies have shown that inhaled grain dust and endotoxin produce similar phys-

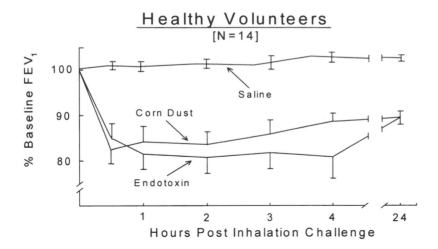

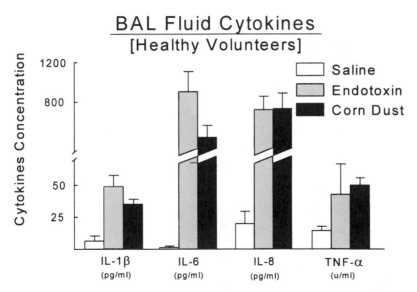

Figure 1 Evidence that inhaled corn dust extract and LPS cause airflow obstruction and airway inflammation. Following inhalation of either corn dust or LPS, healthy, nonasthmatic, nonatopic subjects without airway hyperreactivity develop significant declines in airflow, lasting up to 48 hr, that are associated with a significant increase in the concentration of neutrophils in the bronchoalveolar lavage (BAL) fluid, activated macrophages that produce and release significantly higher concentrations of specific proinflammatory cytokines in the BAL fluid.

iological and biological effects (26,37); the concentration of endotoxin appears to play an important role in the acute biological response to grain dust (26,54,55); a competitive antagonist for LPS (*Rhodobacter spheroides* diphosporyl lipid A) reduces the inflammatory response to inhaled grain dust (56); and genetic or acquired hyporesponsiveness to endotoxin substantially reduces the biological response to grain dust (54). In aggregate, these studies indicate that endotoxin is an important cause of grain dust–induced airway disease.

The alveolar and airway macrophage is likely to play a pivotal role in the initial inflammatory response to inhaled grain dust. Animal inhalation studies have shown that grain dust, like endotoxin, induces a profound neutrophilic response in the lower respiratory tract (31,36,54). This does not appear to be dependent on complement, since inactivation of complement will not affect the influx of neutrophils following exposure to endotoxin (57). Moreover, transfer of macrophages from endotoxin-sensitive mice to endotoxin-resistant mice will render the resistant mice sensitive to the toxic effects of endotoxin (58). Animal studies have also shown that inhalation of endotoxin results in a dose-dependent influx of neutrophils to the alveoli, which can be partially inhibited by prior treatment with TNF-α-specific antibodies (59). Grain dust is directly chemotactic for neutrophils and can induce alveolar macrophages to release factors that have potent chemotactic activity for neutrophils (13). Following inhalation of grain dust, the production and release of specific proinflammatory cytokines (TNF-α, IL-1β, IL-6, IL-8) has been demonstrated in the lungs of humans (22,45).

Epithelial cells may also be involved in recruitment and modulation of the inflammatory response. Interestingly, epithelial cells respond poorly to endotoxin and appear to require a specific host-derived signal (TNF-α or IL-1) for induction of IL-8 (60). The inability to respond to LPS has been demonstrated in vitro in A549 cells (61) and bronchial epithelial cells (62); however, if these cells are exposed directly to either TNF-α or IL-1 they are able to produce and release IL-8. In a baboon model of sepsis, pretreatment with anti-TNF-α antibody significantly reduced the circulating concentration of IL-8 (63), suggesting that TNF-α and/or IL-1 is needed to stimulate other cells to release IL-8 and promote neutrophil chemotaxis. Interestingly, IL-8 is clearly up-regulated in the airway epithelia following inhalation of corn dust extract (22,64) and MIP-2, thought to be the murine homolog of IL-8, is produced and released in the lungs of mice following inhalation of corn dust extract (51). These findings suggest that inhaled grain dust initiates a complex interaction between macrophages and other inflammatory (primarily neutrophils) and structural (bronchial epithelial) cells, and this interaction is mediated by specific proinflammatory cytokines that are initially released by alveolar macrophages.

Chronic Lung Disease

There is increasing evidence that exposure to grain dust leads to the development of chronic lung disease and associated respiratory disability. The evidence is found in a number of epidemiological studies, which can be divided into two categories: studies without detailed exposure assessment and studies that focused on exposure-response relationships.

Studies Without Comparison Groups, or Without Detailed Exposure Assessment

Numerous cross-sectional prevalence studies were conducted on grain workers up to the end of the 1970s, mostly without unexposed comparison groups (65–70). These studies showed a high prevalence of respiratory symptoms and both Tse et al. (68) and doPico et al. (69) showed reductions in pulmonary function compared to population prediction equations. Sheridan et al. (70) also showed a negative relationship between duration of exposure and MMF level. Although detailed information on exposure was not available, some ambient air measurements indicated that exposure levels were often high, ranging from 10 to 800 mg/m^3.

Most cross-sectional studies from the 1980s that included external comparison groups also found increased prevalence rates for respiratory symptoms and many found significantly lower average lung function levels compared to external comparison groups. Most of these studies were conducted among Canadian grain elevator workers or farmers (18,71–75), although similar results were also seen in South Africa (75). In one study (74) the combined effect of both smoking and grain dust exposure resulted in lower mean levels of lung function than either exposure alone.

Follow-up studies were carried out in Canadian grain elevators after 3–6 years. Among grain elevator workers in British Columbia, Chan-Yeung and colleagues (76) found a greater annual decline in airflow rates compared to controls, especially among older workers. This finding was confirmed in a 6-year follow-up study in the same group of workers (77). Broder and co-workers (78) also carried out a 3-year follow-up study of their original cohort, in which the grain workers showed only a slightly more rapid, but not statistically significant, decline in lung function compared to controls. This finding may have been due to a "healthy worker" effect since grain workers who left this employment had significantly more cough and breathlessness at the initial study than those who remained (a difference not seen in the comparison population). A healthy worker effect was also observed in the British Columbia cohort (79,80) favoring the "fit" individuals to remain in the exposed workforce.

Two short-term follow-up studies (81,82) indicated that, among young workers, part of the lung function changes may be reversible with cessation of exposure. However, the results of the longer-duration follow-up studies and the cross-sectional studies indicate that continuous exposure is accompanied by chronic respiratory symptoms and reductions in lung function. This persistence of the effect is further supported by results from a study of retired grain elevator workers (83), which found significant reductions in lung function compared to retired civic workers, even among lifetime nonsmokers. These results are shown in Figure 2. These changes persisted well into retirement, despite cessation of exposure. These retired workers also reported significantly greater breathing-related im-

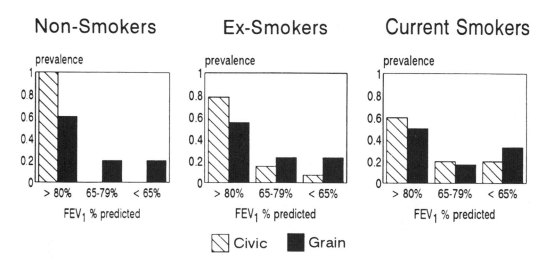

Figure 2 Proportion of grain (solid bars) and civic (hatched bars) retirees with FEV_1 values greater than 80% of predicted ("normal"), between 65 and 80% predicted ("mildly normal"), and less than 65% predicted ("moderately abnormal"), according to smoking status. ($p < 0.05$, FEV_1 impairment category difference between grain and civic retiree groups, controlling for smoking status, Mantel Haentzel chi-square analysis.)

pairment in activities of daily living (unrelated to asthma), indicating that grain dust exposure leads to chronic respiratory disability in some workers.

Studies with Analysis of Exposure-Response Relationships

The weight of evidence from the cross-sectional and follow-up studies discussed above indicates that grain dust has a deleterious effect on the pulmonary system resulting in chronic impairment and, in some cases, disability. Recently a number of well-controlled epidemiological studies have added to this weight of evidence in investigating the nature of the exposure-response relationship. These studies have been carried out primarily among workers exposed to grain dusts in the grain elevator and animal feed industries in Canada and in the Netherlands.

Corey and colleagues (19) found a significant relationship between airflow rates and grain dust level in Ontario grain elevator workers, with Monday morning FEV_1 and flow rates significantly reduced in association with increasing dust exposure among workers who did not wear a dust mask. Enarson and colleagues (84) carried out a nested case-control analysis comparing exposure levels between workers with the largest FEV_1 decline over a 6-year period and those with the smallest FEV_1 decline. The group with the largest FEV_1 decline were significantly more likely to be employed in high-dust jobs. Huy and colleagues (85) used an industry-specific job exposure matrix to compute cumulative and average grain dust exposure values for 454 British Columbia grain elevator workers and found significant exposure-response relationships between average dust exposure and increased prevalence of chronic phlegm and dyspnea, and reductions in both FEV_1 and FVC. In a study of retirees from this same cohort (83), the annual rate of decline in FEV_1 (from 1978 to 1992) in these retired workers was also shown to be significantly greater (-60.7 ml/year) in workers who had a 5% or greater acute cross-shift FEV_1 drop in 1975, compared to -34.2 ml/year in those without an acute cross-shift change in 1975 (86). This effect was most pronounced in workers with the highest dust exposure jobs in 1975.

Studies of animal feed workers have shown results similar to those seen among grain elevator workers. A Dutch study (87) did not find increases in respiratory symptoms among 315 animal feed workers and found that symptom prevalence rates declined with increasing duration of employment (perhaps reflecting a healthy worker effect). However, in this population a strong association was seen between decreased FVC, FEV_1, and MMF levels and increased dust and endotoxin exposure levels. Similarly, Jorna and colleagues (88) found significant exposure-related increases in chronic bronchitis and wheezing and decreases in airflow rates among 194 animal feed workers, also in the Netherlands. Even workers in the lowest exposure group ($0-4$ mg/m^3, on average) had significant reductions in FEV_1 and MMF compared to the non-exposed groups. In a follow-up investigation of the cohort studied by Smid et al. (87), Post and colleagues (89) showed that annual decline in lung function was significantly related to grain dust exposure level.

In a recent collaborative study in which data from the Dutch grain elevator and animal feed workers and Canadian grain elevator and grain loading workers were pooled, Peelen and colleagues (90) found exposure-response relationships of similar magnitude for current grain dust exposure and years employed among these diverse populations when exposure sampling methods and analytical approaches were harmonized.

In summary, when the exposure-response findings from these numerous studies are combined with evidence from earlier studies, there results a strong body of evidence linking grain dust exposure causally with chronic effects on the respiratory system.

The specific nature of this chronic lung disease due to grain dust exposure is unclear. Autopsy carried out on three grain workers who died as a result of the illness showed that the lungs were not only emphysematous, but had diffuse granulomata with fibrosis as well. These findings suggest that grain dust may induce changes in both the airways and the parenchyma (91). Most of the epidemiological studies with detailed pulmonary function measurements showed chronic airflow limitation. Since many grain workers are also smokers, the presenting clinical features (i.e., of chronic airflow obstruction) are difficult to distinguish from those caused by smoking. However, some of the recent studies (19,81,82,85,90) indicated that exposure to grain dust induced changes in FVC as well as FEV_1, suggesting the possibility of parenchymal involvement as well. This needs to be confirmed by more comprehensive clinical and pathological examination of nonsmoking grain workers with chronic pulmonary function abnormalities. The evidence of continued pulmonary disability and impairment in activities of daily living among nonsmoking, retired grain workers (83) also needs to be followed up by additional studies of both nonsmoking grain workers and retired workers to further clarify the nature and consequences of the grain dust−induced chronic lung damage. The possible role of repeated episodes of hypersensitity pneumonitis (see below) also needs further investigation.

Grain Fever

Grain fever, reported in 6−32% of exposed workers in different studies (65−70), is an acute illness occurring during or shortly after exposure to a high concentration of grain dust. The illness is characterized by facial warmth, headache, malaise, myalgia, fever, chilliness, throat and tracheal burning sensation, chest tightness, dyspnea, cough, and expectoration. It is associated with peripheral blood leukocytosis and a left shift of the differential count in most subjects. The pulmonary response is that of diffuse airways obstruction without detectable parenchymal abnormalities. Chest radiography is usually normal. The syndrome was studied in depth by doPico and co-workers (92). They exposed six grain workers and six controls to very high levels of grain dust for 120 min. The mean respirable concentration was 84 mg/m³. All subjects developed symptoms of grain fever. Since controls also developed similar symptoms as grain workers, immunological mechanisms were thought to be unlikely. Moreover, grain fever is not associated with the presence of serum-precipitating antibodies and there is no evidence of alveolitis, as is seen with hypersensitivity pneumonitis. doPico and co-workers (92) postulated that grain fever is due to bacterial endotoxin in the grain dust releasing chemical mediators directly in the airways.

Grain fever has also been classified as an organic dust toxic syndrome, which is associated with exposure to massive concentrations of spores of fungi or thermophilic actinomycetes (93).

Hypersensitivity Pneumonitis

Hypersensitivity pneumonitis is found in farmers usually after exposure to mold spores and has been called farmer's lung. The diagnosis of hypersensitivity pneumonitis is less than straightforward in the clinical setting; in epidemiological studies it is particularly difficult to identify. It is usually acute and self-limited and standardized criteria for its identification have not yet been developed. A useful approach to diagnosis has been proposed by Hentschel and Munt (94). In this schema, the diagnosis is based upon various elements. Three are essential: environmental or serological evidence of exposure, a consistent clinical history, and the presence of an abnormal X-ray during the symptomatic period. In addition, patients should have two of the following: pulmonary crackles, reduced

CO-diffusing capacity, reduced blood oxygen level, consistent histology, or a typical response on bronchoprovocation testing. Because most of these characteristics normalize after a single acute event, it is difficult to detect their presence subsequently. The prevalence of hypersensitivity pneumonitis among grain elevator workers is not known. It is likely to be very low. The distinction between grain fever and hypersensitivity pneumonitis in epidemiological surveys is difficult.

Irritation of Skin and Mucus Membrane

Skin irritation and pruritus are common complaints among grain handlers, barley being the worst offender, followed by oats. Hogan et al. (95) reported that 14.6% of workers had such symptoms. Skin irritation is usually short-lived and is often relieved by washing. The trichome particles of grain dust may play a role in skin irritation. Burning, itchy or watery eyes, and runny nose are also frequent complaints of grain handlers. Direct, nonspecific mechanical irritation is likely to be the reason for such complaints.

PREVENTION

As the dysfunction caused by grain dust exposure affects a relatively high proportion of exposed workers and the abnormalities induced are inflammatory and frequently not allergic, it should be possible to prevent or reduce the severity of the response by controlling the ambient dust levels. Theoretically it is possible to determine the relationship between various levels of exposure and the resulting physiological changes, thereby providing a guide to the permissible concentration for grain dust. This can be done by determining the levels of grain dust in the air at the same time as the physiological measurements are undertaken in a workforce. This would not, however, provide measurements of cumulative exposure. For this purpose, a trend in dust exposure, obtained from a monitoring program, would be required.

Some controlled inhalation studies have suggested a striking inflammatory response in the airways due to peak levels of exposure. In the operation of grain-handling facilities, the pattern of exposure associated with "dusty" areas is frequently a number of high peaks of dust level with intervening low levels. The peaks are often of very short duration. Measurements of an "average" exposure level over a period of 8 hr might not be able to identify these transient levels of high exposure.

Farant and Moore (96) conducted an extensive study of dust concentration in eight terminal and nine transfer elevators in Canada in 1978. A total of 754 work shift dust samples were collected: 434 were personal and 320 were general area samples collected at 14 different worksites in the elevators. The results indicated that grain workers were exposed to total dust concentrations varying from 0.18 to 781 mg/m^3. The respirable fraction of the total dust ranged from nondetectable to 76.3 mg/m^3.

In 1977, Labour Canada implemented a medical and dust surveillance program in the grain industry. Workers are required to have a medical examination including questionnaire, spirometry, and chest X-ray every 3 years. Regular dust monitoring of the elevators is also mandatory. At that time, Labour Canada adopted a permissible concentration of 10 mg/m^3 for grain dust, similar to that for nuisance dust at that time, since there were very few epidemiological studies. A number of epidemiological studies were conducted as part of the medical surveillance program in Canada (18,19,75–78,88,89). All the studies showed that grain workers had more respiratory symptoms and lower lung function compared to the controls even when the dust levels in the elevators were below 10 mg/m³.

Enarson and co-workers (84) showed that workers exposed to levels of dust less than 4 mg/m³ were not at risk for developing rapid decline in lung function. doPico et al. (13) showed a significantly higher prevalence of work-related respiratory symptoms and decrements in lung function over an 8 hr work shift in grain workers compared to controls when the mean level of total dust exposure was below 5 mg/m³ (3.3 ± 7.0 mg/m³). Furthermore, recent studies in which exposure-response relationships have been investigated in detail (85–90) all confirm that the permissible concentration for grain dust should be lowered to at least 5 mg/m³. In fact, a recent Dutch expert committee has recommended a permissible concentration of 1 mg/m³, based on a comprehensive review of the epidemiological literature to date, and including a modest safety factor (97).

SUMMARY

A great deal has been learned about the epidemiology and pathogenesis of grain dust–induced lung diseases. Grain dust has been shown to give rise to a number of clinical syndromes, such as skin and mucous membrane irritation, grain fever, hypersensitivity pneumonitis, asthma, asthma-like syndrome, and chronic lung diseases.

The classic asthma-like syndrome of Monday chest tightness, which was previously thought to occur only in connection with cotton dust exposure, has also been demonstrated among grain workers, workers in swine confinement buildings, in buildings with contaminated air humidifiers, and among poultry farm workers. Organic dusts are complex and consist of many components. They may contain similar microflora and mycoflora depending on the geographic site. It is likely that endotoxin, which can be found in these dusts, is the substance responsible for this syndrome.

There is evidence that chronic lung disease can result from grain dust exposure and that acute changes in lung function over a work shift predict the longitudinal decline in lung function. Although the decline in lung function is clearly dose-related for both acute and chronic exposure, the role of genetic susceptibility has yet to be determined.

ACKNOWLEDGMENTS

The authors wish to thank Mrs. C. Bassett for her assistance in the preparation of this manuscript. The studies on grain elevators in British Columbia were supported over the years by the National Health and Research Development Program, Health and Welfare Canada, British Columbia Terminal Operators Association, British Columbia Health Care Research Foundation, and British Columbia Lung Association. The authors would also like to thank the Grain Workers' Union and the grain workers in British Columbia for their cooperation.

REFERENCES

1. Ramazzini B. De Morbis Articum. Translated by WC Wright. New York: Hafner Publishing, 1964.

2. Farant JP, Moore CF. Dust exposures in the Canadian industries. In: Dosman JA, Cotton DJ, eds. Occupational Pulmonary Disease: Focus on Grain Dust and Health. New York: Academic Press, 1980:477–506.

3. Dashek WV, Olenchock SA, Mayfield JE, Wirtz GH, Wolz DE, Young CA. Carbohydrate and protein contents of grain dusts in relation to dust morphology. Environ Health Perspect 1986; 66:135–143.

4. Lacy J. The microflora of grain dusts: In: Dosman JA, Cotton DJ, eds. Occupational Pulmonary Disease: Focus on Grain Dust and Health. New York: Academic Press, 1980:417–40.

5. Cuthbert OD, Wraith EG, Brostoff J, Brighton ND. The role of mites in hay and grain dust allergy. In: Dosman JA, Cotton DJ, eds. Occupational Pulmonary Disease. Focus on Grain Dust and Health. New York: Academic Press, 1980:469–476.

6. Warren CPW, Cherniak RM, Tse KS. Hypersensitivity reaction to grain dust. J Allergy Clin Immunol 1974; 53:139–149.

7. Chan-Yeung M, Wong R, MacLean L. Respiratory abnormalities among grain elevator workers. Chest 1979; 75:461–467.

8. Broder I, Davies G, Hutcheon M, Leznoff A, Mintz S, Thomas P, Corey P. Variables of pulmonary allergy and inflammation in grain elevator workers. J Occup Med 1983; 25:43–47.

9. Davies RJ, Green M, McSchofield N. Recurrent nocturnal asthma after exposure to grain dust. Am Rev Respir Dis 1976; 14:1011–1015.

10. Warren CPW, Holford-Strevens V, Sinha RN. Sensitization in a grain handler to the storage mite Lepidoglyphus destructor (shrank). Ann Allergy 1983; 50:30–38.

11. Lunn JA, Hughes DT. Pulmonary hypersensitivity to the grain weevil. Br J Ind Med 1967; 24:158–161.

12. Kleine-Tebbe J, Jeep S, Josties C, Meysel U, O'Connor A, Kunkel J. IgE-mediated inhalant allergy in inhabitants of a building infested by the rice weevil (*Sitophilus oryzae*). Ann Allery 1992; 69:497–503.

13. doPico GA, Jacobs S, Flaherty D, Rankin J. Pulmonary reaction to durum wheat: a constituent of grain dust. Chest 1982; 81:55–61.

14. Chan-Yeung M. Grain dust asthma, does it exist? In: Principles of Health and Safety in Agriculture. J Dosman and D Cockcroft, eds. New York: Academic Press, 1990:169–171.

15. Senthilselvan A, Chen Y, Dosman JA. Predictors of asthma and wheezing in adults. Grain farming, sex, and smoking. Am Rev Respir Dis 1993; 148:6676–6680.

16. Senthilselvan A, Pahwa P, Wang P, McDufie HH, Dosman JA. Persistent wheeze in grain elevator workers should not be ignored. Am J Respir Crit Care Med 1996; 153:701–705.

17. Gandevia B, Ritchie B. Relevance of respiratory symptoms and signs to ventilatory capacity changes after exposure to grain dust and phosphate rock dust. Br J Ind Med 1966; 23:181–187.

18. Chan-Yeung M, Schulzer M, MacLean L, Dorken E, Grzybowski S. Epidemiologic health survey of grain elevator workers in British Columbia. Am Rev Respir Dis 1980; 121:329–336.

19. Corey P, Hutcheon M, Broder I, Mintz S. Grain elevator workers show work-related pulmonary function changes and dose-effect relationships with dust exposure. Br J Ind Med 1982; 39:330–337.

20. doPico GA, Reddan W, Anderson S, Flaherty D, Smalley E. Acute effects of grain dust exposure during a work shift. Am Rev Respir Dis 1983; 128:399–404.

21. McCarthy PE, Cockcroft AE, McDermott M. Lung function after exposure to barley dust. Br J Ind Med 1985; 42:106–110.

22. Schwartz DA, Thorne PS, Yagla SJ, Burmeister LF, Olenchock SA, Watt JL, Quinn TJ. The role of endotoxin in grain dust–induced lung disease. Am J Respir Crit Care Med 1995; 152:603–608.

23. Enarson DA, Vedal S, Chan-Yeung M. Fate of grainhandlers with bronchial hyperreactivity. Clin Invest Med 1988; 11:193–197.

24. Clapp WD, Becker S, Quay J, Watt JL, Thorne PS, Frees KL, Zhang X, Lux CR, Schwartz DA. Grain dust–induced airflow obstruction and inflammation of the lower respiratory tract. Am J Respir Crit Care Med 1994; 150:611–617.

25. Clapp WD, Thorne PS, Frees KL, Zhang X, Lux CR, Schwartz DA. The effects of inhalation of grain dust extract and endotoxin on upper and lower airways. Chest 1993; 104:825–830.

26. Jagielo PJ, Thorne PS, Watt JL, Frees KL, Quinn TJ, Schwartz DA. Grain dust and endotoxin inhalation produced similar inflammatory responses in normal subjects. Chest 1996; 110: 263–270.

27. Deetz DC, Jagielo PJ, Quinn TJ, Thorne PS, Bleuer SA, Schwartz DA. The kinetics of grain dust–induced inflammation of the lower respiratory tract. Am J Respir Crit Care Med 1996 (in press).

28. Blaski CA, Clapp WD, Thorne PS, Quinn TJ, Watt JL, Frees KL, Yagla SJ, Schwartz DA. The role of atopy in grain dust–induced airway disease. Am J Respir Crit Care Med 1996; 154:334–340.

29. Olenchock SA, Mull JC, Major PC, Peach MJ, Gladish ME, Taylor G. In vitro activation of the alternative pathway of complement by settled grain dust. J Allergy Clin Immunol 1978; 62:295–300.

30. Olenchock SA, Mull JC, Major PC. Extracts of airborne grain dusts activate alternative and classical complement pathways. Ann Allergy 1980; 44:23–28.

31. Von Essen SG, Robbins RA, Thompson AB, Ertl RF, Linder J, Rennard S. Mechanisms of neutrophil recruitment to the lung by grain dust exposure. Am Rev Respir Dis 1988; 138:921–927.

32. doPico GA, Jacobs S, Flaherty D, Rankin J. Pulmonary reaction to durum wheat. Chest 1982; 81:55–61.

33. doPico GA, Flaherty D, Bhaansali P, Chavaje N. Grain fever syndrome induced by inhalation of airborne grain dust. J Allergy Clin Immunol 1982; 69:435–443.

34. doPico GA, Reddan W, Flaherty D, Tsiatis A, Peters ME, Rao P, Rankin J. Respiratory abnormalities among grain handlers. Am Rev Respir Dis 1977; 115:915–927.

35. Lewis DM, Mentnech MS. Extracts of airborne grain dusts simulate interleukin-1 (IL-1) production by alveolar macrophages. Am Rev Respir Dis 1984; 129:A161.

36. Keller GE, Lewis DM, Olenchock SA. Demonstration of inflammatory cell population changes in rat lungs in response to intratracheal instillation of spring wheat dust using lung enzymatic digestion and centrifugal elutriation. Comp Immun Microbiol Infect Dis 1987; 10:219–226.

37. Clapp WD, Becker S, Quay J, Watt JL, Thorne PS, Frees KL, Zhang X, Lux CR, Schwartz DA. Grain dust–induced airflow obstruction and inflammation of the lower respiratory tract. Am J Respir Crit Care Med 1994; 150:611–617.

38. Von Essen SG, McGranaghan S, Cirian D, O'Neill D, Spurzem JR, Rennard SI. Inhalation of grain sorghum dust extract causes respiratory tract inflammation in human volunteers. Am Rev Respir Dis 1991; 143:A105.

39. Kennedy SM, Christiani DC, Eisen EA, Wegman DH, Greaves IA, Olenchock SA, Ye TT, Lu PL. Cotton dust and endotoxin exposure-response relationships in cotton textile workers. Am Rev Respir Dis 1987; 135:194–200.

40. Haglind P, Rylander R. Exposure to cotton dust in an experimental cardroom. Br J Ind Med 1984; 41:340–345.

41. Rylander R, Haglind P, Lundholm M. Endotoxin in cotton dust and respiratory function decrement among cotton workers in an experimental cardroom. Am Rev Respir Dis 1985; 131: 209–213.

42. Donham K, Haglind P, Peterson Y, Rylander R, Belin L. Environmental and health studies of farm workers in Swedish swine confinement buildings. Br J Ind Med 1989; 46:31–37.

43. Thelin A, Tegler O, Rylander R. Lung reactions during poultry handling related to dust and bacterial endotoxin levels. Eur J Respir Dis 1984; 65:266–271.

44. Schwartz DA, Donham KJ, Olenchock SA, Popendorf W, van Fossen SD, Burmeister LF, Merchant JA. Determinants of longitudinal changes in spirometric functions among swine confinement operators and farmers. Am J Respir Crit Care Med 1995; 151:47–53.

45. Michel O, Ginanni R, Le Bon B, Content J, Duchateau J, Sergysels R. Inflammatory response to acute inhalation of endotoxin in asthmatic patients. Am Rev Respir Dis 1992; 146:352–357.

46. Michel O, Kips J, Duchateua J, Vertongen F, Robert L, Collet H, Pauwels R, Sergysels R. Severity of asthma is related to endotoxin in house dust. Am J Respir Crit Care Med 1996; 154:1641–1646.

47. Cavagna G, Foa V, Vigliani EC. Effects in man and rabbits of inhalation of cotton dust or extracts and purified endotoxins. Brit J Ind Med 1969; 26:314–321.

48. Herbert A, Carvalheiro M, Rubenowitz E, Bake B, Rylander R. Reduction of alveolar-capillary diffusion after inhalation of endotoxin in normal subjects. Chest 1992; 102:1095–1098.

49. Rylander R, Bake B, Fischer JJ, Helander IM. Pulmonary function and symptoms after inhalation of endotoxin. Am Rev Respir Dis 1989; 140:981–986.

50. Michel O, Duchateau J, Sergysels R. Effect of inhaled endotoxin on bronchial reactivity in asthmatic and normal subjects. JAP 1989; 66:1059.

51. Boehlecke B, Cocke J, Bragg K, Hancock J, Petsonk E, Piccirillo R, Merchant J. Pulmonary function response to dust from standard and closed boll harvested cotton. Chest 1981; 79:77S–81S.

52. Castellan RM, Olenchock SA, Hankinson JL, Millner PD, Cocke JB, Bragg CK, Perkins HH, Jacobs RR. Acute bronchoconstriction induced by cotton dust: Dose-related responses to endotoxin and other dust factors. Ann Intern Med 1984; 101:157–163.

53. Castellan RM, Olenchock SA, Kinsely KB, Hankinson JL. Inhaled endotoxin and decreased spirometric values. N Engl J Med 1987; 317:605–610.

54. Schwartz DA, Thorne PS, Jagielo PJ, White GE, Bleuer SA, Frees KL. Endotoxin responsiveness and grain dust–induced inflammation in the lower respiratory tract. Am J Physiol 1984; 267:L609–L617.

55. Jagielo PJ, Thorne PS, Kern JA, Quinn TJ, Schwartz DA. The role of endotoxin in grain dust–induced inflammation in mice. Am J Physol Lung Cell Mol Physiol 1996; 270:L1052–L1059.

56. Jagielo PJ, Quinn TJ, Qureshi N, Schwartz DA. Grain dust induced lung inflammation is reduced by *Rhodobacter sphaeroides* disphosphoryl Lipid A. Am J Physiol (in press).

57. Snella M, Rylander R. Lung cell reactions after inhalation of bacterial lipopolysaccharides. Eur J Respir Dis 1982; 63:550–557.

58. Freudenberg MA, Galanos C. Induction of tolerance to lipopolysaccharide (LPS)-D-galactosamine lethality by pretreatment with LPS is mediated by macrophages. Infect Immun 1988; 56:1352–1357.

59. Kips JC, Tavernier J, Pauwels RA. Tumor necrosis factor causes bronchial hyperresponsiveness in rats. Am Rev Respir Dis 1992; 145:332–336.

60. Strieter RM, Standiford TJ, Rolfe MW, Kunkel SL. Interleukin-8. In: Kelley J, ed. Cytokines of the Lung. New York: Marcel Dekker, 1993.

61. Standiford TJ, Kunkel SL, Basha MA, Chensue SW, Lynch JP, Toews GB, Westwick J, Strieter RM. Interleukin-8 gene expression by a pulmonary epithelial cell line. J Clin Invest 1990; 86:1945–1953.

62. Nakamura H, Yoshimura K, Jaffe HA, Crystal RG. Interleukin-8 gene expression in human bronchial epithelial cells. J Biol Chem 1991; 266:19611–19617.

63. Redl H, Schlag G, Ceska M, Davies J, Buurman WA. Interleukin-8 release in baboon septicemia is partially dependent on tumor necrosis factor. J Infect Dis 1993; 167:1464–1466.

64. Schwartz DA. Grain dust, endotoxin, and airflow obstruction. Chest 1996; 1996:57s–63s.

65. Smith AR, Greenburg L, Siegel W. Respiratory disease among grain handlers. Ind Bull (Dept of Labor, NY State) 1941; 20:1.

66. Williams N, Skoulas A, Merriman JE. Exposure to grain dust. I. A survey of the effects. J Occup Med 1964; 6:319–329.

67. Kleinfeld M, Messite J, Swencicki RE, Shapiro J. A clinical and physiological study of grain handlers. Arch Environ Health 1968; 16:380–384.

68. Tse KS, Warren P, Janusz M, McCarthy DS, Cherniack RM. Respiratory abnormalities in workers exposed to grain dust. Arch Environ Health 1973; 27:74–77.

69. doPico GA, Reddan W, Flaherty D, Tsiatis A, Peters ME, Rao P, Rankin J. Respiratory abnormalities among grainhandlers: a clinical, physiologic, and immunologic study. Am Rev Respir Dis 1977; 115:915–927.

70. Sheridan D, Deutscher C, Tan L, Maybank J, Gerrard J, Horne S, Yoshida K, Barnett GD, Cotton D, Dosman JA. The relationship between exposure to cereal grain dust and pulmonary function in grain workers. In: Dosman JA, Cotton D, eds. Occupational Pulmonary Disease: Focus on Grain Dust and Health. New York: Academic Press, 1979:229–238.

71. Broder I, Mintz M, Hutcheon P, Corey P, Silverman F, Davies G, Leznoff A, Peress L, Thomas P. Comparison of respiratory variables in grain elevator workers and civic outside workers of Thunder Bay, Canada. Am Rev Respir Dis 1979; 119:193–203.

72. Dosman JA, Cotton DJ, Graham B, Li R, Froh F, Barnett D. Chronic bronchitis and decreased forced expiratory flow rates in life time nonsmoking grain workers. Am Rev Respir Dis 1980; 121:11–16.

73. Herbert FA, Woytowich V, Schram E, Baldwin D. Respiratory profiles of grain handlers and sedentary workers. Can Med Assoc J 1981; 125:46–50.

74. Cotton DJ, Graham BL, Li KYR, Froh F, Barnett GD, Dosman JA. Effects of grain dust exposure and smoking on respiratory symptoms and lung function. J Occup Med 1983; 25: 131–141.

75. Yach D, Myers J, Bradshaw D, Benatar SR. A respiratory epidemiologic survey of grain mill workers in Cape Town, South Africa. Am Rev Respir Dis 1985; 131:505–510.

76. Chan-Yeung M, Schulzer M, MacLean L, Dorken E, Tan F, Lam S, Enarson D, Grzybowski S. A follow up study of the grain elevator workers in the port of Vancouver. Arch Environ Health 1981; 36:75–80.

77. Chan-Yeung M, Enarson DA. Prospective changes in lung function in grain elevator workers in large terminals in Vancouver. In: Dosman J, Cockcroft D, eds. Principles of Health and Safety in Agriculture. New York: Academic Press, 1990:131–134.

78. Broder I, Corey P, Davies G, Hutcheon M, Mintz S, Inouye T, Hyland R, Leznoff A, Thomas P. Longitudinal study of grain elevator workers and control workers with demonstration of healthy worker effect. J Occup Med 1985; 27:873–880.

79. Schulzer M, Enarson DA, Chan-Yeung M. Analyzing cross-sectional and longitudinal lung function measurements: the effects of age. Can J Statist 1985; 13:7–15.

80. Chan-Yeung M, Ward H, Enarson DA, Kennedy SM. Five cross-sectional studies of grain elevator workers. Am J Epidemiol 1992; 136:1269–1279.

81. Broder I, Mintz S, Hutcheon MA, Corey PN, Kuzyk J. Effect of layoff and rehire on respiratory variables on grain elevator workers. Am Rev Respir Dis 1980; 122:601–608.

82. Broder I, Hutcheon MA, Mintz S, Davies G, Leznoff A, Thomas P, Corey P. Changes in respiratory variables of grain handlers and civic workers during their initial months of employment. Br J Ind Med 1984; 41:94–99.

83. Kennedy SM, Dimich-Ward H, Desjardins A, Kassam A, Vedal S, Chan-Yeung M. Respiratory health among retired grain elevator workers. Am J Respir Crit Care Med 1994; 150:59–65.

84. Enarson DA, Vedal S, Chan-Yeung M. Rapid decline in FEV_1 in grain handlers—relation to level of dust exposure. Am Rev Respir Dis 1985; 132:814–817.

85. Huy T, De Schipper K, Chan-Yeung M, Kennedy SM. Grain dust and lung function: exposure response relationships. Am Rev Respir Dis 1991; 144:1314–1321.

86. Kennedy SM, Dimich-Ward H, Chan-Yeung M. Relationship between grain dust exposure and longitudinal changes in pulmonary function. In: Human Sustainability in Agriculture: Health Safety and Environment. Michigan: Lewis Publishers, 1995:13–18.

87. Smid T, Heederik D, Houba R, Quanjer PH. Dust- and endotoxin-related respiratory effects in the animal feed industry. Am Rev Respir Dis 1992; 146:1474–1479.

88. Jorna THJM, Borm PJA, Valds J, Houba R, Wouters EFM Respiratory symptoms and lung function in animal feed workers. Chest 1994; 106:1050–1055.

89. Post WK, Heederik D, Houba R. Exposure related lung function decline and selection processes among workers in the animal feed and grain processing industry. Wageningen Agricultural University, Wageningen, 1996.

90. Peelen SJM, Heederik D, Dimich-Ward H, Chan-Yeung M, Kennedy SM. Comparison of dust related respiratory effects in Dutch and Canadian grain handling industries. A pooled analysis. Occup Environ Med 1996; 53:559–566.
91. Cohen VL, Osgood H. Disability due to inhalation of grain dust. J Allergy 1953; 24:193–211.
92. doPico GA, Flaherty D, Bhansali P, Chavaje N. Grain fever syndrome induced by inhalation of airborne grain dust. J Allergy Clin Immunol 1982; 69:435–443.
93. Rask-Andersen A, Malmberg P. Organic dust toxic syndrome in Swedish farmers: symptoms, chemical findings and exposure in 98 cases. Am J Ind Med 1989; 17:116–117 (abstract).
94. Hentschel EF, Munt PW. Management of farmer's lung. Drug Protocol 1988; 3:17–21.
95. Hogan DJ, Dosman JD, Li KY, Graham B, Johnson B, Walker R, Lane PR. Questionnaire survey of pruritis and rash in grain elevator workers. Contact Dermatitis 1990; 14:170–175.
96. Farant JP, Moore CF. Dust exposures in Canadian grain industry. Am Ind Hyg Assoc J 1978; 39:177–193.

33

Hypersensitivity Pneumonitis and Organic Dust Toxic Syndromes

Yvon Cormier
Laval University and Hôpital Laval, Ste-Foy, Quebec, Canada

Hal B. Richerson
University of Iowa, Iowa City, Iowa

Cecile S. Rose
National Jewish Medical and Research Center and University of Colorado, Denver, Colorado

HYPERSENSITIVITY PNEUMONITIS

Introduction

In 1969, Pepys carefully contrasted differences between atopic asthma and hypersensitivity pneumonitis (HP) (extrinsic allergic alveolitis) on the basis of clinical manifestations and presumed, but now obsolete, concepts of pathogenesis (1). Pepys's earlier studies of farmer's lung had established thermophilic actinomyces as causative agents (2). The recognition of other agents responsible for HP in varied and often exotic occupations elevated HP to increasing visibility in modern medical practice as an alternative to asthma in occupation-related hypersensitivity lung disease (3). Inclusion of a chapter on HP is well justified, therefore, in a book on occupational asthma.

Farmer's lung was apparently recognized centuries ago as a disease entity in farmers exposed to stored grains. Olaus Magnus, the last Catholic archbishop of Sweden, published a history of the northern peoples in 1555 that described respiratory difficulties from fine dusts produced during threshing in winter (4). Ramazzini in 1713 recognized respiratory problems in sifters and measurers of grain that probably included both asthma and HP (5).

Although farmer's lung was described in England in 1932 (6), it was not registered in Britain as an industrial disease until 1964, defined at that time as "a pulmonary disease due to inhalation of the dust of mouldy hay or of other mouldy vegetable produce, and characterized by symptoms and signs attributable to a reaction in the peripheral part of the bronchopulmonary-pulmonary system, and giving rise to a defect in gas exchange" (7).

Clinical presentation, causative agent, and pathophysiology essentially define HP as the disease has no pathognomonic marker. Any attempt at definition is simply a description of symptoms and objective findings. HP may be described, therefore, as a pulmonary and constitutional illness with symptoms of dyspnea and cough that results from an immu-

635

nologically induced, noninfectious inflammation of the lung parenchyma involving alveolar walls and terminal airways secondary to repeated inhalation of a variety of antigenic organic dusts and other agents by a susceptible host. The disease is further characterized by a decreased lung-diffusing capacity and increased interstitial markings on chest roentgenograms. Precipitating antibodies (precipitins) to a suspected causative agent are helpful in confirming sufficient exposure to that agent to stimulate an appropriate immunological response. Bronchoalveolar lavage reveals a lymphocytic alveolitis, and pathological study shows an interstitial granulomatous pneumonitis with bronchiolitis (3,8).

Clinical Manifestations

With the ubiquity of potential environmental antigens (often in unsuspected workplace or home environments), the difficulties in identifying and measuring relevant antigenic exposures, the variable disease manifestations, and the often subtle clinical presentation, underrecognition and misdiagnosis of hypersensitivity pneumonitis continue to plague clinicians. Since descriptions of HP may have included cases of organic dust toxic syndromes (see below) this initial confounding diagnosis could explain some of the findings described in references cited in the following subsections. A high degree of clinical suspicion and a careful exposure history remain essential for early disease recognition and successful management.

Signs and Symptoms

HP is frequently classified into three distinct clinical forms—acute, subacute, and chronic—based on clinical presentation and findings, though these forms may overlap. Acute illness typically begins 4–12 hr after exposure, with the patient describing a flulike illness characterized by symptoms of cough, dyspnea, chest tightness, fevers, chills, malaise, and myalgias. Symptoms are usually accompanied by physical findings of fever, tachypnea, tachycardia, and crepitant rales. The acute symptoms of HP typically abate or improve within 24 hr, only to recur hours after repeat antigen exposure.

The subacute and chronic presentations of illness require a high degree of clinical suspicion to confirm the diagnosis and initiate appropriate management. Exertional dyspnea and cough are the predominant symptoms, with sputum production, fatigue, anorexia, and weight loss also reported. Physical examination may be normal or reveal basilar crackles. Cyanosis and right heart failure may be evident with severe fibrotic disease. Digital clubbing is occasionally found in late stages of chronic HP. Clubbing occurred in approximately half of patients in a case series of pigeon breeder's disease and was associated with a poorer prognostic outcome (9).

Physiology

Pulmonary function abnormalities in acute HP are classically restrictive, with a decrease in forced vital capacity, 1-sec forced expiratory volume, and total lung capacity. Impaired gas exchange, as indexed by abnormal diffusing capacity, and hypoxemia are often present. An exercise-induced fall in oxygen tension is an early sign of functional impairment. Four to 6 weeks may be required for complete resolution of these acute abnormalities following removal from exposure (10).

Restrictive, obstructive, or combined defects in pulmonary function occur in chronic HP. In 1965, Pepys and Jenkins reported that 10% of 205 farmer's lung patients showed obstruction alone rather than restriction (11). Decreased diffusion capacity is also commonly observed. Gas exchange abnormalities, particularly with exercise, may be marked.

Methacholine hyperresponsiveness has been described in 22–60% of patients with HP (12,13). The incidence of asthma increased from 1% prior to a diagnosis of farmer's lung disease (FLD) to 7% within 5 years after the diagnosis of FLD in a Finnish study of 1031 farmers with HP (14).

Radiography

In the acute form of disease the chest radiograph may be normal, but typically reveals small, scattered, 1–3-mm nodules (Fig. 1A). Diffuse, patchy infiltrates or a ground-glass appearance may be present. In one study, 4% of acute cases of farmer's lung had normal films and another 40–45% had minimal changes that might easily be overlooked. The extent of radiographic abnormality correlated poorly with the severity of symptoms or functional impairment (15). Chest radiographic abnormalities in acute illness typically regress or resolve over 4–6 weeks if further exposure is avoided.

In chronic HP, linear interstitial markings become more distinct and are often most prominent in the periphery or upper lung zones on plain chest radiograph. There may be progressive loss of lung volume. Pleural abnormalities, hilar adenopathy, calcification, and atelectasis are rarely described.

The computed-tomography (CT) appearance of HP is variable and overlaps with other interstitial lung diseases (16), and the high-resolution CT scan may be normal if disease is diagnosed early (17). Widespread diffuse ground glass opacification, areas of decreased attenuation and mosaic perfusion, and centrilobular micronodules are the most common and characteristic CT manifestations of acute and subacute HP (Fig. 1B) (18–21). Either patchy or diffuse ground glass attenuation was observed in 52% of subacute and 71% of chronic forms of bird breeder's HP (22). Honeycombing is present in more advanced chronic cases, often with concurrent micronodules and/or ground glass attenuation. Emphysematous changes can be seen in both subacute and chronic cases, many of whom are nonsmokers. Pretracheal lymph nodes may be enlarged, but hilar adenopathy is rare (18).

Precipitating Antibodies

The finding of specific precipitating antibodies in the serum of a patient with suspected HP indicates antigen exposure sufficient to generate a humoral immunological response and may be a helpful diagnostic clue (23). Although precipitin testing was previously considered a "gold standard" in confirming an HP diagnosis, its limitations are becoming widely recognized. Specific precipitating antibodies frequently are not demonstrable in patients with HP. False-negatives may occur because of poorly standardized commercial laboratory antigens, insensitive laboratory techniques, use of underconcentrated sera, or the wrong choice of antigen for testing (24). In some patients the antibody response may be too meager to give a precipitin reaction using the traditional Ouchterlony double immunodiffusion technique. More sensitive assays for specific IgG such as ELISA may lead to confusion because of decreased specificity. Serum precipitins may disappear over variable periods of time after exposure ceases and immunosuppressive therapy begins, adding to the difficulty of antigen-specific diagnosis (25). False-positives also occur, and precipitin markers of antigen exposure can be detected in individuals without clinically evident disease (26). Serum precipitins were found in 3–30% of asymptomatic farmers and in up to 50% of asymptomatic pigeon breeders (27,28). The prevalence of positive tests in asymptomatic individuals can fluctuate, with subjects testing variably positive or negative at different times (29).

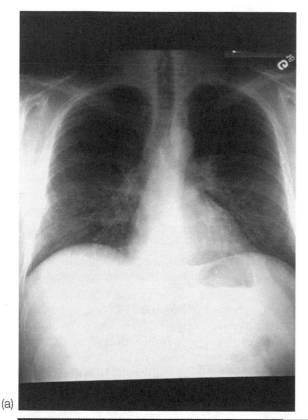

(a)

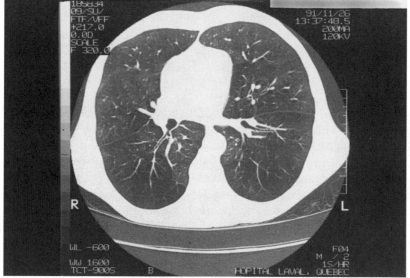

(b)

Figure 1   (a) Posteroanterior chest film of a case of acute HP showing typical scattered micronodules. (b) High-resolution computed-tomography section of a case of acute HP showing patchy
ground-glass infiltrates distributed throughout the lungs.

Other Laboratory Studies

In the acute illness, peripheral blood leukocytosis with neutrophilia and lymphopenia is often present. Eosinophilia is unusual. Mild elevations in erythrocyte sedimentation rate, C-reactive protein, and immunoglobulins of IgG, IgM, or IgA isotypes are occasionally evident, reflecting acute or chronic inflammation. Serum angiotensin-converting-enzyme concentrations may rarely be increased in patients with recurrent acute symptoms (30). Antinuclear antibodies and other autoantibodies are rarely detected. Skin tests have not been useful in the diagnosis of HP (13).

Inhalation Challenge

The use of inhalation challenge in the diagnosis of HP is limited by the lack of standardized antigens and techniques. Inhalation of an aerosolized antigen suspected to be causative is helpful only when acute symptoms and clinical abnormalities are part of the disease presentation and likely to occur within hours after exposure (31). In some patients with acute symptoms, exposure to the suspect environment with postexposure monitoring of symptoms, temperature, leukocyte count, spirometry, and chest radiograph may be preferable to laboratory challenge. Interpretation of results is often difficult, and inhalation challenge is not recommended in most patients with suspected HP except in a research context (32).

Bronchoalveolar Lavage (BAL)

BAL appears to play a useful role in the evaluation of patients with HP and in excluding other conditions that mimic the illness (33), though BAL findings are nonspecific and, by themselves, nondiagnostic. Typically, a marked lavage lymphocytosis without eosinophilia is found. Increased BAL neutrophils are observed shortly after antigen exposure. Total white blood cell numbers are increased, often up to fivefold that of controls. The absolute number of macrophages is similar to controls, although their percentage in lavage is reduced due to the high number of lymphocytes. Mast cells have been reported to be increased in symptomatic patients with hypersensitivity pneumonitis (34), though their pathogenetic role remains unclear. Concentrations of IgG, IgM, and IgA antibodies are typically increased in BAL in subjects with HP (though smoking may mitigate this effect), as are total protein and albumin (35,36). The lavage cellular profile may vary considerably depending on the stage of illness and the time interval between BAL and last antigen exposure (37). The BAL lymphocytosis may persist for years following removal from exposure and despite improvement in other clinical parameters, limiting its utility as a tool to follow the course and progression of disease (38). Asymptomatic farmers may have a BAL lymphocytosis, further limiting the diagnostic utility of lavage (39,40).

Pathology

Lung biopsy may be indicated in patients without sufficient clinical criteria for definitive diagnosis or to rule out other diseases requiring different treatment. Transbronchial biopsies are often sufficient but may sample unrepresentative areas, and thoracoscopic lung biopsy is occasionally required. Special stains and cultures are helpful to distinguish HP from infectious granulomatous conditions such as fungal and mycobacterial diseases.

Histopathology in 60 Wisconsin patients with farmer's lung biopsied during the active phase of their disease showed an interstitial alveolar infiltrate in 100% (consisting of plasma cells, lymphocytes, and occasional eosinophils), granulomata in 70%, unexpectedly mild interstitial fibrosis in 65%, and bronchiolitis to some degree in 50% of the biopsy specimens; no vasculitis was observed in any case (41).

Coleman and Colby (42) studied 27 patients with putative HP and found a "diagnostic triad" of (1) cellular infiltrates of lymphocytes and plasma cells of varying density along airways; (2) interstitial infiltrates of lymphocytes and plasma cells varying from mild to very dense; and (3) single, nonnecrotizing, randomly scattered granulomata in the parenchyma with some in bronchiolar and alveolar walls, but without mural vascular involvement. Eosinophils were scant or absent. About 80% of clinically proven cases were estimated as demonstrating the triad, which may, however, be present in other interstitial diseases.

Sarcoidosis may be particularly difficult to distinguish from HP, but certain histopathologic features may help. In sarcoidosis, but not in HP, granulomata are found in perivascular and intramural areas of blood vessels. Infiltrates of lymphocytes and plasma cells are found only in and around granulomata in sarcoidosis, whereas in HP such infiltrates are also seen involving the parenchyma at sites distant from granulomata. Ultrastructural studies have revealed similar, nonspecific air-blood barrier lesions of alveolar epithelial or endothelial injury and inflammation with type II cell hyperplasia and fibrosis in both HP and sarcoidosis (43).

Diagnostic Criteria and Differential Diagnosis

A number of investigators have suggested diagnostic criteria for HP. Richerson and colleagues (32) proposed the following features to confirm a case of HP: (1) findings of interstitial lung disease by history, physical examination, and pulmonary function testing; (2) a consistent chest radiograph; (3) exposure to a recognized cause of HP; and (4) demonstrable antibodies to the relevant antigen. Terho (44) proposed major and minor criteria for farmer's lung disease; the diagnosis is considered confirmed if the patient fulfills all of the major criteria and at least two additional criteria, and if other diseases with similar clinical findings have been ruled out. A negative chest film is allowed if the biopsy is positive. The major criteria include: (1) exposure to offending antigens revealed by history, by environmental measurements, or by the presence of antigen-specific IgG antibodies; (2) symptoms compatible with HP appearing several hours after exposure; and (3) abnormal chest X-ray. Additional criteria include: (1): basilar crepitant rales; (2) decreased diffusing capacity; (3) decreased oxygen tension or saturation at rest or with exercise; (4) abnormal histology compatible with HP; and (5) positive provocation test by either work exposure or controlled inhalation challenge.

Stringent diagnostic criteria likely underestimate milder cases of HP in which the chest radiograph is normal or when symptoms are subtle or insidious. Hodgson and coworkers (45) showed a decline in the sensitivity of the chest radiograph for diagnosis of HP over the years 1950–1980. Chest X-rays were also less likely to be abnormal when a population-based approach to diagnosis was undertaken. Underrecognition and misdiagnosis of HP probably occur for other reasons as well including: (1) absent or inadequate occupational and environmental history taking; (2) the symptoms and signs of HP are nonspecific and mimic many other diseases such as asthma, influenza, viral pneumonia, and sarcoidosis (Table 1); (3) early disease may be accompanied by normal resting pulmonary function; (4) the microbial antigens that can cause HP proliferate in common environmental niches, complicating the historical identification of a relevant antigen exposure (46); and (5) precipitating antibodies are often difficult to measure and may dis-

Table 1 Differential Diagnosis of Hypersensitivity Pneumonitis

Inhalation fever	Humidifier fever
	Organic dust toxic syndrome (ODTS)
	Silo filler's/unloader's syndrome
	Pontiac fever (nonpneumonic legionellosis)
Granulomatous disorder	Sarcoidosis
	Beryllium disease
	Drug-induced pneumonitis
	Granuloma-vasculitis syndromes
	Lymphatoid granulomatosis
	Eosinophilic granuloma
Immunological disease	Asthma
	Collagen-vascular diseases
	Allergic bronchopulmonary aspergillosis
	Eosinophilic pneumonias
Infection	Viral and *Mycoplasma* pneumonias
	Psittacosis
	Fungal infections
	Mycobacterial infections
Fibrosing lung disease	Idiopathic pulmonary fibrosis (IPF)
	Bronchiolitis obliterans from other causes
	Inorganic dust pneumoconioses
Other	Chronic bronchitis
	Toxic fume inhalation

appear after exposure ceases, so a patient with fibrotic lung disease from previous episodes of HP may not be recognized as such (47).

Hypersensitivity Pneumonitis Versus Asthma in the Workplace

The differential diagnosis of dyspnea and cough in an occupational environment must include asthma and HP, as some sensitizers in the workplace are capable of causing either disease. The two diseases and organic dust toxic syndrome are usually readily distinguishable, as indicated in Table 2, but differentiation is occasionally difficult.

Any attempt to compile a complete up-to-date list of agents reported to be associated with HP in the workplace is both unnecessary and futile in the present age of computer search capabilities. Reports of new agents continue to appear (48). Putative "new" agents are often reported as individual cases or anecdotes, so critical evaluation or verification is needed before they can be considered valid causes of HP.

Without any claim to be exhaustive, Table 3 is organized into reasonably well-documented occupation-related HP and associated environments and antigens including agents that are also capable of inducing occupational asthma.

Epidemiology and Prevalence

The epidemiology of occupation-related HP is meaningful only as it relates to specific types of HP. Definitive prevalence studies are difficult for several reasons (49,50). The diagnosis depends on a group of clinical and laboratory findings, none of which are pa-

Table 2 Differential Diagnostic Features of Hypersensitivity Pneumonitis, Asthma, and Organic Dust Toxic Syndrome

Feature	HP	Asthma	ODTS
Symptoms	Cough, dyspnea, fever	Cough, dyspnea, tightness in chest	Flu-like syndrome with fever
Onset after exposure	Gradual after 4–8 hr	Immediate (early onset) and/or after 4–6 hr (late onset)	Gradual after 3–8 hr
Physical findings	Bibasilar crackles	Expiratory wheezes	None
Chest radiograph	Infiltrates or normal	Hyperlucent or normal	Normal
Pathophysiology	Restrictive pattern	Obstructive pattern	Normal PFTs
Peripheral eosinophilia	No	Yes	No

thognomonic. Symptoms are not specific, and it is impractical in large epidemiological studies to use chest roentgenograms, BAL, lung biopsies, and inhalational challenge studies in either the suspected environment or the laboratory. Serum precipitins and BAL lymphocytosis indicate exposure, not disease. Thus, identification of individuals with clinical HP in any occupational group is tentative, so the accuracy and value of relevant epidemiological studies are questionable.

Variables complicating prevalence studies in individuals and groups include the extent of environmental exposure, geographic location, rainfall and other local conditions, characteristics and hygiene of facilities and processes, safety and control measures, exposure precautions, awareness of the hazard, and host factors. Despite these built-in problems, many epidemiological studies have been carried out, mainly in farmer's lung, bird fancier's lung, and building-related exposures (46) or contaminated humidification devices.

Farmer's lung is primarily a disease of dairy farmers. Early reports of a high prevalence utilized questionnaires only, but more recent studies with strict criteria for diagnosis indicate an annual incidence of 44 per 100,000 farming population in Finland and 23 per 100,000 in Sweden (51). An overall prevalence of 0.42%, or 420 per 100,000, was found in 1400 Wisconsin dairy farmers (52). Differences among various studies have been attributed to geographic location, rainfall, and type of farming as well as to epidemiological methods. Bird fancier's or breeder's lung among populations appropriately exposed has ranged from 3 to 15%. Budgerigar (parakeet) fanciers in Britain have a HP prevalence rate of 0.5–7.5%. Outbreaks of HP from contaminated humidifiers in office buildings have affected 15–52% of exposed individuals. Few useful data are available for other occupation-related HP. Of note is the diminished frequency and even disappearance of a specific HP after the cause is recognized and controlled. Maple bark stripper's lung and bagassosis, for example, have essentially disappeared as occupational diseases.

Pathophysiology

The demonstration of precipitating antibodies to extracts of "moldy" hay and, subsequently, to thermophilic actinomyces in the sera of farmer's lung patients led to the postulation that an immune complex–mediated (Gell and Coombs type III) hypersensitivity reaction accounted for disease pathogenesis. The pathology was not typical of a type III reaction but was rather a granulomatous process suggesting a cell-mediated or delayed hypersensitivity (type IV) reaction. Attempts to correlate antibody levels with the presence or severity of pulmonary disease failed, and animal models demonstrated a role for T-cell-mediated inflammation. Current information overall favors the primary importance of type IV hypersensitivity (3,8,53,54), which has become increasingly complex.

Exploration of cell-mediated (type IV) hypersensitivity mechanisms in human HP has focused largely on cell phenotypes, functional patterns, and cytokine release in BAL fluids. Alveolar lymphocytosis consists predominantly of CD8+ T cells in HP and CD4+ T cells in sarcoidosis in most studies, varying with the stage of disease and causative agent (55). Analysis of the T-cell-receptor, beta-chain-variable region in HP BAL lymphocytes showed overexpression of a particular beta-chain-variable segment reported to belong to the lymphocyte subset that accounts for the alveolitis in HP (CD8+) and sarcoidosis (CD4+), and resolution of alveolitis was accompanied by normalization of the T-cell subsets (56).

Activated CD8+ T cells, macrophages, and resultant cytokines characterize the lymphocyte-rich alveolitis and putatively account for progression to clinical disease. In HP as in many inflammatory processes, including asthma, it would seem that whatever cytokine is in the forefront at the moment is looked for and found. Interleukin-1, tumor necrosis factor alpha, macrophage inflammatory protein-1 alpha, and interleukin-8 are elevated in BAL fluids, synthesized and released by BAL cells (57,58). Other substances increased in HP lungs include fibroblast growth factors, type III procollagen, fibronectin, vibronectin, and hyaluronic acid. Surfactant protein A, associated with macrophage immunomodulatory function, is altered in BAL fluids from HP patients. Serine proteinase inhibitors, alpha one-proteinase inhibitor, secretory leukocyte proteinase inhibitor, and elafin (elastase-specific inhibitor) are present in BAL and may play a role in resolution and control of HP (59). Asymptomatic, exposed individuals may also demonstrate a lymphocyte-rich BAL.

Although increased numbers of CD8+ T lymphocytes in BAL of recently exposed HP patients have been reported by several investigators, others have found no consistent phenotypic preponderance despite increased T-lymphocyte proliferation, activation, and function. Increased populations of CD4+, CD8+, mast cells, and various sorts of cytotoxic cells, including natural killer (NK) cells and MHC-restricted and non-MHC-restricted cytotoxic lymphocytes, have been found in lungs of HP patients (60,61).

Pursuit of antigenic epitopes on the relatively crude extracts of *Saccharopolyspora rectivirgula* or avian proteins has shown that the relevant T lymphocytes recognize a wide range of proteins that induce proliferation (62), but without any clear meaning for pathogenesis (63). An adjuvant effect of the etiological agent itself or a concurrent viral infection may initiate or enhance disease in susceptible individuals, and suppressor cells of lymphocyte or macrophage lineage have been postulated to explain the absence or limitation of inflammation in exposed, asymptomatic individuals. So far none of the cellular humoral, cytokine, mediator, in vitro, or in vivo studies in humans or animal fully explains the pathogenesis of HP. What combination of cells, cytokines, and other substances is both necessary and sufficient for the progression to clinical disease or results in down-regulation without clinical disease remains uncertain.

Because of necessary limitations in using patients in experimental studies and the inadequacies of in vitro techniques for such a purpose, several species of animals have been utilized to help elucidate pathogenesis (53). Recent studies have included adoptive transfer and genetically manipulated mice in attempts to demonstrate the role of the T cell.

Adoptive transfer of HP in animal models has been successful using the transfer of cultured lymphocytes from sensitized, syngeneic strain II guinea pigs (64), LEW rats (65), and inbred mice (66) to naïve recipients subsequently challenged with inhaled or infused intrapulmonary antigen. Athymic nude C57 Black/nu/nu mice were unable to develop

Table 3 Selected Examples of Hypersensitivity Pneumonitis

Occupation	Disease	Source of antigen	Antigen
		Agricultural environment	
Farming	Farmer's lung	"Moldy" hay, silage, grain[a]	Thermophilic actinomycetes
Gardener	Soil fertilizer lung	Soil fertilizer	*Streptomyces albus*
Mushroom hunter	Lycoperdonosis	*Lycoperdon* puffballs	Puffball spores
Mushroom plant worker	Mushroom worker's lung	Mushroom compost	Mushroom spores, thermophilic actinomycetes
Riding stable employee or student	Riding-school lung	Riding stables[a]	Thermophilic actinomycetes
Sugar cane worker	Bagassosis	"Moldy" bagasse (sugar cane)	Thermophilic actinomycetes
		Woods	
Cork workers	Suberosis	Cork dust	Cork dust mold
Fuel chips worker	Fuel chip–induced HP	Wood and peat fuel chips[a]	*Penicillium* species
Greenhouse worker	Orchid grower's lung	Greenhouse bark	*Cryptostroma corticale*
Maple bark stripper	Maple bark lung	Maple bark	*Cryptostroma corticale*
Redwood worker	Sequoiosis	Redwood sawdust[a]	*Aureobasidium* and *Graphium* species
Woodworker	Woodworker's lung	Oak, cedar, pine, spruce, mahogany[a]	Wood dusts and pulp, *Alternaria*
		Animal products	
Bird keeping, handling	Bird fancier's lung	Parakeet, chicken, turkey[a]	Proteins in bird droppings
Feather handling	Feather picker's lung	Duck or goose feathers[a]	Feather dust
Fish meal worker	Fishmeal worker's lung	Fishmeal	Fishmeal dust
Fur worker	Furrier's lung	Animal pelts[a]	Animal fur dust
Mollusk shucker	Mollusk shell HP	Sea-snail shells	Snail antigen
Oyster shell worker	Pearl-oyster lung	Pearl-oyster shells	Shell powder
Pigeon breeding	Pigeon breeder's lung	Pigeon excreta and secretions	Pigeon proteins
Research	Laboratory worker's HP	Laboratory rat, other animals[a]	Antigens in animal urine
Silkworm workers	Sericulturist HP	Silkworm larvae[a]	Silkworm antigens

Worker	Disease	Source	Agent
Humidification and air-conditioning systems			
Humidified factory, plant, office, home	Humidifier lung	Contaminated humidifier water	*Aureobasidium* species, *Amoeba*
Office or plant worker	Ventilation pneumonitis	Humidifier / Air-conditioning	*Aureobasidium pullulans*, other contaminants
Office worker	Office worker's HP	Central air-conditioning	Microorganisms
Milling, making, and manufacturing			
Auto worker, parts manufacturing	Machine operator's lung	Metalworking fluid aerosols	Mixed microbial contaminants
Cheese maker	Cheese washer's lung	Moldy cheese[a]	*Penicillium casei*
Coffee bean worker	Coffee worker's lung	Coffee beans	Coffee bean dust
Detergent maker or user	Detergent lung	Proteolytic enzymes[a]	*Bacillus subtilis* enzymes
Malt worker	Brewer, grower, transporter	Moldy barley[a]	*Aspergillus clavis*, *Aspergillus fumigatus*
Miller	Miller's lung	Infested wheat flour[a]	*Sitophilus granarius* (weevil)
Solderer	HP	Colophony flux-cored solder[a]	Colophony
Stucco maker	Stipatosis	Esparto grass[a] (*Stipatenacissima*)	*Aspergillus fumigatus* / Thermophilic actinomycetes
Metals and chemicals			
Hard metal grinder	Hard metal worker's lung	Coolant for tungsten carbide	Cobalt
Polyurethane production (e.g., auto parts, refrigeration)	Isocyanate-induced HP	Polyurethane foam hardeners, activators[a]	Isocyanates as activators or hardeners
Smelter worker	HP	Zinc fumes	Zinc
Spray painter, roofer, bathtub refinisher, foundry worker	MDI-induced HP	Spray paints, varnishes, foundry castings[a]	Diphenylmethane diisocyanate (MDI)

[a]The source is also potentially asthmagenic.

passively transferred HP from a C57 Black/6 model (67). Depletion of T-cell subsets in the latter murine strain suggested that T cells play a role in the fibrotic process of HP that is detrimental in the early phase but beneficial in the later phase of the experimental disease (68). Concurrent Sendai viral infection has been shown to enhance HP in C57 Black/6 mice receiving repeated intranasal installations of *S. rectivirgula* (69). Cyclosporine, a potent immunosuppressant of T-cell function, has been found to suppress disease in rabbit (70) and murine (71,72) models of HP.

Acceptance of T-lymphocyte mediation of HP pathogenesis has focused interest on individual T-cell subsets and cytokine function. As established primarily in the mouse, the TH1 subset produces predominantly gamma-interferon whereas IL-4 and IL-10 predominate in the TH2 subset, although strict correlation with CD4 and CD8 phenotypes has not held up in either mice or humans (73). In recent experiments using *S. rectivirgula*–sensitized C3H/HeJ mice and CD4+ cell lines with either TH1 or TH2 characteristics based on cytokine production, only TH1 CD4+ cell lines could adoptively transfer experimental HP (66). Other experiments utilized knockout mice on a Balb/c background that were incapable of expressing the gene coding for IFN-γ, and found that IFN-γ was essential for the expression of HP (74).

Animal studies have led to conclusions that TH1 CD4+ lymphocytes and cytotoxic cells are major effector cells of experimental HP. How these findings relate to human disease with CD8+-rich lymphocytosis in BAL, what is responsible for and regulates the influx of effector cells, inflammatory cytokines, and other mediators, and what down-regulates and modulates the responses of the lung that lead to resolution and control are questions motivating further research.

Natural History and Prognosis

Studies on the natural history and prognosis for recovery from HP have been hampered by variable diagnostic criteria, limited duration of follow-up, failure to characterize or control for ongoing antigen exposure, and probably differences in antigen potencies that may affect recovery. While the clinical course of HP is variable, if illness is recognized early and recurrent attacks are avoided, the prognosis for recovery is usually quite good (75). Recurrent illness and ongoing antigen exposure lead to chronic, progressive, and occasionally fatal lung disease (25,76,77).

Following acute attacks of HP, there is usually rapid improvement in lung vital capacity and diffusion capacity in the first 2 weeks, but mild abnormalities in pulmonary function often persist for several months. Generally, single acute episodes are self-limited. Continued symptoms and progressive lung impairment have been reported after recurrent acute attacks and even after a single severe attack (78–80).

The chronic form of HP, with insidious symptoms and more subtle clinical abnormalities, is often recognized later in the course of illness and may have a poorer prognosis (81). Symptomatic pigeon breeders followed for 18 years showed a fourfold average rate of decline in pulmonary function compared to the expected rate (82). In a follow-up study of 33 FLD cases, airflow obstruction with or without emphysema was found in 13, suggesting that asthma and emphysema are more common sequelae of HP than previously recognized (83).

No single functional or biochemical marker exists to predict the probability of developing pulmonary fibrosis in an individual patient with HP. The BAL lymphocytosis is of no prognostic value as it may persist for years following removal from exposure and despite clinical recovery. Precipitating antibodies also have doubtful prognostic significance for the development or persistence of HP. Age at diagnosis, duration of antigen exposure after onset of symptoms, and total years of exposure before diagnosis seem to have predictive value in the likelihood of recovery from pigeon breeder's lung disease (84). Pigeon breeders with HP were more likely to improve or recover completely if they had been in contact with birds less than 2 years. Neither the form of clinical presentation (acute vs. chronic) nor the degree of lung function abnormality at the time of diagnosis was related to recovery in another study of pigeon breeder's disease (85). Rather, younger age at diagnosis (27 vs. 42 years) and exposure to antigen for less than 6 months after symptom onset were associated with complete recovery. Treatment with systemic corticosteroids probably has no positive effect on long-term prognosis.

Treatment and Prevention

Contact Avoidance

Early diagnosis and avoidance of antigen exposure are the mainstays of treatment since accelerated decline in lung function with continued antigen exposure has been demonstrated for most forms of HP. Avoidance can be accomplished in some cases by removing the affected individual from the antigen-containing environment. However, the social consequences and economic disruption to the affected individual may preclude leaving the exposure environment.

There is increasing evidence that some farmers who develop HP can continue their profession if appropriate measures are taken (10,76). Strategies recommended to reduce both FLD recurrence and incident cases include efficient drying of hay and cereals before storage, use of mechanical feeding systems, and better ventilation of farm buildings (86). Studies are ongoing on the efficacy of lactic acid–producing bacteria as grain additives to minimize mold contamination and prevent HP; these additives were found ineffective in preventing molding when used in hay (87). Education of individuals in at-risk occupations about antigen avoidance (e.g, avoidance of very dusty tasks inside dairy barns) and early symptom recognition is helpful (88). A 6-year follow-up study of farmers with HP revealed that 50–60% remained on the farm (25); by 15 years, as many as 70% had returned to farming (76). In such cases, regular follow-up of pulmonary function, radiography, and symptoms is essential to detect clinical deterioration and direct efforts to minimize antigen exposure.

Continued antigen exposure may not lead to clinical deterioration in some cases (89). Bourke et al. found that 18 of 21 pigeon breeders with acute pigeon breeder's lung had continued regular exposure to pigeons 10 years after diagnosis, though many used improved ventilation and respiratory protection; only six of these reported continued respiratory symptoms (90). This phenomenon has been demonstrated in several animal models of disease, where repeated antigen inhalation in sensitized animals results in resolution rather than progression of the pulmonary inflammatory response (91). This modulation of the inflammatory response is not well understood. As yet, no markers are available to predict resolution or progression of disease.

Avoidance of exposure by eliminating the offending antigen from the environment may be difficult. In five homes followed serially after bird removal, antigen levels measured by inhibition enzyme-linked immunoassay declined only gradually despite extensive environmental control measures, with high levels still detectable at 18 months in one home (92). Significant amounts of bird antigens can be found in homes without birds if wild bird excrement is heavily deposited outside the house and tracked in on shoes.

An outbreak of HP traced to fungal contamination of an open water-spray ventilation system was controlled by extensive cleaning of the system and corresponding work areas and replacement of the system with a dry (closed-coil) ventilation system (93). In another large HP outbreak due to microbial contamination of a chilled-water air-conditioning system, a variety of cleaning and water treatment measures were used to reduce antigen concentration. A solid-phase radioimmunoassay method using antiserum from affected workers was used thereafter to assess levels of airborne antigen and monitor the efficacy of control measures (94).

The efficacy of various types of respirators in preventing antigen sensitization and disease progression once sensitization has occurred is largely unknown. Helmet-type powered air-purifying respirators (PAPR) have been used to prevent episodic exposure in individuals with previous acute episodes of farmer's lung (95). Respiratory protection has been examined in bird breeders with HP, many of whom are reluctant to abandon their high-risk hobby. Serial measurements of pigeon-specific IgG antibodies were obtained in 22 pigeon fanciers with HP who had ongoing exposure, 13 of whom wore a PAPR and nine who refused respiratory protection (96). Serum antibody levels declined by 65% over 14 months in those wearing respirators compared to no decline in antibody levels in those without respirators; no data were reported on changes in symptoms or pulmonary function in the two groups. Prolonged wearing of respiratory protection is limited by the fact that most respirators are hot and cumbersome. Dust respirators offer substantial, but in some cases incomplete, protection against organic dusts (31) and are not recommended once sensitization has occurred.

Indoor microbial contamination is often related to problems with control of moisture. Source, dilution, and administrative controls are used to reduce these indoor contaminants (97). Source control includes preventing leaking and flooding, removing stagnant water sources, eliminating aerosol humidifiers and vaporizers, and maintaining indoor relative humidity below 70%. Dilution of contaminants can be effected by increasing the amount of outdoor air in a building, and high-efficiency filters can be added to the ventilation system to clean recirculated air. Complete elimination of indoor allergens is probably impossible, and it is often necessary to relocate immunologically sensitized individuals once hypersensitivity lung disease has occurred.

Personal spore sampling with Burkard personal volumetric air samplers and indirect immunofluorescence testing for spore-specific IgG have been used to assess individual mold sensitization and air quality control (98). However, quantitative bioaerosol sampling for microbial antigens is often difficult to interpret. Negative results should not be used to disprove disease or exposure. Settle plates are unreliable in assessing indoor microbial contaminants.

Drug Treatment

The effect of corticosteroids on the long-term course of various forms of HP has not been adequately investigated. There are many anecdotal reports of the beneficial effects of steroids in acute attacks, but controlled clinical trials are lacking. In cases where pulmonary function abnormalities are minor and spontaneous recovery is likely with removal from exposure, steroids are probably unnecessary. In one study, 36 patients, most having suffered only one acute attack of farmer's lung disease, were randomly assigned to receive prednisolone or placebo for 2 months (99). The steroid-treated group showed more rapid improvement in physiological abnormalities (particularly diffusion capacity) at 1-month follow-up, but no differences were found between the treated and untreated groups 5 years later. Interestingly, the group treated with steroids suffered more frequent recurrences of symptomatic farmer's lung during the 5 year follow-up period, though this finding did not reach statistical significance. In a study of pigeon breeders with HP, there were no significant clinical outcome differences between cases who were treated with steroids and those who were not; the mean time for improvement or normalization of pulmonary function after treatment and removal from exposure was 3.4 months (85).

In cases where disease is progressive despite other measures, an empirical trial of steroids (1 mg/kg/day of prednisone) is indicated, with monitoring of symptoms and pulmonary function 4 weeks after initiation of treatment. If there is objective improvement, a gradual taper to minimum sustaining doses should follow; otherwise, steroids should be tapered and discontinued (100). Monkare showed that 12 weeks of steroid treatment did not produce better results than 4 weeks in patients with farmer's lung disease (101).

Inhaled steroids and beta-agonists may be helpful in patients with HP manifested by symptoms of chest tightness and cough and with airflow limitation on pulmonary function testing (102). No data exist from controlled clinical trials on the efficacy of inhaled steroids in the treatment of HP.

ORGANIC DUST TOXIC SYNDROME

Definition and Clinical Presentation

The term "organic dust toxic syndrome" (ODTS) was coined at the 1985 Skokloster, Sweden workshop on the Health Effects of Organic Dust in the farm environment (103). Prior to that date the disease was variously known as mycotoxicosis (104), atypical farmer's lung, silo unloader's syndrome (105), and inhalation fever (mill fever, humidifier fever, grain fever). Although first described in relation to organic dust exposure on the farm, ODTS can occur wherever abundant organic particles are inhaled. Cases have been reported from exposure to a print shop (106), wood chip compost (107), and recycle processing (108). Manifestations of ODTS include fever, myalgia, chest tightness, cough, headache, and dyspnea that come on 3–8 hr after exposure (105).

Etiology and Mechanisms

ODTS is produced by inhalation of organic dusts or aerosols containing large quantities of microorganisms. What substance or substances are responsible for clinical manifestations is controversial. Immunological mechanisms play no role in the pathogenesis of this condition. Endotoxins and mycotoxins seem to be involved (109); the inhalation of endotoxin itself is able to induce a response similar to ODTS (110). Cases of ODTS have been reported, however, where endotoxin levels in the inhaled air were too low to account for the syndrome, suggesting a combination of factors in pathogenesis (111).

Inhaled "toxins" probably initiate a cascade of mediator release. Cytokines can recruit inflammatory cells to the lung and airways and contribute to systemic manifestations. Inhaled endotoxin (lipopolysaccharide, LPS) and exposure to swine confinement buildings induce release from lung cells of interleukin-1, interleukin-6, and tumor necrosis factor alpha (112,113). Acute swine building exposure, however, induces a transient increase in bronchial responsiveness to inhaled methacholine that is not seen in typical ODTS (105,114,115).

The hypothesis that ODTS is toxic is supported by: (1) a delay between exposure and symptoms that is too short for an infectious process; (2) no need for prior exposure/

sensitization; (3) absence of serum antibodies (precipitins) to the suspected etiological agent or source; (4) the massive quantity of airborne materials incriminated in most cases; (5) susceptibility to ODTS by all similarly exposed individuals (116); (6) spontaneous recovery within 24 hr or so after withdrawal from exposure.

Clinical Evaluation

Except for fever during the acute illness, objective evaluation in most patients with ODTS will include normal physical findings, normal chest radiograms, and normal lung function (105). Although some degree of bronchospasm has been described, no persistent increase in airway responsiveness to methacholine is seen (117,118). Peripheral blood neutrophilia is often present (105). Arterial blood gases are unremarkable, although a mild respiratory alkalosis due to hyperventilation may sometimes be found. Bronchoscopy in the acute stage reveals diffusely inflamed bronchial mucosa, and BAL will contain abundant neutrophils (117,119). BAL done after resolution of the symptoms will retrieve increased numbers of lymphocytes (117).

Treatment and Outcome

The treatment of ODTS is supportive. Analgesics can be given for chest pain and myalgia; antipyretics can be used if needed; cough suppressants may be required if coughing is severe. Antibiotics are not indicated, nor are inhaled or systemic corticosteroids helpful in shortening the duration of symptoms. The best treatment is prevention by educating individuals at risk to avoid unprotected breathing in poorly ventilated, potentially contaminated environments. The usual outcome is spontaneous resolution without sequelae (118). The syndrome will recur with repeated exposure.

Differential Diagnosis (see Table 1)

ODTS may be difficult to differentiate from acute HP (18) or an infectious process. History of exposure, appropriate constellation of symptoms, and paucity of objective findings will help establish the diagnosis of ODTS. The relationship, if any, between repeated bouts of ODTS and the development of HP is unclear (121).

Epidemiology

The incidence of ODTS is difficult to establish, as its prevalence in the farming population varies considerably from one country to another and from one type of farming to another (119,121). This syndrome is, however, much more frequent than farmer's lung in a population at risk. A study of Swedish farmers found the incidence of febrile reactions, the majority of which were considered to be ODTS, to be 100 per 10,000 farmers per year, in contrast to a farmer's lung incidence of 2–3 per 10,000 farmers per year (122).

REFERENCES

1. Pepys J. Hypersensitivity Diseases of the Lungs Due to Fungi and Organic Dusts. Basel: S Karger, 1969:1–19.
2. Pepys J, Jenkins PA. Farmer's lung: thermophilic actinomycetes as a source of "farmer's lung hay" antigen. Lancet 1963; 2:607–611.

3. Richerson HB. Hypersensitivity pneumonitis. In: Rylander R, Jacobs RR, eds. Organic Dusts: Exposure, Effects and Prevention. Boca Raton, FL: Lewis Publishers, 1994:139–160.

4. Rask-Anderson A. Pulmonary reactions to inhalation of mould dust in farmers with special reference to fever and allergic alveolitis. Acta Univ Upsaliensis, Uppsala 1988; 8.

5. Ramazzini B. Diseases of Workers. Latin text of 1713 revised, with translation and notes by WC Wright, ed. Chicago: University of Chicago Press, 1940, available in a special edition for The Classics of Medicine Library, 1983:243–248.

6. Campbell JM. Acute symptoms following work with hay. Br Med J 1969; 2:1143–1144 (1969).

7. Pepys J. Hypersensitivity Diseases of the Lungs due to Fungi and Organic Dusts. Basel: S Karger, 1969:72.

8. Cormier Y. Hypersensitivity pneumonitis. In: Rom WN, ed. Environmental and Occupational Medicine, 3rd ed. Boston: Little Brown, (in press).

9. Sansores R, Salas J, Chapela R, Barquin N, Selman M. Clubbing in hypersensitivity pneumonitis: its prevalence and possible prognostic role. Arch Intern Med 1990; 150:1849–1851.

10. Cormier Y, Belanger J. Long-term physiologic outcome after acute farmer's lung. Chest 87: 796–800.

11. Pepys J, Jenkins PA. Precipitin (FLH) test in farmer's lung. Thorax 1965; 20:21–35.

12. Warren CPW, Tse KS, Cherniack RM. Mechanical properties of the lung in extrinsic allergic alveolitis. Thorax 1978; 33:315–321.

13. Freedman PM, Ault B. Bronchial hyperreactivity to methacholine in farmer's lung disease. J Allergy Clin Immunol 1981; 67:59–63.

14. Kokkarinen JI, Tukiainen HO, Terho EO. Asthma in patients with farmer's lung during a five-year follow-up. Scand J Work Environ Health 1997; 23:149–151.

15. Monkare S, Ikonen M, Haahtela T. Radiologic findings in farmer's lung: prognosis and correlation to lung function. Chest 1985; 84:460–466.

16. Lynch DA, Newell JD, Logan PM, King TE, Muller NL. Can CT distinguish hypersensitivy pneumonitis from idiopathic pulmonary fibrosis? Am J Roentgenol 1995; 165:807–811.

17. Lynch DA, Rose CS, Way D, King TE Jr. Hypersensitivity pneumonitis: sensitivity of high-resolution CT in a population-based study. Am J Roentgenol 1992; 159:469–472.

18. Hansell DM, Moskovic E. High resolution computed tomography in extrinsic allergic alveolitis. Clin Radiol 1991; 43:8–12.

19. Akira M, Kita N, Higashihara T, Sakatani M, Kozuka T. Summer-type hypersensitivity pneumonitis: comparison of high-resolution CT and plain radiograpic findings. Am J Roentgenol 1992; 158:1223–1228.

20. Buschman DL, Gamsu G, Waldron JA, Klein C, King TE. Chronic hypersensitivity pneumonitis: use of CT in diagnosis. Am J Roentgenol 1992; 159:957–960.

21. Hansell DM, Wells AU, Padley SPG, Muller NL. Hypersensitivity pneumonitis: correlation of individual CT patterns with functional abnormalities. Radiology 1996; 199:123–128.

22. Remy-Jardin M, Remy J, Wallaert B, Muller NL. Subacute and chronic bird breeder hypersensitivity pneumonitis: sequential evaluation with CT and correlation with lung function tests and bronchoalveolar lavage. Radiology 1993; 189:111–118.

23. Dalphin JC, Toson B, Monnet E, Pernet D, Dubiez A, Laplante JJ, Aiache JM, Depierre A. Farmer's lung precipitins in Doubs (a department of France): prevalence and diagnostic value. Allergy 1994; 49:744–750.

24. Krasnick J, Meuwissen HJ, Nakao MA, Yeldandi A, Patterson R. Hypersensitivity pneumonitis: problems in diagnosis. J Allergy Clin Immunol 1996; 97:1027–1030.

25. Barbee RA, Callies Q, Dickie HA, Rankin J. The long-term prognosis in farmer's lung. Am Rev Respir Dis 1968; 97:223–231.

26. Burrell R, Rylander R. A critical review of the role of precipitins in hypersensitivity pneumonitis. Eur J Respir Dis 1981; 62:332–343.

27. Roberts R, Wenzel FJ, Emanuel DA. Precipitating antibodies in a midwest dairy farming population toward the antigens associated with farmer's lung disease. J Allergy Clin Immunol 1976; 62:518–524.

28. McSharry C, Banham SW, Lynch PP, Boyd G. Antibody measurement in extrinsic allergic alveolitis. Eur J Respir Dis 1984; 65:259–265.

29. Cormier Y, Belanger, J. The fluctuant nature of precipitating antibodies in dairy farmers. Thorax 1989; 44:469–473.

30. Huls G, Lindemann H, Velcovsky HG. Angiotensin converting enzyme (ACE) in the follow-up control of children and adolescents with allergic alveolitis. Monatsschr Kinderheilkd 1989; 137:158–161.

31. Hendrick D, Marshall R, Faux J, Krall J. Protective value of dust respirators in extrinsic allergic alveolitis: clinical assessment using inhalation provocation tests. Thorax 1981; 36: 917–921.

32. Richerson HB, Bernstein IL, Fink JN, Hunninghake GW, Novey HS, Reed CE, Salvaggio JE, Schuyler MR, Schwartz HJ, Stechschulte DJ. Guidelines for the clinical evaluation of hypersensitivity pneumonitis. J Allergy Clin Immunol 1989; 839–844.

33. Drent M, Mulder PG, Wagenaar SS, Hoogsteden HC, van Velzen-Blad H, van den Bosch JM. Differences in BAL fluid variables in interstitial lung diseases evaluated by discriminant analysis. Eur Respir J 1993; 6:803–810.

34. Laviolette M, Cormier Y, Loiseau A, Soler P, Leblanc P, Hance AJ. Bronchoalveolar mast cells in normal farmers and subjects with farmer's lung: diagnostic, prognostic, and physiologic significance. Am Rev Respir Dis 1991; 144:855–860.

35. Patterson R, Wang JLF, Fink JN, Calvanico NJ, Robert M. IgA and IgG antibody activities of serum and bronchoalveolar fluid from symptomatic and asymptomatic pigeon breeders. Am Rev Respir Dis 1979; 120:1113–1118.

36. Calvanico NJ, Ambegaonkar SP, Schlueter DP, Fink JN. Immunoglobulin levels in bronchoalveolar lavage fluid from pigeon breeders. J Lab Clin Med 1980; 96:129–140.

37. Trentin L, Marcer G, Chilosi M, Zambello R, Agostini C, Masciarelli M, Bizzotto R, Gemignani C, Cipriani A, DiVittorio G, Semenzato G. Longitudinal study of alveolitis in hypersensitivity pneumonitis patients: an immunological evaluation. J Allergy Clin Immunol 1988; 82:577–585.

38. Cormier Y, Belanger J, Laviolette M. Prognostic significance of bronchoalveolar lymphocytosis in farmer's lung. Am Rev Respir Dis 1987; 135:692–695.

39. Cormier Y, Belanger J, Beaudoin J, Laviolette M, Beaudoin R, Hébert J. Abnormal bronchoalveolar lavage in asymptomatic dairy farmers: study of lymphocytes. Am Rev Respir Dis 1984; 130:1046–1049.

40. Cormier Y, Belanger J, Laviolette M. Persistent bronchoalveolar lymphocytosis in asymptomatic farmers. Am Rev Respir Dis 1986; 133:843–847.

41. Reyes CN, Wenzel FJ, Lawton BR, Emanuel DA. The pulmonary pathology of farmer's lung disease. Chest 1982; 81:142–146.

42. Coleman A, Colby TV. Histologic diagnosis of extrinsic allergic alveolitis. Am J Surg Pathol 1988; 2:461–467.

43. Planes C, Valeyre D, Loiseau A, Bernaudin JF, Soler P. Ultrastructural alterations of the air-blood barrier in sarcoidosis and hypersensitivity pneumonitis and their relation to lung histopathology. Am J Respir Crit Care Med 1994; 150:1067–1074.

44. Terho EO. Diagnostic criteria for farmer's lung disease. Am J Ind Med 1986; 10:329.

45. Hodgson MJ, Parkinson DK, Karpf M. Chest x-rays in hypersensitivity pneumonitis: a metaanalysis of secular trend. Am J Ind Med 1989; 16:45–53.

46. Johnson CL, Bernstein IL, Gallagher JS, et al. Familial hypersensitivity pneumonitis induced *Bacillus subtilis*. Am Rev Respir Dis 1980; 122:339–348.

47. Rose C, King TE Jr. Controversies in hypersensitivity pneumonitis. Am Rev Respir Dis 1992; 145:1–2 (editorial).

48. Bernstein DI, Lummus ZL, Santilli G, Siskosky J, Bernstein IL. Machine operator's lung: a hypersensitivity pneumonitis disorder associated with exposure to metalworking fluid aerosols. Chest 1995; 108:636–641.

49. Lopez M, Salvaggio JE. Epidemiology of hypersensitivity pneumonitis/allergic alveolitis. Monogr Allergy 1987; 21:59–69.

50. Fink JN. Epidemiologic aspects of hypersensitivity pneumonitis. Monogr Allergy 1987; 21: 59–69.

51. Malmberg P, Rask-Anderson A, Hoglund S, Kolmodin-Hedman B, Read-Guernsey J. Incidence of organic dust toxic syndrome and allergic alveolitis in Swedish farmers. Int Arch Allergy Appl Immunol 1988; 87:47–54.

52. Marx JJ, Guernsey J, Emanuel DA, Merchant JA, Morgan DP, Kryda M. Cohort studies of immunologic lung disease among Wisconsin dairy farmers. Am J Ind Med 1990; 18:263–268.

53. Richerson HB. Hypersensitivity pneumonitis—pathology and pathogenesis. Clin Rev Allergy 1983; 1:469–486.

54. Richerson HB. Immune complexes and the lung: a skeptical review. Surv Synth Path Res 1984; 3:281–291.

55. Ando M, Konishi K, Yoneda R, Tamura M. Difference in the phenotypes of bronchoalveolar lavage lymphocytes in patients with summer-type hypersensitivity pneumonitis, farmer's lung, ventilation pneumonitis, and bird-fancier's lung: report of a nationwide epidemiologic study in Japan. J Allergy Clin Immunol 1991; 87:1002–1009.

56. Trentin L, Zambello R, Facco M, Tassinari C, Sancetta R, Siviero M, Cerutti A, Cipriani A, Marcer G, Majori M, Pesci A, Agostini C, Semenzato G. Selection of T lymphocytes bearing limited TCR-V beta regions in the lung of hypersensitivity pneumonitis and sarcoidosis. Am J Respir Crit Care Med 1997; 155:587–596.

57. Denis M. Proinflammatory cytokines in hypersensitivity pneumonitis. Am J Respir Crit Care Med 1995; 151:164–169.

58. Denis M, Bedard M, Laviolette M, Cormier Y. A study of monokine release and natural killer activity in the bronchoalveolar lavage of subjects with farmer's lung. Am Rev Respir Dis 1993; 147:934–939.

59. Tremblay GM, Sallenave J-M, Israel-Assayag E, Cormier Y, Gauldie J. Elafin/elastase-specific inhibitor in bronchoalveolar lavage of normal subjects and farmer's lung. Am J Respir Crit Care Med 1996; 154:1092–1098.

60. Drent M, Grutters JC, Mulder PG, van Velzen-Blad H, Wouters EF, van den Bosch JM. Is the different T helper cell activity in sarcoidosis and extrinsic allergic alveolitis also reflected by the cellular bronchoalveolar lavage fluid profile? Sarcoid Vascul Diffuse Lung Dis 1997; 14:31–438.

61. Semenzato G, Trentin L, Zambello R, Agostin C, Cipriani A, Marcer G. Different types of cytotoxic lymphocytes recovered from the lungs of patients with hypersensitivity pneumonitis. Am Rev Respir Dis 1998; 137:70–74.

62. Mendosa F, Melendro EI, Baltazares M, Banales JL, Ximenez C, Chapela R, Selman M. Cellular immune response to fractionated avian antigens by peripheral blood mononuclear cells from patients with pigeon breeder's disease. J Lab Clin Med 1996; 127:23–28.

63. Allen JT, Spiteri M. Pigeon breeder's disease. J Lab Clin Med 1996; 127:10–12.

64. Schuyler M, Cook C, Listrom M, Fenoglio-Preiser C. Blast cells transfer experimental hypersensitivity pneumonitis. Am Rev Respir Dis 1988; 137:1449–1455.

65. Richerson HB, Coon JD, Lubaroff D. Adoptive transfer of experimental pneumonitis in the LEW rat. Am J Respir Crit Care Med 1995; 151:1205–1210.

66. Schuyler M, Gott K, Cherne A, Edwards B. TH1 CD4+ cells adoptively transfer experimental hypersensitivity pneumonitis. Cell Immunol 1997; 177:169–175.

67. Tskizawa H, Ohta K, Horiuchi T, Suzuki N, Ueda T, Yamaguchi M, Ishii A, Suko M, Okudaira H, Shiga J, Miyamoto T, Ito K. Hypersensitivity pneumonitis in athymic nude mice: additional evidence of T cell dependency. Am Rev Respir Dis 1992; 146:479–484.

68. Denis M, Cormier Y, Laviolette M, Ghadirian E. T cells in hypersensitivity pneumonitis: effects of in vivo T cell depletion of T cells in a mouse model. Am J Respir Cell Mol Biol 1992; 6:183–489.

69. Cormier Y, Tremblay GM, Fournier M, Israel-Assayag E. Long-term viral enhancement of lung response to *Saccharopolyspora rectivirgula*. Am J Respir Crit Care Med 1994; 149: 490–494.

70. Kopp WC, Dierks SE, Butler JE, Upadrashta BS, Richerson HB. Cyclosporine immuno-modulation in a rabbit model of chronic hypersensitivity pneumonitis. Am Rev Respir Dis 1985; 132:1027–1033.

71. Takizawa H, Suko M, Kobayashi N, Shoji S, Ohta K, Nogami M, Okudaira H, Miyamoto T, Shiga J. Experimental hypersensitivity pneumonitis in the mouse: histologic and immu-nologic features and their modulation with cyclosporin A. J Allergy Clin Immunol 1988; 81: 391–400.

72. Denis M, Cormier Y, Laviolette M. Murine hypersensitivity pneumonitis: a study of cellular infiltrates and cytokine production and its modulation by cyclosporin A. Am J Respir Cell Mol Biol 1992; 6:68–74.

73. Coffman RL, Weid T. Multiple pathways for the initiation of T helper 2 (TH2) responses. J Exp Med 1997; 185:373–376.

74. Gudmundsson G, Hunninghake GW. Interferon-gamma is necessary for the expression of hypersensitivity pneumonitis. J Clin Invest 1997; 99:2386–2390.

75. Monkare S, Haahtela T. Farmer's lung—a 5 year follow up of eighty six patients. Clin Allergy 1987; 17:143–151.

76. Braun SR, doPico GA, Tsiatis A, Horvath E, Dickie HA, Rankin J. Farmer's lung disease: long-term clinical and physiologic outcome. Am Rev Respir Dis 1979; 119:185–191.

77. Kokkarinen JI, Tukiainen HO, Terho EO. Mortality due to farmer's lung in Finland. Chest 1994; 106:509–512.

78. Barrowcliff DA, Arblaster PG. Farmer's lung: a study of an acute fatal case. Thorax 1968; 23:490–500.

79. Chasse M, Blanchette G, Malo J-L. Farmer's lung presenting as respiratory failure and ho-mogeneous consolidation. Chest 1986; 90:783–784.

80. Greenberger PA, Pien LC, Patterson R, Patterson R, Roberts M. End-stage lung and ultimately fatal disease in a bird fancier. Am J Med 1989; 86:119–122.

81. Grammer LC, Roberts M, Lerner C, et al. Clinical and serologic follow-up of four children and five adults with bird-fancier's lung. J Allergy Clin Immunol 1990; 85:655–660.

82. Schmidt CD, Jensen RL, Christensen LT, Crapo RO, Davis JJ. Longitudinal pulmonary func-tion changes in pigeon breeders. Chest 1988; 93:359–363.

83. Lalancette M, Carrier G, Ferland S, Rodrigue J, Laviolette M, Bégin R, Cantin A, Cormier Y. Long term outcome and predictive value of bronchoalveolar lavage fibrosing factors in farmer's lung. Am Rev Respir Dis 1993; 148:216–221.

84. Allen DH, Williams GV, Woolcock AJ. Bird breeder's hypersensitivity pneumonitis: progress studies of lung function after cessation of exposure to the provoking antigen. Am Rev Respir Dis 1976; 114:555–566.

85. DeGracia J, Morell F, Bofill JM, Curull V, Orriols R. Time of exposure as a prognostic factor in avian hypersensitivity pneumonitis. Respir Med 1989; 83:139–143.

86. Zejda JE, McDuffie HH, Dosman JA. Epidemiology of health and safety risks in agriculture and related industries. Practical applications for rural physicians. West J Med 1993; 158: 56–63.

87. Duchaine C, Lavoie M, Cormier Y. Effects of bacterial hay preservative (Pediococcus pen-tosaceus) on hay in experimental storage conditions. Appl Environ Microbiol 1995; 61:4240–4243.

88. Clark S. Report on prevention and control. Am J Ind Med 1986; 10:267–273.

89. Cuthbert OD, Gordon MF. Ten year follow up of farmers with farmer's lung. Br J Ind Med 1983; 40:173–176.

90. Bourke SJ, Banham SW, Carter R, Lynch P, Boyd G. Longitudinal course of extrinsic allergic alveolitis in pigeon breeders. Thorax 1989; 44:415–418.

91. Richerson HB, Richards DW, Swanson PA, Butler JE, Suelzer MT. Antigen-specific desen-sitization in a rabbit model of acute hypersensitivity pneumonitis. J Allergy Clin Immunol 1981; 68:226–234.

92. Craig TJ. Bird antigen persistence in the home environment after removal of the bird. Ann Allergy 1992; 69:510–512.

93. Woodard ED, Friedlander B, Lesher RJ, Font W, Kinsey R, Hearne FT. Outbreak of hypersensitivity pneumonitis in an industrial setting. JAMA 1988; 259:1965–1969.

94. Reed CE, Swanson BA, Lopez M, Ford AM, Major J, Witmer WB, Valdes TB. Measurement of IgG antibody and airborne antigen to control an industrial outbreak of hypersensitivity pneumonitis. J Occup Med 1993; 25:207–210.

95. Nuutinen J, Terho EO, Husman K, Kotimaa M, Hardonen R, Nousiainen H. Protective value of powered dust respirator helmet for farmers with farmer's lung. Eur J Respir Dis 1987; 152:212–220.

96. Anderson K, Walker A, Boyd G. The long-term effect of a positive pressure respirator on the specific antibody response in pigeon breeders. Clin Exp Allergy 1988; 19:45–49.

97. Macher JM. Inquiries received by the California indoor air quality program on biological contaminants in buildings. Adv Aerobiol 1987; 275–278.

98. Zwick H, Popp W, Braun O, Wanke T, Wagner C. Personal spore sampling and indirect immunofluroescent test for exploration of hypersensitivity pneumonitis due to mould spores. Allergy 1991; 46:277–283.

99. Kokkarinen JI, Tukiainen HO, Terho EO. Effect of corticosteroid treatment on the recovery of pulmonary function in farmer's lung. Am Rev Respir Dis 1992; 145:3–5.

100. Shellito JE. Hypersensitivity pneumonitis. Semin Respir Med 1991; 12:196–203.

101. Monkare S. Influence of corticosteroid treatment on the course of farmer's lung. Eur J Respir Dis 1983; 64:283–293.

102. Carlsen KH, Leegaard J, Lund OD, et al. Allergic alveolitis in a 12-year-old boy: treatment with budesonide nebulizing solution. Pediatr Pulmonol 1992 12:257–259.

103. Rylander R. Lung diseases caused by organic dusts in the farm environment. Am J Ind Med 1986; 10:221–227.

104. Emanuel DA, Wenzel FJ, Lawton BR. Pulmonary mycotoxicosis. Chest 1975; 67:293–297.

105. May JJ, Stallones L, Darrow D, Pratt DS. Organic dust toxicity (pulmonary mycotoxicosis) associated with silo unloading. Thorax 1986; 41:919–923.

106. Mamolen M, Lewis DM, Blanchet MA, Satink FJ, Vogt RL. Investigation of an outbreak of "humidifier fever" in a print shop. Am J Ind Med 1993; 23:483–490.

107. Weber S, Kullman G, Petsonk E, Jones WG, Olenchock S, Sorenson W, Parker J, Marcelo-Baciu R, Frazer D, Castranova V. Organic dust exposure from compost handling: case presentation and respiratory exposure assessment. Am J Ind Med 1993; 24:365–374.

108. Sigsgaard T, Abel A, Donbaek L, Malmos P. Lung function changes among recycling workers exposed to organic dust. Am J Ind Med 1994; 25:69–72.

109. Fogelmark B, Sjöstrand M, Rylander R. Pulmonary inflammation induced by repeated inhalations of beta(1,3)-D-glucan and endotoxin. Int J Exp Pathol 1994;75:85–90.

110. Rylander R, Bake B, Fischer JJ, Helander IM. Pulmonary function and symptoms after inhalation of endotoxin. Am Rev Respir Dis 1989; 140:981–986.

111. Malmberg P, Rask-Andersen A, Lundholm M, Palmberg U. Can spores from molds and actinomycetes cause an organic dust toxic syndrome reaction? Am J Ind Med 1990; 17:109–110.

112. Lewis DM, Olenchock SA. Cellular immune reactions to grain dust and extracts of grain dusts. In: Dosman JA, Cockcroft DW, eds. Principles of Health and Safety in Agriculture. Boca Raton, FL: CRC Press, 1989:72–75.

113. Wang Z, Malmberg P, Larsson P, Larrson B-M, Larsson KA. Time course of interleukin-6 and tumor necrosis factor-alpha increase in serum following inhalation of swine dust. Am J Respir Crit Care Med 1996; 143:147–152.

114. Cormier Y, Duchaine C, Israël-Assayag E, Bédard G, Laviolette M, Dosman J. Effects of repeated swine building exposures on normal naive subjects. Eur Respir J 1997; 10:1516–1522.

115. Larsson K, Eklund AG, Hansson L, Isaksson B, Malmberg PO. Swine dust causes intense airways inflammation in healthy subjects. Am J Respir Crit Care Med 1994; 150:973–977.

116. Britton WT, Vastbinder EE, Greene JW, Marx JJ, Hutcheson RH, Schaffner W. An outbreak of organic dust toxic syndrome in a college fraternity. JAMA 1987; 258:1210–1212.

117. Lecours R, Laviolette M, Cormier Y. Bronchoalveolar lavage in pulmonary mycotoxicosis (organic dust toxic syndrome). Thorax 1986; 41:924–926.
118. May JJ, Marvel LH, Pratt DS, Coppolo DP. Organic dust toxic syndrome: a follow-up study. Am J Ind Med 1990; 17:111–113.
119. Emanuel DA, Marx JJ, Ault B, Roberts RC, Kryda MJ, Treuhaft MW. Organic dust toxic syndrome (pulmonary mycotoxicosis)—a review of the experience in central Wisconsin. In: Dosman JA, Cockcroft DW, eds. Priniples of Health and Safety in Agriculture. Boca Raton, FL: CRC Press, 1989:72–75.
120. Von Essen S, Robbins RA, Thompson AB, Rennard S. Organic dust toxic syndrome: an acute febrile reaction to organic dust exposure distinct from hypersensitivity pneumonitis. Clin Toxicol 1990; 28:389–420.
121. Malmberg P, Rask-Andersen A, Palmgren U, Höglund S, Kolmodin-Hedman B, Stalenheim G. Exposure to microorganisms, febrile and airway-obstructive symptoms, immune status and lung function of Swedish farmers. Scand J Work Environ Health 1985; 11:287–293.
122. Malmberg P, Rask-Anderson A, Hoglund S, Kolmodin-Hedman B. Incidence of organic dust toxic syndrome and allergic alveolitis in Swedish farmers. Int Arch Allergy Immunol 1988; 87:47–54.

34

Building-Related Illnesses

Dick Menzies
McGill University, Montréal, Quebec, Canada

INTRODUCTION

Over the past 30 years, a new man-made ecosystem has developed—the controlled indoor environment within the sealed exterior shells of modern office buildings. This indoor environment may be adversely affected by pollutants that arise from the occupants, their work activities, equipment, plants, furnishings, building materials, and even the ventilation systems themselves. In the vast majority of office buildings in North America, the major mechanism to remove these pollutants, and provide a healthy, comfortable indoor environment, is the heating, ventilation, and air-conditioning (HVAC) systems. These systems are generally highly automated and monitored by only one or two persons. These HVAC operators have no way to monitor pollutant levels in this complex indoor environment and little direct contact with the building occupants.

It is therefore not surprising that a group of health problems related to this ecosystem—termed "building-related illnesses"—have been described in the past two decades. Although in most instances the health effects are relatively mild, the spectrum of illness can range from mild to severe. At present, more than half of the adult workforce in Northern America and Western Europe work in office or "office-like," nonindustrial environments (1), so this new indoor environment may have considerable public health impact. It has been estimated that 20–30% of the occupants of approximately one million buildings in the United States may have symptoms related to work in this environment (2). As a result, this problem has attracted the attention of research scientists from a variety of domains including architecture, engineering, industrial hygiene, biochemistry, and the microbial sciences, as well as epidemiology. It has also attracted the attention of the media, the public, and, increasingly, legislators, all of whom are demanding a solution to this problem.

This chapter will review studies describing the health effects of the nonindustrial, nonresidential indoor environment. The evidence cited has been restricted to outbreak descriptions in which a causative agent could be identified, population-based studies, and experimental manipulations of exposures present in the nonindustrial work environment. Evidence from outbreaks of specific illnesses, as well as from population-based studies, have been used to synthesize a conceptual model of this problem. This evidence has also been used to develop a framework for health professionals in their evaluation of workers with health problems potentially related to this work environment.

DEFINITIONS

The term "building-related illness" (BRI) will be used for illnesses that arise in nonindustrial, nonresidential buildings; the majority of which are office buildings. *Specific BRI* refers to a group of illnesses with a fairly homogeneous clinical picture, objective abnormalities on clinical or laboratory evaluation, and an identifiable source problem or agent(s) known to cause infectious, immunological, or allergic diseases (3). The term *nonspecific BRI* has recently been introduced (4), for a group of heterogeneous and nonspecific work-related symptoms, including irritation of the skin and mucous membranes of the eyes, nose, and throat, headache, fatigue, and difficulty concentrating. These are considered illnesses on the basis of occurrence of symptoms, even though affected workers do not have objective clinical or laboratory abnormalities, and causative agent(s) cannot be found. The symptoms may be considered building-related even if the only supportive evidence is workers' self-report.

The term "sick-building syndrome" (5) will not be used for several reasons. First, this term suggests that buildings are sick and require investigation and treatment, yet it is the workers who develop potentially work-related health problems. The early conceptualization of the problem was that there were two distinct populations of buildings: "sick" buildings, in which many workers had symptoms—these were attributed to the indoor environment; and "healthy" buildings, in which few workers had symptoms, presumed to be non-work-related. This concept has proven incorrect. Epidemiological surveys in office buildings selected without regard to occupant health status have demonstrated that prevalence of work-related symptoms range in a continuous fashion from low (but not zero) to high (6–15). For example, in a study of 47 buildings in Britain, the average number of symptoms reported by the workers in each building ranged in a continuous fashion from 1.5 in the least symptomatic building population, to 5 in highly symptomatic populations. No single cut-point or criterion could distinguish problem from nonproblem buildings. Although, generally nonproblem buildings had a lower average number of symptoms reported, there was considerable overlap with problem buildings (7). Similarly, in a cross-sectional survey of 16 buildings including some considered by the building owners as "problem" buildings, the average number of symptoms (Fig. 1) and carbon dioxide concentrations (Fig. 2) overlapped completely between so-called problem and so-called nonproblem buildings (16). In fact, it is not at all clear how buildings in these population-based studies came to be identified as problem or nonproblem, i.e., sick or healthy buildings. If anything, the concept of "healthy buildings" may be harmful because it suggests that in such buildings, symptoms of affected workers can be disregarded as unrelated to the work environment.

Problems in the definition of "sick building syndrome" or nonspecific BRI are exemplified by procedures of selection in six cross-sectional surveys conducted in Europe and North America involving a total of 267 buildings and more than 14,000 workers. Two surveys selected buildings independent of symptom status (6,9). One survey was entitled "the healthy building study" yet included one known sick building (17). In the remaining three studies, buildings were selected at least in part on the basis of symptom status. One surveyed 11 "sick buildings" (18) while the other two studies included buildings without known complaints, as well as "buildings selected at the request of management" (19) or "known problem buildings" (7).

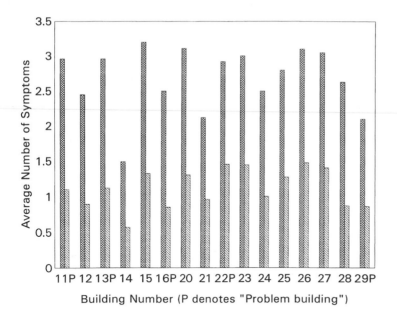

Figure 1 Average number of symptoms reported by workers in 16 buildings studied in a cross-sectional survey. Problem buildings are denoted by the letter "p" following the building number. Buildings are not numbered sequentially, but results from all buildings in the survey are shown. (Taken from Ref. 16 with permission.)

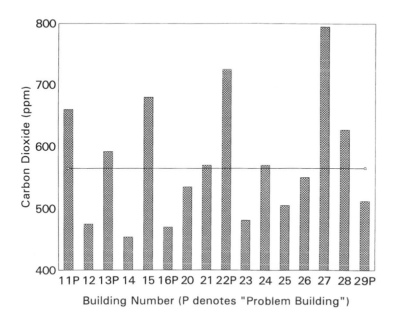

Figure 2 Mean carbon dioxide (CO_2) levels in each of 16 buildings in a cross-sectional survey. The mean CO_2 concentration for all buildings is denoted as a solid horizontal line. Problem buildings are denoted by the letter "p" following the building number. Buildings are not numbered sequentially but results from all buildings in the survey are shown. (Taken from Ref. 16 with permission.)

SPECIFIC BRI

Table 1 summarizes the major specific BRI. There is some evidence that building factors influence the transmission of certain respiratory infections. Low ventilation rates contributed to transmission of tuberculosis within an office building (20). Military recruits housed in mechanically ventilated barracks had significantly increased rates of acute febrile respiratory illnesses (21) while office workers had increased sickness absence due to respiratory illnesses if they shared an office (22). These findings imply that economy measures such as greater recirculation of air, open concept offices, or smaller work stations may actually result in greater transmission of respiratory pathogens with more human illness and net economic loss.

A single causative agent may result in building-related outbreaks with very different manifestations. For example, *Legionella pneumophila*, which has been found in water-cooling towers, humidification, and water supply systems, can result in legionnaires' disease, a pneumonia with case fatality of 10–15% (23,24), or Pontiac fever, a milder, flu-like illness (24,25). Similarly, hypersensitivity pneumonitis and humidifier fever were originally described as separate disorders, but may coexist and result from similar immunological responses to fungi, bacteria, or protozoa contaminating humidifiers or ventilation systems (26–29). Manifestations of both disorders include fever, chills, malaise, and presence of specific antibodies to the microbial agent. Hypersensitivity pneumonitis has additional features of cough, chest tightness, dyspnea, lung function abnormalities, and occasionally radiographic abnormalities.

Outbreaks of asthma related to exposures in office buildings have been reported rarely although the causative agent in such outbreaks was not identified (30,31). Exposure to common indoor allergens such as dust mites, plant products, and passively transported allergens may occur in any occupied building. Challenge tests with photocopier fumes have produced hypersensitivity angiitis (32) and with carbonless copy papers have produced urticaria and laryngeal edema (33,34), or pharyngitis (35).

Dermatitis, conjunctivitis, as well as upper and lower respiratory symptoms may also represent irritant responses from exposure to nonallergic agents. Exposure to man-made vitreous fibers has resulted in itching skin, burning eyes, sore throat, and cough (36,37). Release of glass fibers may occur from ceiling boards through direct physical damage or indirectly through movement of these boards by building vibrations or room pressure changes when doors are opened or closed (36,37).

Carboxyhemoglobin levels of 2.0–3.5% have been measured in nonsmokers exposed to indoor concentrations of carbon monoxide of 4–10 parts per million (ppm). Therefore, exposure to levels of 20–50 ppm from heavy cigarette smoking (38) or intake of exhaust fumes (39) could result in carboxyhemoglobin of 5–10%, which can diminish cognitive function and vigilance (40) and also result in headache and dizziness—so-called "occult carbon monoxide poisoning" (41). Significant exposure to nitrogen dioxide indoors can occur from intake of exhaust fumes or if outdoor levels are high (42,43) and result in mucosal irritation with respiratory symptoms and increased respiratory tract infections. Formaldehyde is well recognized as a mucosal irritant, but there are no well-documented outbreaks of illness related to exposure to this agent in office buildings (44).

The interaction of susceptibility and level of exposure in determining whether the manifestations are mild and self-limited (Pontiac fever, humidifier fever), or severe (legionnaires' pneumonia, or hypersensitivity pneumonitis) is unclear, because airborne concentrations of the causative agents have rarely been measured in these building-related outbreaks.

Table 1 Major Specific Illnesses Known or Suspected to be Related to Buildings

Disease	Study[a]	Ref.	Building	Indoor source	Exposure
Infectious					
Legionnaires' disease and Pontiac fever	Case reports: sporadic or epidemic	23–25	Large buildings (office, hospital, hotel)	Cooling tower, air conditioning, or humidifier, potable water	*Legionella pneumophila*
Flu illness and common cold	Cross-sectional	22	Office buildings	Human source	Respiratory virus
	Longitudinal	21	Military barracks		
Tuberculosis	Index case followed by cross-sectional	20	Office buildings	Human source	*Mycobacterium tuberculosis*
Immunological					
Hypersensitivity pneumonitis and humidifier fever	Case reports	28	Office buildings	Humidifier	Multiple bacteria, fungus, actinomycetes
	Index cases followed by cross-sectional	26, 27, 29	Office buildings Factory	Air conditioning, humidifier Ventilation unit	*Aspergillus, Penicillium* spp. or multiple organisms
Allergy					
Dermatitis, rhinitis, and asthma	Case reports		Office buildings	Surface dust and carpet, clothing	Dust mite, plant product, animal allergen, fungus
	Index cases followed by cross-sectional	30, 31	Office buildings and factory	Humidifier	Unknown
Rhinitis					
Contact urticaria, laryngeal edema	Case reports	32–35	Office buildings	Carbonless copy paper	Alkylphenol novolac resin
Irritant					
Dermatitis, upper and lower respiratory irritation	Case reports	36, 37, 115	Office buildings	Ceiling boards	Fiber glass
	Case report	39	Office buildings	Tobacco smoke, vehicle exhaust, any combustion process	Combustion pollutants: CO, NO_2

[a]Because of space restrictions, references were limited to certain case reports, studies of index cases followed by an epidemiological evaluation, or field studies when available.
Source: Ref. 4.

In outbreaks, when all exposed workers have been carefully examined, prevalence of illness was high and a wide spectrum of manifestations has been described (26,27,29). For example, in one group of 14 workers exposed to levels of *Penicillium* of 5000–10,000 CFU/m^3, one nonsmoking worker developed hypersensitivity pneumonitis, another with history of atopy and cigarette smoking developed asthma, while six others developed nonspecific respiratory symptoms (29). In an industrial setting, 548 workers were exposed to airborne *Aspergillus* species, of whom 152 had positive serum precipitens (26). Among these 152 workers, 29 were asymptomatic, eight had symptoms but did not meet the case definition, and 115 could be classified as cases of hypersensitivity pneumonitis. Less than 10% of these cases had any objective abnormalities; i.e., the vast majority were diagnosed on the basis of symptoms alone. In addition, these cases reported increased occurrence of nonspecific symptoms such as fatigue, headache, and mucosal irritation compared to exposed workers without precipitants (26). In these outbreaks, without the "sentinel cases," workers with less severe responses would have been indistinguishable from, and potentially labeled as, workers with nonspecific BRI.

Exposure to higher concentrations of contaminants results in a higher proportion affected as well as a shift in the spectrum of illness to more severe manifestations. While the evidence for this phenomenon is relatively limited in outbreaks related to the nonindustrial environment, this is supported by epidemiological studies of "farmer's lung" where higher exposures resulted in a higher proportion affected (45,46) as well as more severe symptoms (46).

NONSPECIFIC BRI—ASSOCIATED FACTORS

In cross-sectional surveys in buildings, selected without regard to the occupants' health status, up to 60% of workers reported at least one work-related symptom, and 10–25% reported such symptoms occurring twice weekly or more (9,10,12,14,15,47). The associations, seen in Table 2, with younger age, female gender, and atopic history may reflect greater occupational exposures, as reported by investigators who measured personal exposures directly (48), or result from heightened physiological responses at lower thresholds demonstrated in experimental exposure studies (49–52). Symptoms are also consistently associated with psychosocial factors; this should *not* be taken to mean that "the problem is all in the workers' heads." Psychological testing of symptomatic and asymptomatic office workers are similar (53); it is well known that psychosocial factors are associated with other conditions such as cardiovascular disease (54), and there is evidence that increased stress may be the result, rather than the cause, of health problems (55).

In two cross-sectional studies (56,57) and one experimental study (58), symptoms were significantly associated with relatively small differences in temperatures as shown in Table 3. The temperatures measured were all within the range 22–26°C, traditionally considered acceptable (59). This may be explained by age- and gender-related differences in physiological responses to temperature (50,51). Both low and high humidity have been associated with symptoms (7,58,60–63) (Table 4). This may appear contradictory, but symptoms associated with lower humidity are usually those of mucosal irritation, whereas symptoms associated with high humidity tend to be systemic and/or respiratory suggesting different mechanisms underlying the associations. This association of symptoms with temperature and humidity contradicts the long-standing belief that these are only "comfort parameters" (59,64) and suggests that these factors should be more carefully monitored and controlled.

Table 2 Relationship of Personal/Work/Work Site and Building Ventilation Characteristics and Nonspecific Building-Related Illnesses in Office Workers

	Studies finding an association			Studies finding no association		
	Studies (N)	Subjects (N)	Ref.	Studies (N)	Subjects (N)	Ref.
Personal characteristics						
Female gender	7	23,764	6–8, 10, 15, 56, 92	1	3,948	13
Younger age	4	17,166	7, 13, 15, 56	2	8,450	6, 8
Atopy/allergy/asthma	9	23,662	6, 8–10, 13, 15, 56, 92, 116	0	—	—
Cigarette smoking						
Personal	2	8,433	10, 15	4	13,944	6, 8, 13, 56
Passive	3	15,017	7, 15, 92	2	5,338	10, 13
Psychosocial factors	7	21,762	6, 8, 10, 13, 15, 92, 116	0	—	—
Work characteristics						
Clerical work	3	9,301	6, 7, 10	2	6,489	8, 56
Work with video display terminals	6	22,277	6, 8, 10, 13, 15, 56	1	880	73
Work with carbonless paper	4	16,373	6, 8, 15, 73	0	—	
Photocopiers: work with, or nearby	4	10,720	6, 8, 10, 73	1	3,948	13
Work site characteristics						
Open concept type of office	2	6,489	8, 56	1	3,948	13
Crowding	3	11,430	6, 15, 73	0	—	
Presence of carpets	3	8,335	6, 13, 73	1	4,943	8
Surface dust	2	7,455	6, 13	2	11,986	8, 15
Noise	2	5,338	10, 13	0	—	
Building characteristics						
Ventilation type						
Simple mechanical	3	11,940	11, 17, 72	2	12,977	9, 14
Air conditioning	5	26,838	11, 14, 15, 17, 72	0	—	
Humidification	2	9,721	11, 15	1	11,627	14
Ventilation rate <10 L/sec/person	3	4,959	9, 47, 92	0	—	

Source: Ref. 4.

Table 3 Association of Symptoms of Nonspecific Building-Related Illnesses with Temperature and Humidity

Observational studies, parameter measured (unit)	Symptoms not associated			Symptoms associated		
	Mean	Range	Ref.	Mean	Range	Ref.
Temperature (°C)	23.0	22.4–24.0	63	23.0	21–26	56
				23.3	21–26	57
Relative humidity (%)					10–20%	57
					>40%	7, 60

Experimental studies, parameter varied (unit)	No change in symptoms				Reduction in symptoms			
	Subjects (N)	Baseline level	Post-interv level	Ref.	Subjects (N)	Baseline level	Post-interv level	Ref.
Temperature (°C)					339		1.5° lower	58
Relative humidity (%)								
Field studies					211	24%	33%	61
					339	25%	40%	58
Chamber studies	12	50%	80%	62	12	18%	50%	62
	8	9%	50%	117				

Table 4 Association of Nonspecific Building Related Illnesses with Building Ventilation Type

Author (Ref.)	Year	Population		Comparison of ventilation types	Symptoms associated
		Persons (N)	Buildings (N)		
Mendell (14)	1990	11,627	103	Mechanical vs. natural	None
				Air conditioning vs. natural	CNS (headache/fatigue), mucosal ± respiratory
				Air conditioning and humidification vs. natural	Headache/fatigue, eye, mucosal, respiratory, skin
Zweers (15)	1992	7,043	61	Mechanical vs. natural	Eye, headache/fatigue
				Humidification (evap or steam) vs. none	Skin, mucosal
Harrison (72)	1992	4,610	15	Mechanical vs. natural	Eye, mucosal, CNS
				Air conditioning vs. natural	Eye, mucosal, CNS
Sundell (9)	1993	1,350	27	Exhaust only vs. exhaust and supply	None
Jaakkola (11)	1995	2,678	41	Mechanical vs. natural	Eye, nose, throat, and fatigue
				Air conditioning vs. mechanical	All symptoms
Mendell (12)	1996	880	12	Mechanical vs. natural	Skin, mucosal, respiratory (± headache)
				Air conditioning vs. natural	Eye, skin, mucosal, respiratory (± headache)

The effects of exposure to environmental tobacco smoke in other environments (primarily the home) have been reviewed extensively elsewhere (65), and can be summarized as consistently associated with a number of adverse health effects including lung cancer. It has been suggested (66) that this evidence should be extrapolated to the office environment, in support of a ban on smoking in such buildings, despite the rather limited evidence seen in Table 2.

Surface dust and carpets are reservoirs of fungi (67), volatile organic compounds (63,68), and house dust mites (69), which may be released when disturbed, resulting in health effects. No studies have demonstrated reduction of symptoms following removal of carpets, although symptom reduction following intensive cleaning has been documented (70,71).

As summarized in Table 4, the presence of air conditioning appears to be consistently associated with symptoms (11,14,15,17,72). Whether other building ventilation characteristics such as humidification (11,15) and mechanical ventilation (11,17,72) are independent risk factors for symptoms remains unresolved. These factors can only be studied by comparing health effects in workers in different buildings, a comparison potentially confounded by between-building differences in terms of characteristics of the occupants, their work, and work sites, and potentially biased because of occupants' beliefs regarding the effect of the ventilation system on their health.

Fungi and bacteria have been implicated because of the association of nonspecific BRI with indicators of potential microbial contamination such as high humidity (7,60,63), surface dust (6,13), carpets (6,13,73), and air conditioning (11,12,14,72). Microorganisms and/or their toxins have been detected in high concentrations at sites of localized water damage (74), and in HVAC systems—on cooling coils (75), filters (76), duct work (77,78), humidifiers (79), drip pans (75), and air-cooling units (28,29,75). Despite this, airborne microbial levels have been low and inconsistently associated with symptoms in field studies, as shown in Table 5 (63,72,80–83).

The term "volatile organic compounds" (VOCs) refers to many different compounds produced from a wide variety of sources within office buildings (68). These include new building materials or furnishings (the "new car smell"), cleaning agents, paints, solvents, equipment such as laser printers, photocopiers, and carbonless paper (68). In three single-blind chamber studies (Table 6) of controlled exposures administered to human volunteers, a mix of VOCs commonly found in office environments resulted in mucosal irritation (52,84,85). However, the concentrations of VOCs used (5000 and 25,000 $\mu g/m^3$) were far higher than those detected in most field studies (Table 6) (18,48,63,82,86). In these field studies, associations of symptoms with concentrations of VOCs are inconsistent, although generally, associations were detected in studies where concentrations were higher. Studies of controlled exposures to concentrations of VOCs usually found in the office environment would be of great interest.

Formaldehyde is commonly detected in low concentrations in the indoor office environment. Sources include building materials and furnishings. Exposures in the home environment to concentrations of formaldehyde exceeding 0.3 ppm resulted in symptoms of headache, eye, nose, and skin irritation, in 71% of those surveyed. On the other hand, among subjects exposed to concentrations of less than 0.1 ppm, only 7% reported symptoms—no different from an unexposed control population (49). A similar relationship was seen between mucosal irritative symptoms and levels of formaldehyde exposure in an industrial environment (87). In cross-sectional surveys among office workers (Table 7), exposure levels have been generally low and associations with symptoms rarely detected. In chamber studies, the odor detection threshold has been noted to be very low although

Table 5 Association of Symptoms of Nonspecific Building-Related Illnesses with Airborne Microorganisms

Author, year (ref.)	Study design	Population		Exposure assessment		Concentration measured		Symptom associated
		Persons (N)	Buildings (N)	Type	Microbiological class	Mean (cfu/m³)	Range (cfu/m³)	
Skov 1990 (63)	Cross-sectional	2369	14	Area	Fungi	32	0–111	None
					Bacteria	574	120–2100	None
					Thermo a.		0	None
Nelson 1991 (83)	Cross-sectional	383	3	Personal	Fungi	10	0–100	None
					Bacteria	42	5–240	None
					Thermo a.	7	1–140	None
Menzies 1992 (80)	Case-control	100	6	Personal	Fungi	27	2–200	None
Harrison 1992 (72)	Cross-sectional	4610	15	Area	Total bacteria	342	80–961	None
					Fungi	97	2–978	Nose, skin, throat
Teeuw 1994 (81)	Cross-sectional	1355	19	Area	GM (−) bacteria	17	1–33	SBS—all symptoms
					Fungi	45	28–75	None
Menzies 1996 (82)	Repeated measures	704	2	Area	Fungi	14	8–17	None

Thermo a. = thermophilic actinomycetes; GM (−) = gram-negative; SBS = sick building syndrome.

Table 6 Association of Symptoms of Nonspecific Building-Related Illness with Volatile Organic Compounds (VOCs) and Airborne Dust

Author (Ref.)	Year	Population Persons (N)	Population Buildings (N)	Exposure assessment	VOCs or dust measured Mean ($\mu g/m^3$)	VOCs or dust measured Range ($\mu g/m^3$)	Symptoms associated
VOCs—field studies (all cross-sectional except 82)							
Norback (18)	1990	261	11	Area	380	50–1380	Mucosal + systemic
Skov (63)	1990	215	4	Area	590	70–3190	None
Hodgson (48)	1991	147	3	Personal	1,247		Mucosal + systemic
Sundell (86)	1993	1087	29	Area	70	3–740	None
Menzies (82)	1996	702	2	Area	941	160–2353	Acute mucosal
VOCs—chamber studies:							
Molhave (85)	1986	150		Direct	5,000 25,000		Mucosal ↓ Neurobehavioral performance
Otto (118, 119)	1990	62		Direct	25,000		Mucosal, headache, fatigue No change in performance
Kjaergaard (52)	1991	35		Direct	25,000		Mucosal irritation ↓ FEV_1 ↑ Ocular tears/leukocytes ↓ Neurobehavioral performance
Dust—field studies (all cross-sectional except 82)							
Weber (109)	1984	472		Personal	133	10–962	Eye irritation
Norback (120)	1990	129	6	Area	16	8–24	Eye symptoms
Hodgson (48)	1991	147	5	Personal	52		None
Harrison (72)	1992	4610	15	Area	30	1–110	None
Menzies (82)	1996	704	2	Area	22	13–19	Systemic
Dust–chamber studies							
Weber (109)	1984	33		Direct	58		Eye irritation at lowest level
Walker (89)	1996	17		Direct	217		Nasal, eye irritation, altered respiration Increased eye blink rate

Table 7 Association of Symptoms of Nonspecific Building-Related Illnesses with Formaldehyde and Carbon Monoxide

Author (Ref.)	Year	Population Persons (N)	Population Buildings (N)	Exposure assessment	Formaldehyde level Mean (μg/m³)	Formaldehyde level Range (μg/m³)	Symptoms associated
Formaldehyde—field studies (all cross-sectional except 82)							
Main (121)	1983	21 exposed		Area	0.87 ppm	0.2–1.6	Headache, mucosal, fatigue
		18 not exposed					
Horvath (87)	1988	113		Area		<0.05	4% sore throat
						0.05–0.4	8% sore throat
						0.4–1.0	22% sore throat
						1.0–3.0	33% sore throat
Skov (63)	1990	1018	4	Area	80 μg		None
Norback (18)	1990	261	11	Area	11 μg	0–30	None
De Bortoli (122)	1990	785	10	Area	450 μg	0–139	None
Sundell (86)	1993	1087	29	Area	31 μg	11–59	Usual mucosal skin
Menzies (82)	1996	704	2	Area	0.03 ppm	0.01–0.05	None
Formaldehyde—chamber studies							
Ahlstrom (107)	1986	64		Direct		>60 mcg	Odor
Hempel (88)	1996	10		Direct		>0.88 ppm	Eye irritation

Author (Ref.)	Year	Population Persons (N)	Population Buildings (N)	Exposure assessment	CO level Mean (ppm)	CO level Range (ppm)	Symptoms associated
Carbon monoxide—field studies (all cross-sectional except 82)							
Faust (90)	1981	22	1	Area		5–25	CNS
Robertson (100)	1985	241	2	Area		1–7	None
Hodgson (48)	1991	147	5	Personal	4.5		None
Menzies (82)	1996	704	2	Area	3.9	2–5.5	None

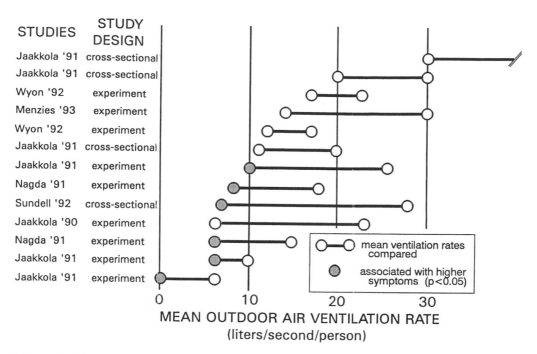

Figure 3 Summary of results from 9 studies of outdoor air ventilation rate and work-related symptoms. Comparison made between estimated mean ventilation rates. (Taken from Ref. 91 with permission.)

there is a considerable range, as shown in Figure 3. Given the very low threshold for odor detection and the unpleasantness of formaldehyde odor, most investigators have found a strong association between detection of formaldehyde odor and symptoms. In an ingenious study with a special apparatus that limited experimental formaldehyde exposure to the corneal surface of one eye, ocular irritation was reported at significantly higher concentrations when the experimental subjects were not able to detect formaldehyde odors (88).

Airborne dust may arise from indoor activity, particularly if there is inadequate cleaning, or from intake of outdoor air if there is inadequate filtration in the HVAC system. In cross-sectional surveys, airborne dust levels have generally been low although there have been some associations with symptoms, particularly eye irritation (Table 6). The association between dust levels and systemic symptoms in one study may have resulted from associated, but unmeasured, contaminants (82). In one chamber study, young, healthy male volunteers were exposed to increasing concentrations of environmental tobacco smoke. Even at the lowest level of exposure, 58 μg/m^3, subjects reported increased eye and nasal irritation and their respiratory pattern was altered. Eye blink rate increased at much higher concentrations (89).

Sources of carbon monoxide in nonindustrial environments include improperly vented combustion such as the heating system (38) and/or intake of automotive exhaust fumes (39) either from outdoor air or from an enclosed garage that is attached to the building. As summarized in Table 7, only one out of four studies detected an association between carbon monoxide levels and CNS symptoms (90). As mentioned earlier, occult carbon monoxide poisoning may give rise to nonspecific symptoms of fatigue, headache, and difficulty concentrating (41). This has only been described in individuals exposed in the home environment, but could occur in the office environment from exposure to high enough levels.

A particularly controversial issue has been the importance of the ventilation rate, by which is meant the amount of outdoor air supplied to the indoor environment. A recent synthesis (91) has largely resolved this by pointing out that in cross-sectional studies (shown in Table 2), symptom prevalence was higher in buildings with outdoor air supply of less than 10 L/sec/person (9,10,47,92). In experimental studies increasing ventilation reduced symptoms [with one exception (93)] if the baseline ventilation rates were below 10 L/sec/person, but had no effect if baseline ventilation rates were higher (56,58,94). This meta-analysis, summarized graphically in Figure 3, was fairly crude, because it considered only statistical significance rather than size of effects. In addition, two more recent cross-sectional studies found that symptom prevalence was lower at higher ventilation rates (9,47). Nevertheless the message from many studies is that symptoms are increased with very low ventilation levels, and the relationship becomes much less consistent at progressively higher ventilation levels. This can be explained by the phenomenon that relatively small changes in ventilation strongly influence indoor pollutant levels when ventilation is at low levels, but have much less effect at higher ventilation rates.

METHODOLOGICAL PROBLEMS OF PAST STUDIES OF NONSPECIFIC BRI

Nonstandardized Symptom Definitions

The following symptom definitions were used in cross-sectional surveys: "Occurrence in the last 6 months" (18), "occurrence often at work" (9), "occurrence at work with improvement away from work" (19), "occurrence at least twice in the past year with improvement away from work" (7), and "work related and often" (6,17). As a result, it is difficult to compare the symptom prevalence reported in these studies. In a cross-sectional survey of workers in 15 different buildings, the ranking of buildings based on average number of symptoms reported changed considerably if these different symptom definitions were used (16) (see Figs. 1 and 2).

Nonstandardized Measurement of Environmental Parameters

Although there are standardized procedures for sample collection and analysis for most of the contaminants commonly found in the indoor nonindustrial environment, these procedures were not developed for measurement in this environment. Therefore, they may not be sensitive enough to accurately characterize the low levels of exposure, or detect differences between workers who are or are not affected. In addition, since the causative agent(s) are unknown, there is no consensus as to which contaminants should be measured, nor the collection and analytical methods, nor even the sampling strategies. Measurement of these contaminants is expensive, time consuming, and requires sophisticated equipment for sample collection and analysis. As a result, in most epidemiological surveys, environmental sampling has been very limited and the methods used, particularly for microbiological and chemical contaminants, nonstandardized. This makes it almost impossible to compare results between studies.

Health Effects Threshold Have Not Been Established

Guidelines for contaminant concentrations in the indoor nonindustrial environment have been issued by authoritative agencies such as the World Health Organization (5), ASHRAE (64), and others (95). However, there is very little information to indicate the true health effects in this population.

Temporal and Spatial Variability

The HVAC systems of large office buildings are designed to provide a stable and constant indoor environment throughout the building. However, postconstruction changes to the ventilation system, or interior space (96), or normal wear and tear may result in malfunctioning of well-designed ventilation systems and substantial reduction in local ventilation effectiveness (97). In addition, there may be important differences in local indoor pollutant sources because of differences in the human occupants themselves (such as perfume use) or because of their work activities and use of equipment. In addition, there may be local pollutant sources such as microbial contamination following water damage, or materials known as "sinks," which trap contaminants such as VOCs and release them slowly later (68). All these factors may result in substantial spatial variation in temperature, air velocity, and indoor pollutant levels between work sites, even those on the same floor of one building (56,98,99). In addition, there may be considerable temporal variation in contaminant concentrations as a result of changes in outdoor air supply, in outdoor air pollutant levels, or in the number and activities of the workers. Spatial variability may have resulted in significant misclassification of exposure in studies where environmental measures were made at only two to seven sites and used to estimate exposure for all workers in an entire building (7,18,63,100). Temporal variability may have resulted in misclassified exposure in studies where environmental measures were not taken at the same time as measures of symptoms (98), or only over a short period (7,63,100).

The unexpected finding of significant spatial variability within large office buildings has given rise to the concept of the "microenvironment" (48). When environmental parameters have been measured directly at the work sites of individual workers—so-called personal measures—associations have been detected between individual contaminants and symptoms although even these results are not consistent. The concept of the microenvironment has provided support for the provision of personal control over the ventilation system to individual workers. This is because in the complex environment of large office buildings, it is simply not possible for a centrally controlled HVAC system to adapt rapidly and effectively to highly variable local conditions, as well as meet the demands or preferences of many workers. Sophisticated automated ventilation systems with electrochemical sensors for a number of environmental parameters could be developed. However, the provision of individual ventilation control offers a more practical solution because it utilizes the most sophisticated, as well as the most relevant sensor—that of the human organism itself. In a cross-sectional British survey of 4373 workers in 46 buildings, those who could regulate temperature and ventilation reported significantly higher productivity and fewer symptoms (101). Among 7043 Dutch workers in 61 office buildings, work absence related to symptoms of nonspecific BRI was 34% lower in buildings where workers could regulate the temperature (102,103). The provision of a personally controlled ventilation system was associated with a significant increase in objectively measured productivity in one study (104) and with persistent and prolonged improvement in symptoms, environmental ratings as well as self-rated productivity in another (105).

Potential Combined Effect of Multiple Agents

Most surveys of the nonindustrial, nonresidential environment have detected many contaminants but all at low concentrations. These same contaminants are known to cause health effects at higher concentrations. It seems plausible that symptoms could result from a combination of two or more agents, but very few studies have examined this hypothesis. In one report, an outbreak of illness among office workers was linked to exposure to carbon monoxide, ozone, and pentane, all at concentrations believed safe. Illness was more common among those with lower body weight, making a toxic effect more plausible (90). In a second report, symptoms were more common in workers in two buildings who were exposed to higher total contaminant load (82). Two experimental studies provide data in support of these observations. Exposure to 0.12 ppm of ozone for 1 hr increased subsequent bronchial reactivity to inhaled allergens (106), while volunteers exposed to 0.82 ppm of formaldehyde had 4 times greater occurrence of mucosal irritation when also exposed to air from a "sick" building (107).

Complex Interrelationship of Indoor Contaminants

In one study, a number of indoor contaminants or pollutants were measured at many sites each week for 6 weeks as outdoor air supply was experimentally varied (82). In the two office buildings studied, VOCs, formaldehyde, dust, NO_2, carbon monoxide, and airborne fungal concentrations varied substantially from week to week and between work sites even on the same floor in the same building. The concentrations of volatile organic compounds and formaldehyde decreased as outdoor air supply was experimentally increased. On the other hand, dust, carbon monoxide, NO_2, and microbial concentrations *actually increased when outdoor air supply was increased* because the major source was outdoors for those contaminants—at that time and in those buildings. An important observation was that outdoor air supply, or ventilation rate, was not the major determinant of any of the contaminant concentrations. More important determinants were changes in outdoor levels, or

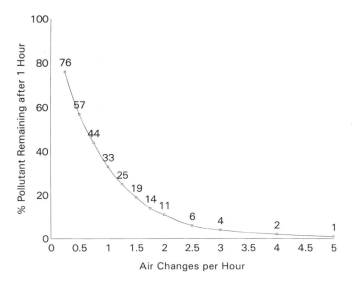

Figure 4 Effect of ventilation rate expressed as air changes per hour on pollutant concentration after 1 hr expressed as a percent of the initial concentration.

changes in indoor pollutant sources related to differences in occupants or work activity, and unexplained, but substantial, spatial variability. These findings help to explain why increasing outdoor air supply to this environment is not a universal panacea as once believed. In addition, the complexity of the indoor environment explains why measurements of a few of these contaminants at a few sites on one or two occasions will almost never detect exposure-response relationships unless exposure is very high such as occurs in outbreaks.

SYNTHESIS OF EVIDENCE REGARDING OFFICE-BUILDING-RELATED ILLNESSES

In summary, a number of personal factors are associated with nonspecific BRI; these may be indicators of increased susceptibility. Symptoms are also associated with markers of individual exposure, such as use of carbonless paper, photocopiers, and VDTs, or presence of carpets and dust, yet the specific agent(s) responsible for the associated health effects have not been identified. The importance of buildingwide factors such as type or presence of mechanical ventilation (9,11,12,14), or humidification (14,15) remains unclear. Studies to examine these factors were confounded by between-building differences in the occupants and their work and may have been biased by occupants' awareness and attitudes. Although symptoms have consistently been associated with temperature, and humidity (56–58), this has not been the case for measured chemical and microbial parameters, despite the indirect evidence implicating them. This may reflect the multiple agents present, their spatial and temporal variability, and that current measurement methods are expensive and insufficiently precise for the low levels usually present in this environment.

Nonspecific BRI may be explained by three phenomena: a wide range in the threshold of response in any population (susceptibility), a spectrum of response to any given agent, and variability in exposure within large office buildings.

Health effects may develop in individuals exposed to an agent or agents at concentrations above their threshold for response. As shown in Figure 5, among healthy adults there is a wide range in the threshold for detection of irritant effects of formaldehyde (87,107); this has also been demonstrated for volatile organic compounds (108) and environmental tobacco smoke (109). Similar variability of the threshold has been demonstrated for physiological response to temperature (50,51), ozone, sulfates, and particulates (110), and endotoxin (111). Although these thresholds show marked variation between individuals, there is much less variation within the same individuals (110). Thresholds for response are lower in workers with asthma (110), or previous building-related symptoms (52), or subjects who are female (49,51), or younger (49,51). In addition, thresholds for physiological response to allergens, organic volatile compounds, and environmental tobacco smoke have been lowered by concomitant exposure to ozone (106), higher temperature (112), and lower humidity (62), respectively.

Although specific BRI initially have been identified when several workers presented with similar clinical manifestations and objective abnormalities, an important but overlooked finding in these outbreaks was the wide spectrum of clinical response to the same agents (26,27,29). The "tip of the iceberg" were the few seriously affected workers with specific clinical abnormalities. Among other exposed workers, a few (often more than the number of initial sentinel cases) had symptoms but no objective abnormalities whereas others were asymptomatic, yet had circulating specific antibodies, (26,27,29). Without the

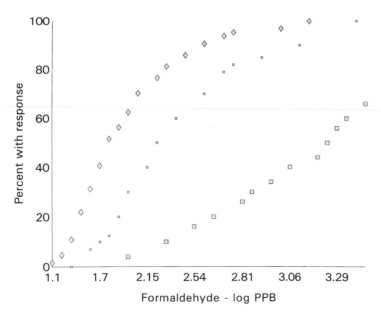

Figure 5 Threshold for response of human volunteers to controlled exposures to formaldehyde. Large squares: Absolute odor threshold (from Ref. 107). Small squares: Odor detection of formaldehyde in all, or 100%, of challenges (from Ref. 107). Triangles: Nasal irritation with formaldehyde (from Ref. 87). (Taken from Ref. 4 with permission.)

sentinel cases the cause for symptoms in these other affected workers may have been missed, or labeled "sick building syndrome."

Modern high-rise office buildings are designed to provide a stable and uniform indoor environment, but as discussed earlier, the actual environment has considerable temporal and spatial variability. This variability may create quite different microenvironments at each work station (82,113). If there was independent variation in the microenvironmental exposures and workers' susceptibility, then individuals could be symptomatic because of localized exposure to one or more agents exceeding their threshold of response. This hypothesis would be difficult to test because of the multiplicity of agents, and symptoms, and the difficulties of accurately characterizing exposure. However, this could explain why past epidemiological surveys failed to identify relationships between environmental parameters measured at a limited number of work sites and symptoms of all workers within these buildings (15,63,100,114). This would provide the rationale for moving affected workers to another work station—a simple solution that has never been evaluated formally. Another potential solution is personal control over ventilation as this would take advantage of highly sophisticated and sensitive monitors located at every workplace—the workers themselves! Individuals who sensed local adverse conditions could mitigate them by changing ventilation—*even if they did not know by what they were affected.*

APPROACH TO THE PATIENT

Given the complexity of the indoor environment in office buildings, and numerous contributing factors, it is difficult to envisage a simple standardized approach to an office worker with health problems that may be work related. However, certain principles can be defined.

A careful history is an essential first step. Workers may fail to recognize the office environment as the source of their symptoms, so it is important to ascertain the onset, course, and temporal relationship of symptoms with the work environment. On the other hand, if workers attribute their symptoms to the work environment, it is still important to exclude nonoccupational causes.

The physical examination is usually normal in nonspecific BRI but may be abnormal with specific illnesses. Additional investigations may be appropriate to diagnose specific entities such as a chest X-ray and lung function tests for hypersensitivity pneumonitis or asthma, allergy skin tests, and serum IgE for those with allergic manifestations.

If a BRI is suspected, a work site "walk-through" is a valuable starting point in the evaluation of the work environment. A team approach including the physician, industrial hygienist, and engineers is best to identify and resolve problems in this complex indoor environment. Clinicians should familiarize themselves with public or occupational health officials at the municipal, state, or federal level who have expertise in evaluation of these problems. An important advantage of contacting such authorities is that they may receive reports of other affected workers in the same building. This should prompt more thorough environmental assessment and may enable workers to receive compensation or similar benefits. Environmental air sampling may be indicated if specific indoor contaminants are suspected, but is expensive and requires considerable expertise, for measurement and interpretation.

Interventions demonstrated to mitigate nonspecific BRI, such as lowering temperature, better control of humidity, or better cleaning, could be suggested although these may not be applicable in all settings. Another possible (although untested) solution for the workers with nonspecific and unexplained symptoms, would be to change micro-environments—by changing work sites—even within the same building.

CONCLUSIONS

Symptoms of nonspecific BRI are common; their heterogeneity suggests they do not represent a single disorder. Although there is little convincing direct evidence to implicate specific causative agents, there is sufficient indirect evidence to support a number of recommendations. For example, it seems prudent to: maintain outdoor air supply rate above 10 L/sec/person; select building materials, furnishings, and equipment that are least likely to release pollutants such as formaldehyde or VOCs; assure proper maintenance and cleaning; and avoid materials that may act as substrates for microbial or mite proliferation.

Workers in the indoor environment of office buildings represent more than half the entire workforce of industrialized countries. A significant proportion have symptoms at work. Given the enormous population apparently affected and our current limited understanding of the health effects of this environment, further research is urgently required. Susceptibility should be assessed in experimental studies of exposures to individual and multiple pollutants at concentrations typically found in the office environment. Proposed interventions should be evaluated in properly designed trials using standardized case definitions, questionnaires, and environmental measurement methods. Such studies could help to ensure that the man-made ecosystem of modern office buildings is a healthy work environment.

ACKNOWLEDGMENTS

This work was supported by a Chercheur-Boursier Clincien award from the Fonds de la Recherche en Santé de Québec. The author thanks Dr. Jean Bourbeau for important contribution and comments for this chapter, as well as Mme. Sylvie Ouimet for secretarial assistance.

REFERENCES

1. Christie B. Human Factors of Information Technology in the Office. New York: John Wiley and Sons, 1985.
2. Woods JE. Cost avoidance and productivity in owning and operating buildings. Occup Med 1989; 4:753–770.
3. Samet JM, Marbury MC, Spengler JD. Health effects and sources of indoor air pollution. Am Rev Respir Dis 1988; 137:221–242.
4. Menzies D, Bourbeau J. Building-related illnesses. N Engl J Med 1997; 337:1524–1531.
5. Indoor Air Pollutants: Exposure and Health Effects. Copenhagen: World Health Organization, 1983.
6. Skov P, Valbjorn O, Pedersen BV, and Danish Indoor Climate Study Group. Influence of personal characteristics, job-related factors and psychosocial on the sick building syndrome. Scand J Work Environ Health 1989; 15:286–295.
7. Burge PS, Hedge A, Wilson S, Bass JH, Robertson A. Sick building syndrome: a study of 4373 office workers. Ann Occup Hyg 1987; 31:493–504.
8. Stenberg B, Hansson Mild K, Sandstrom M, Sundell J, Wall S. A prevalence study of the sick building syndrome (SBS) and facial skin symptoms in office workers. Indoor Air 1993; 3:71–81.
9. Sundell J, Stenberg B, Lindvall T. Associations between type of ventilation and air flow rates in office buildings and the risk of SBS-symptoms among occupants. Environ Int 1994; 20(2): 239–251.
10. Bourbeau J, Brisson C, Allaire S. Prevalence of the sick building syndrome symptoms in office workers before and after being exposed to a building with an improved ventilation system. Occup Environ Med 1996; 53:204–210.
11. Jaakkola JJK, Miettinen P. Type of ventilation system in office buildings and sick building syndrome. Am J Epidemiol 1995; 141(8):755–765.
12. Mendell MJ, Fisk WJ, Deddens JA, Seavey WG, Smith AH, Smith DF, Hodgson AT, Daisey JM, Goldman LR. Elevated symptom prevalence associated with ventilation type in office buildings. Epidemiology 1996; 7(6):583–589.
13. Wallace LA, Nelson CJ, Highsmith R, Dunteman G. Association of personal and workplace characteristics with health, comfort and odor: a survey of 3948 office workers in three buildings. Indoor Air 1993; 3:193–205.
14. Mendell MJ, Smith AH. Consistent pattern of elevated symptoms in air-conditioned office buildings: a re-analysis of epidemiologic studies. Am J Public Health 1990; 80:1193–1199.
15. Zweers T, Preller L, Brunekreef B, Boleij JSM. Health and indoor climate complaints of 7043 office workers in 61 buildings in The Netherlands. Indoor Air 1992; 2:127–136.
16. Menzies D, Pasztor J, Leduc J, et al. The "sick building"—a misleading term that should be abandoned. In: Besch EL, editors. I.A.Q. '94 Engineering Indoor Environment. Atlanta. American Society of Heating Refrigeration Air–Conditioning Engineer (ASHRAE), 1994.
17. Salvaggio JE. Recent advances in the pathogenesis of allergic alveolitis. Clin Exp Allergy 1990; 20:137–144.
18. Norback D, Michel I, Widstrom J. Indoor air quality and personal factors related to sick building syndrome. Scand J Work Environ Health 1990; 16:121–128.

19. Finnegan MJ, Pickering CAC, Burge PS. The sick building syndrome: prevalence studies. Br Med J 1984; 289:1573–1575.

20. Nardell EA, Keegan J, Cheney SA, Etkind SC. Airborne infection: theoretical limits of protection achievable by building ventilation. Am Rev Respir Dis 1991; 144(2):302–306.

21. Brundage JF, Scott RMcN, Lednar WM, Smith DW, Miller RN. Building-associated risk of febrile acute respiratory diseases in army trainees. JAMA 1988; 259:2108–2112.

22. Jaakkola JJK, Heinonen OP. Share office space and the risk of the common cold. Eur J of Epidemiol 1995; 11(2):213–216.

23. Fraser DW, Tsai TR, Orenstein W, Parkin W, Beecham H, Sharrar R, et al. Legionnaire's disease: description of an epidemic of pneumonia. N Engl J Med 1977; 297:1189–1197.

24. Dennis PJ, Taylor JA, Fitzgerald RB, Bartlett CLR, Barnow GI. Legionella pneumophila in water plumbing systems. Lancet 1982; 1:949–951.

25. Kaufman AF, McDade JE, Patton CM. Pontiac fever isolation of the etiologic agent (legionella pneumophila) and demonstration of its mode of transmission. Am J Epidemiol 1981; 114:337–347.

26. Woodard ED, Friedlander B, Lesher RJ, Font WF, Kinsey R, Hearne FT. Outbreak of hypersensitivity pneumonitis on an industrial setting. JAMA 1988; 259:1965–1969.

27. Arnow PM, Fink JN, Schuelter DP, et al. Early detection of hypersensitivity pneumonitis in office workers. Am J Med 1978; 64:236–241.

28. Banaszak EF, Thiede WH, Fink JN. Hypersensitivity pneumonitis due to contamination of an air conditioner. N Engl J Med 1970; 283:271–276.

29. Bernstein RS, Sorenson WG, Garabrant D, Reaux C, Treitman RD. Exposures to respirable airborne *Penicillium* from a contaminated ventilation system: clinical, environmental and epidemiologic aspects. Am Ind Hyg Assoc J 1983; 44:161–169.

30. Hoffman RE, Wood RC, Kreiss K. Building-related asthma in Denver office workers. Am J Public Health 1993; 83(1):89–93.

31. Burge P, Finnegan M, Horsfield N, Emery D, Austwick P, Davies P, Pickering C. Occupational asthma in a factory with a contaminated humidifier. Thorax 1985; 40:248–254.

32. Tencati JR, Novey HS. Hypersensitivity angiitis caused by fumes from heat-activated photocopy paper. Ann Intern Med 1983; 98:320–322.

33. Marks JG, Trautlein JJ, Zwilich CW, Demers LM. Contact Urticaria and airway obstruction from carbonless copy paper. JAMA 1984; 252(8):1038–1040.

34. LaMarte FP, Merchant JA, Casale TB. Acute systemic reactions to carbonless copy paper associated with histamine release. JAMA 1988; 260(2):242–243.

35. Morgan MS, Camp JE. Upper respiratory irritation from controlled exposure to vapor from carbonless copy forms. J Occup Med 1986; 28(6):415–419.

36. Verbeck S, Buise-van Unnik E, Malten K. Itching in office workers from glass fibres. Contact Dermatitis 1981; 7:354.

37. Farkas J. Fibre glass dermatitis in employees of a project-office in a new building. Contact Dermatitis 1983; 9:79.

38. Chappell SB, Parker R. Smoking and carbon monoxide levels in enclosed public places in New Brunswick. Can J Public Health 1977; 68:159–161.

39. Wallace LA. Carbon monoxide in air and breath of employees in an underground office. J Air Pollut Control Assoc 1983; 33:678–682.

40. Horvath SM, Dahms TE, O'Hanlon JF. Carbon monoxide and human vigilance. Arch Environ Health 1971; 23:343–347.

41. Heckerling PS, Leiken JB, Maturen A, Perkins JT. Predictors of occult carbon monoxide poisoning in patients with headache and dizziness. Ann Intern Med 1987; 107:174–176.

42. Turiel I, Hollowell CD, Miksch RR, Rudy JV, Young RA. The effects of reduced ventilation on indoor air quality in an office building. Atmos Environ 1983; 17:51–64.

43. Vanderstraeten P; Muylle E; Verduyn G. Indoor air quality in a large hospital building. 4th ed. Bergund B, Lindvall T, and Sundell J, editors. Stockholm: Swedish Council for Building Research, 1984, 335p.

44. Marbury MC, Krieger RA. Indoor Air Pollution. A Health Perspective. Samet JM, Spengler JD, editors. Baltimore: Johns Hopkins University Press, 1991: 223–251.

45. Maimberg P, Rask-Anderson A, Palmgren U, Hoglund S, Kolmodin-Hedman B, Stalenheim G. Exposure to microorganisms, febrile and airway-obstructive symptoms, immune status and lung function of Swedish farmers. Scand J Work Environ Health 1985; 11:287–293.

46. Malmberg P, Rask-Andersen A, Rosenhall L. Exposure to microorganisms associated with allergic alveolitis and febrile reactions to mold dust in farmers. Chest 1993; 103:1202–1209.

47. Jaakkola JJK, Miettinen P. Ventilation rate in office buildings and sick building syndrome. Occup Environ Med 1995; 52:709–714.

48. Hodgson MJ, Frohliger J, Permar E, Tidwell C, Traven ND, Olenchock SA, Karpf M. Symptoms and microenvironmental measures in nonproblem buildings. J Occup Med 1991; 33(4): 527–533.

49. Ritchie IM, Lehnen RG. Formaldehyde-related health complaints of residents living in mobile and conventional homes. Am J Public Health 1987; 77(3):323–328.

50. Grivel F, Candas V. Ambient temperatures preferred by young European males and females at rest. Ergonomics 1991; 34(3):365–378.

51. Doeland HJ, Nauta JJP, Van Zandbergen JB, Van Der Eerden HAM, Van Dieman NGJ, Bertelsmann FW, Heimans JJ. The relationship of cold and warmth cutaneous sensation to age and gender. Muscle Nerve 1989; 12:712–715.

52. Kjaergaard S, Molhave L, Pedersen OF. Human reactions to a mixture of indoor air volatile organic compounds. Atmos Environ 1991; 25A:1417–1426.

53. Bauer RM, Greve KW, Besch EL, Schramke CJ, Crouch J, Hicks A, Ware MR, Lyles WB. The role of psychological factors in the report of building-related symptoms in sick building syndrome. J Consult Clin Psychol 1992; 60(2):213–219.

54. Karasek RA, Theorell T, Schwartz JE, Schnall PL, Pieper CF, Michela JL. Job characteristics in relation to the prevalence of myocardial infarction in the US Health Examination Survey (HES) and the Health and Nutrition Examination Survey (HANES). Am J Public Health 1988; 78(8):910–918.

55. Klitzman S, Stellman JM. The impact of the physical environment on the psychological well-being of office workers. Soc Sci Med 1989; 29(6):733–742.

56. Menzies RI, Tamblyn RM, Farant JP, Hanley J, Nunes F, Tamblyn RT. The effect of varying levels of outdoor air supply on the symptoms of sick building syndrome. N Engl J Med 1993; 328:821–827.

57. Jaakkola JJK, Heinonen OP, Seppanen O. Sick building syndrome, sensation of dryness and thermal comfort in relation to room temperature in an office building: need for individual control of temperature. Environ Int 1989; 15:163–168.

58. Wyon DP. Sick buildings and the experimental approach. Environ Technol 1992; 13:313–322.

59. American Society of Heating Refrigeration and Air-conditioning Engineers. ASHRAE Standard 55-1981: Thermal Environmental Conditions for Human Occupancy. Atlanta: American Society of Heating Refrigeration and Air-conditioning Engineers (ASHRAE), 1981.

60. Reinikainen LM, Jaakola JJK, Heinonen OP. The effect of air humidification on different symptoms in office workers—an epidemiologic study. Environ Int 1991; 17:243–250.

61. Reinikainen LM, Jaakola JJK, Seppanen O. The effect of air humidification on symptoms and perception of indoor air quality. Arch Environ Health 1992; 47:8–15.

62. Kay DL, Heavner DL, Nelson PR, et al. Effects of relative humidity on non-smoker response to environmental tobacco smoke. Walkinshaw DJ, eds. Proceedings of Fifth International Conference on Indoor Air Quality and Climate, Toronto, July 29–August 3, 1990. Vol 1. Toronto: Canadian Mortgage and Housing; 1993; 275–80.

63. Skov P, Valbjorn O, Pedersen BV, and Danish Indoor Climate Study Group. Influence of indoor climate on the sick building syndrome in an office building. Scand J Work Environ Health 1990; 16:363–371.

64. American Society of Heating Refrigeration and Air-conditioning Engineers. ASHRAE Standard 62-1989: Ventilation for Acceptable Indoor Air Quality. Atlanta: American Society of Heating Refrigeration and Air-conditioning Engineers (ASHRAE), 1989.

65. Surgeon General. The health consequences of involuntary smoking. US Department of Health and Human Services, ed. 1986.

66. Woodward A. Is passive smoking in the workplace hazardous to health? Scand J Work Environ Health 1991; 17:293–301.

67. Gravesen S, Larsen L, Gyntelberg F, Skov P. Demonstration of microorganisms and dust in schools and offices. Allergy 1986; 41:520–552.

68. Brown SK, Sim MR, Abramson MJ, Gray CN. Concentrations of volatile organic compounds in indoor air—a review. Indoor Air 1994; 4:123–134.

69. Wood RA, Eggleston PA, Lind P, Ingemann L, Schwartz B, Gravesen S, Terry D, Wheeler B, Adkinson NF. Antigenic analysis of household dust samples. Am Rev Respir Dis 1988; 137:358–363.

70. Leinster P, Raw G, Thomson N, et al. A modular longitudinal approach to the investigation of sick building syndrome. Walkinshaw DJ, eds. Proceedings of the Fifth International Conference on Indoor Air Quality and Climate, Toronto, July 29–August 3, 1990. Vol 1. Toronto: Canadian Mortgage and Housing, 1990:287–93.

71. Raw GJ, Roys MS, Whitehead C. Sick building syndrome: Cleanliness is next to healthiness. indoor air 1993; 3:237–245.

72. Harrison J, Pickering CA, Faragher EB, Austwick PK, Little SA, Lawton L. An investigation of the relationship between microbial and particulate indoor air pollution and the sick building syndrome. Respir Med 1992; 86:225–235.

73. Fisk WJ, Mendell MJ, Daisey JM, Faulkner D, Hodgson AT, Nematollahi M, Macher JM. Phase 1 of the California Healthy Building Study: a summary. Indoor Air 1993; 3:246–254.

74. Jarvis BB, Zhou Y. Toxigenic molds in water damaged buildings J Nat Prod 1996; 59(6): 553–554.

75. Hugenholtz P, Fuerst JA. Heterotrophic bacteria in an air-handling system. Appl Environ Microbiol 1992; 58(12):3914–3920.

76. Yoshizawa S, ed. Investigation of allergic potential induced by fungi on air filters of HVAC systems. Tokyo: Organizing Comm of 7th Intl Conf of Indoor Air Quality and Climate; Organizing Comm of 7th Intl Conf of Indoor Air Quality and Climate; 1996; 125 p. The Seventh International Conference on Indoor Climate and Air Quality.

77. Smoragiewicz W, Cossette B, Boutard A, Krzystyniak K. Trichothecene mycotoxins in the dust of ventilation systems in office buildings. Int Arch Occup Environ Health 1993; 65:113–117.

78. Pasanen P, Pasanen AL, Jantunen M. Water condensation promotes fungal growth in ventilation ducts. Indoor Air 1993: 3:106–112.

79. Burge PS, Finnegan MJ, Horsfield N, Emery D, Austwick P, Davies PS, Pickering CAC. Occupational asthma a factory with a contaminated humidifier. Thorax 1985; 40:248–254.

80. Menzies RI, Tamblyn RM, Comtois P, et al. Case-control study of microenvironmental exposures to aero-allergens as a cause of respiratory symptoms—part of the sick building syndrome symptom complex. Environments for People. Atlanta; American Society of Heating Refrigeration and Air-conditioning. Engineers, 1992:119–28.

81. Teeuw KB, Vandenbroucke-Grauls CMJE, Verhoef J. Airborne gram-negative bacteria and endotoxin in sick building syndrome. Arch Intern Med 1994; 154:2339–2345.

82. Menzies R, Tamblyn RM, Nunes F, Hanley J, Tamblyn RT. Exposure to varying levels of contaminants and symptoms among workers in two office buildings. Am J Public Health 1996; 86:1629–1632.

83. Nelson CJ, Kollander M, Clayton CA, et al. EPA's indoor air quality and work environment survey: relationships of employees' self-reported health symptoms with direct indoor air quality measurements. IAQ 1991—Healthy Buildings. Atlanta: American Society of Heating, Refrigeration and Air-Conditioning Engineers, 1991:22–32.

84. Otto D, Molhave L, Rose G, Hudnell K, House D. Neurobehavioral and sensory irritant effects of controlled exposure to a complex mixture of volatile organic compounds. Neuro-Behav Toxicol Teratol 1990; 12:649–652.

85. Molhave L, Bach B, Pedersen OF. Human reactions to low concentrations of volatile organic compounds. Environ Int 1986; 12:167–175.

86. Sundell J, Andersson B, Andersson K, Lindvall T. Volatile organic compounds in ventilating air in buildings at different sampling points in the buildings and their relationship with the prevalence of occupant symptoms. Indoor Air 1993; 3:82–93.

87. Horvath EP, Anderson H, Pierce WE, Hanrahan L, Wendlick JD. Effects of formaldehyde on the mucous membranes and lungs: a study of an industrial population. JAMA 1984; 259: 701–707.

88. Yoshizawa S, ed. Eye irritation in humans exposed to formaldehyde—The Seventh International Conference on Indoor Air Quality and Climate. Indoor Air '96. Nagoya: 1996; 325.

89. Yoshizawa S, ed. Perceptual and psychophysiological responses of non-smokers to a range of environmental tobacco smoke concentrations—The Seventh International Conference on Indoor Air Quality and Climate; Indoor Air '96. Nagoya: 1996; 1001.

90. Faust HS, Brilliant LB. Is the diagnosis of "mass hysteria" an excuse for incomplete investigation of low level environmental contamination? J Occup Med 1981; 23:22–26.

91. Mendell M. Non-specific symptoms in office workers: A review and summary of the literature. Indoor Air 1993; B:227–236.

92. Jaakkola JJK, Reinikainen LM, Heinonen OP, Majanen A, Seppanen O. Indoor air quality requirements for healthy office buildings: recommendations based on an epidemiologic study. Environ Int 1991; 17:371–378.

93. Jaakkola JJK, Tuomaala P, Seppanen O. Air recirculation and sick building syndrome: a blinded crossover trial. Am J Public Health 1994; 84:422–428.

94. Jaakkola JJK, Heinonen OP, Seppanen O. Mechanical ventilation in office buildings and the sick building syndrome. An experimental and epidemiological study. Indoor Air 1991; 2:111–121.

95. American Conference of Governmental Industrial Hygienists. Guidelines for the assessment of bioaerosols in the indoor environment. Cincinnati, Ohio. 1989.

96. Tamblyn RT. Healthy Building Manual: Systems, Parameters, Problems, and Solutions. Ottawa: Energy, Mines and Resources, 1988.

97. Lindberg PR. Improving hospital ventilation systems for tuberculosis infection control. Tomasik KM, ed. Plant Technology and Safety Management Series Oakbrook Terrace, IL: Joint Commission on Accreditation of Healthcare Organizations, 1993:19–23.

98. Jaakkola JJK, Heinonen OP. Sick building syndrome, sensation of dryness and thermal comfort in relation to room temperature in an office building: need for individual control of temperature. Environ Int 1989; 15:163–168.

99. Menzies RI, Tamblyn RM, Nunes F, et al. Varying ventilation conditions to provide a more complete assessment of building HVAC operation and indoor air quality. Jaakkola JJK, Ilmarinen R, Seppanen O, eds. Indoor Air '93—Proceedings of the Sixth International Conference on Indoor Air Quality and Climate. Vol. 6. Helsinki, Finland, 1993:551–556.

100. Robertson AS, Burge PS, Hedge A, Sims J, Gill FS, Finnegan M, Pickering CAC, Dalton G. Comparison of health problems related to work and environmental measurements in two office buildings with different ventilation systems. Br Med J 1985; 291:373–376.

101. Raw GJ, Roys MS, Leaman A. Further findings from the office environment survey: Productivity? Walkinshaw DJ, ed. Indoor Air '90—Proceedings of the Fifth International Conference on Indoor Air Quality Climate. Toronto, Ontario, Canada. Canadian Mortgage and Housing Commission, 1990:231–236.

102. Preller L, Zweers T, Brunekreef B, et al. Sick leave due to work-related health complaints among office workers in the Netherlands. Walkinshaw DJ, ed. Indoor Air '90—Proceedings of the Fifth International Conference on Indoor Air Quality and Climate. Toronto, Ontario, Canada, Canadian Mortgage and Housing Commission, 1990:227–30.

103. Walkinshaw D, ed. Health and Indoor Climate Complaints of 7043 Office Workers in 61 Buildings in the Netherlands—Fifth International Air Quality Conference 1990. Toronto; 1990:495.

104. Kroner W, Stark-Martin JA, Willemain T. Rensselaer's West Bend Mutual Study: Using Advanced Office Technology to Increase Productivity. Troy, NY: Rensselaer Polytechnic Institute, 1994:25.

105. Menzies D, Pasztor J, Nunes F, Leduc J, Chan C. Effect of a New Ventilation System on Health and Well-being of Office Workers. Arch Environ Health 1997; 52:360–367.

106. Molfino NA, Wright SC, Katz I, Tarlo S, Silverman F, McClean PA, Szalai JP, Rainzenne M, Slutsky AS, Zamel N. Effect of low concentrations of ozone inhaled allergen responses in asthmatic subjects. Lancet 1991; 338:199–203.

107. Ahlstrom R, Berglund B, Lindvall T, Berglund V. Formaldehyde odor and its interaction with the air of a sick building. Environment International 1986; 12:289–295.

108. Cain W, Cometto-Muniz J. Sensory irritation potency of VOCs measured through nasal localization thresholds. Yoshizawa S, ed. IAQ 96–The Seventh International Conference on Indoor Climate and Air Quality. Nagoya: Organizing Comm. 7th Intl Conf of Indoor Air Quality and Climate; 1996:167–172.

109. Weber A. Annoyance and irritation by passive smoking. Prev Med 1984; 13:618–625.

110. Bascom R, Bromberg PA, Costa DA, Devlin R, et al. Health effects of outdoor air pollution. Committee of the Environmental and Occupational Health Assembly of the American Thoracic Society. Am J Respir Crit Care Med 1996; 153:3–50.

111. Rylander R, Babe B, Fischer FF, Helander IM. Pulmonary function and symptoms after inhalation of endotoxin. Am Rev Respir Dis 1989; 140:981–986.

112. Molhave L, Liu Z, Jorgensen AH, Pedersen OF, Kjaergaard SK. Sensory and physiological effects on humans of combined exposures to air temperatures and volatile organic compounds. Indoor Air 1993; 3:155–169.

113. Hodgson MJ, Collopy P. Symptoms and the micro-environment in the sick building syndrome: a pilot study. IAQ '89—The Human Equation: Health and Comfort. Atlanta: GA. American Society of Heating Refrigeration and Air-conditioning Engineers (ASHRAE); 1989:8–16.

114. Burge PS, Jones P, Robertson AS. Sick building syndrome. Walkinshaw DJ, ed. Proceedings of the Fifth International Conference on Indoor Air Quality and Climate, Toronto, July 29–August 3, 1990. Vol. 1. Toronto: Canadian Mortgage and Housing, 1990:479–483.

115. Schneider T. Manmade mineral fibres and other fibres in the air and in settled dust. Environ Int 1986; 12:61–65.

116. Stenberg B, Eriksson N, Hoog J, Sundell J, Wall S. The sick building syndrome (SBS) in office workers. A case-referent study of personal, psychosocial and building-related risk indicators. Int J Epidem 1994; 23:1190–1197.

117. Andersen I, Lundqvist GR, Jensen PL, Proctor DF. Human response to 78-hour exposure to dry air. Arch Environ Health 1974; 29:319–324.

118. Otto DA, Hudnell KH, House DE, Molhave L, Counts W. Exposure of humans to a volatile organic mixture. 1. Behavioral Assessment. Arch Environ Health 1992; 47:23–30.

119. Otto DA, Hudnell HK, House DE, Molhave L. Exposure of humans to a volatile organic mixture. 2. Sensory. Arch Environ Health 1992; 47:31–38.

120. Norback D, Torgen M, Edling C. Volatile organic compounds, respirable dust, and personal factors related to prevalence and incidence of sick building syndrome in primary schools. Br Med J 1990; 47:733–741.

121. Main D, Hogan T. Health effects of low level exposure to formaldehyde. J Occup Med 1983; 25:896–900.

122. Investigation on the Contribution of Volatile Organic Compounds to Air Quality Complaints in Office Buildings of the European Parliament. 1990; 1990; 695.

35

Tables of Major Inducers of Occupational Asthma

Moira Chan-Yeung
Vancouver General Hospital and University of British Columbia, Vancouver, British Columbia, Canada

Jean-Luc Malo
Université de Montréal and Sacré-Coeur Hospital, Montréal, Quebec, Canada

This compendium consists of a listing of agents known to give rise to occupational asthma, compiled from a selection of key references as it is not possible to include all publications related to each causative agent. The selection was based on the most representative and documented evidence, the number of subjects, study design, and/or tests used. The references were derived mostly from English-language journals, but other languages were also included.

The purpose of this compendium is to provide a list for primary care providers to alert them to the possibility that certain agents have been shown to cause occupational asthma. The diagnosis, however, should be confirmed by objective means if at all possible, as discussed in the text. As new agents are being reported regularly, absence from this list is not against the diagnosis of occupational asthma.

These agents are divided into two broad categories and appear in two sections: high-molecular-weight agents (Table 1) and low-molecular-weight agents (Table 2). The entries are organized by agents and the industry where the cases were reported or studies were conducted and the findings of case reports and prevalence studies are listed. In the case of a prevalence study, the percentage of affected subjects is presented. It should be noted that case definitions for prevalance studies were different. Some were reached according to questionnaire, others according to results of specific bronchoprovocation tests. The number of subjects in each study is presented together with supportive evidence of causative relationship, including evidence of sensitization from results of allergy skin tests, specific IgE antibodies, and other immunological tests. When bronchoprovocation tests were done, the results are presented. Finally, other evidence of work-relatedness is also listed.

Table 1 Agents Causing Occupational Asthma with Key References

Agent	Occupation	Ref.	Subjects (n)	Prevalence (%)	Skin test	Specific IgE	Other immunological test	Broncho-provocation test	Other evidence
High-molecular-weight agents									
Animal-derived antigens									
Laboratory animal	Laboratory workers	(1)	296	13	17%+	34% of 255+	ND	ND	
		(2)	5	NA	100%+	100%+	Neg precipitin	100%+	
Cow dander	Agricultural workers	(3)	49	NA	100%	ND	Immunoblotting	ND	
Monkey dander	Laboratory workers	(4)	2	NA	2+	2+	ND	ND	
Deer dander	Farmer	(5)	1	NA	+	ND	ND	+	
Mink urine	Farmer	(6)	1	NA	+	–	ND	+	
Chicken	Poultry workers	(7,8)		NA	79%+	79%+	ND	1/1+	
Pig	Butcher	(9)	1	NA	ND	+	ND	ND	PEF
Frog	Frog catcher	(10)	1	NA	+	+	Neg precipitin	ND	
Lactoserum	Dairy industry	(11)	1	NA	+	ND	+Basophil degranulation	+	
Bovine serum albumin	Laboratory technician	(12)	1	NA	+	ND	ND	+	
Lactalbumin	Chocolate candy	(13)	1	NA	+	+	ND	+	+Conjunctival
Casein (cow's milk)	Tanner	(14)	1	NA	ND	+	ND	+	
Egg protein	Egg producers	(15)	188	7	34%+	29%+	ND	ND	PEF, 7%+
Endocrine glands	Pharmacist	(16)	1	NA	+	ND	ND	+	
Bat guano	Various	(17)	7	NA	+	+	RAST inhibition	ND	
Ivory dust	Ivory worker	(18)	1	NA	Neg	ND	ND	+	FEV$_1$ at work
Nacre dust	Nacre buttons	(19)	1	NA	+	ND	Neg precipitin	+	
Sericin	Hairdresser	(20)	2	NA	1/1+	ND	ND	ND	
Crustacea, seafoods, fish									
Crab	Snow-crab processors	(21)	303	16	22%+	ND	ND	72% of 46+	PEF, PC$_{20}$
Prawn	Prawn processors	(22)	50	36	26%+	16%+	ND	2/2+	

Allergen source	Occupation	Ref.	No. exposed	No. affected	Skin test	RAST/IgE	Other immunology	Challenge result	Challenge type
Hoya	Oyster farm	(23)	1413	29	82% of 511 with asthma+	89% of ~180 with asthma+	ND	ND	
Clam and shrimp	Food processors	(24)	2	4%	+	+	RAST inhibition	+	PC$_{20}$
Lobster and shrimp	Fishmonger shop	(25)	1	NA	+	+	ND	+	
Cuttle-fish	Deep-sea fishermen	(26)	66	Incidence of 1%/yr	ND	ND	ND	ND	
Cuttle-fish bone	Jewellery polisher	(27)	1	NA	+	ND	ND	+	
Salmon	Processing plant	(28)	291	24 (8%)	ND	15 (9%)	Spec IgG (33%)	ND	PEF
Trout (?)	Trout processors	(29)	5	NA	ND	100% neg	100%+	ND	
Shrimpmeal	Technician	(30)	1	NA	NA	+	ND	+	
Red soft coral	Fishermen	(31)	74	9	2/2+	ND	ND	ND	
Marine sponge	Laboratory grinder	(32)	1	NA	+	ND	Precipitins	ND	Asthma attack at work
Various fishes	Fish-processors	(33)	2	NA	+	+	ND	+	PEF
Anthropods									
Grain mite	Farmers	(34)	290	12	21%+	19% of 219+	ND	ND	
	Grain-store workers	(35)	133	33	25%+	23% of 128+	ND	1/1+	21% of 116 with +PC$_{20}$
Locust	Laboratory workers	(36)	118	26	32% of 113+	done	Specific IgG	ND	Reduced FEV$_1$
Screw worm fly	Flight crews	(37)	15	60	77%+	53%	RAST inhibition	ND	
Cricket	Laboratory workers	(38)	182	25	91% of 11+	ND	ND	ND	
Insect larvae	Fish bait breeder	(39)	2	NA	+	+	Passive transfer	+	
Moth, butterfly	Entomologists	(40)	14	NA	+	+	RAST inhibition	+	
Mexican bean weevil	Seed house	(41)	2	NA	+	ND	ND	ND	
		(42)	2	NA	+	ND	Passive transfer	ND	PEF
Fruit fly	Laboratory workers	(43)	22	32	27%+	27%+	RAST inhibition	21% of 14+	21% of 14+
Honeybee	Honey processors	(44)	1	NA	+	+	ND	+	
L. caesar larvae	Anglers	(45)	14	NA	13/14	13/14	RAST inhibition	7/7+	
Lesser mealworm	Entomologists	(46)	3	NA	Neg	100% of 3+	RAST inhibition	ND	
Mealworm larvae (Tenibrio molitor)	Fish bait handlers	(47)	5	NA	4/5	2/5	RAST inhibition	2/2	

685

Table 1 Continued

Agent	Occupation	Ref.	Subjects (n)	Prevalence (%)	Skin test	Specific IgE	Other immunological test	Broncho-provocation test	Other evidence
Fowl mite	Poultry workers	(48)	13	NA	77%+	60%	ND	1/1+	
Barn mite	Farmers	(49)	38	NA	100%+	~100%	ND	ND	
Mites and parasites	Flour handlers	(50)	12	NA	ND	+	ND	ND	
Acarian (Panonychus ulmi)	Apple growers	(51)	4	NA	+	ND	Neg precipitins	ND	
Tetranychus macdanieli	Vine growers	(52)	35	4/35 (11%)	100%	ND	ND	ND	
Tetranychus urticae	Farmers	(53)	16	16/46 (35%)	100%	100%	ND	ND	
Daphnia	Fish food store	(54)	2	NA	+	+	ND	2/2+	
Sheep blowfly	Technicians	(55)	53	24	ND	67% of 15+	ND	ND	
Grasshopper	Laboratory workers	(56)	16	4 (25%)	7 (44%)	ND	ND	+ in one	
Sewer fly (Psychoda alternata)	Sewage plant workers	(57)	1	NA	+	+	Histamine rel.; PK+	+	
Chironimid midges	Aquarists, fish food	(58)	225	45%	80%	34%	ND	ND	
Beetles (Coleoptera)	Museum curator	(59)	1	NA	+	ND	Passive transfer	ND	
Silkworm	Silk workers	(60)	53	34%	ND	ND	ND	ND	
Larva of silkworm	Sericulture	(61)	5519	0.2	100% of 9 (?)+	1/1 (?)+	P-K reaction	100% of 9+	
Fish feed (Echinodorus larva)	Aquarium keeper	(62)	1	NA	+	+	ND	+	
Arthropods	Technicians	(63)	3	23%	ND	+	ND	ND	
Ground bugs	Bottling	(64)	1	NA	+	+	ND	ND	PEF

								Workplace+	
Mold									
Dictyostelium discoideum (mold)	Technician	(65)	1	NA	+	+	ND	ND	
Aspergillus niger	Technicians	(66)	3	1%	3+	ND	ND	ND	
Aspergillus	Beet sugar workers	(67)	1	1%	+	+	ND	+	
Aspergillus alternaria	Baker	(68)	1	NA	+	ND	Neg precipitins	+	
Aspergillus alternaria	Baker	(69)	1	NA	+	ND	Neg precipitins	+	
Trichoderma koningii	Sawmill worker	(69)	1	NA	ND	ND	Precipitins specific IgG various	ND	PEF
Plasmopara viticola	Agricultural	(70)	1	NA	+	+	ND	+	
Neurospora	Plywood factory worker	(71)	1	NA	+	+	ND	+	
Chrysonilia sitophila	Logging worker	(72)	1	NA	+	+	ND	ND	PEF
Rhizopus nigricans	Coal miner	(73)	1	NA	+	+	+	+	
Algae									
Chlorella	Pharmacist	(74)	1	NA	+	ND	ND	+	PEF
Plants									
Grain dust	Grain elevators	(75)	610	~40	9%+	ND	Neg precipitins	ND	Spirometry pre-post shift FEV$_1$, volumes
		(76,77)	502	47	~50% of 51 exposed+	ND	ND	ND	
Wheat, rye and soya flour	Bakers, millers	(78)	22	NA	0%+	ND	Neg precipitins	27%+	50% PC$_{20}$+
		(79)	279	35	9%+ (cereals)	ND	ND	ND	FEV$_1$, PC$_{20}$
		(80)	7	100	100%+	100%+	100% neg	57%+	
		(81)	9	100	ND	100%+	Western blotting, etc.	ND	
Lathyrus sativus	Flour handler	(82)	1	NA	+	ND	+precipitins	+	
Lathyrus odoratus	Greenhouse worker	(83)	1	NA	+	+	ND	ND	PEF
Saccharomyces cerevisiae	Baker	(84)	1	NA	+	+	ND	+	PEF

Table 1 Continued

Agent	Occupation	Ref.	Subjects (n)	Prevalence (%)	Skin test	Specific IgE	Other immunological test	Broncho-provocation test	Other evidence
Vicia sativa	Farmer	(85)	1	NA	+	+	+Precipitins, passive transfer	+	
Buckwheat	Bakers	(86)	3	NA	100%+	ND	ND	ND	
Gluten	Bakers	(87)	1	NA	+	+	RAST inhibition	+	
Coffee bean	Food processor	(88)	372	34	24%+	12%+	ND	ND	Lung function
		(89)	45	9	9–40%+	ND	ND	ND	Spirometry
		(90)	22	NA	82%+	50%+	ND	67% of 12+	PC$_{20}$+ in 14
Castor bean	Oil industry	(91)	14	NA	100%+	100%+	ND	ND	
Green bean (*Phaseolus multiflorus*)	Homemaker	(92)	1	NA	+	+	Histamine	+	
Carob bean	Jam factory	(93)	1	NA	−	+	ND	+	
Tea	Tea processors	(94)	3	NA	+	+	+PCA with catechin	+	
Herbal tea	Herbal tea processors	(95)	1	NA	ND	neg	ND	+	Tobacco leaf
Tobacco manufacturers	Tobacco manufacturers	(96)	1	NA	+	+	ND	+	
Hops	Brewery chemist	(97)	16	69	ND	ND	ND	ND	PEF
Baby's breath (*Gypsophita paniculata*)	Florist	(98)	1	NA	+	ND	ND	ND	
		(99)	1	NA	+	+	Histamine release	+	
Freesia and paprika	Horticulture	(100)	2	NA	+	+	Histamine release	ND	
Amaryllis	Greenhouse worker	(101)	1	NA	+	+	ND	+	PEF
Limonium tataricum	Floral worker	(102)	1	NA	+	+	ND	ND	PEF
Decorative flowers	Floral worker	(103)	4	NA	+2/4	+2/4	ND	+3/4	

Substance	Occupation	Ref	No.				Immunoblotting	Neg (done 8 months later)	PEF
Spathe flowers	Floral worker	(104)	1	NA	+	+		+	
Herb material	Herbal worker	(105)	1	NA	+	+	Identification of 3 protein fractions	+	
Sarsaparilla root	Herbal tea worker	(106)	1	NA	+	+	ND	+	
Soybean lecithin	Bakers	(107)	2	NA	+	+	ND	+	
Olive oilcake	Oil industry	(108)	1	NA	ND	+	ND	+	
Brazil ginseng (*Pfaffia paniculata*)	Medicinal plant processor	(109)	1	NA	+	+	Neg precipitins	+	
Voacanga africana	Chemist's spouse	(110)	1	NA	+	+	Neg precipitins	+	
Onion	Homemakers	(111)	3	NA	+	+	ND	+	
Onion seeds *Allium cepa*, (red onion)	Seed packing	(112)	1	NA	+	+	Immunoblotting	+	
Fennel seed	Sausage processing	(113)	1	NA	ND	ND	Immunoblotting	ND	
Sesame seeds	Baker	(114)	1	NA	+	+	Immunoblotting	+	
Grass juice	Gardener	(115)	1	NA	+	+	Immunoblotting	+	
Potato	Housewives	(116)	2	NA	+	+	Histamine release	+	
Swiss chard (*Beta vulgaris* L. cycla)	Housewives	(117)	1	NA	+	+	Histamine release	+	
Mushroom	Mushroom soup processors	(118)	8	NA	+	ND	ND	50% of 8+	
Mushroom	Mushroom producers	(119)	1	NA	ND	+	Immunoblotting	ND	
Mushroom *Boletus edulis*	Office worker, cook / Hotel manager	(120)	3	NA	+	+	ND	2+	PEF
Cacoon seed	Decorator	(121)	1	NA	+	ND	ND	ND	
Chicory	Vegetable wholesaler	(122)	1	NA	+	+	Immunoblotting	ND	
Rose hips	Pharmaceutical	(123)	9	NA	67%+	67%+	ND	50% of 4+	
Sunflower	Laboratory worker	(124)	1	NA	+	+	RAST inhibition	+	
Phoenix canariensis	Gardener	(125)	1	NA	+	+	ND	+	

Table 1 Continued

Agent	Occupation	Ref.	Subjects (n)	Prevalence (%)	Skin test	Specific IgE	Other immunological test	Broncho-provocation test	Other evidence
Garlic dust	Food packaging	(126)	1	NA	+	+	ND	+	
		(127)	1	NA	+	+	RAST inhibition	+	
Spices	Spices processing	(128)	1	NA	+	+	ND	ND	
Saffron spice (*Crocus sativus*)	Saffron processors	(129)	5	10%	6%+	26%	Immunoblotting RAST inhibition	+in one	
Aromatic herbs	Butcher	(130)	1	NA	+	+	ND	+	PEF
Lycopodium	Powder	(131)	30	7	ND	ND	ND	2/2+	
Weeping fig	Plant keepers	(132)	84	7	21%+	21%	ND	100% of 6+	PC$_{20}$
Pectin	Christmas candy maker	(133)	1	NA	+	−	Specific IgG4	+	
Henna (conchiolin?)	Hairdressers	(134)	2	NA	+	+	ND	1/2+	
Fenugreek	Food industry	(135)	1	NA	+	+	ND	ND	
Aniseed	Food industry	(136)	1	NA	+	+	ND	+	
Kapok	Sewer	(137)	1	NA	−	−	ND	+	Lung function
Latex	Glove manuf.	(138)	81	6	11%+	ND	ND	ND	PEF
	Health professionals	(139)	72.5%	4.7%+	ND	ND	+	ND	
Biological enzymes									
B. subtilis	Detergent industry	(140)	1642	3.2 (over 7 years)	4.5–75%+	26% of 248+	ND	ND	Lung function
		(141)	38	NA	66%+	ND	Passive transfer 100% of 5+ precipitin (nonspecific)	90%+	Lung function
Trypsin	Plastic, pharmaceutical	(142)	14	29	+	+	ND	75% of 4+	
Papain	Pharmaceutical	(143)	29	45	34%+	34%+	ND	89% of 9+	

Allergen	Occupation	Ref.	No.						Lung function
Pepsin	Pharmaceutical	(144)	1	NA	+	+	ND	+	
Pancreatin	Pharmaceutical	(145)	14	NA	93%+	100% of 3+	ND	ND	100% of 8+
Flaviastase	Pharmaceutical	(146)	3	NA	25%+	+	+Precipitin	ND	
Bromelin	Pharmaceutical	(147)	76	11	+	ND	ND	ND	2/2+ (PEF)
	Pharmaceutical	(148)	2	NA	+	ND	ND	ND	
Egg lysozyme	Pharmaceutical	(149)	1	NA		+	ND	+	
Fungal amylase	Bakers	(150)	118	NA	100% of 10+	2% exposed +34% occup. asthma+	ND	ND	
Fungal amylo-glucosidase and hemicellulase	Bakers	(151)	1	NA	+	+	ND	+	
Bakers		(152)	140	NA	ND	5–24%	ND	ND	
Serratial peptidase and lysozyme	Pharmaceutical	(153)	1	NA	ND	+	Immunoblotting +		
Esperase	Detergent industry	(154)	667	NA	ND	5%	ND	ND	
Xylanase	Laboratory workers	(155)	2	NA	2	2	ND	ND	+ (PFR)
Pectinase	Enzyme factory	(156)	1	NA	1	Neg	ND	+	
Lactase	Pharmaceutical	(157)	207	4%	31%+	ND	ND	ND	
Vegetable Gums Acacia	Printers	(158)	63	19% of 31 (selection)	ND	ND	ND	ND	
		(159)	10	NA	+	ND	Passive transfer (3+)	ND	
Tragacanth	Gum importer	(160)	1	NA	+	ND	ND	ND	
Karaya	Hairdressers	(161)	9	4	+	ND	Passive transfer	ND	
Guar	Carpet manufacturing	(162)	2	162	5%+	8%+	ND	ND	67% of 3+ (PC$_{20}$)
Gutta-percha	Dental hygienist	(163)	1	NA	+	ND	ND	ND	

NA = not applicable; ND = not done; Neg = negative. The number of subjects tested is not specified if it included all subjects; otherwise it is mentioned.
PCA = Passive cutaneous anaphylaxis.

Table 2 Low-Molecular-Weight Agents Causing Occupational Asthma

Agent	Occupation	Ref.	Subjects (n)	Prevalence (%)	Skin test	Specific IgE	Other immunological test	Broncho provocation test	Other evidence
Diisocyanates									
Toluene diisocyanate	Polyurethane	(164)	112	12.5	3%+	0%+	0%+ PCA	45% of 11+	
	Plastics, varnish	(165)	26	NA	ND	19%+	ND	100%+	
		(166)	195	28	ND	5%+	ND	70% of 17+	Specific IgG
		(167)	91	NA	NA	ND	0%+	ND	
		(168)	162[a]	NA	ND	ND	ND	57%+	
Diphenylmethane diisocyanate	Foundry	(169)	11	NA	ND	27%+	36%+	54.5%+	
		(170)	76	13	ND	3%+	7%+ Specific IgG	ND	
		(171)	26	27	4%+	4%+	15%+ Specific IgG	ND	
1,5 Naphthylene diisocyanate	Manuf. rubber	(172)	3	NA	ND	ND	ND	100%+	
Isophorone diisocyanate	Spray painter	(173)	1	NA	ND	ND	ND	+	
Prepolymers of TDI	Floor varnisher	(174)	2	NA	ND	0%+	Specific IgG−	+	
Prepolymers of HDI	Spray painter	(175)	9	45	ND	33%+	56%+	+	
Combination of diisocyanates									
TDI,MDI,HDI,PPI	Paint shop	(176)	51	11.8[b]	ND	ND	ND	60% of 10+ to PPI; 70%+ to TDI; 33%+ to MDI; 33% of 9+ to HDI	
TDI,MDI,HDI	Various indust.	(177)	24	NA	ND	ND	ND		
		(178)	247[†]	NA	60% of 53+ 14%+	ND	ND	ND	
	Paint shop	(179)	62	NA	ND	15%+	47%+ Specific IgG	6%+ to TDI; 16% to MDI; 24% to HDI	

Agent	Use	Ref	N						
TDI,MDI		(180)	28	NA	ND	27% of 22+ TDI-HSA 83% of 6+ MDI-HSA	ND	100%+	
Other hardeners									
Triglycidyl isocyanate	Powder paints	(181)	1	NA	ND	ND	ND	+	
Polyfunctional aziridine	Hardener in paints	(182)	7	NA	33% of 7	ND	ND	+in 7	
Anhydrides									
Phthalic anhydride	Plastics	(183)	1	NA	+	+	ND	+	
	Toolsetter, resin plant agent	(184)	3	NA	ND	ND	ND	100%+	
	Production of resins	(185)	118	28	18% of 11+	ND	ND		
		(186)	60	14	ND	7%+	17%+ Specific IgG	ND	
Trimellitic anhydride	Epoxy resins, plastics	(187)	4	NA	100%+	75%+	100%+	100% of 1+	
Tetrachlorophthalic anhydride	Epoxy resins, plastics	(188)	5	NA	ND	ND	ND	100%+	
Pyromellitic dianhydride	Epoxy adhesive	(189)	7	NA	100%+	100%+	ND	100%+	
		(190)	7	NA	ND	ND	ND	30%+	
Methyl tetrahydrophthalic anhydride (MTHPA)	Curing agent	(191)	1	NA	+	+	–Specific IgG	ND	Improvement with removal
Hexahydrophthalic anhydride	Chemical worker	(192)	1	NA	ND	ND	ND	+	
MTHPA + HHPA	Electrical Plant	(193)	109	5.4	ND	15.4%	ND	6/17	PEF
Himic anhydride	Manufacture of flame retardant	(194)	20	35	ND	40% of 7+	RAST inhibition	ND	

Table 2 Continued

Agent	Occupation	Ref.	Subjects (n)	Prevalence (%)	Skin test	Specific IgE	Other immunological test	Broncho provocation test	Other evidence
Maleicanhydrice	Polyester resin production	(195)	1	NA	ND	ND	ND	+	
Aliphatic amines									
Ethyleneamines									
Ethylene diamine	Shellac handler	(196)	7	NA	100%+	ND	ND	100%+	
	Photography	(197)	1	NA	ND	ND	ND	+	
Hexamethylene tetramine	Lacquer handlers	(196)	7	NA	100%+	ND	ND	100%+	
Aliphatic polyamines	Chemical factory	(198)	12	4/12	ND	ND	ND	100% of 2+	
Triethylene tetramine	Aircraft filter	(184)	1	NA	ND	ND	ND	+	
Mixture of trimethyl-1,6-hexanediamine and isophorondiamine	Floor-covering material salesman	(199)	1	NA	–	ND	ND	+	BAL
Ethanolamines									
Monoethanolamine	Beauty culture	(196)	10	100%+	ND	ND	ND	100%+	
Triethanolamine	Metal worker	(200)	3	2	NA	ND	ND	ND	100% of 2+
Aminoethylethanol-amine	Soldering	(201)	3	NA	ND	ND	ND	100%+	
	Cable jointer	(202)	2	NA	ND	ND	ND	+	
Dimethylethanol-amine	Spray paint	(203)	1	NA	–	ND	ND	+	
Other									
3-(Dimethylamino)-propylamine (3-DMAPA)	Ski manufacture	(204)	34	11.7	ND	ND	ND	ND	Cross-shift
Heterocyclic amines									
Piperazine hydrochloride	Chemist	(205)	2	NA	50%+	ND	ND	100%	

Agent / Occupation	Ref	n						Questionnaire
							PC$_{20}$ / Improvement on removal	
Pharmaceutical	(206)	131	11.4	ND	ND	ND		100% of 1+
Chemical plant	(207)	2	NA	50%+	100%+	ND		ND
	(208)	48	16.6^c	ND	ND	ND		ND
N-Methylmorpholine								
Aromatic amines								
Paraphenylene diamine	(209)	80	37.0	66%+	ND	ND		74%+
Quarternary amine Cleaning product	(210)	1	NA	+	ND	ND		+
(benzalkonium) Manufacture cleaning products	(211)	1	NA	ND	–	ND		+
Mixture of Amines								
EPO 60 Mold maker	(212)	1	NA	ND	ND	ND		+
Fluxes								
Colophony Electronic worker	(213)	34	NA	ND	ND	ND		100%+
Manufacture solder flux	(214)	68 low	4	ND	ND	ND		ND
		14 med	21	ND	ND	ND		ND
		6 high	21	ND	ND	ND		ND
Zinc chloride and ammonium chloride flux Metal jointing	(215)	2	NA	ND	ND	ND		+
95% Alkylarul polyether alcohol +5% polypropylene glycol Electronic assembler	(216)	1	NA	ND	ND	ND		+
Wood dust or bark								
Western red cedar (*Thuja plicata*) Carpentry	(217)	35	NA	ND	ND	ND		ND
Furniture making	(218)	1320	3.4	1.9%+	ND	ND		ND
Cabinet making, carpentry	(219)	22		100%–	ND	100%– Precipitin		82%+
Sawmill	(220)	185		100%–	ND	ND		100%+
	(221)	652	4.1	100%–	ND	ND		ND

695

Table 2 Continued

Agent	Occupation	Ref.	Subjects (n)	Prevalence (%)	Skin test	Specific IgE	Other immunological test	Broncho provocation test	Other evidence
Eastern white cedar (*Thuja occidentalis*)	Sawmill	(222)	3	4–7%	ND	ND	ND	+	PC_{20}
California redwood	Wood carvers	(223)	2	NA	–	ND	– Precipitin	+	+
(*Sequoia sempervirens*)	Carpenter	(224)	1	NA	ND	ND	ND	ND	
Cedar of Lebanon (*Cedra libani*)		(225)	6	NA	17%+	ND	100%– Precipitin	ND	
Cocabolla (*Dalbergia retusa*)		(226)	3	NA	100%–	ND	ND	ND	Improvement on removal
Iroko (*Chlorophora excelsa*)		(227)	1	NA	+	ND	+ Precipitin	+	
Oak (*Quercus robur*)	Carpenter	(228)	1	NA	ND	ND	ND	+	
		(229)	1	NA	–	ND	+ Precipitin	+	
		(230)	3	NA	–	ND	+	+	
Mahogany (*Shoreal sp*)		(229)	1	NA	–	ND	+ Precipitin	+	
Abiruana (*Pouteria*)		(231)	2	NA	+	ND	– Precipitin	+	
African maple (*Triplochiton scleroxylon*)		(232)	2	NA	+	+	+ Precipitin Passive transfer	+	
Sauna builder		(233)	2	NA	100%+	100%+	+	100%+	
(*Tanganyika aningre*)		(234)	3	NA	100%+ Precipitin	100%–	100%–	100%+	
Mukali (*Angineria robusta*)		(235)	1	NA	+	+	ND	+	+

Name	Occupation	Ref	n					Precipitin
Central American walnut (*Juglans olanchana*)		(236)	1	NA	−	−	−	+
Kejaat (*Pterocarpus angolensis*)		(237)	1	NA	+	ND	ND	ND
African Zebrawood (*Microberlinia*)		(238)	1	NA	+	+	ND	+
Ramin (*Gonystylus bancanus*)	Woodworker	(239)	2	NA	+	+	ND	+
Quillaja bark	Saponin factory	(240)	1	NA	ND	+	ND	+
Fernambouc (*Caesalpinia echinata*)	Bow making	(241)	36	33.3	100%−	ND	ND	100% of 1+
Ash (*Fraxinus americana*)	Sawmill	(242)	1	NA	−	−	ND	+
Ash (*Fraxinus excelsior*)	Furniture	(243)	1	NA	−	+	ND	+
Pau marfim (*Balfourodendron riedelianum*)	Woodworker	(244)	1	NA	+	+	ND	+
Capreuva (*Myyrocarpus fastigiatus* Fr. All.)	Parquet floor layer	(245)	1	NA	ND	ND	ND	+
Ebony wood (*Diospyros crassiflora*)		(246)	1	NA	−	ND	ND	+
Kotibe wood (*Nesorgordonia papverifera*)		(247)	1	NA	+	ND	Passive transfer	+
Cinnamon (*Cinnamomum zeylanicum*)		(248)	40	22.5	ND	ND	ND	100% of 1+
Imbuia (Brazilian walnut)	Furniture	(249)	1	NA	ND	ND	+	+
							Precipitin	

Table 2 Continued

Agent	Occupation	Ref.	Subjects (n)	Prevalence (%)	Skin test	Specific IgE	Other immunological test	Broncho provocation test	Other evidence
Unidentified agent	Sawmills of Eastern Canada and USA	(250)	11	NA	ND	ND	ND	+	PEF
Metals									
Platinum	Platinum refinery	(252)	136	29	17%+	21%+	ND	ND	
Nickel	Metal plating	(253)	1	NA	+	ND	− Precipitin	+	
		(254)	1	NA	+	ND	− Precipitin	+	
		(255)	1	NA	+	+	ND	+	
Cobalt	Hard metal grinder	(256)	4	NA	25%+	ND	ND	50%+	
	Diamond polisher	(257)	3	NA	ND	ND	ND	100%+	
Zinc fumes	Solderer	(258)	2	NA	ND	ND	ND	+	
	Locksmith	(259)	1	NA	ND	ND	ND	+	
Tungsten carbide	Grinder	(260)	1	NA	ND	ND	ND	ND	Recovery on removal
Chromium	Printer	(261)	1	NA	+	ND	ND	ND	
	Plater	(262)	1	NA	+	ND	ND	ND	
	Various	(263)	4	NA	+	ND	ND	+	
Chromium and nickel	Welder	(264)	5	NA	ND	ND	ND	100% of 2+	
	Tanning	(265)	1	NA	−	+	ND	+	
	Electroplating	(266)	7	NA	Cr 29%+ Ni 57%+	ND	ND	Cr 100% of 7 Ni 40% of 5	
Cobalt and nickel		(267)	8	NA	75%+ cobalt 62%+ nickel	62%+ cobalt 50%+ nickel	ND ND	100%+ to both cobalt and nickel	

Drugs

Drug	Occupation	Ref					Passive transfer / –Specific IgG	PEF / Improvement off work / Pre-post shift / FEV₁
Penicillins and ampicillin	Pharmaceutical	(268)	4	NA	100%–	ND	ND	75%+
Penicillamine	Pharmaceutical	(269)	1	NA	ND	–	ND	+
Caphalosporins	Pharmaceutical	(270)	2	NA	+	ND	ND	+
	Pharmaceutical	(271)	91	8	71%+	ND	ND	ND
Phenylglycine acid chloride	Pharmaceutical	(272)	24	29	37%+	37%+	ND	100% of 2+
Psyllium	Laxative manuf.	(273)	3	NA	100%+	ND	ND	60%+
Pharmaceutical		(274)	130	4*	19% of 120+	26% of 118+	ND	27% of 18+
	Nurse	(275)	5	NA	80%+	100%+	ND	100%+
	Health personnel	(276)	193	4*	3%+	12% of 162+	ND	26% of 15+
Methyldopa	Pharmaceutical	(277)	1	NA	–	ND	ND	+
Spiramycin	Pharmaceutical	(278)	1	NA	+	ND	ND	+
	Pharmaceutical	(279)	51	8*	100%–	ND	ND	25% of 12+
Salbutamol intermediate	Pharmaceutical	(280)	2	NA	ND	–	ND	+
	Pharmaceutical	(281)	1	NA	–	ND	ND	+
Amprolium	Poultry feed mixer	(282)	1	NA	ND	ND	ND	+
Tetracycline	Pharmaceutical	(283)	1	NA	ND	ND	ND	+
Isonicotinic acid hydrazide	Hospital pharmacy	(284)	1	NA	+	+	ND	+
Hydralazine	Pharmaceutical	(285)	1	NA	–	–	–Specific IgG	+
Tylosin tartrate	Pharmaceutical	(286)	1	NA	ND	ND	ND	+
Ipecacuanha	Pharmaceutical	(287)	42	48	52% of 19+	66% of 18+	ND	25%+
Cimetidine	Pharmaceutical	(288)	4	NA	ND	ND	ND	ND
Piperacillin	Pharmaceutical	(289)	1	NA	+	ND	ND	+
Ceftazidime	Pharmaceutical	(290)	1	NA	ND	ND	ND	+
Opiate compounds	Pharmaceutical	(291)	39	26	+	+	ND	ND
	Pharmaceutical	(292)	4	14	+	+	ND	+
Amoxicillin	Pharmaceutical	(293)	1	NA	–	–	ND	mpl

Table 2 Continued

Agent	Occupation	Ref.	Subjects (n)	Prevalence (%)	Skin test	Specific IgE	Other immunological test	Broncho provocation test	Other evidence
Reactive dyes									
Reactive dyes	Reactive dyes manufacture	(294)	309	25	7%+ orange 8%+ black	17%+ orange 17%+ black	ND	65% of 20+	
	Wool dye house	(295)	6	NA	ND	83%+	100%+	ND	
	Textile dyehouse	(296)	162	NA	NA	80% of 5+	ND	ND	
Levafix brilliant yellow E36	Prep. dye solution	(297)	1	NA	+	ND	ND	+	
Drimaren brilliant yellow K-3GL	Textile industry	(298)	1	NA	+	ND	ND	+	
Black henna (*Indigofera argentea*)	Herbal shop sales	(299)	1	NA	+	+	ND	ND	PEF monitoring+
FD&C blue dye #2	Food industry	(300)	1	NA	−	−	ND	+	
Cibachrome brilliant scarlet 32	Textile industry	(298)	1	NA	+	ND	ND	+	
Drimaren brilliant blue K-BL	Textile industry	(298)	1	NA	+	ND	ND	+	
Lanasol yellow 4G	Dyer	(298)	1	NA	+	ND	ND	+	
Carmine	Dye manufacture	(298)	10	NA	30%+	30%+	ND	100% of 1	
Biocides									
Hexachlorophene (sterilizing agent)	Hospital staff	(302)	1	NA	ND	ND	ND	+	
Chlorhexidine	Nurse	(303)	2	NA	ND	ND	ND	+	
Glutaraldehyde	Hospital endoscopy unit	(304)	9	89	ND	ND	ND	ND	Questionnaire

Agent	Occupation	Ref							
Chloramine T	Endoscopy and radiology	(305)	8	NA	ND	ND	ND	7/8+	PEF monitoring
	Chemical manuf.	(306)	6	NA	100%+	ND	66%+ Passive transfer	ND	
	Brewery	(307)	7	NA	100%+	ND	ND	ND	Recovery with removal
	Janitor, cleaning	(308)	5	NA	100% of 4+	ND	ND	100% of 3+	
Lauryl dimethyl benzyl ammonium chloride	Pharmacist	(309)	1	NA	ND	ND	ND	+	PEF
Isothiazolinono	Chemical plant	(310)	1	NA	ND	ND	ND	+(workplace)	
Fungicides									
Tetracholoro-isophthalonitrile	Farmer	(311)	1	NA	ND	–	+Patch test	+	FEV$_1$ recording at work
Tributyl tin oxide technician	Venipuncutre	(312)	1	NA	–	ND	ND	+	
Captafol	Chemical manuf.	(313)	1	NA	ND	–	ND	+	
Chemicals									
Polyvinyl chloride	Meat wrapper Fumes	(314)	96	69	ND	ND	ND	27% of 11+	History only
	Meat wrapper	(315)	3	NA	ND	ND	ND	ND	PEF
	Manuf. bottle caps Powder	(316)	1	NA	ND	ND	ND	+	
Organic phosphate insecticides	Chemical packaging plant	(317)	1	NA	ND	ND	ND	ND	History only
Persulfate salts and henna	Hairdressing	(318)	2	NA	+	ND	ND	+	
	Hairdressing	(319)	2	NA	+	ND	ND	+	
	Hairdressing	(320)	23	17	4%+	ND	ND	100% of 4+	
	Hairdressing	(321)	1	NA	–	ND	ND	+	
	Hairdressing	(322)	1	NA	ND	ND	ND	+	

Table 2 Continued

Agent	Occupation	Ref.	Subjects (n)	Prevalence (%)	Skin test	Specific IgE	Other immunological test	Broncho provocation test	Other evidence
Diazonium salt	Manuf. of photocopy paper	(323)	1	NA	ND	ND	ND	+	
	Manuf. of fluorine polymer precursor	(324)	45	56	ND	20%+	ND	100% of 2	
Urea formaldehyde	Resin	(325)	2	NA	–	ND	ND	+	
	Resin	(326)	3	NA	ND	ND	ND	100% of 3+	
	Manuf. of foam	(327)	1	NA	ND	ND	ND	+	
Freon	Refrigeration	(328)	1	NA	ND	ND	ND	+	
Furfuryl alcohol (furan-based resin)	Foundry mold making	(329)	1	NA	ND	ND	ND	+	
Styrene	Plastics factory	(330)	2	NA	–	ND	ND	+	
Aziridine	Various	(331)	7	NA	+in 4	ND	ND	+in 7	
Azobisformamide	Plastics, rubber	(332)	151	18.5	ND	ND	ND	ND	Removal with improvement
	Plastic	(333)	2	NA	ND	ND	ND	+	
	Plastics	(334)	4	NA	ND	ND	ND	100% of 2+	
Iso-nonanyl oxybenzene sulfonate	Lab. technician	(335)	1	NA	ND	ND	ND	+	
Tetrazene	Detonator manuf.	(336)	1	NA	ND	ND	ND	+	PEF
Polyethylene	Paper Packer	(337)	1	NA	ND	ND	ND	+	PEF
Tall oil (pine resin)	Rubber tyre manufacturer	(338)	1	NA	–	ND	–Patch test	+	PEF

Agent	Occupation	Ref.	N						Comment
Sulfites	Water plant	(339)	1	NA	–	ND	ND	oral +	
Polypropylene	Food processor	(340)	1	NA	ND	ND	ND	+	
	Bag manufacturer	(341)	1	NA	ND	ND	ND	+	PEF
Polyester	Painter	(342)	1	NA	ND	ND	ND	+	
Glacial acetic acid	Picking	(343)	1	NA	ND	ND	+	ND	Alveolitis
Metabisulfite	Agriculture producer	(344)	1	NA	ND	ND	ND	ND	
Ninhydrin	Laboratory worker	(345)	1	NA	ND	ND	ND	+	PEF
Health care									
Ethylene dioxide	Nurse	(346)	1	NA	ND	+	ND	+	Changes in PC_{20}
Enflurane	Hospital staff	(347)	1	NA	ND	ND	ND	+	
Methyl blue	Hospital staff	(348)	1	NA	ND	ND	ND	+	
Terpene	Hospital staff	(349)	1	NA	ND	ND	ND	+	
Radiographic fixative	Hospital staff	(350)	1	NA	ND	ND	ND	+	
Sulfathiazoles	Hospital staff	(351)	2	NA	–	ND	ND	+	
Formaldehyde	Hospital staff	(352)	28	29[b]	ND	ND	ND	50% of 4+	
	Different indust.	(353)	15	NA	ND	ND	ND	60%+	
		(354)	230	5	ND	ND	ND	5%+	
Methyl methacrylate and cyanocrylates	Adhesive	(355)	7	NA	ND	ND	ND	86%+	PEF 14%+
	Nurse	(356)	1	NA	ND	ND	ND	+	
	Glue	(357)	1	NA	ND	ND	ND	+	PEF monitoring
Synthetic material									
Plexiglass	Factory	(358)	1	NA	ND	ND	ND	+	Pre-post change in FEV_1
Tooth enamel dust	Dentist	(359)	1	NA	ND	ND	ND	ND	
ECG ink	Laboratory nurse	(360)	1	NA	+	ND	ND	+	

Table 2 Continued

Agent	Occupation	Ref.	Subjects (n)	Prevalence (%)	Skin test	Specific IgE	Other immunological test	Broncho provocation test	Other evidence
Unidentified									
(?)	Resp. therapist	(361)	194	19	ND	ND	ND	ND	Questionnaire
(?)	Mineral analysis laboratory	(362)	21	24[c]	ND	ND	ND	ND	Questionnaire PC$_{20}$
(?) Oil mists	Toolsetter	(363)	1	NA	ND	ND	ND	+	PEF recording
(?) Fluorine	Potroom	(364)	52	NA	ND	ND	ND	ND	History
(?) Aluminum	Potroom	(365)	227	7	ND	ND	ND	ND	Questionnaire
	Potroom	(366)	35	NA	ND	ND	ND	ND	History
	Potroom	(367)	57	NA	ND	ND	ND	ND	History
	Potroom	(368)	1	NA	ND	ND	ND	+	PEF monitoring
(?) Pulverized fuel ash	Power station attendant	(369)	1	NA	ND	ND	ND	+	PEF monitoring

[a]Subjects with symptoms.
[b]Based on challenge data.
[c]Presence of bronchial hyperresponsiveness.

NA = not applicable, ND = not done; Neg = negative; the number of subjects tested is not specified if it included all subjects; otherwise it is mentioned; PCA = Passive cutaneous anaphylaxis; PPI = polymethylene polyphenylisocyanate. All proportions including 3 or more as the denominator are expressed as %.

REFERENCES

1. Venables KM, Tee RD, Hawkins ER, Gordon DJ, Wale CJ, Farrer NM, Lam TH, Baxter PJ, Newman Taylor AJ. Laboratory animal allergy in a pharmaceutical company. Br J Ind Med 1988; 45:660–666.
2. Newman Taylor A, Longbottom JL, Pepys J. Respiratory allergy to urine proteins of rats and mice. Lancet 1977; 847–849.
3. Mäntyjärvi J Ylönen R, Taivainen A, Virtanen T. IgG and IgE antibody responses to cow dander and urine in farmers with cow-induced asthma. Clin Exp Allergy 1992; 22:83–90.
4. Petry RW, Voss MJ, Kroutil LA, Crowley W, Bush RK, Busse WW. Monkey dander asthma. J Allergy Clin Immunol 1985; 75:268–271.
5. Nahm DH, Park JW, Hong CS. Occupational asthma due to deer dander. Ann Allergy Asthma Immunol 1996; 76:423–426.
6. Gomez I Jinénez, Anton E, Picans I, Jerez J, Obispo T. Occupational asthma caused by mink urine. Allergy 1996; 51:364–365.
7. Bar-Sela S, Teichtahl H, Lutsky I. Occupational asthma in poultry workers. J Allergy Clin Immunol 1984; 73:271–275.
8. Lutsky I, Teichtahl H, Bar-Sela S. Occupational asthma due to poultry mites. J Allergy Clin Immunol 1984; 73:56–60.
9. Brennan NJ. Pig Butcher's asthma—case report and review of the literature. Irish Med J 1985; 78:321–322.
10. Armentia A, Martin-Santos J, Subiza J, Pla J, Zapata C, Valdivieso R, Losada E. Occupational asthma due to frogs. Ann Allergy 1988; 60:209–210.
11. Moneret-Vautrin DA, Pupil P, Courtine D, Grilliat JP. Asthme professionnel aux protéines du lactosérum. Rev Fr Allergol 1984; 24:93–95.
12. Joliat TL, Weber RW. Occupational asthma and rhinoconjunctivitis from inhalation of crystalline bovine serum albumin powder. Ann Allergy 1991; 66:301–304.
13. Bernaola G, Echechipia S, Urrutia I, Fernandez E, Audicana M, Corres L Fernandez de. Occupational asthma and rhinoconjunctivitis from inhalation of dried cow's milk caused by sensitization to alpha-lactalbumin. Allergy 1994; 49:189–191.
14. Olaguibel JM, Hernandez D, Morales P, Peris A, Basomba A. Occupational asthma caused by inhalation of casein. Allergy 1990; 45:306–308.
15. Smith A Blair, Bernstein DI, London MA, Gallagher J, Ornella GA, Gelletly SK, Wallingford D, Newman MA. Evaluation of occupational asthma from airborne egg protein exposure in multiple settings. Chest 1990; 98:398–404.
16. Breton JL, Leneutre F, Esculpavit G, Abourjaili M. Une nouvelle cause d'asthme professionnel chez un préparateur en pharmacie. Presse Méd 1989; 18:433.
17. El-Ansary EH, Gordon DJ, Tee RD, Newman Taylor AJ. Respiratory allergy to inhaled bat guano. Lancet 1987; 1:316–318.
18. Armstrong RA, Neill P, Mossop RT. Asthma induced by ivory dust: a new occupational cause. Thorax 1988; 43:737–738.
19. Zedda S. A case of bronchial asthma from inhalation of nacre dust. Med Lav 1967; 58:459–464.
20. Charpin J, Blanc M. Une cause nouvelle d'allergie professionnelle chez les coiffeuses: l'allergie à la séricine. Marseille Méd 1967; 104:169–170.
21. Cartier A, Malo J-L, Forest F, Lafrance M, Pineau L, St-Aubin J-J, Dubois J-Y. Occupational asthma in snow crab-processing workers. J Allergy Clin Immunol 1984; 74:261–269.
22. Gaddie J, Legge JS, Friend JAR, Reid TMS. Pulmonary hypersensitivity in prawn workers. Lancet 1980; 2:1350–1353.
23. Jyo T, Kohmoto K, Katsutani T, Otsuka T, Oka SD, Mitsui S, Hoya (Sea-squirt) asthma. In: Occupational Asthma. London: Von Nostrand Reinhold, 1980:209–228.
24. Desjardins A, Malo JL, L'Archevêque J, Cartier A, McCants M, Lehrer SB. Occupational IgE-mediated sensitization and asthma due to clam and shrimp. J Allergy Clin Immunol 1995; 96:608–617.

25. Lemière C, Desjardins A, Lehrer S, Malo JL. Occupational asthma to lobster and shrimp. Allergy 1996; 51:272–273.
26. Tomaszunas S, Weclawik Z, Lewinski M. Allergic reactions to cuttlefish in deep-sea fishermen. Lancet 1988; 1:1116–1117.
27. Baltrami V, Innocenti A, Pieroni MG, Civai R, Nesi D, Bianco S. Occupational asthma due to cuttle-fish bone dust. Med Lav 1989; 80:425–428.
28. Douglas JDM, McSharry C, Blaikie L, Morrow T, Miles S, Franklin D. Occupational asthma caused by automated salmon processing. Lancet 1995; 346:737–740.
29. Sherson D, Hansen I, Sigsgaard T. Occupationally related respiratory symptoms in trout-processing workers. Allergy 1989; 44:336–341.
30. Carino M, Elia G, Molinini R, Nuzzaco A, Ambrosi L. Shrimpmeal asthma in the aquaculture industry. Med Lav 1985; 76:471–475.
31. Onizuka R, Inoue K, Kamiya H. Red soft coral-induced allergic symptoms observed in spiny lobster fishermen. Aerugi 1990; 39:339–347.
32. Baldo BA, Krilis S, Taylor KM. IgE-mediated acute asthma following inhalation of a powdered marine sponge. Clin Allergy 1982; 12:179–186.
33. Rodriguez J, Reano M, vives R, Canto G, Daroca P, Crespo JF, Vila C, Villarreal O, Bensabat Z. Occupational asthma caused by fish inhalation. Allergy 1997; 52:866–869.
34. Cuthbert OD, Jeffrey IG, McNeill HB, Wood J, Topping MD. Barn allergy among Scottish farmers. Clin Allergy 1984; 14:197–206.
35. Blainey AD, Topping MD, Ollier S, Davies RJ. Allergic respiratory disease in grain workers: the role of storage mites. J Allergy Clin Immunol 1989; 84:296–303.
36. Burge PS, Edge G, O'Brien IM, Harries MG, Hawkins R, Pepys J. Occupational asthma in a research centre breeding locusts. Clin Allergy 1980; 10:355–363.
37. Tee RD, Gordon DJ, Hawkins ER, Nunn AJ, Lacey J, Venables KM, Cooter RJ, McCaffery AR, Taylor AJ Newman. Occupational allergy to locusts: an investigation of the sources of the allergen. J Allergy Clin Immunol 1988; 81:517–525.
38. Gibbons HL, Dille JR, Cowley RG. Inhalant allergy to the screwworm fly. Arch Environ Health 1965; 10:424–430.
39. Bagenstose AH, Mathews KP, Homburger HA, Saaveard-Delgado AP. Inhalant allergy due to crickets. J Allergy Clin Immunol 1980; 65:71–74.
40. Stevenson DD, Mathews KP. Occupational asthma following inhalation of moth particles. J Allergy 1967; 39:274–283.
41. Randolph H. Allergic reaction to dust of insect origin. JAMA 1934; 103:560–562.
42. Wittich FW. Allergic rhinitis and asthma due to sensitization to the mexican bean weevil (*Zabrotes subfasciatus boh.*). J Allergy 1940; 12:42–45.
43. Spieksma FTM, Vooren PH, Kramps JA, Dijkman JH. Respiratory allergy to laboratory fruit flies (*Drosophila melanogaster*). J Allergy Clin Immunol 1986; 77:108–113.
44. Ostrom NK, Swanson MC, Agarwal MK, Yuninger JW. Occupational allergy to honeybee-body dust in a honey-processing plant. J Allergy Clin Immunol 1986; 77:736–740.
45. Siracusa A, Bettini P, Bacoccoli R, Severini C, Verga A, Abbritti G. Asthma caused by live fish bait. J Allergy Clin Immunol 1994; 93:424–430.
46. Schroeckenstein DC, Meier-Davis S, Graziano FM, Falomo A, Bush RK. Occupational sensitivity to *Alphitobius diaperinus* (Panzer) (lesser mealworm). J Allergy Clin Immunol 1988; 82:1081–1088.
47. Bernstein DI, Gallagher JS, Bernstein IL. Mealworm asthma: clinical and immunologic studies. J Allergy Clin Immunol 1983; 72:475–480.
48. Lutsky I, Bar-Sela S. Northern fowl mite (*Ornithonyssus sylviarum*) in occupational asthma of poultry workers. Lancet 1982; 2:874–875.
49. Cuthbert OD, Brostoff J, Wraith DG, Brighton WD. "Barn allergy": asthma and rhinitis due to storage mites. Clin Allergy 1979; 9:229–236.
50. Granel-Tena C, Cistero-Bahima A, Olive-Perez A. Allergens in asthma and baker's rhinitis. Alergia 1985; 32:69–73.

51. Michel FB, Guin JJ, Seignalet C, Rambier A, Martier JC, Caula F, Laveil G. Allergie à Panonychus ulmi (Koch). Rev Franç Allergol 1977; 17:93–97.

52. Carbonnelle M, Lavaud F, Bailly R. Les acariens de la vigne sont-ils susceptibles de provoquer une allergie respiratoire? Rev Fr Allergol 1986; 26:171–178.

53. Astarita C, Franzese A, Scala G, Sproviero S, Raucci G. Farm workers' occupational allergy to *Tetranychus urticae*: clinical and immunologic aspects. Allergy 1994; 49:466–471.

54. Meister W. Professional asthma owing to Daphnia-allergy. Allerg Immunol (Leipz) 1978; 24: 191–193.

55. Kaufman GL, Gandevia BH, Bellas TE, Tovey ER, Baldo BA. Occupational allergy in an entomological research centre. I. Clinical aspects of reactions to the sheep blowfly *Lucilia cuprina*. Br J Ind Med 1989; 46:473–478.

56. Soparkar GR, Patel PC, Cockcroft DW. Inhalant atopic sensitivity to grasshoppers in research laboratories. J Allergy Clin Immunol 1993; 92:61–65.

57. Gold BL, Mathews KP, Burge HA. Occupational asthma caused by sewer flies. Am Rev Respir Dis 1985; 131:949–952.

58. Liebers V, Hoernstein M, Baur X. Humoral immune response to the insect allergen Chi t I in aquarists and fish-food factory workers. Allergy 1993; 48:236–239.

59. Sheldon JM, Johnston JH. Hypersensitivity to beetles (Coleoptera). J Allergy 1941; 12: 493–494.

60. Uragoda CG, Wijekoon PMB. Asthma in silk workers. J Soc Occup Med 1991; 41:140–142.

61. Kobayashi S. Different aspects of occupational asthma in Japan. In: Frazier CA, ed. Occupational Asthma. New York: Van Nostrand Reinhold, 1980; 229–244.

62. Resta O. Foschino-Barbaro MP, Carnimeo N, Napoli PL Di, Pavese I, Schino P. Occupational asthma from fish-feed. Med Lavoro 1982; 3:234–236.

63. Lugo G, Cipolla C, Bonfiglioli R, Sassi C, Maini S, Cancellieri MP, Raffi GB, Pisi E. A new risk of occupational disease: allergic asthma and rhinoconjunctivitis in persons working with beneficial arthropods. Int Arch Occup Environ Health 1994; 65:291–294.

64. Lazaro MA Garcia, Muela RA, Irigoyen JA, Higuero NC, Alguacil PV, Gregorio AM de, Senent CJ. Occupational asthma caused by hypersensitivity to ground bugs. J Allergy Clin Immunol 1997; 99:267–268.

65. Gottlieb SJ, Garibaldi E, Hutcheson PS, Slavin RG. Occupational asthma to the slime mold *Dictyostelium discoideum*. J Occup Med 1993; 35:1231–1235.

66. Seaton A, Wales D. Clinical reactions to *Aspergillus niger* in a biotechnology plant: an eight year follow up. Occup Environ Med 1994; 51:54–56.

67. Jensen PA, Todd WF, Hart ME, Mickelsen RL, O'Brien DM. Evaluation and control of worker exposure to fungi in a beet sugar refinery. Am Ind Hyg Assoc J 1993; 54:742–748.

68. Klaustermeyer WB, Bardana EJ, Hale FC. Pulmonary hypersensitivity to alternaria and aspergillus in baker's asthma. Clin Allergy 1977; 7:227–233.

69. Halpin DMG, Graneek BJ, Turner-Warwick M, Taylor AJ Newman. Extrinsic allergic alveolitis and asthma in a sawmill worker: case report and review of the literature. Occup Environ Med 1994; 51:160–164.

70. Schaubschlager WW, Becker WM, Mazur G, Godde M. Occupational sensitization to plasmopara viticola. J Allergy Clin Immunol 1994; 93:457–463.

71. Côté J, Chan H, Brochu G, Chan-Yeung M. Occupational asthma caused by exposure to neurospora in a plywood factory worker. Br J Ind Med 1991; 48:279–282.

72. Tarlo SM, Wai Y, Dolovich J, Summerbell R. Occupational asthma induced by Chrysonilia sitophila in the logging industry. J Allergy Clin Immunol 1996; 97:1409–1413.

73. Gamboa PM, Jauregui I, Urrutia I, Antépara I, Gonzalez G, Mugica V. Occupational asthma in a coal miner. Thorax 1996; 51:867–868.

74. Ng TP, Tan WC, Lee YK. Occupational asthma in a pharmacist induced by *Chlorella*, a unicellular algae preparation. Respir Med 1994; 88:555–557.

75. Chan-Yeung M, Schulzer M, MacLean L, Dorken E, Grzybowski S. Epidemiologic health survey of grain elevator workers in British Columbia. Am Rev Respir Dis 1980; 121:329–338.

76. Williams N, Skoulas A, Merriman JE. Exposure to grain dust. I. A survey of the effects. J Occup Med 1964; 6:319–329.

77. Skoulas A, Williams N, Merriman JE. Exposure to grain dust. II. A clinical study of the effects. J Occup Med 1964; 6:359–372.

78. Chan-Yeung M, Wong R, MacLean L. Respiratory abnormalities among grain elevator workers. Chest 1979; 75:461–467.

79. Musk AW, Venables KM, Crook B, Nunn AJ, Hawkins R, Crook GDW, Graneek BJ, Tee RD, Farrer N, Johnson DS, Gordon DJ, Darbyshire JH, Newman Taylor AJ. Respiratory symptoms, lung function, and sensitisation to flour in a British bakery. Br J Ind Med 1989; 46:636–642.

80. Block G, Tse KS, Kijek K, Chan H, Chan-Yeung M. Baker's asthma. Clin Allergy 1983; 13:359–370.

81. Sutton R, Skerritt JH, Baldo BA, Wrigley CW. The diversity of allergens involved in bakers' asthma. Clin Allergy 1984; 14:93–107.

82. Valdivieso R. Quirce S, Sainz T. Bronchial asthma caused by *Lathyrus sativus* flour. Allergy 1988; 43:536–539.

83. Jansen A, Vermeulen A, vanToorenenbergen AW, Dieges PH. Occupational asthma in horticulture caused by *Lathyrus odoratus*. Allergy Proc 1995; 16:135–139.

84. Belchi-Hernandez J, Mora-Gonzalez A, Iniesta-Perez J. Baker's asthma caused by *Saccharomyces cerevisiae* in dry powder form. J Allergy Clin Immunol 1996; 97:131–134.

85. Picon SJ, Carmona JGB, Sotillos MDMG. Occupational asthma caused by vetch (*Vicia sativa*). J Allergy Clin Immunol 1991; 88:135–136.

86. Ordman D. Buckwheat allergy. S Afr Med J 1947; 21:737–739.

87. Lachance P, Cartier A, Dolovich J, Malo J-L. Occupational asthma from reactivity to an alkaline hydrolysis derivative of gluten. J Allergy Clin Immunol 1988; 81:385–390.

88. Jones RN, Hughes JM, Lehrer SB, Butcher BT, Glindmeyer HW, Diem JE, Hammad YY, Salvaggio J, Weill H. Lung function consequences of exposure and hypersensitivity in workers who process green coffee beans. Am Rev Respir Dis 1982; 125:199–202.

89. Zuskin E, Valic F, Kanceljak B. Immunological and respiratory changes in coffee workers. Thorax 1981; 36:9–13.

90. Osterman K, Johansson SGO, Zetterstrom O. Diagnostic tests in allergy to green coffee. Allergy 1985; 40:336–343.

91. Panzani R, Johansson SGO. Results of skin test and RAST in allergy to a clinically potent allergen (castor bean). Clin Allergy 1986; 16:259–266.

92. Igea JM, Fernandez M, Quirce S, Hoz B de la, Gomez MLD. Green bean hypersensitivity: an occupational allergy in a homemaker. J Allergy Clin Immunol 1994; 94:33–35.

93. vanderBrempt X, Ledent C, Mairesse M. Rhinitis and asthma caused by occupational exposure to carob bean flour. J Allergy Clin Immunol 1992; 90:1008–1010.

94. Shirai T, Sato A, Hara Y. Epigallocatechin gallate. The major causative agent of green tea-induced asthma. Chest 1994; 106:1801–1805.

95. Blanc PD, Trainor WD, Lim DT. Herbal tea asthma. Br J Ind Med 1986; 43:137–138.

96. Gleich GJ, Welsh PW, Yunginger JW, Hyatt RE, Catlett JB. Allergy to tobacco: an occupational hazard. N Engl J Med 1980; 302:617–619.

97. Lander F, Gravesen S. Respiratory disorders among tobacco workers. Br J Ind Med 1988; 45:500–502.

98. Newmark FM. Hops allergy and terpene sensitivity: an occupational disease. Ann Allergy 1978; 41:311–312.

99. Twiggs JT, Yunginger JW, Agarwal MK, Reed CE. Occupational asthma in a florist caused by the dried plant, baby's breath. J Allergy Clin Immunol 1982; 69:474–477.

100. Toorenenbergen AW van, Dieges PH. Occupational allergy in horticulture: demonstration of immediate-type allergic reactivity to freesia and praprika plants. Int Arch Allergy Appl Immunol 1984; 75:44–47.

101. Jansen APH, Visser FJ, Nierop G, Jong NW De, Raadt J Waanders-De Lijster De, Vermeulen A, Toorenenbergen AW van. Occupational asthma to amaryllis. Allergy 1996; 51:847–849.

102. Quirce S, Garcia-Figueroa B, Olaguibel JM, Muro MD, Tabar AI. Occupational asthma and contact urticaria from dried flowers of *Limonium tataricum*. Allergy 1993; 48:285–290.

103. Piirila P, Keskinen H, Leino T, Tupasela O. Tuppurainen. M. Occupational asthma caused by decorative flowers: review and case reports. Int Arch Occup Environ Health 1994; 66:131–136.

104. Kanerva L, Makinen-Kijunen S, Kiistala R, Granlund H. Occupational allergy caused by spathe flower (*Spathiphyllum wallisii*). Allergy 1995; 50:174–178.

105. Park HS, Kim MJ, Moons HB. Occupational asthma caused by two herb materials, *Dioscorea batatas* and *Pinellia ternata*. Clin Exp Allergy 1994; 24:575–581.

106. Vandenplas O, Depelchin S, Toussaint G, Delwiche JP, Weyer R Vande, Sanit-Remy JM. Occupational asthma caused by sarsaparilla root dust. J Allergy Clin Immunol 1996; 97:1416–1418.

107. Lavaud F, Perdu D, Prévost A, Vallerand H, Cossart C, Passemard F. Baker's asthma related to soybean lecithin exposure. Allergy 1994; 49:159–162.

108. Benzarti M, Tlili MS, Klabi N, Hassayoun H, Ammar M Ben, Jerray M, Djenayah F. Asthme aux tourteaux d'olives. Rev Fr Allergol 1986; 26:205–207.

109. Subiza J, Subiza JL, Escribano PM, Hinojosa M, Garcia R, Jerez J, Subiza E. Occupational asthma caused by Brazil ginseng dust. J Allergy Clin Immunol 1991; 88:731–736.

110. Hinojosa M, Moneo I, Cuevas M, Diaz-Mateo P, Subiza J, Losada E. Occupational asthma caused by *Voacango africana* seed dust. J Allergy Clin Immunol 1987; 79:574–578.

111. Valdivieso R, Subiza J, Varela-Losada S, Subiza JL, Narganes MJ, Martinez-Cocera C, Cabrera M. Bronchial asthma, rhinoconjunctivitis, and contact dermatitis caused by onion. J Allergy Clin Immunol 1994; 94:928–930.

112. Navarro JA, Pozo MD del, Gastaminza G, Moneo I, Audicana MT, Corres LD de. *Allium cepa* seeds: a new occupational allergen. J Allergy Clin Immunol 1995; 96:690–693.

113. Schwartz HJ, Jones RT, Rojas AR, Squillace DL, Yunginger JW. Occupational allergic rhinoconjunctivitis and asthma due to fennel seed. Ann Allergy Asthma Immunol 1997; 78:37–40.

114. Alday E, Curiel G, Lopez-Gil MJ, Carreno D. Occupational hypersensitivity to sesame seeds. Allergy 1996; 51:69–70.

115. Subiza J, Subiza JL, Hinojosa M, Varela S, Cabrera M, Marco F. Occupational asthma caused by grass juice. J Allergy Clin Immunol 1995; 96:693–695.

116. Quirce S, Gomez ML Diez, Hinojosa M, Cuevas M, Urena V, Rivas MF, Puyana J, Cuesta J, Losada E. Housewives with raw potato-induced bronchial asthma. Allergy 1989; 44:532–536.

117. Parra FM, Lazaro M, Cuevas M, Ferrando MC, Martin JA, Lezaun A, Alonso MD, Sanchez-Cano M. Bronchial asthma caused by two unrelated vegetables. Ann Allergy 1993; 70:324–327.

118. Symington IS, Kerr JW, McLean DA. Type I allergy in mushroom soup processors. Clin Allergy 1981; 11:43–47.

119. Mlchils A, Vuyst P De, Nolard N, Servais G, Duchateau J, Yernault JC. Occupational asthma to spores of *Pleurotus cornucopiae*. Eur Respir J 1991; 4:1143–1147.

120. Torricelli R, Johansson SGO, Wuthrich B. Ingestive and inhalative allergy to the mushroom *Boletus edulis*. Allergy 1997; 52:747–751.

121. Rubin JM, Duke MB. Unusual cause of bronchial asthma. Cacoon seed used for decorative purposes. NY State J Med 1974; 538–539.

122. Cadot P, Kochuyt AM, Deman R, Stevens EAM. Inhalative occupational and ingestive immediate-type allergy caused by chicory (*Cichorium intybus*). Clin Exp Allergy 1996; 26:940–944.

123. Kwaselow A, Rowe M, Sears-Ewald D, Ownby D. Rose hips: a new occupational allergen. J Allergy Clin Immunol 1990; 85:704–708.

124. Bousquet OJ, Dhivert H, Clauzel AM, Hewitt B, Michel FB. Occupational allergy to sunflower pollen. J Allergy Clin Immunol 1985; 75:70–75.

125. Blanco C, Carrillo T, Wuiralte J, Pascual C, Esteban MM, Castillo R. Occupational rhino-conjunctivitis and bronchial asthma due to *Phoenix canariensis* pollen allergy. Allergy 1995; 50:277–280.

126. Falleroni AE, Zeiss CR, Levitz D. Occupational asthma secondary to inhalation of garlic dust. J Allergy Clin Immunol 1981; 68:156–160.

127. Lybarger JA, Gallagher JS, Pulver DW, Litwin A, Brooks S, Bernstein IL. Occupational asthma induced by inhalation and ingestion of garlic. J Allergy Clin Immunol 1982; 69: 448–454.

128. VanToorenenbergen AW, Dieges PH. Immunoglobulin E antibodies against coriander and other spices. J Allergy Clin Immunol 1985; 76:477–481.

129. Feo F, Martinez J, Martinez A, Galindo PA, Cruz A, Garcia R, Guerra F. Palacios R. Occupational allergy in saffron workers. Allergy 1997; 52:633–641.

130. Lemière C. Cartier A, Lehrer SB, Malo JL. Occupational asthma caused by aromatic herbs. Allergy 1996; 51:647–649.

131. Catilina P, Chamoux A, Gabrillargues D, Catilina MJ, Royfe MH, Wahl D. Contribution à l'étude des asthmes d'origine professionnelle: l'asthme à la poudre de lycopode. Arch Mal Prof 1988; 49:143–148.

132. Axelsson IGK, Johansson SGO, Zetterstrom O. Occupational allergy to weeping fig in plant keepers. Allergy 1987; 42:161–167.

133. Kraut A, Peng Z, BeckerAB, Warren CPW. Christmas candy maker's asthma. IgG4-mediated pectin allergy. Chest 1992; 102:1605–1607.

134. Starr JC, Yunginger J, Brahser GW. Immediate type I asthmatic response to henna following occupational exposure in hairdressers. Ann Allergy 1982; 48:98–99.

135. Dugue J, Bel J, Figueredo M. Le fenugrec responsable d'un nouvel asthme professionnel. Presse Méd 1993; 22:922.

136. Fraj J, Lezaun A, Colas C, Duce F, Dominguez MA, Alonso MD. Occupational asthma induced by aniseed. Allergy 1996; 51:337–339.

137. Kern DG, Kohn R. Occupational asthma following kapok exposure. J Asthma 1994; 31:243–250.

138. Tarlo SM, Wong L, Roos J, Booth N. Occupational asthma caused by latex in a surgical glove manufacturing plant. J Allergy Clin Immunol 1990; 85:626–631.

139. Vandenplas O, Delwiche JP, Evrard G, Aimont P, Brempt X Van der, Jamart J, Delaunois L. Prevalence of occupational asthma due to latex among hospital personnel. Am J Respir Crit Care Med 1995; 151:54–60.

140. Juniper CP, How MJ, Goodwin BFJ. Bacillus subtilis enzymes: a 7-year clinical, epidemiological and immunological study of an industrial allergen. J Soc Occup Med 1977; 27:3–12.

141. Franz T, McMurrain KD, Brooks S, Bernstein IL. Clinical, immunologic, and physiologic observations in factory workers exposed to *B. subtilis* enzyme dust. J Allergy 1971; 47: 170–179.

142. Colten HR, Polkoff PL, Weinstein SF, Strieder DJ. Immediate hypersensitivity to hog trypsin resulting from industrial exposure. N Engl J Med 1975; 292:1050–1053.

143. Baur X, Konig G, Bencze K, Fruhmann G. Clinical symptoms and results of skin test, RAST and bronchial provocation test in thirty-three papain workers: evidence for strong immunogenic potency and clinically relevant "proteolytic effects of airborne papain." Clin Allergy 1982; 12:9–17.

144. Cartier A, Malo J-L, Pineau L, Dolovich J. Occupational asthma due to pepsin. J Allergy Clin Immunol 1984; 73:574–577.

145. Wiessmann KJ, Baur X. Occupational lung disease following long-term inhalation of pancreatic extracts. Eur J Respir Dis 1985; 66:13–20.

146. Pauwels R, Devos M, Callens L, Straeten M Van der. Respiratory hazards from proteolytic enzymes. Lancet 1978; 1:669.

147. Cortona G, Beretta F, Traina G, Nava C. Preliminary investigation in a pharmaceutical industry: bromelin induced pathology. Med Lav 1980; 1:70–75.

148. Galleguillos F, Rodriguez JC. Asthma caused by bromelin inhalation. Clin Allergy 1978; 8: 21–24.

149. Bernstein JA, Kraut A, Warrington RJ, Bolin T, Bernstein DI. Clinical and immunologic evaluation of a worker with occupational asthma from exposure to egg lysozyme. J Allergy Clin Immunol 1991; 87:201 (abstract).

150. Baur X, Fruhmann G, Haug B, Rasche B, Reiher W, Weiss W. Role of *Aspergillus* amylase in baker's asthma. Lancet 1986; 1:43.

151. Birnbaum J, Latil F, Vervloet D, Senft M, Charpin J. Rôle de l'alpha-amylase dans l'asthme du boulanger. Rev Mal Respir 1988; 5:519–521.

152. Baur X, Weiss W, Sauer W, Fruhmann G, Kimm KW, Ulmer WT, Mezger VA, Woitowitz HJ, Steurich FK. Baking components as a contributory cause of baker's asthma. Dtsch Med Wochenschr 1988; 113:1275–1278.

153. Park HS, Nahm DH. New occupational allergen in a pharmaceutical industry: serratial peptidase and lysozyme chloride. Ann Allergy Asthma Immunol 1997; 78:225–229.

154. Zachariae H, Høegh-Thomsen J, Witmeur O, Wide L. Detergent enzymes and occupational safety. Observations on sensitization during Esperase® production. Allergy 1981; 36:513–516.

155. Tarvainen K, Kanerva L, Tupasela O, Grenquist-norden B, Jolanki R, Estlander T, Keskinen H. Allergy from cellulase and xylanase enzymes. Clin Exper Allergy 1991; 21:609–615.

156. Merget R, Stollfuss J, Wiewrodt R. Fruhauf H, Koch U, Bolm-Audorff U, Bienfait HG, Hiltl G, Schultz-Werninghaus G. Diagnostic tests in enzyme allergy. J. Allergy Clin Immunol 1993; 92:264–277.

157. Muir DCF, Verrall AB, Julian JA, Millman HM, Beaudin MA, Dolovich J. Occupational sensitization to lactase. Am J Ind Med 1997; 31:570–571.

158. Fowler PBS. Printers' asthma. Lancet 1952; 2:755–757.

159. Bohner CB, Sheldon JM, Trenis JW. Sensitivity to gum acacia, with a report of ten cases of asthma in printers. J Allergy 1941; 12:290–294.

160. Gelfand HH. The allergenic properties of vegetable gums: a case of asthma due to tragacanth. J Allergy 1943; 14:203–219.

161. Feinberg SM, Schoenkerman BB. Karaya and related gums as causes of atopy. Wisconsin Med J 1940; 39:734.

162. Malo JL, Cartier A, L'Archevêque J, Ghezzo H, Soucy F, Somers J, Dolovich J. Prevalence of occupational asthma and immunological sensitization to guar gum among employees at a carpet-manufacturing plant. J Allergy Clin Immunol 1990; 86:562–569.

163. Boxer MB, Grammer LC, Orfan N. Gutta-percha allergy in a health care worker with latex allergy. J Allergy Clin Immunol 1994; 93:943–944.

164. Butcher BT, Salvaggio JE, Weill H, Ziskind MM. Toluene diisocyanate (TDI) pulmonary disease: immunologic and inhalation challenge studies. J Allergy Clin Immunol 1976; 58:89–100.

165. Butcher BT, O'Neil CE, Reed MA, Salvaggio JE. Radioallergosorbent testing of toluene diisocyanate-reactive individuals using *p*-tolyl isocyanate antigen. J Allergy Clin Immunol 1980; 66:213–216.

166. Baur X, Fruhmann G. Specific IgE antibodies in patients with isocyanate asthma. Chest 1981; 80:73S–76S.

167. Paggiaro PL, Filieri M, Loi AM, Roselli MG, Cantalupi R, Parlanti A, Toma G, Baschieri L. Absence of IgG antibodies to TDI-HSA in a radioimmunological study. Clin Allergy 1983; 13:75–79.

168. Mapp CE, Boschetto P, Vecchio L Dal, Maestrelli P, Fabbri LM. Occupational asthma due to isocyanates. Eur Respir J 1988; 1:273–279.

169. Zammit-Tabona M, Sherkin M, Kijek K, Chan H, Chan-Yeung M. Asthma caused by diphenylmethane diisocyanate in foundry workers. Clinical, bronchial provocation, and immunologic studies. Am Rev Respir Dis 1983; 128:226–230.

170. Tse KS, Johnson A, Chan H, Chan-Yeung M. A study of serum antibody activity in workers with occupational exposure to diphenylmethane diisocyanate. Allergy 1985; 40:314–320.

171. Liss GM, Bernstein DI, Moller DR, Gallagher JS, Stephenson RL, Bernstein IL. Pulmonary and immunologic evaluation of foundry workers exposed to methylene diphenyldiisocyanate (MDI). J Allergy Clin Immunol 1988; 82:55–61.

172. Harris MG, Burge PS, Samson M, Taylor AJ, Pepys J. Isocyanate asthma: respiratory symptoms due to 1,5 naphthylene diisocyanate. Thorax 1979; 34:762–766.

173. Clarke CW, Aldons PM. Isophorone diisocyanate induced respiratory disease (IPDI). Aust NZ J Med 1981; 11:290–292.

174. Vandenplas O, Cartier A, Lesage J, Perrault G, Grammer LC, Malo JL. Occupational asthma caused by a prepolymer but not the monomer of toluene diisocyanate (TDI). J Allergy Clin Immunol 1992; 89:1183–1188.

175. Vandenplas O, Cartier A, Lesage J, Cloutier Y, Perreault G, Grammer LC, Shaughnessy MA, Malo JL. Prepolymers of hexamethylene diisocyanate (HDI) as a cause of occupational asthma. J Allergy Clin Immunol 1993; 91:850–861.

176. Séguin P, Allard A, Cartier A, Malo JL. Prevalence of occupational asthma in spray painters exposed to several types of isocyanates, including polymethylene polyphenylisocyanates. J Occup Med 1987; 29:340–344.

177. O'Brien IM, Harries MG, Burge PS, Pepys J. Toluene di-isocyanate-induced asthma. I. Reactions to TDI, MDI, HDI and histamine. Clin Allergy 1979; 9:1–6.

178. Baur X, Dewair M, Fruhmann G. Detection of immunologically sensitized isocyanate workers by RAST and intracutaneous skin tests. J Allergy Clin Immunol 1984; 73:610–618.

179. Cartier A, Grammer L, Malo JL, Lagier F, Ghezzo H, Harris K, Patterson R. Specific serum antibodies against isocyanates: association with occupational asthma. J Allergy Clin Immunol 1989; 84:507–514.

180. Pezzini A, Riviera A, Paggiaro P, Spiazzi A, Gerosa F, Filieri M, Toma G, Tridente G. Specific IgE antibodies in twenty-eight workers with diisocyanate-induced bronchial asthma. Clin Allergy 1984; 14:453–461.

181. Piirila P, Estlander T, Keskinen H, Jolanki R, Laakkonen A, Pfaffli P, Tupasela O, Tuppurainen M, Nordman H. Occupational asthma caused by triglycidyl isocyanaurate (TGIC). Clin Exp Allergy 1997; 27:510–514.

182. Kanerva L, Keskinen H, Autio P, Estlander T, Tuppurainen M, Jolanki R. Occupational respiratory and skin sensitization caused by polyfunctional aziridine hardner. Clin Exp Allergy 1995; 25:432–439.

183. Maccia CA, Bernstein IL, Emmett EA, Brooks SM. In vitro demonstration of specific IgE in phthalic anhydride hypersensitivity. Amer Rev Respir Dis 1976; 113:701–704.

184. Fawcett IW, Newman Taylor AJ, Pepys J. Asthma due to inhaled chemical agents—epoxy resin systems containing phthalic acid anhydride, trimellitic acid anhydride and triethylene tetramine. Clin Allergy 1977; 7:1–14.

185. Wemfors M, Nielsen J, Schutz A, Skerfving S. Phthalic anhydride-induced occupational asthma. Int Arch Allergy Appl Immunol 1986; 79:77–82.

186. Nielsen J, Welinder H, Schütz A, Skerfving S. Specific serum antibodies against phthalic anhydride in occupationally exposed subjects. J Allergy Clin Immunol 1988; 126–133.

187. Zeiss CR, Patterson R, Pruzansky JJ, Miller MM, Rosenberg M, Levitz D. Trimellitic anhydride-induced airway syndromes: clinical and immunologic studies. J Allergy Clin Immunol 1977; 60:96–103.

188. Schlueter DP, Banaszak EF, Fink JN, Barboriak J. Occupational asthma due to tetrachlorophthalic anhydride. J Occup Med 1978; 20:183–187.

189. Howe W, Venables KM, Topping MD, Dally MB, Hawkins R, Law JS, Taylor AJ Newman. Tetrachlorophthalic anhydride asthma: evidence for specific IgE antibody. J Allergy Clin Immunol 1983; 71:5–11

190. Meadway J. Asthma and atopy in workers with an epoxy adhesive. Br J Dis Chest 1980; 74:149–154.

191. Nielsen J, Welinder H, Skerfving S. Allergic airway disease caused by methyl tetrahydrophthalic anhydride in epoxy resin. Scand J Work Environ Health 1989; 15:154–155.

192. Chee CBE, Lee HS, Cheong TH, Wang YT. Occupational asthma due to hexahydrophthalic anhydride: a case report. Br J Ind Med 1991; 48:643–645.

193. Drexler H, Weber A, Letzel S, Kraus G, Schaller KH, Lehnert G. Detection and clinical relevance of a type-I allergy with occupational exposure to hexahydrophthalic anhydride and methyltetrahydrophthalic anhydride. Int Arch Occup Environ Health 1994; 65:279–283.

194. Rosenman KD, Bernstein DI, O'Leary K, Gallagher JS, D'Souza L, Bernstein IL. Occupational asthma caused by himic anhydride. Scand J Work Environ Health 1987; 13:150–154.

195. Lee HS, Wang YT, Cheong TH, Tan KT, Chee BE, Narendran K. Occupational asthma due to maleic anhydride. A case report diagnosed by inhalation challenge test. Br J Ind Med 1991; 48:283–385.

196. Gelfand HH. Respiratory allergy due to chemical compounds encountered in the rubber, lacquer, shellac, and beauty culture industries. J Allergy 1963; 34:374–381.

197. Lam S, Chan-Yeung M. Ethylenediamine-induced asthma. Am Rev Respir Dis 1980; 121: 151–155.

198. Ng TP, Lee HS, Malik MA, Chee CBE, Cheong TH, Wang YT. Asthma in chemical workers exposed to aliphatic polyamines. Occup Med 1995; 45:45–48.

199. Aleva RM, Aalbers R, Koëter GH, Monchy JGR de. Occupational asthma caused by a hardener containing an aliphatic and cycloliphatic diamine. Am Rev Respir Dis 1992; 145: 1217–1218.

200. Savonius B, Keskinen H, Tuppurainen M, Kanerva L. Occupational asthma caused by ethanolamines. Allergy 1994; 49:877–881.

201. Pepys J, Pickering CAC. Asthma due to inhaled chemical fumes—amino-ethyl ethanolamine in aluminium soldering flux. Clin Allergy 1972; 2:197–204.

202. Sterling GM. Asthma due to aluminium soldering flux. Thorax 1967; 22:533–537.

203. Vallières M, Cockcroft DW, Taylor DM, Dolovich J, Hargreave FE. Dimethyl ethanolamine-induced asthma. Am Rev Respir Dis 1977; 115:867–871.

204. Sargent EV, Mitchell CA, Brubaker RE. Respiratory effects of occupational exposure to an epoxy resin system. Arch Environ Health 1976; 31:236–240.

205. Pepys J, Pickering CAC, Loudon HWG. Asthma due to inhaled chemical agents—piperazine dihydrochloride. Clin Allergy 1972; 2:189–196.

206. Hagmar L, Bellander T, Bergöö B, Simonsson BG. Piperazine-induced occupational asthma. J Occup Med 1982; 24:193–197.

207. Welinder H, Hagmar L, Gustavsson C. IgE antibodies against piperazine and N-methyl-piperazine in two asthmatic subjects. Int Arch Allergy Appl Immunol 1986; 79:259–262.

208. Belin L, Wass U, Audunsson G, Mathiasson L. Amines: possible causative agents in the development of bronchial hyperreactivity in workers manufacturing polyurethanes from isocyanates. Br J Ind Med 1983; 40:251–257.

209. Silberman DE, Sorrell AH. Allergy in fur workers with special reference to paraphenylenediamine. J Allergy 1959; 30:11–18.

210. Bernstein JA, Stauder T, Bernstein DI, Bernstein IL. A combined respiratory and cutaneous hypersensitivity syndrome induced by work exposure to quaternary amines. J Allergy Clin Immunol 1994; 94:257–259.

211. Bernstein J, Stauder T, Bernstein D, Bernstein I. A combined respiratory and cutaneous hypersensitivity syndrome induced by work exposure to quaternary amines. J Allergy Clin Immunol 1994; 94:257–259.

212. Lambourn EM, Hayes JP, McAllister WA, Taylor AJ Newman. Occupational asthma due to EPO 60. Br J Ind Med 1992; 49:294–295.

213. Burge PS, Harries MG, O'Brien I, Pepys J. Bronchial provocation studies in workers exposed to the fumes of electronic soldering fluxes. Clin Allergy 1980; 10:137–149.

214. Burge PS, Edge G, Hawkins R, White V, Taylor AN. Occupational asthma in a factory making flux-cored solder containing colophony. Thorax 1981; 36:828–834.

215. Weir DC, Robertson AS, Jones S, Burge PS. Occupational asthma due to soft corrosive soldering fluxes containing zinc chloride and ammonium chloride. Thorax 1989; 44:220–223.

216. Stevens JJ. Asthma due to soldering flux: a polyether alcohol-polypropylene glycol mixture. Ann Allergy 1976; 36:419–422.

217. Milne J, Gandevia B. Occupational asthma and rhinitis due to western (Canadian) red cedar. Med J Aust 1969; 2:741–744.

218. Ishizaki T, Sluda T, Miyamoto T, Matsumara Y, Mizuno K. Tomaru M. Occupational asthma from western red cedar dust (*Thuja plicata*) in furniture factory workers. J Occup Med 1973; 15:580–585.

219. Chan-Yeung M, Barton GM, MacLean L, Grzybowski S. Occupational asthma and rhinitis due to western red cedar (*thuja plicata*). Am Rev Respir Dis 1973; 108:1094–1102.

220. Chan-Yeung M, Lam S, Koemer S. Clinical features and natural history of occupational asthma due to western red cedar (*thuja plicata*). Am J Med 1982; 72:411–415.

221. Chan-Yeung M, Vedal S, Kus J, MacLean L, Enarson D, Tse KS. Symptoms, pulmonary function, and bronchial hyperreactivity in western red cedar workers compared with those in office workers. Am Rev Respir Dis 1984; 130:1038–1041.

222. Malo JL, Cartier A, L'Archevêque J, Trudeau C, Courteau JP, Bhérer L. Prevalence of occupational asthma among workers exposed to eastern white cedar. Am J Respir Crit Care Med 1994; 150:1697–1701.

223. Chan-Yeung M, Abboud R. Occupational asthma due to California redwood (*Sequoia sempervirens*) dusts. Am Rev Respir Dis 1976; 114:1027–1031.

224. doPico GA. Asthma due to dust from redwood (*Sequoia sempervirens*). Chest 1978; 73:424–425.

225. Greenberg M. Respiratory symptoms following brief exposure to cedar of Lebanon (*Cedra libani*) dust. Clin Allergy 1972; 2:219–224.

226. Eaton KK. Respiratory allergy to exotic wood dust. Clin Allergy 1973; 3:307–310.

227. Pickering CAC, Batten JC, Pepys J. Asthma due to inhaled wood dusts—western red cedar and iroko. Clin Allergy 1972; 2:213–218.

228. Azofra J, Olaguibel JM. Occupational asthma caused by iroko wood. Allergy 1989; 44:156–158.

229. Sosman AJ, Schlueter DP, Fink JN, Barboriak JJ. Hypersensitivity to wood dust. N Engl J Med 1969; 281:977–980.

230. Malo JL, Cartier A, Desjardins A, Weyer R Vande, Vandenplas O, Occupational asthma caused by oak wood dust. Chest 1995; 108:856–858.

231. Booth BH, Lefoldt RH, Moffitt EM. Hypersensitivity to wood dust. J Allergy Clin Immunol 1976; 57:352–357.

232. Hinojosa M, Moneo I, Dominguez J, Delgado E, Losada E, Alcover R. Asthma caused by African maple (*Triplochiton scleroxylon*) wood dust. J Allergy Clin Immunol 1984; 74:782–786.

233. Reijula K, Kujala V, Latvala J. Sauna builder's asthma caused by obeche (*Triplochiton scleroxylon*) dust. Thorax 1994; 49:622–623.

234. Paggiaro PL, Cantalupi R, Filieri M, Loi AM, Parlanti A, Toma G, Baschieri L. Bronchial asthma due to inhaled wood dust: *Tanganyika aningre*. Clin Allergy 1981; 11:605–610.

235. Sotillos MM Garces, Carmona JG Blanco, Picon S Juste, Gaston P Rodriguez, Gimenez R Perez, Gil LA. Occupational asthma and contact urticaria caused by mukali wood dust (*Aningeria robusta*). J Invest Allergol Clin Immunol 1995; 5:113–114.

236. Bush RK, Clayton D. Asthma due to Central American walnut (*Juglans olanchana*) dust. Clin Allergy 1983; 13:389–394.

237. Ordman D. Wood dust as an inhalant allergen. Bronchial asthma caused by kejaat wood (*Pterocarpus angolensis*). S Afr Med 1949; 23:973–975.

238. Bush RK, Yunginger JW, Reed CE. Asthma due to african zebrawood (*Microberlinia*) dust. Am Rev Respir Dis 1978; 117:601–603.

239. Hinojosa M, Losada E, Moneo I, Dominguez J, Carrillo T, Sanchez-Cano M. Occupational asthma caused by African maple (obeche) and ramin: evidence of cross reactivity between these two woods. Clin Allergy 1986; 16:145–153.

240. Raghuprasad PK, Brooks SM, Litwin A, Edwards JJ, Bernstein IL, Gallagher J. Quillaja bark (soapbark)-induced asthma. J Allergy Clin Immunol 1980; 65:285–287.

241. Hausen BM, Herrmann B. Bow-maker's disease: an occupational disease in the manufacture of wooden bows for string instruments. Dtsch Med Wochenschr 1990; 115:169–173.

242. Malo J-L, Cartier A. Occupational asthma caused by exposure to ash wood dust (*Fraxinus americana*). Eur Respir J 1989; 2:385–387.

243. Fernandez-Rovas M, Perez-Carral C, Senent CJ. Occupational asthma and rhinitis caused by ash (*Fraxinus excelsior*) wood dust. Allergy 1997; 52:196–299.

244. Basomba A, Burches E, Almodovar A, Rojas D Hernandez F de. Occupational rhinitis and asthma caused by inhalation of *Balfourodendron riedelianum* (pau marfim) wood dust. Allergy 1991; 46:316–318.

245. Innocenti A, Romeo R, Mariano A. Asthma and systemic toxic reaction due to cabreuva (*Myrocarpus fastigiatus* Fr. All.) wood dust. Med del Lavoro 1991; 82:446–450.

246. Maestrelli P, Marcer G, Dal Vecchio L. Occupational asthma due to ebony wood (*Diospyros crassiflora*) dust. Ann Allergy 1987; 59:347–349.

247. Reques FG, Fernandez RP. Asthme professionnel à un bois exotique. *Nesorgordonia papaverifera* (danta ou kotibe). Rev Mal Respir 1988; 5:71–73.

248. Uragoda CG. Asthma and other symptoms in cinnamon workers. Br J Ind Med 1984; 41:224–227.

249. Jeebhay MF, Prescott R, Potter PC, Ehrlich RI. Occupational asthma caused by imbuia wood dust. J Allergy Clin Immunol 1996; 97:1025–1027.

250. Malo JL, Cartier A, Boulet LP. Occupational asthma in sawmills of eastern Canada and United States. J Allergy Clin Immunol 1986; 78:392–398.

251. Pepys J, Pickering CAC, Hughes EG. Asthma due to inhaled chemical agents-complex salts of platinum. Clin Allergy 1972; 2:391–396.

252. Brooks SM, Baker DB, Gann PH, Jarabeck AM, Hertzberg V, Gallagher J, Biagini RE, Bernstein IL. Cold air challenge and platinum skin reactivity in platinum refinery workers. Chest 1990; 97:1401–1407.

253. McConnell LH, Fink JN, Schlueter DP, Schmidt MG. Asthma caused by nickel sensitivity. Ann Intern Med 1973; 78:888–890.

254. Block GT, Yeung M. Asthma induced by nickel. JAMA 1982; 247:1600–1602.

255. Malo JL, Cartier A, Doepner M, Nieboer E, Evans S, Dolovich J. Occupational asthma caused by nickel sulfate. J Allergy Clin Immunol 1982; 69:55–59.

256. Hartmann AL, Walter H, Wuthrich B. Allergisches berufsasthma auf pektinase, ein pektolytisches enzym. Schweiz Med Wochenschr 1983; 113:265–267.

257. Gheysens B, Auxwerx J, Eeckhout A Van Den, Demedts M. Cobalt-induced bronchial asthma in diamond polishers. Chest 1985; 88:740–744.

258. Malo J-L, Cartier A. Occupational asthma due to fumes of galvanized metal. Chest 1987; 92:375–377.

259. Vogelmeier C, König G, Bencze K, Fruhmann G. Pulmonary involvement in zinc fume fever. Chest 1987; 92:946–949.

260. Bruckner HC. Extrinsic asthma in a tungsten carbide worker. J Occup Med 1967; 9:518–519.

261. Smith AR. Chrome poisoning with manifestations of sensitization. JAMA 1931; 94:95–98.

262. Joules H. Asthma from sensitization to chromium. Lancet 1932; 2:182–183.

263. Park HS, Yu HJ, Jung KS. Occupational asthma caused by chromium. Clin Exp Allergy 1994; 24:676–681.

264. Keskinen G, Kalliomaki PL, Alanko K. Occupational asthma due to stainless steel welding fumes. Clin Allergy 1980; 10:151–159.

265. Novey HS, Habib M, Wells ID. Asthma and IgE antibodies induced by chromium and nickel salts. J Allergy Clin Immunol 1983; 72:407–412.

266. Bright P, Burge PS, O'Hickey S, Gannon PFG, Robertson AS, Boran A. Occupational asthma due to chrome and nickel electroplating. Thorax 1997; 52:28–32.

267. Shirakawa T, Kusaka Y, Fujimura N, Kato M, Heki S, Morimoto K. Hard metal asthma: cross immunological and respiratory reactivity between cobalt and nickel. Thorax 1990; 45: 267–271.

268. Davies RJ, Hendrick DJ, Pepys J. Asthma due to inhaled chemical agents: ampicillin, bensyl penicillin, -6 amino penicillanic acid and related substances. Clin Allergy 1974; 4:227–247.

269. Lagier F, Cartier A, Dolovich J, Malo J-L. Occupational asthma in a pharmaceutical worker exposed to penicillamine. Thorax 1989; 44:157–158.

270. Coutts II, Dally MB, Taylor AJ Newman, Pickering CAC, Horsfield N. Asthma in workers manufacturing cephalosporins. Br Med J 1981; 283:950.

271. Briatico-Vangosa G, Beretta F, Bianchi S, Cardani A, Marchisio M, Nava C, Talamo F. Bronchial asthma due to 7-aminocephalosporanic acid (7-ACA) in workers employed in cephalosporine production. Med Lav 1981; 72:488–493.

272. Kammermeyer JK, Mathews KP. Hypersensitivity to phenylglycine acid chloride. J Allergy Clin Immunol 1973; 52:73–84.

273. Busse WW, Schoenwetter WF. Asthma from psyllium in laxative manufacture. Ann Intern Med 1975; 83:361–362.

274. Bardy JD, Malo JL, Séguin P, Ghezzo H, Desjardins J, Dolovich J, Cartier A. Occupational asthma and IgE sensitization in a pharmaceutical company processing psyllium. Am Rev Respir Dis 1987; 135:1033–1038.

275. Cartier A, Malo J-L, Dolovich J. Occupational asthma in nurses handling psyllium. Clin Allergy 1987; 17:1–6.

276. Malo JL, Cartier A, L'Archevêque J, Ghezzo H, Lagier F, Trudeau C, Dolovich J. Prevalence of occupational asthma and immunologic sensitization to psyllium among health personnel in chronic care hospitals. Am Rev Respir Dis 1990; 142:1359–1366.

277. Harries MG, Newman Taylor A, Wooden J, MacAuslan A. Bronchial asthma due to alpha-methyldopa. Br Med J 1979; 1461.

278. Davies RJ, Pepys J. Asthma due to inhaled chemical agents—the macrolide antibiotic spiramycin. Clin Allergy 1975; 1:99–107.

279. Malo J-L, Cartier A. Occupational asthma in workers of a pharmaceutical company processing spiramycin. Thorax 1988; 43:371–377.

280. Moscato G, Naldi L, Candura F. Bronchial asthma due to spiramycin and adipic acid. Clin Allergy 1984; 14:355–361.

281. Fawcett IW, Pepys J, Erooga MA. Asthma due to "glycyl compound" powder—an intermediate in production of salbutamol. Clin Allergy 1976; 6:405–409.

282. Greene SA, Freedman S. Asthma due to inhaled chemical agents—amprolium hydrochloride. Clin Allergy 1976; 6:105–108.

283. Menon MPS, Das AK. Tetracycline asthma—a case report. Clin Allergy 1977; 7:285–290.

284. Asai S, Shimoda T, Hara K, Fujiwara K. Occupational asthma caused by isonicotinic acid hydrazide (INH) inhalation. J Allergy Clin Immunol 1987; 80:578–582.

285. Perrin B, Malo JL, Cartier A, Evans S, Dolovich J. Occupational asthma in a pharmaceutical worker exposed to hydralazine. Thorax 1990; 45:980–981.

286. Lee HS, Wang YT, Yeo CT, Tan KT, Ratnam KV. Occupational asthma due to tylosin tartrate. Br J Ind Med 1989; 46:498–499.

287. Luczynska CM, Marshall PE, Scarisbrick DA, Topping MD. Occupational allergy due to inhalation of ipecacuanha dust. Clin Allergy 1984; 14:169–175.

288. Coutts II, Lozewicz S, Dally MB, Newman Taylor AJ, Burge PS, Flind AC, Rogers DJH. Respiratory symptoms related to work in a factory manufacturing cimetidine tablets. Br Med J 1984; 288:1418.

289. Moscato G, Galdi E, Scibilia J, Dellabianca A, Omodeo P, Vittadini G, Biscaldi GP. Occupational asthma, rhinitis and urticaria due to piperacillin sodium in a pharmaceutical worker. Eur Respir J 1995; 8:467–469.

290. Stenton SC, Dennis JH, Hendrick DJ. Occupational asthma due to ceftazidime. Eur Respir J 1995; 8:1421–1423.

291. Moneo I, Alday E, Ramos C, Curiel G. Occupational asthma caused by *Papaver somniferum*. Allergol Immunopathol 1993; 21:145–148.

292. Biagini RE, Bernstein DM, Klincewicz SL, Mittman R, Bernstein IL, Henningsen GM. Evaluation of cutaneous responses and lung function from exposure to opiate compounds among ethical narcotics-manufacturing workers. J Allergy Clin Immunol 1992; 89:108–117.

293. Jiminez I, Anton E, Picans I, Sanchez I, Quinones MD, Jerez J. Occupational asthma specific to amoxicillin. Allergy 1998; 53:104–105.

294. Alanko K, Keskinen H, Byorksten F, Ojanen S. Immediate-type hypersensitivity to reactive dyes. Clin Allergy 1978; 8:25–31.

295. Romano C, Sulotto F, Pavan I, Chiesa A, Scansetti G. A new case of occupational asthma from reactive dyes with severe anaphylactic response to the specific challenge. Am J Ind Med 1992; 21:209–216.

296. Nilsson R, Nordlinder R, Wass U, Meding B, Belin L. Asthma, rhinitis, and dermatitis in workers exposed to reactive dyes. Br J Ind Med 1993; 50:65–70.

297. Park HS, Lee MK, Kim BO, Lee KJ, Roh JH, Moon YH, Hong CS. Clinical and immunologic evaluations of reactive dye-exposed workers. J Allergy Clin Immunol 1991; 87:639–649.

298. Topping MD, Forster HW, Ide CW, Kennedy FM, Leach AM, Sorkin S. Respiratory allergy and specific immunoglobin E and immunoglobin G antibodies to reactive dyes used in the wool industry. J Occup Med 1989; 31:857–862.

299. Scibilia J, Galdi E, Biscaldi G, Moscato G. Occupational asthma caused by black henna. Allergy 1997; 52:231–232.

300. Miller ME, Lummus ZL, Bernstein DI. Occupational asthma caused by FD&C blue dye no. 2. Allergy Asthma Proc 1996; 17:31–34.

301. Quirce S, Cuevas M, Olaguibel JM, Tabar AI. Occupational asthma and immunologic responses induced by inhaled carmine among employees at a factory making natural dyes. J Allergy Clin Immunol 1994; 93:44–52.

302. Nagy L. Orosz M. Occupational asthma due to hexachlorophene. Thorax 1984; 39:630–631.

303. Waclawski ER, McAlpine LG, Thomson NC. Occupational asthma in nurses caused by chlorhexidine and alcohol aerosols. Br Med J 1989; 298:929–930.

304. Jachuck SJ, Bound CL, Steel J, Blain PG. Occupational hazard in hospital staff exposed to 2 per cent glutaraldehyde in an endoscopy unit. J Soc Occup Med 1989; 39:69–71.

305. Gannon PFG, Bright P, Campbell M, O'Hickey SP, Burge P Sherwood. Occupational asthma due to glutaraldehyde and formaldehyde in endoscopy and X ray departments. Thorax 1995; 50:156–159.

306. Feinberg SM, Watrous RM. Atopy to simple chemical compounds-sulfonechloramides. J Allergy 1945; 16:209–220.

307. Boume MS, Flindt MLH, Walker JM. Asthma due to industrial use of chloramine. Br Med J 1979; 2:10–12.

308. Dijkman JG, Vooren PH, Kramps JA. Occupational asthma due to inhalation of chloramine-T. 1. Clinical observations and inhalation-provocation studies. Int Arch Allergy Appl Immunol 1981; 64:422–427.

309. Burge PS, Richardson MN. Occupational asthma due to indirect exposure to lauryl dimethyl benzyl ammonium chloride used in a floor cleaner. Thorax 1994; 49:842–843.

310. Bourke SJ, Convery RP, Stenton SC, Malcolm RM, Hendrick DJ. Occupational asthma in an isothiazolinone manufacturing plant. Thorax 1997; 52:746–748.

311. Honda I, Kohrogi H, Ando M, Araki S, Ueno T, Futatsuka M, Ueda A. Occupational asthma induced by the fungicide tetrachloroisophthalonitrile. Thorax 1992; 47:760–761.

312. Shelton D, Urch B, Tarlo SM. Occupational asthma induced by a carpet fungicide-tributyl tin oxide. J Allergy Clin Immunol 1992; 90:274–275.

313. Royce S, Wald P, Sheppard D, Balmes J. Occupational asthma in a pesticides manufacturing worker. Chest 1993; 103:295–296.

314. Andrasch RH, Bardana EJ, Koster F, Pirofsky B. Clinical and bronchial provocation studies in patients with meatwrapper's asthma. J Allergy Clin Immunol 1976; 58:291–298.

315. Sokol WN, Aelony Y, Beall GN. Meat-wrapper's asthma. A new syndrome? JAMA 1973; 226:639–641.

316. Lee HS, Yap J, Wang YT, Lee CS, Tan KT, Poh SC. Occupational asthma due to unheated polyvinylchloride resin dust. Br J Ind Med 1989; 46:820–822.

317. Weiner A. Bronchial asthma due to the organic phosphate insecticides. Ann Allergy 1961; 19:397–401.

318. Pepys J, Hutchcroft BJ, Breslin ABX. Asthma due to inhaled chemical agents-persulphate salts and henna in hairdressers. Clin Allergy 1976; 6:399–404.

319. Baur X, Fruhmann G, Liebe VV. Occupational asthma and dermatitis after exposure to dusts of persulfate salts in two industrial workers. Respiration 1979; 38:144–150.

320. Blainey AD, Ollier S, Cundell D, Smith RE, Davies RJ. Occupational asthma in a hairdressing salon. Thorax 1986; 41:42–50.

321. Pankow W, Hein H, Bittner K, v Wichert P. Asthma in hairdressers induced by persulphate. Pneumologie 1989; 43:173–175.

322. Gamboa PM, de la Cuesta CG, García BE, Castillo JG, Oehling A. Late asthmatic reaction in a hairdresser, due to the inhalation of ammonium persulphate salts. Allergol Immunopathol 1989; 17:109–111.

323. Graham V, Coe MJS, Davies RJ. Occupational asthma after exposure to a diazonium salt. Thorax 1981; 36:950–951.

324. Luczynska CM, Hutchcroft BJ, Harrison MA, Dornan JD, Topping MD. Occupational asthma and specific IgE to diazonium salt intermediate used in the polymer industry. J Allergy Clin Immunol 1990; 85:1076–1082.

325. Cockcroft DW, Hoeppner VH, Dolovich J. Occupational asthma caused by cedar urea formaldehyde particle board. Chest 1982; 82:49–53.

326. Lemière C, Desjardins A, Cloutier Y, Drolet D, Perrault G, Cartier A, Malo JL. Occupational asthma due to formaldehyde resin dust with and without reaction to formaldehyde gas. Eur Respir J 1995; 8:861–865.

327. Frigas E, Filley WV, Reed CE. Asthma induced by dust from urea-formaldehyde foam insulating material. Chest 1981; 79:706–707.

328. Malo JL, Gagnon G, Cartier A. Occupational asthma due to heated freon. Thorax 1984; 39: 628–629.

329. Cockcroft DW, Cartier A, Jones G, Tarlo SM, Dolovich J, Hargreave FE. Asthma caused by occupational exposure to a furan-based binder system. J Allergy Clin Immunol 1980; 66: 458–463.

330. Moscato G, Biscaldi G, Cottica D, Pugliese F, Candura S, Candura F. Occupational asthma due to styrene: two case reports. J Occup Med 1987; 29:957–960.

331. Kanerva L, Keskinen H, Autio P, Estlander T, Tuppurainen M, Jolanki R. Occupational respiratory and skin sensitization caused by polyfunctional aziridine hardener. Clin Exp Allergy 1995; 25:432–439.

332. Slovak AJM. Occupational asthma caused by a plastics blowing agent, azodicarbonamide. Thorax 1981; 36:906–909.

333. Normand J-C, Grange F, Hernandez C, Ganay A, Davezies P, Bergeret A, Prost G. Occupational asthma after exposure to azodicarbonamide: report of four cases. Br J Ind Med 1989; 46:60–62.

334. Malo JL, Pineau L, Cartier A. Occupational asthma due to azobisformamide. Clin Allergy 1985; 15:261–264.

335. Hendrick DJ, Connolly MJ, Stenton SC, Bird AG, Winterton IS, Walters EH. Occupational asthma due to sodium iso-nonanoyl oxybenzene sulphonate, a newly developed detergent ingredient. Thorax 1988; 43:501–502.

336. Burge P Sherwood, Hendy M, Hodgson ES. Occupational asthma, rhinitis, and dermatitis due to tetrazene in a detonator manufacturer. Thorax 1984; 39:470–471.

337. Gannon PFG, Burge P Sherwood, Benfield CFA. Occupational asthma due to polyethylene shrink wrapping (paper wrapper's asthma). Thorax 1992; 47:759.

338. Tarlo SM. Occupational asthma induced by tall oil in the rubber tyre industry. Clin Exp Allergy 1991; 22:99–102.

339. Valero AL, Bescos M, Amat P, Mallet A. Asma bronquial por exposicion laboral a sulfitos. Bronchial asthma caused by occupational sulfite exposure. Allergol immunopathol 1993; 21: 221–224.

340. Malo JL, Cartier A, Desjardins A. Occupational asthma caused by dry metabisulphite. Thorax 1995; 50:585–586.

341. Malo JL, Cartier A, Pineault L, Dugas M, Desjardins A. Occupational asthma due to heated polypropylene. Eur Respir J 1994; 7:415–417.

342. Cartier A, Vandenplas O, Grammer LC, Shaughnessy MA, Malo JL. Respiratory and systemic reaction following exposure to heated electrostatic polyester paint. Eur Respir J 1994; 7:608–611.

343. Kivity S, Fireman E, Lerman Y. Late asthmatic reaction to inhaled glacial acetic acid. Thorax 1994; 49:727–728.

344. Malo JL, Cartier A, Desjardins A. Occupational asthma caused by metabisulphite. Thorax 1995; 50:585–586.

345. Piirila P, Estlander T, Hyrtonen M, Keskinen H, Tupasela O, Tuppurainen M. Rhinitis caused by nihydrin develops into occupational asthma. Eur Respir J 1997; 10:1918–1921.

346. Dugue P, Faraut C, Figueredo M, Bettendorf A, Salvadori JM. Asthme professionnel à l'oxyde d'éthylène chez une infirmière. Presse Méd 1991; 20:1455.

347. Schwettmann RS, Casterline CL. Delayed asthmatic response following occupational exposure to enflurane. Anesthesiology 1976; 44:166–169.

348. Rodenstein D, Stanescu DC. Bronchial asthma following exposure to ECG ink. Ann Allergy 1982; 48:351–352.

349. Seaton A, Cherrie B, Turnbull J. Rubber glove asthma. Br Med J 1988; 296:531–532.

350. Cullinan P, Hayes J, Cannon J, Madan L, Heap D, Taylor A Newman. Occupational asthma in radiographers. Lancet 1992; 340:1477.

351. Rosberg M. Asthma bronchiale caused by sulphathiazole. Acta Med Scand 1946; 126:185–190.

352. Hendrick DJ, Lane DJ. Formalin asthma in hospital staff. Br Med J 1975; 1:607–608.

353. Burge PS, Harries MG, Lam WK, O'Brien IM, Patchett PA. Occupational asthma due to formaldehyde. Thorax 1985; 40:255–260.

354. Nordman H, Keskinen H, Tuppurainen M. Formaldehyde asthma—rare or overlooked? J Allergy Clin Immunol 1985; 75:91–99.

355. Lozewicz S, Davison AG, Hopkirk A, Burge PS, Boldy D, Riordan JF, McGivern DV, Platts BW, Davies D, Newman Taylor AJ. Occupational asthma due to methyl methacrylate and cyanoacrylates. Thorax 1985; 40:836–839.

356. Pickering CAC, Bainbridge D, Birtwistle IH, Griffiths DL. Occupational asthma due to methyl methacrylate in an orthopaedic theatre sister. Br Med J 1986; 292:1362–1363.

357. Chan CC, Cheong TH, Lee HS, Wang YT, Poh SC. Case of occupational asthma due to glue containing cyanoacrylate. Ann Acad Med Singapore 1994; 23:731–733.

358. Kennes B, Garcia-Herreros P, Sierckx P. Asthma from plexiglas powders. Clin Allergy 1981; 11:49–54.

359. Housholder GT, Chan JT. Tooth enamel dust as an asthma stimulus. Oral Surg Oral Med Oral Pathol 1993; 75:599–601.

360. Keskinen H, Nordman H, Terho EO. ECG ink as a cause of asthma. Allergy 1981; 36:275–276.

361. Kern DG, Frumkin H. Asthma in respiratory therapists. Ann Intern Med 1989; 110:767–773.

362. Musk AW, Peach S, Ryan G. Occupational asthma in a mineral analysis laboratory. Br J Ind Med 1988; 45:381–386.

363. Hendy MS, Beattie BE, Burge PS. Occupational asthma due to an emulsified oil mist. Br J Ind Med 1985; 42:51–54.

364. Midttun O. Bronchial asthma in the aluminium industry. Acta Allerg 1960; 15:208–221.

365. Saric M, Godnic-Cvar J, Gonzi M, Stilinovic L. The role of atopy in potroom workers'
      asthma. Am J Ind Med 1986; 9:239–242.
366. Wergeland E, Lund E, Waage JE. Respiratory dysfunction after potroom asthma. Am J Ind
      Med 1987; 11:627–636.
367. O'Donnell TV, Welford B, Coleman ED. Potroom asthma: New Zealand experience and
      follow-up. Am J Ind Med 1989; 14:43–49.
368. Desjardins A, Bergeron JP, Ghezzo H, Cartier A, Malo JL. Aluminium potroom asthma
      confirmed by monitoring of forced expiratory volume in one second. Am J Respir Crit Care
      Med 1994; 150:1714–1717.
369. Davison AG, Durham S, Taylor AJ Newman. Asthma caused by pulverised fuel ash. Br Med
      J 1986; 292:1561.

36

The United States National Occupational Exposure Survey (NOES) Data Base

Joseph A. Seta[†], Randy O. Young, and David H. Pedersen
National Institute for Occupational Safety and Health, Cincinnati, Ohio

I. Leonard Bernstein and David I. Bernstein
University of Cincinnati College of Medicine, Cincinnati, Ohio

INTRODUCTION

Case finding of occupational asthma by both primary care practitioners and specialists is often hampered by the inability of the worker to inform the physician about the specific workplace substance(s) to which there was significant exposure. This information gap may not even be remedied by access to Occupational Safety and Health Act–required material safety sheets, which frequently refer to industrial substances by trade name and generic nomenclature. Although the occupational health specialist has been trained to discover the precise nature of workplace substance(s) by consulting standard toxicological and industrial references, this option often is not possible for many primary care practitioners. Accurate and expeditious diagnosis of workplace asthma would obviously be enhanced if a reasonably accurate and easy-to-use reference source for recognized occupational asthmagens were readily available for all physicians.

Most workers are able to give a reasonable description of the job, the process associated with it, and trade names of job materials. A large, computerized data base containing this information had already been collated by the National Institute for Occupational Safety and Health as a result of the National Occupational Exposure Survey (NOES) conducted from 1981 to 1983. It has been possible to rearrange, classify, and categorize information by job description, industrial process, and generic product identification. This restructuring effort was based on the rationale that access to this type of interactive personalized computer program would enhance early detection and diagnosis of occupational asthma. In addition, in situations where a larger number of workers might be affected, such a data base could provide estimates of the total number of workers potentially exposed to a substance in a specific occupation or job process. Availability of these quantitative indices could also provide the denominators required for determination of prevalence statistics.

[†] Deceased.

With the kind cooperation and personal effort of Joseph A. Seta and Randy O. Young, Division of Surveillance, Hazard Evaluation Field Studies, Surveillance Branch, Hazard Section, National Institute of Occupational Safety and Health, Cincinnati, Ohio, the NOES Data Base was reorganized with these principles in mind. The revised data were transferred to high-density hard disks, which may be used in either IBM- or MacIntosh-compatible personal computers. To illustrate how such data retrievals may be utilized, representative examples of hard-copy tabular data are presented in the following discussion.

DESIGN OF THE SURVEY

Since all data would derive from the NOES Data Base, some background information on the NOES may be useful. The NOES was a nationwide data-gathering effort designed to develop a base of data that would support the development of estimates of the number of workers potentially exposed to various chemical, physical, and biological agents and describe the distribution of those potential exposures. Data relating to in-plant health and safety program were also collected.

Field investigation began in November 1980 and continued for the next 30 months. Trained surveyors conducted on-site visits to each facility in the sample for the purposes of administering a questionnaire to plant management, observing processes and operations, and recording potential exposures of all employees.

Walk-through investigations were conducted in 4490 facilities in 523 different industry types employing approximately 1,800,000 workers in 410 occupational categories. More than 13,000 different potential exposure agents and over 100,000 unique trade name products were seen during the on-site visits.

The set of surveyed facilities was designed to be representative of virtually all nonagricultural, nonmining, and nongovernmental businesses covered under the Occupational Safety and Health Act of 1970. A two-stage sampling strategy was employed to construct the sample of establishments to be surveyed. The first stage resulted in the selection of 98 geographical areas or primary sampling units. The first-stage selection was accomplished by random selection from strata defined by geography, number of employees, and concentration of establishments included in the target population. Second-state selection of establishments employed systemic sampling from a list of establishments ordered by number of employees and Standard Industrial Classification (SIC). The effective refusal rate among establishments selected for inclusion in the survey was 0.3%.

Two stages of ratio estimation were used in the process of projecting survey data to national statistics. Variances of the estimates were calculated using the method of balanced repeated replication. A more detailed explanation of the field guidelines, sampling design, and so forth is provided in Volumes I and II, National Occupational Exposure Survey, Publication numbers 88-106 and 89-102, respectively.

FINDINGS

Potential exposures to the 367 asthmagens observed in the NOES data are presented by major categories (Table 1) and by subcategories within three major categories in the five major headings shown in Table 2. The number of chemicals in each category varies, of course, but a list of individual agents in each is provided on disk.

Table 1 Total Number of Workers and Female Workers Potentially Exposed to Asthmagens by Major Categories

Category	Total employees	Source (%) ACT	Source (%) TRN	Female employees	Female sources (%) ACT	Female sources (%) TRN
Chemicals, other	4,039,856	14	86	1,316,298	15	85
Metals	2,453,012	10	90	370,199	16	84
Plant	2,355,126	25	75	704,350	9	91
Amines	649,104	11	89	127,500	10	90
Foods	604,450	15	85	244,695	11	89
Vegetable gums	503,751	10	90	203,346	9	91
Diisocyanates, polyisocya-nates, and prepolymers	106,373	2	98	33,945	1	99
Anhydrides	163,009	8	92	34,987	8	92
Animal proteins	99,656	19	81	42,273	29	71
Pharmaceuticals	71,218	61	39	46,173	6	31
Medical biological products	54,208	13	87	22,771	1	99
Animal enzymes	35,568	22	78	19,505	18	82
Fragrances	32,660		100	11,135		100
Metallic salts	15,999	75	25	906	43	57
Insecticides	11,772	5	95	1,624	4	96

ACT, actual observation of the chemical being used as a raw material in the workplace.
TRN, refers to whether the material was actually an ingredient incorporated within trade-named products.

Table 2 Total Workers and Female Workers Potentially Exposed in Three Major Categories and Subcategories

Category	Total employees	Source (%) ACT	Source (%) TRN	Female employees	Female sources (%) ACT	Female sources (%) TRN
Plants	2,355,126	25	75	704,350	9	91
Textiles	711,714	10	90	483,839	8	92
Woods	1,672,107	54	46	225,846	35	65
Tobacco	6,897	100		4,021	100	
Foods	604,450	15	85	244,695	11	89
Vegetables and fruits	12,210	86	14	4,660	90	10
Legumes	84,114	27	73	24,869	12	88
Grains	311,312	23	77	64,505	20	80
Animal-derived protein	96,771	44	56	46,442	32	68
Flavors, condiments	271,783	1	99	170,489	1	99
Diisocyanates, polyisocyanate, and prepolymers	206,373	2	98	33,945	1	99
Selected isocyanates	115,670	1	99	19,240		100

A brief description of the data presented in each table illustrates how the data base can be used under specific circumstances. In Table 1, for example, it is estimated that approximately 206,000 workers were potentially exposed to the diisocyanates, polyiso-cyanates, and prepolymers of these chemicals. Of this total, approximately 34,000 were women. It is further noted that the sources of the potential exposures were from actual observation (ACT) of the chemical being used (2%) or as an ingredient in trade-named products (TRN) (98%). The trade-named products were observed being used, and through subsequent direct contact with the manufacturer, a precise formulation was obtained to verify product ingredients.

Three of the major categories were subdivided into more definitive groups. These data are presented in Table 2. The total number of workers and female employees poten-tially exposed to all the agents in the major group, i.e., PLANTS, is presented as well as the number of workers potentially exposed to the agents in the subcategories: textiles, woods, and tobacco. This table has headings similar to those of Table 1 and needs no further explanation.

Table 3 presents the estimated number and percent of workers potentially exposed to selected isocyanates by the major SIC codes. The isocyanates selected for this hard-copy printout were:

> Isocyanic acid, hexamethylene ester (HDI)
> Isophorone diisocyanate (IPI)
> Methylene bisphenyl isocyanate (MDI)
> Polymethylene polyphenylisocyanate (PPI)
> Toluene-2,4-diisocyanate (TDI)
> Toluene-2,6-diisocyanate (TDI)

Table 3 lists the two-digit SIC, the description of that SIC, the total number of workers potentially exposed to the selected isocyanates in that SIC, and the number of workers potentially exposed in the SIC as a percent of the total number of workers potentially exposed in all SICs and the cumulative percentages. It is demonstrated in Table 3 that approximately 75% of the potential exposures to the selected isocyanates were observed in eight of the 25 two-digit SICs.

A more in-depth analysis of workers' potential exposure to the selected isocyanates in SICs 17 (special trade contractors) and 36 (electric and electronic equipment industries) is presented in Table 4, which shows the estimated total number and percent of workers potentially exposed to selected isocyanates by occupation within industry and the percent of the potential exposures controlled by adequate ventilation. The data in Table 4 are interpreted as follows: in SIC 17, special trade contractors, it is estimated that 126 janitors and cleaners (occupation code 453) are potentially exposed to at least one of the selected isocyanates. The 126 workers represent 2.3% of all janitors and cleaners in the SIC. Fifty percent were controlled by ventilation. It should also be noted that occupational code 453 was observed in SIC 36. In this industry, 401 janitors and cleaners, which represents 1.5% of the number of workers having this occupation in this industry, were potentially exposed to at least one of the selected isocyanates.

Other uses for NOES-like data in identifying occupational groups at risk have been developed. The production of relative estimates of health risk for worker groups due to potential occupational exposures by SIC and Census Occupation code was published in 1983 (1). Use of the NOES data to display the geographical distribution of potential occupational exposure to specific chemical agents or groups of agents was also published in 1983 (2).

Table 3 Estimated Total Number and Percent of Workers Potentially Exposed to Selected Isocyanates[a] by Major Industry Classification (NOES 1981–1983)

Code	Description	Total workers	PCT	CUM
17	Special trade contractors	15,626	13.5	13.5%
36	Electric and electronic equipment	12,636	10.9	24.4%
37	Transportation equipment	12,442	10.8	35.2%
45	Transportation by air	11,893	10.3	45.5%
30	Rubber and misc. plastics products	11,219	9.7	55.2%
33	Primary metal industries	8,799	7.6	62.8%
35	Machinery, except electrical	8,547	7.4	70.2%
15	General building contractors	4,839	4.2	74.4%
75	Auto repair, services, and garages	4,004	3.5	77.8%
80	Health services	3,973	3.4	81.3%
22	Textile mill products	3,336	2.9	84.1%
73	Business services	2,855	2.5	86.6%
24	Lumber and wood products	2,298	2.0	88.6%
38	Instruments and related products	2,084	1.8	90.4%
27	Printing and publishing	1,817	1.6	92.0%
44	Water transportation	1,708	1.5	93.4%
28	Chemicals and allied products	1,678	1.5	94.9%
07	Agricultural services	1,472	1.3	96.2%
42	Trucking and warehousing	1,432	1.2	97.4%
34	Fabricated metal products	1,241	1.1	98.5%
31	Leather and leather products	1,013	0.9	99.3%
32	Stone, clay, and glass products	219	0.2	99.5%
39	Miscellaneous manufacturing industries	210	0.2	99.7%
50	Wholesale trade—durable goods	169	0.1	99.9%
25	Furniture and fixtures	153	0.1	100.0%
	TOTAL	115,663		

[a]Isocyanic acid, hexamethylene ester (HDI), isophorone diisocyanate (IPI), ethylene bisphenyl isocyanate (MDI), polymethylene polyphenylisocyanate (PPI), toluene-2,4-diisocyanate (TDI), toluene-2,6-diisocyanate (TD).

The concepts behind this earlier work were combined in a collaborative effort by individuals from the New York School of Medicine and NIOSH's Surveillance Branch, published in 1997 (3). This effort was based on the underlying assumptions that were made in the earlier modeling efforts. First, it was assumed that potential occupational exposure to a chemical agent or group of agents with a common known health effect is likely to elevate the presence of that effect in the workforce, and that the higher the proportion of identified workforces (by industry or occupation) exposed to the agent(s), the greater the likelihood that a given health effect would be noted in that group. Second, it was assumed that national observations of potential occupational exposure (proportions of industrially or occupationally defined workforces potentially exposed) were true at the local level, and could be used to extrapolate national exposure characteristics to the local level.

This effort utilized the NOES files created for Bernstein et al. in 1993 (4) as a starting place to create a working file of potential occupational exposures to one or more of a group of 367 chemicals known to be asthmagens, allergens, irritants, or bronchoconstric-

Table 4 Estimated Total Number and Percent of Workers Potentially Exposed to Selected Isocyanates by Occupations Within Major Industry Classifications and the Percent of Exposures Controlled (NOES 1981–1983)

SIC OCC	Description	Workers		Percent exposures				
		Total	Percent	No CTRL	RESP PROT	PERS PROT	VENT	OTH CTRL
17	Special trade contractors							
453	Janitors and cleaners	126	2.3%	50.0%	0.0%	0.0%	50.0%	0.0%
516	Heavy equipment mechanics	791	3.5%	23.9%	26.1%	26.1%	23.9%	0.0%
558	Supervisors, N.E.C.	207	1.7%	100.0%	0.0%	0.0%	0.0%	0.0%
565	Tile setters, hard and soft	5655	22.5%	100.0%	0.0%	0.0%	0.0%	0.0%
593	Insulation workers	633	5.1%	100.0%	0.0%	0.0%	0.0%	0.0%
595	Roofers	7117	11.2%	0.0%	0.0%	100.0%	0.0%	0.0%
719	Molding and casting machine operators	629	100.0%	50.0%	0.0%	0.0%	50.0%	0.0%
869	Construction laborers	413	0.3%	0.0%	0.0%	100.0%	0.0%	0.0%
887	Vehicle washers and equipment cleaners	56	100.0%	0.0%	100.0%	100.0%	0.0%	0.0%
36	Electric and electronic equipment							
059	Engineers, N.E.C.	23	2.9%	100.0%	0.0%	0.0%	0.0%	0.0%
213	Electrical and electronic technicians	9	0.0%	42.9%	0.0%	57.1%	0.0%	0.0%
327	Other clerks	189	66.3%	100.0%	0.0%	0.0%	0.0%	0.0%
364	Traffic, shipping, and receiving clerks	326	2.1%	100.0%	0.0%	0.0%	0.0%	0.0%

Code	Occupation	Number						
453	Janitors and cleaners	401	1.5%	47.7%	0.0%	52.3%	0.0%	0.0%
593	Insulation workers	117	29.0%	0.0%	0.0%	66.7%	33.3%	0.0%
633	Supervisors, production occupations	78	7.5%	100.0%	0.0%	0.0%	0.0%	0.0%
675	Hand molders and shapers, except jewelers	17	0.6%	0.0%	0.0%	100.0%	0.0%	0.0%
683	Electrical and electronic equipment assemblers	72	0.1%	0.0%	14.9%	70.3%	14.9%	0.0%
719	Molding and casting machine operators	12	0.1%	0.0%	0.0%	83.4%	16.6%	0.0%
723	Metal plating machine operators	1320	7.1%	13.0%	0.0%	0.0%	43.5%	43.5%
725	Miscellaneous metal and plastic processing machine operators	1733	82.6%	77.1%	0.0%	15.3%	7.6%	0.0%
753	Cementing and gluing machine operators	9	0.1%	0.0%	0.0%	50.0%	50.0%	0.0%
756	Mixing and blending machine operators	48	2.0%	20.4%	0.0%	32.6%	32.6%	14.5%
759	Painting and paint spraying machine operators	85	0.7%	0.0%	11.6%	44.2%	44.2%	0.0%
777	Miscellaneous machine operators, N.E.C.	275	0.4%	0.0%	0.0%	100.0%	0.0%	0.0%
779	Machine operators, not specified	467	1.5%	0.0%	0.0%	100.0%	0.0%	0.0%
783	Welders and cutters	194	1.2%	100.0%	0.0%	0.0%	0.0%	0.0%
785	Assemblers	6511	2.2%	57.2%	0.0%	5.2%	37.6%	0.0%
789	Hand painting, coating, and decorating occupations	2	0.3%	0.0%	0.0%	100.0%	0.0%	0.0%
888	Hand packers and packagers	749	3.8%	72.1%	0.0%	26.1%	1.8%	0.0%

CTRL, control; PROT, protection; RESP, respirator; VENT, ventilation; N.E.C., not elsewhere classified.

tors. This information included data on the proportions of industrial production workers potentially exposed to these "asthmagens" by two-digit SIC and three-digit Occupational Code, and whether exposure controls were utilized. These data were extrapolated to a defined local area to tentatively identify occupational groups at elevated risk of asthma-like health effects. The identity of several of the occupational groups highlighted by this surveillance research effort confirmed the results of existing traditional occupational asthma studies, and several other occupational groups were identified as potential targets for additional research.

Similar tables that identify all specific workplace substances can be retrieved according to job descriptions or job process. Directions for these transformations and printouts are included with the disks.

Further information about the availability and cost of this job reference data bank may be obtained by writing to: Mr. Randy O. Young, Environmental Health Specialist, Division of Surveillance, Hazard Evaluation and Field Studies, 4676 Columbia Parkway, R-19, Cincinnati, Ohio 45229-1998. FAX (513) 641-4489.

If these data are referenced in publications by individual users, the following acknowledgment should be cited: Unpublished Provisional Data as of 7/1/90, NIOSH, National Occupational Exposure Survey (1981–83), Cincinnati, Ohio, U.S. Department of Health and Human Services, Public Health Service, Centers for Disease Control, National Institute for Occupational Safety and Health, Division of Surveillance, Hazard Evaluation and Field Studies, Surveillance Branch, Hazard Section.

REFERENCES

1. Pedersen DH, Young RO, Sudin DS. NIOSH Technical Report. A Model for the Identification of High Risk Occupational Groups Using RTECS and NOHS Data. DHHS (NIOSH) Publication no. 83-117, October 1983.
2. Frazier T, Lalich N, Pedersen D. Uses of computer-generated maps in occupational hazard and mortality surveillance. Morbid Mortal Wkly Rep 1983; 33(2SS):27–33.
3. De la Hoz R, Young R, Pedersen D. Exposure to potential occupational asthmagens: prevalence data from the National Occupational Exposure Survey. Am J Ind Med 1997; 31:195–201.
4. Bernstein IL, Chan-Yeung M, Malo J-L, Bernstein DI. Asthma in the Workplace. New York: Marcel Dekker, 1993.

37

Asthma Works: The English Version of the Telematic Information System (Minitel) on Occupational Asthma

Jonathan A. Bernstein
University of Cincinnati College of Medicine, Cincinnati, Ohio

Jean-Luc Malo
Université de Montréal and Sacré-Coeur Hospital, Montréal, Quebec, Canada

Henriette Dhivert-Donnadieu and Philippe Godard
Hoôpital Arnaud de Villeneuve, Montpellier, France

Brigitte Perrin and Jean Bousquet
Respiratory Disease Clinic, Hôpital Arnaud de l'Aiguelongue, Montpellier, France

François-Bernard Michel
University Medical School and Hôpital Arnaud de Villeneuve, Montpellier, France

Occupational asthma is a common respiratory condition in industrial countries. A diagnosis of occupational asthma is often elusive, which has most likely led to underestimation of the true prevalence of this disease. Over 250 agents have now been identified in a variety of different workplaces contributing to causing occupational asthma. Newer agents responsible for occupational asthma are continually being added to the list. The rising prevalence of occupational asthma has generated a significant amount of research. The purpose of the Minitel was to generate a database to help general practitioners detect occupational asthma. The Minitel telephone system has been operating in France for 10 years and became a widely used communication for both professional and private purposes. The authors (Dr. B. Perrin, H. Dhivert, T. Godard, J. Bousquet, and F. B. Michel of the Respiratory Disease Clinic in Montpellier, France) thought that using the Minitel telephone system for health purposes would be an excellent way to detect cases of asthma. As a result, a database on occupational asthma has been created with the aim of making available, to general practitioners using the Minitel telephone system, information on relevant occupations and occupational agents known to cause asthma. Under the direction of Jean-Luc Malo, while he was Chairman of the Occupational Lung Disease Committee for the American Academy of Allergy, Asthma, and Immunology, the Minitel database was translated into English and named "Asthma Works." Asthma Works is available from the American Academy of Allergy, Asthma, and Immunology on IBM or MacIntosh diskette for IBM or MacIntosh or Windows 95–compatible computers. These diskettes can be purchased by calling the AAAAI Information Referral Department at (414) 272-6071. The Asthma Works database diskette costs $20.00.

The Asthma Works main screen is divided into three sections: (1) a list of cards, agents, and occupations; (2) agents; and (3) occupations. Highlighting by using the mouse on one specific topic takes the viewer to another screen where information is given regarding associated occupations. The viewer can identify a specific agent that has been demonstrated to cause occupational asthma, the incidence of the specific cause of occupational asthma, the conditions in which workers are exposed to the specific agent, symptoms that can develop, methods for diagnosis, and a bibliography. For example, if Abietic is clicked, the viewer will be taken to a screen that shows occupations where a worker may be exposed to Abietic, e.g., adhesives industries, beauticians, poulterers, electronics, and tire retreading industries. The agents known to cause asthma include Abietic acid, pyrolysis, aldehyde, and colophony. The incidence of asthma induced by colophony is estimated between 40 and 20%. Subjects who are atopic are more severely affected. No immunological mechanism has been demonstrated to date; however, direct toxicity has been shown in rats. The threshold set by ACGIH for soldered decomposition products is 0.1 mg/m^3 expressed in terms of the formaldehyde concentration. Symptoms may include rhinitis and asthma, which develop after several years of exposure. Fever and myalgia symptoms may also occur. A bronchoprovocation test by inhalation is the only definitive test when studying respiratory parameters in the workplace.

This database is an excellent source of information. It has three limitations: (1) It is current only up until 1995. Efforts are being made to develop a mechanism with which to continuously update the system. (2) The program has been designed so that hard copy cannot be printed for any one particular subject. (3) The bibliography is annotated and references include only the journal, year, volume, and page. Titles are not included. Thus far, 130 occupations and 270 possible sensitizing agents have been listed alphabetically. Sensitizers also indicate the possible connections to proximal synonymous names. Four levels can be selected in the system: (1) general information; (2) information for occupation/workplace; (3) information by occupational agent; and (4) information by occupational agent with evidence, mechanism of action, diagnostic tests, and bibliographic references. The Asthma Work database is intended to be used by health professionals such as allergists and pulmonologists as well as the general public.

Appendix: Occupational History Form

Employment History

1. Demographic information _____

2. Current department _____

3. Current job description _____

4. List chemicals or other substances encountered in the workplace.

Substance	How worker is exposed	Year started	Year ended
a. _____	_____	_____	_____
b. _____	_____	_____	_____
c. _____	_____	_____	_____

5. Date started in current job (month/year)

6. Previous jobs at your current place of employment. Please begin with your most recent job and end with your first job. (Current job *will not* be listed here.)

Department	Job	Year started	Year ended	Duration
7. _____	_____	_____	_____	_____
8. _____	_____	_____	_____	_____
9. _____	_____	_____	_____	_____

10. List prior jobs at previous places of employment as in question 6.

Medical Interview

1. Have you ever been transferred from a job for health reasons?

   Yes _____   No _____

2. What is your usual workshift?_____

3. What shift are you working presently? _____

4. How long have you worked at your current job? _____

5. How long have you been in your current department? (Or, if transferred in and out, when did you first begin working in current department?)

_____

6. While working at your current job, have you had:

    a. Wheezing   Yes _____   No _____

    b. Cough   Yes _____   No _____

    c. Shortness of breath   Yes _____   No _____

If "Yes" to questions 6a, 6b, or 6c, answer questions 7–17.

7. Do these symptoms begin immediately after starting work (less than 1 hour)?

Yes _____   No _____

8. Do these symptoms begin hours after starting work?

Yes _____   No _____

9. If yes, how many hours? _____

10. How many hours do these symptoms last while at work? _____

11. Do these symptoms continue after coming home from work? (example, cough while sleeping)   Yes _____   No _____

12. If yes, for how many hours? _____   Days? _____

13. What time of day do they stop? _____

14. Are these symptoms better on weekends?   Yes _____   No _____

15. Are these symptoms better on vacation?   Yes _____   No _____

16. What month/year did the symptoms start? _____/_____

17. A) Work-related symptoms present?   Yes _____   No _____

_____

B) Are symptoms associated with exposure to a substance or process at work?

Yes _____   No _____

If yes, what process and/or substance? _____

_____

18. While working at your current job, have you had:

   a. Nasal stuffiness   Yes _____   No _____

   b. Itchy eyes or tearing   Yes _____   No _____

   c. Runny nose   Yes _____   No _____

   If "yes" to questions 18a, 18b, or 18c, repeat questions 7–17.

19. A) Occupational-related symptoms present? _____

   B) Are symptoms associated with exposure to process or substance(s) at work?

   Yes _____   No _____

   If yes, what process or substance(s)? _____

   _____

20. While working at your current job, have you had:

   a. Fever   Yes _____   No _____

   b. Chills   Yes _____   No _____

   c. Muscle aches   Yes _____   No _____

   If "yes" to questions 20a, 20b, or 20c, repeat questions 7–17.

21. Impression:

   A) Occupationally-related symptoms present? _____

   _____

   B) Are symptoms associated with exposure to a process or substance(s) at work?
      Yes _____   No _____

   If yes, what process or substance(s)? _____

22. Do you smoke cigarettes?   Now _____   Ex-smoker _____   Never _____

23. How many packs per day? _____

24. How many years have you smoked? _____

25. Do you cough on most days for at least 3 months out of the year?

    Yes _____   No _____

    If yes, how many years have you had this cough? _____

26. Do you have a past history of asthma?   Yes _____   No _____

27. Have you ever been told by a physician that you have emphysema or chronic bronchitis?   Yes _____   No _____

28. Do you have itchy eyes, runny and congested nose during spring, summer, or fall or on a yearly basis?   Yes _____   No _____

29. Have you had a pneumonia seen on a chest x-ray?

    Yes _____   No _____

    If yes, what year? _____

    Did you also have, associated with the pneumonia, any of the following?

    a. Elevated temperature   Yes _____   No _____

    b. Chills   Yes _____   No _____

    c. Fever   Yes _____   No _____

    d. Joint pain   Yes _____   No _____

30. Have you been close to any accidents or spills of substances or chemicals at work?

    Yes _____   No _____

    If so, which substances and how many? _____

    List dates _____

    Associated symptoms: _____

    _____

Index